# Visit our website

to find out about other books from W.B. Saunders
and our sister companies in Harcourt Health Sciences

## Register free at
**www.harcourt-international.com**

and you will receive

- the latest information on new books, journals and electronic products in your chosen subject areas

- the choice of e-mail or post alerts or both, when there are any new books in your chosen areas

- news of special offers and promotions

- information about products from all Harcourt Health Sciences companies including W. B. Saunders, Churchill Livingstone, and Mosby

You will also find an easily searchable catalogue, online ordering, information on our extensive list of journals...and much more!

**Visit the Harcourt Health Sciences website today!**

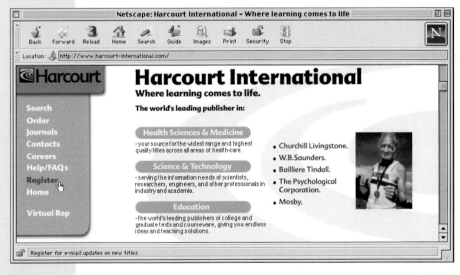

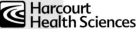

# Veterinary Clinical Examination and Diagnosis

*Commissioning Editor*: Deborah Russell
*Project Supervisor*: Helen Sofio
*Project Manager*: Ian Stoneham

# Veterinary Clinical Examination and Diagnosis

Edited by

*O. M. Radostits*

*I. G. Mayhew*

*D. M. Houston*

**W. B. SAUNDERS**

London • Edinburgh • New York • Philadelphia • St Louis • Sydney • Toronto 2000

WB SAUNDERS
An imprint of Harcourt Publishers Limited

© Harcourt Publishers Limited 2000

 is a registered trademark of Harcourt Publishers Limited

ISBN 0-7020-24767

**British Library Cataloguing in Publication Data**
A catalogue record for this book is available from the British Library

**Library of Congress Cataloging in Publication Data**
A catalog record for this book is available from the Library of Congress

**Note**
Medical knowledge is constantly changing. As new information becomes available, changes in treatment, procedures, equipment and the use of drugs become necessary. The contributors and the publishers have taken care to ensure that the information given in this text is accurate and up to date. However, readers are strongly advised to confirm that the information, especially with regard to drug usage, complies with the latest legislation and standards of practice.

Printed in China

**The
Publisher's
policy is to use
paper manufactured
from sustainable forests.**

# Contents

v

# Contributors

**Jonathon A. Abbott** DVM
Diplomate, American College of Veterinary Internal
Medicine (Cardiology),
Associate Professor, Department of Small Animal Clinical
Sciences, Virginia-Maryland Regional College of Veterinary
Medicine,
Blacksburg, Virginia, USA

**Rodney S. Bagley** DVM
Diplomate, American College of Veterinary Internal
Medicine (Neurology and Internal Medicine),
Associate Professor, Department of Clinical Sciences,
College of Veterinary Medicine
Washington State University,
Pullman, Washington, USA

**Paddy M. Dixon** MVB, PHD, MRCVS
Reader, Department of Veterinary Clinical Studies,
Easter Bush Veterinary Centre,
University Of Edinburgh,
Roslin, Midlothian, UK

**Michael L. Doherty BVM&S (Edin)**, MVM, PHD., MRCVS
Senior Lecturer in Large Animal Medicine,
Department of Large Animal Clinical Studies,
Faculty of Veterinary Medicine,
University College Dublin,
Ballsbridge, Dublin, Eire

**Sue J. Dyson** MA, VETMB, DEO, PHD, FRCVS
Senior Clinician,
Equine Clinical Unit,
Department of Clinical Studies,
Animal Health Trust,
Newmarket, Suffolk, UK

**Gretchen L. Flo** DVM, MS
Professor of Orthopedics,
Michigan State University,
Veterinary Teaching Hospital,
East Lansing, Michigan, USA

**Clive C. Gay** DVM, MVSC, FACVSC
Professor, Department of Veterinary Clinical Sciences,
Director, Field Disease Investigation Unit,
College of Veterinary Medicine,
Washington State University,
Pullman, Washington, USA

**Bruce Grahn** DVM
Diplomate, American Board of Veterinary Practitioners
(Companion Animals),
Diplomate, American College of Veterinary Ophthalmology,
Professor, Department of Veterinary Internal Medicine,
Western College of Veterinary Medicine,
University of Saskatchewan,
Saskatoon, Saskatchewan, Canada

**Doreen M. Houston** DVM, DVSC
Diplomate, American College of Veterinary Internal
Medicine,
Veterinary Medical Diets,
Guelph, Ontario, Canada

**LaRue W. Johnson** BSC, DVM, PHD
Professor of Food Animal Medicine,
College of Veterinary Medicine and Biomedical Sciences,
Colorado State University,
Fort Collins, Colorado, USA

**Thomas R. Kasari** BS, DVM, MVSC
Diplomate, American College of Veterinary Internal
Medicine (Internal Medicine),
Associate Professor, Department of Large Animal Medicine
& Surgery, College of Veterinary Medicine,
Texas Veterinary Medical Center,
Texas A & M University,
College Station, Texas, USA

**Michelle M. LeBlanc** DVM
Diplomate, American College of Theriogenologists,
Professor/Director of Equine Research Program,
Department of Large Animal Clinical Sciences,
University of Florida,
Gainesville, Florida, USA

**I. G. Joe Mayhew** BVSC, PHD, FRCVS
Diplomate American College of Veterinary Internal
Medicine (Neurology and Internal Medicine),
Diplomate European College Veterinary Neurology,
Professor of Veterinary Clinical Studies,
Easter Bush Veterinary Centre,
University of Edinburgh,
Roslin, Midlothian, UK

**Bruce C. McGorum** BSC PHD, CERT EQUINE MED (INT. MED), BVMS,
MRCVS
Senior Lecturer,
Department of Veterinary Clinical Studies,
Easter Bush Veterinary Centre,
University of Edinburgh,
Roslin, Midlothian, UK

**Tim J. Phillips** B.VET.MED., CERTEP, CERTEO, DESTS, MRCVS
Diplomate European College of Veterinary Surgeons,
Specialist of the Royal College of Veterinary Surgeons in
Equine Surgery,
Partner and Surgeon,
The Liphook Equine Hospital,
Liphook, Hampshire, UK

**Klaas Post** DVM, MVETSC
Professor and Head,
Department of Veterinary Internal Medicine,
Western College of Veterinary Medicine,
University of Saskatchewan,
Saskatoon, Saskatchewan, Canada

**Otto M. Radostits**, DVM, MS
Diplomate, American College of Veterinary Internal
Medicine (Internal Medicine),
Professor , Department of Veterinary Internal Medicine,
Western College of Veterinary Medicine,
University of Saskatchewan,
Saskatoon, Saskatchewan, Canada

**Stanley I. Rubin** DVM, MS
Diplomate, American College of Veterinary Internal
Medicine (Internal Medicine),
Professor of Small Animal Medicine,
Department of Veterinary Internal Medicine,
Western College of Veterinary Medicine,
University of Saskatchewan,
Saskatoon, Saskatchewan, Canada

**Jeff W. Tyler** DVM, MPVM, PHD
Diplomate, American College of Veterinary Internal
Medicine (Internal Medicine),
Associate Professor,
Department of Veterinary Medicine and Surgery,
College of Veterinary Medicine,
University of Missouri,
Columbia, Missouri, USA

**James G. W. Wenzel** DVM, MS, PHD
Diplomate, American College of Theriogenologists,
Diplomate, American College of Veterinary Preventive
Medicine (Epidemiology Specialty),
Associate Professor,
Department of Large Animal Surgery and Medicine,
College of Veterinary Medicine,
Auburn University,
Auburn, Alabama, USA

# Preface

A few books have been written and published on clinical examination and diagnosis in veterinary medicine. The third and last edition of *Veterinary Clinical Diagnosis* by W. R. Kelly was published in 1984 by Bailliere and Tindall, London. The sixth and last edition of *Diagnostic Methods in Veterinary Medicine* by G. F. Boddie was published in 1969 by Oliver and Boyd, Edinburgh. *Clinical Examination of Cattle* by G. Rosenberger and his colleagues was published in 1979 by Verlag Paul Parey, Berlin and Hamburg. *Clinical Diagnosis of Diseases of Large Animals* by W. J. Gibbons was published in 1966 by Lea and Febiger, Philadelphia. In 1991, a text entitled *Small Animal Physical Diagnosis and Clinical Procedures* by D. M. Curnin and E. M. Poffenberger was published by W. B. Saunders Co. Philadelphia. This was the first book in many years to be written on the subject of clinical examination of the dog and cat. The *Manual of Clinical Procedures in the Dog and Cat* by S. E. Crow and S. O. Walshaw was published in 1987 by J. P. Lippincott Co. The limited availability of these texts clearly highlights the need for a new textbook devoted to the fundamentals of veterinary clinical diagnosis. Additionally, these earlier books emphasized the physical examination of domestic animals. Diagnostic techniques such as ultrasonography, endoscopy and tests such as cerebrospinal fluid analysis, electrocardiography and electroencephalography have only begun to see routine use since these texts were published.

Many developments have occurred since those earlier books were published. Diagnostic methods have become more sophisticated and new clinical specialties have emerged and private referral veterinary practices are being established in all fields of veterinary medicine. These include small animal medicine and surgery, ophthalmology, dermatology, cardiology, neurology, feline practice, and many others. Clients are more informed about the health and care of their animals and are requesting quality veterinary services. Individual animals have increased in value and their owners are more willing to pay for specialized diagnostic and therapeutic services.

The large amount of information being published in veterinary medical literature and related disciplines presents a challenge for the veterinarian to remain up to date. Fortunately, the rapid developments in computers and software now make it possible to search the literature databases effectively. However, even with the availability of computer technology, veterinarians must first make literature awareness a high personal priority to remain current in the field. Quality veterinary care is best viewed as a moving target. Today's optimal care may be substandard within a decade.

Coincident with the development of clinical specialties a large number of specialized textbooks have been published. There are also many comprehensive textbooks dealing with medicine and surgery of the domestic animals. However, most of these books do not provide sufficient information and instruction on the principles of making a diagnosis and the fundamentals of a complete physical examination. Most veterinary students cannot afford to purchase all of the specialty textbooks. They may buy a few popular ones and complement them with lecture notes and other published materials. A heavy dependence on lecture notes compromises the ability of students to access information in their subsequent practice careers because such notes are cursory and neither indexed nor referenced. As a consequence there is no single book which the undergraduate can use to learn the basic skills of *clinical observation, interviewing clients and taking a history, physical examination, clinical reasoning, and problem-solving.* Veterinary educators may be failing in their responsibility to prepare veterinarians in the most fundamental of all veterinary medical skills: clinical observation and clinical reasoning.

In human medicine it has been stated that graduating medical students lack the basic skills including interviewing, physical examination, and diagnostic skills (Association of American Medical Colleges, 1984). Clinical education is flawed by problems of implementation in that some of the more glaring problems include a lack of clear expectations of student performance, limited emphasis upon clinical reasoning and problem-solving, inadequate feedback to students and inadequate training of mentors, inappropriate role models, and inadequate clinical settings. The General Professional Education of the Physician (GPEP) Report concluded that even though the supervised clinical clerkship is the central element in clinical medical education, the goals, standards of expected performance, and the evaluation of clerkships are not well defined and they recommended a major re-examination of the clerkship so that medical students could master basic skills before graduation.

In veterinary education we must make the content and structure of veterinary medical education more appropriate to the future needs of the student as veterinary practitioners. The diagnostic reasoning processes must be addressed conscientiously in undergraduate education. Diagnostic skills must be taught, and our assumptions underlying such teaching methods must be sound. If we are to teach veterinary medicine the process must first be understood. The study of the diagnostic reasoning process and imparting this process to students has not only implications for the veterinary student but also for the effectiveness of subsequent veterinary practice. We may learn to make better judgements if we can become aware of some of the factors that influence their formation.

We gratefully acknowledge the contributions of all the contributors in this book. We have attempted to have experienced clinicians write individual sections which would reflect the state of the art and science of each of the body systems in accordance with their specialty.

We are also grateful to Juliana Duebner, Department of Veterinary Anatomy, Western College of Veterinary Medicine for her preparation of many of the illustrations throughout the book. Mr David Mandeville, Medical Photography, University of Saskatchewan, took special care in taking most of the photographs and in preparation of the glossy prints from colored slides.

Dr. O. Radostits is very grateful to the Department of Veterinary Internal Medicine, the Western College of Veterinary Medicine, and the University of Saskatchewan for providing the time to write and edit the book, the library resources, the secretarial assistance, the costs of office supplies, the cost of mailing and long distance telephone calls, courier service, assistance with the financing of computers and their maintenance, and all of the other incidental costs associated with such a writing project. Special thanks to Mrs. Linda Kraft for her secretarial assistance in preparation of the manuscript.

Otto M. Radostits, I. G. Joe Mayhew, Doreen Houston, Saskatoon, Canada

# Part One

## Principles

# 1
# Introduction and Orientation

*O. M. Radostits*

*Thinking about thinking processes is never without its difficulties and problems. When the content of the thinking process under study is also especially difficult, then thinking about thinking becomes even more complex. This is particularly the case for the diagnostic thinking processes of doctors and medical students.*

Gale and Marsden, 1983

## INTRODUCTION

Over the past few decades the theoretical and practical aspects of veterinary medicine have changed dramatically. However, the two fundamental intellectual tasks of the veterinarian which have not changed are making a diagnosis and deciding on the best form of therapy or disease prevention for a particular problem in an animal or group of animals. Every day clinicians face three challenges, they must

- reach the correct diagnosis
- select the clinical management that does more good than harm
- keep up to date with useful advances in veterinary medicine.

Some progress has been made in recent years in understanding clinical reasoning and clinical inference. This book is different from the earlier ones on clinical examination in that it also presents the principles of the diagnostic thinking process and diagnostic methods. The importance of clinical reasoning and problem solving in the clinical arena has gained numerous advocates. We, the authors, count ourselves among the ranks of these proponents. This book consequently directs the student and the veterinarian to those diagnostic aids that will yield valuable information after the physical examination has been completed.

Both collectively and as individual clinicians, we must focus our knowledge and experience on solving the problems of an individual animal or group of animals. Thus, rational evaluation of a clinical or laboratory finding in an animal patient demands our critical appraisal of how this finding has influenced the clinical management of many previous patients with the same differential diagnosis. Similarly, the rational selection of a treatment requires our appraisal of how similar patients have responded to various treatments in the past. If, on average, they experienced better clinical outcomes and fewer side effects following one treatment, we will probably prescribe that regimen for the new patient. All of these activities are, unwittingly, in the realm of the strategies and tactics of epidemiology and biostatistics. Further advances in veterinary clinical practice will hinge upon the widespread application of quantitative thought processes.

The scarcity of information about these cognitive activities contrasts with the mountain of information which has accumulated about mechanisms of disease, and the vast array of sophisticated diagnostic equipment and therapy. This book will introduce the cognitive aspects of clinical veterinary medicine. Specifically it will address clinical inference – the legitimate conclusions that can be drawn from information about an animal, obtained directly by physical examination and history taking or indirectly by ancillary testing.

We must focus our attention on the student's future as a practicing veterinarian. There is no more important

> In the absence of critical and quantitative thought our collective experiences will remain unsubstantiated anecdotes.

field in medicine than diagnosis. Without it, we are charlatans or witch doctors treating in the dark with potions and prayers. Yet there is no field more difficult to teach. Strange that this art and science has not attracted innumerable theorists to make it more teachable! Thousands are studying membrane transfer, yet few strive to make a science of diagnosis' (Cutler 1979). Educators within veterinary colleges teach about the collection and interpretation of data, the pathophysiology of disease, and the clinical manifestations and treatment of diseases, yet few colleges, and almost no books, inform the student on how to process or synthesize acquired data into diagnoses or problem lists.

'Clinical veterinary medicine is an art as well as a science.' This is the usual response given by many veterinarians when asked to explain how a certain diagnosis was made. Whether or not this response expresses any deep truth, it surely captures a widely shared perception. In the view of most practicing veterinarians the reasoning processes in clinical medicine are mysterious and inexplicable. Clinical reasoning is perceived as beyond rules, protocols and algorithms. It is thought to involve elements of intuition and creativity that cannot be replaced by mechanistic procedures. The notion that veterinary medicine is an art as well as a science underlies the traditional endorsement of the need to teach clinical veterinary medicine by example, rather than from abstract principles. According to traditional thinking, only when students directly interact with an accomplished practitioner can they learn to perform reliably on their own.

In reality the art and science of veterinary medicine are one. In this sense, the art of veterinary medicine is no different from the art of engineering, architecture or other applied sciences. Some engineers and architects are better than others. Put very simply, they are better 'artists'. Although the art of veterinary medicine is not totally divorced from veterinary science, it is certainly true that some veterinarians are less 'artistic' than others. Some go about their business in an unsystematic manner that not only wastes scarce resources but also threatens the well-being of their patients. Clearly it does little good for veterinary science and technology to make dramatic advances if those advances are applied unwisely.

One of the tenets of this book is that veterinary diagnosis, and treatment and control of disease, is an intelligently planned activity. The basic structure of reasoned goal-seeking action is found in the Aristotelian concept of practical reasoning, a process of answering questions to decide on courses of action to carry out a goal or intention. For example, a technically correct therapeutic action must conform to the best available scientific information and be adjusted to the circumstances of the animal and the client. Clinical decisions are more than instances of scientific principles, or even matters of probability or frequency distribution of characteristics. Instead, clinical decisions are arrived at by a process of optimizing decision and action in the face of uncertainty. By such a continuing process, uncertainty can be reduced but not eliminated.

Knowledge of the diagnostic reasoning process remains at a rather general level. Consequently, teaching strategies used by veterinary educators and veterinary practitioners providing clinical training have been hampered. It is important to understand the diagnostic reasoning process because we learn to make better judgments if we are aware of the factors that influence their formation. Such knowledge should also stimulate a constructive questioning of established applications and a more rigorous self-evaluation. 'Thinking about thinking processes is never without its difficulties and problems. When the content of the thinking process under study is also especially difficult, then thinking about thinking becomes even more complex' (Gale and Marsden 1983). This is particularly true for the diagnostic thinking processes. (The word 'thinking' could be replaced by reasoning, because reasoning involves thinking but thinking does not necessarily involve reasoning.) The problem of diagnosis is especially difficult because there seem to be no rules, boundaries, beginnings or pre-established goals. Diagnosis begins with the owner's complaint and ends when the veterinarian decides that enough information is available to serve as a basis for understanding what action needs to be taken. The problems of diagnosis are not neat and tidy. Each clinical case is different. Each problem requires judgment. There are no externally set criteria against which the accuracy of diagnosis can be measured. A difficult problem such as the Rubik's cube has at least a defined starting point

---

### Veterinary medicine – art, science or both?

The art of veterinary medicine is the skilled application of veterinary science.

---

### Clinical Reasoning

By understanding clinical reasoning, clinicians can modify their approaches in response to each individual clinical situation.

and endpoint, and a set of relevant or possible elements. But diagnostic problems have no such boundaries. To study the diagnostic thinking process is to study a complex problem.

Why did we write a textbook on clinical examination and diagnosis in veterinary medicine? The answer is simple. The clinical examination of an animal patient and making a clinical diagnosis are among the most common daily activities of veterinary practitioners. For the undergraduate veterinary student, learning and acquiring the skills of physical examination and utilizing a diagnostic reasoning process leading to a diagnosis is one of the most rewarding and exciting learning experiences. Diagnosis is central to clinical decision-making activities. It is what we do every day. This book was written because we felt that the rapid growth and development of specialization in the veterinary clinical sciences in the last few decades has de-emphasized the value of clinical examinations.

Veterinary practitioners increasingly depend on the laboratory for making a diagnosis – it is as though there is something much more powerful and diagnostic about laboratory results: there is an almost innate feeling that the laboratory can tell us what is wrong with the animal. If the clinician or veterinary student cannot find an abnormality or a key clue or sign on clinical examination of an animal, or if the diagnosis is not obvious, often the next diagnostic plan is to take blood samples and request laboratory evaluation. There is a myth that 'the laboratory will give us the answers we need!' Only rarely will undergraduate clinical students consider re-evaluating the history and re-examining the animal in an attempt to find clinical clues that may be very helpful in making a diagnosis. This book emphasizes the importance of the clinical or physical examination and the power of observation in making a clinical diagnosis. Part One deals with the principles of diagnosis, diagnostic testing, clinical reasoning and related topics such as developing a prognosis, referral of cases and veterinary information management. Part Two outlines the general aspects of the clinical examination of each species. Part Three describes the detailed clinical examination of each body system, with a description of species differences. The various techniques of physical examination are outlined, along with examples of abnormalities.

## DESIRABLE BEHAVIORAL TRAITS OF THE VETERINARY CLINICIAN

Becoming a good veterinary clinician requires that the person desires to do a good job, strives to do it right the first time, readily admits mistakes in clinical judgment, and develops a learned experience over time. Veterinary curricula should encourage the development of desirable behavioral traits that result in good veterinary practice. Some of these are presented here as prerequisites for becoming a reliable diagnostician and veterinarian who provides good-quality service.

The curriculum that will prepare veterinarians for the 21st century must consist of more than a series of courses that flood the mind with excessive information through too many lectures. It is much more important for students to develop the behavior that exemplifies the skilled and accomplished veterinarian. Dr Lawrence Weed, a pioneer medical educator, has identified four of these behavioral traits; he has determined that clinicians and research scientists must be thorough, reliable, capable of defending the logic of their actions and efficient in completing assigned tasks. Weed's list of behavioral traits applies to veterinary medicine as accurately as it does to human medicine. An examination of the teaching practices that dominate today's veterinary educational process demonstrates that the strategies used actually detract from the development of each of the traits by rewarding their opposites.

### Thoroughness

Thoroughness in didactic learning situations requires a student to read all assignments and handouts and do all assigned problems and exercises. In a clinical setting, thoroughness implies that data obtained from taking a comprehensive history, the results of a physical examination and from laboratory findings are carefully collected and correlated. All of the patient's problems must be identified and considered. Strategies for solving each problem should be developed and progress on their solution recorded. However, it is now impossible for veterinary students

---

### Clinical Examinations

An adequate clinical examination is central to the veterinary practitioner's diagnostic process and health management.

---

### A Good Veterinary Clinician

- wants to do a good job
- tries to do it right the first time
- readily admits mistakes
- learns with experience.

to practice thoroughness as a regular habit throughout the professional curriculum. Analysis of work assignments in any typical week in the first two professional years of a veterinary college indicates that if the student thoroughly and conscientiously attended to these assignments there would not be sufficient time to eat or sleep. Usually such analysis will show 90 to 120 hours per week of assigned work effort. Those who survive these rigorous curricular demands quickly learn to take shortcuts and learn only what might be necessary to pass the course. How often does the teacher hear 'will this be on the examination?' It is clear that superficiality is rewarded in lieu of thoroughness.

## Reliability

Reliability implies that recorded findings are always stated with precision. All the approved medical, surgical and preventive medical procedures employed are faithfully and meticulously followed. No guesswork can be allowed. Any uncertainty about the nature of a finding should be clearly indicated and the highest level at which it can be logically defended clearly stated. Such findings should not be obscured by statements that falsely imply certainty. Yet the predominant type of examination questions given in veterinary courses and on licensing examinations, at least in North America, is multiple choice. Multiple-choice examinations do not allow the expression of partial knowledge and students quite rightly refer to these as 'multiple guess' examinations. Guessing is the antithesis of reliability.

## Critical thought

Critical thought, analytical behavior and logical reasoning comprise the third desirable trait. Critical thought implies that the clinician can defend diagnostic and therapeutic procedures within the context of clinical findings, physiological responses and other clinical problems that may be present in the context of knowledge in the basic and clinical sciences. It also implies that they can draw logical conclusions and adjust plans and procedures as the case progresses. Students who spend most of their time listening to lectures and memorizing information are not given the opportunity to critically analyze the information they are memorizing. Rote memorization is antithetical to critical thought.

## Efficiency

Efficiency implies that the health strategies used are the most efficient and cost effective available for the problem encountered. Students who are afforded little time to practice psychomotor and technical skills in clinical settings often cannot perform rudimentary veterinary tasks at the time of graduation. If they are not given the opportunity to analyze the costs of clinical services rendered they will not perform well in practice. The most frequent criticisms of new graduates by employers are, 'they take too much time,' 'they order too many tests,' or 'they don't understand the economics of practice.'

## COMPONENTS OF CLINICAL CASE MANAGEMENT

Essentially all veterinary practice endeavors to follow a readily recognized course consisting of

- collection of the database
- generation of diagnostic hypotheses
- development of a management plan.

Strict adherence to this process yields tangible benefits, primarily as increased diagnostic accuracy and economy. In ordered sequence, each phase of case management is undertaken and completed prior to the next step. All of these topics will be described in this book, but a brief outline is presented here to permit a better understanding of how these activities are related.

## Database

The database includes information collected from history taking, the physical examination and the results of paraclinical or laboratory testing. This diagnostic cycle will be presented in the sections dealing with making a diagnosis.

### History and signalment

The taking of an adequate history is a critical component of any medical record and, consequently, the development of a diagnosis. Age, sex, species, breed, intended use, diet, immunizations and management factors dramatically affect the probability of disease in an at-risk population as well as the likelihood of a given diagnosis in a particular patient.

The epidemiological characteristics of the patient or the group of animals involved are collected in the database. Epidemiology is the study of the distribution and determinants of health and disease in groups of animals, for example

- left-side displacement of the abomasum occurs most commonly in lactating dairy cattle within the first few weeks after parturition
- eclampsia or hypocalcemia occurs most commonly in heavily lactating bitches in the first few weeks following parturition
- milk fever occurs most commonly in mature lactating dairy cows within 48 hours of parturition
- parvovirus diarrhea occurs commonly in dogs 6 weeks to 6 months of age
- pyometra occurs most commonly in intact female dogs 3 to 4 weeks after estrus.

## Physical examination

The purpose of the physical examination is to detect the clinically significant abnormalities of function and to determine the body system(s) involved. Physical examination includes but is not limited to visual inspection, palpation, auscultation, and assessment of patient responses.

A clinical abnormality of function, or problem, is a deviation from normal which can be detected clinically or with the use of laboratory tests. Examples include dehydration, tachycardia, cardiac arrhythmia, fever, hypothermia, dyspnea, diarrhea, weakness, recumbency, ataxia, convulsions, rumen stasis, fluid-splashing sounds over the abdomen, nystagmus, hematuria, polydipsia, polyuria, pale mucous membranes, and melena.

Ideally all abnormalities should be identified but sometimes they will be missed. In some instances they will be critical to the diagnosis, whereas in others they will be unimportant. The abnormalities are collected and then aggregated into groups related to primary or secondary manifestations of body system or organ disease.

It is important to emphasize that the relative economy of clinical diagnostic procedures supports their preferential use in diagnostic endeavors. With practice and experience, detailed and systematic clinical examinations are rapidly performed, providing a cost-effective way to develop an extensive database that directly monitors the function of diverse organ systems. This early focusing on potential diagnoses raises the de

> **Case Description**
>
> A case description or definition is a concise description of the animals affected and the major clinical findings, the duration of the illness, and any response to treatment that may have been given.

> **Clinical versus Laboratory Tests**
>
> Clinical and laboratory tests are not mutually exclusive. Conscientious history taking and examination procedures will narrow the focus of laboratory testing.

facto prevalence of suspected diseases in the population being studied and enhances the predictive value of any positive or negative test results. Even when patients are referred to specialty centers after exhaustive workups elsewhere, attention is appropriately refocused on the original history and clinical examination.

Many veterinarians would freely admit that they are not up to date with their continuing education. This usually means that they have not studied their veterinary journals and texts on a regular basis and have not attended a conference recently. However, most believe that they can carry out a clinical examination to make a diagnosis. They believe that they can perform a thorough, reliable and accurate clinical examination and detect all of the clinically significant abnormalities in an animal. But it is of greater significance that the level of proficiency be known. It is therefore pertinent to ask how often have clinicians had their clinical examination skills evaluated by their colleagues? In many veterinary colleges there has been a trend away from teaching the essentials of a reliable and accurate clinical examination. This includes the interpretation of clinical findings without resort to sophisticated diagnostic equipment. This has become particularly noticeable in the last decade with the introduction of sophisticated diagnostic aids such as endoscopy and ultrasonography, intensive laboratory testing such as hematology and clinical chemistry, and now computerized tomography (CT) and scintigraphy. Furthermore,

> **Clinical Observation**
>
> Alert clinical observation is essential during the physical examination, it is one of the most basic skills veterinary students must master during undergraduate education. **More mistakes are made for not looking than for not knowing.**

> **Clinical Examination Techniques**
>
> Most clinicians believe that they can perform a reliable clinical examination, not from learning their skills in college, but by trial and error in practice.

most veterinary colleges do not rigorously examine students' abilities in clinical examination technique. When these skills are taught in a laboratory setting, mastery of the material covered is typically not assessed by practical examinations. Most veterinarians have learned their techniques by trial and error on actual patients.

We ought to be educated and humbled when our patient's clinical course demonstrates errors in our original diagnosis. If we systematically document our diagnostic successes and failures we will identify areas in which we need to improve our clinical skills.

The clinical examination is crucial. It serves as the basis for our judgments concerning diagnosis, prognosis, therapy, control and prevention. Typically, clinical observations are more powerful than laboratory evaluations in establishing a diagnosis and prognosis and developing a therapeutic plan. In fact, diagnoses are usually made after the completion of a brief history and clinical examination. On the other hand, one must be aware that errors and inconsistencies in our methods of clinical examination will undermine the power of clinical observations and leads to a misdiagnosis. Such errors and inconsistencies need to be minimized so that the full potential of the clinical examination can be utilized. There is a need for reproducible, reliable clinical observations and we must avoid being misled by poorly collected or biased data. We must come to trust our clinical examination when it is worthy of our trust.

Examples of the power of clinical observation in making a diagnosis include

- the high-pitched ping in the left flank of a recently calved dairy cow with a left-sided displacement of the abomasum
- the enlarged pelvic flexure of the large colon of a horse with impaction of the large intestine
- the inspiratory stridor in a calf with laryngeal disease
- the systolic murmur over the left fifth intercostal space of a mature dog with acquired mitral valvular insufficiency
- the expiratory effort, cough, and wheeze in a cat affected with asthma
- the tell-tale saliva staining of hair on the toes of a dog with contact allergy.

Veterinary medicine deals with both individual animals and herds or groups of animals. A herd involves a group or a population of animals. In farm animal practice the group may be a herd of dairy cattle, beef cattle or pigs, a flock of sheep or goats, a large feedlot, or a band of horses. Groups of small animals such as dogs and cats are also kept in kennels, catteries, and multi-pet households and possess the same herd dynamics.

The examination of the herd assumes primary importance when there are disease outbreaks or productivity problems. The purpose of the herd examination is to define the nature of the problem and identify dysfunctions within the environment that are associated with its occurrence. The ultimate objective in the examination of a group of animals is to establish strategies for the treatment, correction, and prevention of disease problems at both the group and individual level.

---

### Self Improvement?

To advance the art and science in clinical examination, the equipment a clinician most needs to improve is herself or himself.

---

### Paraclinical tests

The history and the results of the initial physical examination will usually localize a suspected disease process to a specific organ system or anatomic site. Additional selective examinations may expedite the localization and confirmation of the lesion. Paraclinical tests are those that can be used to support the historical and clinical findings. Some diagnostic procedures are either too costly or time consuming to be considered a component of a routine physical examination. However, localizing clinical signs increases the likelihood that such examinations will provide useful information. Examples of such specialized examinations include

- thoracic auscultation while using a rebreathing bag to accentuate abnormal lung sounds
- endoscopy of the upper airways
- neurological examination of a patient with a head tilt and nystagmus
- cardiac ultrasonography in a dog patient suspected of mitral valve insufficiency.

There are now a large number of paraclinical tests available to support making a diagnosis. These include medical imaging, endoscopy, biopsy, clinical chemistry, hematology, serology, sophisticated immunological testing, identification of pathogens from tissues and fluids, fecal testing, feed and water analyses, exercise tolerance testing, lung function testing, allergy testing, and toxicological assays. The challenge for the clinician is to decide which tests will be most useful, to interpret the results and to develop management plans based on those results.

> Before undertaking any paraclinical and laboratory testing it should be probable that application of the results will improve the outcome for the patient.

## Diagnosis (generation of diagnostic hypotheses)

Following the collection of the database the clinician moves to the next step of making a diagnosis. The diagnostic reasoning process consists of identifying the key clinical abnormalities, generating hypotheses, and considering each diagnostic possibility using both inductive and hypotheticodeductive reasoning to arrive at a tentative diagnosis.

## Management plan

The management plan includes consideration of additional clinical examinations and laboratory tests, undertaking emergency treatment, taking additional history, making a rational prognosis, developing rationale therapy or control procedures and subsequently evaluating response to treatment and control strategies. The clinician may cycle back and forth between collection of the database, diagnosis and management plan to ensure that all possibilities are considered as the clinical case is being developed. The database, diagnosis and management plan may

### The Importance of Clinician-Client Communication

The provision of advice and recommendations to the client is of paramount importance. Clients should not be left to make medical, diagnostic and therapeutic decisions which are beyond their understanding.

be adjusted as new information becomes available or as new developments occur. Most importantly, all of these deliberations must be communicated to the client, who must be kept informed. The veterinarian is obliged to explain treatment options, including euthanasia or slaughter for salvage, along with their costs and probable outcomes. The veterinarian should assist the client in making a final decision by making a recommendation that considers the goals and values of the client, the welfare of the animal, and the costs of treatment and the probable outcome. By convention the veterinarian is educated and trained to make a diagnosis, provide a prognosis, and recommend rational therapeutic and control procedures. It is the responsibility of the owner to consider the advice and recommendations and make final decisions concerning the care of the patient or herd.

## FURTHER READING

Association of American Medical Colleges. Physicians for the 21st Century. Report of the Project Panel on the General Professional Education of the Physician and College Preparation for Medicine. J Med Educ 1984; 59(11): Part 2. 1–200.

Blood D C, Brightling P. Veterinary information management. London: Baillière Tindall, 1984.

Cutler P. Problem solving in clinical medicine. From data to diagnosis. Baltimore: Williams & Wilkins, 1979.

Gale J, Marsden P. Medical diagnosis from student to clinician. Oxford: Oxford University Press, 1983.

PEW National Veterinary Education Program. Future Directions for Veterinary Medicine. W. R. Pritchard. Study Director. 1–189. Institute of Policy Sciences and Public Affairs. Duke University. Durham, North Carolina. 1988.

Radostits O M, Gay C C., Blood D C, Hinchcliff K. Veterinary medicine. A textbook of the diseases of cattle, sheep, pigs, goats and horses, 9th edn. London: W. B. Saunders, 1999.

Sackett D L, Haynes R B, Guyatt G H, Tugwell P. Clinical epidemiology. A basic science for clinical medicine, 2nd edn. Boston: Little, Brown and Company, 1991.

Weed L A. A new curriculum for education in the medical sciences. Your health care and how to manage it. Vermont: Burlington, 1984.

# 2
# Making a Diagnosis

*O. M. Radostits*
*J. W. Tyler*
*I. G. Mayhew*

*Personally, I have always felt that the best doctor in the world is the veterinarian. He can't ask his patients what is the matter ... he's just got to know.*

Will Rogers

This chapter describes the principles of making a diagnosis, diagnostic testing, the principles of arriving at a prognosis, and veterinary information management. The judicious use of these activities will improve the accuracy and efficiency of making a diagnosis.

## DEFINITION AND PURPOSES OF A DIAGNOSIS

A diagnosis is the label given to a disease with certain clinical or pathologic characteristics applicable to a particular case.

Diagnosis is central to the practice of veterinary medicine. The need to establish a diagnosis places a demand on the veterinarian's education, experience and judgment. The veterinarian assembles and employs clinical data, calls upon scientific theory, and uses reason and experience to arrive at a diagnosis.

Not all diagnoses relate to abnormal or disease states. Pregnancy diagnosis is the process of recognizing a normal physiological state for a breeding-age female. Techniques used for pregnancy diagnosis distinguish between non-pregnancy and pregnancy just as other tests distinguish between normal and diseased states.

To diagnose is to make a diagnosis. A diagnosis means one diagnosis; diagnoses means more than one. The term 'diagnostic' commonly refers to something that may be used to make a diagnosis. A diagnostician is one who makes a diagnosis.

A diagnosis labels the patient. Such labeling has three distinct functions. First, it classifies the patient. In doing so, it facilitates communication with the client and with those responsible for the animal's care. Classification permits focusing on the relevant medical information and theory. Secondly, the diagnostic label provides an explanation of the clinical findings relevant to the patient. The diagnostic label, in effect, assimilates the patient's disease into a known pattern and explains its features. Finally, the diagnosis aids the clinician in arriving at a prognosis for the patient. The recognition that the disease fits into a pattern, plus additional relevant theoretical information, permits the clinician to predict with some degree of certainty both the course of the disease and the response to therapy. None of these three functions of diagnostic labeling can be performed without relying upon a system of disease classification and a body of veterinary medical information and theory. Examples of diagnoses include

- panleukopenia in a young kitten
- foot rot in a cow
- peracute coliform mastitis in a mature dairy cow
- diabetes mellitus in a dog
- Western equine encephalomyelitis in a horse, and
- rabies in all species.

> **Diagnosis**
>
> The word 'diagnosis' is derived from the Greek *dia*, between, and *gignoskein*, to know. Its literal translation means to recognize a disease and to know the difference between it and other diseases.

## Purposes of a diagnosis

The purposes of making a diagnosis include being able to recommend specific treatment, to provide an accurate prognosis, and to make recommendations for cost-effective control and prevention of new cases when groups of animals are at risk. For treatment and control to be of optimum value the diagnosis must be as accurate as possible.

A definitive etiological diagnosis has major implications in clinical research, such as vaccination or therapeutic trials. If the disease outcome cannot be defined it will be difficult to evaluate the efficacy of a vaccine or antimicrobial agent being used. For example, clinical trials to test the efficacy of a pasteurella bacterin for the control of pneumonic pasteurellosis in feedlot cattle depend on the ability of the clinician and pathologist to make a definitive etiological diagnosis in both live affected animals and those that die. If the outcome of measurement is acute undifferentiated bovine pneumonia, the efficacy of the vaccine that is intended for the control of pneumonic pasteurellosis will be unknown. Diagnostic uncertainty is thus the crux of all veterinary problems.

## Types of diagnoses

Types of diagnoses include

- differential
- tentative
- presumptive
- definitive and etiological
- pathoanatomic
- open
- undetermined.

### Differential diagnosis

A differential diagnosis is a list of diseases that may be responsible for the clinical and laboratory findings in a particular circumstance. It is a group of plausible diagnostic possibilities. In most cases the differential diagnostic list consists of 3 to 5 diagnoses, but may be more. Most clinicians do not consider more than a few diagnoses at one time: an overly long list is inefficient and cumbersome. These differential diagnoses should

---

### The Differential Diagnoses for Polydipsia and Polyuria in a Cat

A differential diagnosis list for polydipsia and polyuria in a geriatric cat may include

- hyperthyroidism
- renal failure
- diabetes mellitus
- liver disease.

Although there are a large number of other causes of polydipsia and polyuria in small animals, these are the most common ones in the geriatric cat.

---

be ranked or prioritized relative to their likelihood of occurrence. Development of the differential diagnostic list begins when the clinician takes the history and does the clinical examination. The probability of certain diseases being present or absent will change as new information becomes available.

### Tentative diagnosis

This is the suspected diagnosis based on history or initial clinical examination. Based on a tentative diagnosis and the differential diagnosis list, the clinician will determine which diagnostic tests will improve the accuracy of the diagnosis. It may not be necessary to proceed any further than a tentative clinical diagnosis. An example is a tentative clinical diagnosis of shipping fever pneumonia in beef calves affected with fever, anorexia and toxemia, dyspnea and abnormal lung sounds several days after weaning. The calves may be treated on the basis of the history and the clinical findings, a beneficial response to treatment with antimicrobial agents justifying the assumption that they were affected with pneumonic pasteurellosis. In small animals a tentative diagnosis of sarcoptic mange can be made in a dog affected with intense pruritus whose owner is also itchy. The dog, if not a collie or related breed, can be treated with ivermectin, and a beneficial response to treatment justifies the assumption that the dog was affected with mange.

### Presumptive diagnosis

A presumptive diagnosis is usually made with additional confidence after considering several differential diagnoses and the collection of further clinical and laboratory information. After a more detailed examination of an old cat with polyphagia and weight loss, a

---

### Zoonoses

Many specific diseases of animals are also zoonoses, and their diagnosis is important in order to prevent transmission to humans.

---

presumptive diagnosis of hyperthyroidism may be made if a nodule is palpated in the throat region.

A presumptive diagnosis may also be made by exclusion. For example, a mature cow that calved 8 days ago is examined because of inappetence and decreased milk production. The cow is depressed, with a fever and tachycardia. Common causes of fever, depression and tachycardia in the cow include pneumonia and peritonitis. Clinical examination of the reproductive tract vaginally reveals normal mucus in the vagina and the cervix is closed. The uterus could not be examined by rectal palpation because it is out of reach over the brim of the pelvis. The fever, toxemia and tachycardia may be due to a septic metritis associated with retained fetal membranes, but the abnormality cannot be detected directly. The following day, the cow begins to expel foul-smelling fetal membranes and further examination of the reproductive tract reveals evidence of septic metritis. The clinician presumed a diagnosis of septic metritis by excluding the common causes of fever, toxemia and tachycardia. A presumptive diagnosis of retained placenta and septic metritis was then made when on further questioning of the owner it was revealed that the fetal membranes were not seen to be passed following parturition.

## Definitive and etiological diagnosis

A final diagnosis such as rabies encephalitis requires that the specific cause of a disease be precisely identified based on interpretation of clinical and laboratory findings. If appropriate diagnostic services are available, a definitive and etiological diagnosis may be possible. A definitive diagnosis includes

- a description of the abnormality of structure or function produced by the causative agent or any other event or circumstance that interferes with normal body processes
- an explanation of the clinical manifestations of the abnormalities produced by the causative agent or effect.

Examples of definitive diagnoses include equine *Rhodococcus equi* pneumonia with lung abscesses, and pediatric gastroenteritis due to feline panleukopenia virus.

Often an etiological diagnosis cannot be made because of lack of confirmatory laboratory assistance. Thus, clinical signs (such as bovine chronic diarrhea or canine colitis) or necropsy lesions (such as canine granulomatous meningoencephalitis) are used as the definitive diagnosis. Acute undifferentiated respiratory disease of recently weaned beef calves 6–8 months of age may be caused by multiple viral and/or bacterial pathogens, along with the stress of weaning, mixing of animals from different sources and transportation. The affected animals will respond to treatment with antimicrobial drugs and the definitive etiological diagnosis usually will never be known. Even if such affected calves die and a complete and thorough pathologic and microbiological examination of the tissues is performed a definitive etiological diagnosis may not be possible. The final diagnosis may be viral interstitial pneumonia due possibly to bovine respiratory syncytial virus, or it may be fibrinous pneumonia due possibly to primary or secondary infection with *Pasteurella haemolytica* or *Haemophilus somnus*.

## Pathoanatomic diagnosis

This is a diagnosis based on the pathological findings identifying the affected body system or organ and the morphological description of the lesion (e.g. granulomatous encephalitis).

## Open diagnosis

An open diagnosis is one in which the clinical abnormalities are detected but their cause cannot be determined. An example would be the sudden onset of convulsions and a high case fatality rate in mature lactating cows on pasture. The possibilities include lead poisoning, hypomagnesemic tetany, chlorinated hydrocarbon toxicity and other toxicities. It is usually necessary to continue to examine the history, the animals and the laboratory findings in order to make an etiological diagnosis.

## Undetermined diagnosis

In many cases a diagnosis cannot be made even with extensive epidemiological, clinical and laboratory investigations. Symptomatic therapy or treatment of the clinical abnormalities may need to be initiated. If the response to treatment is unsatisfactory, then cessation of all therapy and close monitoring of the patient over time

### Idiopathic Diseases

Immune-mediated hemolytic anemia in dogs is often classified as idiopathic as no predisposing cause can be determined. The affected animal will usually respond to treatment with immunosuppressive drugs despite the definitive etiological agent not being identified.

may allow some vital clues to be recognized whereby appropriate diagnostic testing may provide a diagnosis. Thus, initial clinical and laboratory evaluation of a dog demonstrating malaise and pelvic limb stiffness may be completely unrewarding, and accepting an undetermined diagnosis and empirical therapy with non-steroidal anti-inflammatory drugs (aspirin) may be rational. With no sustained beneficial response, cessation of therapy and close monitoring may reveal natural biological progression of the disease, with muscle pain, fever and slight joint swellings appearing. This would allow more intensive and focused testing to be performed, including synovial fluid analysis and antinuclear antibody (ANA) and lupus erythematosus (LE) preparation testing to be undertaken. A diagnosis of systemic lupus erythematosus may thus be revealed and appropriate immunosuppressive therapy can be initiated.

## REQUIREMENTS FOR MAKING A DIAGNOSIS

The requirements for making a diagnosis include collection of the information about the animal or herd incorporating the chief complaint; the disease history; examination of the animal or the herd and the environment; the generation of diagnostic possibilities; the selection of laboratory aids to diagnosis; and the interpretation of the results. A management plan usually follows the diagnosis and includes the need for additional history and testing, deciding on a prognosis, and the development of a rational treatment and control program as necessary. Finally, the response to specific treatment and control procedures may also aid in making a diagnosis.

In addition to collecting the data described above, the clinician must possess a body of knowledge about diseases that may be responsible for the abnormalities detected. This is necessary for generating diagnostic hypotheses. An understanding of the knowledge base is necessary for judicious selection of laboratory tests to narrow the list of diagnostic possibilities.

### Data collection and processing

The collection of data begins with the client who describes the chief complaint. This is followed by generation of data from history taking, clinical examination, examination of the environment, laboratory testing, and the results of treatment. Veterinarians collect, collate, search out, investigate, accumulate, record, discard, and finally synthesize a large amount of data into understandable information. The collection and processing of data about a patient is crucial in the process of making a diagnosis, regardless of the diagnostic method used. Data are facts from which conclusions may be drawn and are the building blocks for making a diagnosis. Data also may be clues which can be defined as any information that can guide or direct in the process of problem solving.

Data processing in veterinary medicine is the method by which the database is transformed into diagnostic hypotheses. It is the important step whereby the information collected is critically analyzed and clues are transformed into meaningful problems for evaluation.

The accuracy of the data is critical. Accuracy is simply how well a measurement represents the state it is supposed to be describing. Most errors are due to lack of thoroughness, not to lack of knowledge. Data from the history and from the clinical examination are often more powerful than laboratory data in establishing diagnoses, prognoses and therapeutic plans for most animal patients under most circumstances. The key clinical observations, often the simple ones, must be identified by careful observation and physical examination. In addition, careful observation will identify certain clinical findings that are unimportant.

Clinical measurements must be both accurate and reproducible. The reliability or precision of a measurement is simply its reproducibility. Veterinarians must avoid being misled by biased clinical observations that would lead to an incorrect diagnosis.

A clue is any abnormality in the history or the clinical examination that leads to a diagnosis. The terms key clues, key signs and clinical abnormalities are commonly used interchangeably, but key clues are those that are considered to be most important or pivotal in the diagnostic process.

Positive clues or significant deviations from normal function are generally most useful. Clues may be obtained from the history or the initial physical

---

### A Differential Diagnosis List

Defining the differential diagnosis list is one of the most important aspects of clinical diagnostic reasoning.

---

### Accuracy is the Key to a Correct Diagnosis

There is no substitute for orderliness, thoroughness, and attention to one thing at a time when taking the history and making an adequate clinical examination.

examination of the animal. A history of coughing and labored breathing suggests respiratory tract disease. Abnormal lung sounds and fever in such an animal suggest pneumonia. Tachycardia, fever and a heart murmur suggest endocarditis. The presence of a palpable nodule in the neck of an older cat with a history of polyphagia and weight loss is a positive clue suggestive of hyperthyroidism. A ruminal fluid pH of below 5 in a 10-month-old heifer with weakness, ataxia, dehydration, diarrhea and distension of the rumen are positive clues to carbohydrate engorgement. The presence of fluid-splashing sounds on ballottement of the rumen is further positive evidence that rumen contents are abnormal. The presence of a rumen fluid pH below 5 in the above animal is considered a necessary clue, which indicates that it is present in all cases of the disease. If such a finding is absent the disease can be excluded, unless the animal had just been treated orally with an alkalinizing agent.

Clues may also be primary or secondary. Primary clues are clinical findings related to the disease process itself, while the secondary clues are the resulting physiological changes. An example is carbohydrate engorgement in ruminants, where the primary clues caused by the lactic acidosis are

- rumen fluid pH below 5
- fluid-splashing sounds of the rumen
- rumen stasis
- diarrhea,

and the secondary clues are

- dehydration
- tachycardia
- weakness
- depression.

## Negative Clues

Pertinent negative clues are important in eliminating a suspected diagnosis, for example the presence of a small and easily expressible bladder in a very depressed male cat is an important negative clue excluding a diagnosis of urinary tract blockage.

In dogs with gastric dilatation and volvulus, the presence of a large gas-filled viscus in the cranial abdomen is a primary clinical finding, whereas the tachycardia, weakness and depression are secondary clues or clinical findings.

Most clues have three properties. These are sensitivity, specificity and relative importance. The sensitivity of a clue for a disease is a percentage expression of how often the clue is positive in the presence of that disease (true positive rate). Using defined epidemiologic nomenclature the proportion of animals with this positive clue is equivalent to sensitivity. Because a clue is of necessity either present or absent, it will be absent in, say, 80%, 50% or 10% of cases of the disease in question. These percentages are equivalent to false negative rates. It also indicates how often the clue is not present in the diseased state, because if it is not present it is falsely negative; and the false negative rate equals 100 minus the sensitivity expressed as a percentage. The more sensitive a clue is the more its absence will exclude a disease, as false negatives are rare under such circumstances.

The specificity of a clue for a disease is a percentage expression of how often a clue is absent in the absence of that disease (true negative rate). Likewise, it also indicates how often the clue is present in the absence of that disease (in the presence of health or other diseases), because if it is present it is falsely positive. The false positive rate equals 100 minus the specificity. The more specific a clue is the more its presence will diagnose a disease, as false positives would be rare. In all cases decimals may be used instead of percentages and 100 becomes 1.

The relative importance of a clue is an indication of how significant it is in the diagnostic process. This refers to its role in the pathophysiology of the disease under consideration and the weight the clinician attaches to its presence or absence. A clue that has high sensitivity, high specificity and relative importance is optimal. An excellent example of such a relevant clue is the presence of a rumen pH below 5 in an animal with carbohydrate engorgement. Another example would be a needle biopsy of an enlarged lymph node in a dog with suspected lymphosarcoma. The presence of abnormal lymphocytes is highly sensitive for the diagnosis of lymphosarcoma, and the enlarged lymph node and the abnormal lymphocytes are relevant to the diagnosis.

For some diseases the frequencies of clinical signs or abnormal ancillary test results have been documented and can be readily translated into sensitivities. Unfortunately, most disease processes have not been defined with this degree of analytical rigor.

Information of this type is needed before we can define the specificity of clinical clues. A reasoned diagnostic approach premised upon defined sensitivity and specificity values for all clinical findings should improve the economy and accuracy of diagnosis.

Ranking clinical findings or problems is often difficult to do but is important. Obvious clinical findings, such as icterus, splenomegaly or heart murmur, are clues for which differential diagnoses may be easily established. Many clinical findings, such as anorexia, depression, dehydration and weakness, are, however, non-localizing. These clues have poor relative importance and it is difficult to devise a shortlist of probable differential diagnoses for such findings.

## DIAGNOSTIC METHODS

Making a diagnosis may be a simple or a complex procedure. Some diseases are easy to recognize clinically but others may require detailed clinical examination or ancillary laboratory aids. Examples of simple diagnoses include a papilloma, a fractured distal limb, skin laceration, dystocia with fetus partially delivered, prolapsed uterus, and a prolapsed eyeball. These conditions are obvious on physical examination. Examples of complex diagnoses include acute colic in the horse, neurological disease in any species, and pyelonephritis in small animals. A diagnosis of uterine torsion in a cow may be obvious to an experienced clinician but is likely to be difficult for an undergraduate or novice who has never before encountered one. In some cases the abnormality may be obvious, but additional clinical and laboratory examination is required before a diagnosis can be made. Examples include sudden anorexia in a mature lactating dairy cow, the sudden onset of dyspnea in mature lactating beef cattle on autumn pasture, ataxia and weakness in a 2-year-old Thoroughbred male horse, polydipsia and polyuria in a mature intact female dog, and exercise-associated collapse in a dog.

In some cases, as in surgical colics, the diagnosis may not be made until surgery is done, which is an example of making a diagnosis based on response to treatment: an intussusception is found on exploratory laparotomy, is surgically corrected, the patient recovers, and a diagnosis of acute intestinal obstruction due to intussusception of the ileum is made. Another example is the mature lactating dairy cow which is inappetent and has an enlarged rumen which is contracting normally. On exploratory laparotomy there is no evidence of reticuloperitonitis, but a rumenotomy reveals a large ball of string and rope which has probably caused intermittent obstruction of the reticulo-omasal orifice. In such a case it is unlikely the diagnosis could have been made without surgery, which was also the treatment of choice.

There are different stages in making a diagnosis, based on the clinical and laboratory information that becomes available as the clinician works through a case. Each succeeding stage is characterized by increasing certainty concerning the nature, location and cause of the lesion. In the initial stages the clinician will usually consider a list of possible diagnoses, known as a differential diagnostic list.

There are at least six approaches used to make a diagnosis, described here in order of increasing complexity. Veterinarians use one or a combination of these methods, depending on their experience and the particular circumstances of the case. As a general rule, experienced clinicians use more of the simpler strategies, the novice more of the complex ones. This is because simple methods omit several steps in the clinical reasoning process. The shorter route is taken with confidence only after gaining wide experience and an honest assessment of one's competence as a diagnostician.

### Method 1: pattern recognition

The recognition of syndromes or patterns of disease is probably the most commonly used diagnostic approach. The historical and examination findings are compared with previously diagnosed disease occurrences. A tentative diagnosis is made when the clinical findings observed most closely resemble those usually associated with a particular syndrome or disease.

In pattern recognition, within the first few moments of viewing the patient a diagnosis is made instantaneously and reflexly. Examples include the profuse

**Pattern Recognition**

Pattern recognition is based on comparison of the patient at hand and previous cases in the clinician's memory. One syndrome is recognized as a replica of the other. In the hands of the wise and experienced clinician the method is quick and accurate.

diarrhea of several housed dairy cows with winter dysentery; the skin lesions of contagious ecthyma in a sheep; ringworm in a kitten; and the upright ear position and sardonic grin in a dog with tetanus. The same experience may occur while taking the history. A clinician may have to rely entirely on the history in the case of a dog having a history of epileptic seizures but which is now normal.

Pattern recognition has obvious disadvantages. In the attempt to draw analogies with previously examined individuals or populations, clinicians may subconsciously limit their range of available diagnoses to syndromes they have previously diagnosed. As a consequence, when this method is used routinely only those disease entities that have been previously recognized will be diagnosed. Any factor that limits the veterinarian's base of experience and diagnostic knowledge potentially limits the range of plausible diagnostic possibilities. Older, more experienced practitioners will have seen a greater variety of diseases than recent graduates. However, unless this wealth of experience includes definitive diagnoses the ability to correctly diagnose any disease or syndrome will not be enhanced. Overreliance on this method can yield and perpetuate inaccurate diagnoses because of lack of awareness of advances in veterinary science.

Regional or local differences will also skew the practitioner's basis for forming diagnostic analogies. When veterinarians move into a new geographic area they are frequently confronted by animals that display a pattern of clinical signs outside the realm of their experience. Lacking the appropriate basis to form diagnostic analogies, these practitioners may draw a blank or misdiagnose the disease occurrence. Upon examining a cow with hyperpnea, scleral injection and fever a practitioner might rationally make a tentative diagnosis of pneumonia. However, in another area these same clinical findings could also be consistent with acute anaplasmosis. Examination of the mucous

membranes for pallor and icterus would be second nature for a practitioner in an area with endemic anaplasmosis, whereas these clinical findings might be missed or their significance discounted in an area with a low prevalence of that disease.

Experienced clinicians find pattern recognition a useful and expeditious approach. It is rapid and relatively inexpensive because it involves less iteration of reasoning and hypothesis development, and less diagnostic testing. The basic tenet of this approach is: 'If it walks like a duck, looks like a duck and sounds like a duck, it probably is a duck'. However, it is imperative that pattern recognition be considered inappropriate for veterinary students and practitioners in the early stages of their careers, as such individuals lack the experience to rely on intuitive recognition. For those who may have only seen one duck or only read about ducks, it may be tempting to classify geese, gulls and herons as ducks. Clearly, when this approach does not permit a rapid and accurate diagnosis a more regimented and systemic approach is warranted.

## Method 2: hypothetico-deductive reasoning

The hypothetico-deductive reasoning method of diagnosis is used by experienced clinicians and is probably the most commonly used form of diagnostic reasoning.

As soon as the client begins to relate the presenting signs, usually starting with the key clinical sign, the clinician begins to create a short list of diagnostic possibilities. This is the process of generating multiple plausible diagnostic hypotheses from initial clues. The clinician then begins to ask questions and conduct clinical examinations that test the hypotheses. The questions and examinations may be directed at supporting or discounting the tentative diagnoses (the confirm–exclude technique) but they may lead to the addition of more hypotheses and the deletion of others. Directed questions are used here, aimed at supporting or refuting a hypothesis, and are distinctly different from scanning questions, which are 'fishing expeditions' looking for additional key signs about which to ask search questions. This process of hypothesis and deduction is continued until one diagnosis is preferred to the others. The original list of hypotheses may be expanded, but usually to not more than seven, and in the final stages is usually reduced to two or three. These are then arranged in order of perceived probability and become the list of diagnostic possibilities, or the differential diagnoses.

One of the important characteristics of the hypothetico-deductive reasoning method is the dependence on the selection of pivotal or key clinical findings, or clues, on which to base the original hypotheses. The

### Changes in Disease Patterns over Time

Pattern recognition assumes a static biology of disease, the clinician must therefore be vigilant to changes in diseases over time. There are well-recognized shifts in disease prevalence over the seasons and years. In the late 1970s, for example, practitioners presented with dogs with vomiting and diarrhea rarely considered parvovirus enteritis as a potential diagnosis. Shifts in the disease prevalence rendered accumulated experience less relevant to the diagnosis of an emerging disease problem.

> ### The Hypothetico-deductive Reasoning Approach
>
> This approach depends on the selection of key clues to support or discount a hypothesis. It may falter in complex cases with multiple disease processes.

> ### Algorithm Approach
>
> Algorithms are suitable for inexperienced clinicians as they list the tests to be carried out and clinical cues to be looked for, thus providing the sequential diagnostic steps to be taken.

key sign and additional supporting clinical findings are selected instinctively by experienced clinicians on the basis of prior experience in similar situations. For novices it may be necessary to examine two or more key signs.

## Method 3: multiple-branching or algorithm

This is an extension of the hypothetico-deductive reasoning method but is formalized according to a preplanned program. The hypothetico-deductive reasoning method depends on the clinician remembering and being aware of an all-inclusive list of diagnostic possibilities in the case under consideration. Because memory is unreliable and impressionistic the method is subject to error by omission. The multiple-branching or algorithmic method similarly approaches a listed series of diagnoses and examines each one in turn, with supporting or disproving questions; if they pass the proving test they stay in; if they fail it they are deleted. For example, a key sign of red urine in a cow prompts the question, Has the cow had access to plant substances that color the urine red? If the answer is no, the next question is, Is the red color caused by hemoglobinuria or hematuria? If the answer is hemoglobinuria, all of the diagnoses on the hematuria branch of the algorithm are deleted and the questioner proceeds to the next question, which will attempt to determine whether the cow has postparturient hemoglobinuria or any one of a number of diseases characterized by intravascular hemolysis. In a cat with a sudden onset of a head tilt we need to determine whether the problem is peripheral or central vestibular disease. After examining the cat, the clinician must decide whether it is experiencing vertical nystagmus? If the answer is yes, all of the diagnoses on the peripheral vestibular disease branch of the algorithm are deleted and the clinician then proceeds to the next question, which attempts to determine the cause of the central vestibular disease.

Provided that the list of possible diagnoses is complete and is frequently updated as new diagnoses become available and, just as importantly, as new ways of supporting or discounting each hypothesis are added as soon as they are published, the method works

well. These algorithms are well suited to computerization and can be made readily available.

The algorithmic method is ideal for the clinician who has not had the necessary experience of memorizing long lists of potential diagnoses and the critical tests that confirm or exclude each of them. Because algorithms are likely to include **all** recorded diagnoses having that particular key sign, error by omission is not a risk.

## Method 4: the key abnormality of function

This method is more complex than the previous ones and requires that clinicians rely on their knowledge of normal structure and function to identify and evaluate the key abnormality or clinical cue. When used judiciously it is highly reliable, especially for difficult cases. The method consists of five steps and is summarized in Figure 2.1.

### Step 1: Determination of the abnormality of structure and/or function present

Disease is an abnormality of structure or function that is harmful to the animal or unacceptable to the owner. The first step is to decide what abnormality of function is present. There may be more than one and some insignificant abnormalities may be present, for example a physiological cardiac murmur in a newborn animal. Abnormalities of function are described in general terms as, for example paralysis, weakness, alopecia, pallor of mucous membranes, rumen stasis, diarrhea, dehydration, dyspnea and shock. These terms are largely clinical and their use requires a knowledge of normal physiology. It is at this point that the preclinical studies of physiology, pathology and disease mechanisms merge with the clinical study of medicine. Familiarity with what is normal combined with observations of the clinical case makes it possible to recognize the physiological abnormality present.

### Step 2: Determination of the system or body as a whole or organ involved

Having made a careful physical examination and recognized the abnormalities, it is then possible to consider

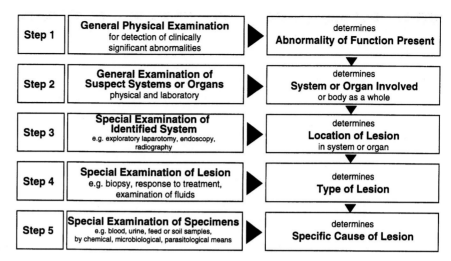

**Fig 2.1**   Making a diagnosis.

which body system or organ is affected. This may not be difficult with some systems: for example, dyspnea may be due to failure of the respiratory or circulatory systems, which are relatively easy to examine. In some cases the body as a whole may be involved. For example, in a recently calved cow weakness and recumbency may be due to hypocalcemia. However, when examining other body systems or organs, such as the nervous system, kidney, endocrine glands and hemopoietic systems, conventional physical examination techniques of palpation, auscultation and percussion may not be rewarding and certain laboratory tests are required. These are described under special examination methods for the various body systems. As a guiding principle, all functions of the body system or organ under examination are observed and any abnormalities noted. For example, if the integrity of the central nervous system is to be examined, the clinician looks for abnormalities of mental state, gait, posture, muscle and sphincter tone and involuntary movements, abnormal posture and paralysis, proprioception and spinal cord reflexes. Knowing the normal physiological functions of systems, one looks for aberrations of them. When only a simple physical examination is possible it may be difficult to choose between two or more systems as the possible location of the abnormality. For example, with a recumbent patient it may be difficult to decide whether the nervous system or the musculoskeletal system or generalized weakness from a systemic illness is the cause of the clinical recumbency.

### Step 3: Determination of the location of the lesion within the system or organ involved

The location of the abnormality within a body system can often be determined by clinical examination. For example, the presence of abnormal lung sounds in an animal with dyspnea suggests the presence of abnormal lung, such as that due to pneumonia or pulmonary edema.

In other cases the location of the lesion within an involved body system may not be obvious and may require special diagnostic techniques and laboratory testing. For example, a detailed neurological examination may be necessary to localize the lesion in an animal with manifestations of disease of the nervous system. This may be combined with radiographic techniques such as myelography. A complete ophthalmologic examination followed by an electroretinogram may be necessary to determine the cause of blindness in a dog. An exploratory laparotomy with intestinal biopsy may be necessary to determine the location of an intestinal lesion thought to be the cause of chronic diarrhea. Medical imaging, including ultrasonograpy and radiography, is often necessary to localize lesions in a body system.

### Step 4: Determination of the type of lesion or the major dysfunction

The abnormality of function may be due to lesions of different types. In general lesions can be divided into morphological or physical, and functional abnormalities. Morphological lesions can be further subdivided into inflammatory, degenerative or space-occupying. These classifications are not mutually exclusive: a lesion may be both inflammatory and space-occupying, such as abscesses in the spinal cord or lung. In these circumstances it is necessary to modify the diagnosis and say that the lesion is space-occupying and may or may not be inflammatory.

> ## Functional Disturbances versus Physical Lesions
>
> The differentiation between functional disturbances and physical lesions is often difficult because the abnormalities produced may be identical, for example
>
> 1. in a case of hypomagnesemia in a cow there is no physical lesion, but differentiation from the encephalitis of furious rabies may be impossible
> 2. a physiological murmur in an anemic puppy may be difficult to differentiate from a congenital subaortic stenosis murmur. As a rule, physiological murmurs will disappear once the underlying predisposing factor is corrected, whereas the congenital murmur will not.

Differentiation between inflammatory, degenerative and space-occupying lesions is usually simpler. Space-occupying lesions result in signs characteristic of pressure on surrounding organs and can often be detected by physical examination. Inflammatory lesions are characterized by heat, pain, swelling and a local or general inflammatory response and, in severe cases, a systemic toxemia. A total white blood cell count and differential is a sensitive but non-specific test for the presence of inflammation. Leukopenia, neutropenia and a degenerative left shift suggest an overwhelming infection, whereas neutrophilia and regenerative shift suggest an active chronic infection. The most common infections of most species that are often not readily obvious clinically are in the thoracic and abdominal cavities, particularly in cattle. These include pleuritis, pulmonary abscesses, pericarditis and peritonitis. Degenerative lesions produce the same loss or abnormality of function as other types but are not usually accompanied by evidence of inflammation unless they are extensive. If the lesion is accessible, biopsy sampling is considered as a means of determining its nature.

### Step 5: Determination of the specific cause of the lesion

If the nature of the abnormality and the type of lesion can be determined the clinician can attempt to identify the specific cause of the abnormality. This may involve examination of laboratory specimens, such as blood, urine, feces, exudate, biopsy material or necropsy examination. For example, in a dog affected with fever and neck pain, a sample of cerebrospinal fluid is obtained and submitted for bacterial culture and drug sensitivity. The results may indicate the presence of meningitis due to staphylococcus infection. In other cases only indirect evidence of the causative lesion is obtained. Thus, if muscular weakness in a well-nourished 2-month-old beef calf was diagnosed as being due to a degenerative lesion of the musculature, only a few causes would be considered as possible diagnoses. Enzootic nutritional myopathy would be highly likely. In many cases it is impossible to go beyond this stage without using additional techniques, particularly laboratory examinations. A high serum creatine kinase activity would provide supporting evidence for a myopathy. It is general practice to make a diagnosis without such confirmatory evidence because of limitations of time or facilities.

It is at this stage that a careful review of the history and examination of the environment yield their real value. It is only by a detailed knowledge of specific diseases, the conditions under which they occur, the epidemiology and the clinical characteristics of each disease, that informed judgments can be made with any degree of accuracy. If the diagnostic possibilities can be reduced to a small number, confirmation of the diagnosis by laboratory methods becomes easier because fewer examinations are needed.

The etiology may also be determined indirectly by response to treatment. In this approach the patient's response following the administration of a treatment specific for a presumptive diagnosis is used to assess the accuracy of that diagnosis. The first readily evident deficiency in this approach is that many clinically ill animals will recover with or without therapeutic intervention. In such cases a response to treatment would be used erroneously to support a presumptive diagnosis which may very well be incorrect. The second weakness is that treatments are usually not entirely specific for a single disease entity. The recovery of a cow following treatment with oxytetracycline for clinical anaplasmosis might be erroneously used to support a diagnosis of pneumonia. Similarly, treatment of a sheep, goat or cow for polioencephalomalacia will often cause a transient response in animals with lead poisoning. In both cases the delays in intervention strategies fostered by misdiagnosis create the potential for continued deaths in the herd.

### Method 5: the exhaustive method

The basis for this method is to take an exhaustive history, examine the patient in great detail and collect as

> ## Accuracy leads to Efficiency
>
> Accuracy in diagnosis means increased efficiency, and this is the final criterion of good veterinary practice.

much baseline laboratory data – screening tests – as is economically justified. Thus the clinician collects as much data as possible then sifts through it all looking for clues to disease. This approach can be very good in diagnosing very rare diseases and for the novice, and should be resorted to when other approaches have failed. Unfortunately, spurious and redundant 'clues' will often be uncovered by this approach. However, all students must be taught how to do this and then to proceed *not* to utilize it very often in practice!

## Method 6: the problem-oriented method

A subcategory of the exhaustive method is the problem-oriented method. The basis of this approach is to carry out a complete clinical and laboratory examination of the patient to acquire a comprehensive database. The problems or key signs in the database are then matched with the knowledge base, in which collections of clinical findings are labeled with diagnoses, to select the best fit.

The method can also be regarded as an expanded version of the hypothetico-deductive method, where the hypotheses are made sequentially as further information becomes available. All diagnostic hypotheses are pursued in parallel because all the possible data have been collected into the database. The source of error in the method is the possibility of undue importance being attached to a chance abnormality in, for example, the clinical biochemistry results. If the abnormality cannot be matched to a clinical finding it should be weighted downwards in value or marked for comment only. The same error may result from the inclusion of an important finding such as diarrhea, which happens either to be present at low intensity or is not diarrhea at all. For example, scant soft feces in cattle with vagus indigestion have been erroneously described as diarrhea.

Following problem identification, potential causes of the abnormalities are identified. The development of a problem list is based on an understanding of potential mechanistic causes of the problems. For example, following history taking and the physical examination, a practitioner identifies the problem of rapid difficult breathing. Understanding the mechanistic or physiologic basis of dyspnea suggests obstruc-

tive airway disease, poor exchange of respiratory gases at the level of the alveolus, compromised blood transport of oxygen, or alternatively respiratory compensation for metabolic acidosis. Identification of these mechanisms readily prompts the listing of potential causes of the patient's condition. For example, decreased blood oxygen transport may occur with anemia, carbon monoxide inhalation and nitrate intoxication. These potential causes are typically referred to as either differential diagnoses or, alternatively, rule-outs, and are introduced *for each problem*.

Each identified problem remains active throughout the diagnosis and management of a case: removal of a problem from the list requires the resolution of that problem, entailing either an effective cure or implementation of a clinical management strategy. In some cases the clinician may relegate one or more problems to inactive status, with a decision being made not to actively pursue a diagnosis.

For each differential diagnosis a test or tests are selected which either increase or decrease the likelihood of that diagnosis. Ideally, tests would confirm rather than merely increase likelihood, and effectively negate the possibility (or rule-out) rather than decrease the likelihood of a diagnosis. Practically, such definitive tests are as much the exception as they are the rule. Progressive cycles of observation and testing permit a more narrow definition of the problem. An initial problem of diarrhea is considered as either a large or a small intestinal problem. Eventually, the repeated testing process permits the framing of a diagnosis. Treatment plans are developed to specifically target the diagnosed disease process. Problems are added or subtracted from the problem list as case management progresses.

The problem-oriented approach inherently resists the temptation to attribute all of a patient's disease manifestations to a single disease process. This method of clinical reasoning is ideally suited to the diagnosis and management of complex cases. The exercise of producing a problem-based medical record has an important instructional role. The importance of this diagnostic method is supported by the American Veterinary Medical Association, which

> ### The Problem-oriented Approach
>
> This approach permits simultaneous investigation of multiple problems and reduces the likelihood of overlooking problems that may be critical to the patient's survival, productivity and quality of life. Each problem is pursued as an independent clinical entity.

requires implementation of a problem-based medical record system as part of its veterinary college accreditation process.

This method also uses the problem-oriented veterinary medical record (POVMR), which is a practical system for the daily recording of clinical and laboratory data in an orderly, systematic and consistent manner that can be followed easily by attending clinicians and their colleagues (see Veterinary Medical Records, pp 67–74).

## DIAGNOSTIC REASONING

Diagnosis is central to clinical veterinary medicine, and the need to establish a diagnostic decision places a demand on the veterinarian's education, experience and judgment. The veterinarian must assemble and employ clinical data, call upon relevant veterinary medical and scientific theory, and use the powers of reason and the lessons of experience to integrate theory and data to arrive at a diagnosis.

If we accept that the generation of diagnostic hypotheses is a crucial step in making a diagnosis, a major question is, How does the veterinarian make the link between the database collected and diagnostic hypotheses? The process of diagnostic reasoning is complex and difficult even for the experienced clinician to describe explicitly. For each of the diagnostic methods described earlier, the clinician had to make a link between the data collected and the generation of diagnostic hypotheses. Just how is that done? Is it necessary for the clinician to have a large knowledge base of the possible diseases, and to compare the essential features of each with the clinical and laboratory findings of the animal for the best fit? What happens if the veterinarian does not have that knowledge base? Is it possible to be sufficiently familiar with a large knowledge base so that diagnostic hypotheses can be generated? Would it be more efficient to attempt to interpret the clinical and laboratory findings with the goal of defining the major dysfunction before generating diagnostic hypotheses?

Diagnostic reasoning can be simply explained as mentally proceeding from data to diagnosis and then to treatment, according to a two-step scheme

The first inference is a matter of arriving at a conclusion about a matter of fact, namely, what is abnormal

> 1. from data, infer diagnosis
> 2. from diagnosis, infer treatment.

about the patient. It is a factual inference. By contrast, the second inference involves arriving at a conclusion about what to do. It is a practical inference. The two-step scheme recognizes that diagnostic reasoning involves a factual and a practical component, separating the two for the purposes of analysis.

The two-step scheme is attractive. Treatment logically follows diagnosis and it would be unwise to treat an animal without some idea of what was abnormal. In addition, once we have a diagnosis we can consult the body of information to determine the treatment of choice.

> Having a diagnosis before instituting therapy seems to be the key to rational treatment.

Yet despite everything favorable that can be said about the two-step scheme, in the end it is an oversimplification of diagnostic reasoning. When a patient is not acutely ill and the diagnosis can be established at little cost or risk, then the scheme represents good clinical practice. However, establishing a diagnosis prior to any treatment is often a clinical luxury. In many cases a diagnosis can only be satisfactorily established by observing the patient's response to treatment.

### A cyclical model of diagnostic reasoning

Six different methods of diagnostic strategies have been described, together with some of the weaknesses that make each of them less than satisfactory. Regardless of which method is used the diagnostic process is cyclical. Patient data prompt diagnostic hypotheses; diagnostic hypotheses prompt tests or treatments; tests and treatments yield new data; new data cause modifications of the diagnostic hypotheses, and so on.

The diagnostic cycle is tentatively represented in Figure 2.2. On initial analysis it can be seen that the clinician cycles through three phases:

> The diagnostic process is potentially so complex that the clinician must make some simplifications in order to proceed at all.

- data generation or gathering (which produces data)
- diagnosis generation (which produces diagnostic hypotheses)
- deliberation about testing or treatment (which produces a management plan for the patient).

The mental and physical actions of the clinician are represented by the arrows, and their products are represented by the boxes. This simple picture is in accord with the two-step scheme: diagnosis generation precedes management in the diagnostic cycle.

### Generation of a diagnosis

Initially we should examine the diagnosis generation portion of the cycle: properly accounting for this will complicate our currently oversimplified simple picture of the process. Obviously, the clinician does not obtain a diagnosis by making inferences from the data alone. Certainly a body of veterinary medical information is involved, especially that defining the features, natural history, etiology and prognosis for various diseases. The current illness might be one not yet recognized, but this possibility is extended by the assumption of completeness. Yet the question remains: How does the clinician deduce a set of diagnostic possibilities from such premises?

One way of explaining such inferences was central to the early diagnostic model developed by Ledley and Lusted (1959) for human medicine. According to the model, medical theory, i.e. the body of medical information, generalizations and scientific laws, associates certain clinical findings with each disease. The association may be effect–cause or cause–effect. It may be logical or merely a statistical association. In any

event, because certain findings are associated with each disease by medical theory, medical theory implies that each finding has certain diseases associated with it. More formally, each finding is associated with a class of diseases we call a disease class. For example, diarrhea is associated with diseases of the digestive tract, even though the lesion causing the diarrhea may be primary (enteritis) or secondary (visceral edema associated with congestive heart failure).

Clinicians are usually portrayed as reasoning from effects to causes. They observe a certain set of manifestations, then deduce one or more possible causes of those manifestations. If they cannot deduce a single cause as the diagnosis, they then perform an experiment designed to eliminate conclusively at least one of the contending hypotheses. The information they acquire may lead them to infer new causes as well, or it may suggest new experiments. Eventually, by repeating this process they deduce the correct diagnosis. The most important observation to make about this style is that it cannot be the complete picture. The reason is basic: causes cannot be deduced from effects – at least, not without employing additional assumptions. Manifestations alone do not imply a particular disease as their cause. In order to make the process work (i.e. in order to get the implication of causes from manifestations) it is necessary to assume that every disease manifestation can be explained by means of current veterinary medical information and theories. This is called the **explanatory completeness assumption**. Given this assumption as a premise, and given that an animal has certain manifestations only if it has some disease or other, it can be deduced that the patient has one of the currently recognized diseases. The body of information contains generalizations to the effect that a certain manifestation is present if – and only if – a

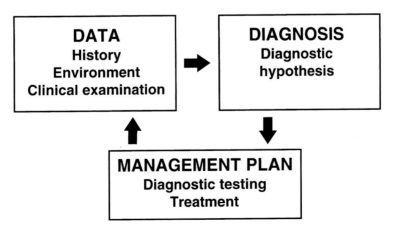

**Fig 2.2** A simplified diagnostic cycle.

certain disease or diseases are present. For example, hemoglobinuria is caused by intravascular hemolysis, of which there are many causes. Similarly, the body of information also contains generalizations to the effect that certain diseases are not present unless certain manifestations are present. For example, in ruminants with carbohydrate engorgement ruminal acidosis is almost always present; the presence of normal ruminal fluid excludes the presence of acute carbohydrate engorgement. Thus if the clinician can establish from clinical data that certain manifestations are absent, then certain diagnostic hypotheses can be excluded.

Thus diagnosticians begin by making observations of certain manifestations. Relying upon the explanatory completeness assumption, they then deductively conclude that the animal has the manifestations because it has one (or more) of the diseases. They then infer that the patient cannot have some of the disease possibilities without certain manifestations. They may then be able to deduce that the patient does not have some of the diseases that are among those possible. But this is as far as they can go deductively. This may be far enough, for they may have eliminated all but one diagnosis. If not, they will have to make additional observations and acquire additional data in the hope of excluding more diagnoses. However, there are at least three shortcomings:

1. the clinical data may be inadequate to eliminate many of the diagnostic possibilities
2. the data available may show that a diagnostic hypothesis under consideration is unlikely, while still failing to eliminate it completely
3. the decisive evidence may be obtainable only at necropsy or by performing a risky diagnostic procedure.

Let us suppose that a patient has certain clinical manifestations. Each of the statements about findings, together with statements from medical theory of the form (**S**) – a patient has finding **F** only if the patient has disease belonging to disease class $D_F$ – entails that the patient has one of the diseases in the disease class associated with that finding. The statements taken together imply that the patient has a disease or diseases belonging to one or more of the disease classes. The explanatory completeness assumption is necessary to assert statements of the form (**S**). Unless the assumption is made, it is possible for a patient to exhibit a finding **F** without having a disease in $D_F$.

At this point the clinician has a list of several possibilities that will include at least some of the diseases the patient may have. The word 'some' is important because the patient may have diseases for which clinical manifestations have not yet been observed. The list

may be long because most findings have many diseases associated with them, and many findings may be present. Some of the possibilities may be eliminated at this stage, if they imply findings that are clearly absent.

It seems reasonable to assume that the patient will have no diseases other than those responsible for the current clinical findings. This assumption will not rule out the recognition of subclinical diseases, provided that the findings contain evidence of them. It will rule out those diseases for which there is no evidence at all. Also, the assumption will not prohibit the introduction of new disease possibilities as additional evidence arises. Each time the clinician goes through the diagnostic cycle, the assumption entails that all the diseases the patient currently has are present on the list derived from the disease classes. This is known as the **no-mere-possibilities assumption**.

The list of possibilities can be narrowed considerably by assuming that the patient has just one disease. Attention can then be centered on those diseases that belong to each disease class associated with the current findings. Assuming the animal has just one disease permits the exclusion of diseases not associated with all current findings. If no disease belongs to all disease classes under consideration, then there is immediate evidence against this assumption. This is called the **one-disease assumption**.

The explanatory completeness assumption is characteristic of ordinary diagnosis. The no-mere-possibilities assumption is part of good scientific methodology. Both can be combined into **background assumptions** (along with current veterinary medical theory) and the one-disease assumption called **simplifying assumptions**.

During diagnostic reasoning the clinician will make background assumptions along with veterinary medical theory and introduce simplifying assumptions. Background assumptions are justified on the basis of being part of diagnostic methodology itself. The simplifying assumptions vary from case to case and their adoption is justified by the situation. Only after the clinician has deduced a range of diagnostic possibilities from the current data and background assumptions will it make sense to consider introducing simplifying assumptions to further narrow the possibilities. Thus Figure 2.2 is revised into Figure 2.3. Here the solid lines represent results arrived at by deductive inference, the dashed lines represent ones resulting from deliberate choices, and the dotted line represents interactions with the animal and client. Thus the initial presentation provides the clinician with a set of data to which is applied background assumptions and current medical theory to deduce an initial set of diagnostic possibilities. At this point the clinician enters the deliberative phase and decides whether to follow a plan of tests or treatments (which might consist of merely continuing to observe the animal for a time) or whether to introduce one or more simplifying assumptions. If tests or treatments are chosen, further data might be awaited before the diagnostic cycle is continued. If the clinician chooses to introduce simplifying assumptions, these will be used to narrow the range of diagnostic possibilities before proceeding to interactions with the patient.

## Diagnostic deliberation

During the course of diagnostic deliberation the clinician chooses a plan for treating the animal or for further determination of diagnosis. There are two kinds of plans, thought plans and management plans. Thought plans involve the introduction of simplifying assumptions to aid the search for the correct diagnosis. They are evaluated in terms of their ability to lead to genuine simplifications, their tendency not to lead the clinician seriously astray, and so on.

Management plans are patient oriented in ways that thought plans are not. They prescribe tests, treatments or observations and are evaluated in terms of how appropriately they deal with what is perceived to be the patient's current situation. However, management plans also include such options as obtaining the opinion of a colleague; acting now rather than thinking further, or thinking now rather than acting. Although these are similar to thought plans, none feeds directly back into the diagnostic-generation phase of the diagnostic cycle. The thoughtful clinician chooses plans, no matter what their type, by weighing them against the other available plans and comparing the potential outcomes of them all. Outcomes are determined partly by the plan and partly by the true state of the patient's health. As the clinician does not usually know the true state, the likelihood of a number of hypotheses must be weighed against the magnitude of the outcomes associated with a plan. These deliberations can be made much more exact by introducing numerical measures of likelihoods and outcome values.

## The acceptance of a diagnosis and closure in making a diagnosis

Clinicians can often proceed without committing themselves to a specific diagnosis. If the diagnostic possibilities can be reduced to a reasonable number, a management plan can be implemented to cover all.

When should clinicians accept a diagnosis and when should they suspend judgment and await further evidence? What are the standards clinicians ought to use in accepting a diagnosis? In science, hypothesis acceptance is usually based upon inductive inferences. Therefore, most hypotheses are never conclusively established, and acquiring more evidence bearing upon the truth or falsity is always possible. The diagnostic process is more promising: it is essentially an exercise in classification which presupposes that the general body of medical knowledge is fixed. Thus there are natural points in which a case can be marked closed. When evidence is pathognomonic, or distinctive or characteristic, then relative to the current veterinary medical classification scheme the evidence suggests the diagnosis deductively and the diagnosis is accepted. The natural histories of diseases provide another means of arriving at closure in diagnosis, and the clinician can make use of them in two ways:

1. when a disease has not run its full course and it is still doubtful whether the animal has it, then the clinician suspends judgment
2. when all diseases under consideration have run their courses and the clinician is still in doubt, then he or she accepts the most likely diagnosis, if any at all is accepted.

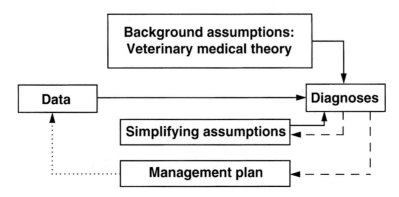

**Fig 2.3**  A complete diagnostic cycle.

When the disease has run its course and all the evidence is in, there is little point in the clinician delaying action on the grounds that more evidence is to be had. However, the quality of evidence is relevant. If there is little evidence and none of the competing diagnoses explains it well, then it is more appropriate for the clinician to acknowledge that fact rather than to accept any diagnosis.

As the clinician works through the differential diagnosis and considers each with the information available, closure of the diagnostic process may be in order. It is important not to close consideration of possible diagnoses too soon. Premature closure on a limited number of problems is an important source of diagnostic error. If the original set of hypotheses was not broad enough to include the patient's problem, the correct diagnosis may never be found during the diagnostic workup. Part of the problem in diagnosis is the limitation on the number of possibilities that can be considered simultaneously. In most cases this ranges from four to seven, which correlates well with the estimates of the capacity of the human short-term memory. However, simple enumeration of the number of possibilities considered simultaneously is misleading, because it fails to recognize the dynamic nature of the diagnostic process. Nevertheless, the total number of hypotheses is usually relatively low and the hypotheses being actively considered profoundly influence subsequent data gathering and interpretation.

The scope of the initial set of hypotheses (the differential diagnostic list) is critical in diagnosis. It should be kept broad and general – 'intestinal obstruction' rather than 'intussusception', for example – in order to generate a net of hypotheses that can encompass all items of information.

## COMPUTER-ASSISTED DIAGNOSIS

In the 1980s there was some interest and activity in the field of computer-assisted diagnosis. It was proposed that the entry of clinical and laboratory data from a case into a computer program could result in the computer providing a differential diagnostic list of diseases from highest to lowest probability. However, despite over 20 years of interest the impact of computer-assisted diagnosis in human medical practice has been slight. Computers have been useful in limited areas such as the differential diagnosis of abdominal pain and the diagnosis and treatment of meningitis, but no program developed for use in a specific localized area of the body has been successfully adapted for generalized use.

Specialists can generate many differential diagnoses in a narrow area of expertise, but the breadth of knowledge required in general practice makes it difficult for generalists to stay current on rare or unusual conditions. If a disease is not considered by the clinician faced with a presenting problem, it is frequently overlooked as a possibility and may not be 'stumbled on' during the diagnostic process. This problem is compounded in veterinary education by the common practice of teaching according to disease entity. The nosology of a disease is presented in a standard format, but in clinical practice the information must then be used in reverse order: the clinician generates a list of diseases based on the history and clinical findings.

The success of a computer-assisted diagnostic program will depend first on the clinician determining the important finding or forceful feature or pivot of the case that can be useful in distinguishing lookalike diseases. The second most important requirement is to know the propensity for a certain clinical finding to occur in a disease syndrome. The algorithm is the center of a computer-aided diagnostic system. Statistical algorithms calculate the most likely diagnosis from explicit statistical analyses of disease probabilities and the frequency of clinical findings in a particular disease. A statistical algorithm is based on the Bayes theorem. The post-test probability that an animal has a given disease can be calculated if one has access to

- the prevalence (pretest probability) of the disease
- the probability of a given clinical finding if the animal has the disease
- the probability of the same clinical finding occurring if the animal has an alternative disease.

After receiving the data, the computer uses this theory to calculate the likelihood of various diseases. However, a major problem with a Bayesian system is the availability of probabilities of the incidence of diseases and clinical findings associated with them. There is a need in veterinary medicine to generate comprehensive databases from which the probabilities of incidence and clinical findings for each disease can be determined from actual clinical practice.

### Textbooks versus Computers for Differential Diagnoses

Textbooks that list differential diagnoses for animals with similar clinical findings are helpful, but they rapidly become outdated because of the many clinical findings which can be associated with a disease. However, the large storage capacity of computer databases, and the ease of access to stored data that can be updated with current findings, make the computer useful for handling this sort of information.

In spite of these limitations, some progress is being made in the development of computer-assisted diagnosis in veterinary medicine, one such program having been developed at Cornell University, Ithaca, New York. The CONSULTANT program was designed by M. E. White and J. Lewkowicz. The clinician enters one or more of the clinical findings in a patient and the computer supplies a list of the diseases in which that clinical finding or combination of clinical findings is present. A complete description can be retrieved for any disease in the list of differential diagnoses. However, a major limitation to date is that the list of differential diagnoses is not in order of probability from highest to lowest. This is because the program does not include the probability of incidence and clinical findings for each disease, information which, as mentioned earlier, is not yet available.

The database is available on the Internet [http://www.vet.cornell.edu/consultant/consult.asp] and contains information on over 6000 diseases of dogs, cats, horses, cattle, sheep, goats and swine.

The initial step in the development of the program was the creation of an exhaustive and exclusive list of clinical signs used in veterinary medicine. This was necessary in order to overcome the problems of syno-nymy and spelling present when signs are entered as free text. Each sign was given an alphanumeric code to facilitate data storage and retrieval, and synonyms were combined under each appropriate code. There are now about 500 separate codes for clinical signs.

After development of the list of signs, a disease database was created by review of the literature. Each disease was given a name, a list of the species affected, a brief description including diagnostic tests and other information useful for diagnosis, a short list of current references and a list of clinical signs seen with the disease. Treatment is not emphasized but is sometimes included in the text. Good review articles are cited so that the user can refer to them for additional details.

CONSULTANT is easy to use. Upon entering the program the user is presented with the choice of accessing information by clinical sign or by disease name. If the clinical sign is chosen, the user is asked to enter the species involved and then one or more clinical signs. Sign codes can be obtained from a printed list, but more often the user enters the name or partial name for the sign and is given the code, which is then entered. More than one sign may be entered, in which case the program searches for only those diseases that have all the indicated signs. As more signs are entered the risk increases that a disease may be inappropriately excluded from the list of differential diagnoses, as human error and disagreements about the definition of diseases makes it impossible that all signs achieve the goal of 100% sensitivity for all diseases.

The CONSULTANT program does not make a diagnosis but merely prompts the clinician to consider possible diagnoses. After all the signs are entered, the program searches the database to find all causes for which that sign or combination of signs has been recorded, and a list of diseases is shown on the screen. Each is numbered and the user may see the entire description in the database by entering the number for that disease. Diseases may also be viewed directly by name, without going through the entire differential diagnosis. The diseases are not ranked in order of probability in the list. Information on diseases in the central database is updated regularly.

Experience with the CONSULTANT program has shown that computer-assisted diagnosis is not used in day-to-day management of routine cases but primarily to provide assurance that a diagnosis was not overlooked when faced with an unusual problem. Computer databases also offer a mechanism for the generalist to search through a complete list of differential diagnoses compiled from the recorded experience of many specialists and kept current as new information is published. Practitioners feel that having access to CONSULTANT is also a significant part of continuing education and a source of references. Experience with a computer-assisted diagnostic system has also confirmed the importance of an accurate history and an adequate clinical examination. If an important clinical finding is not detected, or not adequately recognized, such as neurological weakness of a

---

### The CONSULTANT Program

CONSULTANT was designed to provide differential diagnoses for clinical signs in the seven mammalian species of major veterinary importance and to give current information on diseases of those species. The four major functions of CONSULTANT are

- computer-assisted diagnosis
- review of and access to the clinical literature
- teaching
- diagnostic coding.

---

The CONSULTANT program is best described as an online textbook of differential diagnosis.

limb being misinterpreted as lameness due to musculoskeletal pain, the program will be ineffectual. Disagreement between observers about the meaning of a clinical finding will also continue to be a problem as computer-assisted diagnosis becomes more widely used.

## DIAGNOSTIC TESTING

*It's easier, simpler, and more glamorous to order tests than to talk, examine or think.*

P. Cutler, 1988

### The diagnostic test

A diagnostic test is any procedure used to assist in distinguishing between a normal and an abnormal state in a patient. During the process of making a diagnosis the clinician may select one or more tests to support or possibly exclude diagnostic hypotheses generated by the history and the physical examination. Literally speaking, the use of a stethoscope is a diagnostic test because it can detect the presence of abnormalities. A rectal examination is also a diagnostic test used to diagnose pregnancy in farm animals, and to detect abnormalities of body systems or organs that are palpable by rectal examination. The most commonly employed diagnostic tests are the laboratory tests on fluids and tissues. Diagnostic testing is a critical part of the diagnostic process. Over the past two decades the development of new tests and procedures has increased our ability to reduce diagnostic uncertainty with progressively greater efficiency and lower risk. Until recently human physicians have had virtually a free hand in the use of diagnostic tests, and some order all the tests that may be remotely applicable in a clinical situation. Such a practice may comfort the patient and enhance the physician's belief that all diagnostic avenues have been pursued, but more tests do not necessarily produce more certainty. Veterinary medicine has followed in the footsteps of human medicine with the development of many diagnostic tests, some of which are expensive, and there is some doubt about their validity and applicability. The large number of tests now available is awe-inspiring, but their use is not always in the best interests of the animal.

> ### Diagnostic Tests
>
> More diagnostic tests do not necessarily produce more certainty, but they do incur more expense.

The data generated from diagnostic testing is often less contributory to the case than that obtained from the history and physical examination, but in some cases can be crucial. Some test results are very diagnostic, such as hypocalcemia in a recently calved mature dairy cow which is recumbent or has typical clinical findings of parturient hypocalcemia, hypercalcemia in a mature dog which is experiencing polydipsia and polyuria and has a mass associated with the anal sac. Radiography of the limb of a lame animal may reveal a fractured long bone and is unquestionably a crucial part of developing a diagnosis, prognosis and therapy plan.

Automation and computerization have permitted a large number of tests to be done both quickly and inexpensively. However, many problems have been created by the proliferation of laboratory tests. Evidence provided by each new test may contradict the most likely diagnostic hypothesis, or the test result may be falsely positive or negative. False positive results from unnecessary tests may lead to costly or harmful interventions. Skills in history taking and physical examination may ultimately decline because of overreliance on such testing.

The more information obtained, the more confidence can be felt in the validity of the diagnosis. However, such confidence may not be justified by the quality of information obtained. Despite the limitations of diagnostic procedures, clinicians often run tests excessively, partly because of discomfort with uncertainty.

Absolute certainty in diagnosis is unattainable, no matter how much information we gather or how many tests we perform. Our task is not to attain certainty, but rather to reduce the level of diagnostic uncertainty enough to make optimal therapeutic decisions. Veterinarians have assiduously woven the goal of minimizing uncertainty into the fabric of clinical practice and teaching.

### Kinds of diagnostic tests

Many diagnostic tests are available. Some are expensive, others are inexpensive, some are risky to the animal and others are not. Some are time-consuming whereas others require only a few minutes and can be done in the field.

#### Clinical pathology

A wide variety of laboratory diagnostic tests are in common use as aids to diagnosis. Clinical pathology deals with the laboratory evaluation of body fluids. Clinical hematology deals with measurements such as the hematocrit, white and red blood cell total counts and their differential counts, hemoglobin, plasma proteins, fibrinogen, platelets and clotting factors. Clinical chemistry deals with measurements such as serum electrolytes, trace minerals, lipids, enzymes, glucose, urea, creatinine, blood pH and blood gases. Urinalysis to obtain the specific gravity and measure the constituents of urine is a common diagnostic test.

## Diagnostic microbiology and toxicology

Fluids and tissues may be evaluated in the laboratory for the presence of pathogens in almost any body system. Common examples include the examination of feces for bacteria, viruses, helminths, protozoa and other pathogens. Examination of urine for bacteria is common in small animals. Vacuuming of the haircoat of dogs or cats can aid in the diagnosis of external parasitism and is often performed in conjunction with skin scrapings. Toxic substances can be detected in the feces, stomach contents and body fluids and tissues of poisoned animals. Milk is evaluated for the somatic cell count and the presence of bacterial pathogens causing mastitis.

## Serological tests

Blood samples may be taken from animals with suspected infectious disease and the serum evaluated for the presence of an increase in serum antibody following the infection. A rise in titer between acute and convalescent serum samples indicates that exposure has occurred. This evidence, combined with the presence of clinical findings and isolation of the pathogen from the tissues or fluids, provides supporting evidence for a definitive etiological diagnosis.

## Clinical diagnostic techniques

There are now many clinical diagnostic techniques that are done directly on the animal. They include radiography, ultrasonography, endoscopy, ophthalmoscopy, electrocardiography, electromyography, electroencephalography, scintigraphy, are computerized tomography.

More and more diagnostic procedures are complicated, uncomfortable, expensive or risky. Before resorting to such tests, several factors should be considered.

- What is the likelihood of diagnosis A over diagnosis B?
- Will the test discriminate between A and B?
- If not, what is the incidence of false positives and false negatives?
- What are the risks of the test?
- Will the results of the test alter treatment?
- Is there a choice of treatment?
- What are the risks and possible benefits of the treatment that may result from the test?

## Purposes of diagnostic testing

The most important and common reason for testing is to make a diagnosis. A test or procedure helps to detect, confirm, document or exclude a disease. The aim is to increase certainty and decrease uncertainty.

Diagnostic laboratory data may also assist in making decisions on therapy. An example would be culture and antimicrobial drug sensitivity of bacterial pathogens causing disease. The actual response to therapy can also be measured with some diagnostic tests. Serum electrolytes, blood gases and pH may be determined during hydration therapy of diarrheic and dehydrated animals or those in shock from any cause. The plasma levels of antimicrobial drugs can be measured over time to determine whether minimum inhibitory concentrations have been achieved, and to correlate the levels with clinical response to the treatment.

Prognosis, for example, can be determined by noting the degree of test abnormality, which may be a reflection of the severity of the illness. For example, changes occurring in the leukogram can be used to assist in arriving at a prognosis and following progress in cases of inflammatory disease.

Screening for disease is more complex. Here we search for evidence of illness in healthy animals or look for diseases other than the principal one. The

---

## Clinical Pathology

A combination of laboratory tests of blood and urine can be used to assist in the evaluation of almost any body system or organ.

---

## Reasons for Diagnostic Testing

- to make a diagnosis
- to give a prognosis
- to screen for subclinical disease
- to monitor the clinical course of a patient
- to establish the effectiveness of therapy.

primary purpose of screening for any disease is to alter its natural history by identifying it as early as possible.

The use of tests for monitoring has many purposes. The clinician may desire to measure progression or regression of disease, response to treatment, or drug concentrations of medication being used. Serum levels of copper in grazing animals have been used to monitor their nutritional status and whether or not dietary supplementation is necessary. Monitoring serum electrolytes in previously diagnosed Addisonian dogs, or performing glucose curves in previously diagnosed diabetic animals, aids in therapeutic modification. Somatic cell counts in bulk tank milk samples are a highly reliable method for monitoring the prevalence and incidence of mastitis in dairy herds. Regular serological testing of a herd of animals can be used to monitor the incidence of certain infectious diseases. Saving banks of blood samples from herds of animals is used to retrospectively detect the presence of an infectious disease that may have been present many years before it was recognized as an entity.

## Selection of appropriate diagnostic tests

### Purpose of a test

The major reason for obtaining diagnostic test data ought to be that it is useful for decision making about the animal. The selection of some tests is readily obvious and appropriate, but others are not and may require consideration of the circumstances. Cost is often a major consideration. Determination of the hematocrit, total serum protein concentration and evaluation of the peritoneal fluid in a horse with a suspected intestinal obstruction is clearly indicated.

---

### Diagnostic Tests used for Screening

- Horses hospitalized for major surgical operations may develop salmonellosis, which may be predicted when the leukogram is abnormal, suggesting the early stages of an acute infection.
- The use of metabolic profiles in dairy cattle is intended to detect abnormalities of metabolism associated with the different stages of production in the high-producing dairy cow.
- In breeding dogs, radiography of the pelvis for evidence of hip dysplasia, and blood testing for *Brucella canis* infection and von Willebrand's disease are often performed as screening tests in breeds at risk for such disorders.

---

Performing a Cite test on a fecal sample for the presence of parvovirus in a dog with bloody diarrhea is a reasonable means of obtaining a diagnosis. A sample of ruminal fluid to measure the pH is a powerful diagnostic aid in a ruminant with suspected carbohydrate engorgement. Examination of the semen quality and quantity in a stud animal being evaluated for breeding soundness is necessary. The collection of cerebrospinal fluid from an animal with manifestations of nervous system disease is not routinely indicated unless there is a high probability that the test result will be useful for the selection of treatment.

The criterion for selecting a diagnostic test is whether or not the result can possibly yield any useful information.

### Order of diagnostic testing

Ordinarily the order of testing is from cheap to costly; from less to more risky; and from simple to more complex. For example, measuring of the pH of rumen juice using wide-range pH paper is much simpler and inexpensive than measuring the blood lactic acid level in a ruminant with carbohydrate engorgement. Obtaining cerebrospinal fluid from the lumbosacral space of a heifer with suspected hemophilus meningoencephalitis is more difficult but less risky than obtaining it from the cisterna magna. Within the constraints of time, risk and cost, one usually tries to do the test or procedure with the greatest efficiency as soon as possible, that is, the one with the highest sensitivity, specificity and predicted values.

### Routine testing

Several diagnostic laboratory tests are commonly performed routinely during the diagnostic workup. These include hematology, clinical chemistry, urinalysis, fecal analysis and radiography. Advanced diagnostic laboratory technology has allowed testing of animals for a large number of blood constituents at one time and very quickly; within 1 hour or less if there is access to sophisticated equipment. A group of tests might consist of 10–15 variables, known as small and large animal laboratory panels. These routine tests commonly provide useful evaluation of the blood and blood-forming organs and are considered as part of the clinical examination. In private veterinary practice it is

---

A diagnostic test may be contraindicated because of the degree of risk associated with sample collection.

---

now possible to send blood and other body samples to commercial diagnostic laboratories by courier for testing within hours; the results and interpretation are sent to the practice by facsimile within 24 hours.

## Selective or specific diagnostic testing based on diagnostic hypotheses

In addition to routine testing, there are many elective or special diagnostic tests the use of which is driven by provisional hypotheses. It seems more logical for the clinician to select the tests based on the diagnostic hypotheses that were generated from the history taking and the physical examination, thus

- multiple skin scrapings are recommended on dogs and cats with suspected ectoparasites
- laboratory evaluation of peritoneal fluid is standard practice when evaluating a horse with suspected intestinal obstruction
- coagulation studies are done when bleeding disorders are suspected
- hepatic enzyme determinations are useful when liver disease is suspected
- obtaining pleural fluid from a patient with pleuritis is routine
- the examination of cerebrospinal fluid would be considered routine in animals with suspected disease of the meninges and brain
- in animals with diarrhea, fecal samples may be submitted to determine the presence of enteropathogens
- a transtracheal aspirate or bronchoalveolar lavage may be indicated in animals with pneumonia or disease of the lower respiratory tract.

## Clinical and laboratory measurements

There are three scales to express measurements of clinical and laboratory data: **nominal**, **ordinal**, and **interval.**

Data that can be placed only into categories without inherent order are called **nominal**. Examples include various sounds audible on auscultation and percussion of the abdomen, such as a 'ping' associated with left-side displacement of the abomasum, and the fluid-splashing sounds audible on auscultation and ballottement over the right abdomen of a cow with acute volvulus of the abomasum. A 'ping' may be audible on auscultation and percussion of the cranial abdomen of a dog with gastric dilatation and volvulus. A 'pung' – a low-pitched metallic sound – may be audible on auscultation and percussion of the left abdomen of a cow with an atonic rumen. Normal and abnormal lung

sounds are classified according to a scheme that describes normal breath sounds, crackles and wheezes.

Clinical data that have some inherent order and a consistent measurement scale, such as small to large and good to bad, but for which the size of the intervals cannot be specified, are called **ordinal**. Some clinical examples include mild dyspnea, severe dyspnea, severe distension of the abdomen and a body condition score of 4 out of 5. Deep palpation of the abdomen may reveal an impacted viscus that is described as very heavy, heavy, moderately heavy or light. Lung sounds may be described as being normal breath sounds, loud breath sounds, or loud crackles and wheezes.

Clinical data having an inherent order of rank are known as **interval**. They have also been called numerical or dimensional. The interval scale, used to record quantitative data, represents the highest level of measurement. There are two general types, continuous and discrete. Continuous scales can take on any value in a continuum. Examples include most laboratory values, such as serum chemistry, blood pressure, body weight, body temperature and white and red blood cell counts. Discontinuous or discrete interval scales use only whole numbers: for example, a pen may contain 27 or 28 animals, but not 27.5.

## Test endpoints

In the case of a nominal test result, one test endpoint is often defined as normal. For example, in the case of abdominal percussion and auscultation the absence of a ping is considered normal and its presence is considered abnormal. This type of test result is readily adapted to a black and white presentation of test results in which outcomes are limited to positives and negatives. When ordinal or interval test results are generated by diagnostic testing a threshold or cut-off point is selected and test outcomes are defined relative to this point. Values less than the predetermined level are termed negative and values exceeding this threshold are termed positive.

An alternative strategy often used in the interpretation of interval data is the generation or definition of a normal or reference range. For a test procedure of interest a representative population of normal or healthy animals is screened using the diagnostic test. The mean and standard deviation of the test outcome are calculated. Confidence intervals are calculated (mean $+/- (1.96 \times$ standard deviation$)$). Ideally, 95% of the test endpoints from normal animals will fall within this range; consequently, values that fall outside it are deemed abnormal and suggestive of disease. Theoretically, 2.5% of test results from normal individuals will be lower than the lower confidence limit and 2.5% will exceed the upper confidence limit.

This Gaussian approach is useful but not sacrosanct, as it has a number of inherent problems. The underlying assumption that test outcomes are normally (Gaussian) distributed is probably erroneous under most circumstances: biological data are notorious for their skewed or uneven distributions. Confidence intervals constructed from such data will erroneously place test endpoints from healthy individuals outside the normal range. Consequently, a preliminary analysis of collected test endpoints must be performed to insure a normal or Gaussian distribution prior to the construction of confidence intervals. Such preliminary data screening is rarely performed.

The construction of confidence intervals assumes that 'abnormally low' values (test endpoints less than the lower limit of the confidence interval) are of equal importance to 'abnormally high' values, but in some circumstances this is not true. For example, a high platelet count in horses often occurs with chronic-active infections such as *Rhodococcus equi* pneumonia. However, the activity of many serum enzymes (e.g. sorbitol dehydrogenase, aspartate aminotransferase, serum alkaline phosphatase) below the normal ranges is probably inconsequential. Some positive test results are more positive than others: for example, a rectal temperature of 41.6°C (107.0°F) is more likely to be representative of a real abnormality than one of 40.0 °C (104.0 °F). A serum sodium concentration of 170 mEq/l is more likely to reflect an abnormality than one of 160 mEq/l/l, despite the fact that both exceed the upper limit of established confidence intervals. The further a test result diverges from the reference population values the more likely it is to be indicative of a real organic disease process. When we construct confidence intervals we artificially truncate continuous data and impose a black and white perspective (positive or negative) on test results that are more appropriately viewed as shades of gray.

---

### The Reference Population

The reference population should match the patient as far as possible with regard to age, breed, gender, and use; as differences in these variables will result in entirely different test outcomes. For example, different confidence ranges for hematologic tests are used in warm-blooded horses to those used in cold-blooded horses.

---

### Positive versus Negative Results

The presentation of test results as either positive or negative ignores a basic biological truth – the distributions of test results for diseased and healthy states are not usually mutually exclusive but often overlap.

---

## EVALUATION OF DIAGNOSTIC TESTS

One of the most important determinants in the selection of a diagnostic test is its quality. The criteria for evaluation include validity, reliability, sensitivity, specificity and predictive values.

### Validity

Validity is the degree to which the results of a measurement correspond to the true state of the phenomenon being measured. Another word for validity is accuracy. For clinical observations that can be measured by physical means it is relatively easy to establish validity. The observed measurement is compared to some accepted 'gold' standard. For example, serum sodium can be measured on an instrument recently calibrated against solutions made with known concentrations of sodium. Similarly, the validity of a clinical finding can be established by actual physical examination, surgery, or at necropsy.

---

### Validity

The validity of some clinical observations such as pain, dyspnea or depression cannot be established.

---

### Reliability

Reliability is the extent to which the repeated measurements of a relatively stable phenomenon fall close to each other. Reproducibility and precision are other terms for reliability. It is possible for a laboratory instrument to be on average valid but not reliable, because its results are widely scattered about the true value. On the other hand, an instrument can be very reliable but systematically off the mark or inaccurate.

### Accuracy of a test result

There are four possible interpretations of test results (Table 2.1):

- true positive (a)
- false positive (b)
- true negative (d)
- false negative (c).

Accuracy is the proportion of all test results, both positive and negative (a + b + c + d), that are correct (a + d).

The assessment of a test's accuracy depends on knowing whether or not the disease exists. This is known as the **gold standard,** which is a precise measurement of the truth.

### Test performance

The sensitivity and specificity are used to evaluate a test. It is highly desirable to have a test that is both highly sensitive and highly specific, however this is often not possible. A clear understanding of the principles of test performance is crucial to a reasoned application of diagnostic testing (Table 2.1).

### Sensitivity

The sensitivity of a test is a measure of the proportion of animals with a disease that are positive to the test for that disease (a/(a + c)). A sensitive test will rarely miss animals that have the disease. Sensitive tests are useful during the early stages of a diagnostic workup, when a large number of diagnostic possibilities may be considered, in order to reduce the number of possibilities. Diagnostic tests may be used in these situations to rule out certain diseases, i.e. to establish that certain diseases are unlikely possibilities. Sensitive tests are also useful when the probability of disease is relatively low and the purpose of the test is to discover it.

An example of how this concept could be amplified in a clinical situation is as follows. A mature mid-lactation dairy cow is examined for pelvic limb paresis. Extradural lymphosarcoma caused by the bovine leukosis virus (BLV) is one of the considered differential diagnoses. The agar gel immunodiffusion (AGID) assay is highly sensitive (> 0.95 sensitivity) for infection with BLV. If this cow does in fact have spinal lymphosarcoma caused by BLV the probability of a positive test is 0.95. A negative test under these circumstances effectively negates the possibility of BLV infection, and consequently spinal lymphosarcoma. Using this highly sensitive test the diagnosis of lymphosarcoma is essentially ruled out. Because many cows are virus infected without clinical disease this test has much less application as a procedure to support or confirm the diagnosis of lymphosarcoma. The specificity of AGID serology for lymphosarcoma is inadequate. Stated in more qualitative terms, this test cannot be used as an indicator of lymphosarcoma because virus-infected cows will have positive serology in the absence of lymphosarcoma. Consequently, exclusionary tests place a premium on sensitivity. Such tests may be grossly non-specific, have a high false-positive rate, and still be powerful diagnostic tools. This problem introduces the concept of specificity.

### Specificity

The specificity of a test is a measure of the proportion of animals without a disease that are negative to the test for that disease (d/(b + d)). A specific test will rarely misclassify animals without the disease as being diseased. Specific tests are useful to confirm or 'rule-in' a diagnosis that has been suggested by other data. This is because a highly specific test is rarely positive in the absence of disease, i.e. it gives few false positive results. Consequently, rule-in or confirmatory tests are typically scheduled later in the diagnostic process.

### Probabilities in diagnosis

The probability or likelihood that a disease will occur in a specific animal or herd is usually expressed as a decimal or percentage estimate. For example, the history and the clinical findings may suggest a 0.75 or 75% probability that the animal has a particular disease. The probability of a specific disease in an animal also depends on the prevalence of that disease in the geographical area. In general, diseases restricted to certain foreign geographical areas are usually not considered as probable when generating diagnostic hypotheses.

**Table 2.1. Calculation of selected diagnostic test parameters**

| | Has disease | Does not have disease | |
|---|---|---|---|
| Test positive | a | b | a + b |
| Test negative | c | d | c + d |
| | a + c | b + d | a + b + c + d |

Sensitivity = a/(a + c)
Specificity = d/(b + d)
Prevalence = (a + c)/(a + b + c + d)
Predictive value/positive test = a/(a + b)
Predictive value/negative test = d/(c + d)

As the clinician proceeds along the diagnostic pathway, a most probable diagnosis will emerge, based on an inductive or probabilistic inference. The conclusion is probable relative to the evidence, and additional evidence may make the conclusion more probable. Regardless of how much evidence is acquired, the conclusion will always fall short of mathematical certainty. Clinicians live in a world without certainties and deal with imperfect information. Ideally, probabilities are used to minimize risks and reduce uncertainties. Probabilistic reasoning or inductive inference is practiced in various aspects of veterinary medicine. The pathologist's diagnosis of a biopsied tissue as malignant is based on an inductive inference. Deciding on the effectiveness of an antimicrobial agent, the optimum surgical procedure, the diagnostic relevance of a particular finding, the recommendation of a control procedure such as vaccination of a herd or kennel of animals, the preference for medical or surgical therapy, and the choice of control procedures involves probabilistic estimates.

Probability estimates are obtained from the published data and from estimates clinicians make from their own cases. However, there are limitations to personal experience and so more accurate estimates and monitoring of probability are required.

Prior probability of disease is the proportion of the population that has the disease. The post-test probability of disease or conditional probability is the likelihood that the animal has the disease after the results of the clinical and laboratory examinations are known. As more information is generated about the case the probability can be revised.

In practice, one may start with an animal with an unknown illness knowing that the probability of its having each specific disease equates with the prevalence of each disease. The clinician then aims to use all clues from examinations and tests to raise the likelihood of one or more diseases being present (diagnoses), while reducing the likelihood of other diseases until their probability is negligible (excluded diagnoses). It stands to reason that, if after examination of

a patient the pretest probability of a disease being present (likelihood of a particular diagnosis) is 90%, one should not utilize a particular test that, because of its predictive values, may reduce that likelihood to a post-test probability of 70%. This aspect of diagnostic testing is considered further below.

### Prevalence, prior probability and predictive value

The probability of disease, given the results of a test, is called the predictive value of that test. Positive predictive value is the probability of disease in an animal with a positive or abnormal test result ($a/(a + b)$). Negative predictive value is the probability of not having the disease when the test result is negative or normal ($d/(c + d)$). Predictive value is an answer to the question 'if the test result is positive or negative, what is the probability that the animal does or does not have the disease?' Predictive value is sometimes called post-test probability.

The predictive value of a test is not a property of the test alone. It is determined by the sensitivity and specificity of the test and the prevalence of the disease in the population being tested. Prevalence is the proportion of animals in a given population at a given point in time with the disease in question. Prevalence is also called prior (or pretest) probability.

The following examples illustrate the calculation of the predictive value at varying disease prevalences. An attempt is being made to diagnose disease A. In Table 2.2 the predictive values of positive and negative test results in a population of 10 000 animals with a known disease prevalence of 0.01 (1%) are examined. Test sensitivity and specificity are both 0.95, a reasonable assumption for many commercially available tests.

Although the performance characteristics, sensitivity and specificity of this test are excellent, the predictive value of a positive test is abysmal. Because the test has a sensitivity of 0.95 it will correctly identify 95 of the

### The Use of Statistical Methods

Probabilities are the essence of inductive inference and decision making. Both processes are essential elements of contemporary veterinary medicine. Traditionally, veterinarians made decisions based on accumulated personal experience and reliance on anecdotal information and intuition. However, veterinary medicine has become aware of the significance of analyzed, self-critical experience, and this has encouraged the deliberate use of statistical methods.

**Table 2.2. Example of anticipated test outcomes for a rare disease when using a test with a good sensitivity (0.95) and good specificity (0.95)**

| Test | Disease present | Disease absent | |
|------|-----------------|----------------|------|
| Positive | 95 | 495 | 590 |
| Negative | 5 | 9405 | 9410 |
| | 100 | 9900 | 10 000 |

Prevalence = (95 + 5)/10 000 = 0.01
Sensitivity = 95/(95 + 5) = 0.95
Specificity = 9405/(495 + 9405) = 0.95
Predictive value/positive test = 95/(95 + 495) = 0.16
Predictive value/negative test = 9405/(5 + 9405) = 0.999

100 diseased animals as positive. The remaining 5 will be incorrectly classified as test negative. Because the test has a specificity of 0.95 it will correctly identify 9405 of the 9900 diseased animals as negative, and the remaining 495 will be incorrectly classified as test negative. When dealing with rare or low-prevalence diseases a large proportion of the positive test results represent false positives. Table 2.3 illustrates what happens when an attempt is made to use the same tests in a population with a higher disease prevalence of 0.20. Test sensitivity and specificity remain unchanged at 0.95.

Sensitivity and specificity are properties of the test itself, being static and remaining unchanged as the disease becomes more or less common. Consequently, the proportions of animals correctly identified as disease positive or disease negative by the test remain unchanged. However, the proportion of diseased animals that actually have disease A has increased. As the disease has become more common the number of true positives increases relative to the number of false positives, and the positive predictive value increases. Unfortunately this beneficial change occurs at the expense of a decrease in the predictive value of a negative test. Although this decrease was minimal in our example, substantial reductions in the predictive value of a negative test would occur as the prior probability (prevalence) increases. Consequently, rule-out or exclusionary tests should not be used in animals with a high prior probability of disease.

These examples illustrate four basic truths of diagnostic testing

- decreased prevalence will increase the predictive value of a negative test
- increased sensitivity will increase the predictive value of a negative test
- increased prevalence will increase the predictive value of a positive test
- increased specificity will increase the predictive value of a positive test.

If these concepts are not intuitively obvious the reader should perform similar calculations for different sensitivities, specificities and prevalences. Although these examples are academic exercises, the same properties of sensitivity, specificity and prevalence apply to all test procedures, including clinical examination results, and are therefore of paramount importance to the clinical diagnostic procedure.

Unlike testing, which is performed on a population basis, practitioners have the inherent ability to alter the prior probability of disease. This is one of the factors that amplifies the economy and accuracy of clinical examinations. Although the prevalence of Johne's disease, a chronic wasting disease of cattle, is rela-

**Table 2.3.** Example of anticipated test outcomes for a common disease when using a test with a good sensitivity (0.95 and a good specificity (0.95)

| Test | Disease present | Disease absent | |
|---|---|---|---|
| Positive | 1900 | 400 | 2300 |
| Negative | 100 | 7600 | 7700 |
| | 2000 | 8000 | 10 000 |

Prevalence = (1900 + 100)/10,000 = 0.20
Sensitivity = 1900/(1900 + 100) = 0.95
Specificity = 7600/(7600 + 400) = 0.95
Predictive value/positive test = 1900/(1900 + 400) = 0.826
Predictive value/negative test = 7600/(7600 + 100) = 0.987

tively low, a practitioner can artificially increase its de facto prevalence by limiting testing efforts to animals with an increased likelihood of disease. These will probably be over 2 years of age with chronic diarrhea and weight loss concurrent with a normal appetite. Similarly, the initial diagnosis of Johne's disease in a cow moderately increases the prior probability of the disease in unrelated herdmates, and greatly increases the prior probability in all offspring of the initial case. Therein lies one of the more powerful applications of clinical examinations and diagnostic reasoning. History, signalment and physical examination can be used to decrease the de facto prevalence (prior probability) to the point where the predictive value of a negative test approaches 1. These tests are then used as rule-out procedures. Conversely, these same factors can be used to increase the prior probability of disease, increasing the predictive value of a positive test.

## False positives and false negatives

Each test procedure carries the inherent risk of misclassification, and all tests, including the results of clinical examinations and ancillary or laboratory tests, carry some risk for both false positive and false negative results. Sensitivity and specificity are rarely perfect. As we perform more tests or examinations the potential for an erroneously abnormal false positive result increases. The greatest strength of clinical examination lies in the clinician's intuitive realization that clinically derived data are soft. Clinicians recognize that not all animals with cerebellar disease will have hypermetric gaits, but continue to consciously examine patients for this and other clinical signs in the full knowledge that this observation is neither perfectly sensitive nor perfectly specific. Some patients with cerebellar disease will have a normal gait and some without will have a gait that may be interpreted as hypermetric. Each clinical or laboratory observation either increases or decreases the probability of a specific diagnosis, but neither confirms nor excludes its possibility.

## Rejecting the infallibility of laboratory diagnostic aids

In contrast to the way clinicians question the importance of clinical observation, they often incorrectly overestimate the accuracy and infallibility of laboratory test results. They are often trapped by the authoritative presentation of laboratory data, in which test results are labeled normal, low or high. The process of constructing a 95% confidence interval virtually insures that using most standard laboratory procedures at least 5% of normal, healthy animals will be classified as abnormal or diseased. The specificity of most laboratory procedures is 95%. When 99% confidence intervals are constructed, specificity is enhanced and the false positive rate is decreased. Unfortunately, this increased specificity is usually only achievable by causing a decrease in the sensitivity.

## Serial test procedures and interpretation of test panels

All tests carry an inherent risk of incorrectly identifying a healthy animal as diseased. As the number of tests increases, so does the likelihood that at least one result will be 'abnormal' and fall outside the reference range. This procedure virtually guarantees that a proportion of the normal animals will have abnormal test results. Non-parametrically defined normal ranges have similar problems.

Each measured test outcome has a 5% chance of falling outside the established reference range. If a second test is performed, the probability of at least one false-positive test is 0.0975 (0.05 + (0.95 × 0.05)). If 10 separate tests with a specificity of 0.95 are done, there is a greater than 40% probability that at least one will be abnormal. If a laboratory panel, such as a routine hematology and serum biochemistry screen, contains 33 measured outcomes, there is a greater than 80% probability of at least one false-positive test result, even when the samples tested were obtained from clinically normal individuals. As the number of tests done increases, so does the probability that at least one

measured outcome will be incorrectly labeled as abnormal. These calculations are premised upon the assumption that all test outcomes are independent. This assumption is erroneous; however, this calculation is presented to illustrate the trap of excessive testing. A convenient formula for calculating the probability of at least one false-positive test results is as follows:

$$P = 1 - (\text{specificity})^{(\text{number of tests performed})}.$$

## Parallel testing procedures

The problem of false-positive results is not as monumental as it may at first seem. Clinicians usually de-velop an intuitive knack for interpreting the mass of conflicting test results. Within test panels, safeguards are usually available. If a patient has an increased serum concentration of urea nitrogen, the astute clinician supports a tentative diagnosis of azotemia by assessing the serum creatinine concentration. Subconsciously, the principle of in-series testing is used. Before classifying a patient as azotemic the clinician decided that multiple, independent tests must have outcomes that fall outside the reference range. If two tests with a specificity of 0.95 are used, the probability that both will fall outside the normal range purely by chance drops from 0.05 to 0.0025 (0.05 × 0.05 = 0.0025). In a more general form, if we define a false positive as a case in which multiple, unrelated tests have abnormal results in a clinically normal patient, the probability of multiple abnormal results may be calculated as follows:

$$P_{\text{false positive}} = (1 - \text{specificity}_{\text{test 1}})(1 - \text{specificity}_{\text{test 2}})\ldots 1 - \text{specificity}_{\text{test n}}).$$

## Interpretation of diagnostic test results

Diagnostic test results require assessment and interpretation. Assessments can be easily biased by prior expectations of certain results based on diagnostic hypotheses. This risk is particularly high when the veterinarian who examined the animal, without the aid of an independent observer, interprets the data.

The proper selection and interpretation of diagnostic tests and procedures requires that veterinarians have easy access to up-to-date, readily retrievable

---

**False Positive Results**

By the very method in which reference ranges are constructed, a finite proportion of false positive test results are virtually guaranteed.

---

**Independent Assessment of Test Results is Essential**

Clinicians who interpret their own diagnostic test results without independent confirmation are likely to find exactly what they expect, whether it is there or not.

information about the tests. It is not sufficient to know only the 'range of normal' for an analytical test: it is essential to know the distribution of results in animals with and without the disease in question.

To help exclude the presence of disease a test must be sensitive, whereas to confirm its presence the test must be specific. As one or the other of these characteristics is usually lacking in most tests, few are ideal for both ruling out and confirming the same disease.

## Misuse of laboratory tests and diagnostic procedures

Excessive testing has many causes besides the quest for diagnostic certainty; it may be:

- a function of the forces imposed upon the veterinarian by the system of animal care, for example peer pressure
- the convenience with which tests are ordered
- the demands of a client, or
- the desire to avoid malpractice claims.

The greater availability and variety of tests is a driving force behind excessive diagnostic testing. More and more diseases are being recognized, and their diagnosis and monitoring are aided by laboratory tests. The ability to monitor drug levels and perform toxicologic studies has increased laboratory usage. Other reasons include veterinarians' curiosity about test results, ignorance of the characteristics of tests, financial motives and irrational habits. One of the goals should be to eliminate superfluous diagnostic tests while preserving those that produce substantial benefits. Finally, although the generation of income from laboratory testing is also a cause of misuse of tests, access to diagnostic tests will be restricted because of mounting costs.

Advances in diagnostic technology have allowed the establishment of diagnoses with accuracy and safety beyond the dreams of earlier veterinarians. Some of these tests have sensitivities and specificities that are remarkable. Even the relatively invasive procedures, such as upper gastrointestinal endoscopy and bronchoscopy, can be accomplished with minimal morbidity. Indeed, it is the efficiency and safety of these tests and procedures that compel us to use them.

Some veterinarians may underutilize useful diagnostic tests: such failure has the potential to lead to an increase in the case fatality rate. Accordingly, to promote the optimal use of laboratory tests one must consider not only the factors that are responsible for inappropriate or excessive use, but those that foster underuse as well. The latter include failure to review test results and inability to interpret them. Veterinarians must accept the responsibility for both; when they are uncertain about how to proceed they should consult the clinical pathologist or other specialists. Such an approach can be cost effective and will lead to optimal care.

## Economics of diagnostic testing

Although much is said about the economics of veterinary practice, very little has been published about the economics of the clinical examination and diagnostic testing. It is axiomatic that these should be as efficient and economical as possible: every effort should be made to conduct an efficient but adequate clinical examination at the first contact with the animal. Unnecessary and repeated clinical examinations are costly, particularly if they involve travel to re-examine farm animals. Laboratory tests and specialized diagnostic tests, such as ultrasound and the collection of cerebrospinal fluid, are expensive and add to the total costs of care. In herd epidemics the collection of blood, feces, feed, water and other samples entails considerable time and cost. Laboratory testing should be done only if the history and clinical examination provide substantial evidence that the results will assist in making a diagnosis and in developing rational therapy. The veterinarian should decide which tests are necessary to arrive at the most rational diagnosis, and inform the owner of the cost and request permission to conduct them.

Specialized diagnostic tests should be done if there is a prior probability that the results will be helpful and will improve the outcome.

Owners of companion animals, particularly small animals, will frequently agree to pay for expensive

---

### Excessive Testing

The paramount cause of excessive use of diagnostic tests is the inordinate zeal for certainty.

---

### Economics of Testing

Diagnostic testing must be cost effective for food-producing animals. Livestock producers demand a documented return on their investment for veterinary services, including diagnostic testing, and improvement in profitability is an important objective of veterinarians. The health and production problems of greatest economic importance must be identified and resolved as a priority.

laboratory testing. It may be a matter of professional judgment whether these tests are necessary in order to make a diagnosis or formulate rational therapy.

As a final tenet regarding the economics of diagnostic testing 'if the results of the test or procedure are not likely to alter what is done, or improve the outcome for the animal or client, then it probably should not be done.'

# PROGNOSIS

## Definition and purpose of a prognosis

A prognosis is a prediction about the future clinical course of a disease. The likelihood of recovery and being able to fulfill an intended purpose, such as being a companion animal, performing as a recreation or working animal, being able to produce milk, meat and fiber, or being a breeding animal, is also a part of the prognosis. Giving a prognosis implies predicting the outcome of a clinical case with or without treatment. The prognosis should be rational and based on patient data and clinical findings. The prognosis usually follows the diagnosis and is heavily dependent on it.

The dilemma of whether or not to administer a certain drug or perform a certain surgical procedure in a patient with or without an established diagnosis, or when the outcome is uncertain, is familiar to veterinarians. The owner of an animal expects to receive a reasonably accurate prediction of the outcome and cost of treatment for that animal. However, often there is considerable uncertainty about the presence or absence of a certain disease, or its severity, because confirmatory diagnostic information is not available.

The information required for a reasonably accurate prognosis includes

- probability that the disease in question is present
- expected morbidity and case fatality rates for that disease
- stage of the disease
- whether or not a specific treatment or surgical procedure is either available or possible
- cost of the therapy.

If success depends on prolonged and intensive therapy the high cost may be prohibitive to the owner, who then may select euthanasia as the optimal choice.

Veterinarians have an obligation to inform their clients about all possible outcomes and the treatment which is deemed necessary, and should not hesitate to make clear recommendations regarding the treatment or disposition of a case. Different levels of outcome may affect the prognosis and therapeutic decision making. In farm animal breeding stock, for example,

survival is insufficient and treatment often not undertaken if it is unlikely that it will result in complete recovery and return to full breeding capacity. Slaughter for salvage may be the most reasonable choice. In other cases, such as a pleasure horse or pet, the return of sufficient health to permit companionship may satisfy the owner.

There is little published information on prognosis in clinical veterinary medicine. However, expected morbidity and case fatality rates are available for many specific diseases. Veterinary practitioners make decisions about prognoses every day, and in most cases these are based on clinical experience with similar cases. Making a prognosis could be improved by keeping records and following up cases after they have left the care of the veterinarian.

The diversity of the problems encountered in veterinary practice requires vastly different approaches to prognosis, some of which are outlined below.

- The mature Dachshund dog with acute intervertebral disc herniation may be a candidate for surgery, and the consequences and possible outcomes must be explained to the owner.
- The prognosis for a dog with an uncomplicated fractured femur may be excellent, although the ability of the owner to pay for the surgery may be the most fundamental consideration.
- In a cat with mediastinal lymphoma the prognosis may be reasonably good if the attending veterinarian is knowledgeable about the currently accepted chemotherapy protocol and if the owner is able and willing to pay.
- A valuable breeding bull with a fractured femur has a bad prognosis because of the large size and weight of the animal.
- In a mature dairy cow with left-side displacement of the abomasum of a few days' duration the prognosis is good following surgical correction.
- Conversely, in a mature dairy cow with advanced volvulus of the abomasum the prognosis is often unfavorable even with surgery because of the possibility of ischemic tissue damage, the presence of shock and complicating electrolyte imbalances.
- In a dairy herd with a long history of chronic mastitis due to *Staphylococcus aureus*, the prognosis may be poor if the owner does not fully appreciate the epidemiology of the disease and does not comply with the recommendations of the veterinarian.

## Principles of making a prognosis

An understanding of the natural history of a disease is necessary to make a prognosis. This is the time course of events from the biological onset of the disease, ending with recovery, death, or survival with some disability. The clinical course of the disease is a subset of the natural history that begins when the diagnosis is made and ends with recovery, death or disability. The veterinarian must make judgments about the animal's prognosis, namely, the relative probabilities that it will recover fully with or without treatment; die with or without treatment; or survive with particular level of disability with or without treatment.

In some cases the prognosis is obvious,

- the prognosis in a horse with spasmodic colic is excellent, it will recover and return to normal within hours
- a clinical diagnosis of rabies in an animal dictates a prognosis of certain death
- dairy cattle with acute winter dysentery will recover without treatment
- the prognosis for lymphosarcoma in a cow is nil
- the prognosis for a cure with radioactive iodine in hyperthyroid cats is very good
- the prognosis for a cat with pleural effusion due to feline infectious peritonitis is unfavorable.

In other cases, however, the prognosis is not clear and the veterinarian will have to do some careful clinical reasoning. There are at least three strategies for making a prognosis when there is uncertainty.

1. A reliable up-to-date textbook or a specialist can be consulted.
2. Recent literature on the clinical course and prognosis of the disease may be consulted. This may provide the best guidelines for making a prognosis. Specialists may disagree with one another and their evaluation may not be applicable to other clinical environments.
3. To rely on personal experience and simply recall similar cases and what happened to them under various circumstances. However, such an approach is usually biased towards our recent experiences, and a large number of carefully recorded cases are required in order to have much confidence in our prognostic statements about them.

Making a prognosis depends on accuracy of the diagnosis, the nature of the disease, the animal involved, the herd and facilities, the economical value of the animal and financial capability of the owner and the level of management and expertise of the owner.

## Accuracy of the diagnosis

The fundamental component of making a rational prognosis is the accuracy of the diagnosis.

## The disease

The prognosis will depend on the specific disease, its cause, the stage of the clinical course, the laboratory findings, and whether or not it is curable or incurable. For example

- clinical feline immunodeficiency virus infection is an incurable disease
- pneumonic pasteurellosis in weaned beef calves is a curable disease when treated early in the clinical course
- most cattle with peracute malignant catarrhal fever will die within a few days
- most kittens with panleukopenia will die within a few days
- radiographic evidence of pulmonary edema in a dog with congestive heart failure is a poor prognostic sign
- sarcoptic mange is a treatable disease in the dog and the earlier the diagnosis, the more comfortable for both the animal and the owner.

In many other diseases the prognosis cannot be evaluated until the animal has been treated for a few days to ascertain the response to treatment. A failure to respond to treatment can assist the veterinarian in providing a more reliable prognosis.

## The animal

Characteristics of the animal will affect the prognosis. Young farm animals are more susceptible to infectious diseases than mature animals, especially if they have not received sufficient colostrum. Animals not vaccinated against certain diseases, such as anthrax, tetanus, botulism and distemper, may be more likely to die from these diseases than those that are vaccinated.

## The herd and facilities

Characteristics of the herd and the facilities are critical factors, at least in farm animals. For example, if the owner does not have the facilities to institute procedures for the effective control of acute diarrhea in newborn calves in a large beef herd, the prognosis for

### Economics Influence the Prognosis

The ability of the veterinarian or the practice to provide the therapy required at a cost that the owner is able and willing to pay will influence the prognosis for each particular disease.

effective treatment and control will be substantially decreased. To a certain extent the same principle is true for small animals, in particular dogs housed together in a kennel and cats sharing a cattery environment. If the owner does not have the knowledge or facilities to institute procedures for the effective control of respiratory disease, the prognosis for effective treatment and control will be a problem.

### Level of management and expertise of the owner

These can be major factors in determining the outcome of diseases. When owners do not comply with recommendations of the veterinarian, the morbidity and case fatality rates may be higher than when treatment and control recommendations are followed. In small animal practice the veterinarian provides most if not all of the diagnostic and therapeutic procedures in the veterinary hospital. In large animal practice, the diagnosis is normally made on the farm with the use of diagnostic aids that are done back in the laboratory. Therapy for farm animals is carried out directly on the farm, and any continuous intensive care is usually done by the owner under the indirect supervision of the veterinarian, who may be contacted by telephone to answer any questions.

## Making a prognosis and giving advice

Animal owners want their veterinarians to provide a prognosis, or an estimate of the probability that an animal will recover or not with or without treatment, and how much treatment will cost. They also want an estimate of the likelihood that the animal will recover from the current disease and what the duration of signs and convalescent period are likely to be, so that they are aware of the resources required. The different treatment options should be outlined, along with the estimated prognosis, complications and costs, each being clearly explained.

Whether or not veterinarians should give specific recommendations for treatment is controversial. Some owners want an outline of the various options and then advice as to the best one. Some veterinarians believe that the owner should make the decision from several different options. However, this may place undue onus on the owner, who does not have the same degree of understanding of the disease process and little understanding of clinical reasoning. It is prudent for the veterinarian to explain the circumstances and possible consequences of the various options, and to recommend a best option that considers the welfare of the animal as well as its intended purpose and the eco-

nomics of the situation. Most veterinarians would have no difficulty recommending to an owner that a 500 kg finished beef feedlot animal with a fractured tibia should be slaughtered for salvage. Similarly, it is not difficult to recommend euthanasia for a cow with incurable congestive heart failure due to traumatic pericarditis, as she would be condemned if sent to slaughter for salvage. However, it is much more difficult to recommend euthanasia as the treatment of choice for companion small animals affected with a variety of incurable diseases, or acute or chronic diseases which may require expensive surgery and prolonged convalescent therapy. Many owners of cats and dogs with terminal diseases such as cancer, chronic renal failure or congestive heart failure are willing to have almost anything done to prolong the quality and length of their pet's life.

For some diseases the prognosis is dictated by whether or not the animal is treated. Thus, a cat with urethral obstruction will die without treatment. Similarly, a 10-month-old calf affected with a ruptured urethra and subcutaneous cellulitis due to obstructive urolithiasis will die in several days without treatment. The practical question is what is the prognosis and what are the economic costs and benefits if a urethrostomy is done? Is it economical to perform the surgery and, if so, will the animal survive and be a productive and economic unit?

Ideally, objective quantitative data will be available from published or personal critically evaluated case studies to allow the formulation of a prognosis for a case. Let us assume there was a case study published in which 388 racehorses were operated on for osteochondrosis of the medial trochlear ridge of the distal femur, and 217 were reported to return to racing. One might therefore consider giving a likelihood of 56% that a similar case currently undergoing surgery will be 'successful'. Because of variables such as the severity and

---

### Euthanasia

In veterinary medicine euthanasia is an option for any animal with a condition that is difficult or expensive to treat, for example fractures of the long bones of adult horses and cattle, and deep fungal infections in dogs and cats. Depending on the economic value of the farm livestock affected, euthanasia or slaughter for salvage may be a more economical option than treatment. However the owner of a valuable athletic horse with severe pleuropneumonia requiring prolonged and expensive therapy may request that the veterinarian treat the animal despite the high cost.

## Test Results aid the Prognosis

Laboratory results of clinical cases often assist in developing a prognosis. Cattle with peracute coliform mastitis accompanied by a severe leukopenia and neutropenia have a poor prognosis. A less severe change in the leukogram with an increase in band cells within 24 hours after the onset of the disease is an indication of possible recovery.

duration of the lesion, the experience of the surgeon and the level of racing expected, one may modify such a figure either up or down. Unfortunately, there is often not even this sort of preliminary data available to help formulate a prognosis, and veterinarians frequently resort to 'in my experience … ', which unfortunately relates mostly to how well the last similar case turned out, particularly for the less common diseases – a most unsatisfactory means of arriving at a prognosis.

It is most logical to give a prognosis as a percentage or probability figure. This helps to obviate the terrible confusion inherent in subjective terms such as 'good', 'bad', 'poor', 'fair', 'grave' and even 'excellent', (which may mean 60% to one client and 100% to another). In addition, the nature of the prognosis must be made clear. A prognosis of 80% (100 – mortality rate of 20%) in a racehorse may be misleading if the vast majority of survivors would not be suitable for racing; the real prognosis would be much lower. A disease may have a prognosis for living (100 – mortality rate of 20%), but because the vast majority of survivors would not be suitable for racing the prognosis for the latter would be substantially less.

## REFERRALS IN VETERINARY MEDICINE

*When in doubt, refer it!*

When a veterinarian is unable to make a diagnosis or provide appropriate therapy for whatever reason, consideration must be given to referring the case to a colleague. The case may involve a valuable individual

## Prognosis Figures

It is essential that the client fully understands the prognosis figures. A prognosis of 60% for survival in cases of acute parvoviral gastroenteritis in unprotected puppies may have to be restated more graphically as a 40% chance of death.

animal or a herd affected with an epidemic of uncertain etiology. In some cases the owner may request a consultation with another veterinarian. When the veterinarian is unsure of the diagnosis it may be desirable or necessary to request a consultation, usually from a colleague who has special knowledge of the body system or the species affected. A case which is referred to a specialist for diagnosis and treatment is known as a referral. When a veterinarian requests that a colleague examine a clinical case, or consider the clinical information of a case, such a relationship is designated a consultation. The consulted veterinarian does not usually provide the primary care to the patient. The tradition of referring patients to specialists, or even to other general practitioners with recognized special competency, is not as developed in veterinary medicine as in human medicine.

The increasing numbers of veterinary practitioners with advanced specialty training has created a variety of services available to clients. This variety, combined with rising public expectations regarding the quality of veterinary services, creates a climate wherein a timely referral is also good for public relations. The public has become a sophisticated consumer of medicine, both human and veterinary. People are aware of the roles played by specialists in supporting the veterinary healthcare system: they no longer expect their veterinarians to possess all skills needed to handle the health needs of all animals.

### Advantages of a timely referral

Referral to a specialist provides an opportunity to obtain a second opinion on a difficult or unusual case. A referral can also expedite a diagnosis or treatment that requires specialized equipment or expertise. Many general practitioners recognize it is no longer cost effective or profitable for them to attempt to acquire the skills and equipment required for all veterinary disciplines. Taking advantage of the specialist's skills can expand the practice base, broaden the availability of services and raise the level of practice without requiring major investments in training, equipment or facilities. Also, many veterinarians report that the knowledge gained through referral of a puzzling case is a source of continuing education.

An increasing number of veterinarians are becoming specialists who restrict their activities to referrals from other veterinarians. Until recently, most specialists existed almost entirely in veterinary teaching hospitals. However, specialists for almost all disciplines and all species of animals now exist in private practice. In countries where veterinary clinical specialization is less advanced, more reliance is placed on the traditional second-opinion practices, rather than referral. In some instances, referral practices developed because senior members gradually spent more and more time with certain clinical cases, eventually restricting their practice to one species or one discipline.

## Professional liability

Because of the availability of specialists and subspecialists, the law recognizes that general practitioners should call upon the services of experts to aid in the diagnosis and treatment of complicated illnesses and diseases. In human medicine, malpractice suits have played a significant regulatory role. Human medical generalists may be deemed negligent if a patient's life is lost or their health endangered as a result of failure to involve an appropriate specialist. Failure to discharge one's professional duties with the required skill and attention is malpractice. This may entail doing something in an unskilful manner, or failing to carry out some professional act that should have been performed.

Under the law, generalists and specialists are usually compared with other generalists and specialists. The law currently requires that graduate veterinarians possess and apply the skills of the reasonably well qualified veterinary professional. However, rising expectations as to the standard of practice could conceivably change how the law looks at the 'common denominator' of veterinary medicine.

A client who is aware of alternatives and informed about the benefits of requesting a specialist is in a better position to make an informed decision. With more options available, fewer animals will undergo euthanasia, more lives will be saved, and practice standards will continue to rise – all as a direct result of the exchange of ideas and information between referring veterinarians and specialists.

The referral system has advantages for all who participate.

1. The client and the animal benefit because the case is directed to a veterinarian who is likely to provide the best care available.

2. The referring veterinarian benefits by being able to refer a case in which the diagnosis is unclear, the treatment may be difficult, complex or controversial, and the prognosis uncertain. He/she may also refer severe cases, difficult animals, difficult clients, and cases with a poor prognosis.
3. The referring veterinarian also benefits educationally by having some questions answered and by an improved knowledge base.
4. The specialist veterinarian has the satisfaction of providing a service at a consistently high level of intellectual and clinical skill and at the same time acting as a leader in a particular field.

To be effective, each level of the referral system must contribute. The referring veterinarian must insure that the client has access to the next level in the system – the specialist. Clients are responsible for obtaining the best possible advice and veterinary care for their animals and to provide the funds necessary to accomplish the task. The veterinarian who accepts referrals is required to provide the necessary expertise.

The use of veterinary teaching hospitals as referral centers has the advantage of students being able to see some difficult cases to complement primary accession cases. Referrals are also important for postgraduate clinical training programs.

Communication is a major component to effective referrals. In most veterinary practices a high degree of trust exists between the client and the veterinarian. The client understands that the veterinarian who suggests a referral is not admitting inadequacy, but rather giving a high priority to quality veterinary medicine and patient care. This attitude can only improve client relations and help build a satisfied clientele.

## Referring a case

When referring a case, the referring veterinarian contacts the specialist. The important aspects of the case, can be identified and described and any special concerns of the client can be reviewed and discussed. Taking time to clear the way for the client also reduces

---

### Becoming a Referral Specialist

Clinicians do not become referral specialists merely by acquiring specialist equipment or facilities, rather they must complete specific clinical education programs and acquire the experience of large numbers of clinical cases in a particular field.

---

### Specialist Fees

Specialists usually command a higher professional fee than the primary access veterinarian because referral cases are usually difficult and require a considerable investment in time, technical assistance, laboratory evaluation, and expensive specialized diagnostic testing.

the possibility of future misunderstandings resulting from inadequate communication. In addition, if a referral is not warranted or is not in the best interest of the patient, the client is spared the time and expense of an unrewarding venture.

The referring veterinarian makes the appointment with the specialist in consultation with the client. All relevant information, including a written summary of the case, with radiographs, laboratory tests results, treatments given and dosages prescribed, and other items of interest, is sent to the specialist. This will save time and costs and provides the specialist with useful information upon which to base decisions concerning diagnostic evaluation and patient care. Clients should, however, be informed that it may be necessary to repeat some tests, in order to assess progress or deterioration, or to verify important indicators of disease.

A successful referral depends on good communication. The referring veterinarian, the specialist and the client should be kept informed throughout the referral process, either by telephone or by written word. The specialist's responsibilities include communicating to the referring veterinarian the diagnosis and prognosis, the recommended therapies and the follow-up care, including the schedule for re-examination, if required. Pertinent information is conveyed to the client. Good communication maximizes the likelihood that everyone will be satisfied that the patient received the best possible care based upon the best available information.

In some cases the referring veterinarian will be present at the examination of the case, which is beneficial to all parties because it improves communication and avoids misunderstandings. In herd epidemics the referring veterinarian will usually accompany the specialist to the farm and provide the information that is already known. The history of the farm and its management system, the details of the nutrition of the herd and local knowledge of the herd and surrounding herds have complex interactions that can only be explored by discussion.

The specialist should advise the referring veterinarian as soon as possible when the diagnosis is made and treatment initiated. The specialist should not discharge the animal from the clinic without first notifying the referring veterinarian. The animal may require further treatment, the owner may be concerned about its progress and need further advice, or the disease may recur. Thus it is best for the referring veterinarian to be kept informed of the diagnosis and the treatment and the hospital or discharge status of the animal. It is also good professional conduct for the referring veterinarian to contact the client and express an interest in the animal, and encourage the client to keep the veterinarian informed about the progress of the case.

Immediately upon discharge of the animal the specialist must send the referring veterinarian a detailed report, preferably written, which provides advice about continuing care. The specialist should also advise the client to contact the referring veterinarian regarding continuing care, and inform them that he or she will not treat the animal for any disease other than that involved in the referral, except in emergencies or upon consultation with the referring veterinarian. Each veterinarian will collect his own fee from the client.

It is not only common courtesy to contact the referring veterinarian about a case but in many jurisdictions it is now part of the bylaws of Veterinary Acts. An example of such a bylaw of the Saskatchewan Veterinary Medical Association is as follows:

Saskatchewan Veterinary Medical Association Bylaws 33.5:

Consultation with other members shall be conducted in accordance with the following guidelines:

a) When a member is introduced to a case to consult with the attending veterinarian or to give a second opinion on the case, at the request of the attending veterinarian, the member shall:

 i)  make an effort to review the case with the attending veterinarian
 ii)  cooperate with the attending veterinarian in the spirit of professionalism required to assure the client's confidence in veterinary medicine
 iii)  discuss the findings with the client in such a manner as to avoid criticism of the attending veterinarian
 iv)  inform the attending veterinarian of the diagnosis and treatment recommended
 v)  not revisit the patient or client or communicate directly with the client without the knowledge of the attending veterinarian

b) When consulted by a client dissatisfied with the services of another member or other veterinarian, the member shall observe items (i), (ii), (iii) in (a) above.

### Locating a specialist

The American Veterinary Medical Association directory lists a large number of Boards or Colleges whose

---

### Professional Conduct

The specialist is also prevented by a common tenet of professional conduct to avoid criticizing the behavior or performance of the referring veterinarian.

memberships are composed of veterinary specialists. Some of these, such as the American Board of Veterinary Practitioners and the American College of Veterinary Internal Medicine, are further divided into subspecialties. Specialist registries are also in many other countries, including Europe and Australasia. Admission into these organizations is achieved by successfully passing a qualifying examination and by meeting rigorous practice specifications. Many of these individuals restrict their practice activities to their areas of special competence. Within most urban areas it is becoming common to find the names and qualifications of several veterinary specialists listed under 'Veterinarians' or 'Veterinary Hospitals' in the Yellow Pages of the telephone directory.

Regular attendance at local, state and national veterinary association meetings is a good way to become familiar with available specialists. These individuals are often asked to conduct continuing education courses or to speak on items of topical interest. Attendance at such a course or lecture is an ideal way to evaluate the specialist while learning something new.

The veterinary specialist can elevate the level of patient care by providing access to new treatments and new technologies; however, this can only happen to the extent that the general veterinary practitioner recognizes and utilizes all existing levels of expertise within the profession.

## VETERINARY INFORMATION MANAGEMENT

*Knowledge is best learned when applied to a problem.*

### The need for information

For most veterinarians the working day consists largely of making decisions about sick or injured animals, normal animals presented for health consultations and vaccinations, or about herds or flocks of animals whose performance may be below optimum. Decisions are made about diagnosis, prognosis, treatment and control of disease, and animal management. This multiplicity of tasks makes veterinary practice a rich and

exciting experience. The decisions may be onerous because the life of the animal, the emotional bonding between companion animals and their owners and the financial viability of the owner often depend on the veterinarian's ability to make decisions.

Veterinarians use information to improve the accuracy of their decisions. They must interpret the observations made on each case in the light of their clinical experience (internal experience) and the accumulated experience of the whole profession, available through the veterinary literature (external experience). The ability to find and use the required information is an essential skill.

In all facets of veterinary medicine the body of relevant information is large and growing rapidly. With the volume of new information generated each year, veterinarians find it difficult to keep up to date even in limited areas. The public continues to require higher-quality services and requests more and more knowledge about the veterinary services available.

The body of information developed for professional education and practice and stored on a computer would be equally usable for continuing education. The focus of continuing education could then change from the acquisition of new information to acquiring new methods of problem solving and learning new manual skills.

In a study of information resources used by veterinary practitioners, journals were considered the most important source of up-to-date information on current advances. Although practitioners responding in the study reportedly did not use veterinary medical libraries extensively, many said that they would like more contact with such libraries.

Veterinary practitioners commonly say that lack of time is the reason they do not use the literature to solve clinical problems. The difficulties of using journal literature are at least partly logistical: it takes too long to track down the appropriate information because it is either not immediately at hand or the

### A Successful Referral

A successful referral is a win–win situation, the clinician is happy, the specialist is happy, and the client is happy. Best of all, the patient benefits from specialized care; the second opinion is the key.

### Information Overload

It is unrealistic to expect veterinarians to remember everything they need in order to practice, since only the most commonly used information is readily available from memory. A computerized system can provide the practitioner with more and better-structured information upon which to make decisions. It can also print routine advice on nutrition, vaccination schedules and treatment in a form suitable to be given to the client.

sources are too poorly organized for easy information retrieval. Electronic literature searching promises to reduce these barriers. It is now possible for veterinarians to find applicable references, abstracts and even full articles in a few minutes. Such access to the literature is certainly possible in most veterinary colleges on research university campuses, where many other disciplines use online searching. The major problem for private practitioners is to be able to access online literature searches from the clinic. The use of modems and long-distance telephone connection to literature banks such as the Commonwealth Agricultural Bureau or MEDLINE is currently possible.

Keeping up to date with the literature related to a species or class of livestock is a challenge. Veterinarians generally are not well informed about new and useful information in the literature because clinical practice takes priority over reading journals and filing articles for future reference. How then can a practitioner remain informed about new developments and find the information necessary to solve a problem?

## Finding and critically appraising veterinary literature

Two important objectives of reading the veterinary literature are to keep up to date with new advances in clinical care and to seek new solutions to specific diseases which may be difficult to treat or control. These two objectives call for search strategies.

When faced with a problem in the diagnosis, prognosis, treatment, and control of disease, the veterinarian can access the required information using one or more of the following:

- consultation with a specialist
- personal library
- online computer search of the literature
- online computer-assisted diagnosis.

### Consultation with a specialist

The veterinarian may consult with a colleague in the same practice or another practice, a veterinary specialist, or a former teacher who has expertise and is up to date with the literature and has the clinical experience to provide a consultation. When veterinary practitioners receive advice or information from a specialist they should request the published evidence that forms the basis of the advice. If possible, the original published source of the information should be obtained and critically appraised, so that the one requesting the information can make an independent assessment of the evidence. This is a powerful learning tool, because knowledge is best learned when applied to problem solving. Relying on someone else's interpretation of the literature may be misleading and inappropriate for the clinical problem at hand.

### Personal library

Initial consultation of a textbook of clinical veterinary medicine is immediately appropriate. This can be followed by the use of one's own personal library of reprints of published papers or published proceedings of conferences on the subject. Finally, a search of recent issues of veterinary journals, perhaps aided by a file card/keyword system, to identify an exact issue of the journal.

#### Creating and using one's own library

A personal library has the potential to become the most valuable means of keeping up to date. Because individual practices are different there is no single best system to develop a personal veterinary library. Practitioners usually ask two questions about a personal filing system 'what should I put in my library?' and 'how do I find it when I need it?'

A personal library would contain some or all of the following:

- textbooks
- journal articles filed according to subject headings
- reference cards for recording journal articles, titles of textbooks, and occasional publications
- lecture notes and conference proceedings
- summaries of personal clinical cases.

##### Textbooks

The decision as to which textbooks to purchase, use and rely on can be perplexing. There is now a flood of textbooks, many of which simply repeat information published elsewhere. A good textbook is one that assists the reader in the diagnosis, treatment and control of common diseases.

Authors who are dedicated to mastery of the subject and who have credibility because they practice the discipline write useful and authoritative textbooks. The best test for the quality of a textbook is to use it when questions arise about a clinical case: if the necessary information can be found easily, if it is clear and concise, if it is relevant and really helps the clinician to make a diagnosis, recommend treatment, or explain etiology, epidemiology, and pathogenesis, and does it regularly, then it is a good book. Reviews are also helpful guides to textbooks, but unfortunately many are poor because the reviewer has not read and critically evaluated the entire book. Most are in fact book descriptions. Because many textbooks in veterinary medicine are now written by multiple authors the common weaknesses include gross repetition, lack of uniformity in the subjects covered, omissions of certain subjects, poor indexes, and long delays in publication because contributors do not meet deadlines.

*Journals*
Veterinarians read journals for many reasons:

- to keep abreast of professional affairs
- to understand the pathogenesis of disease
- to determine how other clinicians manage a particular problem
- to determine if a new diagnostic test should be used
- to determine new developments on the etiology or epidemiology of disease
- to obtain new information on therapy
- to learn about new developments in animal production.

The development and maintenance of a personal information system and access to the relevant literature is a necessary prerequisite for the up-to-date veterinary practitioner. It is an activity that veterinarians in general do not do well because they were not taught to read journals critically and to apply the relevant literature to the solution of a problem. The emphasis in veterinary education has been on conveying information to students in the lecture theater.

The practitioner should read and study those particular journals that have been shown to yield the most useful information for their work, and these will soon become obvious. Peer-reviewed journals are considered to be more valid than those publishing non-refereed articles, but there is no assurance that refereed articles are more useful or scientifically valid than non-refereed ones.

Some indication of the journals that yield the most information can be gleaned from an analysis of those that were cited most frequently for the development of the CONSULTANT program (see above): 80% of the citations for large animal diseases were from 17 journals and 90% from 25 journals. The top six journals, ranked from highest to lowest citation frequency, were as follows:

- *Journal of the American Veterinary Medical Association*
- *Veterinary Clinics of North America (Food Animal Practice)*
- *Compendium on Continuing Education for the Practicing Veterinarian*

> Knowledge is best learned when applied to the solution of a problem.

- *Veterinary Record*
- *Australian Veterinary Journal*
- *American Journal of Veterinary Research.*

**Storage and retrieval of journal articles**
Being able to browse through journals and identify quickly and efficiently those articles that contain usable information is vitally important because of the large volume of published information available. In recent years it has been commonly said that there is an 'information explosion', and that it is impossible to remain current in a particular field. However, much of this published literature is of questionable quality and much is redundant. Practitioners must learn to identify the scientifically valid, interesting and useful out of the literature of the entire area of interest. In this way it is possible to keep up to date.

The storage and retrieval of articles requires an indexing and filing system. One recommendation is to tear out articles from journals, and to sort and group them according to subject headings that make sense and reflect an intention to go to the library to access the relevant information. Subject headings may be obtained from a textbook, written on individual file folders, and the sorted papers put into the folders in a filing cabinet. When the file becomes too thick, redundant papers can be discarded or new sections made. If an article belongs in two sections it may be put in the section that makes most sense, or a photocopy can be placed in a second section when cross-referencing is required. Efficient user-friendly computer programs now are available for the storage of bibliographic data.

When a clinical problem is encountered the collection of articles can be consulted and reviewed to obtain the necessary information.

*Online literature search*

Ownership of a personal computer is common in the veterinary workplace and provides the potential for a vast array of library applications. One such application is connection to remote health sciences databases, such as MEDLINE and CAB ABSTRACTS. The most common comprehensive and authoritative database for the biomedical sciences, MEDLINE, provides access to over 3000 periodicals, covering veterinary as well as human medicine. From 1966 to the present day, MEDLINE covers over 60 veterinary journals and is updated monthly. Similarly, CAB ABSTRACTS provides abstracted references to the world's agricultural literature, and BIOSIS PREVIEWS provides references for the interdisciplinary life sciences. PubMed is available on the Internet and provides excellent access to medical and veterinary literature databases.

With the advent of compact disc technology many libraries have chosen to access databases through local microcomputer workstations, in addition to remote databases. As a storage medium CD-ROM proves more economically efficient because it does not require a telecommunication link and its associated fees. Many health science libraries now subscribe to the regular issues of CD-ROM discs that can be accessed free within the library. The user visits the library to perform searches, browse the literature and print citations, with training and assistance provided as needed. Librarians may still serve as intermediaries in the search process through a telephone call. A cost-recovery fee is usually associated with this service, for the telecommunications and the database vendor costs for online searching.

Computers are also used in veterinary practices for accounting, drug inventory, word-processing, writing newsletters, analyzing animal health and production data, decision analysis, computer-assisted diagnosis, online literature searches and accessing other databases.

## Critical appraisal of the literature

After the published papers have been identified and their full texts obtained, they must be critically appraised to determine their validity and applicability to the problem at hand.

In addition to keeping up with the literature, clinical questions about specific patients or herd problems require resolution. Controversy is common in veterinary medicine and frequently an equal number of articles can be retrieved on either side of a question. With critical appraisal skills, the reader has the means to determine whether the methods employed in each study justify the conclusions that have been drawn. Often, the final tally is very different when only articles with valid methodology are counted.

Critical appraisal is also essential to keep up to date with patient management for common problems. Knowing how to evaluate the literature may be the only way to evaluate claims about new approaches to patient management, or animal health management at the herd level. Without the tools to systematically evaluate new information, veterinarians may simply continue to imitate those who taught them, no matter how long ago. The skills of critical appraisal allow them to evaluate which new diagnostic and treatment practices are improvements over the old and should be incorporated into practice, and which are not yet adequately proven.

Reading journals and selecting articles for careful study and filing in a personal library is a task requiring time and discipline. When relevant journals have been browsed and the articles of interest identified, a reference card can be made and filed by subject. If the article is of no interest it is not recorded. If the article appears to be important, it should be read and studied carefully.

The Department of Clinical Epidemiology and Biostatistics at McMaster University, Hamilton, Canada, was among the first to publish a series of articles including a flowchart for guiding critical appraisal. The flow chart has decision nodes specific to the clinical application of the information in an article being read. For example, readers are asked to decide whether the results of the study, if valid, would apply in their own clinical practice. It is also pertinent to know whether their intention in reading the article is to use a new diagnostic technique, to learn the clinical course of a disease, to determine etiology or causation, or to make decisions about therapy or control procedures. Depending on their purpose, readers are referred to a tailored set of questions about the patients and methods used in the study that help them decide whether to accept the findings.

Guidelines for reading journal articles are available and include the following suggestions.

1. Read and consider the title. Is it interesting or useful?
2. Read the summary or the abstract. Would the information be useful in practice? If the summary contains useful information then proceed to read the paper carefully.
3. Read the introduction. Good-quality papers contain a concise up-to-date review of the salient features of the literature of the topic.
4. If it is a clinical research paper, make sure the objectives of the experiment are clearly stated.
5. The materials and methods section should clearly describe the experimental design, and adequate selection and number of **control** animals should be included.
6. Examine the results carefully.

---

### Critical Appraisal Skills

The efficient veterinarian will quickly learn critical appraisal skills to cope with the sheer volume of literature. The pile of unread literature on the desks of veterinarians is silent evidence of its vastness and unmanageability, which doubles every 10 years. Using critical appraisal skills one can quickly eliminate those studies whose methods are inadequate or that are not applicable to one's situation.

7. Read and consider the discussion. Are the conclusions supported by the results of the experiment? If not, discard the paper or file it with your comments noted directly on it. If the results and conclusions can stand critical appraisal, file the article for future reference and attempt to apply the new information in practice at the first opportunity.

The critical appraisal exercise involves the following stages.

1. Defining the problems and identifying the information required to resolve the problems.
2. Conducting an efficient search of the literature.
3. Selecting the best of relevant studies and applying rules of evidence to determine their validity.
4. Being able to present to colleagues in a succinct fashion the content of the article and its strengths and weaknesses.
5. Extracting the clinical message and applying it to the patient problem.

## Evidence-based medicine

In human medicine a new paradigm for practice is emerging. Evidence-based medicine de-emphasizes intuition, unsystematic clinical experience and pathophysiological rationale as sufficient grounds for clinical decision making and stresses the examination of evidence from clinical research. It shifts the emphasis from depending solely on experienced clinicians for information on diagnosis, diagnostic tests and therapy, to the published medical literature based on randomized controlled trials. Evidence-based medicine requires new skills, including efficient literature searching and the application of formal rules of evidence.

An important goal of the medical residency program at McMaster University is to educate physicians in the practice of evidence-based medicine. Strategies include a formal weekly academic half-day for residents, devoted to learning the necessary skills; recruitment into teaching of physicians who practice evidence-based medicine; sharing among faculty of approaches to teaching evidence-based medicine; and providing faculty with feedback on their performance as role models and teachers. The influence of evidence-based medicine on clinical practice and medical education is increasing.

The foundations of this paradigm shift lie in the developments in clinical research over the last 30 years. In 1960 the randomized clinical trial was an oddity. It is now accepted that virtually no drug can enter clinical practice without a demonstration of its efficacy in clinical trials. Moreover, the same randomized trial method is increasingly being applied to sur-

gical therapies and diagnostic tests. Meta-analysis is gaining increasing acceptance as a method of summarizing the results of a number of randomized trials, and ultimately may have as profound an effect on treatment policies as have randomized trials themselves.

A new philosophy of medical practice and teaching has followed these methodological advances, manifested in a number of ways.

- A profusion of articles has been published instructing clinicians on how to access, evaluate and interpret the medical literature.
- The principles of clinical epidemiology are increasingly being utilized in day-to-day clinical practice.
- A number of major medical journals have adopted a more informative, structured abstract format.
- Textbooks are beginning to provide a rigorous review of available evidence, including a Methods section describing both the methodological criteria used to systematically evaluate the validity of the clinical evidence and the quantitative techniques used for summarizing the evidence.
- The American College of Physicians has launched a journal club that summarizes new publications of high relevance and methodological rigor.
- Practice guidelines based on rigorous methodological review of the available evidence are increasingly common. This has resulted in a growing demand for courses and seminars that instruct physicians on how to make more effective use of the medical literature in their day-to-day work.

This new paradigm is called evidence-based medicine.

## Evidence-based veterinary medicine

Evidence-based veterinary medicine is just beginning to emerge in college curricula and in practice. When confronted with clinical problems veterinary practitioners have traditionally depended on personal clinical experience, the use of textbooks and consultations with specialists. Evidence-based veterinary medicine can be taught and practiced. The principles of critical appraisal of the literature can be introduced to

---

### Meta-analysis

Meta-analysis is the use of formal statistical techniques to critically evaluate similar experiments. It provides a quantitative synthesis of all the available data.

undergraduates during their clinical years. Clinical faculty members will have to demonstrate leadership by indicating when their decisions are based on personal experience or on valid published literature. Encouraging students to search the literature for the latest information on diagnostic tests and therapeutic measures for actual patients is a powerful teaching tool.

The relatively small size of the database in veterinary medicine compared to human medicine may impede progress in evidence-based practice. Veterinary medicine has just begun to emphasize the importance of randomized controlled trials for diagnosis, therapy and control procedures such as vaccinations.

# FURTHER READING

Albert DA, Murson R, Resnik MD. Reasoning in medicine. An introduction to clinical inference. The John Hopkins University Press. Baltimore and London, 1988.

Barrows HS, Tamblyn RM. Problem-based learning. An approach to medical education. New York: Springer, 1980.

Blois M. Information and medicine. Berkeley, CA: University of California, 1984.

Cutler P. Problem solving in clinical medicine. From data to diagnosis, 3rd edn. Baltimore: Williams & Wilkins, 1998.

De Dombal FT, Leaper DJ, Staniland JT, McCann AP, Horrocks JC. Computer-aided diagnosis of abdominal pain. Br Med J 1972; 2: 9–13.

Elstein AS, Shulman LS, Sprafka SA. Medical problem solving. An analysis of clinical reasoning. Cambridge MA: Harvard University Press, 1978.

Gale J, Marsden P. Medical diagnosis from student to clinician. Oxford: Oxford University Press, 1983.

Gardner IA, Holmes JC. TESTVIEW: a spreadsheet program for evaluation and interpretation of diagnostic tests. Prev Vet Med 1993;17: 9–18.

Gerstman BB, Cappucci DT. Evaluating the reliability of diagnostic test results. J Am Vet Med Assoc 1986;188: 248–251.

Guyatt JG. Evidence-based medicine. A new approach to teaching the practice of medicine. Evidence-based Medicine Working Group. J Am Med Assoc 1992; 268: 2420–2425.

Kassirer JP. Our stubborn quest for diagnostic certainty. A cause of excessive testing. N Engl J Med 1989; 320: 1489–1491.

Ledley RS, Lusted LB. Reasoning foundations of medical diagnosis. Science 1959; 130: 9–21.

Pelzer NL, Leysen JM. Use of information resources by veterinary practitioners. Bull Med Library Assoc 1991; 79: 10–16.

Sackett DL, Haynes RB, Guyatt GH, Tugwell P. Clinical epidemiology. A basic science for clinical medicine, 2nd edn. Boston: Little, Brown and Co, 1991.

Smith RD. Decision analysis in the evaluation of diagnostic tests. J Am Vet Med Assoc 1993; 203: 1184–1192.

Tyler JW, Cullor JS. Titers, tests, and truisms: rational interpretation of diagnostic serologic testing. J Am Vet Med Assoc 1989; 194: 1550–1558.

Vizard AL, Anderson GA, Gasser RB. Determination of the optimum cut-off value of a diagnostic test. Prev Vet Med 1990; 10: 137–143.

Weed LL. Medical records, medical education, and patient care. Chicago: Yearbook Publishers, 1971.

Weed LL. Knowledge coupling, medical education and patient care. CRC Crit Rev Med Informatics 1986; 1: 55–79.

White ME. Computer assisted diagnosis: experience with Consultant Program. J Am Vet Med Assoc 1985; 187: 475–476.

White ME. Evaluating diagnostic test results. J Am Vet Med Assoc 1986; 188: 1141.

White ME. An analysis of journal citation frequency in the Consultant database for computer-assisted diagnosis. J Am Vet Med Assoc 1987; 190: 1098–1101.

White ME, Lewkowicz J. The Consultant database for computer-assisted diagnosis and information management in veterinary medicine. Automedica 1987; 8: 135–140.

White ME, Lummis MM, Roberts LT. Consultant: Computer-assisted differential diagnosis. Vet Comput 1984; 2: 9–12.

# Part Two

## Evaluation of the Patient

# 3
# Clinical Examination Techniques

*O. M. Radostits*

*Don't touch the patient – state first what you see; cultivate your powers of observation. Teach the eye to see, the finger to feel, and the ear to hear.*

Sir William Osler 1849–1919

## METHODS USED IN THE DETECTION OF CLINICAL FINDINGS

The physical examination is done using the senses of sight, touch, hearing, and smell, and comprises the distant examination and the close physical examination.

The distant examination is done by observation prior to handling or restraining the animal, should never be omitted, and may best be undertaken during the period devoted to obtaining the history and taking note of the environment.

During the general or the systematic examination the outer surface of the body and external orifices are also examined by inspection.

### Distant examination

During the distant examination (also known as the audiovisual inspection) the astute clinician sees and hears abnormalities which are audible and visible from a distance. The skills of observation and listening can be learned by taking the time to inspect the animal from a suitable distance for any abnormal activities or noises associated with breathing or muscle movements. This is known as the distant examination.

The audiovisual inspection of the animal or a group of animals from a distance can often yield important information. There are many good examples. The rapid and deep respirations with an expiratory grunt in cattle on autumn pasture suggest acute interstitial pneumonia. A

> ### Close Physical Examination
>
> Techniques used for the close physical examination are
>
> - audiovisual inspection
> - palpation
> - auscultation
> - percussion
> - simultaneous percussion and auscultation
> - ballottement
> - succussion
> - tactile percussion.

loud inspiratory stridor in a 1-month calf suggests laryngitis. Gross distension of the left abdomen in cattle suggests bloat. A double expiratory effort in the mature horse indicates chronic obstructive pulmonary disease. Abnormalities of posture and gait are associated with disease of the musculoskeletal and nervous systems.

Following the distant examination, a close visual inspection is used to evaluate all body systems or regions. Gross abnormalities are noted, and whether they are symmetrical or asymmetrical. This includes the head and neck, skin, musculoskeletal system (bones, joints and muscles), feet, thorax, abdomen, mammary glands, external genitalia, and the acts of eating, drinking, defecation and urination. The act of parturition can also be inspected and monitored.

### Close physical examination

#### Palpation

Direct palpation with the fingers or indirect palpation with a probe is aimed at determining the size, consistency, temperature and sensitivity of a lesion or organ. Many different abnormalities can be detected by palpation. Light palpation is feeling the tissues gently. Deep palpation is applying pressure to gain more information about the consistency of the tissues, to detect pain or to feel abdominal structures through the adominal wall. The large veins such as the jugular veins can be compressed and filled by palpation. The arterial pulse is palpable. Palpation of the musculoskeletal system is the most commonly used method for the examination of lame animals. The coronary bands and sensitive tissues of the feet are palpated routinely in lameness examinations.

External palpation of the abdominal wall is used to feel abdominal structures such as the rumen of cattle and the kidney of the cat. With suitable restraint and a mouth gag, the oral cavity of most species can be palpated with the hand and fingers. The reproductive tract of mature cattle and horses can be examined directly by vaginal examination of the vagina, cervix and uterus. During exploratory laparotomy the abdominal viscera and organs are palpated for evidence of displacement, the presence of abnormal masses, inflammation, and other abnormalities.

The aim of palpation is to detect the presence of changes in tissues, such as swelling, increased warmth or coolness, and pain on palpation. Important pathological changes that may be detected in an organ or tissue by this means include variations in size, shape, consistency and temperature. The presence of abnormal tissues, such as abscesses, neoplasms and other masses, on any visible or palpable body system is also detectable by palpation. The state of the structures identifiable by palpation may be defined by the following terms:

- resilient – a structure quickly resumes its normal shape after pressure is removed
- doughy – pressure causes pitting which persists for a variable time, as in edema
- firm – resistance to pressure is similar to that of normal liver
- hard – the structure has a bone-like consistency
- fluctuating – an undulating or wave-like movement is produced in a structure by the alternating application of pressure
- emphysematous – the structure is enlarged and puffy and yields on pressure, it produces a crepitating or crackling sound because of the presence of air or gas in the tissue.

### Rectal examination

Rectal examination is a technique in which the abdominal contents can be palpated through the rectal wall.

> ### Light Palpation
>
> Almost all external parts of the body, including the skin, mammary glands, abdominal and thoracic walls, external genitalia, muscles, joints, bones, ears and eyes, can be examined easily by light palpation.

The size of the animal determines how much of the abdomen can be palpated in this way.

In dogs and cats rectal examination is limited to the pelvic part of the abdomen. In mature cattle and horses the pelvic and caudal part of the abdomen can be palpated easily. Rectal examination of the reproductive tract is a common part of monitoring reproductive performance in farm livestock, particularly cattle and horses. The pelvic part of the abdomen may be palpable in swine, sheep, and goats if they are large enough to permit a rectal examination. Rectal examination also allows palpation of the caudal part of the abdomen to assess various parts of the digestive tract, (depending on the species being examined); lymph nodes, blood vessels, urinary tract structures, abnormal masses such as tumors and abscesses, and the bony skeleton of the vertebral column and pelvis. It is also an important aspect of the clinical examination of horses and cattle affected with medical and surgical conditions of the digestive tract.

### Ballottement

Ballottement is a variation of palpation used to detect floating viscera or masses in the abdominal cavity. Using the extended fingers or the clenched fist, the abdominal wall is palpated with a firm push to displace the organ or mass, then allowing it to rebound on to the fingertips. Impaction of the abomasum, large tumors and abscesses of the abdominal cavity may also be detected by ballottement. Ballottement and simultaneous auscultation of the abdomen of cattle is also useful to detect fluid-splashing sounds. Their presence over the left abdomen suggests carbohydrate engorgement and excessive quantities of fluid in the rumen, or left-side displacement of the abomasum. Over the right abdomen, fluid-spashing sounds may indicate intestin-

> ### Clinical Pointer
>
> Edema of subcutaneous tissues is characterized by pitting – a depression left when moderate digital pressure is applied.

al obstruction, abomasal volvulus, cecal dilatation and torsion, and paralytic ileus. Ballottement and simultaneous auscultation of the abdomen of the horse with colic may elicit fluid-splashing sounds indicative of intestines filled with fluid, as in intestinal obstruction or paralytic ileus. A modification of the method is tactile percussion, when a cavity containing fluid is percussed sharply on one side and the fluid wave thus set up is palpated on the other. The sensation created by the wave is called a fluid thrill. It is felt most easily with the palm of the hand placed over the opposite side of the abdomen. A fluid wave is most common in diseases that cause ascites and accumulation of fluid in the peritoneal cavity. (See Tactile Percussion, p.57.)

---

### Ballottement of a fetus

Examination of a fetus is a typical use of ballottement – the fetal prominences can easily be felt by pushing the gravid uterus through the abdominal wall over the right flank.

---

## Succussion

Succussion is the shaking or moving of an animal from side to side while auscultating the abdomen for evidence of fluid-splashing sounds caused by fluid and gas-filled intestines or viscera. Free fluid in the peritoneal cavity will usually not result in fluid-splashing sounds using succussion or ballottement because the cavity is under subatmospheric pressure and there is a relative absence of air space for the fluid to create a splashing sound.

## Auscultation

Auscultation is listening to the sounds produced by the functional activity of an organ located within a particular part of the body, in order to assess its physiological state. It is used to evaluate the normal and abnormal sounds of the respiratory tract, heart and alimentary tract. Crepitating sounds produced by abnormal joints may also be heard by auscultation.

Auscultation is done with a good stethoscope and, with experience, will insure uniform and reliable results. A good stethoscope has the following characteristics.

- Ear tips that fit snugly and painlessly. To get this fit choose ear tips of the proper size, align the ear pieces with the angle of the ear canals, and adjust the spring of the connecting metal band to a comfortable tightness.

- Thick-walled tubing as short as feasible to maximize the transmission of sound, about 30 cm if possible, and no longer than 38 cm.
- A bell and diaphragm with a good changeover mechanism.

The bell and diaphragm, which is acoustically designed, is shaped like an open bell and should have a rubber rim, the purpose of which is to eliminate friction between the chest-piece and the animal's haircoat. For large animals a chest-piece about 2.5 cm or so in diameter is satisfactory, but for cats, puppies and small dogs a chest-piece about 1.5 cm is preferable.

A detailed description of the normal and abnormal sounds that may be heard during auscultation of the various organs will be given later in the appropriate parts of the text.

## Percussion

Percussion is striking a part of the body in order to obtain information about the condition of the contiguous tissues and, more particularly, the deeper-lying parts. The body surface is struck so as to set deep parts in vibration and cause them to emit audible sounds. The quality of sounds produced by percussion varies with the density of the parts set in vibration, and may be classified as

- resonant – characteristic of the sound emitted by air-containing organs, such as normal lungs
- tympanic – the sound produced by striking a hollow organ containing gas under pressure, for example tympanitic rumen or cecum, or a stomach in a dog with gastric dilatation and volvulus.
- dull – the sound emitted by a solid organ such as the liver or heart, or when percussion blows are struck over deep muscle masses in large animals.

The value of the method arises from the vibrations imparted at the point of impact, producing audible sounds that vary in volume, pitch or tone when reflected back, because of differences in density of the tissues.

The quality of the sound elicited is governed by a number of factors. The strength of the percussion blow must be kept constant as the sound volume increases

---

### Uses of Percussion

Percussion is used mainly for the examination of

- the thorax, i.e. the lungs and heart
- the abdomen, and
- to detect abnormalities in paranasal sinuses.

---

with stronger percussion. Allowances must be made for the thickness and consistency of overlying tissues. For example, the thinner the thoracic wall, the more resonant the lung. Percussion on a rib must not be compared with percussion on an intercostal space. The size and body condition of the animal are also important considerations. Pigs and sheep are of a suitable size but the fatness of the pig and the fleece of the sheep, plus the uncooperative nature of both species, make percussion impracticable. In mature cattle and horses the abdominal organs are too large and the overlying tissue too thick for satisfactory outlining of organs or abnormal areas, unless the observer is highly skilled. The lungs of cattle, horses and dogs can be satisfactorily examined by percussion, but it requires practice and experience to become skillful and accurate.

Percussion is done with the fingers or with a plexor (hammer) and pleximeter (percussion plate), which is the traditional method in large animals. The back of the fingers or a pleximeter disc may be placed against the part to be struck.

In small animals percussion is usually done using both hands, the middle finger of one hand acting as a pleximeter and the flexed middle finger of the other as a hammer (finger–finger percussion). If desired the flexed finger may be used to strike a pleximeter, or a hammer to strike the finger. The use of the fingers is always preferable in small animals because they produce little or no additional sound. Percussion is not routinely done in small animals. It is particularly difficult to do and to interpret in cats and small dogs.

### Percussion and simultaneous auscultation

Percussion and simultaneous auscultation of the left and right sides of the abdomen is a useful technique in large animals and may be of benefit in dogs and cats. The stethoscope is placed over the area to be examined and the areas around the stethoscope and radiating out from it are percussed. In the dog it is valuable in the detection of dilatation and volvulus of the stomach. Simultaneous percussion and auscultation of the abdomen of the horse with colic is useful to detect pings indicative of intestinal tympany, associated intestinal obstruction or paralytic ileus. In diaphragmatic hernia the presence of gas-filled intestines in the thorax may be determined by this method. The area being examined is percussed with a flick of the finger,

> ### Types of Percussion
>
> 1. Mediate percussion or acoustic percussion – a finger or pleximeter is placed over the area being struck, no stethoscope is used.
> 2. Immediate percussion – the part is percussed directly with the fingertip or with a plexor, and a stethoscope is used near the part being percussed. This method is used most commonly on the abdomen to detect the presence of gas-filled viscera.

or flexed fingers, or by the use of a plexor while auscultating at the same time. The stethoscope is placed immediately adjacent to the area being percussed and the examiner listens for resonant sounds, which may vary from high-pitched bell-like sounds to a low-pitched bass drum sound. The high-pitched sounds or pings have a musical quality and are associated with intestines and viscera that contain gas, such as in left-sided displacement of the abomasum in cattle. Distended loops of intestine containing fluid and gas will also result in a ping on percussion and auscultation. Lower-pitched sounds such as pungs are audible over viscera containing some gas but probably under less pressure, and in viscera which are thicker walled, such as the rumen in rumen collapse syndrome. The pings and pungs that can be elicited over the right and left abdomen of cattle and horses are described in detail in the sections dealing with clinical examination of the alimentary tract in those species.

To elicit the diagnostic ping it is necessary to percuss and auscultate side by side, and to percuss with a quick, sharp, light and localized force. The obvious method is a quick tap with a percussion hammer or similar object. A gas-filled viscus gives a characteristic clear, sharp, high-pitched ping which is distinctly different from the full, low-pitched note of solid or fluid-

> ### Percussion and Simultaneous Auscultation
>
> This is a valuable diagnostic aid for the detection and localization of a gas-filled viscus in the abdomen of cattle with
>
> - left-side displacement of the abomasum
> - right-side dilatation and volvulus of the abomasum
> - cecal dilatation and torsion
> - intestinal tympany associated with acute obstruction or paralytic ileus
> - pneumoperitoneum.

> ### Clinical Pointer
>
> Percussion may be relatively ineffective in a fat animal.

filled viscera. The difference between the two is so dramatic that it is comparatively easy to define the borders of the gas-filled viscus.

The factors that determine whether a ping will be audible are the force of the percussion, the size of the gas-filled viscus, and its proximity to the abdominal wall. The musical quality of the ping is dependent on the thickness of the wall of the viscus (e.g. rumen, abomasum, small or large intestines) and the amount, nature and tension of the gas present.

### Tactile percussion

Tactile percussion is used to detect a fluid wave, which is an undulation of the abdominal wall created by a sharp percussion of the abdominal wall on the opposite side. A fluid wave may be present when the abdominal cavity or rarely the gastrointestinal tract, contains an excessive quantity of fluid. The tactile impulse of the percussion of one abdominal wall is transmitted across the fluid medium to the other side of the abdominal cavity. The undulation can be both seen and felt. The magnitude of the fluid wave depends on the presence of a certain amount of fluid in the peritoneal cavity: it is estimated that at least the ventral one-third of the abdominal cavity must contain fluid before a fluid wave is detectable. A fluid wave can occur in any disease resulting in an excessive amount of fluid in the abdominal cavity.

### Acoustic percussion of the thorax

Acoustic percussion of the thorax is a low-cost method of assessing the tissue density of thoracic organs that is readily adapted to clinical practice. Indications include any clinical findings of disease of the lungs or heart. When performing acoustic percussion, the clinician strikes the surface of the patient and assesses tissue density based on the pitch, resonance, loudness and duration of induced sound. The technique is done without the use of the stethoscope, as in the thorax the resonant sounds are audible with the unaided ear. The resonant sounds (or lack of them) produced by acoustic percussion are a measurement of the acoustic density of underlying tissue. Air produces lower-pitched tones than do solid tissue or fluid. The useful-

---

> ### Acoustic Percussion
>
> Acoustic percussion permits assessment of tissue density to a depth of approximately 7 cm, and may detect lesions as small as 5 cm in diameter. It is most useful in the examination of the thorax where the large closely related areas of air and fluid allow readily detected contrasts.

ness of this technique is limited by the thickness of the body wall, the degree to which acoustic density of superficial tissues accurately reflects that of deeper tissues, and the extent of the lesion the clinician is attempting to detect.

Radiography and ultrasound provide superior diagnostic imaging in companion animals. Acoustic percussion is particularly attractive as a diagnostic tool in agricultural animals owing to economic constraints.

The following general rules should be observed while applying acoustic percussion.

1. The pleximeter (or the back of the finger) must be pressed firmly against the body surface, so that no air space exists between the pleximeter and the skin.
2. The hand using the hammer must be at a higher level than the hand holding the pleximeter. The handle of the hammer must not be held too firmly, but must rest somewhat loosely between the thumb and first two fingers, in order to deliver a swinging blow. The movement should come from the wrist, and not from the elbow or shoulder. When the finger acts as a striker the hands should be held in the same relative position and the movement should involve the wrist.
3. The blows should fall perpendicularly on to the pleximeter, or directly on to the part of the body being examined, because blows delivered from any other angle will evoke a response that may lead to misinterpretation.
4. The whole of the area requiring examination should be percussed systematically, not just isolated places, otherwise localized pathological changes in the structure of underlying tissues or organs may not be detected.

---

> ### Clinical Pointer
>
> A favorite method for percussing is to 'flick' the front of a first or second finger by suddenly releasing it from behind the thumb.

> ### Clinical Pointer
>
> Acoustic percussion has limitations in sheep and hairy goats as the fleece dampens the induced sound.

5. The pleximeter should be struck only when it is stationary. It is then moved a distance equal to its own width, blows of equal force being delivered at each point.

6. The force of the blows should be as light as possible, the lighter they are, within reason, the easier it is to distinguish differences in tone. Strong percussion is used in the examination of deeply situated structures, especially in large animals, and weak percussion for those more superficially situated. Very gentle percussion (threshold percussion), when applicable, yields particularly accurate information.

These rules are intended for general guidance only. Percussion requires much practice and its value depends on experience and, when instruments are used, familiarity with a particular set is most important. Other general factors, for which allowance must be made in the interpretation of the results, are the thickness of the body wall and the amount of air or gas in the underlying viscus. In the thoracic area, percussion over a rib must not be compared with percussion on an intercostal space.

**Anatomical landmarks and techniques**

The thoracic fields identified by acoustic percussion have readily identified boundaries. The triceps brachii muscle forms the cranial border of the percussable lung field. Although the lungs extend further forward, the mass of the triceps muscle makes meaningful percussion difficult. The dorsal extent of the lung field is defined by a line immediately ventral to the transverse processes of the thoracic vertebrae. The diaphragm forms the caudal border of the percussable lung field, and its location will vary between species. The cardiac shadow comprises the cranioventral portion of the lung field.

Instruments are available for performing acoustic percussion (Fig. 3.1), specifically small mallets or hammers (plexors) and metal plates (pleximeters), which are held against the patient's side and then struck with the hammer. Pleximeters are held firmly in an intercostal space, then struck with a loosely held plexor. Tablespoons are often substituted for pleximeters. Many clinicians prefer to use their hands as both plexor and pleximeter. In this case, the index (and third) finger is extended and held against the patient's side, then tapped sharply with three or four fingers of the opposite hand. The frequency (pitch), intensity (loudness) and duration of the induced sound are then assessed. Generally, one begins at the craniodorsal aspect of the thoracic field and sequentially percusses each intercostal space, moving in a ventral direction.

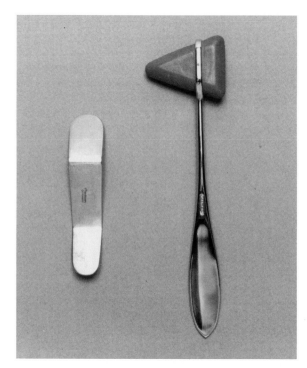

**Fig 3.1** Instruments commonly used in acoustic percussion. Left = pleximeter; right = plexor.

**Abnormal percussion patterns**

The most common abnormality observed when performing acoustic percussion of the thorax is an enlarged area of dullness in the cranioventral area. The most common abnormality detected on acoustic percussion of the thorax is an enlarged area of dullness in the cranioventral area of the thorax on one side or both sides. Potential causes include pleural effusion, anteroventral consolidation of lungs, pericardial effusion, cardiac enlargement, and a space-occupying lesion of the thorax. A pleural effusion commonly results in an area of dullness over the ventral aspect of the thorax with a horizontal border dorsally known as a fluid line.

---

### Sounds Heard with Acoustic Percussion

The sounds which may be heard are:

- Normal resonance associated with normal lung
- Dullness associated with pleural effusion, consolidation of lung, space-occupying mass in thorax, cardiac enlargement, pericardial effusion
- Hyper-resonance in pneumothorax or pulmonary emphysema.

---

## Clinical Pointer

Percussion is often a sensitive indicator of pleural inflammation. Individuals with pleural inflammatory disease may show severe signs of pain (pleurodynia) and may flinch, kick, bite, bellow, or grunt during percussion.

Ancillary clinical findings and diagnostic tests, including transtracheal wash, bronchoalveolar lavage, pericardiocentesis, pleurocentesis, electrocardiography, radiography and ultrasonography may permit narrowing of the differential diagnosis. Test selection will be governed by the presence or absence of other clinical signs.

## EQUIPMENT NEEDED FOR CLINICAL EXAMINATION

The equipment needed for a clinical examination is simple and relatively inexpensive. Some pieces, such as the stethoscope and thermometer, are basic for the examination of any species. The hoof knife is required only in large animal practice. The equipment required includes

- a stethoscope with the characteristics described earlier
- a watch with a second hand
- a thermometer – rapid electronic thermometers are now popular for taking the temperatures of large numbers of animals
- a flashlight or penlight
- a plexor and pleximeter for acoustic percussion and to test reflexes in a neurological examination
- an ophthalmoscope and otoscope
- a ruler and flexible tape measure marked in centimeters for the measurement of lesions
- gloves and protective sleeves for oral, rectal and vaginal examinations
- a hoof knife for the examination of feet in large animals
- a pair of hemostats for a neurological examination
- paper and pen for recording information
- a camera to photograph affected animals and the environment if civil litigation is a possibility
- pail, soap, water, and paper towels
- hypodermic needles and tubes for blood sampling
- sample containers and bags for collection of urine and feces
- cotton-tipped swabs for nasal and ocular discharges.

## DETECTION OF CLINICAL ABNORMALITIES

The physical examination is carried out by looking, listening, touching and smelling. The student is encouraged to cultivate powers of observation, auscultation, palpation, percussion, and smelling. The purpose of the examination is to identify clinically significant abnormalities related to the animal's current illness. It must be done carefully, methodically, and thoroughly to avoid missing any important abnormality.

A clinically significant abnormality of function or structure, also known as a clinical finding or clinical sign, is a deviation from normal which can be detected clinically. Examples include dehydration, diarrhea, vomiting, polydipsia, polyuria, tachycardia, bradycardia, cardiac arrhythmia, fever, hypothermia, dyspnea, epistaxis, intra-abdominal masses on rectal examination, lameness, weakness and recumbency, distension of the abdomen, ataxia, convulsions, rumen stasis, fluid-splashing sounds over the abdomen, nystagmus, hematuria, pale visible mucous membranes, and melena.

The clinical findings are identified and then aggregated into groups related to primary or secondary manifestations of body system or organ disease. For example, acute diarrhea, dehydration, depression, cool extremities, weak peripheral pulse, weakness and recumbency probably represent hypovolemic shock.

When groups of animals are affected with abnormalities it is important to define the case. A case definition is a precise description of the clinical abnormalities affecting a group of animals, including the pattern of occurrence, such as who is affected and when and where it is occurring. Ideally, all clinical abnormalities should be identified.

The diagnosis depends on being able to detect the significant abnormalities and to determine which body systems are involved. However, some abnormalities may not be detectable clinically. In some cases undetectable abnormalities are critical to the diagnosis, whereas in others they may be merely incidental. For example, an enlarged and impacted stomach in a horse with colic cannot usually be detected on clinical examination alone, but detection is critical for the diagnosis. Similarly, it may be difficult to detect evidence of the presence of septic metritis associated with a retained placenta in a large mature dairy cow that calved 6 days ago. Anorexia, fever and tachycardia may be present, but because the cervix is closed and no foul-smelling uterine discharges are detectable on vaginal examination, and because the uterus may not be easily palpable on rectal examination because it is out of reach over the brim of the pelvis, it is difficult to identify the major primary clinical abnormality. In such cases the animal must be monitored over the next few days for evidence of the expulsion of a foul-smelling necrotic placenta with large quantities of uterine exudate.

In most cases animal patients are examined once and a diagnosis is made, but multiple examinations of the same patient are not uncommon. In some cases the abnormalities may not be detectable on initial examination, and re-examination may be necessary. The clinician may be uncertain about particular clinical findings at the first examination but more certain in later examinations. Some clinical findings which were apparently not present on initial examination may become obvious on re-examination, having simply been overlooked the first time. Conversely, one or more abnormalities may not be detectable on careful re-examination. This is particularly true if a consultation is requested; another clinician may decide that there is no abnormality. Repeated physical examinations may be required when the progress of a patient is being monitored over hours or days. For example, a horse with a history of unrelenting abdominal pain may have to be examined repeatedly over several hours before a tentative diagnosis is made. The same animal may have to be examined repeatedly following corrective abdominal surgery in order to identify any complications that may arise.

## THE DIAGNOSTIC POWER OF CLINICAL FINDINGS

Most diagnoses are made after the clinical examination and history taking. Some clinical findings are powerful or convincing determinants of the diagnosis, prognosis and therapy. Others may not be so convincing. Thus, recognition of the key or pivotal clinical abnormalities is a crucial part of the diagnostic cycle. Clinical findings must be reproducible, reliable and unbiased. A mature bull with an obvious hard localized immovable swelling of the mandible probably has lumpy jaw due to actinomycosis. It is unlikely there will be any inconsistency between clinicians in the detection, description and interpretation of the abnormality. However, in an animal with dyspnea there may be significant inconsistencies between clinicians in the type of respirations observed and the breath sounds

---

### Clinical Pointer

By cultivating the powers of observation for the physical examination, the clinical findings should be accurate, reproducible and unbiased.

---

### Primary and Secondary Clinical Findings

It is important to distinguish between primary and secondary clinical findings during the diagnostic process.

- Profuse acute diarrhea in a newborn calf is probably a primary clinical finding.
- Dehydration, weakness, depression, tachycardia and acidosis are clinical findings secondary to the loss of fluids and electrolytes caused by the diarrhea.

---

audible on auscultation. The findings on rectal examination of a horse with acute surgical colic may vary widely between clinicians.

## RELATIVE MERIT OF CLINICAL AND LABORATORY EXAMINATIONS

*When you hear hoof beats, think first of horses, not zebras.*

Coupled with a conscientious history, physical examination will permit a relatively accurate diagnosis in most individual and herd problems. Laboratory tests and other ancillary examinations are best viewed as adjuncts to traditional, low-technology diagnostic approaches. In an ideal diagnostic environment, clinical and laboratory examinations are viewed as parts of a single cohesive whole. The tendency to rely heavily on laboratory diagnostic aids should be resisted. This is not to say that practitioners should reject all technological advances as negative or unnecessary; rather, the strengths of clinical examinations deserve close consideration. The advantages include low cost, ability to

---

### Case Definition

An example of a case definition is the occurrence of acute, highly fatal, diarrhea in beef calves 6 to 8 weeks of age during the calving season, characterized clinically by

- profuse diarrhea
- progressive dehydration and weakness
- failure to respond to treatment with fluid and electrolyte therapy and antimicrobials.

The case definition could be extended to include the pattern of occurrence by indicating whether the calves were born from first-calf heifers or mature cows, and the vaccination history of the dams.

---

pursue multiple lines of reasoning with a single set of tests, repeatability, immediacy of results, and relative diagnostic acuity.

## Cost

First and foremost, clinical examinations are economically more sound than laboratory test procedures. A conscientious history and physical examination includes many separate observations, and these are typically completed during the course of several minutes. These data are broad based, permitting initial, tentative recognition of abnormalities in virtually all organ systems and disease states. Cost considerations are straightforward. Thought and reasoning are relatively inexpensive. In a horse with pneumonia, thoracic auscultation and acoustic percussion can be done for a fraction of the cost of radiography and ultrasonography. Manual vaginal examination of the cow with septic metritis is obviously more efficient than a complete blood count. Based on observed abnormalities, problems are identified and diagnostic hypotheses framed. If ancillary tests are ordered they focus on previously identified problems.

Although clients vary, most have a limit to the financial resources they are willing to devote to the care of an agricultural, performance or companion animal. As diagnostic and treatment efficiency are increased this creates the potential to increase the practitioners financial remuneration, we also improve the cost-efficiency of the services and permit a larger cadre of clients to support optimal care. Consequently, efficient diagnosis creates an environment in which client, patient and practitioner all benefit.

## Synchronous, multiple testing

One of the greatest strengths of the routine physical examination is that it permits the collection of a broad base of medically relevant data. No single laboratory test permits such broadly focused data collection. Consequently, a detailed history and physical examination are the logical first steps in any clinical investigation.

The use of a routine database (CBC, serum chemistry, urinalysis and fecal examination) should be

> Of all the available diagnostic aids, the traditional clinical examination is probably the most underrated.

questioned. Unlike data derived from clinical examination, laboratory test results are often erroneously perceived as 'hard data', or data that really tell the truth. However, most laboratory tests have defined normal ranges, based on confidence intervals derived from a reference population. Reference populations may or may not accurately reflect the group comprising animals at risk. Furthermore, a significant proportion of normal animals will have test results that fall outside established reference ranges. Abnormal test results are not only anticipated, but are actually programmed into this approach.

The perception that physical examination results are soft data is actually a strength because no single observation will typically determine a diagnosis. A single clinical finding is viewed as suggestive, and supporting observations or test results are sought. The skepticism with which we process the results of the clinical examination becomes a significant strength.

As previously discussed, one of the greatest strengths of clinical examination procedures is their ability to alter the prior probability, or de facto prevalence, of disease. As examinations decrease the likelihood of disease, the predictive value of negative test results increases for any laboratory or ancillary tests performed. Maximizing the predictive value of negative tests permits the clinician to effectively rule out low-probability differential diagnoses. In a similar vein, as more and more clinical findings support a diagnostic hypothesis, the prior probability, and consequently the predictive value of positive tests, increases. This permits the clinician to select test procedures with the goal of definitive or confirmatory testing in mind.

## Repeatability and immediacy

The results of the physical examination are readily obtained and are immediately available: there is no time lag for sample collection, submission, processing and reporting, and the clinician can move on to specific diagnostic testing and immediate care. Laboratory testing is not undesirable but waiting for results slows the diagnostic process, which can be life-threatening in critically ill patients. An emphasis on clinical examination permits the clinician to continue the diagnostic process pending the return of confirmatory laboratory test results.

The immediacy of the results highlights the strength of historical and clinical examination data. Following

## Variation in Clinical Findings

Much of the variation between clinicians in the detection of clinical abnormalities is due to the previous experience of the clinicians.

### Speed of the Results

The clinical examination is fast, its results are immediately available; in contrast the clinician must wait for laboratory test results.

auscultation, palpation and observation, test results are integrated and the clinician frames diagnostic hypotheses. The short turnaround time accelerates the diagnostic process. Hypotheses are rejected or more narrowly defined during the examination process. In contrast, laboratory or ancillary testing enforces a halt in the diagnostic reasoning process. During the interval in which samples are obtained, submitted and processed, and results are reported, the diagnostic process is frozen.

Clear definition of clinical problems may in many cases permit life-saving intervention pending the return of definitive test results. For example, recognition of blindness, ataxia, head-pressing, and odontoprisis in a group of young cattle grazed in proximity to a refuse dump strongly suggests lead poisoning. In these circumstances early intervention may reduce the potential intoxication of healthy herdmates pending the return of blood lead determinations. As laboratory results may not be available for several days, the first priority is clearly to move the cattle to a different pasture.

### Acuity

The power of clinical examination is often overlooked. Meticulously cataloged clinical findings will create a strength of evidence which is difficult for laboratory tests to match. For example, the presence of peripheral edema, tachycardia, distension and a marked jugular vein pulse, a right-sided cardiac murmur, and cyclic fevers in a cow provides far more information than a complete blood count for roughly an equivalent expenditure of client resources. The described findings provide strong evidence for bacterial endocarditis of the tricuspid valve. If definitive diagnostic testing is requested or required, highly specific tests, such as blood culture and echocardiographic examination, are selected. It is imperative that practitioners approach cases in a relatively regimented manner. History and physical examination are our most powerful tools, and consequently are performed first. Ancillary test procedures are undertaken only to evaluate diagnostic hypotheses generated by these preliminary exercises.

The specificity and diagnostic value of historical and physical findings often create nearly perfect diagnostic acuity. For example, the recognition of a high-pitched ping in the left paralumbar fossa of a recently calved anorexic dairy cow is a powerful clinical finding. This observation has a test specificity approaching 100%. No laboratory procedure or ancillary examination can reliably achieve the specificity of these observations. Consequently, further diagnostic testing is probably of academic interest only.

### Summary

Ancillary diagnostic testing is right, proper and necessary when the results will

- meaningfully alter treatment to the benefit of the patient
- permit accurate assessment of prognosis and, consequently, aid clients in making informed decisions
- permit the client and clinician to provide better quality care to other animals in the herd or household.

When testing supports these goals it should be strongly encouraged. When it does not it should be discouraged.

Clinical examination procedures have real and distinct advantages over laboratory-based ones. The reasoned application of examination results accelerates the diagnostic process, reduces the cost of ancillary tests, and permits the more definitive interpretation of subsequent test results. Ideally, diagnostic testing is performed to support or reject diagnostic hypotheses raised in response to the history and physical examination.

## ERRORS AND INCONSISTENCIES IN THE CLINICAL EXAMINATION

Consistency is the extent to which multiple examinations of the same patient or specimen agree with one another. Consistency is desirable but insufficient; accuracy also is needed. There is not much consistency in most clinical observations. The clinician must also avoid being misled by poorly collected or biased clinical observations into making an incorrect diagnosis that may lead to inappropriate diagnostic testing and patient management.

Accuracy is the closeness of clinical observation to the true clinical state. The gold standard for a disease is the actual definitive diagnosis determined by an independent test. For example, the presence of characteristic histopathologic changes in the intestinal tissues along with the presence of *Mycobacterium paratuberculosis* is the gold standard for the diagnosis of Johne's disease in cattle. For most clinical assessments

## Consistency versus Accuracy

Consistency – agreement between multiple examinations.
Accuracy – agreement between the clinical observation and the clinical state.

## Some Essential Diagnostic Techniques

1. Simultaneous auscultation and ballottement of the right abdomen is necessary to elicit the fluid-splashing sounds caused by distended loops of intestine associated with acute intestinal obstruction in a mature cow.
2. The passage of a nasogastric tube in a horse with acute colic is necessary to detect a gastric reflux due to a distended fluid-filled stomach that could be fatal unless relieved.
3. A rectal examination is a necessary part of the clinical examination of a horse or cow with abnormalities related to the abdomen.

there is no gold standard of accuracy. Bias is any systematic deviation of an observation from the true clinical state.

Errors in the clinical examination and inconsistencies between veterinarians may occur in the history taking, in the physical examination, and in the interpretation of the findings. Errors often occur because of inadequate clinical examination, more mistakes are made for not looking than for not knowing.

Abnormalities may not be detected on routine physical examination. For example, a reduction in the intensity of the breath sounds over the thorax of an animal with a pleural effusion may not be detected on the initial physical examination. If this is the case the possibility of a pleural effusion may not be considered and the abnormality may simply be missed. The same clinician may re-examine the same lung fields some time later – maybe only minutes later – and detect the abnormality. The failure to perform a thorough clinical examination appropriate for the case is a major cause of error. Auscultation of only one side of the thorax of a cow with suspected respiratory disease may result in failure to detect the absence of breath sounds due to a pleural effusion on the other side. Another reason for missing abnormalities is the failure to carry out certain simple diagnostic techniques. A rectal examination in a 2-year-old heifer that is anorexic and has a fever 10 days following an apparently successful cesarean section, is essential to detect the presence of diffuse peritonitis and intra-abdominal abscesses also a novice may do such a rectal examination but fail to feel the abnormalities because of lack of experience.

## Clinical disagreement

Clinical disagreement is the difference between two or more clinicians about any aspect of a case. It may be about the history, clinical findings, test interpretation, diagnosis, prognosis, or therapeutic decisions.

### History

No two clinicians will obtain the same history about an animal from the same client. Although there may be agreement about the principles of history taking, the facts obtained will often vary between clinicians.

### Clinical findings

Clinicians who examine the same patient often disagree, and the clinician who examines the same patient twice often disagrees with previous findings. One will detect a certain number of abnormalities, whereas another may detect different abnormalities or characterize them differently. This is known as interobserver and intraobserver disagreement. There are many examples to illustrate this problem. One clinician may examine a patient and not detect an abdominal mass on palpation of the abdomen which was detected by a second clinician. One may decide that there is a heart murmur in a young calf with dyspnea whereas another will claim that the abnormal sound is not a heart murmur but a pleural–pericardial friction rub. The changes in the absolute intensity of the heart sounds in an animal with congestive heart failure may not be detectable by some clinicians. A subtle degree of skeletal neurogenic muscle atrophy may not be recognizable by some clinicians, but easily recognizable by one who has taken an interest in that particular disease. Whether or not a mature cow has a grunt on deep palpation of the xiphoid sternum may be controversial. The assessment of the state of the rumen, and its frequency and amplitude of contractions, will vary widely between clinicians.

### Interpretation of diagnostic tests

Clinical disagreements about the interpretation of diagnostic tests are common and include the results of laboratory testing, necropsy findings, and diagnostic techniques such as medical imaging and endoscopy.

The interpretation of subtle changes on radiographs can vary between clinicians.

## Diagnosis

Clinical disagreements are usually most striking when they apply to diagnostic or management decisions. When the diagnosis is not obvious, such as mild, bilateral hind limb lambness, mild liver disease or gastric impaction, clinical disagreement can be common. The differentiation between surgical and medical colic in the horse can be difficult, and disagreement between two clinicians examining the same animal is common.

## Prognosis and therapy

Prognoses and treatment methods commonly vary between clinicians.

## Causes of errors in the clinical examination and clinical disagreement

The causes of errors and disagreements in clinical examinations may arise from the examiner, the animal, or the examination procedure.

### Examiner

Inaccuracies and incompleteness of the history can be a major cause of errors in clinical diagnoses. Some clinicians may obtain more relevant information simply because of previous experience and knowing what to ask.

The thoroughness and reliability of a clinician's findings may vary from one physical examination to another because of fatigue, mood, or lack of care in the examination.

The urge to infer first, rather than identify then interpret the evidence, is a common cause of error and disagreement. For example, being able to palpate a firm and pitting enlargement of the pelvic flexure of the large colon in the horse is clinical evidence; but to conclude in the first instance that the large colon is impacted is to make an inference that may be incorrect. The first is simple evidence, the second is inferential.

Lack of clinical experience and knowledge is a common source of error in the clinical examination. Veterinary students must examine many normal animals so that the normal state of all body systems is recognizable, including the biological variations between different animals according to age, sex, breed, stage of pregnancy and production, and environment. It is difficult to encourage veterinary undergraduates to examine a sufficient number of normal animals so that abnormalities can be readily recognized.

> ## Avoid Preconceived Ideas
>
> Preconceived ideas can be a major cause of errors in the clinical examination. Clinicians tend to find those abnormalities which they expect, based on the original encounter with the animal and its owner.

### Animal being examined

Biological variations in the body systems of different species can affect the results of the clinical examination. For example, major anatomical and physiological differences in the digestive tract of dogs, cattle, and horses can result in variations in how clinicians detect and interpret certain clinical findings. An experienced bovine clinician may not appreciate certain abnormalities of the equine abdomen which may be obvious to the equine clinician.

The owner or attendant may change the details of the history after thinking about it for a time. Major changes in the history may affect the diagnostic hypotheses and the management plan. Different clinicians may elicit different histories from the same animal owner.

### Examination procedure

A disruptive or inadequate environment for examination, or the lack of proper facilities or equipment, can result in important clinical clues being missed. Fractious animals which are difficult to restrain may not be examined fully and important diagnostic abnormalities go undetected.

Disruptive interactions between the examiner and the animal are common causes of incomplete examinations.

An incorrect function or use of diagnostic tests can affect the results of the examination procedure. Most diagnostic techniques require some learned skill to perform them consistently and accurately. Endoscopy, ultrasonography, simple examination of the eye, rectal examination, and percussion of the thorax and abdomen, for example, all require some clinical acuity.

## Minimization of clinical disagreements and learning from one's mistakes

Several strategies are available to minimize the occurrence of clinical disagreements, and to resolve them when they do occur.

1. Match the diagnostic environment to the diagnostic task. As far as possible, the location of the examination should be conducive to conducting an appropriate examination.

2. Seek corroboration of key findings:

   - repeat key elements of the physical examination
   - corroborate important findings with documents and witnesses
   - confirm key clinical findings with appropriate tests
   - ask colleagues to examine the patient. Do not inform them of your findings.

3. Report evidence as well as inference, making a clear distinction between the two.

4. Use appropriate technical aids. Use precise measurement devices and specific anatomical locations when possible, rather than reporting that a certain abnormality is similar to a well known object such as an apple, plum, etc.

5. Make 'blind' assessments of raw diagnostic test data. This means asking someone to interpret the results of the diagnostic testing without revealing the suspected diagnostic hypotheses.

6. Examine at necropsy as many cases as possible that die, and correlate the pathological findings with

---

**Clinical Pointer**

Always consider the effects that the course of the illness and medications already given may have on the clinical findings.

---

**Clinical Pointer**

For a fractious animal always use proper handling and restraint techniques to insure that all body systems are fully examined.

---

the clinical and laboratory findings. This is an effective learning method that requires clinicians to admit their mistakes.

'To advance the art and science in clinical examination, the equipment a clinician most needs to improve is himself.' We ought to be educated as well as humbled when our animal's clinical course, surgery or necropsy shows that we erred in our original diagnosis. If we were to carry out a systematic documentation of our own successes and failures in diagnosis we could identify areas in which we need to improve our clinical skills, and find out whether we are making progress in reducing our rate of clinical disagreement.

## FURTHER READING

Roudebush P, Sweeney CR. Thoracic percussion. J Am Vet Med Assoc 1990;197: 714–718.

Tyler JW, Angel KL, Moll HD, Wolfe DF. Something old, something new: Thoracic acoustic percussion in cattle. J Am Vet Med Assoc 1990;197: 52–57.

Sackett DL, Haynes RB, Guyatt GH, Tugwell P. Clinical epidemiology. A basic science for clinical medicine, 2nd edn. Boston: Little, Brown and Co, 1991.

# 4

# Veterinary Medical Records

*D. M. Houston*
*I. G. Mayhew*
*O. M. Radostits*

## IMPORTANCE

A veterinary medical record contains the information about a patient, or herd of animals, including laboratory reports, radiographs and clinical notes. It reveals how veterinarians assess their patients, what plans they make and the actions they take, and how the patient responds to their efforts. According to the American Animal Hospital Association (AAHA), veterinary medical records provide 'documentary evidence of a patient's illness, hospital care, and treatment, and serve as a basis for review, study, and evaluation of medical care rendered by the hospital.' Veterinary medical records also 'serve as a basis for planning patient care and as a means of communication among hospial staff.' Record management systems vary from simple to complex, according to the needs of veterinary hospitals. The AAHA standard for medical records of AAHA-approved hospitals states that a 'legible individual record must be maintained for every patient to which the hospital administers' and that the problems 'under medical or surgical management must be identified.'

The AAHA suggests that the hospital administrator 'frequently review medical record files with a critical view for ease of information retrieval.' Regarding the retention of medical records of member hospitals, the AAHA declares that 'Records should be purged frequently (yearly). Old records should be kept for compliance with federal, state, or provincial statutes of limitations (usually 3–10 years).' In the teaching hospitals of veterinary colleges the records often become very detailed and extensive because of the teaching component and the use of records for long-term retrospective clinical research.

A good record is the result of the veterinarian taking the patient data, organizing them, evaluating the importance and relevance of each item, and constructing a clear, concise, yet comprehensive report.

Regardless of the system used, certain principles will help to organize a good record which is user friendly

- order is imperative
- the information must be presented consistently and obviously, so that other readers, including the original writer, can find the information quickly
- headings should be clear, indentations and spacing should be used to accentuate organization, and important points should be underlined
- the information should be presented in chronological order.

Although several different record formats are used successfully in veterinary practices the reasons for keeping records and the common characteristics of good records are outlined here.

## CHARACTERISTICS OF VETERINARY MEDICAL RECORDS

### Patient data

The most important reason for keeping records is to keep patient information, such as the history, clinical

---

### Clinical Records

An accurate, clear, well organized clinical record reflects and facilitates sound clinical reasoning.

---

and laboratory findings, diagnosis, treatment administered, and disease control procedures recommended, especially when dealing with herds of animals. The record should be written as soon as possible either during or after the examination. All data, both positive and negative, should be recorded. The clinician must attempt to be as objective as possible when making observations. No diagnosis should be made, no problem identified, unless the basis for the diagnosis or the problem has been recorded.

Useful records permit practitioners to monitor disease progression and response to treatment. Large animal practitioners can now keep a computerized record of the disease control recommendations they make to their clients. If a question arises about which vaccine was recommended and dispensed for a particular herd in previous years, it is a simple task to retrieve the record and determine which vaccine was recommended for which class and age of animals in that particular herd, including the date it was recommended. Any adverse reactions to drugs or vaccines are also recorded and reported as appropriate.

## Costs of veterinary service

Records are necessary so that the owner can be charged the appropriate fees for professional services and for the costs of materials and supplies. A good record will contain details of

- clinical examinations
- diagnostic tests
- drugs and materials used
- telephone consultations related to the case
- intensive care provided.

Ideally the costs are recorded so that they can be easily tabulated at the termination of the case. Computers can now monitor the costs of veterinary services on an ongoing basis, with the total charges available when the animal is discharged and the case closed.

## Legal implications

Written evidence of the clinical case is necessary in the event that the owner makes a legal claim of malpractice.

### Malpractice Claims

It is amazing how a seemingly insignificant clinical case can turn into a malpractice claim by a disgruntled client. Failure to keep good records can result in dire consequences.

When veterinarians are called to investigate outbreaks of disease in herds it is wise to record as much detail as possible regarding the animals, the feeds and feeding systems used, the facilities, the drugs the owners may have used, the results of necropsy examinations, recent climatic changes, and any other notable item. It may be highly desirable to take photographs of the circumstances for future reference.

## Avoidance of drug residues

In food-producing animal practice it is of paramount importance to maintain treatment records in order to avoid drug residues in meat and milk. This applies both to animals the veterinarian treats and to those the owner may treat under the direction of the veterinarian. The recommendations must be clear and explicit.

## Prospective studies

Good clinical case records provide a bank of information that can be analyzed either prospectively or retrospectively to determine one's own performance in diagnosis and treatment. They can also provide valuable information about the prevalence of certain diseases in households, herds, or particular geographical areas, their common clinical findings, and responses to treatment. Veterinary medicine needs information on prospective and retrospective clinical studies of the common diseases and how they respond to various therapies under different circumstances. The techniques of veterinary epidemiology are now readily available to analyze clinical studies of disease under naturally occurring conditions.

## Communication

A colleague should be able to visualize the patient and understand the practitioner's clinical approach after reading a record. This characteristic is particularly important in group practices, or when patients are referred to a specialist. A logical presentation of the practitioner's thought processes will permit a more rational extension of the initial exploration of the problem and will expedite the processes of diagnosis and treatment. The results of consultation with colleagues should be recorded, preferably by the consultant.

## Terminology and legibility

Simple ordinary terminology is used so that records are understandable. Legibility is essential. Redundacies, such as those in parentheses that follow should be avoided: pink (color), resonant (by percussion), audible (on auscultation of the lungs), and (bilaterally) symmetrical. The emphasis should be on what the clinician observed, rather than what they did. Abbreviations and symbols should be used only if they are commonly used and understood. Diagrams add to the clarity of a record and should be used where appropriate. Precise description of anatomical locations of abnormalities is desirable. Exact measurements of abnormalities should be made, rather than making comparisons with certain objects, e.g. 'pea-sized', 'walnut-sized' and so on.

# COMPONENTS OF VETERINARY MEDICAL RECORDS

## Signalment or patient identification

In the case of individual records the patient must be clearly identified. The signalment is the description of the animal for identification purposes. It may also provide clues about risk factors that may be related to species, breed, sex, age, color, and weight. In companion animals the patient's name, birth date, breed, sex, and color pattern are often adequate to maintain adequate identification.

Color pattern is sometimes a useful identifying characteristic. Cattle breeds such as Holstein-Friesians and Shorthorns have a wide array of possible color patterns. However, if the patient is a member of a breed with a defined, consistent phenotype, physical descriptions will be of limited value. Stating that an Aberdeen Angus cow is black and polled (naturally hornless) provides little useful information because all Aberdeen Angus cows are black and polled.

In small registered herds owner recall may be sufficient for identification, but the use of registration tattoos and brands, numbered ear tags, or patient descriptions associated with breed registry requirements is preferable because these forms of identification are more definitive. Definitive, permanent identification is of paramount importance in two settings.

1. The treatment of food-producing livestock. In many countries, extralabel drug use requires permanent individual animal identification. This permits the practitioner to establish reasonable meat and milk withdrawal times and prevents contamination of the human food chain. Identification also permits the veterinarian to document a paper trail in which withdrawal times have been communicated to livestock owners.

Consequently, it is recommended that all food-producing animals examined and treated by a veterinarian be permanently identified. Metal ear tags are a cheap way to fulfill this responsibility.

2. When legal concerns or litigation arise. An insurance examination, health papers, or lawsuit all create an obligatory requirement for permanent, definitive identification. It is imperative that each clinical record be maintained as a legal document. Adverse drug reactions, the unexpected demise of a patient, or deep emotional attachments between the client and patient can all create circumstances in which definitive documentation of diagnosis and treatment becomes obligatory. The veterinarian is morally and ethically bound to maintain factual and complete medical records.

### Patient Identification in Households with Several Pets

In multiple-pet households, particularly in the case of clients with impaired or faulty memory, a definitive identification system may be required such as tattoos or implanted microchips.

## History, signalment and physical examination

Information recorded in an initial client interview includes the signalment, previous health problems, diagnoses and treatments, current problem or clinical signs, diet, vaccinations, and recent health problems in other animals in the same group or household. The content of this history will vary with the species under consideration. Forms incorporating a checklist are often used because they permit standardized and complete data collection. However, care should be exercised not to restrict the client's potential responses. Ideally, this information is obtained through an oral interview, rather than a written survey which the client completes without direction. Any history or interview should conclude with a consciously open-ended ques-

### Keep Records as the Case Progresses

Records display the veterinarian's logical approach to a disease and should be recorded in real time as the information is generated. Retrospective or corrected record entries are biased by the case outcome and are inappropriate.

tion, such as 'is there any thing else you would like to tell me?' This part of the clinical examination is addressed in greater depth in other chapters. If a case has been referred the referring practitioner is identified. If an animal is insured, the agent and underwriter are identified. Most insurance underwriters prefer to be contacted immediately when an animal comes under the care of a veterinarian.

---

### Clarity of Records

Use short words rather than long ones when they mean the same thing, for example

- use felt, not palpated
- use heard, not auscultated.

---

## Daily record entries

Each page of the record should be clearly identified using the owner's name and the patient's unique identification. Each entry must include the date and time, and be signed by the person recording the information. Records lacking this information quickly become disorganized. If pages fall out of a record it may become impossible to return information to it so that it can be read, interpreted and understood.

Record entries should be legible and use proper syntax, grammar and spelling. Deficiencies in these areas will directly undermine the credibility of the practitioner if records are examined at a later date.

## TYPES OF DAILY RECORDS

Unfortunately, many daily entries in veterinary medical records are sparse and disorganized, with more subjectivity than objectivity. By following a set format the clinician can record clearly and accurately what clinical progress is being made with a case. Indeed, such records can guide and teach.

## Problem-oriented veterinary medical records (POVMR)

This type of record is based on four phases of action

- database collection
- problem definition
- plan formulation
- follow-up plans.

---

### Avoid Jargon

Non-standard or local jargon, abbreviations and acronyms should be avoided in records.

---

### Database collection

The database is the source of problem formulation and always includes data from the history and physical examination. The initial database may include screening laboratory data, such as a hemogram and urinalysis.

### Problem definition

A problem can be defined as something that concerns the patient, the owner, or the veterinarian. It is anything that has, does, or may require healthcare management or which affects a patient's wellbeing.

The initial problem list is not synonymous with tentative diagnoses: it contains all problems identified in the database. All problems are listed, even if there are no immediate plans to solve them, as such a decision should be made after analyzing the patient as a whole.

Problems are stated at their highest level of refinement and defined in such a way that their refinement can be defended with reasonable certainty on the basis of current knowledge about the patient. There are four levels of refinement. From highest to lowest these are

1. a clinical finding, such as vomiting, dyspnea or diarrhea
2. an abnormal laboratory finding, such as hypocalcemia, leukopenia, hyperkalemia, hypokalemia or hypoproteinemia
3. a pathophysiological syndrome, such as shock or congestive heart failure
4. a diagnostic entity, such as bilateral pyelonephritis or diabetes mellitus.

When formulating the problem list, clinical findings or problems should be aggregated according to the body system or organ to which they are related. This localizes the problem.

The construction of a meaningful problem list requires disciplined thought and reasoning. Clinical manifestations of disease are often a combination of primary clinical findings induced by disease, such as diarrhea caused by enteritis, and the secondary clinical findings of dehydration and the weakness and depression associated with the acidosis. Several manifestations of a disease may be listed as a single problem, provided it is probable that they are related.

In summary, the initial problem list should be as accurate and complete as possible. Problems should be refined to the highest degree possible by the database, but they should not be overstated.

## Plan formulation

### Initial plan

Each problem on the problem list is analyzed in terms of the need for further diagnosis and therapy. A priority list should be formulated so that the most important problems are evaluated first.

### Diagnostic plan

The diagnostic plan for each problem should always state what cause(s) is/are to be ruled out (R/O) and by what tests. This is analogous to the tentative diagnosis of older systems of clinical diagnosis. The rule-outs (tentative diagnoses) are listed so that the most probable causes are evaluated first, and the least probable last.

One of the most frequent errors made by inexperienced diagnosticians is the premature consideration given to hypothesizing specific disease entities without first localizing problems to the appropriate body system or organ, and secondly, considering what basic disease mechanisms might be involved.

Following the establishment of the most probable causes of a problem, appropriate clinical and laboratory testing is selected to rule them in or rule them out.

### Therapeutic plan

Each problem is evaluated according to the necessity or desirability of therapy. The therapeutic plan should state the goal of therapy, and whether the therapy is specific, supportive, symptomatic or palliative in nature.

---

### Re-evaluation of Therapeutic Plans

The frequency of re-evaluation depends on the significance of the problem to the patient and the rate at which it is changing, for example

- the diagnostic and therapeutic plans for a patient in hypovolemic shock due to acute intestinal obstruction require constant re-evaluation because of the rapid changes associated with the problem, while
- a horse with chronic obstructive lung disease of 3 months' duration can be evaluated at intervals of weeks.

---

## Follow-up plans (Progress notes)

Each unresolved problem is re-evaluated at appropriate intervals. This phase is referred to as the follow-up plans or progress notes. Follow-up plans incorporate new information obtained during the course of investigation and management of a problem, and the subsequent addition or modification of diagnostic and therapeutic plans based on this new information. It also includes plans for client education.

In order to be organized and complete, problem-oriented progress notes should be divided into four sections, commonly referred to as the SOAP format: Subjective, Objective, Assessment and Plan.

### Subjective data entries

These entries include those observations that also require interpretation. Most clinical examination results are subjective, for example

- the recognition and location of a cardiac murmur
- gait abnormalities
- mucous membrane color
- the degree of scleral injection
- enlargement or displacement of abdominal viscera on palpation of the abdominal wall or rectal examination.

In the hands of an astute diagnostician subjective assessments may assume the characteristics of objective observations. However, it must be recognized that in subjective assessments the practitioner actively serves as a filter between the patient and the clinical record.

### Objective data entries

Objective data entries are clinical observations or test results which are readily quantified. Most laboratory test results fall into this category. Measurements of temperature, heart rate, respiratory rate and, in cattle, rumen motility are usually considered objective because different observers should measure and record the same results. Obviously, the dividing line between subjective and objective assessments often becomes blurred.

### Assessments

Assessments are the portion of the record documenting the practitioner's reasoning processes and conclusions. The significance of various subjective and objective observations is assessed and interpreted. As the results of additional historical facts, clinical examination results and laboratory tests become available, additional assessments are added to the record. These entries will be used to attempt to reach conclusions regarding the status (correct or incorrect) of diagnostic hypotheses.

### Plans

Plans include all anticipated diagnostic, treatment, or preventive procedures for the individual patient or the herd of origin. When each task is completed it is dated, timed and signed. The substance of communications with clients and referring veterinarians is likewise summarized and entered in the record.

**Advantages and disadvantages of SOAPS**

In the database diagnostic approach, separate entries are often made for each clinical problem identified. The inherent strength of this approach is that problems are not overlooked. The recognition of separate problems and the development of subjective and objective observations, assessments and plans tends to insure that each is fully explored and appropriate intervention undertaken. The downside of maintaining separate SOAPs for each problem is that the mass of the clinical record tends to become overwhelming, particularly in complex cases with multiple problems.

As a general rule, records are maintained and updated at least once daily. In critically ill or intensively managed patients, multiple daily SOAPs will become necessary. Each entry builds on previous findings, the spectrum of likely differential diagnoses becomes progressively narrower, the prognosis becomes more definitive and responses to treatment are noted.

*Example of the problem-oriented method of making a diagnosis*

A 14-year-old spayed female Siamese cat is presented with a problem of weight loss despite a voracious appetite. Clinical examination reveals a thin cat with tachycardia (heart rate > 260 bpm)(see Table 4.1.).

Differential diagnoses for weight loss despite a voracious appetite include:

- inadequate diet
- increased metabolic rate (e.g. hyperthyroidism)
- catabolic disorders (e.g. diabetes mellitus, hyperadrenocorticism, cancer, chronic inflammation)
- malabsorptive disorders (e.g. exocrine pancreatic insufficiency, inflammatory bowel disease, lymphangiectasia, giardiasis, protein-losing enteropathy).

Differential diagnoses for tachycardia are:

- anemia
- stress
- fever
- pain
- hyperthyroidism.

Reasonable and common causes for the defined problems are identified and tests selected for their ability to either increase or decrease the likelihood of the specific differential diagnosis.

**Table 4.1. Problem list on day 1**

| Problem no. | Date or day of illness recognized | Problem | Day resolved | Update to problem no. |
|---|---|---|---|---|
| 1 | 1 | Weight loss | | |
| 2 | 1 | Voracious appetite | | |
| 3 | 1 | Thin | | |
| 4 | 1 | Tachycardia | | |

The initial diagnostic plan included:

- complete diet history
- complete blood cell count
- serum chemistries, including blood urea nitrogen (BUN), creatinine, liver enzymes (serum alkaline phosphatase (SAP), alanine amino transferase (ALT), $\gamma$-glutamyl transferase (GGT), glucose electrolytes and protein
- urinalysis
- electrocardiogram (ECG).

The complete blood cell count was ordered to rule out anemia, a potential cause of a 'physiological' heart murmur and tachycardia. Serum chemistry tests were ordered to assess the potential for diabetes, hyperthyroidism (elevation in SAP is very common), and hypoproteinemia, as occurs with protein-losing enteropathies. The urinalysis was selected to rule out the glucosuria often seen in cats with diabetes mellitus. The electrocardiogram (ECG) was ordered to assess cardiac rhythm. Tachycardia can be sinus, atrial or ventricular in origin, and an ECG is necessary to distinguish between them.

The initial test results revealed an elevated SAP and ALT. These 'new' problems were added to the problem list. Elevations of these liver enzymes support a diagnosis of hyperthyroidism, but could also be indicative of liver disease. The ECG revealed a sinus tachycardia. Tachycardia (problem no 4) can now be updated to problem no 7 (see Table 4.2.).

To further investigate the elevations in SAP and ALT and the tachycardia, a serum $T_4$ was submitted. This was markedly elevated, confirming a diagnosis of hyperthyroidism (Table 4.3).

Hyperthyroidism causes an increase in metabolic demand and was thought to be the cause of the weight loss, despite a voracious appetite. Hyperthyroidism is the most common systemic disturbance to affect cardiac function in cats: the excessive thyroid hormone exerts both direct and indirect effects on the heart, causing

| Table 4.2. | | Problem list on day 2 | | |
|---|---|---|---|---|
| Problem no. | Date or day of illness recognized | Problem | Day resolved | Update to problem no. |
| 1 | 1 | Weight loss | | |
| 2 | 1 | Voracious appetite | | |
| 3 | 1 | Thin | | |
| 4 | 1 | Tachycardia | 2 | 7 |
| 5 | 2 | ⬆ SAP | | |
| 6 | 2 | ⬆ ALT | | |
| 7 | 2 | Sinus tachycardia | | |

both increased contractility and increased heart rate. The master problem list is refined as shown in Table 4.3.

Radioactive iodine was administered as treatment for the hyperthyroidism. The clinical signs resolved within 1 month of therapy.

## Modified objective, assessment and plans (OAP) records

The POVMR system can be modified to be less laborious by writing OAP daily notes on the whole patient, as opposed to SOAP notes on every problem. Thus

| Table 4.3. | | Problem list on day 3 | | |
|---|---|---|---|---|
| Problem no. | Date or day of illness recognized | Problem | Day resolved | Update to problem no. |
| 1 | 1 | Weight loss | | 8 |
| 2 | 1 | Voracious appetite | | 8 |
| 3 | 1 | Thin | | 8 |
| 4 | 1 | Tachycardia | | 7 |
| 5 | 2 | ⬆ SAP | | 8 |
| 6 | 2 | ⬆ ALT | | 8 |
| 7 | 2 | Sinus tachycardia | | 8 |
| 8 | 3 | Hyper-thyroidism | | |

there is an opportunity to record the Objective data of cardinal signs, physical findings and laboratory test results; to give an Assessment of these findings and evaluate the progress of the case; and then to arrive at a future Plan, as in the POVMR system.

## Systems review records

A method of record keeping based on reviewing each important body system and monitoring parameters pertinent to the type of case can be used, particularly for more intensive patient monitoring practices. This insures that nothing is overlooked and that objective data are separated from their interpretation. Patient evaluation and case notes follow a set routine, and for a neonatal intensive care unit might be recorded as objective data followed by interpretation under the following headings:

- integument
- umbilicus
- eyes, nose, throat
- respiratory
- heart
- gastrointestinal
- orthopedic
- urinary
- neuromuscular
- catheters
- hematology
- clinical chemistry
- blood gases.

## DISCHARGE INSTRUCTIONS AND CASE SUMMARIES

When the animal is returned to the client's primary care, or at the conclusion of a period of veterinary care, clients should be given a synopsis of relevant events. This case summary provides a diagnosis and details the steps or tests that led to that diagnosis; it also makes treatment and preventive recommendations, both for the individual patient and for other animals in the herd or group. The discharge notes outline explicitly the instructions to the owner for convalescent therapy, the clinical signs of a continued favorable or an unfavorable response, and under what circumstances the owner should again consult the veterinarian regarding the present illness. A copy of the report is kept in the medical record, and in the case of referred cases a copy is forwarded to the referring veterinarian. For agricultural animals, slaughter and milk withdrawal times should also be clearly specified. Recommendations for specific vaccination schedules are recorded clearly and explicitly and kept in the veterinarian's computer file for quick and easy reference when needed.

## RECORD STORAGE AND RETRIEVAL

There is a clear dichotomy between the needs of companion or pleasure animal practice and agricultural practice. An optimal medical record would ideally be restricted to a single individual patient. For companion animals, a separate record is usually developed for each pet in a household. A record is created and the animal assigned an accession number the first time it is examined or treated. Each subsequent visit is appended to this record, providing a complete and sequential medical history.

In agricultural practice a single client's farm may have several thousand animals in residence. Maintaining separate medical records for each is clearly unreasonable and unworkable. Consequently, all medical records from a single herd are typically maintained as a single record according to the owner's name. Individual entries are clearly identified with the unique identification of each animal examined and treated.

Records must be retrievable and should be accessible by

- client name
- patient identification
- accession number
- species
- diagnoses.

Although hard copy or physical record systems can function in a practice setting, most veterinary clinics are shifting to computerized record systems which can sort and scan the database for the record of interest, permitting the hard copy record to be filed under a standardized accession number. The development of expanded-memory computers and practice management software has facilitated efficient record retrieval. In the near future many practices are expected to eliminate permanent paper records. Online records will replace hard copy in many, if not most, practices.

Diagnoses on each animal are typically entered using a standardized and restricted set, based on anatomic site, the nature of the disease process and the etiologic agent. Several codifications of diagnoses have been developed and most currently available systems are modifications of the SNOVET scheme (Standard Nomenclature of Veterinary Medicine).

## RETENTION OF VETERINARY MEDICAL RECORDS

One legal authority states that veterinarians should maintain medical records for at least 10 years, and longer if litigation arises.

Active records should be archived indefinitely because many pets and livestock have extended life-spans. The medical history from an earlier visit will expedite the delivery of healthcare services at subsequent visits. Inactive records should be maintained for a minimum of 5 years.

There is little agreement between national, state, and veterinary college policies regarding the retention periods for medical records. One survey revealed a wide variation in retention periods between veterinary teaching hospitals and the recommendations of state veterinary boards and veterinary associations. Some universities recommend a 10- to 20-year retention period. Most maintain their veterinary medical records beyond the legally required duration. Most records of routine procedures do not need to be maintained for lengthy periods. The recommendations of the state boards of veterinary medical examiners vary widely, from no guidelines to several years. The longer the records are kept, the more costly they are to store and the less likely they will be used for research. There is a need for a collaborative effort between veterinary colleges and state or provincial boards of veterinary examiners to establish guidelines for common record-retention periods.

## FURTHER READING

Rosenblatt DJ, Lee TNP. Retention patterns for veterinary medical records. J Am Vet Med Assoc 1995; 206: 1217–1219.

---

### Discharge Notes

Insure that discharge notes are clearly written, dated, explicit, easy to read, preferably typed, and signed by the veterinarian. Many different forms of discharge notes are now available that provide the name, address, and telephone number of the veterinary practice for ease of use by the client.

# 5
# Handling and Restraint of Animals for Clinical Examination

*D.M. Houston*
*I.G. Mayhew*
*O.M. Radostits*

Because animals often object to clinical procedures it may be necessary to employ a suitable means of restraint, in order to carry out an examination safely and without risk of injury to the clinician, assistants, or the animal itself. Animals can kick with their hindlimbs, strike with their forelimbs, bite, scratch, step on someone's feet, squeeze handlers against walls, and jump on top of a person. All of these actions can inflict injuries ranging from mild to serious and crippling. With the decline in the percentage of veterinary students who have significant farm animal background, learning the principles of handling and restraint of large animals assumes major importance.

Restraint has been defined as the restriction of an animal's activity by verbal, physical (using various techniques or instruments) or pharmacological means (the use of drugs to induce varying degrees of sedation or immobilization) so that the animal is prevented from injuring itself or people. This section will describe some of the techniques used to handle and restrain animals for the purpose of an adequate clinical examination.

## METHODS OF RESTRAINT

There is no one method of restraint that is equally effective in every case, because individual animals react to different methods in different ways. Well trained animals may be very easy to handle and examine. Others may be fractious or apprehensive towards the clinician, (even when examined in their own environment) hyperexcitable in clinic surroundings, and in some cases very dangerous to handle because of the injury they are capable of inflicting. Therefore, one should always have at hand several means of restraint in order to achieve the desired effect.

Physical or chemical restraint should if possible not be applied prior to such preliminary procedures as general observation of the patient, taking the pulse and noting the character of the respirations. It is important to perform all the physical manipulations in a quiet and gentle manner in order to avoid seriously disturbing the patient, otherwise its physiological functions and behavior will be altered, adding to the problem of diagnosis.

Sometimes the animal is so difficult to handle because of fear or pain that, even with the aid of physical restraints examination is unsafe or impracticable. Use must then be made of special aids such as muzzles, twitches and stocks, or the administration of sedative, psychotropic (tranquilizing), narcotic or immobilizing drugs – chemical restraint.

Recommendations for dosage rates for chemical restraint can be obtained from textbooks on veterinary pharmacology, or in the relevant datasheets provided by the pharmaceutical manufacturers. Some

> **Restraint of Animals**
>
> It is incumbent upon every veterinary student to learn the behavioral patterns of each species of animal and to become familiar with the commonly used methods of restraint and handling.

> **Mechanical Restraints**
>
> Mechanical restraint techniques must be used correctly to avoid injuries.

recommendations for chemical restraint for each species are provided in this chapter.

## RESTRAINT OF THE DOG

A dog bite can be very serious and precautions should be taken to avoid injury. The amount of restraint necessary will vary depending on

- the animal's behavior
- the veterinarian's approach to the animal
- the environment
- the degree of discomfort caused by the examination.

A dog's behavior is determined largely by breed, training, previous experience and degree of human contact. The owner cannot always be relied upon to give an accurate assessment of their pet's behavior, particularly when the animal is injured or ill. The animal should be observed on the floor or in its cage, and its initial reaction to the examiner determined. Most dogs are not happy to be at the veterinarian's office and will express varying degrees of apprehension, fear, excitement, or anger. An animal that is totally oblivious to a strange environment is abnormal. Family dogs usually enjoy human contact and approach the veterinarian with the tail wagging. They are generally easy to handle and examine. A nervous dog, guard dog, fear biter, or a dog that is not used to being handled will be easily frightened, and can be recognized by an anxious expression, rapid head movements, and constant pricking of the ears in response to sound or movement. The head is often held low, the lips may be pulled back in a grimace, and the animal may cower in a corner. These animals may also be boisterous and undisciplined, and attempt to bite the handler and veterinarian. A vicious, aggressive dog holds its head low and avoids looking directly at the examiner. Such an animal may attack without warning. Stray dogs should be handled with caution. If such an animal appears aggressive, gloves should be worn as rabies is a possibility.

Before the dog is handled an attempt should be made to socialize with it. The dog is approached slowly from the side, called by name, and continually spoken to in a friendly manner with a soft, low-pitched and soothing voice. The back of the hand can be extended toward the dog's nose and the dog allowed to sniff it. If no aggressive tendencies are noted, the veterinarian can pat the dog's head and scratch its back to relax it prior to the examination. An outstretched hand should not be offered to a nervous dog; instead, it may help for the examiner to sit close to the dog and speak calmly to it until the dog relaxes and approaches the

veterinarian. If the animal is perceived as aggressive, or if the owner states that the dog will bite, adequate restraint should be used.

Whenever possible, the owner should be allowed to stay with their animal and assist in lifting, holding, and comforting their pet. A veterinary assistant may be needed to handle a difficult dog.

To lift a medium-sized to large dog on to the examination table, the examiner kneels next to the dog and places one arm in front of the forelegs and the other hand behind the hindlegs or under the abdomen. If possible, the owner should assist by lifting the forequarters while the veterinarian lifts the hind end. The dog is pulled toward the lifter's body, the lifter stands up and places the dog on the table. Giant-breed dogs are best examined on the floor.

### Restraint on a table

The animal must always be held on the table and never left unattended. In general, small animals are restrained by placing them on a table in the standing position, with the owner holding and talking to them. The owner or assistant stands on the opposite side of the dog from the examiner and places both hands on its head and shoulders. If more restraint is needed, the holder places one arm under the dog's neck, with the forearm cradling the head securely in such a manner that the dog cannot bite the handler or examiner. The other arm is placed underneath the abdomen or thorax, which prevents the dog sitting down. The dog is pulled close to the chest of the holder, as this gives them more control (Fig. 5.1).

If lateral recumbency is needed, the examiner reaches across the standing dog's back and takes hold of both forelegs in one hand and the hindlegs in the other. Two people may be needed for a large dog. The dog's legs are gently lifted off the table or floor and its body allowed to slide slowly against the holder's body to a position of lateral recumbency. The restrainer's forearm is positioned over the side of the dog's head and neck, which exerts pressure and immobilizes the head. The index finger of each hand is positioned between the two limbs being held, proximal to the carpus and tarsus, thus insuring a good grip (Fig. 5.2).

> ### Clinical Pointer
>
> To remove an aggressive dog from a cage, the loop of a leash can be tossed over its head, the dog pulled off balance, and the head held away from the handler while the dog is grasped. A muzzle should be applied prior to placing an aggressive dog for examination.

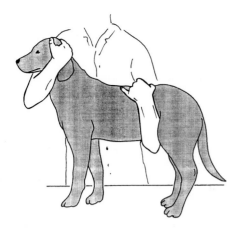

**Fig. 5.1** Restraint of a dog in the standing position. One arm is placed under the dog's neck so that the forearm holds the animal's head securely, and the other is placed underneath the animal's abdomen or thorax.

## Handling and restraint of puppies

Most puppies can be handled with ease by placing one hand under the abdomen and chest to give support, and holding them close to the body. If properly socialized, puppies enjoy human contact and have not learned to fear strangers.

## Muzzling

When muzzles are needed, either a 1 meter strand of 2 inch gauze, or commercial leather or plastic muzzles may be used. Commercial muzzles need to fit the animal well or should not be used. Placing a muzzle on a fractious dog requires at least two people: one holds the leash and distracts the dog while the other applies the muzzle. The animal should be on a leash prior to fitting the muzzle to prevent it from backing away when approached. To insure rapid placement of a gauze muzzle and to minimize the length of time the opera-

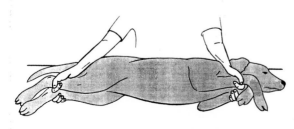

**Fig. 5.2** Restraint of a dog in lateral recumbency. The restrainer's forearm is positioned over the side of the dog's head and neck. The index finger of each hand is positioned between the two limbs being held, proximal to the carpus and tarsus.

tor's hands must be near the animal's mouth, a loop about twice the diameter of the snout should be made with one-half of a square knot. The loop is slipped over the dog's nose and mouth, with the half-square knot on the dorsal surface of the snout, and quickly tightened by pulling on the ends (Fig. 5.3 A, B). The hands should be kept as far away from the dog's mouth as possible while the muzzle is applied. The free ends of the muzzle are crossed, but not tied, under the dog's lower jaw, brought up behind the dog's ears and tied in a bow (Fig. 5.3 C, D). The muzzle is removed by simply untying the bow and pulling on one end. The muzzle should be removed if the animal has difficulty breathing, becomes cyanotic or is vomiting.

### Elizabethan collars

These plastic collars prevent the dog from licking or chewing at wounds or bandages on the body or legs. They may also be used to keep the animal from biting the handler. Some dogs find it difficult to drink and eat with the collar in place.

### Chemical restraint

For vicious animals, snares and rabies poles are used to corner the animal before chemical restraint is administered. Several different analgesics, tranquilizers and

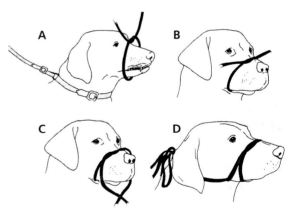

**Fig. 5.3** Applying a muzzle to an aggressive dog. One person holds the leash and distracts the dog while a second person applies the muzzle. (A) A loop of gauze is made with one half of a square knot so that the diameter of the loop is about twice the diameter of the dog's snout. The loop is slipped over the dog's nose and mouth with the half-square knot on the dorsal surface of the snout, and tightened quickly by pulling on the ends. (B) The free ends of the muzzle are crossed, but not tied, under the dog's lower jaw and brought up behind the dog's ears and tied in a bow (C,D).

> ### Problems when using a Muzzle
>
> - the mouth cannot be examined
> - abdominal palpation becomes difficult, as the animal tends to splint when muzzled
> - panting and tongue movement are inhibited, as these are the normal cooling mechanisms of the dog, thus hyperthermia and dyspnea may result
> - the tongue may become lacerated if the muzzle is too tight.

sedatives are available (Table 5.1). In general, these are indicated whenever their use will result in increased safety and efficiency for the clinician and owners, and the greatest comfort, safety, and humaneness for the animal.

## RESTRAINT OF THE CAT

Of all domestic animals, the cat is one of the most unpredictable and difficult to handle. Cats defend themselves by biting and scratching. They have retractable claws that are capable of inflicting serious and debilitating wounds. Cat scratch disease in humans, commonly known as cat scratch fever, is thought to be caused by a Gram-negative bacterium that causes dermal or conjunctival lesions, peripheral lymphadenopathy, an array of non-specific clinical signs, including lethargy, fever and myalgia.

A cat should remain in its carrier and an unrestrained cat should be kept in the owner's arms until the time of examination. If cats are allowed to roam the examination room prior to evaluation, residual animal odors may cause them to become irritated or hostile. The owner, rather than a veterinary assistant, may be better able to coax a cat out of its cage and restrain it. It takes some time before a cat will accept handling by a new person, and some never tolerate manipulation by a stranger. Cats often exhibit territorial characteristics and can be quite aggressive even in their cage. An unfriendly cat positions its ears backwards and hisses, spits and growls at the person nearing the cage, and may strike out with a paw or attempt to bite an encroaching hand. A non-aggressive cat will usually come out of the cage on its own and, if approached calmly, will allow examination. Some cats are initially approachable, but behavior can change quickly.

The veterinarian's first contact with the cat is critical and will determine the ease with which the examination proceeds. If the cat is not hissing or growling, the examiner can extend a hand and the cat, being naturally curious, will advance towards it for initial interaction. Scratching the dorsum of the head establishes a positive rapport between veterinarian and patient. Each cat has a different area of critical distance that can be approached only with time and patience. If the cat remains hostile, the owner should position the cat so it is facing them, allowing the clinician to attempt to scratch the cat's head from the rear. If the cat will still not allow contact additional restraint techniques are recommended.

### Restraint on a table

Cats should be handled with a minimum of restraint and the examination should be carried out as quickly as possible. The windows and doors of the examination room should be closed before opening the cat's

| Table 5.1. | Analgesics, sedatives and tranquilizers commonly used in dogs | |
|---|---|---|
| *Drug* | *Indication* | *Adverse effects* |
| Acepromazine 0.025–0.2 mg/kg IV 0.10–0.25 mg/kg IM | Sedation | Hypotension, bradycardia |
| Diazepam 0.5–1 mg/kg IV | Mild sedation | Paradoxical excitement, aggression |
| Oxymorphone+ 0.05–0.1 mg/kg IV 0.1–0.2 mg/kg IM, SQ | Sedation, analgesia | Respiratory depression, bradycardia, panting |
| Butorphanol 0.2–0.4 mg/kg IM, IV, SQ | Analgesia, mild sedation | Panting |
| + Oxymorphone in combination with acepromazine is a commonly used sedation in dogs. | | |

cage, which should be placed on the table and the cat allowed to come out on its own, or be removed by the owner. No blanket or towel should be placed on the stainless steel table, as the smooth and slick surface will force the cat to try and maintain stability and it is less likely to use its claws for scratching. For sternal recumbency, firm but gentle pressure is applied to the cat's back with both hands. To immobilize the cat, the forearms are placed against each side of the cat's body, with the head facing away from the restrainer, and the head is held with both hands. If more restraint is necessary the scruff or loose skin over the back of the neck can be grasped, this prevents the cat from turning its head around and biting. The cat can then be pressed on to the table with one hand over the neck and the other stretching out the hindlimbs (Fig.5.4). This prevents the cat from lashing out with either the front or the back paws. To place a cat in lateral recumbency, the holder reaches across the cat's back and takes hold of both forelimbs with one hand and both hindlimbs with the other. The cat's limbs are gently pulled off the table and its back is allowed to slide against the holder's body to a position of lateral recumbency. One hand is then used to hold all four legs and the other is placed around the cat's head, so that the palm of the hand surrounds the dorsal part of the head and the jaws are held closed by the fingers and thumb. Alternatively, the paws are held immobile using both hands and the head is restrained by placing the forearm over the neck (Fig 5.4).

If a cat becomes unmanageable, the skin on the neck may be scruffed and the cat picked up and held away from the examiner. With scruffing, the paws curl up and the cat becomes somewhat limp and immobilized.

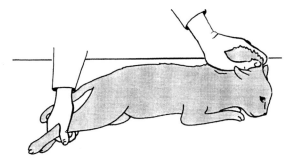

**Fig. 5.4**  Restraint of a cat in sternal recumbency. The scruff or loose skin over the back of the neck is grasped and the cat is pressed on to the table with one hand over the neck and the other stretching out the hindlimbs.

## Handling and restraint of kittens

Most kittens can be handled with ease by placing one hand under the abdomen and chest to give support, and holding them close to the body. If properly socialized, kittens enjoy human contact and have not learned to fear strangers.

## Other means of restraint

A cat may be restrained with a commercial cat muzzle, a towel, cat bag or heavy gloves. The use of a towel or cat bag prevents damage from the claws. To use the cat bag, the cat is picked up by the scruff of the neck and placed in the bag. This limits the extent of physical examination but allows the head or any limb to be left outside for manipulations.

| Table 5.2.   Analgesics, sedatives and tranquilizers commonly used in cats | | |
|---|---|---|
| *Drug* | *Indication* | *Adverse effects* |
| Ketamine+ 11–33 mg/kg IM 2.2–4.4 mg/kg IV | Sedation | Increased muscle activity, seizures |
| Diazepam 0.05–0.15 mg/kg IV | Sedation | |
| Midazolam 0.066–0.22 mg/kg IM, IV | Sedation | Respiratory depression |
| Acepromazine 0.05–1.0 mg/kg | Sedation | Hypotension, bradycardia |
| + Ketamine should not be used alone because of increased muscle activity and the risk of seizures. It is usually combined with diazepam or midazolam for use in cats. | | |

> **Clinical Pointer**
>
> When heavy gloves are used to hold a cat, more force is applied and the risk of injury to the cat is increased. Gloves do not deter biting.

## Elizabethan collars

These plastic collars prevent the cat from licking or chewing at wounds or bandages on the body or legs. They may also be used to keep the animal from biting the handler. Some cats find it difficult to drink and eat with the collar in place.

## RESTRAINT OF THE HORSE

Horses vary in size from minature horses which may weigh only 50 kg to large draft horses weighing up to 1200–1400 kg. The horse can kick backwards with one or both hindlimbs and strike forward with the forelimbs with absolutely no warning. The bite of a horse can be very serious: it can fracture the bones in the hand of a mature person.

For examination of the halter-trained horse it may be sufficient to have the owner or attendant hold the animal with a lead shank attached to the halter (Fig. 5.5). The safest place for the handler to stand is next to the left forelimb, close to the body, to prevent kicking, striking, and biting. Horses are startled by quick movements and loud noises but respond to voice commands. Continually speaking to the animal and maintaining physical contact by stroking the skin firmly will soothe most horses. Examination of the limbs and feet of the horse usually require that the limbs be manipulated and lifted.

## Twitch

The twitch is the most commonly used method of physical restraint in the horse. A twitch consists of a wooden handle about 50 cm in length with a loop of chain attached to one end. The loop is placed over the upper lip with one hand, while the other twists the handle so that the lip is twisted into a firm grasp but not painfully tight (Fig. 5.6). At the same time the halter lead shank is used to pull the head and neck to the left side. The twitch distracts the animal's attention away from the clinician and the part of the body being examined. Once the lip twitch is applied, a gentle rocking motion with the handle will focus the animal's attention on the twitch while it is being examined or treated. Removal of the twitch must be quick and

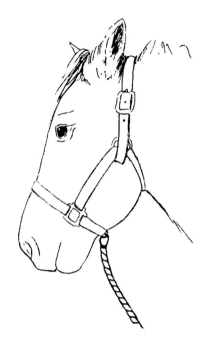

**Fig. 5.5** Simple halter on a horse.

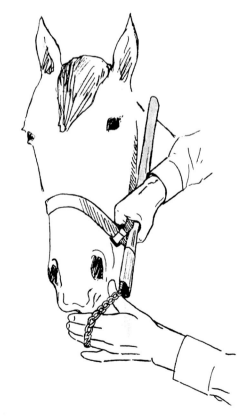

**Fig. 5.6** Application of nose twitch on a horse.

careful to avoid the animal jerking it out of the operator's hand. A hand twitch may be applied to the ear or nose. The animal may strike with the forelimbs when a nose twitch is applied and the operator must always stand to the side, preferably near the left shoulder, to avoid injury. It is sometimes effective to distract the patient by covering the eyes with the hands, or to place a cloth sack over the head as a hood or blind.

## Stocks

Diagnostic techniques such as

- rectal examination
- passage of a nasogastric tube
- abdominocentesis
- standing laparotomy
- dental examination
- endoscopy of the respiratory tract

are commonly performed with the animal in stocks. Stocks are a restraint device or chute for horses, constructed of wood or metal. They consist of four corner posts, two solid side-bars or doors, and usually a door at either end. The back door of the stocks should be well padded to prevent injury should the horse kick. Depending on the size of the patient the top of the back door should not be higher than 1 meter above the ground, which is low enough to avoid injury to the clinician if the animal goes down during a rectal examination. Stocks must be of smooth construction, have a good non-slip ground surface for footing, be easily cleaned and disinfected and be designed for quick release of the animal if it becomes recumbent. Stocks are efficient, safe for handlers, and horses generally tolerate them well.

## Walls, corners and stalls

These structures can be used in the restraint of the horse to limit its potential for movement. Many procedures can be effectively undertaken with the horse placed up against a wall, particularly in a stall, where the animal may also be backed into a corner. Examples of procedures that are often conducted under these circumstances include

- examination of the head, eyes and oral cavity
- passage of a stomach tube
- injections
- blood sampling
- general physical examination.

Under the proper circumstances a reasonably safe rectal examination can be conducted by backing a horse into an open doorway and using the door jamb for protection. Rectal palpation over a low stall door can also be accomplished safely.

## Breeding hobbles

Breeding hobbles are commonly used in the hand breeding of horses to prevent the mare from kicking the stallion. They can also be used as a restraint device for rectal and vaginal examinations. Breeding hobbles should always be applied snugly so that the mare or stallion cannot become tangled in the ropes. The hobbles should be designed to be applied to the hocks and not to the fetlocks. This again helps minimize the chance of entanglement.

Side lines and breeding hobbles should never be applied unless the animal is in a secure enclosure. An animal that escapes wearing such a device is potentially subject to severe injury.

Breeding hobbles should be purchased as a properly constructed piece of equipment from an appropriate supplier, but a temporary set may be fashioned out of soft cotton rope.

## Cradles

A cradle is a collar that prevents the horse from licking or chewing a wound or a bandage on the body or limbs. The size of the device used depends upon the size of the animal. Properly applied, it will keep the horse from lowering the head and neck and turning the neck to either side. For this reason, feed and water must be placed at the level of the horse's mouth when a cradle is in place.

## Surcingle and side pole

This device is used to prevent the horse from reaching caudal parts of the body with the mouth. It gives more freedom than the cradle so that the animal can eat and drink normally, but it may not prevent it reaching a wound on the forelimbs with the mouth.

## Cross-tie

The cross-tie prevents the horse from licking or chewing a wound on the limbs or body, and will also prevent it from rubbing a wound on the head or a painful eye. The cross-tie is also useful in transporting animals. This method is frequently used in large horse vans where horses must be transported standing next to one another. When cross-tied the horses cannot get at each other with their teeth.

## Blindfolds

Blindfolds are useful in loading a shy horse into a vehicle, stall or enclosure that it is afraid to enter. They may also be useful in testing VIIIth cranial nerve function during the neurological examination. A towel or cloth is eased gently over the eyes and tucked into the halter on either side of the head. It must be possible to remove the blindfold in a single pull, should the horse react adversely to it. The horse must be under the complete control of an experienced handler when the blindfold is in place.

## Handling and restraint of foals

A newborn foal up to a few weeks of age is usually easy to restrain by simply grasping the tail with one hand and the neck with the other hand and arm. This will usually allow the clinician to carry out a clinical examination. A foal can be made to lie down by pulling the tail between the hindlegs and maintaining pressure: the foal will relax and slump to the ground. The foal can be held in the lateral recumbent position by pulling the tail between the hindlimbs are in front of the stifle and placing pressure on the neck.

## Handling the recumbent horse

Proper physical examination is difficult on the recumbent horse. Recumbent horses commonly lie on their weak side and turn to get up on their strong side. Coaxing the recumbent horse to stand can be done by slapping it on the rump or knudging it in the ribs with the knees.

## Slings

Slings are used to assist the recumbent horse to its feet or to give a weak animal some assistance or support while standing. They are not suitable for use with animals that cannot bear their full body weight on the limbs once standing.

The best horse sling is made by Liftex from woven polyester. It has chest, belly and butt pieces. Simple slings consisting only of a belly band placed around the girth may help some weak horses stand, but very weak animals slip out.

> ### Clinical Pointer
>
> With a recumbent horse, take care must be taken not to become trapped against the wall if the horse makes an attempt to stand and then falls.

> ### Adjusting a Sling
>
> With the horse in the standing position the sling should be adjusted so that a hand may be slipped between the belly band and the ventral abdominal wall. Constant pressure at any one point will lead to pressure sores or necrosis at that point.

In emergencies a rope sling may be needed to lift a horse. Two long lengths of thick cotton rope are ideal. A non-slip collar is made using both lengths of rope and the free ends are passed between the front limbs and under the collar. The free ends are then crossed over the back before being led down between the hindlimbs and up next to the root of the tail. The ropes should not cross underneath the horse as the udder or urogenital organs may be injured. The ropes are then led back under the collar. If the sling is to remain in place for more than a few minutes, the ropes should be padded where they pass under the limbs to stop them cutting into the flesh. The free end of the rope can then be tied under the standing part to complete the sling.

## Chemical restraint of the horse

In recent years a number of reliable tranquilizers have been developed that are extremely useful in the horse (Table 5.3). These drugs provide an important adjunct to physical restraint and every practitioner should be thoroughly acquainted with their use. When to use sedatives and tranquilizers as an aid to restraint is very much a matter of personal choice and style on the part of the clinician. However, these drugs are indicated whenever their use will lead to increased safety and efficiency for the clinician and handler, and greater comfort and safety for the animal. All tranquilizers and sedatives have some side effects and occasionally cause adverse reactions, of which the clinician should be constantly aware (Table 5.3).

# HANDLING AND RESTRAINT OF CATTLE

Cattle resist restraint in various ways. The horned animal is capable of quick thrusts sideways and forward with the horns and may fatally gore an individual. A handler working around the head of a horned animal must be continually conscious of the swinging arc of the head and the extent of the reach of the horns.

Both polled and horned animals may butt. They may rush at people and knock them down, or crush them against fences or walls. Cattle may also push against people with their bodies, squeezing them against walls, fences, or other animals.

## Table 5.3. Analgesics, tranquilizers and sedatives commonly used in horses

| Drugs | Recommended IV dosage | Analgesic potency | HR | Cardio-pulmonary effects BP | RR | Adverse effects |
|---|---|---|---|---|---|---|
| **Narcotic agonists and partial agonists** | | | | | | |
| Morphine | 0.05–0.1 mg/kg | 1 | – | ↑ | ↓ | Excitement, respiratory depression |
| Meperidine | 0.5–1.0 mg/kg | 0.1 | – | ↑ | ↓ | Excitement, respiratory depression |
| Oxymorphone | 0.02–0.1 mg/kg | 10 | – | ↑ | ↓ | Excitement, respiratory depression |
| Pentazocine | 0.4–0.8 mg/kg | 0.25 | – | ↑ | ↓ | Excitement, respiratory depression |
| Butorphanol | 0.05–0.1 mg/kg | 5 | – | – | – | Excitement with higher doses |
| **Tranquilizers** | | | | | | |
| Acetylpromazine | 0.02–0.05 mg/kg | None | ↓ | ↓ | ↓ | Hypotension |
| **Sedative – hypnotics** | | | | | | |
| Xylazine | 0.5–1.0 mg/kg | Good | ↓ | ↑↓ | ↓ | Bradycardia, respiratory depression |
| Romifidine | 40–80 µg/kg | Good | ↓ | ↑↓ | ↓ | Bradycardia, respiratory depression |
| *Detomidine | 10–20 µg/kg | Good | ↓ | ↑ | ↓ | Bradycardia, respiratory pauses |
| **Drug combinations** | | | | | | |
| Xylazine-morphine | 0.5–1.0 mg/kg (xyl) 0.3 mg/kg (mor) | Good | ↓ | ↑↓ | ↓ | Bradycardia, respiratory depression, hypotension |
| Xylazine-acetylpromazine | 0.5 mg/kg (xyl) 0.025–0.05 mg/kg (ace) | Good | ↓ | ↑↓ | ↓ | Bradycardia, respiratory depression, hypotension |
| Meperidine-acetylpromazine | 0.5 mg/kg (mep) 0.05 mg/kg (ace) | Good | ↑ | ↓ | ↓ | Hypotension |
| Xylazine-butorphanol | 0.5–1.0 mg/kg (xyl) 0.05–0.1 mg/kg | Good | ↓ | – | – | Bradycardia |
| Xylazine-pentazocine | 0.5–1.0 mg/kg (xyl) 0.3–0.5 mg/kg (pent) | Good | ↓ | ↓ | – | Bradycardia |
| Xylazine-acetylpromazine-pentazocine | 0.5 mg/kg (xyl) 0.025 mg/kg (ace) 0.3 mg/kg (pent) | Good | ↓ | ↑↓ | ↓ | Bradycardia, respiratory depression, hypotension |
| Detomidine-butorphanol | 10 µg/kg (det) 0.05 mg/kg (but) | Good | ↓ | ↑↓ | ↓ | Bradycardia, respiratory depression, hypotension |

* Detomidine should not be used in association with intravenous sulfonamides, particularly combinations with trimethoprim.

IM dosage is 2–3 times recommended IV dosage.
HR = heart rate
BP = arterial blood pressure
RR = respiratory rate
↑ = increase
↓ = decrease
↑↓ = initial increase followed by a decrease

Cattle seldom use the front feet as weapons, though they may paw the ground to display anger. However, being stepped on is a hazard of working with cattle: even small calves can inflict pain if they step on a toe, and heavier animals may severely bruise or fracture the toes and feet.

Cattle are adept at kicking with the hindlimb. The kick is usually forward and out to the side in an arc reaching some distance. They are less likely to kick directly backward, although they are able to do so. Usually only one limb kicks at a time, in contrast to the equine species where both hindlimbs habitually kick simultaneously. The safest place to stand is probably at the shoulder, but cattle can kick forward past the shoulder with the hindlimb.

Breeds of cattle differ markedly in their reactions to manipulation. Dairy cows are usually accustomed to being handled by milkers and handlers, and as a result are likely to be more docile than other breeds. However, the dairy cow can become extremely agitated and may vigorously resist handling if not treated gently. Dairy bulls, however, are extremely dangerous and special restraint practices must be observed when working with them. In general, all bulls should be handled with care and caution: no bull should be trusted. Ideally, every mature bull should have a nose ring and should be handled with an excellent chute and stocks or, if individually, with a bull staff attached to the nose ring. Cattle which have had little association with people are easily frightened. Techniques used to handle them must involve chutes and stocks, where movement can be restricted before they are approached. Beef cattle are usually grazed on pastures and handled less frequently, and therefore will exhibit a frightened reaction when approached.

## Methods of physical restraint of cattle

The veterinarian in bovine practice is commonly

---

### Bovine Tails

The tail is used to swat flies and switches in response to any touch on the skin. The tail may be a source of annoyance to the clinician during restraint procedures and may also contaminate a prepared surgical field. Furthermore, it may inflict personal injury if the tail hair flicks the eyes, and it becomes an awesome weapon when it is filled with foreign bodies such as burrs or grass awns. Bovine tails are fragile and therefore must be tied or attached only to the animal's own body when restriction is required.

---

judged by the handling techniques used during the clinical examination. The desired results are more likely to be achieved by a confident approach, rather than shouting, hitting, or kicking, which are commonly used when the handler becomes frustrated with uncooperative animals.

The temperament of each animal must be considered before approaching it for examination. Dairy animals can usually be approached if confined in a stanchion or tied to a fence. With beef cattle it is likely that one will have to either rope the animal or put it into a squeeze chute or stock to halter it or approach closely enough to conduct an examination. Horned cattle can be restrained by holding both horns or tying them to a strong post. A twitch applied to a hindleg above the hock can also be used. In the horse and ox, in order to obtain protection against kicks from the hindlimb, the forelimb is held up in a flexed position on the side on which the clinician is standing.

When working with cattle the handler must make the animals aware of any prospective movements. Quick motions usually startle animals; firm, slow, deliberate actions should be the rule. Speaking to animals lets them locate your position and avoids startling them with an unexpected touch. Any animal should not be approached directly from the front unless it is secured in a stock. It is natural for an animal to charge forward and butt anyone who makes such an approach. It is most desirable to approach the animal from either the left or the right shoulder. Placing a firm hand on the shoulder lets it know the handler's presence and confidence. Then, if necessary, the head can be approached.

### Halter

A rope halter is the basic tool of restraint for cattle. It is important to place the halter correctly. Parts of a standard cow halter include the permanent V, which contains a closed loop, the nose rope, the chin rope, the poll rope, and the lead or shank. It is standard practice to place the halter on the animal from the left side.

Frequently a halter is put on upside down, or is improperly placed with the rope behind the horns but not behind the ears. This results in the rope crossing over or near the eye, endangering the eye.

Placing the halter on an animal which is already restrained in a chute or a stanchion is easy. An animal loose in a box stall may present some difficulty. However, if the nose loop is made slightly larger than the poll loop, one can flip it over the nose and then over the poll and behind the ears very easily. This may require that the handler walk beside the left side of the animal as the animal walks away from the handler. If it is impossible to approach the animal in this manner, it may be necessary to first place a lariat around its neck. Once the animal is subdued, the halter is placed over the head.

Once haltered, the animal can be tied to a post, a ring, or any other secure object to carry out additional procedures. It is usually necessary to fix the head by pulling it tightly to the side or upward, or both, and snubbing it to the post with a halter tie. Many procedures, such as withdrawing blood, giving injections or examining the teeth, can be carried out by controlling the head in this manner. If the halter is to be left on an unattended animal, be certain that there is sufficient lead rope so that the animal can lie down.

### Leading cattle with a halter

Both young and adult cattle should be led by means of a halter. The person leading an animal walks on its left side and a short distance in front. The animal can be prevented from going too fast by pulling back on the halter or by light hand blows on the bridge of the nose.

Cattle that do not respond to leading can be encouraged to walk forward if the handler moves back towards the shoulder and allows the animal to walk forward without being led or pulled. The handler will then have to attempt to direct the movement of the animal by pulling back on the halter. If a mature cow 'gets her head', i.e. she can put her head down and walk forcefully ahead, she will be difficult to control. The handler can pull the head and neck to one side in an attempt to stop the animal walking forward, but if this is unsuccessful and the animal begins to move forward quickly, the handler may have to release the lead shank of the halter and let the animal go.

When animals resist being led with a halter, some prodding and goading by an assistant behind the animal will often get them to move. The use of an electric

### Leading Animals with a Halter

When leading an animal never wrap the lead shank of a halter around the hand, this can result in injury from being dragged away if the animal runs away.

### Clinical Pointer

A pair of nose tongs is an effective restraint for cattle.

prod can assist in getting animals to move, but these devices must be used humanely and judiciously. In some cases they will frighten animals and make them much more fractious. Cattle can be coaxed to move ahead by a slight twist of their tails. Excessive force must not be used because it is possible to fracture the coccygeal vertebrae.

### Nose tongs

Cattle have an unusually sensitive nasal septum. A routine restraint practice is to grasp this between the thumb and finger via the nostrils, forming a manual nose tong. A large animal is difficult to hold by hand because one cannot maintain sufficient pressure for more than a few seconds. For more permanent and more secure restraint, mechanical devices acting on the septum are available. Commercially available nose tongs look like a pair of pliers with two metal balls at the end of the jaws. When fully closed, a space of approximately 3.5 mm should remain between the two balls to prevent necrosis of the nasal cartilage. The surface of the metal balls must be smooth to avoid scrapes or lacerations.

Placement of the nose tongs is not always easy, particularly if the animal has experienced the device previously, as it frequently darts its head about in an attempt to prevent placement. To place tongs on an animal in a squeeze chute or stock

- grasp the animal's head or nose with one hand and arm
- using the other hand place one side of the tongs into one nostril
- apply the other side of the tongs into the other nostril
- quickly close the tongs and hold secure with the lead of the tongs.

To keep the tongs in place tension must be maintained on the lead part. An assistant must hold the tongs, or the rope can be tied above and to the side of the stanchion or chute.

Cattle will respond to the placement of nose tongs by holding their head and neck outstretched and will attempt to pull backwards, and/or rotate the head and neck in attempt to resist the restraint. Some animals will bellow and become quite excitable. Others will yield to the restraint and walk forwards if the handler pulls on the tongs.

The nose tongs should not be left unattended. If they are not attached to a solid object or are not being held tight by the handler the animal may butt its head and neck and the tongs will become dislodged and can inflict injury on nearby personnel.

### Tail-jack (lift-grip of the tail)

Manipulation of the tail as a diversionary tactic can be an excellent method of restraint while performing minor surgical or diagnostic techniques, such as abdominal paracentesis or minor teat surgery. It is applied primarily to dairy cows accustomed to being handled. However, it can be used for beef animals and other species of tailed bovids if they are restricted in lateral movement in a squeeze chute. Although an excellent restraint, one must be cautious that pressures are properly applied, otherwise the tail can be fractured and permanently disfigured. To apply the tail-jack, the animal is tied up or put in a stanchion and, standing directly behind the animal, the restrainer lifts the tail with one hand and reaches under and grasps its base with the other. The tail is then held as close to the base as possible with both hands, pressing the tail upward, straight over the back. When this technique is carried out properly, the pressure will not break the tail but will make the animal relax and ignore manipulation elsewhere. Once the animal has settled down the pressure can be released, to be reapplied only when a particular procedure requires the animal to stand quietly. It is important for the pressure to be exerted at the base of the tail, not further along it.

### Handling recumbent cattle

Lateral recumbency means lying on one side or the other with all four limbs extended parallel to the ground. Sternal recumbency means sitting upright on the sternum with the forelimbs flexed towards the sternum and the hindlimbs tucked under the abdomen. In sternal recumbency the animal is lying on its left or right side. If it is lying on its right side, the left hindlimb (uppermost limb) is visible and the right hindlimb (lowermost limb) is not. However, the hoof of the right hindlimb will usually be visible from the left side. Sternal recumbency is the usual resting position for cattle, although they occasionally lie in lateral recumbency.

> ### Clinical Pointer
>
> Weak recumbent animals, such as mature cattle down with milk fever, can be assisted to stand by grasping the tail and lifting it up towards the base. Once the animal is standing it may be steadied by holding on to the tail for a few minutes.

> ### Clinical Recumbency
>
> In clinical recumbency the animal is unable to stand. The reasons may include
>
> - generalized weakness: (hypocalcemia or milk fever), peracute coliform mastitis
> - painful conditions of the musculoskeletal system, such as fractured limbs
> - diseases of the nervous system.
>
> A complete and thorough clinical examination is necessary to determine the cause of recumbency.

Recumbent cattle should be rolled from one side to the other several times daily to minimize the ischemic necrosis that occurs as a result of compression of the limb muscles. Rolling an adult cow requires that the uppermost hindlimb be flexed, placed, and held next to the lateroventral abdomen which is uppermost at the time. Two or three people are then required to roll the animal over. As the animal is being rolled over it is important to ensure that the hindlimb it has been lying on is pulled out and exposed and made comfortable on the side which is now uppermost. The forelimbs are usually not a problem. If the animal is on pasture or a natural ground surface, bedding is not a concern. If on a solid barn floor surface, such as wood, concrete or other slippery surfaces, liberal quantities of straw should be placed under her while it is being rolled over and repositioned. One person may be able to roll over an average-sized cow by tying a rope around the fetlock of the uppermost limb and pulling the rope under the cow's abdomen to the other side. This brings the distal part of that limb next to the lateroventral aspect of the abdomen. The rope is then brought over the cow's back and pulled slowly and deliberately in the direction of the handler.

Recumbent cattle can be moved from one point to another by placing them on a flat bed made of rubber or other strong material. A piece of plywood measuring 1 × 3 m is useful if the animal is not too large. The flat bed can be dragged along the ground and the animal moved without causing injury. In veterinary teaching hospitals, low steel-plated wheeled trolleys are commonly used to move recumbent animals. In some cases recumbent cattle must be lifted and moved with the aid of a front-end loader on a tractor. Ropes are placed around the animal at the level of the thorax and caudal abdomen and made into a sling. Care and caution must be used when moving recumbent cattle with such a powerful force.

## Coaxing and assisting recumbent cattle to stand

If animals are able to stand but need some coaxing, a nudge in the ribs with the handler's knees will often stimulate them to do so. A slight jolt with an electric prod can provide the same stimulus.

If the animal makes no attempt to rise, or appears to creep along the ground, all attempts to stimulate it to stand should be postponed until there is evidence that it has the ability.

In animals that are unable to stand successfully it may be necessary to provide assistance with hip-lifters, or other commercially available lifting devices. These include slings made of ropes and/or material similar to automobile seatbelts. These are placed around the animal's thorax and abdomen and, using a winch, the animal is lifted and allowed to stand for several minutes to ascertain whether it can stand on its own. The hip-lifters are applied across both tuberscoxae, which provides the lifting points. Considerable tissue damage below the tuber-coxae can occur if hip-lifters are not used carefully, humanely and judiciously.

## Catching cattle which have escaped from confinement

Occasionally individual animals or groups of cattle escape from confinement because the gates were left open, the chute system collapsed, or the doors of the clinic were left open. Escape usually occurs when animals are being handled. Fractious animals and those which are not halter broken – especially beef animals – which escape will commonly run randomly and wander for up to several hours. They will run across fields, into bushes, across highways, into urban areas among houses, over lawns and gardens, and wherever they can find freedom. The more one chases them, the more wildly they run. Continued pursuit can result in exhaustion, possible capture myopathy, recumbency, and death of the animal. The simplest method of capture is herding the animal back into an enclosure, but this is not usually possible. A lariat can be used if someone can get close to the animal from the back of a truck or from horseback. A capture gun, which can fire a bolus of a rapidly acting tranquilizer, also can be used. In some cases uncontrollable animals which are potentially very dangerous, such as large bulls, may have to be killed by gunshot if they cannot be captured alive. When working in veterinary clinics, every effort must be made to insure that animals cannot escape confinement.

## Chemical restraint of cattle

When to use sedatives and tranquilizers is very much a matter of personal choice and style on the part of the attending clinician. In general, these drugs are indicated whenever their use will result in increased safety and efficiency for the clinician and owners, and the greatest comfort, safety and humaneness for the animal.

All tranquilizers and sedatives have some side effects and occasionally cause adverse reactions, of which the clinician should be constantly aware. Table 5.4 summarizes those commonly used in cattle for chemical restraint. They provide an extremely important adjunct to physical restraint, and it is no longer necessary to possess and use brute strength and elaborate roping techniques to restrain cattle.

**Table 5.4. Analgesics, sedatives, and tranquilizers commonly used in bovids**

| Drug | Indication | Adverse effects |
|---|---|---|
| Acepromazine 0.05–0.1 mg/kg IM IV | Mild sedation | Hypotension |
| Xylazine 0.05 mg/kg IV; 0.1 mg/kg IM; 0.07 mg/kg in 7 ml saline epidurally | Standing sedation, analgesia | Bradycardia, hypotension, rumen stasis, hypoventilation, abortion in last trimester, regurgitation |
| Xylazine 0.1–0.2 mg/kg IV or IM | Recumbent sedation, analgesia | As above |
| Detomidine 10 μg/kg IV | Standing sedation, analgesia | Bradycardia, hypersalivation, hyperglycemia, increased urination |
| Pentobarbital 2–3 mg/kg IV/IM | Standing sedation | Short-acting (15–20 min), may decrease pain threshold |
| Butorphanol 0.1mg/kg IV or IM alone, or in combination with a sedative or tranquilizer | Analgesia | Potential excitation |
| Chloral hydrate 80–90 mg/kg IV (10% solution) | Recumbent sedation | Bradycardia, respiratory depression, irritation, dermal slough with perivascular administration |

## RESTRAINT OF SHEEP

Sheep are one of the easiest of the domestic animals to restrain for a clinical examination. Sheep do not bite, kick, or strike. Well trained sheepdogs are used to move groups of sheep on the farm. Sheep should be crowded into alleyways or narrow chutes for mass medication, examination, and vaccinations. An individual sheep is easiest to catch if left with the group, where it can be approached slowly and quietly. One hand is placed under the chin or brisket, which stops its forward motion, and the other hand over the perineum. The animal can then be guided into any desired position. Sheep will usually remain upright. The wool should never be grasped as a means of restraint. Mature ewes and rams can be set up on their haunches (setting up a sheep) for examination of the abdomen and reproductive tract as follows:

- hold the animal by the neck and the rump from the left side
- the operator places the right knee in the left flank of the animal and grasps the right flank with the right hand
- the animal's head and neck are then twisted to the right with the left hand
- at the same time the handler's knee is pressed into the right flank and the animal is whirled around and set down.

This quick, coordinated movement forces the animal to sit down on its left hip, and an additional twirling motion will place it on its rump (haunches). The back of the animal is cradled between the handler's legs, which are slightly spread. The animal should be sitting at approximately 60° to the vertical. If it is too perpendicular it may struggle to free itself. If the animal is properly balanced, both of the handler's arms will be free to examine the feet, trim the hooves, and examine the abdomen, mammary glands, prepuce, and testicles.

Lambs are easily handled by supporting them under their thorax and abdomen with the arms.

## RESTRAINT OF GOATS

Goats do not kick, bite or strike, but are usually active. They vocalize and stamp their feet as threats. Once they are caught they are easy to handle. Horned goats may use their heads for butting. Goats can be handled similarly to sheep, except that they cannot be set up on their haunches. Halters are commonly used in dairy goats or those that are companion animals on hobby farms. The feet and limbs of a goat can be picked up

easily. Adult goats can be placed in lateral recumbency for special examinations. Goat kids are handled as easily as lambs.

## HANDLING AND RESTRAINT OF PIGS

The major weapon of the pig is the teeth. The boar has long canine teeth known as tusks which can inflict serious injury; a sow with a litter may attack a person and bite. Both boars and sows are unpredictable and may attack without warning.

It is difficult to capture or handle an adult pig in a large enclosure, and it is necessary to move them into a small pen where movement is restricted.

Most sows in farrowing crates can be examined if the clinician moves carefully, talks to the animal and strokes the udder firmly. Lively, fractious or timid animals will need to be restrained, as this allows a more thorough examination. Sucking and weaned piglets are best held by the hindlimbs with the head down to minimize squealing. Hindfeet can be examined easily with the animal held in this position. However, if all four feet are to be considered, it is possible for a person to sit and hold the piglet on the lap in a dorsal position with a thoracic and a pelvic limb in each hand. Weaned and growing pigs can be restrained in lateral recumbency by firmly grasping the forelimb and flexing and slightly adducting the limb. Growing and finishing pigs can be cast with a rope and restrained. A loop is placed around the snout, the free end of the rope is then passed around a hindlimb above the tarsus in a half-hitch and pulled so that the snout and tarsus are drawn together as the pig is pulled off balance. A simple slipknot is used to secure the ropes while the pig's feet are examined. Larger finishing pigs, sows, and boars can be restrained using a criss-cross or half-hitch method of casting, however the half-hitch method is less strenuous for casting a mature pig.

Pigs naturally pull back when pressure is applied around the upper jaw. Restraint is achieved by means of a wire or rope twitch, or a pair of blunt tongs applied to the upper jaw or snout, or by confining the pig in a corner with a small gate or hurdle. A cable snare (hog snare) placed around the upper jaw behind the tusks can be used to restrain a pig for a short time for exam-

> ### Clinical Pointer
>
> One way to control a placid sow is to stroke the udder while talking to her softly.

ination, palpation, and manipulation of extremities. If the foot is to be examined it must be picked up to examine the polar aspect; this can be facilitated by a firm manual grip on the tendon of the gastrocnemius, or placement of a noose above the tarsus for examination of the hindfoot. Usually at least two people are required to restrain larger pigs.

For pigs up to 50 kg in weight, simple V-shaped cradles consisting of sawhorse frames and a wooden or canvas hammock suffice to hold them on their backs. However, two people are required to lift the pig into the cradle. More sophisticated crates, which can be turned manually or semiautomatically, have been made to hold finishing pigs and even sows and boars. These cradles and crates can be used for bleeding pigs from the cranial vena cava and jugular vein and for simple surgery, as well as for examination and treatment of the feet. Areas that are to be scrutinized should be cleansed at this stage. When manual restraint is too difficult, it is as simple, expedient, and humane to use chemical restraints in the form of either tranquilizers or general anesthetic.

## FURTHER READING

Bishop Y. The veterinary formulary, 4th edn. London: Pharmaceutical Press, 1998.

Crow SE, Walshaw SO. Manual of clinical procedures in the dog and cat. Philadelphia: JB Lippincott, 1987.

Fowler ME. Restraint and handling of wild and domestic animals, 2nd edn. Ames, Iowa: Iowa State University Press, 1983.

Hardy RM. General physical examination of the canine patient. In: Bistner SI (ed) Symposium on physical diagnosis. Vet Clin North Am (Small Anim). Philadelphia: WB Saunders, 1981; 11: 453–467.

Leahy JR, Barrow P. Restraint of animals, 2nd edn. Ithaca: Cornell Campus Store Inc., 1953; 30–85.

Stein BS. Physical examination of the cat. In: Bistner SI (ed) Symposium on physical diagnosis. Vet Clin North Am (Small Anim). Philadelphia: WB Saunders, 1981; 11: 469–479.

Vaughen JT, Allen R. Physical restraint of the horse. In: Colahan PL *et al* (eds) Equine Medicine and Surgery, 4th edn. Goleta, California: American Veterinary Publications, 1991; 219–228.

Wear DJ, English CK, Margileth AM. Cat scratch disease. In: Greene CE (ed) Infectious diseases of the dog and cat. Philadelphia: WB Saunders, 1990; 632–635.

# 6

# The Clinical Examination

*D. M. Houston*
*O. M. Radostits*

*More mistakes are made for not looking than for not knowing.*

O.M. Radostits

## INTRODUCTION

A thorough clinical examination consists of taking the history, evaluating the environment, and physical examination of the animal. Inadequate performance of any of these may lead to errors. Examination of the animal represents only a part of the complete investigation. Careful questioning of the owner or attendant can yield information about the diet, recent vaccinations or surgery, or the introduction of other animals into the group, that may provide clues to a diagnosis. However, in some circumstances, for example lead poisoning in cattle, the most thorough examination of the animal and the most careful questioning of the owner may fail to elicit the necessary evidence: only a careful physical search of the environment can provide this information. Thus neglect of one aspect of the clinical examination can render valueless a great deal of work on the other aspects and result in an error in diagnosis. Although the actual environment is seldom investigated in dealing with individual dogs and cats, this information can be obtained by taking the history. To minimize errors in the clinical examination, and ultimately in the diagnosis and prognosis, every reasonable effort should be made to do a thorough examination of the history, the environment, and the animal on the first examination. In difficult cases the clinician may have to obtain some additional history and repeat the clinical examination to obtain new information. However, taking the time for an adequate history and clinical examination when first presented with the animal will often improve the efficiency of diagnosis and avoid the costs of excessive testing.

This chapter describes the fundamentals of history-taking, examination of the environment, and the actual clinical examination of the animal. Other chapters describe the clinical examination of dogs and cats, horses and foals, cattle, pigs, sheep and goats, and llamas and alpacas. Details of the clinical examination of each body system are presented in Part III.

## HISTORY TAKING

History taking can be the most important of the three aspects of a clinical examination.

History taking is an important key to diagnosis, and to be useful it must be both accurate and complete. However, various factors can affect the quality of a history: there may be insufficient time, the importance of particular facts may not be appreciated by the owner, and there may be misunderstanding. To avoid being misled, it is essential to assess the accuracy of the history by careful examination of what the owner relates about the animal.

The protocol for history taking varies considerably depending on the species involved, whether one animal or a herd is being examined, and the number of animals affected. Taking a history from the owner of a dog or cat in a small animal hospital is heavily

> **Listen Carefully to the Owner's Description**
>
> Animals are unable to describe their clinical abnormalities and we depend on their owners to describe them for us.

91

dependent on the owner's ability to describe the situation. Taking a history on a farm may be much more complex because a herd of animals may be involved, many animals may be affected, and questioning about the environment is an integral part of evaluating the history. However, often the veterinarian will make observations of the environment or other animals which may lead to important questions about the history that might not otherwise be asked. Rarely would a small animal practitioner be required to evaluate the home environment of a dog or cat. The history taking described here is therefore generic, to include most (but not all) situations encountered in veterinary medicine.

The history should suggest not only the diagnostic possibilities but also the probabilities.

---

### Taking the Animal's History

The animal's history is of prime importance and adequate time should be devoted to this stage of the examination, this time also allows the patient to adapt to the presence of strangers.

---

### History-taking method

Successful history taking involves veterinarian–client relationships that are learned by experience. Some guidelines are suggested here.

1. The veterinarian should introduce himself or herself to the owner, and the usual greetings of the day will help to establish a relationship. Asking the owner 'how can I help you?' is an effective opening question which gives owners the opportunity to relate their concerns about the animal.
2. The owner or attendant must be handled with diplomacy and tact. The use of nonmedical terms is essential, as owners are likely to be confused by medical terminology or be reluctant to answer a question when confronted with terms they do not understand.
3. Test statements for accuracy, particularly those concerned with time, by restating the facts to the owners and asking them to confirm them. Owners – and more especially herdsmen and agents – may attempt to disguise their neglect by condensing time or varying the chronology of events. If a detailed cross-examination causes antagonism it is advisable to forgo further questioning and be content with estimating the dependability of the history.
4. Distinguish the owner's **observations** from **interpretations**. A statement that the cow has diarrhea may, on closer questioning, mean the feces were soft but also scant, which is an important distinction. Often, however, it is impossible to avoid the use of leading questions, such as 'did the cow pass her placenta?', or 'did the dog or cat vomit?', but it is necessary to weigh the answers according to the credibility of the owner. The absence of a sign can only be determined by enquiring whether or not it occurred. Simply asking the owner for a history invariably results in incompleteness.
5. Assume the leadership role and ask appropriate questions in a logical sequence. Consider the answers carefully, repeat what the owner said for confirmation, then ask appropriate additional questions. This is the process of active listening. Owners usually do not relate the animal's abnormalities in the sequence in which they actually occurred, and part of the task is to establish the chronology of events.

For completeness and accuracy in history taking a logical system is desirable. The system outlined here includes patient data, disease history and management history. The order in which these are taken will vary between species.

### Patient data

Patient data may be kept in a records system. Accurate identification of the patient is essential. An animal's previous history can be retreived, the disease status of a herd can be examined, and specimens for laboratory examination can be submitted with the knowledge that the results can be related to the correct patient. Accurate records are also necessary for the submission of accounts for veterinary services rendered, and the details of the owner's address and of the animals examined and treated must be accurate. The relevant data include

- owner's name and initials
- postal address and telephone number
- signalment of the animal.

The **signalment** of an animal is its description for identification purposes and includes breed (or estimate of parentage in a crossbreed), sex, age, identification number (tattoo, eartag etc.), color markings and other identifying marks, and body weight. Such a list

---

### Clinical Pointer

When history taking it is best to take the disease history first. The psychological effect is good as the owner appreciates the desire to get down to the facts about the animal's illness.

may appear formidable, but many of the items, such as age, sex, breed, type (use made of animal, e.g. beef, dairy, mutton, wool) and, in small animals, whether the animal is a family pet or a hunting dog, are often important in the diagnosis. A case history of a particular animal may suggest that further treatment is likely to be uneconomic because of age, or that a particular disease is assuming sufficient importance in a herd for different control measures to be warranted.

Computers are now used for recording the details of clinic office calls, farm calls, the animals examined and treated, the amounts charged for travel and professional services, the costs of laboratory services, the drugs used and dispensed, and the diseases that occur on a particular farm on an ongoing basis.

## History of the present disease

### The primary complaint

The primary complaint (also called the presenting complaint) is the concern expressed by the owner and it must be established and verified by questioning. The complaint, along with the signalment, can often help to generate diagnostic hypotheses early in the clinical examination. For example

- an 8-month-old kitten with a history of diarrhea is unlikely to have hyperthyroidism
- an 8-year-old cat with a history of diarrhea is much more likely to have hyperthyroidism than ascariasis
- a 1-year-old heifer with diarrhea is unlikely to have clinical Johne's disease
- a recumbent adult cow is more likely to have parturient paresis than a first-calf heifer
- a recumbent first-calf heifer is more likely to have maternal obstetric paralysis than is an adult cow.

The history may indicate that convulsions occurred in the affected animals several hours ago, but that now the animals are normal. For example, in hypovitaminosis A in beef calves from 6 to 10 months of age the animals may be seen when they are clinically normal, and the only means of reaching a diagnosis may be consideration of the history of the clinical findings and the nutritional status.

### Chronology of abnormalities

The details of the clinical abnormalities observed by the owner should be determined in the sequence in which they occurred. If more than one animal is affected a typical case should be chosen and the variations in history of other cases noted. Variations from the normal in feed or water intake, milk production,

growth rate, respiration, defecation, urination, sweating, activity, gait, posture, voice, and odor should be noted. There are many specific questions that need to be asked in each case, that are variations on the questions already suggested.

If a number of animals are affected information may be available from laboratory examinations already done, or necropsy examinations on fatal cases. The behavior of animals before death, and the period of time elapsing between the first observable signs and death or recovery, are important facts. Prior surgical or medical procedures, such as castration, docking, shearing, or vaccination, may be important factors in the production of disease.

### Morbidity, case fatality and population and mortality rates

The morbidity rate is the percentage of animals that are clinically affected compared to the total number exposed to the same risks. The case fatality rate is the percentage of affected animals that die. The population mortality rate is the percentage of all exposed animals that die.

### Prior treatment

Information on all prior treatments is desirable. Owners may be reluctant to admit they have treated the animal or, more commonly, have forgotten about certain treatments. Precise details of the drugs and dosages used may be of value in

- eliminating or considering some diagnostic possibilities
- assessing the probable efficiency of the treatment
- assessing the significance of laboratory tests
- prescribing additional treatment.

Drug withdrawal regulations now require that treated animals or their products, such as milk, be withheld from slaughter or market for varying lengths of time

---

**Clinical Pointer**

Determine if the owner has been affected with similar clinical manifestations to their pet's

- if both the dog and the owner are scratching, sarcoptic mange is a possibility
- if the family dog and owner have diarrhea, suggest fecal cultures from both, *Camplylobacter*, *Salmonella* and *Yersinia* spp. affect dogs, cats, and humans.

to allow drug residues to reach tolerable limits. This necessitates that owners reveal information about the drugs they have used.

## Preventive and control procedures

The control procedures used in the herd or for the individual animal should be known. These include vaccines and vaccination schedules and specific control procedures. In outbreaks of parvovirus infection in a canine kennel the owners should be asked about disinfection methods, isolation procedures, and the type of protective clothing being worn by handlers.

## Previous exposure

When examining a group of animals it is important to know when particular animals were added to the group. Is the affected animal one of the group, or has it been introduced; if so, how long ago? If it has been in the group for some time, have there been recent additions? Is the herd 'closed' or are animals introduced at frequent intervals? Not all additions are potential disease carriers, they may have come from herds where control measures are adequate, they may have been tested before or after sale or kept in quarantine for an adequate period after arrival, or they may have been vaccinated or received mass medication with antimicrobials. They may have originated from areas where a particular disease does not occur, although a negative history of this type is less reliable than a positive history of derivation from an area where a particular disease is endemic.

## Transportation and mixing of animals

Prolonged continuous transportation can be a risk factor for diseases such as pneumonia in cattle and horses. The mixing of animals from different origins followed by transportation to a feedlot is a potential risk factor for certain diseases, such as shipping fever pneumonia.

## Recent travel to other geographical regions

Animals that have recently been to other geographical regions in which certain infectious diseases are endemic may become infected and return to their current home. This applies for all species, but is particularly common in dogs and cats, and horses used in racing and other competitive sports. Ruminants and swine may have been taken to livestock shows and become infected with certain diseases that become clinical after their return to the home farm.

## Culling rate

The reasons for previous culling of animals from the herd may provide clues about the diagnosis.

## History of any previous disease

Information about previous diseases is often useful. Questions should be asked about clinical observations, necropsy findings, morbidity, case fatality rates, the treatments and control measures used and the results obtained. Enquiries should be made about herds from which introduced animals originated, and also about herds to which other animals from the same source have been sent. If dealing with a cattery or a multicat household, enquiries should be made about previous testing for feline leukemia and feline infectious peritonitis, and what control measures have been used to prevent these diseases.

# Management history

The management history includes nutrition, breeding policy and practice, housing, transport, and general handling. It is important to know if there has been any change in the prevailing practice prior to the appearance of disease. The fact that a disease has occurred when the affected animals have been receiving the same ration, originating from the same source over a long period, suggests that the diet is not at fault, although errors in the preparation of concentrate mixtures, particularly with the current practice of introducing additives to feeds, can cause variations which are not immediately apparent.

## Nutrition

The nutritional history includes the quantity and quality of the diet compared with the nutrient requirements recommended for a similar class of animal. In some situations it may be necessary to submit feed and water samples for analysis. For dogs and cats, it is important to question the owner about the

---

### Misleading Terminology

Terminology can be misleading: 'treats' may mean purchased pet treats, such as milkbones and rawhide bones, or it can mean cheese, toast, and milk. This information may be invaluable, particularly in dealing with a dog or cat with gastrointestinal or dermatological signs of disease.

feeding of table food. If asked, some owners will say that they do not give 'table scraps' but do feed left-overs from family meals.

### Livestock at pasture

Grazing animals are on a diet which is less controlled and thus more difficult to assess. The risk of parasitic infestation and nutritional deficiencies may be much greater. Questions should be asked about

- the composition of the pasture
- its probable nutritive value with particular reference to recent changes brought about by rain or drought
- whether rotational grazing is practiced
- the fertilizer program and whether or not minerals and trace elements are provided by top-dressing or mineral mixtures.

The origin of mineral supplements, particularly phosphates which may contain excess fluorine, and home-made mixtures which may contain excessive quantities of other ingredients, should receive attention. An actual field examination of the pasture is more rewarding than a description of it.

### Handfed or automated livestock feeding systems

Animals receiving controlled feed may be affected by a dietary mistake because of an error in feed preparation. Types and amounts of feeds fed should be determined. Cattle introduced to carbohydrate-rich diets too quickly may develop lactic acidosis.

The sources of the dietary ingredients may also be of importance. Because the digestive enzyme capacity of newborn farm animals is most efficient in the digestion of whole milk, the use of nonmilk sources of carbohydrates and proteins in the formulation of milk replacers may result in indigestion and nutritional diarrhea.

### Changes in diet

In both handfed and grazing animals any changes in diet should be determined. The removal of animals from one field to another, from pasture grazing to

cereal feeding, from unimproved to improved pasture, may precipitate disease. Periods of sudden dietary deficiency can occur due to inclement weather, transportation, or during a change to unfamiliar feeds. Rapid changes are more important than gradual alterations, particularly in pregnant and lactating ruminants, when metabolic diseases, including those caused by hypocalcemia, hypoglycemia and hypomagnesemia, may occur. An acute onset of diarrhea is common in dogs and cats experiencing sudden diet changes.

### Drinking water supply

The availability of drinking water must be determined and water analysis may be indicated.

### *Reproductive management and performance*

In the examination of a single animal the breeding and parturition history may suggest or eliminate some diagnostic possibilities. Pregnancy toxemia occurs in late pregnancy in ewes. Acute septic metritis is a possibility a few days after parturition in any species, but unlikely several weeks later. Pyometra should be considered in any bitch with a mucopurulent vaginal discharge occurring 4–12 weeks after standing heat, whereas hypocalcemic tetany or eclampsia occur primarily 3 to 4 weeks after parturition.

The examination of herd reproductive history involves comparing past and present reproductive performance with certain optimum objectives. The mean length of the interval between parturition and conception, the mean number of services per conception, and the percentage of young animals weaned relative to the number of females that were originally exposed for breeding (calf or lamb crop, pigs weaned) are general measures of reproductive performance and efficiency. Using cattle as an example, other important reproductive performance objectives include

- percentage of abortions
- length of the breeding season
- percentage of females pregnant at specified times after the onset of the breeding period
- bull : cow ratio
- size and topography of breeding pastures
- fertility status of the females and males at breeding time.

The percentage of females that need assistance at parturition and the percentage of calves that die at birth are also indices of reproductive performance indicative of the level of management provided. The breeding history may also be of importance with regard to inherited disease. The existence of a graphic relationship between sires and dams should be noted.

### General management

There are many items in the proper management of livestock which if neglected can lead to the occurrence of disease. Some of the more important include

- hygiene, particularly in milking parlors and in parturition and rearing stalls
- adequacy of housing in terms of space, ventilation, draining, location, and suitability of feed bunks
- opportunity for exercise and the proper management of milking machines to avoid udder injury.

The class of livestock under consideration is also important: for example, clostridial enterotoxemia is most common in finishing lambs, parturient paresis in cows in the peripartum period, obstructive urolithiasis in lambs and steers in feedlots, and shipping fever pneumonia in recently arrived beef calves in the feedlot.

## CLIMATE

Many diseases are influenced by climate and season.

- Parvovirus infection in dogs has a peak incidence during the warm months.
- Rocky Mountain Spotted Fever, a tick-borne rickettsial disease affecting dogs and humans, has a higher incidence in areas supporting deciduous forests, with high humidity and warm temperatures.
- Foot-rot in cattle and sheep reaches peak incidence in warm, wet summers and is relatively rare in dry seasons.
- Diseases spread by insects are encouraged when climatic conditions favor the propagation of the vector.

### Respiratory Tract Disease in Catteries

Respiratory tract disease is a common problem in catteries. Proper hygiene, isolation procedures, ventilation, separation of cages by at least 1.5 m, and removal of affected carrier queens are all measures to reduce the problem.

- Internal parasites are similarly influenced by climate.
- Cool, wet seasons favor the development of hypomagnesemia in pastured cattle.
- Anhidrosis in horses is specifically a disease of hot, humid countries.
- The direction of prevailing winds is important in many disease outbreaks, particularly in relation to the contamination of pasture and drinking water by fumes from factories and mines, and the spread of diseases carried by insects.

## EXAMINATION OF THE ENVIRONMENT

Examination of the environment is a necessary part of any on-farm clinical investigation because of the possible relationship between environmental and managemental risk factors and the incidence of disease. It requires an adequate knowledge of the management of the species being examined, as well as its environmental needs.

Animals may be kept outside year round, housed part of the year, or kept in total confinement. For animals raised on pasture the effects of topography, plants, soil type, ground surface, and protection from extremes of weather assume major importance. For animals housed indoors, hygiene, ventilation, and avoiding overcrowding are a major concern. Each observation should be recorded in detail so that reports can be submitted to the owner when necessary.

### Suspected Poisoning

Detailed records and photographs of environmental characteristics assume major importance when poisonings are suspected and where litigation is possible.

### Outdoor environment

#### Topography and soil type

The topography of grasslands, pastures and wooded areas can contribute to disease or inefficient production. Low marshy areas facilitate the spread of insect-borne diseases and soil-borne infections requiring damp conditions, such as leptospirosis. Liver fluke infestation and lungworm pneumonia are more prevalent in such areas. Dogs allowed to roam in heavily wooded areas are much more likely to be exposed to ticks and tick-borne diseases.

The soil type may provide important clues to the detection of nutritional deficiencies

- copper and cobalt deficiencies are most common on littoral sands
- the copper deficiency/molybdenum excess complex usually occurs on peat soils.

The ground surface and its drainage characteristics are important in highly intensive beef feedlots, and in large dairy herds where finishing cattle and dairy cows are kept and fed under total confinement. Where beef cows are calved outdoors during cold and wet spring seasons, excessive surface water, mud and fecal-contaminated bedding increase the spread of infectious disease and result in a marked increase in neonatal mortality.

## Stocking rate (population density)

Overcrowding is a common risk factor for infectious disease. An excessive build-up of feces and urine increases the infection pressure. Under such conditions the relative humidity is commonly increased and more difficult to control. Overcrowding in catteries is a risk factor for respiratory disease outbreaks. Overcrowding also makes it difficult to detect and identify animals for whatever reason, such as illness, estrus and impending parturition.

## Feed and water supplies

On pasture the predominant plant types, both natural and introduced, may be associated with certain soil types and may be the cause of actual disease. The presence of specific poisonous plants, evidence of over-grazing, or the existence of a bone- or bark-chewing habit are usually obvious if the environment is inspected.

Vital clues in the investigation of possible poisoning in a herd may be the existence of a garbage dump or ergotized grass or rye in the pasture, or the chewing of lead-based painted walls in the barn. The possibility that the forage may have been contaminated by environmental pollution from nearby factories or highways should be examined. Lush legume pasture, or heavy concentrate feeding with insufficient roughage, can cause a serious bloat problem.

The feed supplies for animals raised in confinement outdoors must be examined for evidence of moulds, contamination with feces and urine, and excessive moisture due to lack of protection from rain and snow. Empty feed troughs may confirm a suspicion that the feed delivery system is faulty.

The **drinking water** supply and its origin may be important in the cause of disease. Water in ponds may be covered with algae containing neurotoxins or hepa-

totoxic agents, and flowing streams may carry effluent from nearby industrial plants. In a feedlot water may suddenly be unavailable because of frozen water lines or faulty water tank valves, but should not go unnoticed if one recognizes the anxiety of a group of cattle trying to obtain water from a dry tank.

## Waste disposal

The disposal of feces and urine is a major problem for large intensified livestock operations. The application of slurry on pastures is a risk factor for the transmission of certain infectious diseases in animals that subsequently graze those pastures. Lagoons can provide ideal conditions for the propagation of flies.

## Indoor environment
### Housing and ventilation

Inadequate housing and ventilation, overcrowding and uncomfortable conditions can have detrimental effects on housed animals, making them more susceptible to infectious disease and less productive. Thus it is important to examine and assess all aspects of an indoor environment that may be a risk factor for disease.

### Sanitation and hygiene

The level of sanitation and hygiene is usually a reliable indicator of the standard of management. Poor hygiene is often associated with a high level of infectious disease

- the incidence of lice and coccidiosis in puppies may be high in kennels where the level of sanitation and hygiene is low
- dogs housed on wet straw or improperly cleaned concrete runs may develop skin disease due to *Strongyloides stercoralis* infection
- the incidence of diarrhea in piglets may be high because the farrowing crates are not suitably cleaned and disinfected before the pregnant sows are placed in them. A similar situation applies to lambing sheds, calving pens and foaling boxes.

### Preweaning Mortality in Piglets

More piglets die from chilling and crushing in the first few days of life, than from infectious disease. This is caused by

- poorly designed farrowing crates
- slippery floors
- inadequate heating
- overcrowding of the farrowing facilities.

## Ventilation

Inadequate ventilation is a major risk factor contributing to many diseases of the respiratory tract. Primary infections may have minimal effects on the animal, but inadequate ventilation may precipitate outbreaks of disease. Ventilation is assessed by determining

- number of air changes per unit of time
- relative humidity during the day and night
- presence or absence of condensation on the haircoats of the animals or on the walls and ceilings
- presence of drafts
- building and insulation materials used
- positions and capacities of the fans and the size and location of the air inlets.

Measuring the concentration of noxious gases in animal barns, such as ammonia and hydrogen sulfide, may be a valuable aid in assessing the effectiveness of a ventilation system.

## Population density

Overcrowded conditions can be a risk factor for infectious diseases, and measurements of population density and observations of animal behavior in such conditions assume major importance. When pigs are raised indoors in crowded conditions with inadequate ventilation their social habits may change drastically, and they begin to defecate and urinate on the clean floor and on their pen mates, rather than on the slatted floor over the gutter. This can result in outbreaks of diseases which are transmitted by the fecal–oral route.

## Floor quality

The quality of the floor is often responsible for diseases of the musculoskeletal system and skin. Poorly finished concrete floors with an exposed aggregate can cause severe foot lesions and lameness in adult swine. Recently calved dairy cows are very susceptible to slipping on slippery floors in dairy barns, a common cause of the downer cow syndrome. Dirt floors in dog kennels and runs are risk factors for internal parasites. The quality and quantity of bedding used should also be noted. The use of sawdust and shavings in loose-housing systems for dairy cattle may be associated with outbreaks of coliform mastitis.

## Floor plan

The floor plan and general layout of an animal house must be examined for evidence that the routine movements of attendants, the movements of animals and the feeding facilities may actually be spreading disease. Communal gutters running through adjacent pens may promote the spread of disease through fecal or urinary contamination. The nature of the partitions between pens, whether solid or open grid type, may assist the control or spread of infectious disease. The building materials used will influence the ease with which pens, such as farrowing crates and calf pens, can be cleaned and disinfected for a new batch of piglets or calves. Fomite transmission of respiratory tract pathogens is an important risk factor in catteries.

## Lighting

The amount of light available in a barn should be noted. With insufficient light it may be difficult to maintain a sufficient level of sanitation and hygiene, sick animals may not be recognized early enough, and general errors in management are likely to occur.

# EXAMINATION OF THE PATIENT

A complete clinical examination of every patient is unnecessary because of the obvious nature of some diseases. In most cases, in all sectors of clinical veterinary medicine the diagnosis will be obvious after taking the history and examining the animal. As experience is gained the veterinarian will know the extent to which a clinical examination is necessary. In this section we describe a general approach to the complete examination of an animal patient. There are major differences between species in the ease with which this is done and the amount of information that can be obtained. More detailed examination techniques are presented under the individual body systems in Part III.

The examination of a patient consists of three parts:

- distant examination or general inspection
- particular distant examination of body regions
- close physical examination.

## Distant examination or general inspection

Standing back at a convenient distance and looking and listening can provide valuable information about the state of the animal. The examiner must stay a reasonable distance away from animals unaccustomed to frequent handling to prevent excitement.

### Behavior and general appearance

The general behavior and appearance of the animal are evaluated from a distance.

## Behavior and demeanor

The behavior and demeanor are reflections of the animal's health and its response to other animals or observers. Separation of an animal from its group is often an indication of illness. If it responds normally to external stimuli such as sound and movement, the mentation is known as bright and alert.

## Depression states

Depression states are common and their severity varies widely. If the reactions are sluggish and the animal is indifferent to the movements of the examiner and surrounding external noises, it is dull or apathetic. Cattle with carbohydrate engorgement are commonly depressed and reluctant to move. A cat hiding under the bed or a dog growling as its owner approaches may indicate illness. A pronounced state of indifference in which the animal remains standing and does not respond to external stimuli is referred to as the 'dummy' syndrome, for example

- subacute lead poisoning
- listeriosis
- encephalomyelitis
- hepatic cirrhosis.

The terminal stage of apathy or depression is coma, in which the animal is unconscious and cannot be roused.

## Excitation states

Excitation states vary in severity. A state of anxiety or apprehension is the mildest form. The animal is alert and looks around constantly but is normal in its movements. Such behavior suggests moderate constant pain or other abnormal sensations, such as early parturient paresis or recent blindness. A more severe manifestation is restlessness, in which the animal moves constantly, lies down and gets up, and may go through other abnormal movements, such as looking at its flanks, kicking at its belly and rolling and bellowing. Such behavior is indicative of pain. Abdominal pain in the dog due to gastric dilatation and volvulus (GDV) may be associated with restlessness, a tendency to lie down and get up frequently, and extension of the head and neck. More extreme degrees of excited demeanor include mania and frenzy. In mania the animal performs abnormal movements with vigor. Violent licking at its own body, licking or chewing inanimate objects, and pressing against obstacles with the head are typical examples. In frenzy the actions are so wild and uncontrolled that the animal is a danger to anyone approaching.

### Mania and Frenzy

In both mania and frenzy there is usually excitation of the brain, as in rabies, acute lead poisoning, and some cases of nervous acetonemia.

A dog in epileptic seizures will often be in lateral recumbency and paddle uncontrollably with all four limbs. Postictally it may appear blind and bite at anyone who approaches.

## Voice

Abnormalities of voice are noted. In dogs with laryngeal paralysis the larynx does not abduct during inspiration, resulting in a change in the bark.

The voice may be hoarse in rabies, or weak in gut edema of pigs. Continuous lowing may be heard in cattle with nervous acetonemia, or persistent bellowing indicative of acute pain. Bellowing and yawning occur in rabid cattle, and yawning often occurs in horses with hepatic encephalopathy.

## Appetite and eating

The owner can usually provide information about feed intake if it is known. Appetite is evaluated by observing the animal's reaction to being offered food, or by the amount of food available which has not been eaten. The total amount of feed being consumed per day is important information. In a patient which has retained its appetite there may be abnormalities of prehension, mastication or swallowing and, in ruminants, of belching and regurgitation.

### Prehension

Prehension, or the ability to grasp feed, may be interfered with by

- an inability to approach the feed
- paralysis of the tongue (cattle)
- masseter myopathy
- osteomyelitis of cervical vertebrae or other painful conditions of the neck.

If there is pain in the mouth, prehension may be abnormal and affected animals may be able to take only certain types of feed.

### Mastication

Mastication or chewing may be slow, one-sided or incomplete when oral structures, particularly teeth, are affected. A cat with a tooth root abscess may no longer be willing to chew hard food but still able to eat soft canned food. Periodic cessation of chewing when food is still in the mouth occurs commonly in the 'dummy' syndrome, of cerebral diseases such as space-occupying lesions or encephalomyelitis.

### Swallowing

Swallowing may be painful because of inflammation of the pharynx or esophagus, as may occur in strangles in the horse, in calf diphtheria, and where improper use of balling and drenching guns has caused laceration of the pharyngeal mucosa. Attempts at swallowing, followed by coughing up of feed or regurgitation through the nostrils, can also be the result of painful conditions but are most likely to be due to physical obstructions such as esophageal diverticula or stenosis, a foreign body in the pharynx, or paralysis of the pharynx. It is important to differentiate between material that has reached the stomach and ingesta regurgitated from an esophageal site.

### Regurgitation and eructation

Regurgitation is the passive retrograde movement of food or fluid from the oral cavity, pharynx or esophagus, typically, the contents have not reached the stomach. In ruminants, however, regurgitation is a normal activity. Congenital megaesophagus due to a vascular ring anomaly (persistent right aortic arch), esophageal agenesis or esophageal deviation (Bulldogs and Shar Peis) is a cause of regurgitation in young animals, whereas acquired megaesophagus is a cause in older dogs.

In ruminants there may be abnormalities of rumination and eructation. Absence of cudding occurs in many diseases of cattle and sheep.

There may be inability to control the cud, 'cud-dropping', due to pharyngeal paralysis or painful conditions of the mouth. Failure to eructate is usually manifested by bloat in cattle.

### Vomiting

Vomiting is an active process whereby material is ejected from the stomach, and possibly the duodenum.

---

**Clinical Pointer** ✳

1. Partial esophageal obstruction is usually manifested by repeated swallowing movements, often with associated flexion of the neck and grunting.
2. Vigorous efforts to regurgitate with grunting suggests esophageal or cardiac sphincter obstruction.

---

### Excretion

Defecation may be abnormal. Constipation is a decrease in the frequency of defecation and the passage of feces with an increase in dry matter concentration. It is usually associated with impaction of the feces in the rectum and must not be mistaken for scant feces due to functional or physical obstruction of the intestinal tract. In constipation, rectal paralysis or stenosis of the anus, defecation may be difficult and be accompanied by straining or tenesmus.

In small animals with colorectal tumors the animal often appears constipated and passes ribbon-like stools. If there is abdominal pain or laceration of the mucocutaneous junction at the anus, defecation may cause obvious pain.

Diarrhea is an increase in the frequency of defecation and the passage of feces with an increase in concentration of water. Involuntary defecation occurs in severe diarrhea and when there is paralysis of the anal sphincter.

Urination may be difficult when there is partial obstruction of the urinary tract, or painful when there is inflammation of the bladder or urethra. In cystitis and urethritis there is increased frequency with the passage of small amounts of fluid, and the animal remains in the urination posture for some time after flow ceases.

Incontinence, with constant dribbling of urine, is usually due to partial obstruction of the urethra or incompetence of its sphincter.

---

**Constipation versus Scant Feces**

Impaction of feces in the rectum results in constipation
Functional or physical obstruction of the intestinal tract results in scant feces.

---

## Abnormal postures

An abnormal posture is not necessarily indicative of disease, but when associated with other signs it may indicate the site and severity of a disease process. One of the simplest examples is resting a limb in painful conditions of the extremities.

- A horse continually shifting its weight from limb to limb may indicate the presence of laminitis.
- Dogs with panosteitis may have alternating limb lameness.
- Dogs with immune-mediated joint disease affecting multiple joints may be reluctant to move or stand, and walk as if 'walking on eggshells'.

- Arching of the back with the limbs tucked under the body usually indicates mild abdominal pain. Downward arching of the back and 'sawhorse' straddling of the legs is characteristic of severe abdominal pain, usually spasmodic in occurrence.
- In the horse severe abdominal pain can be manifested by a 'dog-sitting' posture, and repeated uncontrollable episodes of lying down, rolling, lying quietly for a few moments and then standing quickly.
- A dog with abdominal discomfort may assume a 'sawhorse' stance and be reluctant to move despite an owner's commands.
- A dog with acute pancreatitis may assume a 'praying position', in which the head rests on the front limbs on the ground while the hindquarters are elevated.
- Elevation and rigidity of the tail, and rigidity of the ears and limbs, suggest tetanus in all species.
- Abduction of the elbows indicates thoracic pain or difficulty in breathing. A dog with congestive heart failure may stand with the elbows abducted and the head and neck extended. The animal may not be able to sit or lie down in one position for any length of time.

---

### Clinical Pointer

If an animal urinates during the inspection, take a sample for visual and laboratory analysis.

---

**Abnormal postures in recumbency**

Abnormalities of posture may occur in recumbent animals. The head may be held in the flank in parturient paresis in cows and in colic in horses. Sheep affected with hypocalcemia, and cattle with bilateral hip dislocation, often lie in sternal recumbency with the hindlegs extended behind in a frog-like attitude. Inability or lack of desire to rise is usually indicative of muscle weakness or of pain in the extremities, as in nutritional myodegeneration or laminitis.

### Gait

Limb movements are usually described according to rate, range, force, and direction. Abnormalities may occur in one or more of these categories.

1. In true cerebellar ataxia all modes of limb movement are affected.
2. In arthritis because of pain in the joints, or in laminitis because of pain in the feet, the range is diminished and the patient has a shuffling, stumbling walk. The direction of progress may be affected.
3. Walking in circles can be associated with rotation or deviation of the head. It may persist in listeriosis or occur spasmodically, as in acetonemia and pregnancy toxemia.
4. Compulsive walking, or walking directly ahead regardless of obstructions, is part of the 'dummy' syndrome, characteristic of encephalomyelitis and hepatic insufficiency in the horse.
5. A cat with peripheral vestibular disease will circle to the side of the lesion and may use a wall to lean on for balance while walking. In the acute phase the cat may fall and appear disorientated.
6. Cats with thromboembolic disease affecting the aortic bifurcation may walk on the front limbs but drag the hindlimbs.
7. Dogs with disc disease affecting the thoracolumbar junction may have a normal gait in the forelimbs but be ataxic in the pelvic limbs.

### Body condition

Body conditioning scoring is now used to assess the body condition numerically. Body condition may be obese, normal, thin or emaciated. The difference between thinness and emaciation is one of degree. Thin animals can be physiologically normal. Emaciation is severe loss of body condition usually accompanied by other signs of illness, or due to severe undernutrition.

The difference between fatness and obesity is of the same order. Weight loss is considered significant in dogs and cats when a 10% decrease in normal body weight occurs unassociated with loss of body fluids. Weight loss of 30% to 50% of lean body mass is usually fatal. Obesity, the most common nutritional disorder in small animal practice, is defined as a body weight 15% to 20% or more above the ideal body weight.

### Conformation

The assessment of conformation or body shape is based on the symmetry and the shape and size of the different body regions relative to other regions. An abdomen which is very large relative to the thorax and hindquarters can be classified as an abnormality of conformation.

---

### Cachexia

Cachexia is a state of extreme weight loss and ill health: the haircoat is lustreless, the skin is dry and leathery, and work performance reduced.

---

## Skin

Abnormalities of skin can usually be seen from a distance. They include

- changes in the hair or wool
- the presence of discrete or diffuse lesions
- evidence of discharges and itching.

The normal lustre of the coat may be absent, it may be dry, as in most chronic debilitating diseases, or excessively greasy as in seborrhea. In debilitated animals the long winter coat may be retained past the normal time. Alopecia may be local or diffuse. Bilateral symmetrical alopecia in the dog is most commonly due to endocrinopathies, particularly hyperadrenocorticism and hypothyroidism. Alopecia of the flank and ventral body wall in the cat may be self-induced. Sweating may be diminished, as in anhidrosis of horses; patchy as in peripheral nerve lesions; or excessive as in acute abdominal pain. Hypertrophy and folding of the skin may be evident, hyperkeratosis being the typical example. Discrete skin lesions range in type from urticarial plaques to the circumscribed scabs of ringworm, pox and impetigo. Discrete lesions include papules, nodules, pustules, vesicles and wheals. Diffuse lesions include scales, parakeratosis, and excoriations. Diffuse enlargements include subcutaneous edema (anasarca), hematomas, and subcutaneous emphysema. Enlargements of lymph nodes and lymphatics may be also evident when examining an animal from a distance.

## Particular distant examination of body regions

The particular distant examination consists of inspection of each body region for evidence of abnormalities. With clinical experience this is usually done along with the general distant examination.

## Head

The facial expression may be abnormal, for example
- the sardonic grin of tetanus owing to contraction of the facial muscles
- the cunning leer or maniacal expression of rabies and acute lead poisoning
- the open mouth of a dog with trigeminal nerve paralysis.

The symmetry and configuration of the bony structures of the head are noted. Doming of the forehead occurs in some cases of congenital hydrocephalus and in chondrodysplastic dwarfs, and in the latter there may be bilateral enlargement of the maxillae.

Swelling of the maxillae and mandibles may occur in horses with abscessed teeth. In cattle, enlargement of the maxilla or mandible is common in actinomycosis. A soft-tissue swelling below the eye and associated with the maxilla is often seen in the dog or cat with an abscess of the upper carnassial tooth. Asymmetry of the soft structures may be evident and is most obvious in the carriage of the ears, degree of closure of the eyelids and situation of the muzzle and lower lip. Slackness of one side of the face and a pulling to the other are constant features in facial paralysis. Tetanus is accompanied by rigidity of the ears, prolapse of the third eyelid and dilatation of the nostrils.

The carriage of the head is observed for abnormalities

- rotation of the head and neck is usually associated with defects of the vestibular apparatus on one side
- deviation of the head and neck suggest unilateral involvement of the medulla oblongata or cervical spinal cord
- opisthotonos is an excitation phenomenon associated with tetanus, strychnine poisoning, acute lead poisoning, hypomagnesemic tetany, polioencephalomalacia, and encephalitis.

The eyes and eyelids are inspected from a close distance

- entropion is inversion of the eyelid
- ectropion is eversion of the eyelid.

Ocular discharges are usually obvious. Spasm of the eyelids and excessive blinking (blepharospasm) indicates pain or peripheral nerve involvement.

Exophthalmos or protrusion of the eye may suggest a retro-orbital mass, such as a tumor or abscess. Enophthalmos or retraction of the eye occurs in dehydration. Prolapse of the nictitating membrane (third eyelid) suggests central nervous system involvement, e.g. tetanus in the horse.

Protrusion of the third eyelid also occurs if the eye is actively retracted, as in painful conditions or if it retracts in the orbit due to atrophy of the muscles of mastication, as with trigeminal nerve paralysis or

## Horner's Syndrome

Horner's syndrome consists of enophthalmos, protrusion of the third eyelid, miosis and ptosis, and is not uncommon in small animals. It is commonly due to

- a cranial mediastinal mass
- injury to the cervical sympathetic trunk
- brachial plexus injury
- cranial thoracic spinal cord disease, or
- otitis media.

chronic myositis. In cats, bilateral protrusion of the third eyelid is seen with severe systemic disease and depression (Haws syndrome). A reddened eye is often seen with glaucoma, corneal ulceration, conjunctivitis and uveitis. Dilatation of the nostrils and nasal discharge suggest the advisability of closer examination of the nasal cavities at a later stage.

Excessive salivation suggests a painful condition of the mouth or pharynx. Frothing saliva is associated with 'chewing gum' fits associated with nervous system irritation.

Swellings below the jaw may be inflammatory, as in actinobacillosis and strangles, or edematous as in acute anemia, protein starvation or congestive heart failure. Swellings below the jaw in the dog may be due to salivary secretion accumulation (sialocele) due to injury to the mandibular or sublingual salivary gland duct. Unilateral or bilateral swelling of the cheeks in calves usually indicates necrotic stomatitis.

### Neck

Any enlargement of the proximal part of the neck region must be more closely examined to determine whether lymph nodes, salivary glands (or guttural pouches in the horse) or other soft tissues are involved. Goiter causes a discrete local enlargement of the neck in some species and not in others. A prominent jugular pulse, jugular vein engorgement and brisket edema may be present. A cylindrical enlargement of the neck may be due to esophageal distension.

### Thorax and respirations

The respirations or breathing movements are examined from a distance, preferably with the animal standing as recumbency is likely to modify them considerably. Allowance should be made for the effects of exercise, excitement, high environmental temperatures and fatness of the subject.

## Clinical Pointer ✳

The respiratory rates of obese cattle can be two to three times those of normal animals.

The variables of breathing to be noted from a distance are rate, rhythm, depth, type, symmetry of the thoracic wall movements and the presence of any respiratory noises.

**Respiration rate**
In normal animals under average conditions the respiratory rate per minute should be within the ranges given in Table 6.1. Many dogs pant when hyper-excitable and being examined, thereby making it difficult to determine the resting respiratory rate. An increased respiratory rate is designated as polypnea or tachypnea; decreased rate as oligopnea; and complete cessation as apnea. The rate may be counted by observation of thoracic wall or nostril movements, by feeling the nasal air movements, or by auscultation of the thorax or trachea. A significant rise in environmental temperature or humidity may double the normal respiratory rate.

**Rhythm**
Normal breathing consists of three phases of equal length: inspiration, expiration and pause; variation in the length of one or all phases constitutes an abnormality of rhythm.

Prolongation of inspiration is usually due to obstruction of the upper respiratory tract, especially the larynx.

Prolongation of expiration is usually due to disease of the lower respiratory tract. In most lung diseases there is no pause and the rhythm consists of two phases instead of three. There may be variation between cycles.

- Cheyne–Stokes respiration, characteristic of advanced renal and cardiac disease, is a gradual increase and then a gradual decrease in the depth of respiration

## Heat Stress and Respiratory Rate

Animals that are acclimatized to cold outdoor temperatures are susceptible to heat stress when exposed to warmer temperatures. Indoors the respiratory rate may increase six to eight times the normal rate, and panting open-mouth breathing may be evident within 2 hours.

**Table 6.1.** Physiological vital signs for domestic animals

| Species/age | | Body temperature (°C) | Heart rate and pulse (beats/min) | Respiratory rate (breaths/min) |
|---|---|---|---|---|
| | | Range | Range | Range |
| Dog | | | | |
| | Small breeds | 38.5–39.2 | Toy breeds up to 180 | 24–36 |
| | Large breeds | 37.5–38.5 | 60–140 | 18–30 |
| | Puppies | 38.5 by 4 weeks | up to 220 | 20–30 |
| Cat | | 37.8–39.2 | 120–240 | 20–30 |
| Horse | | 37.5–38.5 | 28–46 | 8–16 |
| Foal | | | | |
| | 1 week–6 months | 37.5 – 38.9 | 40–60 | 10–25 |
| | Foal < 1 week | 37.2–38.9 | 60–120 | 20–40 |
| Cow/bull | | 37.8–39.2 | 60–72 | 20–30 |
| Calf | | 38.5–39.5 | 80–120 | 24–36 |
| Ewe/ram | | 38.5–40.0 | 70–90 | 20–30 |
| Lamb | | 39–40.0 | 80–90 | 36–48 |
| Sow/boar | | 37.8–38.5 | 60–90 | 10–20 |
| Piglet | | 38.9–40.0 | 100–120 | 24–36 |
| Goat | | 38.6–40.2 | 70–90 | 20–30 |
| Goat kid | | 38.8–40.2 | 100–120 | 36–48 |

- Biot's breathing, which occurs in meningitis affecting the medulla oblongata, is characterized by alternating periods of hyperpnea and apnea, the periods often being of unequal length.
- Periodic breathing occurs commonly in animals with electrolyte and acid–base imbalances: there are periods of apnea followed by short bursts of hyperventilation.
- Animals with acidosis, such as dogs with diabetic ketoacidosis, may have compensatory hyperventilation (Kussmaul's breathing). Persistent acidosis may ultimately lead to depression of the respiratory center.

**Depth**

The depth of breathing may be reduced in painful conditions of the thorax or diaphragm and increased in any form of hypoxia. A moderate increase in depth is called hyperpnea, and labored breathing is dyspnea. In dyspnea the accessory respiratory movements become more prominent, there is

- extension of the head and neck
- dilatation of the nostrils
- abduction of the elbows
- breathing through the mouth
- increased movement of the thoracic and abdominal walls
- loud respiratory noises, especially expiratory grunting, may also be heard.

Pneumothorax as a cause of dyspnea is common in small animals.

**Type**

In normal breathing there is movement of the thoracic and abdominal walls. In painful conditions of the thorax, such as acute pleurisy, and in paralysis of the intercostal muscles there is relative fixation of the thoracic wall and a marked increase in the movements of the abdominal wall. There may also be an associated pleuritic ridge caused by thoracic immobility with the thorax expanded. This syndrome is usually referred to as abdominal-type breathing, causing the costochondral junction to be more visible than usual. The reverse situation is thoracic-type breathing, in which the movements are largely confined to the thoracic wall, as in peritonitis, particularly when there is diaphragmatic involvement.

### Symmetry of thoracic wall movements

Normally both sides of the thorax move uniformly. In painful diseases of the thorax and in pneumothorax, one side of the thorax may not move as much as the other. These movements are evaluated by looking down on the animal from above.

### Respiratory noises

Abnormal respiratory noises include

- coughing due to irritation of the pharynx, larynx, trachea and bronchi
- snorting due to nasal irritation
- wheezing due to stenosis of the nasal passages
- snoring when there is pharyngeal obstruction due to pharyngitis
- stridor when there is constriction of the larynx
- roaring in paralysis of the vocal cords
- grunting, a forced expiration against a closed glottis, which occurs in many types of painful and labored breathing
- wheezes can be occasionally heard in asthmatic cats without the use of a stethoscope.

## Abdomen

Variations in the size of the abdomen are obvious during the distant examination.

### Distension

Distension, or an increase in size, may be due to the presence of excessive feed, fluid, feces, flatus or fat, or the presence of a fetus or a neoplasm. Further differentiation is usually possible only on close examination. In advanced pregnancy in cattle fetal movements may be visible over the right flank. Intestinal tympany usually results in uniform distension of the dorsal abdomen, whereas fluid in the peritoneal cavity results in increased distension of both sides of the vertical abdomen (pear-shaped abdomen). Distension may be bilaterally symmetrical, asymmetrical, or more prominent ventrally or dorsally. Normal and abnormal

ruminal movements can be seen in the left paralumbar fossa of cattle and require additional examination using auscultation, palpation and percussion, which are described in Chapter 17.

### Gaunt

Gaunt refers to an obvious decrease in the size of the abdomen, seen most commonly in starvation, severe diarrhea and in many chronic diseases in which appetite is reduced.

### Ventral edema

Ventral edema is commonly associated with impending parturition, gangrenous mastitis, congestive heart failure, infectious equine anemia, and rupture of the urethra due to obstructive urolithiasis.

## External genitalia

Gross enlargements of the preputial sheath or scrotum are usually inflammatory in origin, but varicoceles or tumors can also be responsible. An umbilical hernia, omphalophlebitis, or dribbling of urine from a patent urachus may be apparent on inspection of the ventral abdominal wall. Degenerative changes in the testicles may result in a small scrotum. Discharges of pus and blood from the vagina indicate infection of the genitourinary tract. A cryptorchid dog may have a small scrotum. Examination of the reproductive tracts is described in Chapter 22.

## Mammary glands

A disproportionately sized udder suggests acute inflammation, atrophy or hypertrophy of the gland. These abnormalities can be differentiated only by further palpation and examination of the milk or secretions. See Chapter 23.

## Limbs and feet

Symmetry of the musculoskeletal system is important. Enlargement or distortion of bones, joints, tendons, sheaths and bursae should be noted, and so should any enlargement of peripheral lymph nodes and lymph-atic vessels. The feet are examined for evidence

---

**Clinical Pointer**

A grossly enlarged asymmetrical swelling of the abdomen suggests herniation of the abdominal wall.

of overgrown hooves or nails, and evidence of swelling or lesions of soft tissues surrounding the digits. Detailed examination of the musculoskeletal system is described in Chapter 21.

## Close physical examination

The close physical examination consists of audiovisual inspection, palpation, ballottement, auscultation, percussion, tactile percussion, succussion and percussion and simultaneous auscultation, which are described in Chapter 3.

### Examination method and sequence

The close physical examination is done as gently as possible to avoid disturbing the patient and prevent increases in resting heart and respiratory rates. At a later stage it may be necessary to examine certain body systems more closely after exercise, but resting measurements should be done first. If possible the animal should be standing, as recumbency may restrict the complete examination of some body systems.

The sequence in which the body systems are examined will vary depending on the species and on the results of the history and the diagnostic hypotheses. A systematic examination ensures that all body systems are examined. Not every case requires this, but when the diagnosis is uncertain or not obvious it may be necessary. Special examinations, such as a neurological examination, are usually done after the general clinical examination.

The sequence of examination of body systems or regions described here is as follows:

- vital signs (temperature, pulse, respirations), commonly referred to as the TPR
- peripheral circulation and state of hydration
- thorax, including the heart and lungs
- abdomen and gastrointestinal tract
- head and neck

- urinary system
- reproductive tract
- mammary glands
- musculoskeletal system and feet
- skin including ears, feet, hooves, nails, and horns
- nervous system

### Vital signs

The vital signs include the body temperature, peripheral circulation and hydration, and respirations. The respirations are evaluated in the particular distant examination.

**Body temperature**

Taking the temperature with a rectal thermometer is the accepted method of determining core temperature. Traditional clinical thermometers contain a column of mercury and have interval gradations in both Celsius and Fahrenheit, usually from the lowest level of 35 °C to a high of 43 °C. Most mercury thermometers will record the maximum temperature when placed in the rectum for up to 1 minute, but it is commonly recommended that up to 2 minutes be allowed. In a maximum thermometer the mercury column will remain at the maximum reading until the thermometer is 'shaken down' to return the mercury column to its lowest minimum level. This is achieved by a wrist-flicking action with the thermometer held between the thumb and first two fingers.

Electronic and digital thermometers are now available which provide the maximum temperature within seconds, some having a red light or other device, such as a beeping sound, to indicate when the maximum temperature has been reached. Available models include

> ### Procedure for Taking a Rectal Temperature
>
> 1. Lubricate the bulb end of the thermometer and gently insert it, with a rotary action, through the anal sphincter into the rectum. Ensure that the bulb is inserted to a relative constant depth in each species and that it makes contact with the mucous membrane of the rectum.
> 2. Leave the thermometer in situ for 2 minutes. If there is any doubt about the accuracy of the reading the temperature should be taken again.
> 3. An air-filled rectum, makes an accurate reading difficult, try to obtain a consistent reading.
> 4. Wipe the thermometer clean before storage and use on the next patient.

## Electronic Thermometers

Electronic thermometers give the animal's temperature in seconds and reduce the time required to examine large groups of animals individually. For example, the rectal temperatures of every animal arriving in a beef cattle feedlot can be determined quickly and provide an indication of early pneumonia.

## Clinical Pointer ✳

Regularly cross-check thermometer readings against standards to ensure accurate recordings.

handheld, desk-top and wall-mounted units, all with probes which are inserted rectally.

Either mercury bulb or electronic thermometers are adequate in a clinical setting. Continuous-reading thermometers will record the actual rectal temperature of the animal as it fluctuates up or down over a period of time. These are useful for continuous recording of core body temperature during prolonged surgical procedures.

All thermometers are potentially fallible: quality control is therefore necessary and must be monitored. Mercury thermometers which are left in a high ambient temperature often become non-functional. At high temperatures the bulb may break, or a gas bubble may become trapped in the mercury column. These problems are often not easily recognized and erroneous measurements are often accepted as accurate. Electronic thermometers are also prone to error and must be regularly checked against standards. Clinicians are encouraged to maintain a stock of thermometers and to frequently cross-check measured temperatures. Disposal of broken thermometers and the mercury is now an environmental and toxicological concern that must be considered by veterinarians.

Measurement of body core temperature is a common component of the clinical examination in all species. Taking the rectal temperature is usually done early in the course of the physical examination, after the distant and particular distant examination. It is part of monitoring the vital signs and is done early for two reasons.

1. Increased activity may cause spurious increases in rectal temperature.
2. Rectal examination, a common component of an extensive clinical examination will often cause a decrease in the measured rectal temperature. If a rectal examination is done prior to the measurement of rectal temperature, the vaginal temperature may be used as an acceptable proxy in female patients. If vaginal temperature measurements are used, they should be duly noted and recorded as such in the clinical record because they may be lower than rectal temperatures.

In hospitalized patients the temperature is commonly taken daily in the morning, when the animals are re-examined for their specific illnesses. In severely ill animals the temperature and other vital signs may be recorded more frequently over an extended period of time. In intensive care units the vital signs, including body temperature, may be recorded and evaluated hourly. In farm animals under veterinary care or being treated by an animal attendant for specific diseases, for example pneumonia, the temperature is often taken and recorded at least once daily to monitor the progress of the patient and the response to treatment.

In normal animals under average conditions the rectal temperature should be within the ranges in Table 6.1. These temperatures are not appropriate for use in all patients, climates, and circumstances. Rather, they should be used as guides, with empirical adjustments made for extenuating factors.

The temperature values given in Table 6.1 are applicable only when the animal is at rest, the environmental temperature and humidity moderate, and the ventilation satisfactory. As a general rule, the smaller the species the higher the normal body temperature. Female, pregnant and young animals have a higher normal temperature than male, non-pregnant and old animals. Some animals appear to possess a protective tolerance to low environmental temperatures, consisting of a mechanism that permits their body temperature to fall, thereby reducing the temperature gradient. Provided they have obtained colostrum, neonatal lambs when subjected to cold have been shown to survive low body temperatures for 48 to 72 hours, probably by readjustment of the hypothalamus. Young piglets affected with neonatal hypoglycemia characteristically have subnormal body temperatures.

## Interpreting Body Temperature

Body temperature represents a clinical finding and is not a diagnosis, it must be interpreted along with the results of other examination procedures. A body temperature fluctuation may represent a normal host response, rather than a clinical expression of disease states.

## Physiological variations of body temperature

Physiological variations in the body temperature of homeothermic animals may be due to age, sex, season of the year, time of day, environmental temperature, exercise, eating, digestion, and drinking of water. Before a rectal temperature is considered abnormal, these influences should be considered and the significance of an increased or decreased temperature interpreted accordingly.

Diurnal variations in body temperature are related to the time of day. In animals that are active during the daytime, maximum temperatures are usually found in the early afternoon and minimum temperatures early in the morning, whereas animals that are active at night have a reversed temperature rhythm. The degree of diurnal variation varies in different species. In mature cattle the rectal temperature is regularly higher in the afternoon than in the morning, with a difference of about 0.5°C.

Ambient temperatures and humidity can cause marked changes in body core temperatures. In general, healthy animals will maintain body core temperature over a broad range. At lower ambient temperatures protective mechanisms, such as increased metabolic rates and shivering, will offset heat losses to the environment. At high ambient temperatures sweating and panting will promote cooling. Despite these adaptive responses, animals will tend to have lower rectal temperatures in cold environments and at sufficiently high temperatures will begin to have increased rectal temperatures. At sufficiently high ambient temperatures, not only may their ability to dissipate heat to the environment be decreased, but under severe enough conditions they will actually begin to absorb kinetic heat from the environment. Excessive humidity will further compromise an animal's ability to prevent excessively high body temperatures. Evaporative cooling, either from the respiratory tract or in conjunction with sweating, becomes far less efficient as ambient humidity increases.

Physical activity will usually result in an increase in the rectal body temperature. This includes planned activity such as a lameness examination, and unplanned activities which the veterinarian may be unable to control. Such unplanned physical exertions included the pursuit, capture and restraint of fractious farm animals and the nervous responses of livestock or pets when placed in an unknown or threatening environment. The handling and processing of recently weaned beef calves will result in an increase in their rectal temperatures which may be erroneously interpreted as fever associated with the early stages of acute pneumonia.

Dark-colored animals will tend to have higher temperatures when exposed to bright sunlight because they absorb radiant heat more efficiently. A heavy fleece or haircoat also insulates the animal, decreasing the efficiency of heat exchange with the environment. Under most circumstances animals with heavy coats will have a higher rectal temperature than those with less hair.

In animals accustomed to a cold climate a marked increase in body temperature will often occur when they are placed in a warm environment. This is most common when livestock or outside pets are brought into heated barns, homes, or veterinary facilities during the winter months.

Subnormal temperatures are often observed immediately prepartum in cows, sows and mares.

## Abnormal variations in body core temperature

In addition to normal physiological and adaptive responses to environmental influences there are general categories of abnormal or pathological deviations from established ranges for rectal temperature. These include hyperthermia, fever, and hypothermia.

### Hyperthermia

Hyperthermia (or pyrexia) is a systemic state in which the body temperature is increased above critical for that species. The underlying mechanisms are physical factors, such as excessive heat absorption or production, or deficient heat loss. The term hyperthermia is commonly used to refer to the effects of non-inflammatory circumstances. Common causes include

- high ambient temperature
- convulsions
- exercise
- damage to the thermoregulatory center of the hypothalmus
- dehydration
- intoxication
- malignant hyperthermia.

If animals which have been acclimatized to cold outside temperatures are brought indoors to a warmer temperature their body temperatures may exceed the critical temperature within 2 to 4 hours. Many other causes of hyperthermia have been identified, including the ingestion of endophyte-infected grass pastures in otherwise healthy cattle.

## Clinical Pointer

To improve the reliability of rectal temperature measurements minimize the psychic stressors associated with handling and restraint.

Excessive heat absorption occurs during exposure to high environmental temperature. High environmental humidity and temperature and exercise will cause temperature elevation: the deviation may be as much as 1.6°C (3°F) in the case of high environmental temperatures and as much as 2.5°C (4.5°F) after severe exercise; in horses, after racing, 2 hours may be required before the temperature returns to normal.

The effect of such exposure in animals is likely to be exaggerated by

- high humidity
- muscular exertion, especially in severe exercise
- strychnine poisoning
- obesity
- a heavy haircoat or fleece
- confinement, particularly with inadequate ventilation as on board ship.

Animals in a state of dehydration are slightly more prone to hyperthermia because heat loss by evaporation of tissue fluids is correspondingly reduced. Neurogenic hyperthermia occurs occasionally as the result of damage to the hypothalamus, which could result from spontaneous hemorrhage. Other causes of hyperthermia include the porcine stress syndrome and levamisole poisoning.

In general hyperthermia is an undesirable state because the metabolic rate may be increased up to 50%, with a rapid depletion of liver glycogen stores and an increased metabolism of endogenous protein as a source of energy. The severity of the metabolic disturbance is indicated by the degree of hypoglycemia and rise in blood non-protein nitrogen that occurs. Dehydration will lead to dryness of the mouth and this, together with the respiratory embarrassment, will cause anorexia, with considerable loss of body weight.

The dry mouth causes increased thirst. The heart rate is increased directly by the rise in body temperature and indirectly by the fall in blood pressure induced by the peripheral vasodilatation. Polypnea is due directly to the effect of high temperature on the respiratory center.

*Fever*

Fever or pyrexia, or being in the febrile state, refers to those hyperthermic states caused by systemic manifestations of toxemia or mediators of inflammation. Septic fevers are most common, and are caused by inflammation due to infections such as bacterial, viral, protozoal or fungal disease. The inflammatory process may be localized in the form of an abscess, or an

> **Clinical Signs of Hyperthermia**
>
> Clinical signs of hyperthermia, detectable when the recorded rectal temperature is above 39.5°C, consist of
>
> - an increase in heart and respiratory rates, with a large-amplitude soft pulse
> - salivation
> - initial sweating which is absent later
> - restlessness which is quickly replaced by dullness, stumbling gait and recumbency.
>
> In most species, when the rectal temperature reaches 41°C (106°F) dyspnea and general distress are evident, with collapse, convulsions, and coma. Death is likely if the temperature rises as high as 41.5 to 42.5°C.

empyema involving a body cavity, or it may occur in a generalized form, as in bacteremia or septicemia. Aseptic fevers may occur in diseases associated with immune mechanisms, including allergy and anaphylaxis, angioneurotic edema, and isoerythrolysis, and when there is severe and extensive tissue damage or necrosis, as in severe hemoglobinemia associated with intravascular hemolysis, extensive infarction, or diffuse neoplasia.

The recognition of a fever should not necessarily prompt the automatic use of antimicrobials. Rather, the clinican should perform detailed examinations that will serve to localize the disease process and permit a more accurate diagnosis. A fever of undetermined origin is one in which the cause cannot be determined, often even with extensive laboratory testing.

Although a fever usually indicates the presence of inflammation, the absence of fever in an animal with evidence of clinical disease does not preclude the presence of inflammation. The body temperature may be persistently normal in animals with clinical evidence of an inflammatory lesion such as chronic pneumonia. In such cases there is usually laboratory evidence of inflammation, such as a change in the leukogram and a hyperfibrinogenemia and hypergammaglobulinemia.

A fever is commonly accompanied by

- shivering in the early stages
- tachycardia and polypnea
- varying degrees of depression and anorexia
- decreased milk production in lactating animals
- irregular body surface temperature
- decreased intestinal motility
- decreased urinary output.

> ### Levels of Fever
>
> In a fever the body temperature is elevated above normal:
>
> mild fever 1°C (2°F).
> moderate fever 1.7 to 2.2°C (3 to 4°F)
> severe fever 2.8 to 3.3°C (5 to 6°F)

*Hypothermia*

Hypothermia is a reduction of rectal body temperature below the normal range for that species. Exposure to environmental conditions that promote heat loss (cold, wet and windy) will result in a decreased body core temperature unless losses are minimized by protective responses or offset by increased metabolic activity. The physiological responses and clinical manifestations of hypothermia include increased blood viscosity, shivering, hypotension, cardiac arrhythmias, hypoxemia and acidosis. Shivering may persist for a long time, depleting the skeletal muscle and liver glycogen reserves and causing a fall in the glycogen content of cardiac muscle. Concomitant with the fall in body temperature there is gradual slowing of the heart rate and a hemoconcentration as the result of fluid shift from the blood to the tissues. The lethal low body temperature level varies between species and among individuals of the same species. In both humans and dogs, cardiac arrest followed by respiratory depression and death may occur at a rectal temperature of approximately 25°C. Considerably lower levels of rectal temperature have, however, been observed in surviving humans and animals.

Circumstances that reduce the protective responses of animals to cold environments include

- shearing, clipping or grooming
- inanition
- inadequate dietary carbohydrates and lipids
- general anesthesia
- hypocalcemia in cattle
- anemia
- dehydration
- hypoproteinemia
- administration of vasodilating agents.

Neonates are especially suceptible to hypothermia, particularly if ingestion of colostrum and/or milk is delayed. Newborn piglets are particularly sensitive to hypothermia and will typically die of fatal hypoglycemia if inanition persists longer than 24 hours.

Neonatal puppies and kittens have lower body temperatures than adults. Healthy kittens will often have body core temperatures as low as 37.5°C in the first 3

weeks of life, and temperature will increase progressively until the 7th week (mean 38.5°C). In puppies rectal temperature increases from 34°C on the first day of life to 37.5°C on day 10. The existence of physiological or normal hypothermia should not be misconstrued to mean that hypothermia in general is benign. Bitches and queens may cull hypothermic neonates, restricting their maternal efforts to warmer ones, and puppies that die in the neonatal period have consistent and significantly lower core temperatures than those that survive. Calves and foals appear to resist the negative effect of inanition to a greater extent than neonatal swine or companion animals, however, they are not immune to fatal hypothermia.

> ### Clinical Pointer
>
> In severely ill patients an abrupt and dramatic fall in body temperature may occur immediately before death: this should be considered a grave prognostic indicator.

*Peripheral circulation and hydration*

The peripheral circulation and state of hydration are determined by inspection and palpation of the skin and the visible mucosae and examination of the arterial pulse and the state of the peripheral veins.

**Inspection and palpation of skin and appendages**

The temperature of the skin is best assessed by palpation. The palmar surface of the hand is applied to the ears, horns in cattle if present, neck, trunk, and extremities of the fore- and hindlimbs. Feeling the temperature of the skin of various parts of the body, especially the ears, limbs, feet, tail, and over the thorax and abdomen, provides an indication of normal warmth, increased warmth, or coolness. Skin temperature is partly dependent upon the degree of dilatation of the cutaneous capillaries, but physical activity, the environmental temperature and the functional activity of the heat-regulating areas in the hypothalamus all have a much more significant effect by influencing the internal temperature.

In shock, the temperature of the skin will be reduced and it may be cool and clammy. In white-skinned animals such as pigs with iron-deficiency anemia, changes in skin color are readily obvious. Cyanosis and deep purple blotching of the skin over the ears and abdomen may occur and are associated with vascular lesions of the skin caused by septicemias. In the early stages of local gangrene the skin will appear blue and cool and lack elasticity. Cold injury or frostbite of the ears in cats and calves or the distal extremities in newborn animals occurs when these animals are exposed to cold outdoor temperatures during the winter months in temperate climates. In newborn animals the feet of the hindlimbs are most commonly affected. The skin just above the coronary bands of the feet is usually swollen, painful and cool to touch initially. If the animal is brought indoors and the feet gradually warmed the affected skin will become moist. Dry gangrene may follow, with ultimate sloughing of the affected tissues, including the claws.

Irregular variation of skin temperature occurs in febrile states, and in most severe illnesses affecting the cardiovascular system. The extremities of the body (ears, feet, horns, tail, vulva) are either cooler or warmer than normal. A generalized rise in skin temperature occurs during exertion, after unaccustomed exposure to sunlight (heatstroke in pigs), or high environmental temperatures, and in the fastigium stage of fever. The temperature over the whole body surface is usually lowered, and shortly before death the skin feels cool and clammy. This also occurs in states of extreme emaciation, and following severe hemorrhage and other forms of shock. A local rise in skin temperature occurs adjacent to areas of localized inflammation of the skin and subcutaneous tissues. A local fall occurs where there is local ischemia, as in frostbite of the extremities of calves and in ergot toxicity. Interference with the arterial blood supply due to thrombus or embolus in the related artery (such as in iliac thrombosis) will also result in decreased temperature of the skin of the affected part.

### State of hydration

The state of hydration and degree of dehydration are evaluated by inspection and palpation of the skin, and examination of the eyes for the degree of enophthalmos or sunken eye. The depth of the recession of the eyeball can be measured with a plastic ruler in millimeters. Normal skin is elastic and when picked up or 'tented' with the fingers it returns to its previous position when released.

### Visible mucous membranes

These include the mucosae of the conjunctivae, nasal and oral cavities, vulva, and the prepuce. They represent the arteriolar–capillary–venous circulation, and along with the circulatory and hydration state of the skin represent the important parts of the peripheral circulation which are easily examined. Monitoring the color and capillary refill time of the oral mucous membranes is a useful aid in the diagnosis and prognosis of animals with hypovolemic and endotoxemic shock. The mucous membranes of the oral cavity can be examined along with the state of hydration, or later in the examination of the various parts of the oral cavity.

### Arterial pulse

This is taken at the middle coccygeal or facial arteries in cattle, the facial artery in the horse, and the femoral artery in sheep, goats, dogs, and cats. With careful palpation the rate, amplitude and rhythm of the pulse are determined.

#### Rate

The pulse rate is dependent on the heart alone and is not directly affected by changes in the peripheral vascular system. It may or may not represent the heart rate; in cases with a pulse deficit, where some heartbeats do not produce a pulse wave, the rates will differ. Normal resting pulse and heart rates in beats per minute (bpm) for the various species are given in Table 6.1.

Although there are significant differences in rate between breeds of dairy cows, and between high- and low-producing cows, the differences are not noticeable during a routine examination. In newborn thoroughbred foals the pulse rate is

- 30–90 bpm in the first 5 minutes
- 60–200 bpm up to the first hour
- 70–130 bpm up to the first 48 hours after birth.

The pulse is not readily palpable in the pig but the comparable heart rate is 60–100 bpm.

### Amplitude

Pulse amplitude is determined by the amount of digital pressure required to obliterate the pulse wave. It is a measure of the difference between diastolic and systolic blood pressures and may be considerably increased, as in the 'waterhammer' pulse of aortic semilunar valve incompetence, or decreased as in most cases of myocardial weakness and shock.

### Rhythm

The rhythm may be regular or irregular. All irregularities must be considered abnormal except sinus arrhythmia, the phasic irregularity coinciding with the respiratory cycle. There are two components of the rhythm, namely the time between peaks of pulse waves, and the amplitude of the waves. These are usually both irregular at the one time, variations in diastolic filling of the heart causing variation in the subsequent stroke volume. Regular irregularities occur with constant periodicity and are usually associated with partial heart block. Irregular irregularities are due to ventricular extrasystoles or atrial fibrillation. Most of these, except that due to atrial fibrillation, disappear with exercise. Their significance lies chiefly in indicating the presence of myocardial disease. Although premature ventricular contractions (PVCs) induced by trauma, acid–base or electrolyte disturbance usually resolve with management of the predisposing causes, they may persist in dogs with severe underlying heart disease such as dilated cardiomyopathy.

### Peripheral veins

The state of the large superficial veins is examined by inspection and palpation. The jugular veins may be engorged in right-side congestive heart failure, or collapsed and difficult to raise by digital pressure in shock. A jugular pulse is normal in all species. Abnormal jugular pulses are prominent and usually related to valvular disease.

## Examination of body regions

After the vital signs, peripheral circulation, and state of hydration have been determined, the various body systems are examined. The thorax and abdomen are examined before other body systems so that any changes in the heart rate due to handling and excite-

ment may be minimized. However, in some situations it may be desirable or necessary to examine a particular body system or region before the thorax and abdomen. The order of the examination will vary depending on

- the experience of the clinician
- the prevalence of certain diseases in the area
- the state of the animal from a distance
- the species and the historical findings.

The sequence outlined here can be modified to meet most circumstances.

### Thorax

Close physical examination of both sides of the thorax is done primarily by auscultation of the heart and lungs. Palpation of the thoracic wall and acoustic percussion of the cardiac area and the lungs may also be indicated. The wide variations between species in the thickness of the thoracic wall, the size of the animal and the respiratory rate require careful and methodical examination. For example, in the adult horse the thick thoracic wall and the normally slow breathing rate contribute to an almost soundless respiration on auscultation of the thorax.

### Heart auscultation

Auscultation is performed to determine the heart rate, the character of normal heart sounds and the presence of abnormal sounds. Optimum auscultation sites are the fourth and fifth intercostal spaces, and because of the thick shoulder muscles that topographically cover the cranial border of the heart, the use of a flat stethoscope chest piece pushed under the triceps muscles is necessary. Areas where the various sounds are heard with maximum intensity are not directly over the anatomical sites of the cardiac orifices because conduction of the sound through the blood in the chamber gives optimum auscultation at the point where the fluid is closest to the thoracic wall.

---

### Clinical Pointer

Manual extension of the forelimbs can facilitate auscultation of the heart..

---

### Heart sounds

1. The first (systolic) sound is heard best over the cardiac apex, the tricuspid closure being most audible over the right apex, and mitral closure over the left apex.

2. The second (diastolic) sound is heard best over the base of the heart, the aortic semilunar closure caudally and the pulmonary semilunar cranially, both on the left side. The variables to be noted are

- rate
- intensity
- rhythm
- presence of abnormal sounds.

Comparison of the heart and pulse rates will determine whether there is a pulse deficit due to weak heart contractions failing to cause palpable pulse waves: this is most likely to occur in arrhythmic states.

*Heart rate*
The normal ranges of heart rates for the different species according to age, and in some cases breed, are given in Table 6.1.

- Tachycardia, or a marked increase in the heart rate, is common and occurs in septicemia, toxemia, circulatory failure, pain and excitement. Counting should be done for at least 30 seconds. Large-breed dogs with dilated cardiomyopathy may have supraventricular tachycardia or atrial fibrillation. Cats with hypertrophic cardiomyopathy due to hyperthyroidism often present with sinus tachycardia.
- Bradycardia, or marked slowing of the heartbeat, is unusual unless there is partial or complete heart block, but does occur in cases of space-occupying lesions of the brain; in respiratory and gastrointestinal diseases of the dog and cat, where vagal tone may be high; in cases of vagus indigestion in cattle; or when the rumen is much emptier than normal. In small animals drug history is important, as phenothiazine tranquilizers, digoxin, β-blockers, calcium channel blockers and lidocaine are all capable of causing sinus bradycardia.

*Intensity*
The absolute or relative intensity of the heart sounds may vary. The absolute intensity may be increased in excitement states, as in hypomagnesemia of cattle. The heart sounds are usually muffled when the pericardial sac is distended with fluid. The relative intensity may be increased in states of increased outflow, as in pulmonary hypertension (cor pulmonale), where the second heart sound is much louder than the first.

*Rhythm*
Normally the rhythm of the heartbeat is in three-time and described as LUBB-DUPP-pause, the first sound being dull, deep, long, and loud, and the second sharper and shorter. As the heart rate increases the cycle becomes shortened, mainly at the expense of diastole, and the rhythm assumes a two-time quality.

More than two sounds per cycle is classified as a 'gallop' rhythm, and may be due to reduplication of either the first or the second sounds. Gallop ryhthms due to the presence of $S_3$ (early ventricular filling) or $S_4$ (atrial systole) heart sounds are abnormal in small animals and warrant further investigation of myocardial function. Reduplication of the first sound is common in normal cattle, and its significance in other species is explained in Chapter 14.

*Abnormal heart sounds*
These are sounds which either replace one or both of the normal sounds or accompany them. Abnormal sounds related to events in the cardiac cycle are **heart murmurs**, caused mainly by

- endocardial lesions such as valvular vegetations or adhesions
- insufficiency of valve closure
- abnormal orifices such as a patent interventricular septum or ductus arteriosus.

Abnormal sounds not related to the cardiac cycle include **pericardial friction sounds**, which occur with each heart cycle but are not specifically related to either systolic or diastolic sounds. They sound superficial, are heard more distinctly than murmurs and have a to-and-fro character.

*Palpation of the heartbeat*
The size of the cardiac impulse can be evaluated, and detection of palpable thrills may on occasion be of more value than auscultation of murmurs. Palpation is most easily done with the palm of the hand and on both sides. In dogs and cats both sides of the thorax can be palpated at the same time. The point of maximum intensity, i.e. the point where the heartbeat can be palpated best, is generally at the 5th intercostal space on the left side. An increased cardiac impulse, or the movements of the heart against the thoracic wall during systole, may be easily seen on close inspection of the left precordium and can be felt on both sides. It may be due to cardiac hypertrophy or

---

**Clinical Pointer**

Take care to distinguish local pleuritic friction sounds from pericardial friction sounds, especially if respiratory and cardiac rates are equal.

dilatation associated with cardiac insufficiency or anemia, or to distension of the pericardial sac with edema or inflammatory fluid. Care should be taken not to confuse a readily palpable cardiac impulse due to cardiac enlargement with one due to contraction of lung tissue and increased exposure of the heart to the chest wall. Normally the heart movements can be felt as distinct systolic and diastolic thumps. These are replaced by 'thrills' when valvular insufficiencies or stenoses or congenital defects are present. When the defects are large the murmur may not be very loud but the thrill is readily palpable. Early pericarditis may also produce a friction thrill.

Acoustic percussion to determine the boundaries of the heart is of little value in large animal practice and is not routine in small animals. The area of cardiac dullness is increased in cardiac hypertrophy and dilatation, and decreased when the heart is covered by more than the usual amount of lung, as in pulmonary emphysema.

**Lungs**

The lungs are examined by auscultation, acoustic percussion of the thorax, and palpation of the thoracic wall.

*Auscultation*

The normal breath sounds are heard over most of the lungs, particularly in the middle third cranially over the base of the lung. The sounds are heard with variable ease, depending on the thickness of the thoracic wall and the amplitude of the respiratory excursion. In well-muscled horses and fat beef cattle the sounds may

be only barely audible at rest. The amplitude, or loudness, of the breath sounds is increased in dyspnea and in early pulmonary congestion and inflammation. It is decreased or totally inaudible when there is pleural effusion, and with space-occupying lesions in the lung or pleural cavity. Abnormal lung sounds include crackles, wheezes and pleuritic friction sounds.

To auscultate the lungs of a dog, it is often necessary to calm the animal and stop it panting. Auscultation should always be done in a quiet room. It may help to have the owner petting the dog's head or holding its muzzle. To force a deep inspiration, the muzzle is held closed with one hand and both nostrils are blocked with the other. The nostrils are then released and the lungs auscultated. In cats purring can interfere with ausculation. Many cats will stop purring if they hear running water (turn a tap on) or if they are annoyed by tapping or blowing on their nose.

Sounds of peristalsis are normally heard over the lung area in cattle and in horses. In cattle these sounds are due to forestomach contractions, and in horses to colonic motility. Their presence is of little significance in these species unless there are other signs. In cattle the sounds of swallowing, eructation, and regurgitation may be confused with peristaltic sounds: to identify these, ruminal movements and the esophagus should be observed simultaneously for the passage of gas or a bolus.

*Acoustic percussion of the thorax*

This is done to detect areas of increased dullness or resonance, especially related to the lungs and pleural cavity. Increased dullness may indicate the presence of

- a space-occupying mass
- a consolidated lung
- an accumulation of fluid in the ventral half of the pleural cavity.

In a pleural effusion the upper limit of the area of dullness can be determined by percussion, and the fluid line can be delineated and used to assess the progress of therapy.

*Palpation of thoracic wall*

Palpation of the thoracic wall may reveal the presence of pleural pain (pleurodynia), a pleuritic thrill associated with pleuritis, bulging of the intercostal spaces when fluid is present in the pleural cavity, or narrowed intercostal spaces and decreased rib movement over areas of collapsed lung.

**Abdomen and gastrointestinal tract**

The contour of the abdomen is noted during the particular distant examination, and any marked changes

## Clinical Pointer

1. Tissue containing more air than normal creates an overloud normal percussion note, e.g. an emphysematous lung.
2. Pneumothorax or a gas-filled viscus penetrating through a diaphragmatic hernia elicits a tympanitic note.

are considered in the close examination. Close examination of the abdomen and gastrointestinal tract is done by palpation, auscultation of gastrointestinal sounds, simultaneous percussion and auscultation, tactile percussion, rectal examination, passage of a nasogastric tube, and abdominocentesis. The techniques used depend on the species being examined and the diagnostic hypotheses. Examination of the abdomen of cattle and horses depends much more on auscultation and percussion than it does in small animals. Rectal examination of cattle and horses is also an important part of the examination of the digestive tract and abdomen compared to small animals. Passage of a nasogastric tube and abdominocentesis are important in large animals, but not part of the routine examination of the abdomen in dogs and cats. Special examinations of the abdomen include

- gastroscopy
- laparoscopy
- ultrasonography
- radiography.

### Auscultation

This is an essential part of the clinical examination of cattle, horses, and sheep. The characteristics of the gastrointestinal sounds and their frequency and amplitude can be valuable aids in clinical diagnosis. The intensity, duration and frequency of the sounds are noted and interpreted. The intensity and frequency will be increased following eating and excitement.

*Cattle and sheep* Auscultation of the rumen of cattle and sheep in the left paralumbar fossa is a necessary part of any clinical examination. Primary cycle reticulorumen contractions occur at the rate of 1–2 per minute, and involve the reticulum and the dorsal and ventral sacs of the rumen, depending on the amount of time elapsed since feeding and the type of feed consumed. Secondary cycle contractions of the dorsal and ventral sacs of the rumen occur about 1 per minute and are commonly associated with eructation. Along with the sounds of the contractions there are move-

ments of the abdominal wall, which reflect the contractions of the rumen sacs.

The intestinal sounds audible on auscultation over the right middle to lower abdomen of cattle and sheep consist of frequent faint gurgling sounds which are difficult to interpret. The contraction of the abomasum and the intestines results in a mixture of sounds which are difficult to distinguish.

*Horse* The intestinal sounds of the horse are clearly audible and their evaluation is one of the most vital parts of the clinical examination and surveillance of horses with suspected abdominal disease. For auscultation purposes the abdomen of the horse is divided into four quadrants: ventral and dorsal left abdomen, and ventral and dorsal right abdomen. Over the right abdomen, loud booming sounds (borborygmi) of the colon and cecum are audible at peak intensity about every 15–20 seconds. Over the left abdomen there are the much fainter, rushing gurgling peristaltic sounds.

*Dog and cat* Auscultation of the abdomen is of limited value in the dog and cat.

### Palpation of the abdomen

Because of the thickness and weight of the abdominal wall in mature cattle and horses, palpation of the abdomen to evaluate the viscera and organs has limited value compared to its usefulness in the dog and cat.

*Dog and cat* Palpation of the abdomen in the dog and cat is relatively easy and informative. It is possible to feel several intra-abdominal organs, including parts of

### Changes in Abdominal Sounds in the Horse

1. Enteritis causes an increase in the intensity and frequency of sounds, with a distinct fluid quality.
2. Spasmodic colic has loud, almost crackling, sounds.
3. Impaction of the large intestine is indicated by a decrease in the intensity and frequency of the borborygmi.
4. In thromboembolic colic due to verminous aneurysm and infarction of the colon there may be a complete absence of sounds.
5. Intestinal obstruction decreases the peristaltic sounds markedly, they may be absent and replaced by fluid tinkling sounds.

the small and large intestine, kidneys, and bladder. In the cat the kidneys are easily palpable. Although the stomach, liver, and uterus are generally not palpable they may be if they are enlarged or displaced from their normal position.

*Horse* In the horse no viscera or organ can be felt by palpation, with the exception of the gravid uterus and fetal prominences in advanced pregnancy.

*Cattle* In cattle the rumen and its contents (rumen pack) can be palpated in the left paralumbar fossa. Ruminal distension is usually obvious, whereas an inability to palpate the rumen may be due to a small or relatively empty rumen or to medial displacement, as in left-side displacement of the abomasum. In cattle in advanced pregnancy the fetal prominences are palpable over the right lower abdomen. A markedly enlarged liver in cattle may be palpable by deep palpation immediately caudal to the middle third of the right costal arch.

*Sheep* In sheep the normal rumen, an impacted abomasum and a gravid uterus are usually palpable through the abdominal wall.

*Pig* The abdomen of pigs is difficult to examine by palpation because they are seldom sufficiently quiet or relaxed, and the thickness of the abdominal wall limits the extent of deep palpation. In late pregnancy the gravid uterus may be balloted, but it is usually not possible to palpate fetal prominences.

### Simultaneous percussion and auscultation

Simultaneous percussion and auscultation of the abdomen can elicit the presence of gas-filled viscera near the abdominal wall.

In left-side displacement of the abomasum, percussion and simultaneous auscultation over the upper third of the costal arch between the 9th and 12th ribs of the left side will elicit the typical high-pitched musical sound or 'ping'. A lower-pitched ping, or 'pung', may be present in ruminal atony. Using a combination of palpation, percussion and simultaneous auscultation over the right paralumbar fossa and caudal to the entire length of the right costal arch, it may be possible to detect any of the following in cattle:

- right-side dilatation and displacement and/or volvulus of the abomasum
- cecal dilatation and torsion
- intestinal obstructions, including torsion of the coiled colon, all of which also are associated with 'pings' due to fluid- and gas-filled viscera.

> **Clinical Pointer**
>
> The viscera can be palpated more easily by positioning the sheep on its hindquarters.

The ease of hearing the ping depends on the proximity of the gas-filled viscus to the abdominal wall, the size of the distended viscus, and the amount of force used in percussion. A percussion hammer provides a sufficient and consistent level of percussion to elicit pings; slight tapping with the fingertips may be insufficient.

### Ballottement and simultaneous auscultation

This technique consists of pushing the clenched hand into the abdominal wall while auscultating with the stethoscope in the immediate area. Fluid-splashing sounds are commonly audible if the intestines or a hollow viscus such as the abomasum is filled with fluid.

### Tactile percussion

This aids in the detection of an excessive quantity of fluid in the peritoneal cavity, such as in ascites, urine due to a ruptured bladder, transudate in congestive heart failure and exudate in diffuse peritonitis. A sharp blow is struck with the open hand on one side of the abdomen and a fluid wave, a 'blip' or undulation of the abdominal wall, can be seen and felt on the opposite side. The peritoneal cavity must be about one-third full of fluid before a fluid wave can be elicited.

### Detection of abdominal pain

In cattle, the site of abdominal pain may be located by deep palpation of the abdominal wall. Deep palpation with a firm uniform lift of the closed hand, or with the aid of a horizontal bar held by two people under the animal immediately caudal to the xiphoid sternum, is a useful aid for the detection of a grunt associated with traumatic reticuloperitonitis. In cattle or horses superficial pain may be elicited by a firm poke of the hand or extended finger. In cattle and horses, pain may be elicited over the right costal arch when there are liver lesions, or generally over the abdomen in diffuse peritonitis.

The response to palpation of a focus of abdominal pain in cattle is a grunt, which may be clearly audible without a stethoscope. If it is not, simultaneous auscultation of the trachea will detect a perceptible grunt when the painful location is palpated. In calves with abomasal ulceration a focus of abdominal pain may be present on deep palpation over the area.

In dogs and cats with abdominal pain even gentle palpation will evoke muscle tensing and arching of the back. The animal may cry or whine, or turn and attempt to bite the examiner.

In severe abdominal distension (ruminal tympany in cattle, torsion of the large intestine) it is usually impossible to determine by palpation and percussion only which are the distended viscera. Pneumoperitoneum is rare, and thus gross distension of the abdomen is usually due to distension of viscera with gas, fluid, or ingesta.

## Nasogastric intubation

An important part of the examination of the abdomen and gastrointestinal tract of large animals, especially cattle and horses, is the passage of a nasogastric tube, into the rumen of cattle and into the stomach of horses. Gastric reflux is common in the horse with colic and it is important to determine whether the stomach is distended with fluid, and to relieve it as necessary. In cattle, when disease of the rumen is suspected the nasogastric tube is passed into the rumen to relieve any distension and to obtain a sample of rumen juice for determination of pH and the presence or absence of live protozoa.

## Rectal examination

Rectal examination is a vital part of the complete examination of the abdomen of large animals, especially cattle and horses, and in small animals with evidence of gastrointestinal disease. It is also recommended when examining intact male dogs over 4 years of age to assess the size of the prostate gland. Sedation is usually required to perform a rectal examination in cats. In all species unexpected abnormalities may be found on rectal examination which may be the cause of illness when no other significant clinical abnormalities have been found. Special care is necessary to avoid injuring the patient and causing it to strain.

Rectal examination enables evaluation of the normal and abnormal palpable parts of the alimentary tract,

---

**The Use of Nasogastric Tubes in Small Animals**

The passage of a nasogastric tube is not indicated as part of the examination in small animals, except for

- dogs with a history of ingestion of toxic substances that require gastric lavage
- dogs with gastric dilatation, in which relief of gaseous distension is indicated
- anorexic cats needing supplemental nutrition.

---

urinary and genital tracts, large blood vessels, lymph nodes, peritoneum and pelvic structures. The amount and nature of the feces in the rectum is always noted. Important abnormalities of the gastrointestinal tract are

- distension of viscera
- displacement or absence of viscera
- presence of tight mesenteric bands.

---

**Clinical Pointer**

To avoid injury to the patient during a rectal examination

- restrain and control the patient
- use ample lubrication
- avoid force.
- use sedation, parasympathetic drugs or local anesthetics, as necessary.

---

## Abdominocentesis

Paracentesis of the abdomen includes obtaining a sample of peritoneal fluid when peritonitis or inflammation of the serosae of the intestines or other viscera of the abdomen is suspected. Aspiration of fluid from a distended abdominal viscus is also possible and may aid in the diagnosis.

**Head and neck**
The head and neck may be examined in detail after the other body systems in order to minimize the effects of handling and excitement on the vital signs. However, if the history suggests a primary abnormality of the head and neck regions these may be examined after determining the vital signs.

*Eyes*
The eyes are examined using a light source to illuminate the eyes, eyelids, and the pupillary light reflexes. Both eyes are examined and compared.

---

**Severe Abdominal Distension**

To determine the cause of severe abdominal distension it may be necessary to use a combination of

- rectal examination
- passage of a stomach tube
- abdominocentesis
- exploratory laparotomy.

---

*Eyesight and blindness* Tests for eyesight include the menace reflex and an obstacle test. In the menace reflex a threatening blow at the eye is simulated with the extended fingers, care being taken not to cause air currents. The objective is to elicit reflex closure of the eyelids. This does not occur in peripheral or central blindness, and in facial nerve paralysis there may be withdrawal of the head but no eyelid closure. An obstacle test allows the animal to walk in unfamiliar surroundings and its ability to avoid makeshift obstacles is assessed. The results are often difficult to interpret if the animal is excited. A similar test for night blindness (nyctalopia) is arranged in subdued light, either at dusk or on a moonlit night. Nyctalopia is one of the earliest indications of avitaminosis A. Total central blindness is amaurosis; partial central blindness is amblyopia.

*Ocular discharges* Ocular discharges are usually readily evident: they may be

- watery in obstruction of the lacrimal duct
- serous in the early stages of inflammation, and
- purulent in the later stages.

A unilateral discharge may be due to local inflammation; a bilateral discharge suggests a systemic disease.

*Eyelids* Abnormalities of the eyelids include abnormal movement, position, and thickness. The size of the palpebral fissure or opening is noted. Movement may be excessive in painful eye conditions or in cases of nervous irritability, including hypomagnesemia, lead poisoning, and encephalitis. The eyelids may be kept permanently closed when there is pain in the eye, or when the eyelids are swollen, as in local edema due to photosensitization or allergy. The third eyelid, or membrana nictitans, may be located across the eye or prolapsed, due to pain in the orbit, dehydration states, tetanus, and encephalitis, and in cats may occur with a variety of systemic illnesses. Prolapse of the third eyelid also occurs as part of Horner's syndrome especially in small animals. Tumors may also be present on the eyelids.

*Conjunctiva and sclera* Examination of the conjunctiva provides a good indication of the state of the periph-

eral circulation. The upper eyelid is everted with the aid of the index finger and simultaneous compression of the eye with the thumb. Congestion of the conjunctiva is common in endotoxic shock, and pallor in anemia. In jaundice the sclera is yellow. Engorgement of the scleral vessels, petechial hemorrhages, edema of the conjunctiva, as in gut edema of pigs or congestive heart failure, and dryness due to dehydration and fever, are all readily observable.

*Cornea* Responses to corneal injury include edema, vascularization, scar formation, pigmentation, cellular infiltration, and accumulation of abnormal material within the cornea, all of which appear as opacity. Advanced inflammation of the cornea or keratitis is often associated with vascularization, ulceration, and scarring. Increased convexity of the cornea is usually due to increased pressure within the eyeball, and may be due to glaucoma or hypopyon.

*Size* The size of the eye does not usually vary except in congenital microphthalmia, when it is smaller than normal. Exophthalmos (protrusion of the eye) occurs and, when unilateral, is in most cases due to pressure from behind the orbit or following traumatic injury. Periorbital lymphoma in cattle, retrobulbar abscesses or tumors in small animals, dislocation of the mandible, and periorbital hemorrhage are common causes. A decrease in the size or retraction of the eye (sunken eyes or enophthalmos) is a common manifestation of dehydration and the loss of periorbital fat in starvation.

*Abnormal eye positions and movements*
1. Nystagmus is due to hypoxia or lesions of the cerebellum or vestibular tracts and is characterized by periodic involuntary eye movements, with a slow component in one direction and a quick return to the original position. The movement may be horizontal, vertical or rotatory. In paralysis of the motor nerves to the orbital muscles there is restriction of movement and abnormal position of the eyeball at rest.
2. Strabismus is deviation of the eye which the animal cannot overcome. Dorsal rotational strabismus occurs commonly in polioencephalomalacia and with other cerebral diseases in ruminants. Convergent strabismus, in which the visual axes converge (cross-eye) is a normal finding in Siamese cats.

*Pupils* The pupils are examined with the aid of a strong light source such as a penlight or ophthalmoscopic illuminator. Pupil size and shape varies between species. Under normal conditions shining a light into

---

### Conditions of the Eyelid

- ectropion – eversion of the eyelid
- entropion – inversion of the eyelid
- ptosis – drooping of the upper eyelid.

one pupil causes constriction of that pupil (direct) and constriction of the opposite pupil (consensual).

Mydriasis, or bilateral excessive dilatation of the pupils, occurs

- with local lesions of the central nervous system affecting the oculomotor nucleus
- in diffuse lesions including encephalopathies
- in functional disorders such as botulism and anoxia.

Peripheral blindness due to bilateral lesions of the orbits may have a similar effect.

Excessive constriction of the pupils (miosis) is unusual in large animals unless there has been overdose with organic phosphate insecticides or parasympathomimetic drugs. Miosis is commonly seen with uveitis. It is also a feature of Horner's syndrome but may be seen also with any unilateral ocular disorder that causes pain, such as corneal ulcers and keratitis.

*Deep structures of the eye* The deep structures of the eye are examined with an ophthalmoscope, but gross abnormalities may be observed by direct vision. Pus in the anterior chamber – hypopyon – appears as a yellow to white opacity, often with a horizontal upper border obscuring the iris. The pupil may be abnormal in shape or position, as a result of adhesions to the cornea or other structures. An abnormal degree of dilatation is an important sign, unilateral abnormality usually suggesting a lesion of the orbit such as glaucoma. Opacity of the lens is readily visible, especially in advanced cases.

*Nostrils (external nares)*
The nostrils or external nares are examined by direct inspection and preferably with a source of light. In cattle, the first part of the mucosa of the nasal cavities can be viewed directly with the aid of a flashlight. In the horse the alar fold must be retracted in order to view the nasal mucosa. Normally, a small amount of serous fluid occurs in the external nares.

*Nasal discharge*
A nasal discharge is an abnormal amount of nasal secretions present in the external nares that commonly accumulates over the muzzle. Nasal discharges may be restricted to one nostril in a local infection, or be bilateral in systemic infection. In the early stages of inflammation it will be a clear, colorless fluid, which later turns white-yellow as leukocytes accumulate in it. A rust or prune-juice color indicates blood originating from the lower respiratory tract, as in pneumonia and in equine infectious anemia in the horse.

In all species vomiting or regurgitation caused by pharyngitis or esophageal obstruction may be accompanied by the discharge of food material from the nose or the presence of food particles in the nostrils. In some cases the volume of nasal discharge is intermittent, often increasing when the animal is feeding from the ground, and with infection of the cranial sinuses. Erosion and ulceration of the nasal mucosa is often apparent in dogs afflicted with nasal aspergillosis.

The nasal discharge can be sampled using cotton-tipped swabs and submitted for laboratory analysis.

Epistaxis or bleeding from the nose may be caused by lesions of the nasal mucosa, hemorrhagic diseases or pulmonary hemorrhage. Blood from the upper respiratory tract or pharynx may be present in large quantities, or as small flecks only. In general

- blood from the upper respiratory tract is unevenly mixed with any discharge
- blood from the lower tract comes through as a uniform color.

The discharge may consist of bubbles or foam. Coarse bubbles suggests that the discharge originates in the pharynx or nasal cavities; fine bubbles like a foam originate in the lower respiratory tract.

*Lesions of nasal mucosa*
Inflammation of the nasal mucosa varies from simple hyperemia, as in allergic rhinitis, to diffuse necrosis, as in bovine malignant catarrh and mucosal disease, to deep ulceration as in glanders. In hemorrhagic diseases variations in mucosal color can be observed and petechial hemorrhages may be present.

*Odor of breath*
The odor of the expired breath is noted. Halitosis is an offensive odor. There may be a sweet sickly smell of acetonemia in cattle, or a fetid odor which may originate from several different sources, including gangrenous pneumonia, necrosis in the nasal cavities, or the accumulation of nasal exudate. Odors originating in the respiratory tract are usually constant with each breath and may be unilateral. The odor of eructated ruminal gas may occasionally be detected. Odors originating in the mouth from abscessed teeth or necrotic stomatitis in calves may be detectable on the nasal

---

**Clinical Pointer**

The color and consistency of a nasal discharge will often indicate its source.

breath but are stronger on the oral breath. In the dog or cat there may be the sweet smell of diabetic ketosis or the ammonical smell of renal failure originating from the nasal breath or oral cavity.

*Volume of breath*

The volume of breath from each nostril may assist in determining possible obstruction of the nasal cavities. Variation in volume between nostrils, as felt on the hands, may indicate obstruction or stenosis of one nasal cavity. This can be examined further by closing off the nostrils one at a time: if there is obstruction in one nostril, closure of the other causes some respiratory embarrassment.

*Mouth*

The external aspects of the mouth are examined by direct inspection of the lips, and the oral cavity is examined by inspection and palpation with the aid of a light source.

*Saliva*

Strings of saliva drooling from the lips, commonly accompanied by chewing movements, occur when a foreign body is present in the mouth and with inflammation of the oral mucosa, including the tongue. Actinobacillosis of the tongue, calicivirus infection of the tongue or oral mucosa in the cat, foot-and-mouth disease and mucosal disease are typical examples of diseases causing drooling of saliva from the mouth. Excessive salivation may also occur in diseases of the central nervous system, as in acute lead poisoning in young cattle, and in cats with hepatic encephalopathy.

*Oral mucosa*

Inspection of the oral mucous membranes is best done in natural daylight or with the aid of a flashlight. The lips are retracted to expose the mucosa of the gingiva, which are easiest to examine. The oral mucosa is normally pale pink.

The capillary refill time of the oral mucous membranes is a useful indicator of peripheral tissue perfusion and the state of the cardiovascular system. The gingiva over the incisor teeth is compressed with the ball of the finger to blanch the mucosa. The time required for the blanched area to return to its original color is the capillary refill time. The capillary refill time is an indicator of various conditions, for example

- the normal refill time is between 1 and 2 seconds
- in dehydrated animals the refill time increases to 2–4 seconds
- with severe dehydration it may increase to 5–6 seconds.

In the horse with surgical colic the prognosis generally worsens as the oral mucosa becomes cool, congested, cyanotic and drier, and as capillary refill time increases. A refill time of 3 seconds or more, accompanied by cyanotic oral mucosae, indicates a poor prognosis, and a refill time of 10 seconds or more indicates potentially fatal peripheral circulatory failure.

Abnormalities of the oral mucosa include

- hemorrhages in purpuric diseases
- discolorations of jaundice and cyanosis
- the pallor of anemia.

Care must be taken to clearly define the appearance of lesions in the mouth, especially in cattle, because differentiation between erosions, vesicles, and ulcerative lesions is of diagnostic significance in mucosal diseases of this species. Immune-mediated disease affecting the oral mucocutaneous junction in dogs and cats is not unusual. In particular, about 90% of dogs and cats with pemphigus vulgaris have oral lesions at the time of diagnosis, and they are present as the initial sign in

**Clinical Pointer**

Monitor the color and capillary refill time of the oral mucous membranes closely and carefully in a horse with suspected acute intestinal obstruction.

**Clinical Pointer**

When examining a cat with a history of vomiting, inappetance, or drooling, check the undersurface of the tongue for string or thread embedded at the base.

about 50% of cases. Feline immunodeficiency virus (FIV) can cause diffuse gingivitis and gingival hyperplasia in affected cats.

*Teeth*
Examination of the teeth can yield useful information. Delayed eruption and uneven wear may signify mineral deficiency, especially calcium deficiency in sheep. Excessive wear with mottling and pitting of the enamel is suggestive of chronic fluorosis. Retained deciduous teeth are not uncommon in young small animals and extraction is often indicated. Tartar accumulation and periodontal disease are common problems in small animals, and dental prophylaxis is now commonly performed. A number of veterinarians have undertaken advanced training in dentistry and offer a variety of dental procedures for dogs and cats (root canals, capping and bridging).

*Tongue*
The tongue is examined for local edema or inflammation as in actinobacillosis of cattle, or shrunken and atrophied in postinflammatory or neurogenic atrophy. Lesions of the tongue surface, such as erosions, vesicles, and ulcers, are part of the general oral mucosal response to injury. Most horses require prophylactic dentistry twice yearly.

*Pharynx*
Examination of the pharynx in large animals requires some dexterity and the use of an appropriately sized speculum. The oral cavity and pharynx of calves, lambs, and goat kids can be examined by holding the mouth open and depressing the base of the tongue with the fingers or a tongue depressor; the pharynx, the glottis, and the proximal part of the larynx and arytenoid cartilages can then be viewed. In adult cattle a metal or plexiglass cylindrical speculum, 45 cm in length and 4 cm in diameter, placed in the oral cavity and over the base of the tongue will allow viewing of the pharynx and the larynx. Foreign bodies, diffuse cellulitis, and pharyngeal lymph node enlargement can also be detected by this means. The use of a speculum wedged between the upper and lower molar teeth in cattle allows manual exploration and evaluation of lesions of the pharynx and proximal part of the larynx. Examination of the pharyngeal

region in small animals generally requires sedation or general anesthesia. In the horse the pharynx cannot be viewed from the oral cavity and manual exploration requires general anesthesia. Endoscopy is a useful method of examination in this species, and the modern fiberoptic endoscope has made it possible to visualize lesions in the caudal nares, pharynx esophagus, larynx-trachea in the standing, conscious horse and cattle.

*Submandibular region*
Abnormalities of the submandibular region may include enlargement of lymph nodes due to local foci of infection, subcutaneous edema as part of a general edema, local cellulitis with swelling and pain, enlargement of salivary glands, or guttural pouch distension in the horse. Thyroid gland enlargement may be mistaken for other abnormalities, but its site makes it characteristic.

**Neck**
An important part of the examination of the neck of cattle and horses is to determine the state of the jugular veins.

*Jugular veins*
Bilateral engorgement of the jugular veins may be due to obstruction of the veins by compression or constriction, or to right-sided congestive heart failure. A jugular pulse of small magnitude moving about one-third of the way up the neck is normal in most animals, but must be differentiated from a transmitted carotid pulse, which is not obliterated by digital compression of the jugular vein at a lower level. Variations in size of the vein may occur synchronously with deep respiratory movements but bear no relation to the cardiac cycles. When the jugular pulse is associated with each cardiac movement it should be determined whether it is physiological or pathological. The physiological pulse is presystolic and due to atrial systole and is

**Clinical Pointer**

To enhance visualization of the jugular veins clip the haircoat and/or apply water to the neck.

normal. The pathological pulse is systolic and occurs simultaneously with the arterial pulse and the first heart sound; it is characteristic of an insufficient tricuspid valve.

*Esophagus*

Local or general enlargement of the esophagus associated with vomiting or dysphagia occurs in esophageal choke, diverticulum, stenosis and paralysis, and in cardial obstructions. The passage of a stomach tube or endoscope can assist in the examination of esophageal abnormalities.

*Trachea*

The trachea is examined by palpation and auscultation. In dogs and cats the cervical trachea is easily palpated. A cough can usually be elicited by palpation of animals with narrowed or collapsing trachea or inflamed trachea. Auscultation is a useful diagnostic aid. Normally, the tracheal breath sounds are louder and more distinct than those audible over the lung. In laryngitis and tracheitis the sounds are louder and harsher and may be whistling (stridor). Loud stenotic tracheal sounds on inspiration are characteristic in calves with tracheal collapse. Abnormal tracheal sounds, regardless of their cause, are usually transferred to the major bronchi and are audible over the lungs, primarily during inspiration. They are commonly confused with abnormal lung sounds due to pneumonia, which are usually present on both inspiration and expiration.

**Urinary system**

Examination of the urinary tract consists of

- observations of the act of urination
- evidence of difficult and painful urination
- evidence of abnormal urine
- collection of urine and urinalysis, and
- depending on the species, palpation of the kidneys, bladder and urethra.

**Reproductive tract**

The reproductive tract of all domestic animals is routinely examined for evidence of abnormalities that may cause infertility, and for pregnancy. Pregnancy diagnosis is a major veterinary practice activity, especially in farm animal practice.

*Postpartum examination of large animals*

Examination of the reproductive tract in females is necessary in the immediate postpartum period. The vagina, cervix, and uterus should be examined carefully by vaginal palpation for evidence of gross abnormal-

ities, such as lacerations of the vagina and cervix, retained placenta, and ruptured uterus. The involuting uterus can also be palpated by rectal examination, but it is not as reliable for the determination of metritis, retained placenta, and other abnormalities of the cervix and uterus, which can be palpated vaginally, particularly if the cervix is open and the uterus can be examined.

*External and internal genitalia of large animals*

The external and internal genitalia of male cattle and horses are readily examined for evidence of abnormalities. The external genitalia of both female and male sheep, goats, and swine can be examined by inspection and palpation, but the internal genitalia are not accessible by routine clinical examination techniques.

*Genitalia of small animals*

In small animals (particularly dogs) the external genitalia (vestibule of the vagina in the female; prepuce, penis, and scrotum in the male) are easily examined. The cervix is not palpable on vaginal examination in the normal dog.

**Mammary glands**

*Symmetry and consistency*

The mammary gland is inspected for symmetry and consistency, and palpated for evidence of abnormalities. An asymmetrical udder may be due either to a unilateral increase or a decrease in the size of the mammary gland. Acute inflammation, edema, and abscessation will result in enlargement of the udder. However, edema will typically be a diffuse symmetrical swelling. End-stage fibrosis of the mammary gland due to chronic infection may cause atrophy of single or multiple mammary glands.

*Temperature*

Changes in the temperature of the mammary gland should be noted, particularly if restricted to a single gland or half of the udder. Inflamed glands are often warm. When gangrene is present the gland feels cool or cold, and a clear border of erythema and warmth often defines the border of necrotic and viable udder parenchyma.

*Skin of udder and teats*

The skin of the udder is examined closely by direct inspection. Several viral diseases are associated with vesicular or erosive lesions of the teats and udder.

*Gross examination of milk or secretions*

Examination of the mammary gland secretions is a component of the clinical examination of all lactating animals. After washing with soap and water if excessively soiled, the teat ends are swabbed with alcohol-soaked gauze and the teat sphincters examined both visually and by palpation. The external orifice is visually appraised for eversion of the streak canal, traumatic lesions, and verrucous growths.

Inspection of the milk or secretions is a standard component of many clinical examinations of the udder and of vital importance in lactating ruminants. The milk is first inspected grossly using a strip cup. The California Mastitis Test solution is used to evaluate the degree of inflammation in the mammary gland of cattle.

*Mammary glands of small animals*
Examination of the mammary glands of dogs and cats begins with inspecting the glands to determine their number, size, color, and the presence of any overlying skin lesions or discharges. Any milk secretion should be evaluated visually for color and consistency, and cytologically. This is followed by manual examination of each gland, associated lymph nodes, overlying skin, and surrounding tissues. Swellings or nodules are characterized in terms of size, firmness, attachment to surrounding tissues, and overlying skin, and by whether pain is elicited by palpation. It may be difficult to differentiate between swelling of normal glandular tissue and the development of neoplasia. Neoplastic growths are less often painful than inflammatory disorders, with the exception of inflammatory mammary carcinoma in the bitch.

**Musculoskeletal system and feet**
Examination of the musculoskeletal system and feet is necessary when there is lameness, weakness, or recumbency. The gait is inspected during walking and trotting to determine the origin of the lameness. The muscles, joints, ligaments, tendons, and bones are inspected and palpated to determine abnormalities. The feet are examined by inspection, palpation, and the trimming of hooves in farm animals, to identify lesions associated with lameness. Medical imaging is commonly used to define lesions not readily recognizable by routine clinical examination.

## Detection of Mammary Gland Tumors

Palpation of the mammary glands and associated lymph nodes is indicated in all general physical examinations of dogs and cats, since mammary gland tumors are often detected during routine office visits.

**Skin**
It is necessary to examine the skin systematically to avoid misinterpretation of any lesions. Inspection of the behavior of the animal and of the skin and hair, and palpation and smelling of the skin are the most common physical methods used. The important prerequisites for an adequate skin examination are good lighting, such as natural light or day-type lamps, clipping the animal's hair when necessary to visualize lesions adequately, magnification of the lesions with a hand lens to improve visualization of the changes, and adequate restraint and positioning of the animal. Palpation can be used to assess

- the consistency of lesions
- the thickness and elasticity of skin, and
- to determine the presence of pain associated with diseases of the skin.

Close inspection and palpation of the skin and haircoat are necessary to identify and characterize lesions. Magnifying spectacles or an illuminated magnifying glass may prove useful. The dorsal aspect of the body is inspected by viewing it from the rear, as elevated hairs and patchy alopecia may be more obvious from that angle. All parts of the head, including the nose, muzzle, and ears, are examined. The lateral trunk and the extremities are then examined. The feet of large animals need to be picked up to examine the interdigital clefts and parts of the coronary bands. The ventral aspect of the body is carefully examined, using a light source to illuminate the underside of adult cattle and horses.

Every centimeter of the skin needs to be examined by sight, touch and smell for the presence of lesions in different stages of development. The presence or absence of some ectoparasites can be determined by direct inspection. For example, in cattle, lice and ticks are usually easily visible. Fleas are the most common cause of skin disease in the dog and cat, and haircoat brushings should be part of every examination of the skin. In some diseases the odor of the skin may be abnormal: dermatophilosis in cattle is characterized by a foul and musty odor.

The length of the hairs and broken hairs, changes in color and the accumulation of exudative material on hair shafts are noted. The texture and elasticity of the skin must be assessed by rolling it between the fingers. Careful digital palpation of the haircoat, which may appear normal on visual inspection, may reveal underlying lesions such as pustules. In some cases tufts of hairs may be seen protruding through an accumulation of exudate. A combination of visual inspection of the wool coat of sheep is done carefully and systematically by parting the wool and evaluating the condition of the fibers and the underlying skin.

Clinical manifestations of diseases of the skin include primary and secondary lesions and combinations of both.

1. A primary lesion is defined as the initial reaction that develops spontaneously as a direct reflection of underlying disease.
2. A secondary lesion evolves from a primary lesion, or is induced by the patient scratching or rubbing, or by external factors such as trauma and treatment.

Other manifestations of skin diseases include

- abnormal coloration
- pruritus or itchiness
- evidence of pain
- abnormalities of sweat and sebaceous gland secretion
- changes in elasticity, extensibility and thickness
- abnormalities of hair and wool fibers
- abnormalities of footpads, nails, hooves, coronary bands, and horns.

There are also secondary effects of diseases of the skin such as dehydration, toxemia, and loss of body weight or chronic wasting.

The important observations to make are

- the distribution pattern of the lesions
- the configuration of the lesions
- the morphological appearance of the lesions.

## Clinical Pointer

Examine the haircoat closely by parting the hairs with the fingers or by gently blowing them.

## Clinical Pointer

Do not clip, groom, or wash the haircoat before identifying the lesions.

### Nervous system

Veterinarians will commonly include some components of a neurological examination in a thorough clinical examination. However, it may be necessary to conduct a complete neurological examination, which may reveal additional clinical findings necessary for diagnosis and prognosis.

A complete neurological examination includes examination of

- mental status
- head posture and movement
- cranial nerve function
- gait and posture
- function of the neck and forelimbs
- function of the trunk and hindlimbs
- palpation of the bony encasement of the central nervous system
- examination of cerebrospinal fluid
- medical imaging of the bony skeleton of the head and vertebral column.

## SPECIAL DIAGNOSTIC AND LABORATORY TESTING

Special diagnostic techniques and laboratory analysis of samples are available to aid in the diagnosis of diseases of each body system. These are presented in the sections dealing with each body system in Part Three.

# 7

# Clinical Examination of Dogs and Cats

*D. M. Houston*

## INTRODUCTION

A good history and an appropriate physical examination are important to the small animal practitioner. They provide the information necessary to make a diagnosis, to select appropriate diagnostic tests, to give a prognosis and to make recommendations about therapy. An inadequate history or a physical examination that is not thorough may result in a misdiagnosis, failure to use certain diagnostic tests, the use of unnecessary and expensive testing, and delays in appropriate clinical management of the patient. History taking is described in Chapter 3.

Unlike humans, animals cannot explain their problems and the owner may not be able to provide a complete history. Consequently, in veterinary medicine a general physical examination of every patient is recommended. The clinician develops a fixed routine for performing the physical examination. Most start at the head and work towards the tail, taking time to evaluate every system in between. For patients with obvious problems the client will be more at ease and appreciative of your concern if the problem area is investigated first. The nature of the illness will dictate which body system warrants further examination.

- For an animal with a history of acute vomiting, a thorough examination of the abdomen is indicated. This may necessitate palpation with the animal in a variety of positions.
- A lame dog will require an orthopedic and possibly a neurological examination.
- An animal in acute respiratory distress or shock requires emergency therapeutic intervention at the time of presentation and a general physical examination once it is stabilized.

The owner should be present during the physical examination, allowing additional history to be gathered as needed.

## DISTANT EXAMINATION

This is the observation of the animal from a distance – the 'no hands on' part of the examination. It allows the clinician to make observations about the animal's behavior, level of mentation, posture and gait, body conformation and condition, coat condition, and voice abnormalities.

### Behavior and mentation

The animal is observed as it enters the examination room. A bright and alert animal shows interest in the new environment and responds normally to external stimuli such as sound, movement and new people; if it is oblivious and uninterested it is said to be dull or apathetic. A dog in pain may be reluctant to move, or may cry out when it does. Abdominal pain in the dog due to gastric dilatation and volvulus may be associated with obvious restlessness, a tendency to lie down

---

**Practice makes Perfect**

Every physical examination is an opportunity for the clinician to improve their diagnostic accuracy. Techniques of inspection, palpation, auscultation, percussion, and ballottement are learned through practice and experience.

and get up frequently, and extension of the head and neck. An animal presenting after an epileptic seizure may appear blind, stunned, or demented.

## Voice

Abnormality of the voice is noted. Dogs with laryngeal paralysis, where there is failure of the larynx to abduct during inspiration due to recurrent laryngeal nerve damage or disease, often experience a change in bark, which may be of different pitch or muted. Congenital laryngeal paralysis is uncommon but has been reported in the Siberian Husky and the Bouvier des Flandres breeds. Acquired bilateral paralysis is most commonly encountered in elderly dogs of the larger breeds as the result of a neurogenic atrophy of the laryngeal musculature.

## Eating

The appetite of an animal is usually assessed in the client interview but can also be observed by offering food and noting the animal's response

- the inappetent dog will turn away from food
- a dog with dysphagia may sniff the food but not be able to prehend it
- a cat with a tooth root abscess may no longer be willing to chew hard food but still is interested in eating soft canned food.

## Defecation

Observing the animal defecate may provide clues to the origin of diarrhea. Small animals with colorectal tumors often appear constipated and pass ribbon-like stools.

## Urination

If the animal urinates in the examination room a sample should be obtained. Animals with cystitis or urethritis often have increased frequency of urination with the passage of small amounts; those with bladder stones may have hematuria and crystalluria. A dog with polydipsia and polyuria may void large amounts of dilute urine, in contrast to the cat with urethral obstruction, which despite continual attempts is unable to void at all.

## Posture and gait

The dog is observed walking around the examination room and cats observed while on the examination table.

1. Puppies with panosteitis often have alternating limb lameness.
2. A mature dog with a ruptured cranial cruciate ligament will carry the affected limbs.
3. A dog with disc disease may present with an arched back and a reluctance to move, or the pelvic limbs may be paralyzed.
4. An animal with peripheral vestibular disease will circle to the side of the lesion and may use a wall to walk along for balance.
5. A dog with congestive heart failure may stand with the elbows abducted and the head and neck extended; it may not be able to sit or lie down in one position for any length of time.
6. Cats with thromboembolism of the aortic trifurcation will have normal function of the forelimbs but will drag the hindlimbs.
7. A dog with severe abdominal discomfort may assume a 'sawhorse' stance and refuse to move despite the owner's command, or may assume a 'praying posture', in which the head rests on the forelimbs, which are extended on the ground while the pelvis is elevated.

## Body condition

The animal may have normal body condition or be obese, thin, or emaciated. Weight loss is considered significant in dogs and cats when a 10% decrease in normal body weight occurs unassociated with loss of body fluids. Emaciation is extreme weight loss due to severe undernutrition. Weight loss of 30%–50% of lean body mass is usually fatal. Cachexia is a state of extreme ill health. A body condition score system for small animals is now available.

---

### Clinical Pointer

Cats with pharyngeal polyps occasionally have an altered meow.

---

### Obesity

Obesity, the most common nutritional disorder in small animal practice, is defined as a body weight 15%–20% or more above the ideal. Inability to palpate the ribs suggests obesity.

## Skin

Some skin abnormalities, including hair loss, pruritus, and evidence of seborrhea, can be appreciated from a distance. A dog or cat that constantly scratches may have ectoparasites or allergies. Bilateral symmetrical alopecia in the dog is most commonly due to endocrinopathies, particularly hyperadrenocorticism and hypothyroidism. Flank and ventral alopecia in the cat may be self-induced. Localized alopecia, such as periorbital alopecia in a young dog, may indicate demodectic mange. Periauricular alopecia is a normal finding in cats. A cat that fails to groom is usually sick. Many dogs require grooming, and failure to do so results in hair matting, particularly at the base of the ears and on the limbs. Fear and stress induce excessive shedding.

# PARTICULAR DISTANT EXAMINATION OF BODY REGIONS

An inspection of the various body regions is recommended prior to handling the animal.

## Head and neck

The facial expression should be observed. The dog with tetanus may have a 'sardonic grin' due to contraction of the facial muscles. A dog with trigeminal nerve paralysis will be unable to close the mouth. Asymmetry of the soft tissues of the head may be evident, and is most obvious in the carriage of the ears, the degree of closure of the eyelids and the situation of the muzzle and lower lip. Unilateral facial nerve paralysis causes slackness of one side of the face and is seen most frequently in the Cocker Spaniel. A soft tissue swelling below one eye and associated with the maxilla is often seen with an abscess of the upper carnassial tooth. Exophthalmus occurs in small animals with retrobulbar abscesses or masses. Prolapse of the nictitating membrane may be seen in several diseases. Horner's syndrome, consisting of enophthalmus, protrusion of the third eyelid, miosis, and ptosis, is not uncommon in small animals and is most often due to

- a cranial mediastinal mass
- injury to the cervical sympathetic trunk
- brachial plexus injury
- cranial thoracic spinal cord disease, or
- otitis media.

The third eyelid also protrudes if the eye is actively retracted, as in painful conditions and tetany, or if the eye retracts in the orbit due to atrophy of the muscles of mastication, as with trigeminal nerve paralysis or chronic masseter myositis. In cats, bilateral protrusion of the third eyelid is seen with severe systemic disease and depression (Haws syndrome). A red eye may indicate glaucoma, corneal ulceration, conjunctivitis, or uveitis. Excessive salivation in the cat with a non-painful mouth has been identified with hepatic encephalopathy.

Enlargement of the submandibular and prescapular lymph nodes may cause the neck to appear grossly enlarged. Injury to the mandibular or sublingual salivary gland duct results in noticeable swelling below the jaw owing to the accumulation of secretions (sialocele, mucocele).

## Thorax and respirations

The respiratory rate, rhythm and depth are determined with the animal standing and the examiner positioned a few feet away.

### Rate

The rate is counted by observing the movement of the thorax with each breath. The respiratory rate in dogs and cats is normally between 20 and 40 breaths/minute. Exercise, excitement, anxiety, obesity, and a high environmental temperature will result in an increase in the respiratory rate, termed tachypnea. Many dogs pant when nervous, making it difficult to determine the respiratory rate with any accuracy.

### Rhythm

Normal respiration consists of an inspiratory phase, an expiratory phase, and a pause. Abnormalities in the length of one or all phases constitutes an abnormality of rhythm. Prolongation of inspiration and inspiratory stridor due to obstruction of the upper respiratory tract occurs with an elongated soft palate and laryngeal paralysis in the dog, and obstruction due to a nasopharyngeal polyp or lymphoma in the cat. Prolongation of the expiratory phase of respiration may be due to failure of the normal lung to collapse, as occurs with chronic bronchitis and bronchiectasis in the dog and asthma in the cat.

> ### Clinical Pointer
>
> Examine the region from the neck to the thoracic inlet in all cats older than 6 years for thyroid nodules.

## Depth

The amplitude or depth of respiratory movements should be assessed. They may be reduced in painful conditions of the thorax or diaphragm, for example with fractured ribs, or increased in any condition leading to anoxia, for example smoke inhalation. Labored breathing or difficulty in breathing is known as dyspnea, and is common in small animals with pleural effusion and in those with pneumothorax. Orthopnea is difficult breathing in certain positions. The dog with congestive heart failure may be able to breathe comfortably while standing, but is unable to lie down for any length of time. With severe congestion in the lungs a dog may present with extension of the head and neck, abduction of the elbows and open-mouth breathing.

## Respiratory noises

In addition to the inspiratory stridor mentioned under 'Voice abnormalities', animals with respiratory tract disease may cough, sneeze, or wheeze.

Cough receptors are located on the major airways, including the trachea and bronchi, and will be stimulated by a variety of irritants. Dogs with mitral valve insufficiency and left atrial enlargement may cough because of compression of the left main stem bronchus caused by the enlarged left atrium. Small-breed dogs with a collapsing trachea are described as having a 'goose honking' cough.

Snorting occurs with nasal irritation and is common with foreign bodies lodged in the turbinate structure, environmental irritants such as smoke and, in the cat, feline rhinotracheitis and calicivirus infections. Reverse sneezing occurs in dogs and consists of short periods (1–2 minutes) of rapid, repeated, difficult inspiratory efforts (dyspnea), characterized by extension of the neck, abduction of the elbows and bulging of the eyes. Swallowing or massaging the pharyngeal area causes the attack to stop.

## Abdomen

The contour of the abdomen is examined by visual inspection. An increase in the size may be due to enlargement of any abdominal viscera or organ, and excessive quantities of fluid, feces, gas, or fat. An obvious decrease in the size of the abdomen is referred to as a 'gaunt' appearance and occurs most commonly in states of chronic malnutrition resulting from

- starvation
- protein-losing enteropathy
- cancer cachexia
- chronic diseases where appetite is reduced.

An umbilical hernia may be apparent on general abdominal inspection. Ventral edema is occasionally seen in a dog with right heart failure or hypoproteinemia.

## External genitalia

In the male dog the scrotum and prepuce are examined and in the female the vulva. Gross enlargement of the scrotum is usually due to a tumor in older animals. A small scrotum may be the result of degenerative changes in the testicles or cryptorchism, in which one or both testicles failed to descend into the scrotum. In the intact dog a small amount of cloudy, non-odorous discharge from the penis is normal. Swelling of the vulva is normal in the intact female dog in proestrus. Discharges of pus and blood from the vagina are indicative of genitourinary tract infection.

## Mammary glands

Enlargement of one or several mammary glands may be due to pregnancy, false pregnancy, inflammation, infection, hyperplasia or tumor.

## Limbs

General abnormalities in the inspection of posture and gait have been described. The forelimbs and hindlimbs should be compared and any abnormality of bone, joint, tendon, or bursa recorded. In an outdoor cat, the limbs should be carefully inspected for swellings, bite wounds, and dried blood or pus indicative of abscessation.

---

### Wheezes

Wheezes are generated by the vibration of airway walls as air passes through narrowed airways. Wheezes are commonly heard in cats with asthma. Occasionally wheezes can be heard without the use of a stethoscope.

---

## CLOSE PHYSICAL EXAMINATION

When handling a dog or cat the examiner needs to be gentle and quiet. Sudden movements may startle the animal, resulting in someone getting scratched or bitten. Restraint and positioning for the purposes of physical examination are described in Chapter 5.

## Vital signs

Vital signs include temperature (T), pulse rate (P) and respiratory rate (R), commonly referred to as the TPR. Body weight and hydration status are usually also obtained. Some veterinarians obtain the vital signs at the beginning of the examination; others obtain the respiratory rate during the inspection of the thorax and take the temperature and pulse after examination of the head and neck region. Vital signs should not be taken at the end of examination as all may be falsely elevated by the associated stress and anxiety. The animal's weight can be taken at the beginning or at the end of the examination. The vital signs are described here and are mentioned in the course of the physical examination as they are obtained.

### Temperature

The body temperature is taken rectally with an automated digital or mercury thermometer. The mercury column should be shaken down, the thermometer bulb lubricated, and the thermometer inserted gently into the rectum and held against one side of the rectal mucosa for approximately 2 minutes. A false low reading will occur if

- the temperature is read immediately after defecation
- the thermometer is placed centrally into a fecal mass
- the thermometer is left in the rectum for insufficient time.

If there is doubt as to the accuracy of the reading, the temperature should be taken again. The normal temperature for a dog is 37.8–39.3°C (100.2–102.8°F) and in the cat is 38.0–39.2°C (100.5–102.5°F). In small animals, temperatures above 39.5°C (103.0°F) are generally considered abnormal (febrile) and a temperature greater than 40.0°C (104°F) is considered critical and potentially life-threatening. Temperatures above 40.0°C result in cell dysfunction and death. Hyperthermia is defined as a simple elevation of the temperature past the critical point, as occurs in heat stroke. The body temperature is often increased with physical activity, excitement and high environmental temperatures. It is not unusual for highly excitable cats and dogs to have elevated temperatures at the time of the physical examination.

Hypothermia, defined as a temperature below the normal range, occurs in a number of conditions, including shock and circulatory collapse. Twelve to twenty-four hours prior to whelping the bitch and queen may experience a drop in body temperature of about 1°C. An astute owner may monitor this as an indication of impending birth.

### Arterial pulse

The arterial pulse is obtained by palpating both femoral arteries for a period of 15–30 seconds. The examiner stands behind the animal or to one side and places the four fingers of each hand on the medial surface of the upper thigh. Only light pressure is required. The pulse rate, rhythm, and amplitude should be assessed.

**Rate**
The normal pulse rate for an adult dog is 70–160 bpm; for giant breeds 60–140 bpm; and for toy breeds up to 180 bpm. Puppies have a pulse rate of up to 220 bpm. The normal pulse rate for a cat is highly variable (120–240 bpm).

**Rhythm**
The rhythm may be regular or irregular. Sinus arrhythmia is a common and normal rhythm disturbance in which the heart rate increases with inspiration and decreases with expiration. All other irregular rhythms are abnormal. Simultaneous palpation of the pulse and auscultation of the heart will reveal pulse deficits. Premature ventricular contractions and atrial fibrillation are common causes of pulse deficits. Although premature ventricular contractions (PVCs) induced by trauma and, acid–base or electrolyte disturbances usually resolve with management of the predisposing causes, in dogs with severe underlying heart disease they may persist.

**Amplitude**
The pulse pressure is a reflection of cardiac stroke volume and the difference between diastolic and systolic pressures generated

- a bounding pulse is typical of a patent ductus arteriosus
- a weak pulse is often palpated with subaortic stenosis.

### Respirations

The respiratory rate is obtained by observing the thoracic wall and counting breaths for a period of 15–30 seconds. Normal respiratory rates in the dog and cat are highly variable. In a relaxed environment it is approximately 20–40 breaths/minute.

### Hydration status

To assess hydration status the skin between the scapulae is picked up with the fingers of one hand, forming a 'tent', and its elasticity is then determined. Normally, tenting the skin and then releasing it results in a rapid return of the skin to its normal position. With significant dehydration (10% or more) the skin remains tented.

## Examination of body regions

### Skin

As the animal is first approached and petted, the skin may be examined. The skin over the head, thorax, abdomen, and limbs is examined for the presence of ectoparasites, alopecia, seborrhea, masses, erythema, and pruritus. Any lesion should be defined according to its location, size, shape, depth, color, texture (soft, hard, dry, greasy, moist, powdery), and the presence of exudate (hemorrage, serum, pus).

### Head and neck

#### Eyes

The size and direction of the eyeballs and pupillary size should be assessed. The eyes should be similar in appearance, look in the same direction and have equal-sized pupils. The size of the eyeball does not usually vary, but pressure from a retrobulbar abscess or mass may cause unilateral protrusion.

*Anisocoria*

Anisocoria is an inequality of the diameter in the pupils that can occur with a number of disorders of the optic nerve, oculomoter nerve, or retina. An abnormal degree of dilation in one eye suggests a lesion of the orbit, such as glaucoma. The pupil may be small or miotic, with uveitis due to ciliary muscle contraction. A unilateral miotic pupil may also be seen with Horner's syndrome or any unilateral ocular disorder that causes pain.

*Nystagmus*

This is the involuntary rhythmic movement of the eyes, seen most often with acute vestibular disease. Vertical nystagmus signifies central vestibular disease.

*Strabismus*

A deviation of the globe, may be indicative of a brainstem lesion; it is a normal finding in Siamese cats.

*Ocular discharge*

Any ocular discharge, unilateral or bilateral, should be noted; it may be clear, as in obstruction of the lacrimal duct, or purulent with inflammation and infection. The eyelids should be observed for the presence of entropion (rolling in of the eyelid), ectropion (rolling out of the eyelid), aberrant eyelashes, cysts, and

tumors. Closure of the eyelids is common with painful eye conditions and with ocular irritation.

*Third eyelid*

The third eyelid is usually not apparent on examination but may protrude or prolapse if the eye is actively retracted due to pain or tetany, or it sinks in the bony orbit owing to atrophy of the muscles of mastication. This could occur with trigeminal nerve paralysis, chronic myositis or severe dehydration. In cats, bilateral protrusion of the third eyelid, or Haws syndrome, is seen with severe systemic disease and depression. Prolapse of the third eyelid also occurs as part of Horner's syndrome and may be due to a cranial mediastinal mass, injury to the cervical sympathetic trunk, brachial plexus injury, cranial thoracic spinal cord disease or otitis media.

*Ocular sclera and conjunctiva*

The ocular sclera and conjunctiva should be examined. The conjunctival tissue may be used to assess the state of the peripheral vascular system. The pallor of anemia and the yellow coloration of jaundice may be visible.

*Cornea*

The cornea must be examined closely because small abnormalities are difficult to see on cursory examination. Corneal reactions to disease include

- edema
- vascularization
- scar formation
- pigmentation
- cellular infiltration
- accumulation of abnormal material within the cornea.

A red eye may indicate conjunctivitis, corneal ulceration, glaucoma or uveitis.

*Deep structures of the eye*

Although examination of the deep structures of the eye can be satisfactorily carried out only with an ophthalmoscope, some gross abnormalities may be observed by direct observation. Looking from the side, the anterior chamber can be examined with a penlight. With uveitis the anterior chamber may be filled with blood, pus, or cells.

*Pupillary light reflexes*

The direct and consensual pupillary light reflexes (PLRs) are examined. Direct PLRs are assessed by shining a bright light into one pupil, medially and laterally, and observing it for a prompt contraction. The process is repeated in the opposite eye. The consensual PLRs are assessed by shining a bright light source into one eye while observing the contralateral pupil for contraction. The process is then repeated in the other eye. Direct and consensual PLRs require functional cranial nerves II and III and bilateral iris constrictor muscles. For an animal presenting with an ocular abnormality a complete ophthalmologic examination should be performed.

### Ears

The symmetry of the ears is examined by visual inspection. The pinna and skin around the base of each ear is examined and any erythema, alopecia, crusting or skin lesions noted. All cats have a normal area of alopecia in the area between the eye and the base of the ear. The pinna is a region of the body prone to numerous skin diseases. The prevalence of otitis externa in dogs is 10–20%, and in cats, 2–10%. The pinna can be gently stretched dorsally and each ear canal visually inspected with a penlight for signs of irritation or increased wax production. Any odor, discharge, discoloration, or evidence of pain should be recorded. The normal ear canal has no foul odor, is light pink in color and has no discharge.

A normal animal will move the ears in response to noise. If this does not occur the examiner should stand behind the animal and make a loud noise. If there is no response a hearing test may be recommended.

### Nose

The nares are examined for symmetry, patency, color, and discharge. The external portion of the nose, including the overlying skin, the palanum nasale, nostrils, cartilage, and bone, can all be palpated. This aids in detection of areas of tenderness, or defects resulting from bone loss or swelling secondary to bone proliferation, neoplasia, or soft tissue inflammation.

Erosion and ulceration of the nasal mucosa is often apparent in dogs afflicted with nasal aspergillosis, or in dogs and cats with chronic nasal discharge. Rhinitis due to feline rhinotracheitis or calicivirus is very common in cats. Squamous cell carcinoma of the nasal planum is also common in the cat. Dogs and cats with nasal foreign bodies, such as grass awns, usually present with snorting and excessive pawing at the nose.

The patency of each nostril can be determined with a dental mirror, glass slide or stainless steel table. The head is gently held toward the table, or a mirror or glass slide and the condensation pattern elicited by breathing through each nostril (fogging) is noted.

### Mouth

The lips, mucous membranes, teeth and gingival tissues, hard and soft palates, tongue and tonsils are evaluated.

*Lips*

The lips are examined for symmetry, pigmentation, and the presence of blood, masses or other lesions. An animal with unilateral facial nerve paralysis may have a drooping lip on one side. Depigmentation and ulceration of the oral mucocutaneous junction may be seen with immune-mediated diseases. About 90% of dogs and cats with pemphigus vulgaris have oral cavity lesions at the time of diagnosis, with oral cavity lesions being the initial sign in about 50% of cases. If the animal is drooling, protective gloves are recommended in countries where the possibility of rabies exists.

---

**Clinical Pointer**

Look at the mucous membranes to assess hydration. They are normally moist but become tacky with dehydration.

---

*Oral mucous membranes*

The oral mucous membranes are examined for color (normally pink), capillary refill time (normally less than 2 seconds), moisture (normally wet) and the presence of any lesions. Icterus, cyanosis, and anemia may be reflected in the color of the mucous membranes.

---

**Clinical Pointer**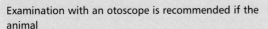

Examination with an otoscope is recommended if the animal

- shakes its head
- scratches its ears frequently
- resents examination of the ears.

If painful, sedation will be required

---

**Nasal changes and immune-mediated disease**

Immune-mediated disease can affect the nasal philtrum and mucosa, causing

- ulceration
- excoriation
- depigmentation.

*Teeth and gingival tissues*
The teeth and gingival tissues are examined for evidence of tartar accumulation and periodontal disease, common problems in small animals. By gently touching the teeth with a dental probe areas of sensitivity can be identified. The base of each tooth is examined for blood, pus, and embedded hair. Retained deciduous teeth are not uncommon and extraction is usually indicated.

*Hard and soft palates*
Occasionally cleft defects, ulcers, erosions, and foreign bodies are identified on the hard or soft palates.

*Tongue*
The tongue is examined for symmetry, color, texture, and movement. The cat's tongue is rougher than that of the dog to assist in normal grooming behavior. It is important, particularly in a cat with a history of vomiting, inappetence or drooling, to examine the underside of the tongue for string, wool, or thread, which may be embedded at the base.

> ## Clinical Pointer
>
> Gently pull on the tongue and note the animal's efforts to retract it, failure to retract indicates a neurological problem.

*Tonsils*
The tonsils are not visualized in the normal cat. Gentle pressure on the base of the tongue with the index finger allows the tonsils to be visualized in the dog. Sedation or general anesthesia is recommended for thorough examination of the pharyngeal region.

## Salivary glands
The salivary glands are not readily palpable, although the mandibular salivary gland may be palpated as a firm structure ventral and medial to the angle of the mandible.

## Lymph nodes
The submandibular lymph nodes are located just ventral to the mandibular salivary glands; the prescapular lymph nodes are located in front of the shoulders. Normally these nodes are small and may not be palpable. Lymphadenopathy occurs with tumor infiltration or as a result of a reactive process, as occurs in response to systemic fungal or bacterial infection.

> ## Clinical Pointer
>
> Take care to distinguish the mandibular salivary glands from the submandibular lymph nodes. The salivary glands are deeper and more dorsal than the nodes, bilobed, and generally softer.

## Jugular veins
With the head gently extended, the jugular veins are examined. The hair may need to be clipped or, if the haircoat is short, alcohol applied to the neck to allow better visualization of the vessels. Normally the jugular veins are not visible without occluding the thoracic inlet. A jugular pulse of small magnitude, moving about one-third of the way up the neck, is normal in small animals.

## Trachea
The trachea is examined by palpation and auscultation. In the presence of tracheitis or a collapsing trachea gentle palpation and compression will commonly induce a cough. In the cat both sides of the trachea are palpated, from the pharynx to the thoracic inlet, for the presence of a thyroid nodule. In the normal dog or cat the thyroid gland is not palpable. Hyperthyroidism due to adenomatous hyperplasia of one or both thyroid glands is common in middle-aged and older cats and commonly results in a palpable thyroid nodule.

The larynx, trachea and lungs are auscultated in sequence.

## Esophagus
In a normal dog or cat the esophagus is not visible or palpable in the neck region. It may become visible with distension due to the accumulation of food, fluid, or gas, as occurs with megaesophagus.

## Clavicle
The cat has a well developed clavicle which can be palpated at the distal end of the spine of the scapula. It is occasionally mistaken for a foreign body.

> ## Engorgement of the jugular veins
>
> An obstruction to the vein → unilateral engorgement.
> Right heart failure or pericardial effusion → bilateral engorgement.

## Forelimbs

The forelimbs are inspected for symmetry and palpated for evidence of pain, crepitus and swellings. Each joint is inspected and palpated. Passive flexion and extension of the joints will reveal evidence of abnormal movement or pain. The feet are picked up and examined and any interdigital smell, discoloration, or lesions recorded. The nails, nailbeds, and footpads need to be evaluated for depigmentation, tenderness, or injury.

If any problem is found a more complete examination of the area is indicated.

## Thorax

Examination of the thorax includes palpation, auscultation, and percussion of both the cardiac area and the lungs.

### Palpation

With one hand on each side of the thoracic wall the thorax is palpated for the presence of

- masses
- asymmetry of the ribcage
- old rib fractures, or
- swellings.

Lipomas – benign collections of fat – are often found in the axillary region and on the ribcage. Any mass should be aspirated and cytological examination performed. An animal in good body condition will have palpable (but not visible) ribs, in an obese animal ribs will not be palpable.

In the cat the cranial thoracic region requires gentle compression. With the thumb on one side of the thorax and the fingers on the opposite side, the ribs should have a spring-like resiliency and allow for moderate compression of the cranial thorax. This compressibility is lost with the presence of a cranial mediastinal mass such as lymphoma.

The point of maximum intensity (PMI) of the heart is palpated. A palpable thrill is felt with a grade V–VI/VI murmur.

### Auscultation

Auscultation of the heart is aimed at determining the character of normal heart sounds and detecting the presence of abnormal sounds. Auscultation of the right and left sides of the heart is best done in the standing animal. Extension of the left forelimb will facilitate auscultation. Both the diaphragm (high and medium frequency) and bell (low frequency) of the stethoscope are used. The first heart sound S1 or LUBB, is generated by the closure of the right (tricuspid) and left (mitral) atrioventricular valves. The mitral valve is located on the left side about the level of the 5th intercostal space, below the costochondral junction. The tricuspid valve is located on the right side between the 3rd and 5th intercostal spaces. The first heart sound tends to be louder, longer, and lower pitched than the second. The second heart sound, S2 or DUBB, is generated by the closure of the aortic and pulmonic valves, located over the heart base. The aortic valve is at the level of the left 4th intercostal space at the costochondral junction; the pulmonic valve is located slightly cranial and ventral to the aortic valve at the level of the 3rd intercostal space. In small dogs and cats the valve areas are difficult to auscultate separately as a great deal of overlap occurs because of the size of the stethoscope and the small size of the patient. Occasionally split S1 or split S2 sounds are heard owing to asynchronous closure of the associated valves.

The normal cardiac rhythm consists of LUBB-DUBB-pause, LUBB-DUBB-pause. The presence of third or fourth heart sounds is abnormal in small animals. The third sound (S3) is a low-frequency sound generated by the sudden cessation of rapid ventricular filling with distension and vibration of the ventricular wall, papillary muscles and chordae tendinae. This 'gallop' rhythm may be heard in animals with dilated cardiomyopathy and heart failure. The fourth heart sound (S4) is the result of atrial contraction ejecting blood into the ventricles. It indicates ventricular diastolic dysfunction with filling of an already over-distended ventricle on atrial contraction. Cats with hypertrophic cardiomyopathy and reduced diastolic distensibility often have this 'gallop' rhythm.

### Heart murmurs

Heart murmurs are common in dogs and cats. Innocent murmurs tend to occur in young animals, have no known cause, are soft, low-amplitude sounds, occur early in systole, vary in intensity with a change in

---

### Clinical Pointer

The point of maximum intensity of the heart (PMI) is usually on the left chest wall between the 4th and 6th intercostal spaces in the region of the apex of the heart.

---

### Clinical Pointer

It is not possible to differentiate S3 from S4 sounds, but it is important to know that their presence is abnormal in small animals.

heart rate or body position, and generally disappear by 6 months of age. Physiological murmurs have a known cause, such as fever, anemia, or hypoproteinemia, and disappear as the underlying cause is corrected. Pathological murmurs are caused by underlying heart or vessel disease, such as stenosis or valve insufficiency. Congenital subaortic stenosis is common in a number of dog breeds and causes a systolic murmur heard best over the left heart base. Mitral valve insufficiency is the most common cause of a murmur in the older, small breed dog. It causes a systolic murmur heard best over the apex of the heart on the left side. Murmurs are classified according to

- their location on the thorax
- the time of occurrence in the cardiac cycle (systolic, diastolic or continuous)
- duration and position (holosystolic if occurs throughout all of systole)
- intensity (grades I–VI, with I being barely audible and VI audible without a stethoscope)
- quality, frequency, and configuration on a phonocardiogram.

*Sinus arrhythmia*
In the normal dog and cat the LUBB-DUBB-pause occurs with a set regularity. Sinus arrhythmia is a normal rhythm disturbance associated with respiration in which heart rate increases with inspiration and decreases with expiration.

*Bradycardia and tachycardia*
Bradycardia is a heart rate less than normal and tachycardia is defined as a heart rate greater than normal. Bradycardia occurs with partial or complete heart block, with space-occupying lesions of the cranium, and occasionally in respiratory and gastrointestinal conditions where vagal tone is high. In small animals drug history is important, as phenothiazine tranquilizers, digoxin, β-blockers, calcium channel blockers, and lidocaine are all capable of causing sinus bradycardia. Tachycardia is common in small animals and occurs with pain, stress, and anxiety. Sustained tachycardia is pathological and needs to be addressed. Large-breed dogs with dilated cardiomyopathy may present with supraventricular tachycardia or atrial fibrillation. Cats with hypertrophic cardiomyopathy due to hyperthyroidism often present with sinus tachycardia.

*Pulse abnormalities*
While the heart is being auscultated, the femoral pulse should be palpated. Normally, a pulse is generated with each heart contraction.

- Hypokinetic or weak pulses are due to decreased cardiac output or slower rate of rise due to delayed emptying of the left ventricle. This may occur with heart failure or shock.
- Hyperkinetic or strong, exuberant pulses rise and fall quickly, and are due to large left ventricular stroke volumes with rapid diastolic runoffs. Hyperkinetic pulses are common in animals with patent ductus arteriosus (PDA) or aortic insufficiency, and are occasionally felt in animals with fever or anemia.
- Pulse deficits are common with rhythm disturbances, such as premature ventricular contractions and atrial fibrillation.

**Auscultation of the trachea, larynx and lung**
Auscultation is performed in a quiet room as respiratory sounds are often subtle and difficult to hear. Panting and sniffing in the dog and purring in the cat are a hindrance to auscultation. Talking to the animal or holding the muzzle closed helps stop panting and sniffing. Cats will usually stop purring if a water tap is turned on, the nose is gently tapped with a finger, or someone blows on its nose.

The lung field is divided into sections or grids and auscultated dorsally to ventrally, listening for a few seconds in each area. In the cat at least four sites of auscultation are made, whereas in the dog nine sites are attempted. Normal breath sounds are blowing in character and are created by air passing through the sinuses, larynx, trachea, and major bronchi. These sounds are first listened for over the hilus of the lung. The stethoscope is moved in a circular manner farther and farther peripherally until the sounds are lost. They are best heard over the cervical trachea. The inspiratory and expiratory sounds are loud and of equal duration.

Decreased lung sounds, including 'silent lung', and abnormal lung sounds, including crackles, wheezes, and pleural friction rubs, are suggestive of pulmonary pathology.

Decreased lung sounds may occur in normal cats, in animals that are breathing shallowly, are obese, have pleural effusion, pneumothorax, diaphragmatic hernia or thoracic masses. Dogs and cats with severe diffuse airway disease may also have decreased lung sounds.

---

### Clinical Pointer

To encourage the animal to make a deep inspiration, hold its muzzle with one hand and block both nostrils with the other, then release the nostrils and auscultate the lungs.

*Crackles*

Crackles are popping or crackling sounds generated by the sudden opening of airways or the bursting of bubbles in airway secretions. They are similar to the sound produced when Velcro strips are slowly pulled apart, or when someone pops holes in cellophane wrap. They occur when there is edema or exudate within airways, or when airways are snapping open at different times owing to uneven lung inflation. Crackles may occur in the dog or cat with

- pulmonary edema
- bronchopneumonia
- tracheal collapse, and
- inflammatory or neoplastic interstitial lung disease.

*Wheezes*

Wheezes are musical, continuous sounds that commonly occur with diseases such as asthma, bronchoconstriction, bronchial wall thickening, external airway compression, and other forms of obstructive lung disease when airway narrowing occurs. Wheezes are heard best on expiration.

*Stridor*

Stridor, a high-pitched sound, occurs during inspiration and is usually associated with laryngeal disease.

*Stertor*

Stertor, a harsh, snoring sound, is heard when the pharyngeal area is partially obstructed, as occurs with an elongated soft palate in the dog or a pharyngeal polyp in the cat.

*Pleural friction sounds*

Pleural friction sounds are not common in small animals. They are caused by inflamed parietal and visceral pleura rubbing against each other and are associated with septic pleural effusions.

Simultaneous auscultation and percussion of the lung may be of some benefit in the diagnosis of pleural effusion, lung lobe consolidation or an intrathoracic mass. In such cases the percussion note is dull and heart and lung sounds are muffled.

**Acoustic percussion of the thorax**

Acoustic percussion of the thorax may be valuable in the diagnosis of pleural effusion, lung consolidation or an intrathoracic mass.

## Abdomen

Examination of the abdomen includes palpation, auscultation, percussion, and ballottement. Rectal examination is also recommended in any animal pre-

---

**Clinical Pointer**

Take time to recognize the common artifactual or extraneous sounds

- hair moving across the diaphragm of the stethoscope
- muscular trembling
- sniffing and purring.

---

senting with signs of gastrointestinal disease or systemic illness of unknown cause.

**Palpation**

Abdominal palpation is diagnostically useful in small animals. In the cranial abdomen intestinal loops (duodenum) may be palpable. The liver, stomach, and pancreas are not usually palpable except in cases of diffuse hepatomegaly or mass lesions, or with gastric dilatation and volvulus. In the middle abdomen loops of the small intestine are readily palpable. In the cat both kidneys are palpable, with the right one cranial to the left and the left slightly more movable than the right. The spleen and kidneys are variable as to the ease with which they are palpable in normal dogs. The left kidney, because of its more caudoventral location, can occasionally be palpated, particularly in large dogs. In the caudal abdomen loops of small intestine, colon, and bladder may be palpated. The urinary bladder lies just cranial to the symphysis pubis and is easily palpable when distended with urine. The reproductive organs are not usually palpable unless distended with a fetus or with fluid as in the case of pyometra. The cervix is not palpable on abdominal palpation in most dogs and cats, although in proestrus or estrus in the dog it may be palpated as a firm, walnut-shaped organ in the caudal abdomen.

Altering the position of the animal may assist in abdominal palpation

- raising the forelimbs allows cranial abdominal contents to fall back, so that the caudal liver margins, spleen and cranial intestinal structures come within reach
- raising the hindlimbs allows caudal abdominal organs to come cranial. This facilitates palpation of the pelvic structures, including the bladder, prostate, uterus, and colon.

Left and right lateral recumbency or dorsal recumbency may also assist in palpation if an abnormality is suspected.

**Auscultation, percussion and ballottement**

These techniques are of limited value in the clinical examination of the dog and cat and are not routinely performed.

### Perineal region

Once the abdomen has been palpated the tail should be lifted, tail tone assessed and the perineal region examined. The anus is a mucocutaneous junction and may be affected by immune-mediated skin disease. The perianal region should be inspected for tapeworm segments, perineal hernias, perianal fistulae, and masses.

### Hindlimbs

The hindlimbs are inspected for symmetry and palpated for evidence of pain and swellings. Each joint is inspected and palpated for evidence of swellings, crepitus, and pain. Passive flexion and extension of the joints will reveal evidence of abnormal movement or pain. The feet are picked up and examined, and any interdigital smell, discoloration, or lesions recorded. The nails, nailbeds, and footpads need to be evaluated for depigmentation, tenderness, or injury.

If any problem is found on examination of the limbs, a more complete examination is indicated.

**Popliteal lymph nodes**
The popliteal lymph nodes are often palpable in dogs and cats. These nodes lie in the fat depots in the popliteal space just caudal to the stifle joint, between the medial border of the biceps femoris and the lateral border of the semitendinosus muscles.

### Reproductive and urinary systems

Particularly in dogs, the external genitalia (vestibule in female; prepuce, penis and scrotum in male) are easily examined. In the female any discharge, redness, vulvar swelling, infolding of the mucocutaneous junction, or the presence of masses are recorded.

In the male the scrotum, testicles, and epididymides are palpated and assessed for symmetry and consistency. Cryptorchidism – the failure of one or both testicles to descend into the scrotum by 6 months of age – is a hereditary defect in the dog and affected males should not be used for breeding. The penis is palpated both within the prepuce and extruded from the prepuce to assess for the presence of frenula or fibrous bands attaching the penis to the sheath. A small amount of odorless mucoid discharge at the preputial orifice is a normal finding in male dogs. An excessive amount or an odorous discharge is abnormal and a sample should be taken for cytology. In the cat, protrusion of the penis is more difficult and many cats will not tolerate it. In the intact male cat the penis is covered with minute spiny papillae which atrophy and disappear with neutering.

The kidneys, bladder, and uterus are described under abdominal palpation. The prostate gland is further described under rectal examination.

### Rectal examination

A rectal examination is indicated in an animal with evidence of gastrointestinal disease. It is also recommended in intact male dogs over 4 years of age to assess prostate size. In the cat sedation is often required to perform a rectal examination.

In the dog the rectum, distal colon, pelvic bones, urethra, anal sacs, uterus and vagina in the female, and prostate gland in the male, are palpated. Rectal palpation may be combined with abdominal palpation to assist in evaluation of the prostate gland. The normal prostate gland is smooth, symmetrical, and painless on palpation. In the cat the rectum, distal colon, pelvic bones, urethra, and anal sacs are usually accessible to palpation.

Tumors, polyps, rectal and colonic mucosal roughening, and enlarged sublumbar lymph nodes are abnormalities that may be palpable on rectal examination in the dog.

If necessary the anal sacs may be emptied at the end of the rectal examination.

Once the history and physical examination have been completed and recorded, it is important to summarize abnormal findings to the owner and then make recommendations for further diagnostics or therapy.

---

**Clinical Pointer**

Rectal examination is normally done at the end of the close physical examination.

---

## PHYSICAL EXAMINATION OF THE NEONATE

The clinician requires a knowledge of the normal development of a kitten and puppy (Table 7.1). Most healthy puppies and kittens are first examined by a veterinarian at 6 to 8 weeks of age. If examination is necessary prior to this time, the dam should be present, if possible, to calm the puppy or kitten. Neonates are examined on a warm surface and kept warm throughout the examination. A neonate with a history of failure to thrive is examined for the presence of congenital defects, such as a cleft palate, imperforate anus, or heart murmur.

Table 7.1. Age-related developmental stages of the puppy
Reprinted, with permission, from Hoskins JD. (editor)
Veterinary Pediatrics: Dogs and Cats from Birth to Six Months, 2nd ed. Philadelphia: WB Saunders Co., 1995.

| Body system | Age | Developmental stages |
|---|---|---|
| Eyes | Birth–13 days | Eyelids are closed, but puppies respond to a bright light with a blink reflex. This reflex disappears at 21 days, probably due to development of accurate pupil control. Palpebral reflex is present at 3 days, becoming adult-like by 9 days. |
| | 5–14 days | Menace reflex is present but slow. Eyelids separate into upper and lower lids. Pupillary light responses are present within 24 hours after eyelids separate. Reflex lacrimation begins when eyelids separate. Corneal reflex is present after eyelids separate. |
| | 3–4 weeks | Vision should be normal. |
| Ears | Birth–5 days | External ear canals are closed. Hearing is poor. |
| | 10–14 days | External ear canals open (should be completely open by 17 days). For the first week after the ear canals are completely opened there is an abundance of desquamated cells and some oil droplets, which is normal as the ear canals remodel to the external environment. |
| Teeth | 4–6 weeks | Deciduous incisors erupt, followed by deciduous canines. |
| | 4–8 weeks | Deciduous premolars erupt. |
| Circulatory | Birth–4 weeks | Lower blood pressure, stroke volume and peripheral vascular resistance present. Increased heart rate (>220 bpm), cardiac output and central venous pressure present. Heart rhythm is regular sinus. |
| Respiratory | Birth–4 weeks | Respiratory rate is 15–35 breaths/minute. |
| Neuromuscular | Birth | Flexor dominance is present at birth, with extensor dominance starting as early as 1 day. Seal posture reflex can last up to 19 days. Sucking reflex is present, but disappears by 23 days. Anogenital reflex disappears between 23 and 39 days. Cutaneous pain perception is present, but withdrawal reflex is noticeable at about 7 days. Tonic neck reflexes are present until 3 weeks of age. Puppy can raise head. Righting response is present. Myotatic reflexes are present at birth, but difficult to elicit in newborns. Panniculus reflex is present at birth. |
| | 5 days | Nystagmus associated with rotary stimulation appears at the end of the first week. Cross extensor reflex ends between 2 and 17 days; persistence indicates upper motor neuron disease. Direct forelimb support of body weight. |
| | 14–16 days | Puppies are crawling. Rear limb support of body weight. |
| | 20 days | Puppies can sit and have reasonable control of distal phalanges. |
| | 22 days | Puppies are walking normally. Vestibular nystagmus becomes adult-like. |
| | 23–40 days | Puppies are climbing and have air righting response. |
| | 3–4 weeks | Hemiwalking response, but may not be fully developed in rear limbs until 6 weeks old. |
| | 6–8 weeks | Postural reactions are fully developed. Time frames for normal development are approximate as variances occur in some individuals. |

## FURTHER READING

Edwards NJ. Bolton's handbook of canine and feline electro-cardiograph, 2nd edn. Philadelphia: WB Saunders, 1987.

Griffin CE. Otitis externa and otitis media. In: Griffin EC, Kwochka KW, MacDonald JM (eds) Current veterinary dermatology. Philadelphia: Mosby Year Book, 1993; 245.

Kruth SA. History and physical examination of the dog and cat. In: Allen DG (ed) Small animal medicine. Philadelphia: JB Lippincott 1991; 7–11.

LaFlamme DP, Kealy RD, Schmidt DA. Estimation of body fat by body condition score. J Vet Int Med 1994; 8: 154A.

Lusk RH. Thermoregulation. In: Ettinger SJ (ed) Textbook of veterinary internal medicine, 3rd edn. Philadelphia: WB Saunders, 1989; 23–26.

Muller GH, Kirk RW, Scott DW. Small animal dermatology, 4th edn. Philadelphia: WB Saunders, 1989; 347–357.

Peiffer RL. Small animal ophthalmology: a problem-oriented approach. Philadelphia: WB Saunders, 1989.

Root MV, Johnston SD. Basis for a complete reproductive examination of the male dog. Semin Vet Med Surg (Small Animal) 1994; 9: 41–45.

Scott DW. External ear disease. J Am Anim Hosp Assoc 1980; 16: 426–433.

Tilley LP. Essentials of canine and feline electrocardiography, 3rd edn. Philadelphia: Lea and Febiger, 1992.

Van Pelt DR, McKiernan BC. Pathogenesis and treatment of canine rhinitis. In: Rosychuk RAW, Merchant SR (eds) Ear, nose and throat. Vet Clin North Am (Small Animal) 1994; 24 (5): 789–806.

White SD. Diseases of the nasal planum. In: Rosychuk RAW, Merchant SR (eds). Ear, nose and throat. Vet Clin North Am (Small Animal) 1994; 24 (5): 887–895.

# 8

# Clinical Examination of Horses and Foals

*I. G. Mayhew*

## INTRODUCTION

Despite comments made by people unfamiliar with handling domesticated equids, the veterinary physical examination of domestic horses is a safe procedure in almost all circumstances. Although their size and power can be awesome at times, horses are usually easily controlled and their relatively large size does offer advantages. Large organ size and body areas make many procedures, such as endoscopy and evaluation of thoracic movements quite easy compared to small patients. Body orifices, being relatively large, are easier to evaluate and instrument, as well as making rectal palpation easier and extremely useful. Finally, large sample volumes of body fluids and tissues are usually available for analysis.

## APPROACHING THE PATIENT

Notwithstanding the above advantages, a good understanding of how to approach, handle, and restrain horses and foals is necessary for the clinical examination to proceed effectively, efficiently and safely (Figs 8.1, 8.2). Horses tend to flee when upset, and in a confined space may turn to face away from an approaching person and accurately kick out sideways or backwards with the hindlimbs. When encountering such behavior one must take care to maneuver towards the head without cutting off a personal escape route. Sometimes if a broom or stick is held in one hand this may help prevent the horse turning and allow a rope to be placed around its neck or a halter applied. In any event it is worth uttering soft-spoken, repeated words or phrases, or whistles to help calm the patient. Only rarely will a rogue horse (usually a stallion) attack an approaching person by biting and/or rearing to strike with the front feet (Fig. 8.1). A whip is usually necessary to approach such a patient in a lion-taming fashion. More often than not, once a rope has been placed around the upper neck or a halter applied, horses usually will give clear warning of any further biting, striking, or kicking actions. Once the halter or bridle is applied it is safest initially to hold the reins or lead rope close to the head, so that head movements can be clearly felt before the horse is able to bite the handler's arm. When led, some horses have a tendency to rush through doorways and past unfamiliar obstacles. This

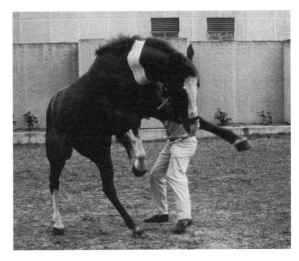

**Fig. 8.1** The safest place to stand when near any horse is close to the left shoulder. If the horse is unhandled, unpredictable, in great pain (as shown), or a rogue stallion, one still should attempt to remain at this site to maintain control.

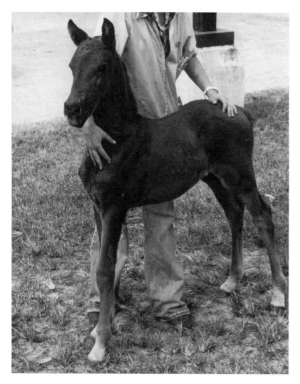

**Fig. 8.2** The vast majority of unhandled foals can be restrained with quiet verbal assurances and one hand placed in front of the thorax, with the other over or behind the rump.

activity should be predicted and firmness applied on the halter or bridle prior to leaving a box or passing an unusual object. Slight jerking movements will usually attract the horse's attention and a firm voice can give added control.

Young foals tend to show similar behavioral characteristics in trying to flee from an approaching examiner. Although their kicks may not have the force of an adult horse, they can certainly injure, and their ability to turn and kick in one motion can be as fast as that of a donkey or zebra!

If unhandled, it is safest to restrain the young foal with a hand around the base of the neck and another round the rump (Fig. 8.2). It is common for neonatal foals to show jerky, twitchy movements on handling. In approaching a neonatal foal it is worth recalling the

---

## Clinical Pointer

Take care in handling young foals, unexpected contact over the rump can trigger the foal to lash out.

---

natural expected behavior so that this is not misinterpreted as abnormality. A newborn foal will usually lie quietly after being delivered and this should be encouraged for a period of 20–30 minutes to allow placental blood to re-enter the foal's circulation. Unless membranes or fetal fluids are interfering with respiration they should not be touched. There is no need to attend to the umbilicus until the foal has risen and the cord has ruptured spontaneously. A newborn foal should stand up within 30–120 minutes, and after a few shaky steps should immediately begin searching for the mare's udder. After a prolonged delivery this initial effort may be delayed, but if suckling has not been successful within 2–4 hours then close inspection of both mare and foal should be undertaken with a mind to supplying colostrum (the mare's or stored), via nasogastric tube if necessary. A healthy newborn foal will always follow the mare and usually needs no handling to do so. If approached when lying down, a newborn foal should get up quickly and, if not disturbed to the point that it tries to flee, it should take time to stretch, like most kittens. Newborn foals are exceedingly responsive to tactile, auditory, and visual stimuli, and all these should therefore be minimized.

Not all equine patients presented for veterinary attention require a complete and detailed physical examination. Thus with a client complaint of a solitary skin lesion, in the absence of any evidence of illness and with normal vital signs present, one may proceed immediately to an examination of the integument. Likewise, when the purpose of the examination is not for diagnosis and treatment, modified physical examinations are most appropriate, for example

- for examination for insurance purposes
- as part of the prepurchase examination
- as part of a vaccination and anthelmintic program.

Finally, although most re-examinations are focused on the problems at hand, it cannot be overemphasized that if at any stage the diagnostic process is floundering it is best to undertake another complete physical examination and detailed examination of all systems that might potentially be involved.

## INITIATING THE EXAMINATION

It is extremely useful to consciously sum up the general situation before proceeding with the examination. Along with the brief history contained in the client's complaint one needs to quickly sum up

- the urgency of the case
- the nature of the patient

- the general environment
- the capabilities of the owner and handler
- any professional or legal implications that may be evident.

If a foal does not rise when a stranger enters its stall this often indicates some degree of urgency to the case. However, it may be sensible to observe the situation quietly, noting eye and ear movements, chest movements, any evidence of hemorrhage or body discharges, and disturbances to the bedding, before proceeding with a speedy examination and instituting clinical care. A colicky horse with clearly distended abdomen, and a gravid mare showing forceful straining may both require immediate restraint and sedation, the passage of a nasogastric tube and a rectal examination on the one hand and perineal, rectal, and vaginal examination on the other.

The nature of the patient and the handler's comments and approach to it usually give one an excellent idea as to how it may be handled.

The immediate environment often indicates the standard of management. A quick inspection of the barn, and particularly the feed manger and watering facilities, as well as the state of the bedding, or evaluation of the quality of pasture and state of fencing, often indicates how well the owner and handler understand and care for the animal. Inspection of the environment should be made for evidence of feces, noting their consistency, amount, color, and the presence of sand, whole grain, undigested fiber, and worms. Areas of urine soiling should be looked for and inspected, and any evidence of blood or discharges on bedding, walls, or manger noted. Badly disrupted or flattened bedding may indicate that the patient has been recumbent, rolling, or pawing.

Professional and legal complications arise only rarely associated with the examination of horses. However, at this early stage the examiner may take mental note of such things as

- evidence of previous veterinary attention
- extremely poor condition of other horses on the premises
- a patient whose identity or obvious illness does not seem to fit the description given.

## GENERAL DISTANT EXAMINATION

A fleeting evaluation of the patient is necessary to sum up the general situation as discussed above. Suffice it to say that a critical, mainly visual, evaluation of the horse in its own environment can be most rewarding in highlighting diagnostic cues that may not be evident on closer inspection. Continuing to discuss historical information with the client before the patient is disturbed is a useful ploy to achieve this. Useful diagnostic cues that may well be missed during later stages of the examination include:

- a young foal arising quietly after resting without stopping to stretch
- an adult horse remaining in a dog-sitting posture for some time while rising
- a horse shifting weight repeatedly on its pelvic limbs while resting
- a mare hanging her head down over her sick foal while her contemporaries are away grazing in the paddock
- a slightly abnormal head posture before the patient is disturbed.

The general demeanor and response of the patient to its environment and its handler should be noted. Observing the passing of feces and urine can be useful, and the opportunity to collect freshly voided urine should not be missed, particularly if there is the possibility of a generalized or metabolic illness.

An evaluation of the patient's general body condition and conformation is useful and may give an indication as to general nutrition and the severity and duration of illness. Most patients, if free, will move, and some indication as to the nature of the gait should be evident from a distance. The examiner may be able to observe abnormal movement and activities such as

- rubbing on objects because of localized pruritus
- straining to pass urine or feces
- pawing the ground due to impatience or colic
- packing bedding under the heels because of foot pain
- abdominal contractions due to synchronous diaphragmatic flutter
- subtle head trembling or muscle tremors due to various metabolic toxic, systemic, or neuromuscular disorders.

Finally, from a distance the general condition of the hair and skin can be noted, detecting gross abnormalities and perhaps soiling of the haircoat with mud or bedding material, urine scald, or fecal contamination.

## Clinical Pointer

Suggest that the usual handler approach the horse first because 'the horse is more used to you than me'.

## PARTICULAR DISTANT EXAMINATION

This aspect of the examination allows the clinician to prepare mentally for the detailed close physical examination that follows by focusing on the head, neck, trunk, limbs, feet, and external genitalia.

### Head and neck

With experience the clinician will be able to determine the general demeanor of a patient by observing characteristics of the head and neck that will give a very good indication as to the general severity of any illness present. In horses a normal flexed head and elevated neck posture, erect ears, bright eyes, and being alert to the environment are all healthy signs. A patient with the head held low, ears drooping, eyes sunken and partly closed, poor expression on the face, and little response to the environment has a substantial problem.

General symmetry, particularly of muzzle, nares, eyes and ears, should be noted, along with any irregularities. It is not uncommon for horses to have single or multiple, symmetric or asymmetric, small bony anomalous protuberances covered with intact skin on the frontal region and on the ventral mandible. These may be a few millimeters or up to 2 cm in diameter and height. If the horse is eating there will be the opportunity to observe its ability to prehend, chew and swallow.

### Thorax and abdomen

Inspection of the trunk allows confirmation of respiratory rate, depth, and rhythm. Observing for abdominal movement during expiration may be the only way to determine respiratory rate in a patient breathing quietly.

> ### Abdominal distension
>
> Degrees of abdominal emptiness or distension are significant and comparison of the left and right sides is useful, particularly with abdominal distension. Accumulation of gas in the large intestine is often most prominent in the cecum on the right dorsal side.

### Genitalia and mammary glands

The female external genitalia and mammary glands are normally not evident from a distance unless a mare is lactating, when evidence of mammary distension and even dripping or squirting of milk might indicate that her foal is sick and not sucking. If observed for some time many stallions and even some geldings will protrude the penis during an examination This can signal the beginning of urination. Most patients will resent this organ being handled.

### Distant examination of a recumbent horse

In evaluating a recumbent patient it is critical that the general circumstances and distant examination be undertaken quietly but rapidly. If there is overt evidence of marked respiratory dysfunction, such as froth at the nares, or evidence of severe hemorrhage, or of a fracture of either the axial skeleton or proximal long bones, then emergency measures will be required. These may include a decision for rapid intervention, including euthanasia.

At this stage evidence of struggling, prior passage of feces and urine, and evidence of self-trauma, particularly to the head and to pressure points such as the hip, needs to be noted. It is important to observe the willingness and ability of a recumbent horse to regain sternal recumbency and to attempt to stand, but it is also wise to examine such a patient quietly before it does make these attempts; a particular distant examination may thus initially be bypassed. An adult horse that attempts to rise and reaches a sternal posture with the thoracic limbs extended ('dog-sitting' posture) and remains so for half a minute or longer will often have a disorder caudal to the brachial region. This includes the thoracolumbar region of the vertebral column, the sacrum, pelvis, and bilateral pelvic limbs.

## HANDLING FOR THE CLOSE PHYSICAL EXAMINATION

As previously noted, a calm approach, slow movements, and quiet voice on the part of the handler and examiner are always useful in allowing the examination to proceed successfully. It can be useful to observe the handler approach the horse and (usually) apply a halter for routine restraint.

> ### Clinical Pointer
>
> With low-grade abdominal pain partial and repeated penile protrusion is common.

Further restraint may be necessary if the horse is

- dangerous
- very difficult to handle
- unpredictable, or
- in an unstable state, as with profuse bleeding, a fractured limb, or being cast in a ditch.

Examination of a suckling foal may require someone to restrain the mare and a second handler to restrain the foal. Unless a young foal is used to being handled with a halter applied it may require restraint by the handler placing one hand around the base of the neck and another around the rump (Fig. 8.2). Tightly gripping the base of the tail in a horizontal position is useful for added restraint, and further extension of the tail without twisting may also be useful in quieting a fractious foal.

A horse may be dangerous to handle because it is completely unbroken, because it is rabid or because it is showing violent behavior resulting from medical problems. The safest place to be near such an animal is close to the left thoracic limb while holding a bridle lead or lunge line attached to the horse's head (Fig. 8.1). Such patients need to be approached carefully and chemical restraint should be seriously considered. With dangerous or very difficult horses it is still necessary to control the head, and in addition to a halter or bridle additional means of restraint must be considered such as

- holding up and perhaps tying up a thoracic limb
- grasping and twisting a handful of loose skin on the caudal neck
- grasping and twisting the base of the ear
- applying a chain or rope twitch to the muzzle
- applying a muzzle clamp
- using a rearing chain, rearing bit, or lip chain.

Any or all of these should be accompanied by continued calming verbal commands of moderate intensity.

As stated above the vast majority of equine patients can be handled with minimal restraint; however, there are several very practical rules that should always be applied.

1. The person restraining the head will by preference initially stand on the left side, and then preferably either near the head or the shoulder on the same side as the examiner.
2. Unless it is obvious by familiarity, the examiner should always indicate to the handler what procedure is to be performed next, such as 'I am just going to lift up this left hindlimb'.
3. If the horse becomes slightly unruly the handler should always draw the head towards the side that he/she and the examiner are standing.

4. In a confined box it is often better to direct an unruly or restless horse straight forward into a wall to prevent compulsive forward movement.

If these approaches along with continued reassuring verbal commands are insufficient then further restraint, including chemical restraint, needs to be considered.

Adult horses should always be approached from the front, and it is wise to reassure the patient with gentle rubbing of parts of the face and neck, particularly the muzzle, giving it the opportunity to smell the examiner. While the horse is still standing quietly with the handler at the head closer general inspection from the head to the neck, the thoracic limb, thorax, abdomen and hindlimb, can be made on each side.

---

### Clinical Pointer

While reassuring the horse by rubbing its face and neck, palpate the facial or transverse facial artery for a pulse, noting its rate and quality, and record the respiratory rate.

---

The scene is now set for a thorough close physical examination or an abbreviated or a specific examination, as appropriate. At this stage one should be in possession of sample containers for urine and feces in case the opportunity arises to collect them.

## CLOSE PHYSICAL EXAMINATION

Because of the size of an adult horse it is sensible to perform the examination by proceeding around the patient, rather than purely on a body systems basis. Because one usually approaches the equine patient at the head it may be reasonable to begin at that point. However, it is also convenient to place a rectal thermometer early, so that this can be removed a few minutes later.

The order for the close physical examination described here begins with placement of a rectal thermometer and proceeds clockwise around the horse. This allows one to move calmly from the head to the tail region, sliding a hand along the dorsal trunk and pelvic region to reassure the horse and to get a feeling for its responsiveness.

### Left pelvic limb

With the thermometer in place, and preferably clipped to the tail hairs, evaluation of the left rump and hip can begin, proceeding down the left hindlimb. Specific palpation should be applied to the joints of the stifle, hock, and fetlock, as well as the calcaneal and digital flexor tendons, continuing to slide the hand down to the pastern, palpating digital pulses but pausing over the coronary region to determine coronary and hoof wall superficial temperature. The horse may be induced to pick up the left hindlimb by gently pinching the digital flexor tendons. The foot should be inspected for symmetry and balance, usually requiring the use of a hoof pick to remove impacted bedding from the sole. The condition and smell of the hoof wall and sole give a strong indication as to whether or not the attendant has cleaned the feet regularly and had the hooves trimmed and balanced appropriately. Unattended cracks in the hoof wall, a crumbling sole and a putrid (anerobic) smell all indicate degrees of neglect of the feet. Many owners (even of thoroughbred horses), by design as well as neglect, will allow the hooves to be overgrown at the toe and low at the heel, resulting in an acute pastern/hoof to ground axis.

The hand can then be slid up the medial aspect of the limb, palpating the saphenous vein and the skin in the inguinal region and groin that is not visible. Some horses will resent this, but with gentle persuasion and slow hand movements it is tolerated in most cases. This gives the opportunity to palpate

- the inguinal canals
- inguinal lymph nodes (if enlarged)
- mammary tissue or scrotum and testes as applicable,

before moving to the prefemoral region, palpating for prefemoral lymph node enlargement. Normally the

### The Umbilical Region

Deep palpation of the umbilical region may reveal firm, painful tissue indicating sepsis, and it may be necessary to cast the foal on its side to examine this region adequately. Umbilical hernias, even with ring sizes up to three fingertips in diameter, often resolve as the foal grows, but should be inspected regularly for such resolution.

latter are a cluster of flattened, 0.5–1.0 cm nodules under the fascia lata. Most important in foals, particularly neonates, is palpation of the umbilical stump for any evidence of pain, heat, and swelling and drainage of serum, urine, or pus.

## Left abdomen

The left hand can then be swept over the ventral abdomen cranially to the sternal region, checking for skin lesions, ventral edema, and other swellings while stethoscopic auscultation in cranial and caudal, dorsal and ventral quadrants of the abdomen is undertaken. Occasionally the fluid-rushing sounds of small intestinal activity can be distinguished in the dorsal flank from the generally louder, lower-pitched explosive sounds (borborygmi) of colonic activity in the midflank. In most adult horses, however, the latter predominates. Simultaneous finger percussion and auscultation also should be undertaken in each quadrant, occasionally revealing small areas of resonance ('pings') that usually change in tone rapidly with time and intestinal motility.

## Left thorax

Auscultation is then moved to the thorax, usually beginning with the heart. Identification of the site of the apex beat with the fingers holding the stethoscope head is the best point to start. This is normally palpated at the ventral third of the fifth to sixth ribs, and mitral valve sounds are normally loudest halfway up the ribs at this site. The aortic and pulmonic outflow sites are slightly dorsal to this over the fifth and fourth ribs, respectively. Normally when two heart sounds are heard these are in the form of 'lub-dup' (S1–S2); three or four heart sounds may be heard, the latter resembling 'ba lub-dup bup' (S4–S1–S2–S3), and may include a split second heart sound. By beginning with determining the apex beats it is easier to relate systolic and diastolic phases, and consequently systolic and diastolic murmurs, which can at times be difficult. At the same time one can observe the ventral neck region for normal, low-intensity caudal jugular pulsations, palpate the facial pulse, or even palpate the caudal jugular groove deeply for a carotid pulse (which can be difficult), again to confirm the phases of the cardiac cycles.

Before undertaking pulmonary auscultation it is worth determining the airway sounds at the ventral cervical trachea. Similar, large airway breath sounds can be expected to be conducted through to the thoracic wall to a greater or lesser extent, depending on the amount of air moving and particularly depending on the condition of the animal. These can be inaudible in normal horses. These normal breath sounds can be mimicked by almost completely closing one's lips and breathing deeply and evenly in and out. They perhaps resemble 'veep-pause-eeep', with the former, louder sound being inspiration. Breath sounds are loudest over the larger airways and decrease as the stethoscope is moved to the peripheral fields. Both inspiratory and expiratory movements usually are biphasic at rest. After each there is a pause, particularly after expiration. Abnormal lung sounds may consist of

- small explosive sounds without resonant tones (crackles), and
- various resonant or musical tones (wheezes).

Crackles can be so low pitched as to resemble thumping, or high pitched and staccato as a distant machine-gun. Wheezes also may be low pitched, as in groaning sounds, and high pitched so as to resemble a cooing dove or tin whistle. To exaggerate both normal breath sounds and any abnormal sounds it often is convenient to hold off the nostrils at the end of inspiration for approximately 30 seconds and listen carefully over both sides of the thorax immediately the nostrils are released. Alternatively, a plastic rebreathing bag (5–10 litre volume) may be held over, but not occluding, the nostrils to induce deep breathing while the lung fields are auscultated. It is extremely useful to determine that breath sounds can be heard both ventrally and dorsally, and that the heart sounds fade quite rapidly as one moves away from the hilar region.

Radiation of heart sounds dorsally is often indicative of pleural filling. Sometimes in normal horses, particularly if thin or if the heart rate is elevated, slightly thumping pulsations can be heard dorsally that may be due to radiation of flow murmurs from great blood vessels. In addition, on both sides of the thorax, but particularly the left side in the diaphragmatic region, low-pitched crackling sounds can be heard in normal horses. These appear to relate neither to air movement nor necessarily to movement of the thoracic wall under the stethoscope head. Whether these are muscular movements in the intercostal regions, or passive movement of lungs or of intestinal contents unrelated to peristalsis, but perhaps to diaphragmatic movement, is unclear. Auscultation with percussion, ballottement and other techniques is usually reserved for cases in which thoracic or possibly abdominal disease is suspected.

## Left thoracic limb

While listening to the thorax the proximal left thoracic limb can be visually and manually examined for swellings involving muscles, tendons, and joints, and the cranial sternal region can be palpated for edema or other enlargements or skin lesions.

The distal musculoskeletal structures of the left thoracic limb can be evaluated while the horse is weight bearing, and also after the limb is picked up, as for the left pelvic limb.

## Left neck

The superficial caudal cervical (so-called prescapular) lymph nodes, which are impossible to find in the normal horse, and the deep caudal cervical and cranial thoracic lymph nodes, which are occasionally palpable deeply in the ventral, caudal jugular groove, can be investigated manually. The jugular vein should be observed for normal filling up to approximately a third of the neck (with the head in a normal alert position) with each phase of systole. Occlusion of the jugular vein in its groove should result in very slow filling, which is best appreciated when the vein is released and the distended vessel quickly collapses.

Attention should then be paid to the neck region and any long mane flipped to the other side to give an appreciation of the nuchal region; this is very prominent in stallions and particularly obese horses, and especially ponies. Being a common site for intramuscular injections the dorsal and caudal neck musculature should be closely inspected and palpated deeply for evidence of adverse injection reactions.

## The head

Arriving at the head, the examiner can better consider all aspects by standing directly in front of the horse, comparing the symmetry of the two sides. Thus, both hands may be used to begin by palpating the pharyngeal

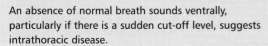

## Clinical Pointer

An absence of normal breath sounds ventrally, particularly if there is a sudden cut-off level, suggests intrathoracic disease.

## Clinical Pointer

Visible and palpable evidence of jugular vasculitis, perivasculitis, and even thrombosis or occlusion is usually indicative of previous intravenous medication and must be noted.

and laryngeal region, including the dorsal hyoid apparatus at the base of the ear. Guttural pouch swellings, salivary gland enlargements and lymphoid masses are usually clearly evident. Many horses resent deep palpation of the internal pinnae and the temporohyoid region, which can make it difficult to interpret an apparently exaggerated avoidance response.

Inspection of the ears often reveals evidence of aural plaque formation, although it is usually unnecessary to inspect the external auditory canal manually, a procedure resented by most horses. Facial, eye, jaw, nose and lip symmetry and movement can be clearly appreciated, both visually and palpably.

Discharge from the eye as well as the nose and mouth is usually readily apparent. Hydration status can be determined by the degree of wetness of the conjunctival, nasal, and oral membranes, and particularly by how well the eye is held forward in its bony orbit and by the turgidity of the palpebral skin. A fold of this skin is held tented for a few seconds and upon release normally returns to its flat contour within a second or so. With dehydration the tented skin will remain so for about 3 seconds (~5% dehydration) to 6 seconds (~10% dehydration), and the eyes will be dry and sunken within the bony orbits (~12–15% dehydration).

The frontal and maxillary sinuses can be percussed either by tapping with the end of a bent finger or by a finger-flick maneuver. In either case it is better if the examiner's other hand lies in the interdental space to cause the horse to open the mouth, allowing greater resonance of these air-filled structures. However, interpretation of these clearly inducible sounds can be problematical.

Further inspection of the nasal cavities can be achieved by placing the right hand flat on the dorsal nasal region, using the thumb to elevate the dorsolateral aspect of the nostril and enlarging the nasal ostium. This can be repeated with the left hand applied from the right side of the patient, using the left thumb. A penlight can then be used to illuminate

the rostral nasal region, looking particularly for any discharge from the nasal cavity or the nasolacrimal puncta in the ventral region, but also from the dorsolateral region and the nasal septum itself. The nasal septum can be transilluminated by applying the penlight into the opposite nasal cavity.

Most horses will allow the upper muzzle to be grasped, exposing the membranes of the dorsal gum and lip, and allow a hand to be placed in the interdental spaces (Fig. 8.3) to cause chewing movements and allowing inspection of the rostral oral cavity and lower gums. At this stage the examiner can smell the oral cavity for abnormal odors. Presumably because of oral commensal organisms, the normal equine mouth (and saliva) has a distinct, slightly pungent odor. However, with anorexia from any cause this will become very powerful and persist on the examiner's hand. Thus, the detection of anerobic processes (such as dental caries or periodontal disease) by noting a pungent (anerobic bacterial-like) odor from the mouth is problematic. The mouth can be viewed by grasping the tongue firmly but without pulling it rostrally, and rolling it to one side or flexing the tip dorsally with one hand (Fig. 8.4). Retracting the commissure of the lips and directing a penlight into the mouth with the opposite hand will allow easy inspection of the rostral dental arcades and midlingual region.

Routine palpation of the intermandibular and laryngeal regions for normal structures, symmetry, and any inducible cough should then be undertaken.

Place one to three fingers just lateral to the larynx on each side, to palpate this structure for symmetry.

In the majority of tall (over 16 hands) horses and in a large proportion of normal medium-sized horses, asymmetry to the dorsal and lateral intrinsic laryngeal musculature will be palpable. Although this finding may reflect degrees of recurrent laryngeal neuropathy it does not mean that the horse has any clinically evident laryngeal inspiratory embarrassment ('roaring'). Firm palpation of the larynx may induce normal horses to cough, but gentle palpation will not usually do so unless there is irritation to the upper respiratory structures, such as with rhinotracheitis.

While palpating the laryngeal region it is sometimes easy to detect the two freely mobile lobes of the thyroid glands, which move anywhere from dorsal to ventrolateral to the larynx and cranial tracheal rings on either side. These glands vary from 2 to 5 cm in diameter, but

---

### Examination of the eyes

Inspect each eye with a bright light, observing

- the clear anterior structures
- the pupillary responsiveness to light
- a view of the fundus by looking along the shaft of light directed through the pupil at the retina and optic disc (this will take practice)
- scleral and conjunctival color (interpret mild degrees of apparent pallor and jaundice very cautiously, particularly under artificial light).

---

### Clinical Pointer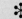

While inspecting the nasal cavity note any abnormal breath odor.

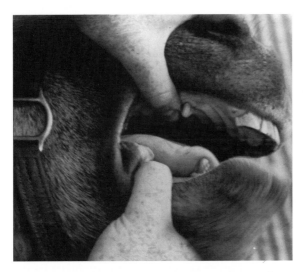

**Fig. 8.3** A horse can be prompted to open the mouth with one or more fingers in the interdental space, so that teeth and membranes can be viewed.

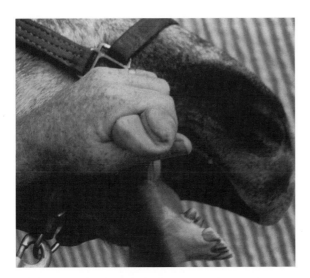

**Fig. 8.4** By gently grasping the tongue, without pulling it rostrally but rotating it between the molars, the jaws can be held open to allow better inspection of the rostral oral cavity.

may be somewhat asymmetric and may even be greatly enlarged without any clinical signs of thyroid dysfunction.

The air-filled guttural pouches medial to the mandible and parotid salivary gland are not palpable. Distension of these pouches with air, which usually occurs in foals and yearlings, results in a tympanitic swelling caudal to the mandible. The retropharyngeal lymph nodes are not normally palpable, but if enlarged will push the overlying parotid salivary glands laterally; deep palpation of this region will then reveal enlarged glands, or at least evidence of a localized painful response.

### Right thorax

The examination now proceeds down the right side of the neck, the thoracic limb, thorax, abdomen, and pelvic limb in a fashion similar to that undertaken on the left side. Some horses are more suspicious when approached on the right side and it is usual to have the handler move to that side as the examination proceeds. Notable differences on this side compared to the left thorax include

- absence of a cardiac apex beat
- much quieter heart sounds
- heart sounds loudest over the tricuspid region deep under the triceps muscle.

### Right abdomen

As well as the rumbling sounds of borborygmi on the right side there are frequently higher-pitched fluid and gas sounds in the right paralumbar fossa, relating to cecal activity. Often these sounds are audible without the use of a stethoscope in a quiet environment, depending partly on the condition of the horse and partly on its diet. Horses on lush pasture may have considerable splashing and tinkling fluid cecal sounds, whereas those on a high-fiber diet may have more lower-pitched rumblings. Simultaneous finger percussion and auscultation over the cecal area produces small (a few cm) to large (25 cm) areas of variable, dull to high-pitched resonance ('pings') which in normal horses change in tone quite quickly, indicating cecal motility.

---

### Submandibular lymph nodes

Normal submandibular lymph nodes are palpated as a sheet of coalescing small nodes up to 1 cm in diameter in the intermandibular space.

### Clinical Pointer

Foals may have benign goiter because of oversupplementation of the mare with iodine during pregnancy, but this usually abates with time.

Examination of the right side of the patient concludes with inspection of the musculoskeletal structures and with lifting up each right limb. The examiner then arrives back at the tail and will be able to register the rectal temperature on removal of the thermometer if this has not already been done. The anus and skin of the perineum and tail should be inspected for melanomas. This is an appropriate time to consider whether rectal examination is indicated.

## Rectal examination

If up to this stage there is any indication of systemic disease or of gastrointestinal, hepatic, genitourinary, or bilateral hindlimb disorders then a rectal examination should be undertaken. For various reasons many equine practitioners prefer to use the left arm for this procedure. The tail can then be held to the left side of the left arm and either held in place by an assistant, or the tail hairs held with the right hand on the dorsum of the pelvic region. Horses are more susceptible to iatrogenic rectal tears than are cattle and these can occur extremely rapidly. For the safety of both horse and examiner there are three very important factors that must be attended to in undertaking a rectal examination

- adequate restraint (chemical if necessary) of the patient
- use of a large amount of non-irritant lubricant
- patience on the part of the examiner.

In a proportion of cases previous scarring can be identified histologically at the site of an iatrogenic rectal tear, usually in the dorsal quadrant. Because of potentially fatal consequences it is important that pressure on the rectal lumen is minimized, especially by the examiner's knuckles, by

- holding the wrist and hand extended with the fingers and thumb close together
- minimizing the diameter around the examiner's metacarpophalangeal joints
- never forcing the hand against a contracted rectum.

A routine sequence of events should be undertaken for abdominal palpation per rectum. Because palpation of the reproductive tract is so frequently undertaken by equine practitioners it is sensible, because of familiarity, that this is undertaken first while the rectum is emptied of feces and adequate lubrication is applied. One can begin in the left caudal quadrant, proceeding along the left side of the abdomen to pass across the midline and back through the contents of the right cranial and caudal quadrants. The urinary bladder can usually be palpated if there is a liter or more of urine

present, as it bulges either in the pelvic inlet or just over the pelvic brim. The inguinal regions should be palpated and are easiest to recognize in stallions, when the inguinal vessels can be palpated on the ventrolateral aspect of the abdominal wall before they disappear into the slit-like inguinal rings. If the hand is then passed along the left abdominal wall it will reach the caudal aspect of the base of the spleen, which usually lies against this abdominal wall. The dorsal extent of the spleen can usually be reached and it is usually a short distance medially from there to the caudal pole of the left kidney, the region of the so-called nephrosplenic ligament. During palpation of this region and as the hand is drawn caudally the medial surface of the pelvic flexure can often be identified.

If an attempt is made to palpate the more cranial abdomen, then considerable patience may be required because of peristalsis and abdominal straining by the patient. From a functional point of view there does appear to be a sphincter effect between the small colon and rectum, which is approximately 40–50 cm cranial to the anus. To pass through this region and be able to palpate the midabdominal region, and even sometimes the right kidney in an average-sized horse, one must allow the cranial rectum to move along the fingers and hand rather than attempting to push through this region. This requires good lubrication, narrow knuckles, and patience. While waiting in this position the cranial mesenteric root often can be touched with the tips of the fingers in the midline or slightly to the right side. On the medial (left) aspect of this structure often one or more pulsating vessels can be palpated. As the examination proceeds caudally in the right middle quadrant the cranial and medial aspect of the cecum is usually palpated, and one or more cecal bands are usually prominent traveling from the right dorsal to the left ventral region of the abdomen. Medial to the cecum in the mid- to ventral abdomen fecal balls in the small colon will usually have been apparent, and any distended small intestine may be palpable dorsally. Returning to the dorsal midline, the terminal aorta and its quadrification into external and internal iliac arteries is usually apparent. Approximately 3 cm caudal to this on the dorsal midline a ventral bony protuberance representing the lumbosacral intervertebral disc will be

### Clinical Pointer

The pelvic flexure can be felt when drawing the hand caudally, if this is attempted while proceeding cranially the pelvic flexure often will fold on itself and be difficult to identify.

palpable, and a similar distance caudally the S1–S2 junction is usually less evident. In the region of the origin of the iliac arteries any enlargement of iliac lymph nodes may be palpable.

In concluding the abdominal and pelvic examination per rectum the pelvic cavity is palpably scanned and note taken of any irregularities to the surface of the rectal mucosa. Exiting the rectum, small mucosal defects, sand embedded on the mucosa and mucosal edema may all be evident. Anal tone should still be quite strong as the hand is removed, and the glove must then be inspected for abnormal material such as sand or blood. If blood is detected a new glove should be applied and, with or without the aid of sedation and/or epidural analgesia, the rectum examined extremely carefully for the site and extent of any mural or deeper defects.

## EXAMINATION DURING MOVEMENT

At this stage the patient may be taken out of its box to evaluate movement. While outside in daylight it can be worth reinspecting membranes, particularly vulval, conjunctival, nasal, and oral membranes, for any evidence of discoloration such as pallor or jaundice.

The animal may be observed moving around freely, especially if it is a foal that has not been handled. By this stage any normal foal will usually have proceeded to be observed suckling and will readily follow its dam. It is appropriate to observe how the horse moves while walking or trotting freely. In addition, a decision should be made whether to observe the horse working under tack and performing its expected duties.

## FURTHER READING

Baxter GM, Schlipf JW Jr. Handling, restraint and clinical evaluation. In: Colvic CN, Ames TR, Goer RJ (eds) The horse: diseases and clinical management. Philadelphia: WB Saunders, 1995; 23–34.

Koterba AM. Physical examination. In: Koterba AM, Drummond WH, Kosch PC (eds) Equine clinical neonatology. Philadelphia: Lea & Febiger, 1990; 71–83.

Madigan JE. Manual of equine neonatal medicine, 2nd edn. Woodland CA: Live Oak Publishing, 1991; 45–52.

Pinsent PJN, Fuller CJ. Outlines of clinical diagnosis in the horse, 2nd edn. Oxford: Blackwell Science, 1997.

Rose RJ, Hodgson DR. Manual of equine practice. Philadelphia: WB Saunders, 1993;1–23.

Rose RJ, Wright WD. Principles of patient evaluation and diagnosis. In: Colahan PT, Mayhew IG, Merritt AM, Moore JN (eds) Equine medicine and surgery, 4th edn. Vol 1. Goleta, CA: American Veterinary Publications, 1991; 51–81.

Speirs VC. Clinical examination of horses. Philadelphia: WB Saunders, 1997.

Taylor FGR, Hillyer MH. Diagnostic techniques in equine medicine. London: WB Saunders, 1993.

# 9
# Clinical Examination of Cattle and Calves

*O. M. Radostits*

Young heifers, mature cows, bulls, or calves are relatively easy to examine because the body systems are easily accessible clinically. The digestive tract, the cardiovascular system, the respiratory tract, the mammary gland, the reproductive organs, the urinary tract, the musculoskeletal system, the nervous system, and the skin can be examined easily in the field. In recumbent cattle a reliable examination may be difficult because the musculoskeletal and nervous systems are often difficult to examine adequately.

This chapter outlines a systematic method of clinical examination of cattle which will yield the most useful information necessary to make a diagnosis. The extent of the examination will depend on the nature of the complaint: a case of ringworm, for example, does not require a detailed examination. In cattle with suspected pneumonia, the emphasis is on examination of the respiratory tract. However, when presented with a mature lactating dairy cow that calved 10 days ago and is now anorexic and whose milk production has suddenly decreased markedly for no obvious reason, a detailed clinical examination is warranted.

## RESTRAINT OF CATTLE FOR CLINICAL EXAMINATION

Cattle are examined under many different circumstances and the veterinarian must ensure that adequate restraint is provided. Serious personal injuries and even death can occur from cattle kicking or trampling, and especially from bulls squeezing people against solid obstacles, which may happen in box stalls or handling chutes or even in an open field.

Before examining any animal the veterinarian must assess the circumstances to predict its behavior and

> ### Clinical Pointer
>
> Before handling cattle
>
> - assess the circumstances
> - ensure there is adequate restraint
> - approach the animal in its field of view.

what might happen, and make appropriate arrangements to avoid injury. Walking behind a fractious mature beef cow which is tied to a post or in any restraint device is potentially hazardous because cattle can kick both backwards and sideways. Cattle which are restrained by a halter or in a restraint device should always be approached within their angle of vision, so that they know the examiner is present. Once a presence has been established the examiner may proceed to touch the animal, gently at first and then more firmly while talking to it. The placing of a stethoscope over the thorax or abdomen of a beef cow, dairy bull or weaned beef calf may create sufficient apprehension and fright that the animal will jump from side to side. With some patience and perseverance most of these animals will adjust their behavior accordingly.

Most dairy cows are relatively easy to handle and restrain with a halter or if placed in stanchion-type handling stock. However, dairy cattle that are not halter trained will have to be coaxed into handling stocks. Modern dairy farms have good handling facilities and the attendants usually provide suitable restraint. Dairy cattle that are housed indoors and kept in stanchions are usually examined with no additional restraint, except for special circumstances when the feet need to be examined. Dairy calves can usually be examined by simple manual restraint, aided by holding them against a wall or in a corner.

Beef cattle are usually restrained in fixed handling facilities consisting of a chute and stocks, which restrains the animal and allows for maximum restraint of the head and neck with a head gate. A wide variety of chutes and head gates with many different supplementary features are now available. Many stocks are equipped with sides which can be adjusted for maximum restraint of the animal for examination and treatment procedures. The use of prolonged maximum restraint in a handling device can be stressful, and care must be taken not to use this equipment too harshly. The excitement and stress of being restrained can also result in an increase in body temperature by one or two degrees within 15 minutes.

Examination of the feet of all classes of cattle for lameness requires lifting the limbs, which is done effectively using ropes made into slings and pulleys, with the animal suitably restrained in a holding stanchion or similar device. Some large animal clinics have hydraulically operated surgical tables which can handle large bulls and cows for detailed examination of their feet. Lame cattle can also be allowed to walk freely and can be chased around several times in an enclosure for observation of abnormal gait.

In some situations groups of cattle can be inspected from a distance with no restraint. For example, when investigating epidemics in beef herds the first part of the examination may be to view the affected group or pen of animals from a distance. The veterinarian can walk among the animals, make some preliminary observations and identify and select certain animals for detailed clinical examination or necropsy. In the feedlot industry, cattle are commonly handled in groups in a handling chute and individually in restraint stocks.

## THE CLINICAL EXAMINATION

### History taking and examination of the environment

The principles of history taking and examination of the environment were discussed in earlier chapters.

> ### Clinical Pointer
>
> Never trust bulls over 6 months of age, and especially mature bulls. They require effective handling techniques and ideally, should possess a permanent nose ring which, along with suitable halters, assists their handling.

## Animal identification

All relevant information on the specific identification of the animal (eartag, tattoo, brand), its age, breed, sex, diet and stage of production cycle, including time of recent parturition or recent activities, such as bulls during the breeding season, should be obtained and recorded. In special circumstances, such as the certification of pedigree animals for sale or breed association registration, the color markings of the animal may have to be recorded.

## DISTANT EXAMINATION

### General inspection

This is done from a suitable distance, usually a few steps away, so that the entire animal can be seen. General observations are made and any abnormal noises noted. When cattle or calves are examined indoors with subdued light, or in dark barns at any time or outdoors during the night, it is important to use a flashlight to examine the various parts of the body.

### Demeanor

This is a reflection of the animal's mental state and its reaction to its internal and external environment. What is the animal doing? Is it bellowing, groaning or grunting? Is it eating and drinking, or does it ignore the feed and water available? Is the animal ruminating while being observed? Does it notice the observer? Is it indifferent? It may be bright and alert, apathetic, appear like a dummy, in a coma, restless or anxious, or be separated from the rest of the herd.

### Defecation and urination

The acts of defecation and urination are observed for evidence of difficulty and to determine the amounts of feces and urine passed. Difficult defecation may be accompanied by groaning. Difficult urination in a cow is often accompanied by a marked arching of the back, paddling of the hindlimbs, kicking out with the

> ### Clinical Pointer
>
> A recumbent animal that does not attempt to stand when approached suggests an abnormal situation requiring further investigation.

hindlimbs, and groaning. Difficult urination in a bull is characterized by a sawhorse stance, visible pulsations of the perineal urethra, holding up the tail and the passage of small amounts of urine or dribbling.

## Feces

Gross examination of the feces includes noting the amount passed in the previous several hours, the odor and consistency, and the presence of abnormal substances such as blood, fibrin or undigested feed particles.

## Attitude or posture

Does the animal stand normally and hold its head and neck normally? Are the ears, eyelids and tail normal? Does the animal lean against the wall? Abnormal postures are not necessarily indicative of disease: a dog-sitting position in a mature bull may be due to spondylosis or a behavioral attitude.

Some examples of abnormal postures in the standing animal are:

- alternate and frequent resting of limbs in laminitis, myositis or arthritis
- the 'sawhorse' attitude seen in tetanus and some forms of abdominal pain
- extension of the head and neck in severe pulmonary disease
- slight arching of the back and disinclination to move, as in acute traumatic reticuloperitonitis in cattle a disinclination to move may also indicate myositis, arthritis, or a fractured long bone
- kicking at the belly and swishing of the tail, as in cystitis and obstructive urolithiasis.

If the animal is recumbent, the following questions should be considered.

- Is the animal in sternal or lateral recumbency?
- Can it move itself from lateral to sternal recumbency?
- How long has it been recumbent?
- In what positions are the head and neck held?
- What is the position of the legs in the recumbent animal?

Normally, in sternally recumbent cattle the upper hindleg is clearly visible and the distal aspect of the lower hindleg is visible under the abdomen. The hindlegs may be rigidly outstretched in milk fever, broken femur, meningitis, and in spinal cord injury. In mature cattle with rupture of the adductor muscles, the hindlegs may be held in extension and directed forwards at about a 45° angle to the body. In spinal cord injury the hindlegs may assume a criss-cross pattern, or a frog-leg pattern because of flaccidity. Are the legs stretched out perpendicular to the long axis of the body? Is there any evidence of opisthotonos? Does the recumbent animal have the ability or the desire to rise? Does it struggle to rise and eventually get up or fall back down again?

## Gait

The animal is observed as the animal walks. Some examples of abnormal gaits include:

- ataxia or incoordination – inability to walk in a straight line, as in cerebellar ataxia or carbohydrate engorgement
- stiffness of limbs – lack of normal flexion and extension of the limbs when the animal walks. This is commonly associated with arthritis or myositis in calves and lambs, or degenerative joint disease in mature cattle
- shuffling or stumbling – shuffling gait and dragging toes on the ground as in laminitis or spondylitis
- walking in circles – often in one direction with deviation of the head and neck as in listeriosis.

## Body Condition Score

Body condition scoring (BCS) is a subjective method of assessing the amount of metabolizable energy stored in fat and muscle (body reserves) on a live animal. BCS in dairy cows is done using a variety of scales and systems. There is difficulty in interpreting the literature because of variability in the way authors apply scoring methods. In Australia an 8-grade system is used and a similar 10-point system is used in New Zealand. Body condition

---

### Thin versus emaciated

An animal that is physiologically thin usually has

- a good appetite
- a smooth shining haircoat, and
- works well.

An animal that is emaciated usually has

- an erect dry haircoat
- leathery dry skin
- prominent ribs and bones, and
- a dull demeanor.

scoring in the US is generally done according to a 0–5 scale. This method involves palpating the cow to assess the amount of tissue under the skin.

Figures 9.1a–f are schematic drawings of cows with body condition scores from 0 to 5. Figure 9.2 indicates the anatomical areas which are evaluated in scoring body condition in Holstein cows. Details of the scoring system are summarized in Figure 9.3.

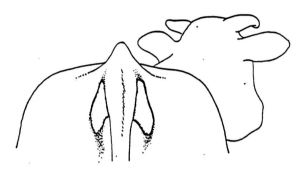

9.1a)
Score:            0
Condition:        Very poor
Tailhead area:    Deep cavity under tail and around tailhead. Skin drawn tight over pelvis with no tissue detectable in between.
Loin area:        No fatty tissue felt. Shapes of transverse processes clearly visible. Animal appears emaciated.

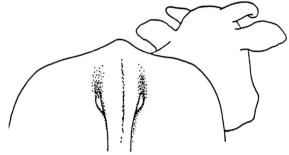

9.1c)
Score:            2
Condition:        Moderate
Tailhead area:    Shallow cavity lined with fatty tissue apparent at tailhead. Some fatty tissue felt under the skin. Pelvis easily felt.
Loin area:        Ends of transverse processes feel rounded but dorsal surfaces felt only with pressure. Depression visible in loin.

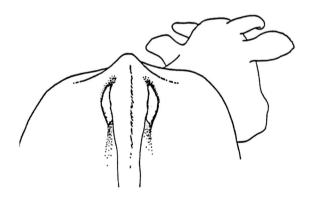

9.1b)
Score:            1
Condition:        Poor
Tailhead area:    Cavity present around tailhead. No fatty tissue felt between skin and pelvis, but skin is supple.
Loin area:        Ends of transverse processes sharp to touch and dorsal surfaces can be easily felt. Deep depression in loin.

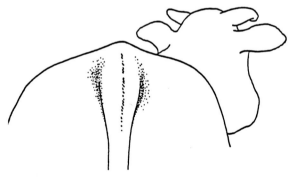

9.1d)
Score:            3
Condition:        Good
Tailhead area:    Fatty tissue easily felt over the whole area. Skin appears smooth but pelvis can be felt.
Loin area:        Ends of transverse processes can be felt with pressure but thick layer of tissue dorsum. Slight depression visible in loin.

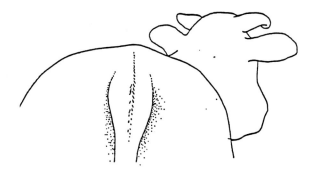
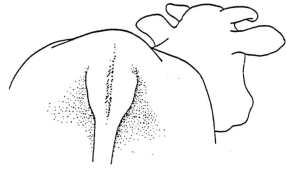

9.1e)
Score:       4
Condition:   Fat
Tailhead area:   Folds of soft fatty tissue present.
                 Patches of fat apparent under skin.
                 Pelvis felt only with firm pressure.

Loin area:       Transverse processes cannot be felt
                 even with firm pressure. No
                 depression visible in loin between
                 backbone and hip bones.

9.1f)
Score:       5
Condition:   Grossly fat
Tailhead area:   Tailhead buried in fatty tissue. Skin
                 distended. No part of pelvis felt even
                 with firm pressure.
Loin area:       Folds of fatty tissue over transverse
                 processes. Bone structure cannot be
                 felt.

**Figure 9.1 a–f**   Body Condition Scoring

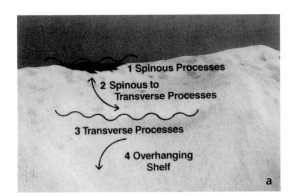
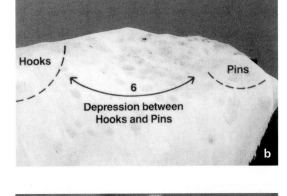
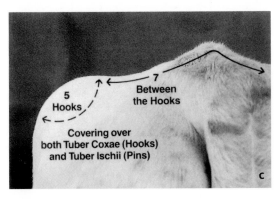
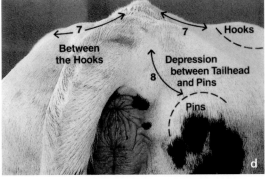

**Fig. 9.2 a–d.**   Anatomical areas evaluated in scoring body condition of Holstein cows (see Fig. 9.3). Figures courtesy of Upjohn International Animal Health. The Upjohn Company, Kalamazoo, MI. 49001. USA

Body condition scoring chart for Holstein cows.

| | | 1 Spinous processes (SP) (anatomy varies) | 2 Spinous to Transverse processes | 3 Transverse processes | 4 Overhanging shelf (care – rumen fill) | 5 Tuber coxae (hooks) & Tuber ischii (pins) | 6 Between pins and hooks | 7 Between the hooks | 8 Tailhead to pins (anatomy varies) |
|---|---|---|---|---|---|---|---|---|---|
| SEVERE UNDERCONDITIONING (emaciated) | 1.00 | individual processes distinct, giving a saw-tooth appearance | deep depression | very prominent, >1/2 length visible | definite shelf, gaunt, tucked | extremely sharp, no tissue cover | severe depression, devoid of flesh | severely depressed | bones very prominent with deep "V" shaped cavity under tail |
| | 1.25 | | | | | | | | |
| | 1.50 | | | | | | very sunken | | |
| | 1.75 | sharp, prominent ridge | | 1/2 length of process visible | | | | | bones prominent "U" shaped cavity formed under tail |
| FRAME OBVIOUS | 2.00 | individual processes evident | obvious depression | between 1/2 to 1/3 of processes visible | prominent shelf | prominent | | | |
| | 2.25 | | | | | | thin flesh covering | definite depression | first evidence of fat |
| | 2.50 | sharp, prominent ridge | | 1/3-1/4 visible | | | | | |
| | 2.75 | | | <1/4 visible | moderate shelf | | | moderate depression | |
| FRAME & COVERING WELL BALANCED | 3.00 | | smooth concave curve | appears smooth, TP's just discernable | slight shelf | smooth | depression | | bones smooth, cavity under tail shallow & fatty tissue lined |
| | 3.25 | smooth ridge, the SP's not evident | smooth slope | distinct ridge, no individual processes discernable | | | | slight depression | |
| | 3.50 | | | | | covered | slight depression | | |
| | 3.75 | | | smooth, rounded edge | | | sloping | | |
| FRAME NOT AS VISIBLE AS COVERING | 4.00 | flat, no processes discernable | nearly flat | | none | rounded with fat | flat | flat | bones rounded with fat and slight fat-filled depression under tail |
| | 4.25 | | | edge barely discernable | | | | | |
| | 4.50 | | | | | | | | |
| | 4.75 | | | | | buried in fat | | | bones buried in fat, cavity filled with fat forming tissue folds |
| SEVERE OVERCONDITIONING | 5.00 | buried in fat | rounded (convex) | buried in fat | bulging | | rounded | rounded | |

This chart was developed by A.J. Edmondson, I.J. Lean, L.D. Weaver, T. Farver, and G. Webster. It is reproduced courtesy of the *Journal of Dairy Science*.

**Fig. 9.3** Body condition scoring chart for Holstein cows.

## Conformation

The symmetry of the head and neck, limbs, thorax, and abdomen is inspected. Are there any obvious abnormalities?

## Haircoat, skin and subcutaneous tissues

### Haircoat

The lustre of the haircoat and any discoloration are noted. Shedding of hair is seasonal. If there is alopecia (loss of hair). Is it general or local? Is there any evidence of ectoparasites, such as lice, which are best seen over the dorsum of the withers and the back?

### Skin

The state of hydration and the degree are assessed. The skin is inspected for evidence of hypertrophy, wrinkling, discoloration, hemorrhages, eruptions, injuries and pruritus, and staining by feces as in calves with diarrhea or mature cows with Johne's disease.

### Subcutaneous tissues

The subcutaneous tissues are examined for evidence of edema, urticaria, hematomas, abscesses, inflammatory swellings, emphysema and peripheral lymph node enlargements.

## Unusual odor

Unusual odors are noted. An acetone odor may be present around the mouth and on the breath of dairy cattle with acetonemia. A necrotic odor may emanate from the breath of an animal with gangrenous pneumonia. A foul odor is common around the hind quarters of a recently calved cow with septic metritis.

# PARTICULAR DISTANT EXAMINATION

Each body region is inspected from a suitable distance.

## Head and neck and associated structures

### Mental status

When assessing the animal's mental status consider if the animal is

- bright and alert
- depressed
- lethargic
- dejected
- in a state of stupor.

### Symmetry of head

The head is examined for any obvious abnormalities such as swellings and bony enlargements. Are there any obvious abnormalities of the horns? Has the animal been dehorned recently?

### Ears

The ears are observed for their normal carriage. One or both ears may be drooped, which in calves may indicate otitis externa. In hypomagnesemia the ears may be flickering. Does the animal use its ears when turning towards an extraneous sound?

### Eyes and eyelids

The eyes are observed for normal opening. Are the eyes closed? Does the animal attempt to keep the eye closed because it appears painful? Ocular discharges commonly accumulate at the medial canthus and stream down the face, and may be copious and serous or mucopurulent. The upper eyelid of one eye may be drooped, as in unilateral facial paralysis in listeriosis. The nictitating membrane is noted for evidence of protrusion, the presence of abnormal masses, discoloration and inflammation. The state of the eyeballs is inspected for size, evidence of retraction as in dehydration, and obvious abnormalities of the cornea, sclera or pupils.

The degree of dehydration can be assessed by the amount of space between the eye and the orbit (the sunken eye). See Table 14.1, Chapter 14.

### Muzzle

The muzzle is normally moist with beads of moisture. Abnormalities from a distance include

- a dry muzzle indicating systemic illness or cardiovascular collapse, for example hypocalcemia in recently calved lactating cattle or dehydration in diarrheic calves
- an inflamed muzzle indicating photosensitization or infections of the oral cavity, for example mucosal disease
- abnormal nasal discharges that accumulate on the surface of the muzzle resulting in the formation of a muzzle crusting which eventually peels, these have various causes

### The pupillary light reflex

While examining the eyes, test the pupillary light reflex using a strong, pointed light such as a flashlight or penlight.

- the presence of rumen contents in the nostrils indicating recent regurgitation of rumen contents, for example a cow with third-stage milk fever.

### Nostrils (external nares)

The nostrils are normally coated with a thin film of serous discharge which normal animals regularly lick off. The accumulation of an excessive quantity or abnormal discharge may indicate disease of the respiratory tract or the failure to lick off the discharge if the animal is depressed for any reason. The nasal discharge may be abnormal in amount or character including the presence of blood in one or both nostrils. The nares normally dilate and constrict slightly with each respiration and excessive movements are associated with dyspnea.

### Mouth

Inspection of the external aspects of the mouth may reveal that the mouth is held open slightly, the presence of excessive saliva drooling from the mouth, slight protrusion of the tongue, excessive jaw or chewing movements, and all of which suggest abnormalities of the oral cavity which must be examined as part of the close physical examination.

### Appetite and prehension

Cattle with a normal appetite, grasp feed with their tongues and bite grass with their incisors and dental pad. A cow attempting to grasp feed without the use of its tongue is suggestive of the presence of a painful condition of the oral cavity. Cattle which appear hungry and push their muzzle into a source of feed as if to eat but are unable to protrude their tongue may have a painful lesion of the oral cavity such as glossitis or paralysis of the tongue due to a cranial nerve lesion. Cattle normally suck water through their lips; if they lap water with their tongues, painful conditions of the teeth such as fluorosis may be present.

### Mastication

Mastication or chewing can easily be observed from a distance. Rapid and incomplete mastication with dropping of feed suggests a painful condition of the oral cavity. Slow mastication may suggest the presence of encephalopathy. Bruxism or grinding of the teeth occurs in states of increased intracranial pressure, encephalomalacia and abdominal pain.

---

### Clinical Pointer

A fractured mandible may be manifested by a dropped jaw with the mouth held partially open.

---

### Swallowing

Painful swallowing manifested by alternate extension and flexion of the neck, gagging, and drooling of saliva mixed with feed may be associated with the presence of a foreign body in the pharynx or esophagus, or the existence of pharyngitis or laryngitis. Regurgitation and dropping cuds on the ground suggests disease of the esophagus or the cardia of the reticulorumen.

### Neck

The entire length of the neck and submandibular region is inspected. Normally the jugular veins are not visibly full and a jugular pulse is visible about one-third the distance of the neck from the thoracic inlet. Abnormalities of the jugular veins include

- engorgement
- venous pulsations which extend up to the proximal part of the neck at the angle of the jaw
- diffuse enlargements of one or both jugular grooves due to thrombophlebitis associated with previous intravenous injections or prolonged intravenous catheterization.

There may be enlargement of the brisket or submandibular space due to edema or abscessation. The prescapular lymph node region is inspected for evidence of enlargement. Other enlargements of the neck may indicate tumors, abscesses, lymphatic enlargements, or periesophageal fistulae as a sequela to traumatic pharyngitis caused by careless use of a balling gun.

Abnormal swallowing movements, manifested as undulations of the skin due to esophageal motility, may be visible on the left side of the neck.

## Thorax

### Respirations

#### Rate

The normal respiratory rates (breaths/minute) of different classes and ages of cattle are as follows:

- mature beef cow 12–30
- mature dairy cow 20–30
- housed dairy calf 24–36.

Considerable variation in the respiratory rate can occur without any pathological change in the respiratory tract. The rate increases when animals are standing in the sun for long periods, when they are excited or handled, in obese animals, in states of acid–base imbalance, during restraint, after long transportation, and in the holds of ships and cabins of airplanes. The rate usually decreases during the cold winter months.

## Clinical Pointer

To inspect the respirations of cattle stand behind and slightly to the side of the animal. Note the movements of the thoracic and abdominal walls during each respiration and determine the respiratory

- rate
- type
- depth, and
- rhythm.

## Type

Respirations may be abdominal or thoracic (costal) which reflects the relative movements of the thoracic wall (costal breathing) or the abdominal wall (abdominal breathing). In cattle they are normally costoabdominal, with the thoracic and abdominal walls participating equally.

## Rhythm

The normal rhythm is inspiration, expiration, pause.

- Prolonged inspiration indicates upper respiratory tract disease causing reduction of the diameter of the upper airways, especially the larynx.
- Prolonged expiration indicates lower respiratory tract disease, such as pneumonia, pulmonary edema and pulmonary emphysema.

## Depth

The depth of respirations is an assessment of the length of inspiration and expiration. Respirations may be shallow or deep, and are assessed by observing the movements of the abdominal and thoracic walls:

- polypnea is rapid shallow respirations
- tachypnea is very rapid shallow respirations similar to panting

## Abdominal and thoracic breathing

- Prominent **abdominal** wall movements suggest painful conditions of the thorax such as pleurisy, which restrict thoracic wall movements and exaggerate those of the abdominal wall.
- Prominent **thoracic** wall movements may occur in severe pulmonary disease, as in severe pulmonary edema, pneumonia, and pulmonary emphysema. The accessory muscles of respiration are used and respirations become exaggerated, with marked movements of the intercostal muscles.

- hyperpnea is an increase in the depth of respirations
- dyspnea is labored respirations, usually associated with varying degrees of extension of the head and neck, excessive dilatation of the nostrils, abduction of the elbows, excessive abdominal or thoracic movements, accompanied by an expiratory grunt, mouth breathing, and prominent activity of the intercostal muscles.

### Respiratory noises

Respiratory noises are those which are audible without the aid of a stethoscope and may be audible several steps or more from the animal. They include

- coughing due to irritation of the pharynx, trachea and bronchi
- snorting due to nasal irritation
- wheezing due to stenosis of the nasal passages
- snoring due to pharyngeal obstruction
- inspiratory stridor due to laryngeal or tracheal lesions
- expiratory grunting and groaning associated with the thoracic pain of advanced pulmonary disease, especially pleural pain.

## Abdomen

Abnormalities of the abdomen and associated structures in cattle and calves are visible by careful inspection from a distance. Variations in abdominal size are usually noted during the general inspection of the animal. Distension of the abdomen may be due to the presence of excess feed, fluid, feces, flatus, or fat, or the presence of a large fetus or intra-abdominal neoplasms. Further differentiation is usually possible only on close examination, although fetal movements may be visible in the right flank of cattle. Gaseous distension of the intestines usually results in uniform distension of the dorsal portion of the abdomen, whereas excess fluid in the peritoneal cavity or in the uterus causes distension ventrally. The term 'gaunt' is often used to describe a decrease in abdominal size. It occurs most commonly in starvation, in severe prolonged diarrhea, and in many chronic diseases where appetite is reduced.

Inspection of the ventral abdomen may reveal the presence of an umbilical hernia or an enlarged umbilicus associated with omphalophlebitis in the calf. Ventral body wall edema is commonly associated with approaching parturition in dairy cattle, gangrenous mastitis, congestive heart failure, and rupture of the urethra due to obstructive urolithiasis.

> ### Clinical Pointer
>
> Ruminal movements are observable over the left abdominal wall from a distance, but are better examined at a later stage.

## External genitalia

### Male

Gross enlargements or prolapse of the prepuce are readily visible. Abnormalities of the scrotum, including asymmetrical enlargements, are obvious. Degenerative changes in the testicles may result in a small scrotum.

### Female

The vulva of the female is observed for lesions of the skin, gross swellings and edema, which may be associated with impending parturition or result from dystocial injuries. Discharges of purulent material and blood from the vulva may accumulate below the vulva or on the tail, and may indicate abnormalities of the genitourinary tract.

### Mammary gland

The mammary gland is inspected from both the side and the rear. Special attention is given to the symmetry of the four quarters and the shape and state of the teats. The skin of the udder and teats is visually inspected for evidence of lesions. A disproportionate size of the quarters of the udder suggests acute inflammation, atrophy or hypertrophy of a gland. These conditions can be differentiated only by palpation. The shape of the teats is noted.

## Limbs and feet

Abnormalities of posture and gait are noted. The symmetry of the locomotor system is important and pairs of limbs and feet should be compared when there is doubt about the significance of an apparent abnormality. Enlargement or distortion of bones, joints, tendons, sheaths and bursae should be noted, as well as any enlargement of peripheral lymph nodes and lymphatic vessels. The feet of all four limbs are inspected for evidence of overgrowth or abnormalities of the hooves, excessive wear of the toes of the claws, and abnormalities of the interdigital cleft.

## CLOSE PHYSICAL EXAMINATION

The close physical examination of a cow begins at the rear of the animal, where several observations and evaluations can be made quickly and efficiently. Before examining the cow, especially a lactating dairy cow which may have acetonemia, a **urine** sample is usually easily obtained by manually stroking the skin just below the vulva, which usually initiates urination. The entire stream of urine flow can be observed and a sample taken.

Next, the **rectal temperature** is taken. During this procedure the **vulvar mucous membranes** may be everted and examined for discoloration and the presence of discharges and lesions. The **pulse rate** can be counted and assessed using the middle coccygeal artery of the tail at about the level of the tip of the vulva. The rate and character of the **respirations** may be noted again at this time. The **haircoat** and skin are assessed for evidence of dehydration, loss of hair and skin lesions. The area over the **tailhead** and the perineal region are inspected for any evidence of skin lesions, such as mange, and genital discharges. The amount and nature of **feces** in the immediate vicinity of the animal are noted, and any abnormalities should be further investigated by obtaining more history.

## CLOSE EXAMINATION OF BODY REGIONS AND SYSTEMS

The various body regions and systems are then examined systematically in the following sequence:

- left side – thorax, neck, abdomen (rumen), prescapular and prefemoral lymph nodes
- right side – thorax, neck, abdomen (abomasum and intestines), prescapular and prefemoral lymph nodes
- ventral abdomen (umbilicus)
- head and mouth
- mammary gland
- rectal examination – reproductive tract, urinary tract (bladder, ureters, urethra and kidneys), alimentary tract, bony skeleton, blood vessels and lymph nodes
- genitourinary system
- musculoskeletal system
- nervous system
- hair and skin.

## Left side

The animal is examined on the left side in the following systematic manner.

### Left thorax and neck

Examination of the thorax includes palpation, auscultation and percussion of the cardiac area and the lungs, and inspection and palpation of the neck and associated structures.

## Heart

The heart is examined by auscultation. The points to be noted are the rate, rhythm, intensity and quality of heart sounds, and whether abnormal sounds are present. Comparison of the heart and pulse rates will determine whether there is a **pulse deficit** due to weak heart contractions failing to cause palpable pulse waves: this is most likely to occur with cardiac arrhythmias. While auscultating the heart, the pulse may be evaluated simultaneously by palpation of the median artery in the medial aspects of the forelimb.

## Lungs

Auscultation and acoustic percussion of the thorax are the primary methods for examination of the lungs. Auscultation of both lung fields for the presence of normal breath sounds and abnormal breath sounds is an important part of the examination of the thorax of cattle. Auscultation of the dorsal, middle and lower thirds of both lung fields is a reliable method to evaluate the differences in breath sounds in different parts of the lung. As most cases of pneumonia in cattle are bronchogenic the cranioventral aspects of both lung fields will be affected first and most severely.

Acoustic percussion of the thorax is a valuable diagnostic aid if the lung sounds are muffled over the ventral aspects of the thorax, suggesting the presence of a pleural effusion (see Chapter 16). Palpation of the thoracic wall, including deep digital palpation of the intercostal spaces while auscultating over the trachea, may elicit a grunt, which indicates thoracic pain associated with pleuritis.

---

### Pericardial friction sounds

Pericardial friction sounds are abnormal sounds not related to the cardiac cycle. They occur with each heart cycle but are not specifically related to either systolic or diastolic sounds. They are more superficial, more distinctly heard than murmurs, and have a to-and-fro character. Local pleuritic friction sounds may be confused with pericardial sounds, especially if respiratory and cardiac rates are equal. Additional details for the examination of the heart are given in Chapter 14.

---

### Clinical Pointer

To auscultate the anteroventral aspects of the lungs depress the triceps muscle and insert the stethoscope into the axilla (see Chapter 16).

---

## *Left neck and associated structures*

### Brisket, jugular veins, and trachea

The left neck is inspected and palpated for evidence of enlargements, such as brisket edema, abscesses or other swellings. An important part of the examination of the neck of cattle is to determine the state of the jugular veins. Normally these appear almost collapsed. A pulse of small magnitude moving up the jugular vein about one-third of the way up the neck is normal in most animals but must be differentiated from a transmitted carotid pulse, which is not obliterated by compression of the jugular vein at a lower level. When the jugular pulse is associated with each cardiac movement it should be determined whether it is physiological or pathological:

- a normal jugular pulse is presystolic and due to atrial systole
- a pathological jugular pulse is commonly systolic and occurs simultaneously with the arterial pulse and the first heart sound; it is characteristic of an insufficient tricuspid valve.

If the jugular vein is compressed digitally in the middle of the neck, the vein should fill above the point of compression and be empty distal to that point. If the jugular vein is obvious and feels tense then it is full and engorged. When an engorged jugular vein is compressed digitally, the vein below the point of compression will remain full: this is known as the positive venous stasis test. Bilateral engorgement of the jugular veins may be due to obstruction by compression or constriction from a space-occupying mass in the thoracic inlet, or to right-sided congestive heart failure. Further details on examination of the jugular veins in cattle are given in Chapter 14.

**Tracheal auscultation** is a useful diagnostic aid. Normally, the sounds which are audible are louder and more distinct than breath sounds audible over the lungs. In upper respiratory tract disease such as laryngitis and tracheitis, the sounds are louder and harsher and may be whistling in the presence of stenosis. Very loud stenotic tracheal sounds are characteristic in calves with tracheal collapse. Abnormal tracheal sounds regardless of their cause are usually transferred down the major bronchi and are audible on auscultation over the thorax, primarily during inspiration.

### Left side of abdomen

This particularly includes examination of the left paralumbar fossa and the left lateral abdominal wall.

#### Left paralumbar fossa and lateral abdominal wall

The left paralumbar fossa and the rumen are examined by inspection, auscultation, palpation and ballottement, and percussion and simultaneous auscultation. Movements of the left abdominal wall caused by contractions of the rumen can be seen, felt, and heard at the same time.

*Inspection*

The left paralumbar fossa and the movements of the rumen are best evaluated by viewing the area from a slightly oblique angle. The concavity of the left paralumbar fossa or the hollow of the flank is inspected. The fossa may be deep because of a relatively empty rumen, it may be bulging because of a full rumen, or it may be markedly distended as in bloat or rumen overload.

The alternate rising and sinking of the left paralumbar fossa in healthy cows is associated with the concurrent contraction and relaxation of the dorsal sac of the rumen. It occurs more frequently and is seen more easily in the dairy cow during and after eating and during rumination, and is apparent in both standing and recumbent animals. The movements are best seen in dairy cattle with a well groomed haircoat: a rough haircoat may obscure the movements.

*Palpation*

The **rumen pack** is the mass of rumen contents which can be palpated through the abdominal wall in the left paralumbar fossa. It is normally doughy and pits on digital pressure. Normally the rumen contractions can be felt while the rumen is being auscultated in the fossa, and can be correlated with the audible rumen sounds associated with the primary and secondary contractions. The presence of palpable rumen contractions without concurrent sounds is significant. The presence of 3–5 ripples per minute in the left paralumbar fossa and left lower flank region, without

---

**Clinical Pointer**

Abnormal tracheal sounds are commonly confused with abnormal lung sounds due to pneumonia. However in pneumonia the abnormal sounds are usually present on both inspiration and expiration.

---

being able to hear the concurrent typical sounds of the rumen contractions, suggests hyperactivity of the rumen associated with vagus indigestion, in which the rumen contents may be homogeneous and frothy.

*Auscultation*

The ruminal movements should be auscultated for a total of at least 3 minutes. During the first part of the primary cycle of rumen motility (during the contraction of the dorsal sac after the biphasic contraction of the reticulum), the fossa rises and loud booming thunderous crackling sounds are audible with the stethoscope over an area extending from the middle of the fossa cranially to the upper third of the area of the 10th to 13th ribs. The sounds associated with the contraction of the dorsal sac gradually become louder, reach a crescendo and then fade away, over a period of about 5–8 seconds. This is quickly followed in about 2–4 seconds by the second part of the primary contraction, in which the ventral sac contracts and produces sounds which are similar to but not as loud as those of the dorsal sac. The frequency of complete primary contractions ranges from three per 2 minutes to four per 3 minutes.

The secondary cycle of rumen motility involves contraction of the dorsal sac and then the ventral sac, not preceded by contractions of the reticulum. Secondary contractions occur approximately every 2 minutes between primary contractions, and are usually associated with a concurrent eructation. Primary contractions are usually longer and louder than secondary contractions. Rumen stasis or **atony** is characterized by either a lack of audible sounds or weak sounds that may be normal in frequency or occur only once every few minutes. Weak sounds with normal frequency may indicate the presence of a viscus between the rumen and the abdominal wall, as may occur in left-side displacement of the abomasum. The presence of fluid-tinkling or splashing sounds over the rumen suggests stasis along with excessive quantities of fluid, as in carbohydrate engorgement. Spontaneous percolating or tinkling sounds may be audible over the ruminal area when there is left-side displacement of the abomasum.

*Percussion and simultaneous auscultation*

This is performed over the dorsal third of the left abdominal wall between the 10th and 13th ribs, extending caudally up into the left paralumbar fossa. Its purpose is to detect the presence of a '**ping**', which may indicate the presence of a gas-filled viscus such as left-sided displacement of the abomasum, or a low-pitched '**pung**' indicating an atonic rumen.

*Ballottement and simultaneous auscultation*

Ballottement of the left ventral abdominal wall just ventral to the left paralumbar fossa while auscultating with the stethoscope over the 13th rib may elicit fluid-splashing sounds, which may indicate excessive quantities of fluid in the rumen, as in carbohydrate engorgement or the presence of a left-sided displacement of the abomasum containing fluid.

## Left prescapular and prefemoral lymph nodes

These are located and palpated for evidence of enlargement, this may be difficult if the animal is obese.

## Right side

### Right thorax and neck

The right side of the thorax, neck, jugular veins, brisket and trachea are examined in the same way as the left side. The right prescapular and prefemoral lymph nodes are inspected and palpated for evidence of enlargement.

### Right side of abdomen

The right side of the abdomen is examined by inspection, palpation, percussion, and simultaneous auscultation, ballottement, succussion, and tactile percussion.

### Right paralumbar fossa and right lateral abdominal wall

*Palpation*

The right lateral abdominal wall is palpated behind the right costal arch from the dorsal to ventral aspects for evidence of distended viscera, gravid uterus, and an enlarged liver.

*Percussion and simultaneous auscultation*

This is used to detect the presence of 'pings' associated with the following:

- cecal dilatation and cecal volvulus
- abomasal dilatation and abomasal volvulus
- intestinal tympany due to paralytic ileus or fluid-filled intestines due to acute intestinal obstruction
- pneumoperitoneum following a laparotomy
- postpartum pings (due to local intestinal tympany and occurring most commonly in lactating dairy cattle within a few days after calving).

*Ballottement of the right lateral abdominal wall*

Ballottement is used to detect the presence of firm masses in the right abdomen. After 7–8 months

> ### Enlarged liver
>
> An enlarged liver may be palpable as a firm structure immediately behind the costal arch, extending from the dorsal aspect of the right paralumbar fossa to the ventral right flank. The area of liver dullness can be outlined using acoustic percussion and a liver biopsy may be taken for special examination.

gestation the gravid uterus is easily ballotted. The procedure may reveal **fluid-splashing sounds**, indicating the presence of fluid-filled intestines in acute intestinal obstruction or fluid-filled viscera such as in abomasal dilatation or abomasal volvulus or cecal dilatation and cecal volvulus.

*Tactile percussion*

This is sharp percussion of one side of the abdomen while observing and palpating for the presence of an undulation of the opposite side, which is known as a **fluid wave**. This suggests the presence of excessive quantities of fluid in the peritoneal cavity, or ascites.

**Detection of abdominal pain**

Cattle with acute local or diffuse peritonitis may **grunt** with almost every expiration or if they walk a few steps. In the recumbent position the grunt may be exaggerated. Grunting may also be caused by severe pneumonia, pleurisy, and diffuse pulmonary emphysema and pericarditis. Careful auscultation and percussion of the lungs is therefore necessary to exclude the presence of pulmonary disease.

Not all grunts occur spontaneously. Deep palpation of the cranial part of the abdomen using the closed hand or knee is often necessary to elicit a grunt. The objective is to locate painful sites over the ventral abdomen most closely associated with the reticulum, because of the common occurrence of traumatic reticuloperitonitis as a cause of abdominal pain. Simultaneous auscultation with a stethoscope over the trachea may be necessary to hear a grunt.

The ventral aspect and both sides of the abdomen should be examined, beginning at the level of the xiphoid sternum and moving caudally to a point distal to the umbilicus. A grunt usually means the presence of a lesion of the peritoneum, pleura or pericardium (stretching, inflammation, edema).

The absence of a grunt does not preclude the presence of a peritoneal lesion. In acute traumatic reticuloperitonitis the grunt may be absent or barely audible, or inconclusive, within 3–5 days after the initial penetration of the reticulum.

---

### Deep palpation of the abdomen to locate painful abdominal sites

- auscultate over the trachea for inspiratory and expiratory sounds over the trachea for a few breaths
- apply deep palpation pressure to the abdomen with the closed fist or a knee
- apply the pressure at the end of inspiration and beginning of expiration
- make several attempts to elicit a grunt before assuming its absence
- start palpation just caudal to the xiphoid sternum and extend to both the left and right sides of the abdomen.

---

**Pinching of the withers** is also used to elicit a grunt. In the average-sized cow pinching the withers causes the animal to depress its back. In an animal with a lesion of the peritoneum, pleura or pericardium the pinch will commonly result in a grunt, which may be audible without auscultation over the trachea, but auscultation is usually necessary. Pinching the withers is difficult in very large mature cows and bulls.

### Paracentesis

Fluid can be obtained from the peritoneal cavity, pleural cavity, pericardial sac, joint cavities and subcutaneous swellings for laboratory analysis. These samples are useful for the diagnosis of peritonitis, pleuritis, pericarditis and cellulitis.

## Head and associated structures

The head, including the eyes, nostrils and nasal cavities and mouth, is examined in detail if the initial examination indicates the presence of abnormalities.

---

### Clinical Pointer

In large mature cows and bulls it may be necessary to use a horizontal rigid bar or wooden pole to elicit a grunt. The bar is held by two people in a horizontal position just behind the xiphoid sternum; a third person auscultates over the trachea as the bar is quickly lifted up into the abdominal wall. The process is repeated several times to ensure that a grunt, if present, can be elicited and heard.

---

### Eyes

The eyes and eyelids are examined for evidence of ocular discharges and abnormalities.

**Ocular discharge**
The nature of the ocular discharge is noted and whether it is unilateral or bilateral.

**Abnormalities of the eyelids**
These include abnormal movement, position and thickness. Movement of the eyelids may be excessive in painful eye conditions or in cases of nervous irritability, including hypomagnesemia, lead poisoning, and encephalitis. The lids may be kept permanently closed when there is pain in the eye, or when the eyelids are swollen, as for instance in local edema due to photosensitization or allergy. The membrana nictitans may be displaced across the eye when there is pain in the orbit, or in tetanus or encephalitis. There may be tumors on the eyelids.

**Examination of the conjunctiva**
This provides an indication of the state of the peripheral circulation. The pallor of anemia and the yellow coloration of jaundice may be visible, although they are more readily observed on the oral or vaginal mucosae. Engorgement of the scleral vessels, petechial hemorrhages, edema of the conjunctiva – as in gut edema of pigs or congestive heart failure – dryness due to acute pain or high fever are all readily observable abnormalities.

**Corneal abnormalities**
These include opacity varying from the faint cloudiness of early keratitis to the solid white of advanced keratitis, often with associated vascularization, ulceration and scarring. Increased convexity of the cornea is usually due to increased pressure within the eyeball and may be caused by glaucoma or hypopyon.

**Size of the eyeball**
This does not usually vary, but protrusion is relatively common and when unilateral is due in most cases to pressure from behind the orbit. In cattle periorbital lymphoma, dislocation of the mandible and periorbital hemorrhage are common causes. Retraction of the eyeballs is a common manifestation of reduction in volume of periorbital tissues from

- starvation when there is disappearance of fat, or
- dehydration when there is loss of fluids.

### Abnormal eyeball position and movements

These include nystagmus and abnormal positioning of the eyeball. In nystagmus there is periodic involuntary movement with a slow component in one direction and a quick return to the original position. The movement may be horizontal, vertical, or rotatory. In paralysis of the motor nerves to the orbital muscles there is restriction of movement and abnormal position of the eyeball at rest (strabismus).

### Pupillary light reflex

The pupillary light reflex – closure of the pupil in response to light is best tested with a strong flashlight. An abnormal degree of dilatation is an important sign, unilateral abnormality usually suggesting a lesion of the orbit. Bilateral excessive dilatation (mydriasis) occurs in local lesions of the central nervous system affecting the oculomotor nucleus, or in diffuse lesions including encephalopathies, or in functional disorders such as botulism and anoxia. Peripheral blindness due to bilateral lesions of the orbits may have a similar effect. Excessive constriction of the pupils (miosis) is unusual unless there has been overdose with organo phosphate insecticides or parasympathomimetic drugs. Opacity of the lens is readily visible, especially in advanced cases.

### Deep structures of the eye

These can be examined satisfactorily only with an ophthalmoscope, but gross abnormalities may be observed by direct vision. Hypopyon – pus in the anterior chamber – is usually manifested by yellow to white opacity, often with a horizontal upper border obscuring the iris. The pupil may be abnormal in shape or position owing to adhesions to the cornea or other structures.

### Tests of vision and ocular reflexes

A number of such tests are easily carried out and, when warranted, should be done at this stage of the examination. Tests for blindness include the **menace reflex** and an **obstacle test**. In the former a manual threat to the eye is simulated, care being taken not to cause air currents. The objective is to elicit the eye preservation reflex, manifested by reflex closure of the eyelids. This does not occur in peripheral or central blindness.

An obstacle test in unfamiliar surroundings should be arranged and the animal's ability to avoid obstacles assessed. The results are often difficult to interpret if the animal is nervous. A similar test for night-blindness (nyctalopia) should be arranged in subdued light, either at dusk or on a moonlit night. Nyctalopia is one of the earliest indications of avitaminosis A. Total central blindness is called amaurosis; partial central blindness is called amblyopia.

> **Clinical Pointer**
>
> In facial nerve paralysis the animal's response to the menace reflex test may be withdrawal of the head but no eyelid closure.

## Nostrils and nasal cavities

The nostrils and nasal cavities are examined for the presence of discharge, lesions of the mucosa and abnormalities of the breath.

### Nasal discharge

Discharges may be restricted to one nostril in a local infection, or be bilateral in systemic infection. The color and consistency of the exudate will indicate its source. In the early stages of inflammation the discharge will be a clear, colorless fluid which later turns to a white or yellow exudate as leukocytes accumulate in it. In Channel Island cattle the color may be a deep orange, especially in allergic rhinitis. Blood from the upper respiratory tract or pharynx may be in large quantities, or appear as small flecks. In general blood from the upper respiratory tract is unevenly mixed with any discharge, whereas that from the lower tract may be evenly mixed with other secretions. The consistency of the nasal discharge will vary from watery in the early stages of inflammation, through thick, to cheesy in long-standing cases.

Regurgitation caused by pharyngitis or esophageal obstruction may be accompanied by the discharge of feed material from the nose or the presence of feed particles in the nostrils. In some cases the volume of nasal discharge varies from time to time, often increasing when the animal is feeding from the ground, especially with inflammation of the paranasal sinuses.

Inflammation of the nasal mucosa varies from simple hyperemia, as in allergic rhinitis, to diffuse necrosis, as in bovine malignant catarrh and mucosal disease, to deep ulceration as in glanders. In hemorrhagic diseases variations in mucosal color can be observed and petechial hemorrhages may be present.

> **Clinical Pointer**
>
> - large bubbles of nasal discharge usually originate in the pharynx or nasal cavities
> - fine bubbles originate in the lower respiratory tract.

### Lesions of the nasal mucosa

These can usually be seen by direct inspection of the first several centimeters of the nasal mucosa using a strong light. They are common in cattle with diseases such as infectious bovine rhinotracheitis and summer snuffles (allergic rhinitis).

*Odor of breath*

The nasal breath may be odorous because of

- gangrenous pneumonia
- necrotic lesions in the nasal cavities
- rumen contents that have been regurgitated into the nasal cavities.

The volume of breath expired can be evaluated by holding the back of the hand over each nostril to determine the amplitude of flow.

## Mouth

Examination of the oral cavity (buccal cavity) is an important part of the clinical examination because oral lesions are common in cattle. Excessive salivation, with ropes of saliva hanging from the mouth and usually accompanied by chewing movements, occurs when there is a foreign body in the mouth, and also in many forms of inflammation of the oral mucosa or the tongue. Excessive salivation may also occur in diseases of the central nervous system, as in acute lead poisoning in young cattle and in rabies.

### Abnormalities of the buccal mucosa

These include local lesions, for example

- hemorrhages in purpuric diseases
- discolorations of jaundice and cyanosis
- the pallor of anemia and shock.

Care must be taken to define the exact nature of lesions, as differentiation between **vesicles**, and both **erosive** and **ulcerative lesions** is of diagnostic significance in differentiating the mucosal diseases of cattle.

### Teeth

The teeth are examined by inspection and palpation with the aid of an oral speculum. Delayed eruption and uneven wear may signify mineral deficiency; excessive wear with mottling and pitting of the enamel is suggestive of chronic fluorosis. Malalignment of the cheek teeth is associated with actinomycosis.

### Tongue

The tongue may be

- enlarged and firm due to inflammation, as in actinobacillosis, or

- shrunken and atrophied as in postinflammatory or neurogenic atrophy.

Distinct lesions of the surface of the tongue occur along with lesions of the mucosa of the oral cavity.

### Pharyngeal region

This examination requires some dexterity and the use of an appropriately sized speculum. The oral cavity and pharynx can be visualized by holding the mouth open, depressing the base of the tongue with the fingers or a tongue depressor, and viewing the pharynx, the glottis and the proximal part of the larynx and arytenoid cartilages.

Foreign bodies, diffuse cellulitis and pharyngeal lymph node enlargement can also be detected by this means. The use of a speculum wedged between the upper and lower molar teeth allows manual exploration and evaluation of lesions of the pharynx and proximal part of the larynx. Use of the fiberoptic scope has now made it possible to visualize lesions in the caudal nares and pharynx-esophagus/larynx-trachea in the standing conscious animal.

Local or general enlargement of the esophagus associated with vomiting or dysphagia occurs in esophageal diverticulum, stenosis and paralysis, and in cardial obstructions. Passage of a stomach tube can assist in the examination of the esophagus for obstructions.

### Submandibular region

Abnormalities of the submandibular region include

- enlargement of lymph nodes due to local foci of infection
- subcutaneous edema as part of a general edema
- local cellulitis with swelling and pain
- enlargement of the salivary glands.

## Ears

The external and internal aspects of the pinnae are inspected for evidence of lesions or ectoparasites. The external auditory meatus, which normally contains some wax-like secretion, should be gently compressed between the fingers and thumb of one hand at the base of the ear as close to the head as possible. A squelching

---

**Clinical Pointer**

Place a metal or plexiglass cylindrical speculum, 45 cm in length and 4 cm in diameter, in the oral cavity and over the base of the tongue to allow viewing of the pharynx and the larynx.

sound indicates the presence of a fluid exudate and is indicative of otitis externa, which may occur in calves and yearlings.

## Mammary gland

The mammary gland is inspected and palpated for enlargement of the quarters, increased or decreased temperature and firmness. The skin of the teats and udder is inspected for lesions. The teat cistern, streak canal, and teat end are palpated for evidence of stenosis or blockages. The supramammary lymph nodes are palpable deep in the subcutaneous tissues on the dorsal lateral aspects of the hind quarters of the udder.

### Gross examination of milk

Milk from each quarter should be examined with the aid of a strip plate or strip cup on to which streams of milk are directed so that its consistency can be evaluated. Clots, purulent material, blood and other abnormalities are easily visible. The California Mastitis Test is used extensively as a cowside test to evaluate subclinical mastitis in dairy cattle. Suitable milk samples may be taken for culture of mastitis pathogens.

## Rectal examination

A rectal examination is indicated when abnormalities of the abdomen are detected by physical examination or when the diagnosis is not obvious. For purposes of diagnostic orientation and information recording the abdomen can be divided, as viewed from the animal's rear, into four quadrants: left dorsal and ventral, and right dorsal and ventral. The abnormalities palpable can be localized to a quadrant.

The amount and consistency of the feces, and the presence of any blood or other unusual substances in the rectum are initially noted.

Abdominal structures that are palpable in their normal state include:

- the pelvic bony skeleton
- the caudal part of the dorsal sac of the rumen
- the abdominal aorta and iliac arteries and associated lymph nodes
- the left kidney

- the deep inguinal lymph node
- the internal genitalia of both female and male
- the bladder distended with urine.

Abdominal structures that are commonly palpable by rectal examination when abnormal include:

- dilated cecum (distended with gas and/or fluid)
- distended loops of small or large intestine (fluid and/or gas)
- enlarged abomasum (dilated with fluid and gas or impacted with ingesta), an impacted abomasum cannot be palpated rectally in advanced pregnancy
- enlarged omasum (usually due to impaction)
- intussusception
- enlarged liver
- enlarged left kidney and both enlarged ureters
- fibrinous peritoneal adhesions and abnormal masses such as tumors, abscesses and fat necrosis of the caudal abdomen
- abnormalities of the reproductive tract, bony skeleton, lymph nodes and bladder.

### Hemetest for occult blood in feces

The hemetest is used to detect the presence of occult blood in the feces. **Melena** or **black tarry feces** is highly suggestive of hemorrhage in the proximal parts of the alimentary tract including the abomasum. When the feces are scant they may be darker than normal but melena is not present.

## Genitourinary system

The genitourinary system is examined by inspection of the vulva, the vulvar mucous membranes and palpation of the vagina, cervix, uterus, bladder, ureters, and kidneys through the vagina and rectum as appropriate.

### Reproductive tract of the cow

In the recently calved cow, the vagina and cervix can be palpated manually by vaginal examination with the aid of a protective sleeve and glove. The vulva and perineal skin area are thoroughly cleansed with antiseptic soap and water. Within a few days after parturition the cervix may still be sufficiently open to allow manual exploration of the uterus for evidence of retained fetal membranes and foul-smelling exudate, indicating the presence of metritis. Even if the cervix is closed the vagina can be palpated for evidence of a foul-smelling exudate which indirectly indicates the presence of a postpartum septic metritis and possibly a retained placenta. The presence of slightly serosanguineous mucus with a normal odor suggests that the uterus is involuting normally and that septic metritis is not present. Such information cannot be deduced by rectal examination of the postpartum uterus. The vagina and cervix can also be visualized with the aid of an illuminated vaginoscope.

### Urinary bladder

A full bladder can be palpated by rectal examination. The small contracted ruptured bladder of the steer with obstructive urolithiasis can also be palpated as a small firm pouch at the brim of the pelvis. The cow has a suburethral diverticulum and, with some dexterity, the urethra can be catheterized relatively easily in order to obtain a urine sample if the cow cannot be stimulated to urinate by stroking the area immediately below the vulva.

### Reproductive tract of bull

The scrotum and testicles are inspected and palpated for evidence of skin lesions and for abnormalities of the testicles, including abnormal size and changes in the morphology of the epididymis. The external penis and prepuce are examined for evidence of swellings. The internal genitalia, including the seminal vesicles, pelvic urethra and prostate gland, are examined rectally.

---

**Clinical Pointer**

A urine sample may be obtained from bulls or steers by gently massaging the prepuce with paper towels soaked in warm water.

---

### Urine

Gross examination of the urine for the presence of red blood cells, turbid and cloudy material or hemoglobin is easily done in the field. Paper test strips can be used to determine variations in concentrations of ketones, glucose, protein, pH and blood in urine. Cattle affected with hypochloremic metabolic alkalosis due to right-sided dilatation and torsion of the abomasum may be in a state of paradoxic aciduria and the urine pH will be below 6.

The detailed physical examination of the external and internal genitalia of cattle is described in Chapter 22. For details of rectal palpation of the reproductive tract of cattle for the purposes of reproductive performance and pregnancy diagnosis readers are referred to the appropriate textbooks.

## Musculoskeletal system

The musculoskeletal system includes the bony skeleton, muscles, joints, ligaments, bursae and tendons. The animal is examined while recumbent, during the act of rising from recumbency, and while standing and walking.

### Inspection

Is the animal able to stand and walk? In the standing position the limbs, trunk, head and neck are inspected for evidence of gross enlargements, severe lameness, or asymmetry due to dislocations of joints or fractures of long bones. In the recumbent animal each limb is examined for evidence of gross enlargements or decreases in size (atrophy). Does the animal exhibit a desire to stand? Does it drag itself along the ground surface? Does it sit up in the dog-sitting position?

### Close physical examination

The muscles, bones, joints, ligaments, tendons and feet are examined by a combination of inspection, palpation and passive flexion and extension. Each limb and joint must be palpated and passively flexed to identify areas of pain, swelling or crepitus. Severe myopathy is characterized by hardness of muscle. Acute arthritis is characterized by severe lameness, distension and sometimes thickening of the joint capsule, severe pain on palpation, and restriction of movement of the joint on passive flexion and extension. Arthrocentesis to obtain joint fluid for laboratory examination is indicated when the joints are enlarged.

## Musculoskeletal examination in recumbent cattle

1. Inspect, palpate, and passively flex and extend each limb, and examine carefully for evidence of fractures, swellings, or pain. In large cows and bulls examination of the pelvic limbs is difficult because of their sheer size.
2. Passively abduct, adduct and rotate each limb in a large circle distally while noting any excessive movements at any level of the limb, or at the coxofemoral joint in the case of coxofemoral joint luxation.
3. Roll the animal from side to side to ensure that every part of the musculoskeletal system is examined.

### Feet

Examination of the feet of cattle consists of inspection of the external aspects of the digit, which are visible in the standing animal, and close inspection of the bearing surfaces of the digit, which requires that the feet be picked up and examined closely. Suitable restraint is required for close examination.

Most of the lesions causing lameness in cattle occur in the lateral claw of the hindfeet. The feet of mature dairy cattle which are accustomed to being handled can usually be raised manually for a cursory examination, provided the animal is restrained and movement restricted.

The bovine digit can be divided into anatomical zones, which provides a means to relate lesions to anatomical structures. It is important to record the precise location of lesions in the digit so that diagnostic terms can be standardized.

1. The **abaxial external wall and bulb** consists of the coronary band, the dorsal border of the wall, the abaxial wall, the horizontal grooves of the wall, the distal abaxial border of the wall, the abaxial face of the bulb, and the abaxial border of the wall.

### Examination of the feet of cattle

The ideal situation for both dairy and beef cattle is to raise the hindlegs with the aid of ropes secured just above the hock joints and hoisted to a solid structure such as a beam or horizontal bar above the animal. This allows the leg to be suspended for extended periods of time so that the foot can be examined in detail and any necessary treatments given. The availability of a foot-trimming table or restraint stocks is the ideal situation.

2. The **weight-bearing surface** is composed of the wall, sole and bulb. These are divided into the abaxial angle of the sole, the axial angle of the sole, the body of the sole, the apex of the sole, the base of the bulb, the apex of the bulb, the white line, and the hoof wall.
3. The **axial external wall and bulb** are composed of the axial hoof wall, the distal axial border of the wall, the axial groove, and the axial face of the bulb.

The measurable traits of the hoof are

- toe length
- sole length
- height of the caudal wall
- sole breadth.

Each foot is examined initially from a distance in the standing animal to identify any obvious abnormalities and to determine if the animal is not bearing weight on any foot.

In the standing animal the coronary band and the external walls of each digit can be examined visually. Dirty feet should be washed to permit an adequate examination. The coronary band may be enlarged and appear inflamed. The hoof walls of both the lateral and medial digits can be examined by direct visual inspection for normal length or an overgrown state. The shape of the hooves can be examined from the front and side. Abnormal shapes may be due to overgrown hooves or inherited defects, such as scissor claws. The angle between the front of the hoof and the sole should be about 50°. The lateral digit of the hindfoot is larger than the medial digit and more vulnerable to lesions, and so should be examined more closely. The digits are also examined from the rear, which will provide an indication of the health of the bulbs of the foot and the relative weight bearing and wearing of the medial and lateral digits. Lesions of digital dermatitis can be seen by examining the caudal aspect of the interdigital cleft. The horn of the hoof should be solid and smooth and the horizontal growth rings obvious.

Obvious abnormalities of the hoof walls include

- overgrown toes
- the deformed overgrown hoof of chronic laminitis
- sand cracks (vertical crack in the hoof wall) extending from the coronet in the direction of horn growth
- defects such as 'corkscrew claws', which are thought to be inherited.

Abnormalities of the horn include horizontal or vertical discontinuities and defects with loss of horn substance, such as vertical sand cracks and laminar rings associated with laminitis.

The interdigital clefts can be examined visually from the dorsal and ventral aspects for the presence of lesions. Common lesions of the interdigital space include the dermatitis associated with viral diseases such as bovine virus diarrhea and foot-and-mouth disease, interdigital necrobacillosis (foot-rot), interdigital fibromas and traumatic injuries.

Examination of the bearing surfaces of the digits requires that the limb be raised and held so that all parts of the foot can be examined (see above). The undersurface of each digit is cleaned out with a hoof knife and washed with water and a brush if necessary in order to obtain a clear view of the sole, the bulbs, the white line, the bearing surfaces of the walls and the interdigital cleft. Hoof testers are used to apply pressure from the sole to the external wall to evince pain indicating the presence of deeper lesions. Percussion of the sole and the external walls using a plexor may identify painful points. Trimming or paring the horn of the sole and walls may be necessary to locate deep lesions which are not obvious on superficial examination. When lesions are found it may be necessary to determine their extent by using a metal probe.

Some of the common lesions of the weight-bearing surfaces which are important causes of lameness include

- sole ulceration
- overworn soles
- bruised sole
- sole overgrowth
- chronic laminitis
- white-line abscess
- white-line separation
- horn erosion
- heel erosions
- solar abscesses
- underrunning of heel and sole
- foreign bodies
- infections of the deep structures of the foot.

## Nervous system

The neurological examination includes examination of gait, cranial nerve function, spinal reflexes and the collection of cerebrospinal fluid. The basic principles are the same for all species. It is often more difficult to test some of the reflexes in recumbent mature cattle. Cerebrospinal fluid can be obtained with relative ease by puncture of the cisternomedullary cavity or the lumbosacral space. Cerebrospinal fluid must be examined within minutes of collection because the cells degenerate quickly. When collected in the field a drop of the fluid sample may be smeared and dried on a glass slide and examined later for the presence of cells. However, this often is of poor quality.

## Examination of recumbent cattle

Cattle may be recumbent and unable to stand for many different reasons. The downer cow syndrome, which is a complication of milk fever in the recently calved cow, is probably the most common cause. A recumbent mature cow or bull is difficult to examine because their large size prevents easy access to all parts of the musculoskeletal system, it is difficult to carry out a reliable neurological examination, and the mammary gland of the cow is difficult to access.

A general examination of the recumbent animal includes routine evaluation of the mental status, appetite, temperature, heart and lungs, alimentary tract and genitourinary systems. A urine sample should be obtained for routine urinalysis, and particularly for proteinuria and globinuria associated with ischemic myonecrosis. A rectal examination should always be done to detect abnormalities of the uterus, soft tissues, dystocial injuries of the pelvic cavity, bony skeleton of the pelvic girdle, or any other abnormality that might account for the recumbency.

Severe injury of the adductor muscles in recently calved cows may modify the flexor withdrawal reflexes of the pelvic limbs, making it difficult to decide whether the recumbency is due to spinal cord injury or muscle injury.

For examination of the mammary gland the cow must be rolled into lateral recumbency and each quarter of the udder examined for swelling and skin discoloration. The milk must be grossly examined for abnormalities indicating acute or peracute mastitis, which is a major cause of recumbency in cattle.

Daily re-examination of recumbent animals may be necessary for a few days in order to make a diagnosis and provide a prognosis.

---

### Care of recumbent cattle

Recumbent cattle should be kept on a heavily bedded ground surface, preferably soil or sand, and should be rolled from side to side every 4–6 hours, more often if possible.

---

# CLINICAL EXAMINATION OF THE CALF

## The calf at birth

A full-term calf is covered with amniotic fluid and unable to stand. Occasionally it is stained by yellowish-tan-colored meconium, which suggests partial fetal anoxia associated with dystocia. The umbilical cord is obvious and varies in length from 10 to 30 cm. It will remain moist for up to 4 days after birth, then becomes dry, dark, and contracted, and falls off after about 14 days, leaving behind a prominent scab. Within minutes after birth the dam will begin smelling and licking the calf, and make efforts to protect its offspring from anyone attempting to handle it. The dam will continue to lick the calf vigorously over its entire body for 30 minutes or more, by which time the calf may attempt to stand.

At birth the full-term calf has at least six and usually all eight temporary incisors, which appear overlapped like tiles on a roof. They are extensively covered by the gums, which recede from the central incisors by the 12th day; this recession spreads outwards to the medial and lateral incisors until at 3 weeks these and the corner incisors are exposed from their neck outwards. At 4 weeks of age the temporary incisors form a regular arc. The **fetal claw cushions** are clearly obvious at the distal ends of the claws and are shed within a few days after the calf walks. The menace reflex is not fully developed until several days of age.

Some calves will begin to attempt to stand about 15–45 minutes after birth. After standing the calf will appear very ataxic, and will commonly fall several times before it remains standing and begins to walk. Others will not attempt to stand for up to 60 minutes. Calves with traumatic injuries and fetal hypoxia associated with parturition may not attempt to stand for several hours or days. Traumatic injuries include fractured ribs, fractures of the long bones such as the femur, metatarsus and metacarpus, and the mandible. A calf left with its dam will begin to seek the teats within 30 minutes of standing. Normal vigorous calves may be sucking within an hour; others may not suck successfully for up to 2–6 hours after birth. Edema of the head and neck associated with prolonged parturition may be accompanied by protrusion of the tongue, which may be markedly edematous and interfere with the ability to suckle for several hours. The weak calf syndrome is characterized by weakness, lethargy, lack of a suck reflex, inability to stand even when assisted, and high case fatality within several hours of birth.

Congenital defects are usually obvious and are most common in the musculoskeletal system, nervous system and eyes.

> ### Clinical Pointer
>
> Calves that do not begin sucking within a few hours, regardless of the reason, must be force-fed liberal quantities of colostrum, usually by stomach tube.

## Clinical examination

Clinical examination of the newborn calf or the young calf up to several months of age is similar to that for adult cattle. A thorough clinical examination does not usually take as long as in the mature cow because some systems, such as the reproductive tract and mammary gland, are not examined. Also, until the calf is a ruminant, ruminal contractions will not be detectable. Nor is it possible, because of the small size, to examine the abdomen rectally. The examination of the calf which is described here is intended to emphasize those aspects which are important in calves from birth to about 2 months of age.

### History taking

Some aspects of history taking assume more importance than in adult cattle. These include:

- the age of the calf – in hours, days, or weeks
- the ease or difficulty of its birth
- the calf's behavior immediately after birth and the time it took to stand
- if, when, and how much colostrum the calf ingested.

A calf might have been born several hours before it was seen by the attendant. In herds in which calves are born on pasture, the time and circumstances of the birth may not be precisely known, nor the onset of any abnormality such as dyspnea. Was the abnormality present at birth or did it begin several hours afterwards? If a calf is found in a state of weakness and recumbency several hours after birth it may be impossible to determine whether the weakness was already present or is associated with some postnatal environmental influence, such as cold weather. If the calf is presented within 2 days of birth it is important to determine whether it has passed any meconium. Questions should be asked about the appetite and whether there is a suck reflex: a completely absent suck reflex must be noted and the cause explored during the clinical examination.

The breed, sex and age of the calf are noted. If it is less than a few days old the circumstances of the birth should be determined. Was it born unassisted or with obstetrical assistance? The parity of the dam is also important: calves born from first-calf heifers are more likely to

- suffer traumatic injuries associated with dystocia
- acquire infectious diseases because their colostral immunity may be poor (mature cows have more colostrum and usually exhibit more effective maternal behavior than first-calf heifers).

The vaccination history of the dams may influence the occurrence of diseases in calves and must be evaluated. The medications used for the treatment of any previously affected calves should be determined.

## Presenting complaint

Some common clinical manifestations of diseases of various body systems in newborn calves include the following:

The body as a whole

- dullness or depression
- refusal to suck for several hours or more
- weakness and recumbency
- inappetence and anorexia
- dehydration.

Abdomen and alimentary tract

- hemorrhage from umbilical cord
- enlarged and painful umbilicus
- diarrhea
- dysentery
- complete absence of feces
- atresi ani
- distension of the abdomen
- abdominal pain or colic
- bruxism (grinding of teeth).

Respiratory system

- dyspnea
- coughing
- respiratory noises (stridor).

### Clinical Pointer

When examining hand-fed calves note the nature of the diet. Cow's whole milk and milk replacers are used after the colostral feeding period until the calves are weaned. The quality of milk replacers varies widely and must be evaluated as part of the history.

Musculoskeletal system

- weakness and inability to stand
- recumbency
- reluctance to move.

Nervous system and eyes

- depression and somnolence
- convulsions
- ataxia
- blindness
- ocular abnormalities (cataracts, hypopyon)
- inability to stand or walk.

Skin and haircoat

- absence of hair at birth
- abnormal skin and skin lesions.

## Distant examination

The distant examination can be done quickly and efficiently. The following observations should be made.

*Habitus*
What is the calf doing? Standing? Walking? Will it follow its dam?

*Recumbent*
If recumbent, can the calf stand on its own or with assistance? Does the recumbent calf stand when approached or coaxed?

*Overall body condition*
Is the body size of the calf within the normal range for its age? Is there any evidence of dehydration, for example sunken eyes?

*Demeanor and behavior*
What is the calf's mental state? Bright and alert or depressed? Is it grinding its teeth?

*Eyesight*
Can the calf see normally when it walks?

*Suck reflex*
Can the calf suck? Is it sucking now? Does it appear to be hungry and will it suck a finger?

## Particular distant examination

The particular distant examination notes any obvious abnormalities of body regions.

*Head and neck*

Are there any abnormalities of posture? Any evidence of drooling from the mouth? What is the condition of the face and external features of the mouth and eyes? Any abnormalities of the ears such as complications associated with frostbite?

*Thorax*

The respirations are characterized for rate, rhythm, and depth. Are there any respiratory noises such as wheezing, sneezing, or inspiratory stridor?

*Abdomen*

What is the contour of the abdomen? It is distended? Which side? Is the abdomen gaunt? What is the state of the umbilicus and the umbilical cord? Are any feces being passed? Are there any abnormalities of the tail such as complications from frostbite?

*Limbs and feet*

Is there any evidence of lameness or any obvious swellings of the limbs, joints, or soft tissues of the feet?

## Close physical examination

The routine for the close physical examination of the calf can be similar to that used for a mature cow. However, depending on the clinical status of the calf on presentation it may be more appropriate to examine certain parts of the animal first. For example, if presented with a calf in a state of collapse associated with a history of diarrhea, it may be more appropriate to examine the hydration status and peripheral circulation first by looking at the eyes, the skin and the mucous membranes of the oral cavity, followed by the remainder of the examination. In a standing calf the standard orderly routine used in mature cattle can be used.

## Mental attitude

The calf may be bright and alert or depressed and somnolent. Mental attitude is a reflection of the presence or absence of toxemia, the degree of acidosis and dehydration, hypoglycemia, anemia, hypothermia or fever, or other systemic states that can affect cerebral function. The sucking reflex is a good indicator of mental status and is tested by inserting one's finger deep into the calf's mouth and stroking the soft palate.

In newborn animals the suck reflex is an innate physiological one. The normal newborn calf will suck a finger: a depressed calf which is dehydrated and acidotic or toxemic may not have a suck reflex.

**Clinical Pointer**

Testing the sucking reflex with a rubber nipple attached to a milk bottle is not totally reliable, a calf which has sucked its dam for a few days will have a suck reflex to a finger but not to a rubber nipple.

### Hydration and dehydration

The state and degree of dehydration are assessed by examining the eyes and the elasticity of the skin. Dehydration is expressed as an approximate percentage of body weight, such as 6%, 10%, 12% or higher. Dehydration results in varying degrees of enophthalmos and loss of postorbital fat, which makes the eyes appear smaller than normal with a circumferential space between the eye and the orbit.

Skin elasticity is evaluated by tenting the skin of the upper eyelid and over the neck. The number of seconds the skin remains tented before returning to normal can be an approximation of the degree of dehydration (See Table 14.1, Chapter 14).

### Mucous membranes of oral cavity and conjunctivae

The oral mucous membranes are examined for degree of wetness or dryness, discoloration and temperature on digital palpation. In dehydrated and hypothermic calves they will be dry and cool to touch. The presence of lesions such as erosions, petechiae and ulcers is usually readily obvious on inspection of the oral cavity.

### Temperature

The rectal temperature is recorded. Care must be taken to ensure that the thermometer is held against the mucosa of the rectum, particularly in diarrheic calves, when the anus and rectum may be slightly dilated, resulting in a reading lower than actual body temperature. The normal temperature of the newborn calf ranges from 38.5 to 39.5°C. A temperature above 39.5°C suggests the presence of fever. Systemic infec-

**Clinical Pointer**

Examine the conjunctivae for discoloration and evidence of petechiae or episcleral hemorrhages, these can occur in newborn calves as a result of dystocial injuries.

tions of newborn calves under a few days of age may not result in fever. Temperatures below 38.0°C are regarded as hypothermia and may be as low as 35.0°C in calves exposed to cold weather for more than a few hours, especially if dehydrated and diarrheic.

## Cardiovascular and lymphatic systems

The normal heart rate of the newborn calf in the first few days after birth ranges from 80 to 100 bpm. After this age it will range from 72 to 84 bpm, and will gradually decline to adult values as the calf becomes older. In toxemia due to septicemia, bacteremia, and with some of the common infections of the newborn calf, the heart rate will range from 110 to 120 bpm. Tachycardia in the range of 160–200 bpm suggests myocardial disease, such as enzootic muscular dystrophy due to vitamin E and selenium deficiency. Bradycardia at 40–60 bpm suggests severe acidosis and hyperkalemia, which occurs in diarrheic calves.

The jugular veins are examined by inspection and palpation. In dehydrated calves they are commonly collapsed and may not fill proximally when compressed at the midcervical area as in normal animals.

The prescapular and prefemoral lymph nodes are palpated for enlargement. Calves with congenital lymphomatosis may have enlarged peripheral lymph nodes, along with the skin lesions typical of the congenital disease in calves.

## Respirations

The respiratory rate of the newborn calf in the first few days of life ranges from 24 to 36 breaths/minute. In the normal calf respirations are primarily abdominocostal. On auscultation of the lungs of a calf under a few days of age the breath sounds are clearly audible, as in the adult.

In diarrheic calves under 30 days of age the severe acidosis and dehydration may be accompanied by marked variations in the depth and rate of respiration. There may be hyperpnea and polypnea, or very shallow and slower than normal respirations. These variations are considered to be related to acid–base and electrolyte imbalances.

An **inspiratory stridor** in a young calf which is clearly audible without a stethoscope is commonly due to a laryngeal lesion, such as necrotic laryngitis. The loud stenotic sound is audible on inspiration, which is prolonged and hyperactive, resulting in a falsely exaggerated expiration. An expiratory grunt with an exaggerated expiration indicates diffuse or advanced disease of the lungs.

---

### Pneumonia in the calf

Pneumonia in a calf is characterized by

- an increased rate and depth of respirations, which are markedly abdominocostal
- louder than normal lung sounds and audible abnormal lung sounds (crackles and wheezes).

Milk aspiration pneumonia is characterized by marked hyperpnea and exertional respirations in the calf under a few days of age.

---

## Abdomen

Examination of the abdomen consists of visual inspection of the contour, palpation, and percussion and ballottement with simultaneous auscultation, plus the passage of a nasogastric tube to determine the status of the rumen. Abdominal pain or colic, characterized by kicking at the abdomen, stretching, lying down and bellowing, is also observed and heard in calves with distension or painful lesions of the abdominal viscera.

The contour of the abdomen of the normal calf is similar to that of the adult, except that the left abdomen is not as prominent because of the relatively small size of the rumen in the preruminant calf. The contour of the right abdomen may appear to be prominent in some calves immediately after ingesting large quantities of milk or fluid, which causes distension of the abomasum. On palpation, the abdomen of the calf under 30 days of age feels resilient and no specific part of the gastrointestinal tract, such as the intestines or normal abomasum, can be felt through the abdominal wall. As the calf becomes a ruminant the rumen pack can be felt in the left paralumbar fossa.

A gaunt or 'drawn in' abdomen occurs commonly in calves with diarrhea of a few days' duration, or if they have failed to suckle or eat recently.

Distension of the abdomen is a common occurrence in calves from birth up to about 4 months of age. It should be inspected for symmetry, asymmetry, anatomical location of the greatest prominence (left or right), and degree. In mild distension the skin of the abdomen can usually be picked up and held between the fingers, indicating that the abdominal wall is not being stretched. Such mild or moderate distension may not represent an emergency.

Determination of the cause of abdominal distension in a calf requires a combination of inspection, palpation, percussion and ballottement, and simulta-

## Clinical Pointer

If the abdominal skin is very tense like a board it indicates severe abdominal distension and represents an emergency situation.

neous auscultation of the abdomen. The objective is to determine the anatomical location of maximal distension and then to diagnose the possible causes. Simultaneous percussion and auscultation, and ballottement of both sides of the abdomen, will reveal areas of resonance, pings, and fluid-splashing sounds, which indicate the abnormal accumulation of fluid and gas in gastrointestinal viscera.

Determination of the presence or absence of feces in the calf is an important aspect of the examination. A complete absence of feces over a period of several hours and the failure to obtain any feces by digital examination of the rectum may suggest the presence of an acute intestinal obstruction. However, the presence of intestinal ileus due to peritonitis, which results in the failure of peristalsis and absence of feces for several hours, may also resemble acute intestinal obstruction. The most important objective is to decide whether the abdominal syndrome can be treated medically or surgically. Examination of the abdomen must be combined with examination of the cardiovascular system to evaluate the possibility of impending shock and dehydration, which may indicate the presence of a surgical lesion.

Some common causes of abdominal distension in suckling beef calves over 8 days of age and under 2 months are as follows:

- dilatation of the abomasum
- volvulus of the abomasum
- torsion of the root of the mesentery
- torsion of the coiled colon
- rupture of abomasal ulcer with diffuse peritonitis
- diffuse peritonitis causing adynamic ileus.

Fluid-splashing sounds audible by ballottement and auscultation over the **left** abdomen suggest an abnormal quantity of fluid and gas in the preruminant rumen. Percussion and simultaneous auscultation may reveal low-pitched pings. Such findings could be due to the presence of fermented milk in the rumen in calves that have consumed too much too quickly. The passing of a stomach tube into the rumen can aid in determining whether the rumen is distended with fluid or gas, and can aid in differentiation from other abnormalities causing abdominal distension. Failure to relieve the distension following passage of the tube into the rumen suggests that other viscera, such as the abomasum and intestines, may be responsible.

## Atresia ani and atresia coli

Atresia of the intestines (atresia ani or atresia coli) is one of the most common causes of abdominal distension in calves under 8 days of age. The signs are

- gross symmetrical distension of the abdomen
- no feces passed since birth
- examination of the anus may reveal atresia.

If an anus is present and no feces have been passed in the first 24–48 hours then atresia coli may be the problem. Digital examination of the rectum will fail to detect any meconium or feces and only mucus will be present. Determination of the location of the atresia can be assisted by contrast radiography. Passage of a tube into the rectum cannot ascertain the location of most cases of atresia coli, which requires exploratory laparotomy.

Fluid-splashing sounds audible by ballottement and auscultation over the **right** abdomen suggest an abnormal quantity of fluid and gas in the small or large intestines or in the abomasum. This may be due to distension of the abomasum or intestines regardless of the cause. Because of the relatively large size of the abomasum in the preruminant, compared to the size of the rumen, distension of the abomasum will result in bilateral symmetrical distension of both the right and left sides of the abdomen.

Dilatation of the abomasum, regardless of the cause, will result in distension of the right abdomen, increased tenseness of the abdominal wall over the affected viscera, and increased resonance, with pings on percussion. Some degree of abdominal pain may also be elicited by deep palpation over the distended abomasum. Causes of intestinal fluid and gas distension include

- acute enteritis
- acute intestinal obstruction
- ileus associated with peritonitis.

Abdominocentesis to obtain peritoneal fluid can be an aid to the diagnosis of acute intestinal obstruction with ischemic necrosis of intestines, and in peritonitis.

Inspection and palpation of the external and internal aspects of the umbilicus are necessary to determine the state of the umbilicus and whether there are complications of an omphalitis, such as inflammation and abscessation of the umbilical vein to the liver, or of the urachus or the umbilical arteries to the bladder. Deep palpation above the umbilicus may reveal the presence of masses in the abdomen which will require surgical intervention. Ultrasonography can assist in the identification of lesions of the umbilicus that cannot be palpated.

### Feces

The newborn calf will pass tan-colored meconium within the first 24 hours. Healthy normal calves receiving cow's whole milk will pass only small quantities of feces daily for the first several days. The digestibility of milk is over 95% and some calves will not pass feces for intervals of up to 24 hours for the first several days. Beginning at about 7–10 days of age the intake of milk in suckling calves will increase and the amount of feces passed will increase: their consistency will be soft and formed and they may be odorous. As the calf becomes older the feces become dark brown and assume the characteristics of adult feces.

An absence of feces in the first 24–48 hours suggests atresia of the anus or colon (described above).

The feces in calves under 30 days of age with acute diarrhea can vary in consistency from being soft and formed, to large quantities of free-flowing liquid. The odor will also vary widely and is often foul.

The characteristics of the feces in diarrheic calves are not highly reliable indicators of the cause of the diarrhea, but there are some general indicators of possible causes.

1. The presence of fibrinous casts suggests severe inflammation of the intestines, such as in salmonellosis.
2. A profuse liquid diarrhea in calves under 3 days of age suggests enterotoxigenic colibacillosis.
3. A profuse liquid diarrhea with green mucoid feces in calves 3–4 weeks of age suggests a coronavirus diarrhea.
4. Blood from hemorrhage in the abomasum or small intestine (melena) may cause black tarry feces.
5. Hemorrhage in the large intestine will result in feces which are uniformly red.
6. Hemorrhage in the rectum will result in feces with chunks of bright red colour.

In diarrheic calves under 30 days of age small flecks and streaks of blood may occasionally appear in the feces and in most cases is inconsequential. The presence of large quantities of frank bright red blood in the feces of calves older than 3–4 weeks suggests the possibility of coccidiosis, or infection with attaching and effacing *Escherichia coli*.

### Urine

Every reasonable attempt should be made to observe urination and to collect a sample from a calf patient.

Stroking the vulva will usually yield some urine in female calves. In males wetting the prepuce and waiting patiently for it to urinate is the only available method.

### Musculoskeletal system and feet

Newborn calves that have experienced a difficult birth may have fractures of long bones, especially the femur and the metacarpal and metatarsal bones, and fracture of the ribs and mandible. With displacement of long bone fractures the abnormality may be obvious on initial examination, as the calf is usually lame or unable to stand. In a recumbent newborn calf the musculoskeletal system should be examined systematically by

- careful palpation of long bones
- passive flexion and extension of the limbs
- careful palpation of each rib
- palpation of the mandible.

Congenitally contracted flexor tendons of the thoracic limbs occur occasionally in newborn calves. The contractures are obvious at birth and most will resolve over a period of days.

The large movable joints, such as metacarpal, metatarsal, stifle, hock, elbow, and shoulder, coxofemoral and fetlock, should be examined by inspection and palpation and passive flexion and extension. Polysynovitis is common in newborn calves and is difficult to detect by direct visual inspection and palpation.

The limb muscles are examined by visual inspection and palpation. The muscles masses of the calf are normally moderately firm. Acute nutritional muscular dystrophy is characterized by a stiff gait, weakness and recumbency, and firmer than normal muscle masses. However, a remarkable increased firmness and pain on palpation of the large muscle masses in calves with muscular dystrophy is uncommon.

The fetal claw cushion is present on all four feet of the calf at birth and falls off within hours or a day after the calf stands and begins to walk. Examination of the feet of lame calves consists of inspecting the coronary bands and the skin and soft tissues above them.

In temperate climates where calves are born in cold weather, cold injury of the extremities, such as the

### Omphalophlebitis

Omphalophlebitis may be associated with urachitis and cystitis in calves under 2 weeks of age.

## Frostbite

Even the experienced clinician may not detect frostbite as the haircoat and pigmentation mask its early signs.

## Ophthalmitis

This is a common acquired abnormality of the young calf under 30 days of age. It is due to neonatal infection with the common opportunist pathogens. Affected calves have unilateral or bilateral hypopyon, with the gray exudate clearly visible in the anterior chamber of the eye.

hindfeet, ears and tail, may occur. The clinical finding of frostbite of the feet of calves is not readily obvious even to the experienced observer, as the normal hair covering and skin pigmentation often masks the early changes of frostbite. The distal parts of the limbs are cool and clammy on palpation, and the soft tissues above the coronary bands are swollen, edematous, and may have well demarcated limits. After several hours of warming indoors the feet remain cool and close examination reveals some moistness and dark redness to bluish discoloration. The affected skin will become pink, red or purplish-blue. If the frostbite is not severe, complete recovery may occur within a few days. In more severe cases the affected skin will slough and the hooves may become detached several days later. Palpation of the affected tissues is painful.

### Nervous system

The newborn calf will usually attempt to stand within an hour of birth; some vigorous animals will stand within 30 minutes, whereas others may not stand for a few hours and some cannot stand even after several hours. The spinal reflexes and the flexor withdrawal reflexes of the limbs are intact at birth. Cranial nerve function is present at birth.

The suck reflex is functional at birth and is tested by inserting a finger deep into the oral cavity and stroking the soft palate: this results in the calf sucking the finger with its tongue and creating a sucking sensation with the mouth.

Neurological examination of the calf is similar to that for adult animals. Common clinical abnormalities associated with congenital or acquired diseases of the nervous system in the first few days of life include

- mental depression
- skeletal muscle weakness and recumbency
- blindness
- absence of the suck reflex
- ataxia due to congenital cerebellar hypoplasia
- involuntary movements such as tremors and convulsions.

### Eyes

The newborn calf appears to be able to see at birth but the menace reflex is not fully developed until several days of age. The pupillary light reflex is fully functional within the first day. Congenital abnormalities of the eyes which are obvious at birth include bilateral cataracts, microphthalmia, and blindness due to retinal disease associated with fetal infection with the bovine diarrhea virus. Ophthalmitis is also common in calves affected with bacteremia and/or pepticemia.

### Skin and haircoat

At birth the haircoat of the calf is covered with the slimy fetal fluids which are quickly licked off by the dam; the coat then dries within a few hours. The haircoat of the young calf is sleek and glossy and the skin is pliable. Abnormalities of the haircoat and skin of calves under a few weeks of age are uncommon. Congenital abnormalities include alopecia and the absence of skin (epitheliogenesis imperfecta). Some common acquired skin lesions include excoriations of the perineum associated with constant wetting by feces in prolonged diarrhea, and frostbite injury to the feet, ears, and tail.

## FURTHER READING

Edmonson AJ, Lean IJ, Weaver LD, Farver T, Webster G. A body condition scoring chart for Holstein Dairy Cows. Journal of Dairy Science 1989;72: 68–78.

Ferguson JD, Galligan DT, Thomsen N. Principal descriptors of body condition score in Holstein cows. Journal of Dairy Science 1994;77: 2695–2703.

Mills LL, Leach DH. A revised/proposed nomenclature for the external anatomical features of the bovine foot. Canadian Veterinary Journal 1988;29: 444–447.

Mills LL, Leach DH, Smart ME, Greenough PR. A system for the recording of clinical data as an aid in the diagnosis of bovine digital disease. Canadian Veterinary Journal 1986;27: 293–300.

Naylor JM, Bailey JV. A retrospective study of 51 cases of abdominal problems in the calf: etiology, diagnosis and prognosis. Canadian Veterinary Journal 1987;28: 657–662.

# 10
# Clinical Examination of Sheep and Goats

*C. C. Gay*

## INTRODUCTION

Sheep and goats, also referred to as small ruminants, are reared for diverse reasons and under diverse conditions. In all countries sheep and goats are managed as flocks and herds and are reared for commercial reasons. In North America and some other countries, sheep are reared as family pets and a single goat may be kept by a family to provide milk. The approach to the clinical examination of individual sheep and goats is similar to that for companion animals, and incorporates a physical examination of the individual animal coupled with an examination of the history of the problem, the environment and appropriate laboratory tests. The purpose of clinical examination of an individual is to arrive at a diagnosis and a strategy for treatment and correction of the problem.

## IMPORTANCE OF EPIDEMIOLOGY IN GROUPS OF SMALL RUMINANTS

Most sheep and goats are managed in groups (bands, mobs, herds, flocks). The approach used to determine the nature and cause of disease in flocks or herds is similar to that used for individual animals, but the epidemiology of the problem is also examined to assist in making a diagnosis.

Many diseases have specific circumstances of occurrence and patterns of attack. Making a diagnosis can be assisted by determining the epidemiology as well as the age- and class-specific incidences of the problem, coupled with an examination of management practices and potential environmental influences. The final diagnosis requires integration of the epidemiological findings with the findings from clinical, laboratory and possibly postmortem examination. The clinical examination of the group also provides an opportunity for the early detection of disease and the risk of spread to normal animals.

The structure of a group of sheep will vary with the size and management of the farm flock. On farms with small numbers of sheep, the whole farm flock may be run as one group, whereas on farms with large numbers of sheep the flock is usually divided into different subgroups, based on age, type of sheep and other circumstances. For example, an enterprise with a large flock may run mature ewes, maiden ewes, weaned sheep, and, in the case of wool breeds, wethers, as separate groups.

### Risk factors

Many diseases of sheep occur in particular age groups, and there are certain risk factors for most diseases. For these reasons, and because sheep managed in groups are subject to the same management influences, most diseases of sheep affect more than one animal and occur as outbreaks.

A knowledge of the risk factors for each of the diseases of sheep, their relative importance and the relative risk for a given disease occurring in association

> ### The aim of diagnosis
>
> The aim of the diagnosis in sheep and goats is to
>
> - determine the treatment strategy for the affected animals
> - establish intervention strategies to maintain or restore the health of the group.

179

with the management practice being observed, is important as it allows the formulation of a list of possible diseases and diagnostic rule-outs. A clinician will consider this list while conducting further clinical examination of the flock and of individual sheep. For example, each of the clostridial diseases in sheep has specific management practices that are determinants for disease occurrence, and almost without exception each has an age-specific and/or management-specific time of occurrence. Thus these diseases have a distinct tendency to occur under a known set of circumstances. Nearly every highly productive pasture has some risk, such as

- hypomagnesemia
- rye grass staggers
- phalaris toxicity
- fescue hyperthermia
- clover disease

but their manifestation requires specific management circumstances. A further example is hypocalcemia in sheep, which is uncommon but can occur when pregnant – or occasionally lactating – ewes are subjected to a period of food restriction coupled with exercise or other movement stress. Thus it may occur following the yarding of late pregnant sheep for crutching or vaccination, or as a sequela to the transport of late pregnant sheep. Hypocalcemia in sheep is very rare in other circumstances except in association with osteoporosis in young lambs and early weaned sheep on inadequate calcium and trace element diets.

There is also a relationship between risk of the occurrence of disease and age and management practices in goats, and this knowledge is equally valuable to clinical examination and diagnosis. It is more difficult to apply where goats are managed as small farm herds or as single family pets, as occurs in much of the western hemisphere.

## COMPONENTS OF A CLINICAL EXAMINATION OF A FLOCK OF SHEEP OR HERD OF GOATS

A complete examination of a flock of sheep or a herd of goats requires

- the identification of sick animals
- a distant and a close physical examination
- an examination of the management and environment of the group
- an examination for risk factors that will predispose the conditions under consideration.

In large populations necropsies are a routine part of the examination. The sequence of these various aspects will vary from problem to problem, but it is important that all are completed. This chapter describes the distant and close physical examination components of the general clinical examination of sheep and goats. Details of the environmental and epidemiological examinations can be found in the Further Reading list.

## Distant examination

### Behavior of groups of sheep

Minor changes in behavior occur in many diseases but may be masked if the sheep are distracted and disturbed. A distant examination is particularly informative where there are diseases of the central nervous and the musculoskeletal systems.

Sheep with myopathy are depressed and stand with the back arched and the head held low. Because of its value in the detection of certain clinical abnormalities, where possible, sheep should initially be examined from a sufficient distance that they are minimally disturbed by the presence of the clinician. A distant examination can be expected to be more informative clinically with sheep at pasture, as there are more opportunities for sheep kept extensively to display abnormalities in innate patterns of social behavior than for those kept in intensive conditions. The distant examination concentrates on abnormality in behavior and on determining the prevalence of the problem, as well as helping to identify affected sheep.

The behavioral examination concentrates on deviations from normal activity. Grazing is the dominant behavior in pastured sheep, and clinically normal sheep alternate between periods of grazing and periods of rest. Sheep graze for 8–9 hours a day, and for as long as 14 hours if feed supply is limited. Grazing generally occurs in bouts that last from 20 to 90 minutes, each followed by a rest period where the sheep lie down and ruminate. Another 8 to 10 hours is spent ruminating in periods that vary from a few minutes to 2 hours. During rumination there is rapid side-to-side chewing in one direction, with the bolus being held on one side of mouth during the whole of

> **Clinical Pointer**
>
> The behavioral changes that are the initial indication of the onset of scrapie are best observed by distant examination.

any one chewing period. Grazing is not common during the night, but in hot climates it may be concentrated in the hours immediately before dusk and around dawn. The patterns of grazing over a pasture are influenced by

- breed
- preferred plant distribution
- site of water
- day and night rest spots
- ambient temperature.

Merino sheep camp together at specific sites, whereas hill breeds generally keep separate at night and sleep on the higher portions of the pastures, moving to the lower parts during the morning and returning higher in the late afternoon and evening. Whereas abnormalities in grazing and flocking behavior may be apparent to the clinician, abnormalities and changes in grazing patterns are only likely to be detected by an astute shepherd.

Sheep have a highly developed flocking instinct, exhibiting flocking/following behavior when moving; flocking when resting, sleeping or when disturbed; and a strong group flight reaction with close disturbance.

Vision is the dominant factor in social organization in sheep, and the dispersal of a group of healthy sheep in a field is determined by their ability to see each other. However, there is breed variation in the intensity of gregariousness and flocking response

- Merino sheep have short individual distances and small social distances, consequently they are highly gregarious and graze and move close together even in a large paddock
- British lowland breeds of sheep, and most goat breeds, tend to disperse evenly over a confined area and may be found in subgroups
- hill breeds of British sheep, such as the Scottish Blackface, are highly individualistic and disperse widely over a hill area.

Sheep have a limited binocular vision which is approximately 40° wide in the plane in which they face. The remainder of the visual field is monocular, except for the caudal sector, which a sheep cannot see without turning its head. Normal sheep disturbed by the approach of a human will turn their head to face the approach and show an alert and attentive posture.

Further encroachment on the **flight zone** may result in a kick (upward movement of a stiff foreleg), a head threat (head moved sharply down and towards the examiner), possibly a snort of aggression, but invariably an alarm and flight reaction, where the sheep moves sideways or away from the examiner with the head raised and a stiff rigid gait. When observing a flock, the greater the number facing away the closer the group is to flight or movement. An aberration of this behavior is seen in ewes with systemic or central nervous disease.

A distant examination includes an examination of the group with minimal disturbance followed by a slow approach so as to allow flocking with its associated behavior. Following this there should be a further slow approach to cause a gentle flight reaction, which induces the group to move slowly away from the observer.

### Detection of abnormalities from a distance

The distant examination of sheep at pasture can detect abnormalities that may not be easily detected in closely grouped and highly disturbed animals. Also, although this examination by itself seldom leads to a definitive diagnosis it does identify individuals for closer physical examination. It is of particular value in determining those body systems that need a very careful and special examination during the individual physical examination. Such a necessary focus might not be so evident if the initial examination is only of mustered and disturbed sheep, or of a sheep preselected and presented to a clinic for examination. Examples are abnormality in prehension, resulting from painful or physical impairment, as occurs with actinobacillosis, orf and facial eczema, or that resulting from centrally initiated impairment, as occurs with central nervous system disease. A further example could be the observation of a low prevalence of hind limb lameness in lactating ewes, coupled with mild depression, both disappearing following the onset of rapid movement of the flock. This could be due to mastitis and indicates that udders must not be excluded from the physical examination.

---

### Clinical Pointer

Although there is a common belief that sick sheep will separate from the rest of the flock, this behavior varies with the breed and the circumstances of management.

---

### Pregnancy toxemia

Ewes affected with pregnancy toxemia can hear the approach of the clinician and so turn towards the sound, giving the impression that they can see, but because of their visual defect they can be approached to the point of physical capture before they turn and flee.

## Estimation of morbidity

The distant examination also provides an estimate of the morbidity in the flock and of the number of individuals that may need to be physically examined. Further, coupled with the history of the management of the sheep and the examination of the environment, it provides information for the epidemiological input to diagnosis. An example is in the distant examination of lameness in a flock. This allows an estimate of

- the percentage of lame animals in the group
- the percentage of animals lame in one limb only
- the percentage lame in the forelimb rather than the hindlimb
- the differences in age- and class-specific incidence.

This information, combined with the season of occurrence and the past history of the flock, may provide a tentative diagnosis and differential diagnosis list, including foot scald, contagious foot-rot, toe abscess, heel abscess, tick pyemia, erysipelas arthritis, chlamydial polyarthritis and post-dipping lameness. It certainly will dictate the nature and scope of the individual animal physical examination and the sampling for laboratory testing. During this phase components of the environmental examination are also conducted, such as those relating to pasture, its composition and utilization.

## Observation of the group while walking

Following distant examination with minimal disturbance the group should be quietly walked for a period of 5–15 minutes. Often this can be accomplished by moving the flock from the pasture to a yard for further examination. This procedure is valuable in the detection of the early signs of many diseases and will often identify sheep for subsequent examination, as most sick sheep will show some evidence of exercise intolerance along with more specific signs of the disease problem.

---

### Aberrant behavior associated with skin disease

Aberrant behavior associated with parasitic skin disease is best examined at a distance. Evidence includes

- itchiness and rubbing against inanimate objects
- restlessness
- stamping
- attempts at wool licking and chewing
- areas of fleece loss or irregularity.

---

1. Sheep with musculoskeletal disease exhibit a low exercise tolerance, are reluctant to travel, and consequently fall behind the moving group.
2. Sheep with polyarthritis will be lame; those with a primary myopathy will exhibit a stiff gait with knuckling at the fetlocks; both, if pushed, will collapse to lie in sternal or lateral recumbency.
3. Sheep with respiratory disease will show exercise intolerance, a labored respiration and will separate to the tail of the moving group.
4. The disorientation and locomotor disorders that occur with central nervous system diseases such as polioencephalomalacia or swayback, or disorders of neuromuscular transmission such as botulism, become particularly evident in a moving flock, as do the early behavioral abnormalities and locomotor disorders of scrapie.
5. Some diseases, such as the stagger and tremorogenic syndromes, may not be evident while the sheep are undisturbed but result in dramatic locomotor abnormality precipitated by activity.

## Observation in confinement

Movement of the sheep should be followed by a period of further observation while they are confined and relatively at rest, usually in a yard or pen. This allows further close observation of individuals prior to the physical examination. Several animals will pass feces at this time. Normal feces in both sheep and goats have a firm consistency and are passed as small balls or pellets. The passage of putty-like or fluid feces is abnormal: it is often accompanied by fecal staining and matting of the wool (dags) in the perineal region, and indicates the need for specific clinical and laboratory examination.

At this time there should be a careful and systematic visual examination of the conformation of members of the group. This allows the detection of innate or acquired abnormalities in conformation, such as the long spider-like limb with its medial deviation at the carpus and tarsus associated with hereditary chondrodysplasia; other bone abnormalities, such as those associated with bent leg and rickets; and defects such as the high tail of sheep with clover disease. These abnormalities can be further examined during later individual examination.

The opportunities for the clinician to detect subtle behavioral aberrations are fewer when sheep are held and reared in yards or pens. Nevertheless, the same sequence and purpose of examination is followed. Thus housed sheep should be observed quietly from a distance before moving closer and finally entering the pen to conduct a close examination.

## Close physical examination

### Examination of individual animals

Following the distant examination, selected animals are caught for individual physical examination. The degree of restraint required and the limitation this places on the conduct of the examination differs between sheep and goats, and also with age and the degree of domestication of the animals. Most of the physical examination of sheep can be performed with the animal held standing. The sheep should be confined to a small pen or a race (chute), and an individual is caught as it faces away by moving forward quickly to grasp a hindleg above the hock, or by hooking it with a shepherd's crook. Sheep in a yard will circle if approached, and the circling can be allowed to continue until the wanted sheep is toward the back of the group, when it can be caught as above. **Sheep should not be caught or restrained by holding the wool.** Once caught, movement is minimized by holding the sheep with the open hand under the jaw to keep the head elevated above the back line, and by backing it against a wall or into a corner, where it can be restrained with one hand under the jaw.

In normal sheep, the examination of the udder and feet and palpation of the abdomen are best performed with the sheep cast in full restraint sitting on its rump, with its withers between the clinician's knees. If a separate handler holds the sheep the clinician needs to be careful not to be raked by the claws if standing in front of the sheep.

Goats are more used to being handled than sheep, are often domesticated, and have frequently been neck tied and tethered. They can be restrained by holding firmly around the neck behind the head or by attaching a collar. Goats are not usually cast during an examination: instead they can be gently rolled over on to their side for examination of the underbelly and the feet, or the feet can be lifted.

### Vital signs, age, body condition score

Once the sheep is caught and restrained the rectal temperature and pulse rate are determined. The pulse rate is taken at the femoral artery. The respiratory rate can be taken at this time but is better observed prior to catching and restraining the animal. Sheep may have rapid respiratory rates, especially in high ambient temperatures or following minor exercise, and the significance of an altered respiratory rate in a suspected sick animal can best be determined by comparing it with the respiratory rate of healthy flock mates. The age of the animal is usually determined at this time by a quick inspection of the incisor teeth (see below). It is advisable to determine the condition of the animal early in the examination, as this can give an indication of the acuteness or chronicity of a problem. Again, this should be measured against the condition of healthy flock mates. The body condition of shorn sheep and of goats can be determined visually; however, visual assessment can be misleading in sheep with any degree of wool cover, and in these animals body condition should be determined by palpation. The British Meat and Livestock Commission has developed a scoring system which is detailed in Table 10.1.

Bone quality is subjectively examined by determining the 'spring' of the ribs and their resistance to bending from lateral pressure, and the resistance of the frontal bones to thumb pressure. The measure is not sensitive but will detect the osteoporosis of calcium and copper deficiency in lambs. Local softening of the frontal bone also occurs in sheep infested with *Coenurus cerebralis*.

### Examination of fleece and skin

Following the determination of body condition the fleece and the underlying skin are examined visually for the presence of a breakpoint in the fleece, for signs of bacterial infection and parasitic infestation, and also examined by palpation. Similarly the hair, skin and superficial lymph nodes of goats are examined visually and by palpation. In both species this examination should be over the entire skin surface.

---

**Clinical Pointer**

In general, sheep will become passive once they are caught, but those with neurological disease, such as early listeriosis, may continue with frenetic attempts to escape.

---

**Determining body condition by palpation**

Palpate immediately behind the last rib to determine

- the prominence of the spinous and transverse processes of the lumbar vertebrae
- the amount of muscular and fatty tissues underneath the transverse process
- the fullness of the eye muscles and its fat cover in the supra-orbital fossa.

**Table 10.1.   Body condition scoring of sheep (Adapted from Russel, A. 1984. In Practice 6:91–93)**

Score

0. There is no detectable muscular or fatty tissue between the skin and the bone. Extremely emaciated.

1. Spinous and transverse processes are prominent and sharp. It is easy to feel between each process. The eye muscle areas are shallow with no fat cover.

2. Spinous and transverse ventral processes are prominent but smooth and rounded. It is possible to pass the fingers under the ends of the transverse process with a little pressure. The eye muscle areas are of moderate depth but have little fat cover.

3. Spinous processes are detected only as small elevations and are smooth and rounded. The transverse processes are smooth and well covered and firm pressure is required to feel the edges. The eye muscle areas are full and have a moderate degree of fat cover.

4. The spinous processes can just be detected with pressure as a hard line between fat-covered muscle areas. The ends of the transverse processes cannot be felt. The eye muscles are full and have a thick covering of fat.

5. The spinous processes cannot be detected even with firm pressure and there is a depression between the layers of fat in the position where the spinous processes would normally be felt. The transverse processes cannot be detected. The eye muscle areas are very full, with very thick fat cover. There may also large deposits of fat over the rump and the tail.

---

**Wool-breaks**

Wool-breaks reflect the occurrence of a serious disease or period of poor nutrition in the past history of the animal, that compromised the nutrition of the wool follicle and produced a defect in wool growth. A wool-break is common following diseases such as pregnancy toxemia and blue tongue. Although it is not of concern to the current health of the sheep, the presence of a wool-break significantly downgrades the commercial value of the wool.

---

With sheep the fleece is initially examined by parting it in the area of its greatest quality, which is behind the shoulder. The presence of a breakpoint is indicated by a horizontal line of thinning of the wool fiber and a change in the crimp at this site on the staple. Commonly dust accumulates in this area, resulting in a dark line in the fleece. The wool is tender at this spot and will break when the staple is snapped, either between the fingers or spontaneously on the sheep, resulting in shedding of the wool at this point.

Clinical signs of parasitic infestation, common to different parasites, include

- irritation
- head shaking
- stamping
- dermatitis
- fleece damage
- wool and hair loss.

Some, such as the sheep ked, are easily visible and also produce staining in the wool. Similarly, tick infestations and the presence of cutaneous myiasis – fly strike – are easily determined. Sucking lice on the head and lower body also can be relatively easily detected. *Damalinia ovis* are barely visible to the naked eye but can be observed if the examination is concentrated in the dorsum of the body close to the skin, which is the area where they are most commonly present. The parasites associated with sheep scab (*Psoroptes ovis* or *Sarcoptes scabiei*) and the equivalent infestation in goats (*Psoroptes cuniculi*) cannot be seen macroscopically but their presence is suggested by the occurrence of severe pruritus, the presence of small pustules in the skin and the presence of a hard yellow crust at the skin surface or in the wool. Persistent ear irritation should be investigated for the presence of psoroptic mange mites. Any increase in scurf seen during parting the fleece to the skin level suggests a parasitic infestation and indicates that a skin scraping should be taken.

Palpation is part of the examination of the fleece and skin. The fleece should be palpated for evidence of mycotic dermatitis (lumpy wool disease). The hard scabs associated with this infection can be palpated at skin level or in the wool, and are usually present along the back line of the sheep with 'ribs' of infection running down the sides. The skin should be palpated for evidence of thickening and dermatitis associated with infection, or inflammation from other causes, such as photosensitivity, and the subcutaneous lymph nodes palpated for abnormality. The subcutaneous lymph nodes that are normally palpable include the

- mandibular
- parotid (palpated in conjunction with the parotid salivary gland)
- superficial cervical (prescapular)
- subiliac (prefemoral), and
- in the young lamb and kid, the popliteal and the axillary.

Small subcutaneous hemal lymph nodes are also commonly detected while palpating the skin in both sheep and goats. Swelling of a lymph node occurs as the result of infection or trauma in its drainage area. Swellings of the parotid and mandibular lymph nodes are quite common in sheep, but a common cause of enlargement and abscessation of lymph nodes in both sheep and goats is caseous lymphadenitis. This is associated with fluctuant abscesses in the lymph nodes in the early stages of the disease, which may rupture to discharge green-yellow pus into the wool or on to the skin, or may progress to inspissation, with the occurrence of hard, swollen lymph nodes. Lymphatic tumors are rare in both species. Subcutaneous dependent edema may also be detected during palpation. This pits on pressure like putty, but there is no pain or heat associated with its occurrence. Subcutaneous edema may result from congestive heart failure, but in sheep and goats it rarely results from hypoproteinemia. Ventral edema can also be the result of urethral rupture as a consequence of urolithiasis.

The fleece of lambs frequently contains more hair (kemp and gare) fibers than that of the adult and, depending upon the breed, these are particularly noticeable on the rump and the limbs. They are shed within a few weeks of birth.

A particularly hairy coat coupled with the presence of halo hairs projecting above the fleece, especially around the neck and thorax, and the presence of pigmented areas in the fleece, are strongly suggestive of congenital infection with pestivirus (Border disease, Hairy shaker disease). Wool loss may be associated with non-parasitic diseases such as scrapie and wool slip.

### Head and neck

The face should be examined both visually and by palpation. It is common to find small (2–5 mm) gray crusty scabs in the non-wooled part of the face. These are chronic lesions of mycotic dermatitis and provide the site of perpetuation of this infection. Similar lesions are on the haired parts of the feet. Larger lesions can occur on the ears and face when conditions favor the spread of the infection. Larger white crusty lesions around the eyes and elsewhere on the face can also be caused by ringworm fungus infections. Inflammation of the skin in the periorbital area suggests periorbital eczema, a disease caused by *Staphylococcus aureus*, in which infection results in dermatitis that progresses to deep necrotic ulceration with overlying scab formation. Lesions may also occur elsewhere on the skin of the head. Sheep, but not goats, have small invaginations – face or tear glands – beneath the eyes. Goats have wattles hanging from both sides of the upper neck.

Swelling of the mandible may be associated with dentigerous cyst infections in the tooth roots, fibrosarcoma or, rarely, hypertrophic osteopathy in the newborn. The area between the mandibles should also be specifically palpated for the presence of edema (bottle jaw). Edema resulting from hypoproteinemia is commonly first evident at this site, and its detection indicates the need for further specific and laboratory examination for the causes of hypoproteinemia. Edematous swelling of the ears and of the subcutaneous tissue all over the face occurs with blue tongue and photosensitivity. An inflammatory edema of the head also occurs in rams, associated with *Clostridium novyi* infection (big head).

The salivary glands can be examined by palpation. They include the mandibular gland, which is found medial to the angle of the mandible. Its duct opens on the floor of the mouth beneath the tip of the tongue on the papillus. The parotid salivary gland is caudal to the mandible and below the ear. Swelling in this area may also be due to lymphadenitis of the parotid lymph node, which is in the same region. The parotid salivary duct discharges opposite to the fourth upper cheek tooth. The sublingual gland is beneath the tongue and between the rami of the mandible, and consists of two parts: the dorsal part empties via several ducts on the floor of the mouth beside the tongue, and the ventral part has a single duct which joins the mandibular duct. These salivary glands are examined quickly, as abnormality is extremely rare. Salivary cysts involving the ducts occur occasionally in goats and present as large visible fluctuating swellings. Swellings on the face of goats are also commonly associated with caseous

---

**Clinical Pointer**

Subcutaneous edema in the neck of newborn lambs, accompanied by palpable enlargement of the thyroid gland, is indicative of primary or secondary iodine deficiency.

---

**Photosensitivity**

Photosensitivity is accompanied by pain, heat, irritation, and exudation, followed by necrosis of the skin and hair loss, and, in severe cases, by sloughing of the necrotic skin. Lesions may also occur on the forelimbs, scrotum, and perineum, and in goats can occur in any non-pigmented part of the body.

lymphadenitis. The frontal sinus is large, especially in horned breeds of sheep, and can be examined by percussion: clinically detectable abnormality is rare.

### Examination of eyes and conjunctivae

The mucous membranes of the conjunctivae and the eyes should be inspected visually. The conjunctiva and sclera are generally the best sites to assess the presence of anemia, such as occurs with hemonchosis and epery-throzoonosis, as in black-faced sheep the oral mucous membranes are often pigmented. Jaundice can also be detected at this site.

Small white heaped-up follicles on the conjunctivae occur following pink eye caused by chlamydial or rickettsial infection, and may be the site for carriage of these organisms. Lacrimation and blepharospasm are indicative of abnormality in the eye, and blepharospasm and epiphora may be seen at the distant examination. If the problem is unilateral the eye should be examined for the presence of a foreign body, particularly a grass seed, which will commonly be lodged under the third eyelid. Conjunctivitis and neovascularization of the dorsal cornea suggest the occurrence of infectious keratoconjunctivitis. Entropion is a common defect in newborn lambs and is easily recognized by the inversion of the lower eyelid. Blindness can be assessed with the menace response, and may be central or due to retinal atrophy associated with the ingestion of bracken fern. Defects in vision indicate the need for special and ophthalmoscopic examination of the eye. Bilateral epiphora accompanied by nasal discharge also indicates that the upper respiratory tract should be particularly examined for infection.

Unilateral paralysis of an ear, the lip, cheek, eyelid, and nostril results from unilateral facial nerve disease, which in sheep commonly is due to listeriosis. A detailed and specific examination of cranial nerve function is usually not conducted unless there are signs of CNS and/or cranial nerve dysfunction.

### Oral cavity

Following examination of the head and eyes the oral cavity is next examined. The lips are thin, mobile, have a well marked philtrum in the upper lip, and are prehensile and thus subject to trauma and infection. Actinobacillosis in sheep affects the upper and/or lower lip, causing swelling and fibrous thickening with pustules and fistulae, which periodically discharge purulent material. Salivation with wetting of the hair around the lips is not normal but occurs in lambs that are hypothermic and hypoglycemic, and in lambs that have enteric infections and watery mouth. Less commonly excessive salivation results from a lesion in the mouth or from nervous dysfunction.

Next the lips should be elevated and the mucous membranes of the mouth examined for color and the presence of abnormality. At this time it is common to smell the breath for ketone and the saliva for an ammoniacal smell associated with azotemia. In both cases direct biochemical testing of blood and urine is more objective. The lips are the site of linear erosive lesions in blue tongue disease, and these are usually most evident at the mucocutaneous junction of the upper and lower lips and at the commissures, as are the proliferative and scabby lesions of contagious ecthyma (orf).

The hard palate is prominent in its rostral part and forms the dental pad. The transverse ridges of the hard palate are smooth on their edges and do not extend across the width of the palate, but alternate at the median line. The part of the hard palate caudal to a line between the first molar teeth has no ridges but contains orifices of the ducts of the palatine glands. The cheeks are studded with large papillae which are pointed. The tongue of sheep and goats has a pointed end, is narrower than that of cattle, and its base is not as prominent. The dorsal surface is covered by filiform and fungiform papillae. Erosive lesions occur on the tongue and hard palate with blue tongue.

*Teeth*

Sheep have 32 permanent teeth and the dental formula is:

2 (I 0/4, C 0/0, P 3/3, M 3/3) = 32.

There are 20 deciduous teeth, all of which erupt within a few days of birth and all of which are functional by 2–4 weeks of age. The eruption time of the permanent teeth is quite variable but is nevertheless the major method by which sheep are aged. The permanent central incisors erupt at 10–12 months of age and are well exposed by 15 months. The middle permanent incisors erupt at 18–24 months (two-tooth), the third

---

### Clinical Pointer

Severe jaundice can result in yellow discoloration of the skin in white sheep.

---

### Foot-and-mouth disease

Vesicular lesions on the tongue are highly suggestive of foot-and-mouth disease and should be reported to the relevant authority.

incisors at 2–2.5 years and the lateral incisors at 3–4 years (full mouth). Sheep have no incisors on the upper jaw and the lower incisors impact against a dental pad. The incisors can be examined by retracting the lips. Clinical examination of the cheek teeth requires the use of a gag and a flashlight, and even with these there is only superficial vision of the angle of the tables of the teeth and the spaces associated with absent teeth. Further examination is made by palpating the outside cutting edge of the upper molars and the ventral and lateral aspect of the mandible through the cheek, which will allow the detection of gross abnormalities.

The shape of the incisor teeth changes with age. Healthy mature sheep should have closely packed, short, spade-shaped incisors. Peg-like teeth are quite common in normal sheep and may result from natural tooth-to-tooth wear. Excessive wear is a problem both in the individual and in the flock, and can reduce the incisors to pebble-like structures, which severely reduces grazing efficiency and the lifetime productivity of the ewe. The normal gingiva is pink and closely applied to the teeth. Gingivitis may be found in almost all sheep but is commonly slight and localized around the gingival margin of one or two teeth. Extensive and severe gingivitis and periodontitis is present where there is premature loss of incisor teeth, and may be present as a prelude to tooth loss in flocks where this is a problem. Premature loss of the incisor teeth (broken mouth) is a major cause of early culling of ewes and predisposes to a number of diseases associated with suboptimal nutrient intake.

*Larynx and trachea*
The larynx, trachea, and esophageal area are examined by palpation. Choke is rare, but balling gun injuries, suspected from the presence of dysphagia coupled with swelling and pain on palpation in the retropharyngeal area, can occur, with inexperienced labor.

## Thorax (heart and lungs)

In goats and shorn sheep the thorax is examined using auscultation, percussion, and percussion with auscultation, but the wool cover of sheep negates percussion. Auscultation of the heart and lungs in sheep is also made difficult by the presence of wool. The heart may be auscultated by placing the stethoscope on the non-wooled skin under the elbow, which is sufficiently mobile that it can be moved to auscultate the area of the heart. The lungs are more difficult to auscultate and can only be approached by parting the wool. The techniques of examination are the same as for the cow, but the anatomy of the thorax differs in sheep and the area of auscultation of lung sounds is larger. In sheep the reflection of the pleura from the diaphragm to the ribs extends from the sternum along the 7th and 8th costal cartilages, and does not occur dorsal to the costochondral cartilage until the 9th rib. It continues along the ventral ends of ribs 10–12, and crosses the 13th rib at its midpoint to end dorsally midway between the last thoracic and first lumbar vertebra.

**Breath sounds in sheep**
The normal breath sounds on auscultation are of a higher pitch than those in cattle. In sheep of condition score 3 they are normally heard over the ventral half of the thorax at resting respiratory rates, and are most intense over the bronchial hilus. The intensity of the sounds and the area of the thorax over which they can be heard increases with lower condition scores and decreases as the animal gets fatter.

Lower respiratory tract infections are common in sheep during the first year of life, and chronic respiratory disease from progressive pneumonia, pulmonary adenomatosis or pulmonary infections with *Actinomyces pyogenes* is common in older sheep. The viral and bacterial lower respiratory tract infections of young sheep and goats particularly affect the cranial lobes of the lung, producing an exudative bronchopneumonia with consolidation. The abnormal increase in intensity and pitch of the airflow sounds that occurs with these infections is best heard by auscultation over the bronchial hilus and cranial and ventral to it. The changes are usually greatest on the right side. The pneumonias of older sheep, such as maedi, produce a more diffuse change in the auscultative findings, as does pulmonary adenomatosis. In the latter there is considerable fluid production in the lung, with associated coarse fluid sounds on auscultation and the pouring of many ml of fluid from the nostrils when the

> ### Clinical Pointer
>
> To make a sheep cough, pinch its larynx or rostral trachea, the increase in air flow will allow brief auscultation of sounds in the more distal parts of the lung, and may also allow the detection of exudate in the airways. Alternatively, a rebreathing bag can be used for a more prolonged increase of air movement.

> ### Clinical Pointer
>
> Any bony swelling above the cheek teeth suggests serious tooth damage.

hind end of the sheep is elevated. Auscultatory findings associated with lungworm are concentrated in the diaphragmatic lobe and can be induced by pinching the trachea and eliciting a cough. Abnormal sounds on auscultation may suggest the need for further laboratory examination of fluid obtained by tracheobronchial aspiration.

### Heart sounds

The apex beat of the heart is palpable on both sides of the chest in moderate to thin body-conditioned sheep, but more palpable on the left. Displacement of the apex beat or of the area of maximal audibility of heart sounds indicates the presence of an intrathoracic mass, which in sheep and goats is usually an abscess associated with generalized caseous lymphadenitis. The heart may be auscultated on both sides but is more audible on the left. The area of maximal audibility of the left atrioventricular valve is in the 5th intercostal space at the level of the point of the elbow. The aortic valve is most audible in the 4th intercostal space on the left side at the level of the scapulohumeral joint, and the pulmonic valve is most audible slightly ventral to this and in the 3rd intercostal space. The right atrioventricular valve is most audible in the 4th intercostal space on the right side at the level of the point of the elbow.

Cardiovascular disease is comparatively uncommon (or unrecognized) in sheep and goats. When a heart murmur is detected, it most commonly will be a systolic heart murmur and due to anemia or hypoproteinemia. Otherwise the detection of a heart murmur most commonly indicates the presence of endocarditis. The murmur is usually systolic because these infections in sheep and goats have a predilection for the right and/or left atrioventricular valve. Cardiac arrhythmias may be detected in animals with nutritionally induced or associated cardiomyopathies, such as selenium/vitamin E deficiency, ionophore poisoning and acute phalaris poisoning. Atrial fibrillation occurs in goats and sheep that develop cor pulmonale as a consequence of chronic pulmonary disease.

### Abdomen

The examination of the abdomen is conducted as in cattle and will not be repeated here. The anatomical locations of the gastrointestinal organs are briefly described for reference.

The rumen has a capacity of approximately 3 gallons and occupies almost all of the abdominal cavity left of the median plane. When full it extends to the right of the median plane. The reticulum is relatively larger than that in the cow and is situated mostly to the left of the median plane, between the diaphragm and the cranial part of the rumen, omasum and abomasum, and to the left of the liver. It contacts the sternal part of the diaphragm and extends forward to the 6th rib. The omasum is the smallest of the four compartments, is dorsal to the abomasum and has no contact with the abdominal wall. The abomasum contacts the abdominal floor and is situated mostly to the right of the medial plane. Its cranial blind end is situated dorsal to the xiphoid cartilage, the body extends caudally to the right costal arch, and the pylorus is opposite the ventral part of the 11th intercostal space. The rest of the abdomen is occupied by the intestine. The small intestine is about 24m long. The cecum is 25–30 cm long, is dorsal to the colon and extends backward, with the blind end pointing toward the pelvic cavity and occasionally within the pelvic inlet.

There are some examination techniques that can be used in small ruminants that are not used in cattle. Rectal palpation is not possible in sheep because of their small size.

### Palpation of the abdomen

In young animals and thin adults the contents of the abdomen can be palpated through the abdominal wall. The technique is to palpate with both hands at the same time with one on either side of the abdomen. This is done both with the animal standing and with it cast and lying on its back. Succussion can also be used in lambs and kids, and may assist in detecting the fluid and gas accumulation in the stomach and intestines seen with diseases such as watery mouth.

### Urinary tract

Examination of the urinary system is largely by laboratory testing of blood and urine. The presence of crystalline calculi clinging to preputial hair is evidence of a potential risk for urolithiasis, and animals with this disease are distressed, strain to urinate and pass small

---

**Clinical Pointer**

When counting back from the last rib it should be recognized that some sheep have 14 ribs.

---

**Clinical Pointer**

The left kidney is mobile and can be palpated in the mid-abdomen in thin sheep. It should not be mistaken for an abnormal mass.

amounts of bloodstained urine or none at all. Female sheep and goats have a suburethral diverticulum that impedes urethral catheterization for the collection of urine, and collection is usually attempted by inducing fright-induced urination via temporary smothering. The vulva is examined for vulvitis and distortion, which can result in urine staining of the wool. The vulva and perineal area is a site for squamous cell carcinoma, which can occur with significant prevalence in sheep that have had skin removed from the region to reduce fecal soiling of the perineum ('mulesed sheep') with short-docked tails. The nose is also a site of predilection.

### Reproductive tract

The contents of the scrotum of the ram are examined by palpation with particular reference to the size and consistency of the testicles and the size, shape and consistency of the head, body, and tail of the epididymis. The purpose of the examination is to detect

- congenital abnormality
- atrophy for any reason
- the presence of inflammatory disease, particularly epididymitis.

This examination is conducted with the ram standing and the clinician crouching behind it. In any ram suspected as being infertile as a result of the physical examination of the testicles, the semen should be tested. The surface of the scrotum should also be examined for evidence of parasite infestation. Lesions of *Dermatophilus congolensis* infection are commonly present on the scrotum of rams.

### *Examination of limbs and udder*

The sheep is turned over for this stage of the examination and the limbs and udder, and the prepuce in wethers and rams, are examined. It is also convenient to take blood for laboratory examination while the animal is thus restrained.

Limb abnormalities which may have been detected at the distant examination should now be examined in more detail. The presence of swelling and heat in the joints and/or tendon sheaths and bursae should be determined by palpation. Abnormalities are more likely to be detected in the larger joints.

The claws and interdigital skin area are examined by palpation for heat, by pressure for pain, and visually for abnormality. The presence of inflammation and exudate in the interdigital space is suggestive of foot scald. Particular attention should be given to the health of the skin–horn junctions in the interdigital space, as this is the site of the early lesions of contagious foot-rot.

Separation at the skin–horn junction in the interdigital cleft and underrunning of the horn are the lesions that occur in foot-rot and, if found, the foot may need to be pared further to confirm the presence of under-running, to determine its severity and to obtain material for laboratory examination. The detection of heat on palpation and pain on pressure is most commonly associated with the presence of an abscess in the foot, which usually manifests with severe lameness. Toe abscesses most commonly involve one claw of the front foot and can be confirmed by paring the horn at the toe, which will result in the release of pus under pressure. Heel abscesses most commonly involve the medial claw of a hind limb.

Sheep have skin invaginations forming a pouch that opens near the top of the cleft between the two toes. In the front feet of goats this is absent or only vestigial. Short wool fibers project from these invaginations and they have a sebaceous secretion. They can be the site for grass seed penetration. Inflammation of the skin in the region of the coronet is most commonly associated with infection with contagious ecthyma virus and with foot louse. Blue tongue produces hemorrhage in this area. Vesicular lesions at the coronary band and in the interdigital skin suggest foot-and-mouth disease.

> ### Balanoposthitis
>
> Balanoposthitis is a common disease in wethers on a high-protein diet. It is indicated by the presence of pustules and a foul-smelling exudate around the opening of the prepuce, palpation over the prepuce can determine the degree of internal infection.

The udder should be palpated and the milk examined for evidence of mastitis, in the same way as for cattle. A firm distended udder at the time of parturition, but which has very little milk, is suggestive of lentivirus infection in sheep and goats (hard bag). Lesions of contagious ecthyma can be present on the skin of the udder when there is this infection in sucking lambs, and may also be present on the feet above the coronet and, less commonly, around the vulva. Warts are also occasionally present on the skin of the udder.

## EXAMINATION OF NEONATES

Physical examination of the newborn should include those body systems at particular risk for congenital defects. The examination of a sick lamb or kid should particularly include palpation of the umbilicus for evidence of navel ill and a thorough examination of the joints for joint ill and polyarthritis.

## FURTHER READING

Arnold GW. Grazing behavior. In: Morley FWH (ed) Grazing animals. Amsterdam: Elsevier Scientific Publications, 1981;79–104.

Bruere AN, West DM. The sheep. Health, disease and production. Veterinary Continuing Education, Massey University, New Zealand, 1993.

Crofton HD. Nematode populations in sheep on lowland farms. VI Sheep behavior and nematode infections. Parasitology 1958; 48: 251–260.

Hecker JF. The sheep as an experimental animal. London: Academic Press, 1983.

Hindson JC, Winter AC. Outline of clinical diagnosis in sheep. London: Wright, 1990.

Linklater KA, Smith MC. Color atlas of diseases and disorders of the sheep and goat. Wolfe Publishing, 1993.

Lu CD. Grazing behavior and diet selection of goats. Small Ruminant Research 1988; 1:205–216.

May NDS. The anatomy of the sheep. University of Queensland Press, 1954.

Morley FWH. Management of grazing systems. In: Morley FWH (ed) Grazing animals. Amsterdam: Elsevier Scientific Publications, 1981; 379–400.

Pearce GR. Rumination in sheep. The circadian pattern of rumination. Australian Journal of Agricultural Research 1965;16:635–648.

Radostits OM, Blood DC, Gay CC. Veterinary medicine, 8th edn. London: Baillière Tindall, 1994.

Sherman DM, Robinson RA. Clinical examination of sheep and goats. Veterinary Clinics of North America 1993; 5(3):409–426.

# 11

# Clinical Examination of Llamas and Alpacas

*L. Johnson*

## INTRODUCTION

From the outset the reader should be aware of the marked similarities between these two domestic members of the South American camelids. Because of this, in most cases details of the physical examination procedure will be applicable to both. The most striking differences between the two are in their body size/weight, fineness of wool, body conformation and temperament. The alpaca is expected to be smaller, with fine wool, having a normal conformation characterized by marked rounding of the rump and generally a herd temperament, making it somewhat more excitable when isolated. Except for unusual animals, a clinical examination will necessitate the use of a restraining chute or at least some manual restraint, and occasionally chemical restraint. Their reluctance to cooperate with minimal restraint (e.g. a halter) is traced to their social/herd behavior, which includes extreme dominance and subordinate relationships. These are established by body language and sparring, the latter including either playful or serious biting at the limbs, ears and even gonads.

Most animals will be presented for clinical examination as individuals. They may be on their own turf, or be presented off their turf (e.g. at a clinic). In either case a degree of apprehension is to be expected, but is likely to be more exaggerated in a strange setting.

> ### Clinical Pointer ✳
>
> Be aware, when examining camelids, that they are very sensitive about parts of their body and they will protect themselves fiercely.

There will, from time to time, be a need for herd evaluation. On such occasions it is well to be aware that camelids are extremely visual, innately curious, but cautious. As such, a normal herd will have animals that range considerably in response to the veterinarian's presence. Once this has been recognized, there will be some that retreat and others that show their usual curiosity. Llamas that approach and seem very 'friendly' are not usual and in most cases will be found to have abnormal behavior towards humans. The clinical examination of either llamas or alpacas should be conducted in an organized repetitive fashion, similar to that performed on cattle and horses.

## EVALUATION OF OWNER, MANAGEMENT AND THE ENVIRONMENT

In addition to taking a detailed history of the present problem, the client's reasons for owning the animal(s) are to be considered, along with establishment of the economic value. Moreover, familiarity with existing management and environmental factors will distinctly influence interpretation of the subsequent clinical examination.

## DISTANT EXAMINATION

### Mentation

Unless extremely ill, most camelids will be alert and very aware of the presence of people. Whether restrained or not, many will demonstrate apprehension by voluntarily producing a near ectropion of the lower lid that results in a 'worry wrinkle' (Fig. 11.1), accompanied by a tightening of the lips. Animals that are truly defensive will posture themselves to face the examiner, lay their ears back and raise their heads. Unless it is aggressive the usual way of approaching a defensive animal is to avoid eye contact and casually attempt to make contact by touching the back of your hand on the animal's body, encircling the neck with your right hand from the animal's left side, moving forward to place your right hip against the animal's left shoulder, and gently placing a halter in position. Under farm conditions this would presumably be done by the owner.

Camelid owners and experienced veterinarians will agree that patient stoicism is a factor to acknowledge in assessment by inspection. As such, it appears that even neonates may present an impression of wellbeing in spite of serious health alterations. Close physical inspection or subsequent laboratory tests will aid in pinpointing the severity of any problems.

Whether the animal is free in a stall or presented with halter and lead, conformation should be assessed.

## Conformation

The most common limb conformation abnormality is carpus valgus; however, cow hock and sickle hock conditions are observed. Abundant leg wool in alpacas and some llamas makes evaluation of leg conformation somewhat difficult. Repeated standing posturing may be essential in order to make a final judgment on limb conformation, as the animals have a tendency to be somewhat erratic in limb placement. Alpacas will generally tend to appear somewhat sickle-hocked, with a 'camped under' result owing to their normal rounded

> ### Limb conformation
>
> Normal limb conformation of camelids is quite similar to horse conformation, with the exception that most camelids will normally toe-out slightly with the forelimbs.

rump. Evaluation of normal walking gait reveals a near pace, with only the slightest delay in the same-side forelimb touching the ground after the rear. Varying according to width of chest, the tracking may be wide or narrow; however, use of the llama as a packing animal favors a narrow track. The observed gaits of a free camelid include walking, pacing, galloping and pronking. Generally during a prepurchase examination the animal will be led at a walk, and only when assessing cardiac and respiratory function would there be indication to perform more vigorous exercise.

## Integument and hair

In their native habitat camelids would be regularly shorn for their fiber; however, in North America great variability is to be expected in their presented grooming state. Many llamas will rarely, if ever, be shorn, with their natural shedding building up as a thatch, mats of which will occasionally pull off. In contrast, others will be regularly groomed to remove some of their fine underfibers, leaving the long coarse guard hairs. Others, especially in hot humid climates, will be shorn completely or be given a 'poodle cut'. Alpacas are more likely to be shorn at regular intervals, but may be kept in a well groomed show condition. The

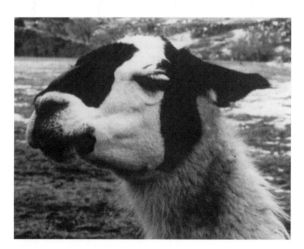

**Fig. 11.1** An apprehensive llama, with tight lips, worry wrinkle and ears pinned back.

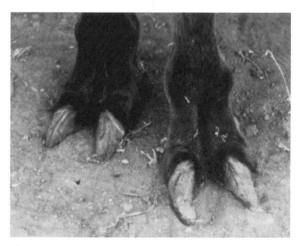

**Fig. 11.2** Llama toenails in need of trimming.

examiner should therefore be prepared to observe wide variations in normal fiber presentation. Camelids have two toes and their respective nails, which will wear adequately with exercise on a rough surface. However, most North American camelids will need periodic toenail clipping, as with inadequate attention they will tend to elongate and curl (Fig. 11.2), often resulting in permanent alteration of growth as well as distortion of the digit tendon and ligament configuration.

Because of the extensive wool cover of most camelids visual inspection of specific anatomical locations is rather limited, in many cases excluding limb conformation, perineal genitalia and body condition. Consequently, other than an assessment of head anatomy and suggested conformation, the examiner may have to delay conclusions until a hands-on evaluation can be accomplished.

### Urination, defecation and rumination

Normal functions, including urination, defecation, and the various phases of rumination, are unlikely to be observed at clinical examination. Camelids have a usual dunging area, which is why they are less likely to perform under such circumstances. However, if the examiner is able to observe the animal(s) on their home turf these functions would be observed if healthy. If this observation were to be deemed essential for the presented case, the owner could be asked to provide a 'seed sample' of the animal's dung pile, which will often prompt the subject to defecate and urinate upon exposure. Upon hospitalization, these functions should be a part of daily observation and would be anticipated to normalize.

## CLOSE PHYSICAL EXAMINATION

### Rectal temperature

Without the influence of exercise, anxiety, or unusual ambient temperatures, the resting body temperatures of camelids would be expected to be in the range of 99.5–102 °F (37.5–38.9 °C). During extremely hot weather, many animals that appear normal are found to have core temperatures approaching 104 °F (40 °C), which predisposes them to heat stress upon exertion.

### Pulse

In a practical sense there is but one location to reliably ascertain a peripheral pulse in camelids, that being the medial saphenous artery, located on the inside of the rear leg at mid-femur level. If the animal is restrained in a chute evaluation is best accomplished by, for example, first making contact with the fiberless area of the left abdomen and gradually moving the left hand to the inside of the left rear leg, where the artery will readily be detected. Avoid contact with the lower limb as this will usually create uneasiness. The pulse rate will vary with degree of excitability from the procedure, but should fall in the range of 60–90 bpm.

### Respirations

A resting respiratory rate may best be determined by observation of nostril flaring, but during normal clinical examination can be determined by stethoscopic auscultation over the trachea in the caudal neck region. Normal rates tend to have a wide range of 10–30/min, with the effort being combined thoracic and abdominal. Exaggerated abdominal involvement would be deemed abnormal.

### Body condition score

A subjective assessment of body condition is important for the current physical examination as well as for subsequent nutritional considerations. A scale of 1 (thin) to 10 (fat), with 5 being ideal, has been utilized. Principal locations for assessment include the mid-back (T8–L2) region, as well as the fiberless area of the thorax behind the point of the elbow. Palpation over the dorsal pelvis tends to suggest poor body condition in all camelids. In addition, particularly for those deemed to be over-conditioned, assessment of the brisket and perineal region has proved valuable. Guidelines for assessment are given in Figure 11.3.

### Visible mucous membranes

As with most species, sites for the assessment of mucous membranes are limited to the oral mucosa and the conjunctivae, except for the female where the vaginal mucosa is utilized. Many camelids have variable degrees of oral pigmentation, making evaluation challenging; however, a pink color will indicate normality. Attempts to assess capillary refill time will first be made from the orolabial mucosa, but the vaginal mucosa is also of value.

### Wool

Departures from normal wool condition include areas of alopecia, stiff wool and reduction of pigmentation.

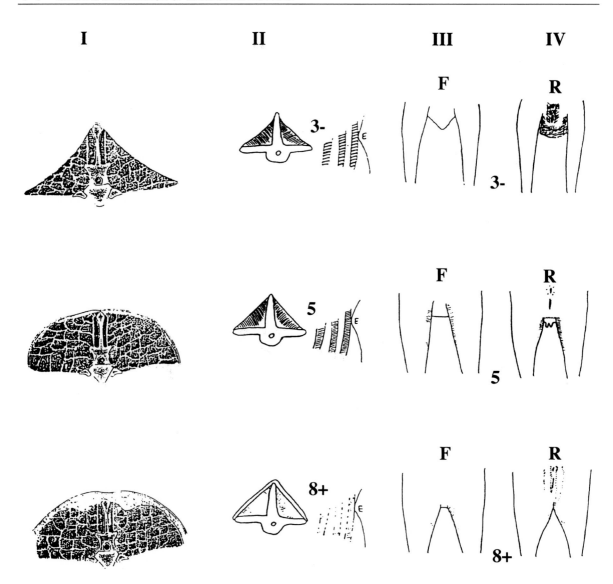

**Fig. 11.3** Guidelines for body condition scoring of camelids. I (Muscle/vertebral column cross-section at level of T12. II The elbow (E) and the degree of presence of ribs just caudal. III Appearance of animals from front (F) view. IV Appearance of animals from rear (R) view. (Numbers 3, 5 and 8 represent example BSCs.)

Certain llamas tend normally to have biannual shedding of the neck and shoulder regions. Camelids have occasionally been observed to undergo the condition referred to in sheep as 'woolslipping'. in response to high fever or major alterations in nutrition.

## Skin

Considering the extensive wool covering of most of the camelid body, true evaluation of the skin requires a hands-on approach. Skin on the head and ears is normally covered with fine hair, but many animals will have rubbed the hair from the dorsum of their nose (dorsal nasal alopecia) and ears as they respond to summertime insects. The areas of perineum and brisket, as well as the underbelly and a small area behind the point of the elbow, are available for evaluation without parting the wool. Parting of wool over the dorsum will generally yield a variable amount of debris trapped in the wool, making assessment of ectoparasites and dryness as well as dandruff somewhat more challenging.

**Clinical Pointer**

- lice are located along the dorsum, making this a prime area for inspection
- mange is present initially over the fiberless areas of the perineum, brisket, and lower limbs.

## Eyes

Relatively large expressive eyes characterize the camelids, which gives the impression of having extremely well developed eyesight. Unique normal features include

- long eyelashes
- extremely prominent corpora nigra
- variable pigmentation of the iris
- pronounced retinal vascular pattern
- no fovea
- no tapetum.

Unfortunately, because their eyes are so prominent, the most common presenting complaint is eye injury. Close examination of the eyes is best facilitated by adequate physical restraint, including cross-tying as well as chemical restraint using butorphanol (0.02–0.04 mg/kg) either intravenously or intramuscularly.

## Ears

Another small difference between llamas and alpacas is found in the normal length of the ear, with alpacas generally having shorter ones. As with eye examination, most camelids will respond to examination of the ears with resistance. A true otoscopic examination is difficult because of the small ear canal diameter (3–5 mm), which is characterized by a sharp bend making visualization of the tympanic membrane virtually impossible without using a very small endoscope. External ear problems include lacerations, usually caused by fighting, and sloughage due to frostbite. Internal abnormalities include the presence of foreign bodies, notably foxtails and seasonal ticks, both of which may contribute to neurological presentations.

## Nares

Visual inspection will reveal a pair of well defined external nares characterized by moistness due to normal nasolacrimal duct drainage. Any departure from a clear moistness, including dryness and serous, mucous, purulent or sanguinous discharge, and combinations thereof, would be regarded as abnormal. Uniform air flow from each nostril is to be expected. Exceptions indicating abnormality are upper airway involvements, including unilateral infections, nasal bots and partial to complete unilateral choanal atresia.

**Clinical Pointer**

An accumulation of plant material in the external nares suggests cleft palate.

## Oral cavity

When there is abnormal mastication, weight loss or jaw lesions, or in the assessment of a geriatric case, a detailed inspection of the oral cavity is indicated. To accomplish this successfully, minimal sedation may be used ideally anesthesia using ketamine at 4.4 mg/kg bw and xylazine at 0.44 mg/kg bw, are required owing to the extremely narrow space between arcades, the small range of jaw opening and the extremely sharp premolars and molars, as well as the fighting fangs if present. Irregular wear of cheek teeth, as well as broken or missing teeth, can be detected visually by gently displacing the tongue laterally. The permanent tooth dental formula is:

$$I_{1/3}{}^*, C_{1/1}, PM_{1-2/1-2}, M_{3/3} \times 2.$$

*The rostral maxillary fighting tooth is regarded as a vestigial incisor. The base of the tongue is characterized by a thick dome whose dorsal surface has many papillae, some of which normally appear pitted. The extremely narrow oropharyngeal space is normal, and the long soft palate accounts for these animals being near-obligatory nasal breathers.

## Jaw alignment and teeth

Normal jaw alignment would have the three pairs of lower incisors in a relative vertical plane contacting the rostral margin of the maxillary jaw dental pad. With age the incisors tend to become more horizontal, causing a slight forward protrusion. Unfortunately, jaw malalignment is relatively common, with either maxillary or mandibular disproportion contributing. An

## Clinical Pointer

The condition of the molars and premolars of camelids can be assessed to some degree by external palpation of the arcades through the lateral buccal tissue.

## Palpation of the testicles

Testicular palpation is difficult, especially if the testicles have been drawn upward by cremaster muscle contraction, as the scrotum of camelids is not pendulous. However it can be achieved by raising the tail and massaging the perineum, gradually approaching the scrotum, the presence of two uniformly sized and textured testicles is deemed normal. Heat-stressed males will tend to have a pendulous, edematous scrotum.

abnormality occurring in degrees is referred to as 'wry face', which involves maxillary jaw distortion and is generally regarded as a genetic defect; inheritance is currently unknown. Examination of the dentition beyond the incisors and canine 'fighting teeth' require chemical restraint because of the narrow oral cavity, as well as the extremely sharp points of the outside upper and inside lower premolars and molars. Understandably, when jaw malalignment occurs dental malocclusion also occurs. Only with a history of quidding would floating of the premolars and molars be indicated.

## Lymph nodes

Except in the very young, normal peripheral lymph nodes are not found to be readily palpable. Young animals will often show lymphadenopathy in a regional lymph node in response to a vaccination. Recent reports indicate a significant incidence of lymphoma in llamas and alpacas, which would be the most likely explanation for a generalized lymphadenopathy. Dental abscesses or oral lesions due to *Actinobacillus* sp. will often produce a submandibular lymphadenopathy.

## Genitalia

During the course of a close physical examination some emphasis is needed on external genitalia. It can be surprising to the examiner that even a lactating female will have a relatively small udder, which, in combination with abundant wool, makes visual inspection difficult without displacing wool for a lateral view, or elevation of the tail to view between the legs. Generally four small (3 x 1 cm) teats will be uniformly spaced on the four separate quarters, with the cranial two quarters generally being slightly larger. Upon gentle palpation the udder will be found to be soft and pliable; however, on occasion mastitis will be encountered, as evidenced by firmness, pain, and swelling. If mastitis is acute in onset there will often be accompanying edema of the ventral abdomen. Chronic mastitis will tend to cause firmness of the affected quarter, with reduction of size and minimal or no milk production. Except when a female is urinating or defecating, the wool-laden tail tends to cover the perineum. It will therefore usually be necessary to elevate the tail

to assess the size and status of the labia. In spite of post-pubertal females having follicular/estrogen waves, the external genitalia do not reflect an elevated level of estrogen by either discharge or swelling. Some late-gestation females may show vulvar tumification, but this is extremely unpredictable.

Wool cover also makes visualization of the male external genitalia somewhat difficult. The relaxed prepuce will normally point backward, but with sexual arousal points forward owing to stimulation of the strong protractor prepuce muscles. Despite being somewhat pendulous, injury or posthitis is fortunately rare. Palpation of the prepuce will prompt a twitch response. The shaft of the penis can be traced on its sigmoid course through the prepuce towards the ischial arch. In cases of obstructive urolithiasis urethral pulsations may be palpated along the course of the penis.

## Auscultation of thorax

Although the camelids are approachable from either the right or the left side, auscultation procedures generally proceed from the left in an orderly fashion, listening first to the breath sounds detected in the caudal cervical trachea while observing the character of effort. Cardiac auscultation is initiated in the left axillary space by folding the gravid wool covering out of the way and carefully advancing the stethoscope forward, being careful to not touch the lower leg. At the level of the third to fifth intercostal spaces rhythmic heartbeats will be detected, which often reduce in rate after initial excitement. Sinus arrhythmia is occasionally detected, as well as third beats; both tend to disappear with exercise. Holosystolic murmurs, characteristic of ventricular septal defects, are the most common abnormality detected by auscultation, being heard from either the left or the right axillary region. Although the lung field of camelids is relatively small, only the cranio-ventral one-third is free of wool cover, making it necessary to part the wool carefully and seat the stethoscope head firmly for any chance of hearing the normal muted lung sounds. Upon exercise, normal breath sounds will be detectable normally.

## Auscultation of abdomen

Continuing with the auscultation examination, gastric motility is best appreciated by dorsally reflecting the wool from the wool-free abdominal area located just cranial to the left stifle. Normal gastric motility will be 3–5/min, with a new contraction quickly following the former. As the first stomach compartment (C1) contains little gas, percussion and auscultation is generally unrewarding. Because of normal abdominal tone, gastric motility is not readily detected by palpation as can be done in the cow. Over the comparable right abdomen, intestinal borborygmi would be slight, except in the case of diarrhea. On the right ventral abdomen, with patient auscultation the flow of gastric contents through the third compartment (C3) will be detected as it passes through the duodenal ampulla. Comparable thoracic and cardiac auscultation is performed on the right side to complete the examination.

## Rectal examination

Although not all camelids will be of adequate size, nor all examiners have a small enough hand, a manual rectal examination should be carried out if indicated. Clinical findings suggesting the location of lesions in the digestive tract, urinary system, reproductive tract, and hindlimb incoordination would justify a rectal examination.

Good physical restraint and possibly chemical restraint or a sacrococcygeal epidural (2 ml 2% lidocaine) will facilitate examination. It is imperative to lubricate both rectum and sleeved/gloved hand adequately before attempting a gradual entry. Removal of fecal pellets to the depth of the operator's forearm will at least facilitate exploration somewhat forward of the cranial pelvic brim. The contents of the pelvic canal, including the female genital tract, the urinary bladder, femoral arteries and iliac lymph nodes are thus accessible. Many male llamas have a relatively

tight rectum and pelvic canal, making rectal palpation less feasible; however, when it is possible the paired bulbourethral glands will be found just inside the rectum at 5 and 7 o'clock; the pelvic urethra will be located in the midline and, upon following cranially, will appear to dilate owing to the presence of the prostate gland near the neck of the bladder. If deeper palpation is possible the medial/dorsal surface of C1 can be palpated, above which the left kidney should be found. Palpation of the lower right quadrant will reveal the intestinal pack, including the spiral colon, a common site for impaction. To facilitate interpretation of palpated organs, as well as those just out of reach, transrectal ultrasound is useful.

## Musculoskeletal and nervous systems

If neuromuscular function appears impaired or there is skeletal compromise, locomotor assessment is indicated. The process is the same as for an equine lameness evaluation but the animal will probably be less halter trained. If, after observing the patient both walking and at a faster gait, there appears to be a focal area of concern, joint manipulation and deep palpation can be attempted, but most camelids will be somewhat limb sensitive. Camelids present no unique features as regards a neurological examination.

## Urinary tract

Examination of the camelid urinary tract includes

- observation of urination
- collection of urine
- urinalysis
- close inspection of visible anatomy
- rectal palpation
- ultrasound, both transrectal and transabdominal. (laparoscopy has occasionally been used)

Gender differences relate principally to the lower urinary tract. The relatively large female urethra exits at the ventral junction of the vagina and vulva. It can be visualized with the aid of a vaginoscope or palpated digitally. The suburethral diverticulum can cause confusion and difficulty during urethral catheterization.

Examination and catheterization of the penile urethral opening presents several challenges. It is virtually imperative to anesthetize the male, as any attempt to exteriorize the penis of an awake individual will cause spasms of the retractor penis muscles, as well as much uneasiness. The procedure for exteriorizing the penis includes manual extension of the sigmoid flexure while applying caudal force to the external prepuce. As the glans penis emerges, a 4 x 4 gauze sponge is used to grasp it while another is gently tied at the level of the preputial reflection. The short urethral process is observed caudal to the prominent cartilaginous tip.

Even with anesthesia many geldings will be found to have limited preputial sheath mobility, which is usually related to castration at an early age. Surgical exteriorization of the penis may therefore be necessary. A rectal examination, if possible, will allow assessment of bladder tone and wall thickness, but will be enhanced by transrectal ultrasound. Ultrasound can also be used to observe the pelvic urethra, bulbourethral glands and prostate of the male, as well as at least the more caudally placed left kidney. Cystocentesis and renal biopsy have been performed with ultrasound guidance and could be done by laparoscopy.

## Reproductive tract

The male reproductive tract has been described relative to the urinary tract. Once the penis has been exteriorized the glans and prepuce should be examined for lesions, including lacerations, ulcers, scars and strictures that would affect libido and intromission. The shaft of the penis should be uniform in

size throughout the sigmoid flexure, except at the attachment of the retractor muscles. Palpation and measurement of the testicles is facilitated during sedation/anesthesia. Ultrasound imaging of the scrotum has proved valuable in ascertaining

- scrotal edema
- hydrocele
- testicular scarring
- cysts.

Semen evaluation is essential for a complete fertility examination, but the procedure has major drawbacks owing to inconsistent success in obtaining samples. Techniques employed include

- an artificial vagina in a dummy mount
- intravaginal condoms
- electroejaculation under anesthesia
- semen retrieval from a bred female.

The last is the most practical, reliable, and well accepted procedure, but requires a receptive female and microscopic interpretation of vaginal components, including elliptical erythrocytes, epithelial cells, and microbes. The advantages include observation of libido, mounting, and intromission ability, and the fact that ejaculation is natural. The fact that llama semen is extremely viscous makes for a challenge in motility evaluation as well as morphological staining.

Interpretation of morphology is no different than for other species; however, any elliptical erythrocytes might be interpreted as separated heads. If after extensive routine male fertility tests the production of normal sperm remains in doubt, the more invasive option of testicular biopsy remains. This can be done either by surgical wedge biopsy or via needle aspiration, followed by microscopic assessment of normal progressive maturation or lack thereof.

The female genital tract will by necessity require internal inspection. After appropriate perineal scrubbing and tail restraint, a digital vaginal examination can be performed with a lubricated and gloved hand. A nulliparous female will normally have a slight stricture at the level of the former hymen, but most multiparous females will permit up to a three-finger exploration to the level of the stricture. Based on anticipated diameter for passage, the largest diameter vaginoscope is lubricated and passed through the vulvar lips, initially upward and slightly rotating the scope. After approximately 10 cm of forward progress the scope is directed more ventrally and a light source inserted for visualization of the vaginal mucosa and subsequent location of the cervical external os. Except under the influence of higher levels of estrogen, the external os will appear quite small and closed. A female

---

### Catheterization of the male urethra

The very small diameter (3–5 mm) of the distal male urethra makes catheterization difficult but not impossible. An extremely small catheter (5 Fr) must be used and advanced slowly, however it will not pass beyond the ischial arch owing to the presence of a urethral recess. If stranguria is included in the presentation catheterization is indicated, especially in the male, as obstructive urolithiasis may well be the diagnosis and catheterization will facilitate location of the site.

at maximal ovarian follicular development, which is
accompanied by maximal circulating estrogen, will tend
to show a more relaxed and open cervix. Discharges in
the vagina or cervix should be considered abnormal
unless within the first 7–10 days postpartum, or for
several days after breeding. Abnormalities that would
be suspected or confirmed by this procedure include

- vaginitis
- cervicitis
- double cervix
- segmental aplasia of the vagina
- imperforate hymen
- septal hymen
- neoplasia
- abcessation of the vaginal vault.

After the vaginal examination, rectal palpation should
be attempted as described earlier. A left-handed
examiner will, after locating the cervix on the mid-floor
of the pelvis, follow the tract forward, detect a small
uterine body with distinct bifurcation, having only a
suggestion of an intercornual ligament. The left hand
will comfortably follow the right horn for approximately 10–12 cm, when it ends abruptly. Careful thumb
and forefinger palpation will allow the fallopian tube to
be traced to the right ovary, which is approximately 10 x
15 mm in size without luteal or follicular structures.
When present, graafian follicles 5–12 mm in size should
be detectable by their relative fluctuation. A corpus
luteum may vary from an initial soft depression (corpus
hemorrhagicum) 5–7 mm in diameter to a protruding
firm structure up to 15–20 mm in diameter. Ultrasound
imaging is ideal for these structures. Retracing the right
uterine horn to the bifurcation and subsequent
palpation of the left structures is facilitated by a slightly
back-handed approach, whereupon a comparable

examination is accomplished to the left side.

Uterine tone does not change dramatically under the
influence of estrogen, but will tend to be slightly more
firm. An early pregnant uterus will become more fluctuant and, with progression, cause increased cornual
asymmetry, as well as causing the cervix to become
more readily palpable and to tend to tip forward.
Depending on the degree of severity, uterine pathology
may be detected by firmness and subinvolution.

Ultrasound evaluation of the genital tract has
proved invaluable. Even in animals that are too small
to palpate it is possible to carry out near-thorough
evaluation of the genital tract using an ultrasound
probe guided by a rigid extender into a well-lubricated
rectum (Fig. 11.4).

## SPECIAL DIAGNOSTIC PROCEDURES

Certain of the procedures described here require that
wool be clipped: this should be minimal and the area
masked with duct tape before surgical scrubbing (Fig.
11.5).

### Urine collection

For both genders a free catch of urine is possible but the
timing is not always convenient. One should attempt to
collect urine when the individual wakes in the morning,
when a trip to the dunging area is a ritual. On their
normal turf this is somewhat easier than in a hospital
stall. However, a cup on a stick is suggested, as the close
proximity of the collector will often result in cessation of
flow. Catheterization of a female is possible by physical

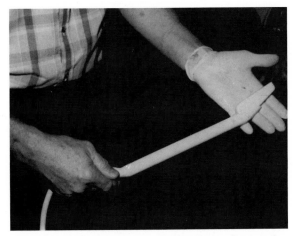

**Fig. 11.4** Polyvinyl adapter for 5 MHz linear ultrasound
transducer.

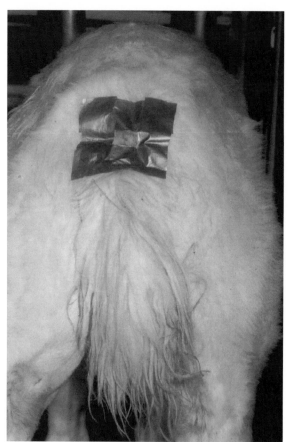

**Fig. 11.5** Tape-masked site for administration of an epidural anesthetic.

restraint, perineal hygiene and the placement of a blunt object in the suburethral diverticulum while passing a 5 Fr polyethylene catheter over the top and into the urethra for approximately 15 cm. A vaginoscope with a ventral slit facilitates the procedure.

## Gastric contents

Animals presenting with inappetence, diagnosed with gastric acidosis would be likely candidates for C1 content sampling and analysis. Cross-tying an animal with a loose-fitting noseband on the halter will allow placement of a PVC speculum (2.4 cm OD x 25 cm length) in the oral cavity and allow the safe passage of a gastric tube into C1 for aspiration of the contents. Determination of pH, methylene blue reduction and the microscopic appearance of the organisms, as is done in bovines, is indicated. Lack of a normal pH (6.5–7.5) and diminished as well as lack of variety of observed microbes, including diverse protozoa and

> ### Urine samples from male camelids
>
> Bladder catheterization is not possible in a male camelid, but urine samples can be obtained by
>
> 1. waiting for a free catch
> 2. placing a triangular-shaped plastic bag (17 x 26 x 17 cm) over the prepuce, and securing it with tape or gauze wraps over the abdomen. The animal will object at first, then often lie down. When it gets up the animal will visit the dunging area to urinate, even if some urine escapes from the bag sufficient will be retained for urinalysis.

bacteria, suggest the animal is in need of transfaunation (transfaunation is the transfer of fauna from the rumen of a normal animal to an animal whose rumen has been defaunated, for whatever reason). The use of rumen contents from fistulated cows or a local slaughter plant has proved effective.

## Liver biopsy

When the history, clinical examination and biochemistry suggest liver dysfunction, liver biopsy is indicated. The procedure can be performed in the standing or sternally recumbent animal. The preferred site is the 9th intercostal space approximately 10–12 cm below the transverse spinous process. After adequate site preparation and local anesthesia the biopsy needle is inserted through a skin incision and directed slightly caudoventrally. Initially there will be contact with the diaphragm, producing movement of the needle synchronous with respiration. Further advancing the needle (2–3 cm) will result in liver penetration and allow the biopsy to proceed.

## Transtracheal wash

Camelids present no major alterations for transtracheal wash procedures. However, the trachea is well vascularized, increasing the possibility of hemorrhage, with resultant coughing, hemoptysis, and likely alteration of cytology interpretation.

## Peripheral blood sampling

Although there are many options as regards sampling sites, many examiners will have a preference. Under adequate physical restraint the head is extended upward and to the left, allowing the left hand to occlude the internal jugular vein medial to the fifth or sixth ventral vertebral process. The right hand is then used to thump the jugular furrow at the level of the second to third vertebrae. The transmitted pulse is detected by the left thumb, confirming the location of the vein. An 18- or 20-gauge 1.5 inch needle is inserted just above the left thumb while negative pressure is applied to the syringe. The vein is not deep, but the longer needle facilitates visualization of blood flow. Other anatomical sites include the internal jugular at the level of the mandibular ramus, the auricular veins and the middle coccygeal vein. All have their advantages and disadvantages.

## Arterial blood sampling

The most accessible site for taking arterial blood for blood gas determination is the auricular artery. Using a heparinized 3 ml syringe and a 22-gauge 1 inch needle, an adequate sample can be secured if proper restraint is applied. In neonatal, recumbent, anesthetized or cooperative animals the medial saphenous artery is large and very accessible.

## Abdominocentesis

Some indications for abdominocentesis include

- fever of unknown origin
- non-responsive diarrhea
- melena
- suspected obstructive bowel disease
- gastric/duodenal ulcers
- chronic weight loss.

The principles of abdominocentesis in camelids are comparable to those in the cow or horse, with the exception that the site is rather specific. In the standing animal this should be exactly on the midline, just caudal to the umbilicus. Going caudal to the umbilicus will reduce the interference of flow through the teat cannula from the omentum. In laterally recumbent animals the site should be at least 20 cm from the midline on the dependent side.

## Bone marrow sampling

As a follow-up to information gained from a leukogram, or in an anemic patient, a bone marrow sample may be obtained. Although a number of theoretical site options exist (wing of ileum, ribs), the preferred site for reliable sampling is the midsternum, avoiding the cutaneous normal callosity. Because aspiration is painful, deep sedation or general anesthesia is advised unless the patient is at extra risk for chemical restraint.

### Clinical Pointer

As most camelids have a thick (6 cm) layer of retroperitoneal fat that extends laterally from the midline for up to 20 cm, but which parts at the midline, the site for abdominocentesis is exactly on the midline.

## Lymph node biopsy

There are relatively few situations that indicate lymph node biopsy; however, an incidence of lymphoma as well as juvenile llama immunodeficiency syndrome (JLIDS) is well recognized. Peripheral lymph nodes are normally not readily detectable, but may well be so in lymphoma. In the presence of lymphadenopathy a needle aspiration will be adequate without the additional effort of a wedge biopsy or node extirpation. As a result of the lymphoid depletion that characterizes JLIDS locating a node to biopsy is often difficult. Under anesthesia, however, an inguinal node can often be located.

## THE NEONATE

The normal camelid neonate is precocious and as such is expected to be vigorous, alert, and generally up and suckling within a few hours of birth. Although the first attempts at standing and ambulation are not always successful, they are amazingly so considering the length of the limbs and neck. Immediately postpartum the rectal temperature will generally be 0.5–1 °C above that of the dam; however, depending upon its new thermal environment this will commonly lose up to 2 °C normally. Once the animal is dry and active the normal rectal temperature will be approximately 37.5–38.5 °C. The normal heart rate immediately postpartum is 80–120 bpm, but will slow to 60–100 after several hours. Respiratory rate should be in the range of 15–30/min.

A newborn camelid neonate will put up minimal physical resistance to restraint, but is often best examined initially in sternal recumbency. This can be accomplished by an assistant gently straddling the animal. Because of the relatively high incidence of congenital defects in camelids, each neonate should be evaluated for the more important common problems, including

- choanal atresia
- atresia ani
- polydactyly
- syndactyly

- cleft palate
- maxillary distortion (wry face)
- cardiac abnormalities.

Varying degrees of umbilical hernia are encountered: some require immediate repair, whereas others are worth watching for spontaneous closure. Tendon laxity and contracted tendons are the more common limb problems observed, both of which tend to respond to conservative therapy unless severe.

Special examinations and procedures may be necessary if the neonate is considered at high risk. Any one of a combination of factors will suggest this, such as problems of the dam during late gestation, or a previous history of problem neonates. Problems during birth, notably dystocia, as well as the conclusions of the current physical examination, may well signify a high-risk neonate. Such individuals would be at high risk for

- in utero sepsis
- pulmonary immaturity
- failure of passive transfer
- postpartum sepsis

and subsequent complications that may arise. In addition to inspection and a close physical examination, a complete blood count, arterial blood gas analysis, blood culture and an assessment of immune status 24–36 hours postpartum are indicated.

As discussed, the major differences in the clinical examination of camelids rest with certain relatively unique anatomical, physiological and behavioral

---

### Premature camelids

A combination of factors indicate prematurity, birth weight is an obvious one, others include

- tendon laxity
- fine wool
- floppy ears
- failure of incisors to erupt
- domed skull
- relative lack of vigor.

---

features. Beyond those, most of the common examination procedures and techniques used in the domestic species are also applicable to camelids.

## FURTHER READING

Cebra CK, Garry F, Powers B, Johnson LW. Lymphosarcoma in New World camelids: 10 cases. Journal of Veterinary Internal Medicine 1995; 9: 381–385.

Fowler ME. Clinical diagnosis: examination and procedures. In: Fowler ME (ed) Medicine and surgery of South American camelids. Ames: Iowa State University Press, 1989; 35–50.

Fowler ME. Digestive system. In: Fowler ME (ed) Medicine and surgery of South American camelids. Ames: Iowa State University Press, 1989; 224–260.

Gionfriddo JR. Ophthalmology. In: Johnson LW (ed) The Veterinary Clinics of North America Food Animal Practice: Update on Llama Medicine, 10:2 Philadelphia: WB Saunders July 1994: 371–382.

Hutchison JM, Garry F. Ill-thrift and juvenile llama immuno-deficiency syndrome. In: Johnson LW (ed) The Veterinary Clinics of North America Food Animal Practice: Update on Llama Medicine, 10:2 Philadelphia: WB Saunders July 1994: 331–343.

Leipold HW, Hiraga TH, Johnson LW. Congenital defects in the llama. In: Johnson LW (ed) The Veterinary Clinics of North America Food Animal Practice: Update on Llama Medicine, 10:2 Philadelphia: WB Saunders July 1994: 401–420.

Rosychuk RAW. Llama dermatology. In: Johnson LW (ed) The Veterinary Clinics of North America Food Animal Practice: Llama Medicine, 5:1 Philadelphia: WB Saunders March 1989: 203–215.

---

### Birth weight

Birth weight is an objective parameter used to assess prematurity and subsequent performance.

- normal alpaca birth weight is 5.5–9.5 kg
- normal llama birth weight is 10.0–15.5 kg.

Small neonates suggest prematurity and extremely large neonates are often slow starters, both should be included in a high-risk neonate category.

# 12

# Clinical Examination of Pigs

*C. C. Gay*

Clinical examination of a single sick pig, for example a sow, is similar to that for an individual of any species and involves a physical examination, an examination of the history of the problem, an examination of the animal's environment if indicated, and appropriate laboratory examination. When individual sick pigs are examined the prime purpose is to arrive at a diagnosis and a strategy for treatment and correction of the problem.

Clinical examination in pigs also has an additional purpose. Most pigs are reared in herds and managed as groups. Diseases therefore commonly involve more than one animal because the group determinants of disease are associated with the management and environment of that group. Because of this, the clinical examination must establish a diagnosis with sufficient precision to allow both an estimate of the risk of occurrence of the disease in others in the herd, and the establishment of effective preventive measures.

Diseases that have implications for the health of the herd may require a more precise diagnosis than would be required to direct the treatment simply of an individual complaint. Certainly there are significant economic consequences if the diagnosis is incorrect. In order to maximize the likelihood of correct diagnosis all information that might have a bearing on the problem becomes part of the clinical examination. This includes a distant and a physical examination of the animals, examination of their management and nutrition, examination of the environment in which they are kept, and relevant sampling for laboratory examination. This, along with a knowledge of the risk of disease within certain age groups and of the risk that management practices and environmental influences have on disease occurrence, is considered specifically in relation to the health history of the herd.

---

### Postmortem examinations

Postmortem and associated laboratory examinations are a valuable adjunct to clinical examination in the determination of a diagnosis because physical examination has limited diagnostic utility in pigs. Where large groups of young or growing pigs are at risk it is common to sacrifice a sick pig for this purpose.

---

Programmed clinical examination of groups of pigs is also used as a monitor of health status to allow early detection of an impending problem and the early implementation of an intervention strategy. In open herds that have frequent intakes of new pigs, such as those that buy weaners for fattening, clinical examination is used to monitor the health of pigs entering the premises so that strategies for disease prevention and amelioration can be determined immediately.

This chapter is concerned primarily with the distant and physical examination component of the general clinical examination of pigs.

## DISTANT EXAMINATION

### Mentation and behavior

The pigs should be examined at a distance, initially as unobtrusively as possible, so that natural behavioral activities can be observed. As a rule pigs in groups play together and sleep together. Healthy pigs are bright and alert and have an inquisitive demeanor. When awake there is continual activity in the group, including feeding, drinking, nosing, darting, exploration, and play fighting. Huddling is common during sleep in growing pigs of all ages. When a group of sleeping pigs is disturbed the observant animals within the group will give an explosive bark and the whole group will erupt to activity and stand to face the observer. During the distant examination the clinician is looking for aberrations in these behavioral activities. The distant examination also looks for changes in demeanor, mental state, and movement in individual pigs. Pigs which are depressed and lack normal alertness are noted for closer examination. Depression is usually an indication of systemic disease. Depression and disorientation also occur in diseases involving the central nervous system. These and other signs of nervous system disease, such as dementia, seizure, head pressing, circling, incoordination, and ataxia, indicate that a special neurological examination is required. Excitatory and localizing signs may be seen where there is either bacterial or viral infection of the brain. With several diseases these signs are intermittent, and when pigs in a group exhibit signs of central nervous dysfunction the group should be observed without disturbance for several minutes so that this expression can be observed. The clinical syndrome in growing pigs caused by salt poisoning is one such disease.

---

### Clinical Pointer

Sick pigs show abnormal behavior in these ways:

- they move slowly with the head held low
- they are often bumped by their pen mates when there is rapid movement in the pen
- their ears droop or are held flat against the head
- they prefer to lie down and will burrow under straw if possible
- traditionally a sick pig loses the curl in its tail, although this is seldom seen now because of the practice of docking tails at birth.

---

Changes in patterns of defecation within a pen suggest the presence of enteric disease. A higher than normal prevalence of scratching and rubbing indicates that the close physical examination should include sampling for mange. Paroxysms of coughing in the period immediately following the sudden awakening of a group of pigs, or the recognition of sporadic but noticeable coughing and/or sneezing in the piggery during the course of a visit, suggest the need for further special examination for lower and upper respiratory disease, particularly

- enzootic pneumonia
- inclusion-body rhinitis
- atrophic rhinitis.

Clinical indices are numerical values assigned to the frequency of signs observed during distant examination and, for diseases such as sarcoptic mange and enzootic pneumonia, can provide quantitative measures of severity and economic significance.

## Piglet behavior

Piglet behavior can be an important indication of disease in the sow, as most sows will develop hypogalactia or agalactia if they become sick. On average piglets suck every 1–2 hours. In the first 1–2 days after farrowing the suckling process is usually initiated by the sow calling, but after that it is generally initiated by the piglets vocalizing, combined with their physical activity on the udder. At the start of sucking activity there can be considerable vocalization as the piglets sort out their order on the teats. Piglets rapidly establish a sucking order such that a given piglet sucks the same teat at each suckling. During this sorting-out period, and for a short time afterwards, the piglets vigorously bunt and nuzzle the teats and udder, which stimulates oxytocin release. This vigorous bunting lasts for 1–2 minutes. The period of milk letdown is quite short and during it the piglets become very quiet and suck lying quietly with their ears held flat along the side of the head. There follows a period where the piglets will gently nose the udder, after which, one by one, they leave the udder or even fall asleep still attached to a teat.

Where the sow has hypo- or agalactia the piglet activity never progresses from the active vocalization period to the quiet sucking period. Piglets will continue to vocalize and will attempt to knock other piglets off adjacent teats. Consequently, an initial sign of sickness in the sow is a noisy litter which shows continuous, not vigorous, activity, compared to a normal litter where the piglets, at least during the first few days of life, tend to either suckle, sleep, or show brief periods of active play. Piglets that are not receiving sufficient milk will seek a source of nutrients from other areas on the sow, from the pen walls, and from surface water on the pen floors. With continuing milk deprivation they become progressively weaker and develop the typical facial, gait, and neurological signs of hypoglycemia. Abnormal behavioral and activity patterns in litters suggest that the sow should also be part of a closer physical examination.

The conformation and body regions of the pigs are also examined from a distance. One of the most

## Runt pigs

1. Runt pigs are small for their age and have a large head in relation to body size.
2. There is poor muscle development and the bones of the hips, head, and shoulder tend to be prominent.
3. The haircoat is coarse and prominent and there is pallor of the skin.
4. Examination seldom gives an indication of cause of the runting, as the inciting condition will have occurred several weeks prior to examination.

common conformation abnormalities relates to severe growth depression, i.e. the runt pig. This is usually the result of a past disease process.

The distant examination should be conducted systematically and include the haircoat and skin. Most skin abnormalities are best observed on closer physical examination, but the discoloration associated with septicemic/toxemic disease can be observed from a distance and large diffuse lesions, such as those produced by *Microsporum nanum* in adult pigs, are more easily seen from a distance and can actually be missed on close physical examination. The head and neck are examined for carriage and symmetry. Asymmetry may be due to cranial nerve dysfunction, such as facial paralysis or middle ear infection, or may be due to local lesions. Edema is often most obvious in the neck of the pig and the early stages of iron deficiency anemia may be manifest by edema in this area.

The observations on the thorax concentrate on the rate and nature of respiration. The most prominent abnormality occurs in pigs with respiratory disease, where there is a forceful expiration with abdominal breathing resulting in a thumping action during expiration. The abdomen is examined for symmetry, abnormalities include

- a slab-sided gaunt abdomen that is associated with several diseases including swine dysentery
- a distended abdomen that may be caused by ascites or by intestinal abnormalities such as rectal stricture.

Distant examination may also detect swellings in the

## Clinical Pointer

Observe respiratory rates at a distance before the pigs are disturbed, vocalization masks the true rate.

joints, as occurs with polyarthritis, or in the tendon sheaths as occurs with Glasser's disease. In adults abnormalities of the claws of the feet are also apparent.

## CLOSE PHYSICAL EXAMINATION

A detailed physical examination should be deferred until after the assessment of behavior and the distant examination.

There are two main constraints on the conduct and utility of physical examination in pigs:

1. anatomy – the thickness of the skin, the subcutaneous fat cover and the muscularity and compactness of the animal limit the diagnostic information that can be obtained by techniques such as auscultation and palpation, which have considerable utility in other domestic animal species
2. temperament – pigs normally object to any imposed physical restraint by struggling violently and voicing their displeasure. This also significantly limits the information that can be obtained by techniques such as palpation or auscultation.

### Restraint for examination

For this reason, the physical examination should when possible be conducted without restraint. This requires a considerable investment of time and patience but is generally possible in adults: sows will tend to quieten when talked to and touched. In many piggeries sows are housed in crates or stalls or equivalent systems that restrict their movement. Because they are used to such confinement a physical examination can be successfully conducted with patience. However, there is an increasing move to loose housing or outdoor housing for adults. In herds with good stockmanship it is usually possible to conduct much of the physical examination of loose-housed sows with minimal restraint, and this may be facilitated by providing feed during the examination. A pig board may also help in limiting movement.

Restraint will, however, be required in many instances. The methods that can be used will vary according to the size of the pig. Newborn and young piglets can be held in the palm of the hand or on the forearm against the crook of the elbow, or can be held suspended by the front or hind limbs. Effective and prolonged restraint is limited to pigs under 60 lb for most handlers. Larger pigs can be restrained using snout loops. These methods of restraint allow simple examinations, such as

- taking the rectal temperature
- superficial examination of skin lesions
- palpation of joints

but are almost useless for more complex sensory examinations. Pigs that are restrained by any method other than snout loops will object, attempt to escape, and will scream for much of the restraint period. Pigs restrained with snout loops will lean backwards against the loop but will still scream. Because of this as much as possible of the examination should be conducted with no restraint, with the caveat that safety of the examiner must be paramount.

## Vital signs

The temperature, pulse, and respiratory rates are taken at the start of the examination. The temperature is taken at the rectum and the pulse rate at the femoral artery on the medial side of the hind limb in younger animals. Pulse rate can also be taken from the ventral coccygeal artery or the rostal rim of the ear in older pigs, or the heart rate by palpation of the apex impulse, or auscultation at the left 5th intercostal space. In pigs not used to close human contact the pulse/heart rate will not be a resting one. Respiratory rates are best taken by observation of thoracic wall movement prior to restraint of the animal.

## Body surfaces and skin

Following the determination of the vital signs, a systematic examination is conducted of all the body surfaces, including the limbs, joints, and feet. In the examination of newborn piglets the sites of predilection for congenital abnormalities are a particular part of this examination. These include an examination for the presence of inguinal and scrotal hernias and atresia ani.

The skin surface should be examined for external parasites and the skin inspected both visually and by palpation. The haircoat of the pig is sparse and consists of 60–70% bristles, with the remainder a fine downy hair. In healthy animals the hair lies flat and smooth. The skin is at its thickest on the dorsal aspect of the body.

Traumatic lesions on the face are common in piglets as a result of fighting, and occur especially in litters where the canine teeth are not clipped after birth. The initial skin abrasions bleed, rapidly become infected, and there is usually a large scab. Lesions occur between the mouth and the eyes and on both sides of the face. Wrinkling of the skin over the nose of young growing pigs occurs where there is facial deformity, shortening and rotation of the snout associated with atrophic rhinitis, and occasionally bull nose.

In older pigs traumatic lesions may be found on the tips or lobes of the ears at the ventral border, these lesions occur in association with the vices of ear sucking and ear, flank, and tail biting. The tail is the more common site for attack. The inside of the ear of older pigs should be specifically examined for lesions associated with chronic infestation with *Sarcoptes scabiei*. The lesions are white and crusty in nature and occasionally accompanied by a hematoma resulting from irritation, head shaking, and ear scratching.

Areas of hyperkeratosis which may progress to superficial necrosis are common on the dorsum of the carpal area and on the caudal surface of the hocks in baby pigs reared on abrasive floors, especially new cement floors. This type of skin necrosis may also occur on the elbows, at the coronets, on the soles of the feet, and at the base of the tail. Similarly, trauma from abrasive floors and slatted or otherwise perforated floors, may result in hypertrophy of the skin, with underlying fibrosis and callus formation over joints and bony prominences in older pigs, around the coronary band, and on the accessory digits. Swelling with necrosis of the teats and the tip of the vulva occurs in some litters, possibly associated with the ingestion of estrogenic diets by the sow. Splayleg may predispose to teat necrosis of the cranial teats in newborn piglets.

Thickened hyperkeratotic and parakeratotic areas occur in the skin over the joints of grower pigs with zinc deficiency. Parakeratosis and apparent hyperkeratosis with excess skin scaling occurs on the skin of adults kept in confinement such that they cannot groom themselves or be groomed by others. Excessive keratinization with a thickened and wrinkled skin occurs with chronic infestations with *Sarcoptes scabiei*. Hair loss and skin changes also occur with different vitamin B

---

### Clinical Pointer ✳

Many diseases affecting the skin are localized in their distribution and if necessary the pig should be lifted or turned over so that lesions, such as those associated with pityriasis rosea, can be visualized.

---

### Clinical Pointer

- lice and flea infestations can be determined by visual examination
- infestations with *Sarcoptes scabiei* require microscopic examination of skin scrapings.

deficiencies, although these are not common. Infestations with external parasites are accompanied by dermatitis. Pruritus is a feature of sarcoptic mange but can occur also with flea infestations, and the associated trauma contributes to the dermatitis seen with these diseases.

Bacterial and viral diseases of the skin generally produce distinctive focal lesions that are widely distributed over the skin surface. The same is true for fungal infections associated with *Microsporum* and *Trichophyton* spp., although these seldom involve the skin of the mammary gland. A detailed examination and definition of the nature of lesions associated with infectious skin disease will commonly allow a diagnosis to be made on clinical examination alone.

In all ages of pig erythema of the skin, especially on the ears, the snout, under the neck, along the underline, and in the perineal area, occurs in association with systemic infections. There may be a more severe purple discoloration in areas where there is vascular damage, such as occurs with salmonellosis and erysipelas, and this may progress to superficial necrosis. The lesions of erysipelas are often rhomboid in shape and in pigs with colored skin can be palpated. Patchy reddening of the skin occurs in some pigs associated with restraint and handling, but can also be the early signs of the porcine stress syndrome. Erythema, especially in the thin-skinned areas of the body, is present with mange infestation and in the early stages of greasy pig disease. Pallor of the skin may be observed in iron deficiency anemia and in diseases with hemorrhagic tendencies, such as esophogastric ulceration and the hemorrhagic enteropathies. The pallor associated with

---

### Clinical Pointer

The presence and extent of dehydration is not easily assessed by clinical examination. Some indication of the state of hydration in pigs can be obtained from the plasticity of the skin behind the ear and by the extent to which the eyeball occupies the orbit.

---

anemia is most easily seen where there is direct light, and is not clinically evident until the hemoglobin concentration in the blood falls below 7 g/dl.

## Musculoskeletal system and feet

The limbs, joints, and feet should be examined visually and by palpation, with special attention if lameness or defects in conformation were observed during the distant examination. The joints and tendon sheaths are palpated for heat and increased fluid. The joint capsule may be visibly and palpably distended with fluid in the polyarthritis associated with streptococcal, hemophilus and mycoplasmal infections, but this may be less apparent in other diseases, such as erysipelas.

The lateral claw of the foot is normally larger than the medial claw, and this difference predisposes the lateral claw to disease. The foot should be lifted for examination, particularly if there is lameness. The individual claws are palpated for heat and by a pinch test for pain. Dark discolored areas with hyperkeratinization on the weight-bearing surface of the heel and on the sole are usually a reflection of trauma and bruising, and may be followed by sole erosion. The white-line area should be examined for erosion and separation, with an appreciation that the separated region may be impacted with feces and other material. Swelling and the presence of discharging sinuses at the coronary band suggests the presence of a chronic and deep infection of the claw, indicating the need for further examination of this region.

The clinical differentiation of lameness in adult pigs not associated with lesions of the claws is very difficult. Degenerative joint disease – cartilaginous necrosis of the articular joint surface – is often accompanied by a knuckling forward posture of the carpal and fetlock

---

### Edema in pigs

Subcutaneous edema, although an uncommon clinical finding in pigs, can indicate a variety of disorders

- edema at the base of the ear, in the subcutaneous tissues of the frontal area, and the eyelids may be present in cases of gut edema (edema disease)
- pharyngeal edema is a major presenting sign of anthrax in pigs
- edematous swelling, usually with gas and crepitation, occurs with clostridial wound infections
- sunburn in pigs reared outdoors is manifest with erythema and edema on the dorsal surfaces
- tenosynovitis associated with Glasser's disease can result in edematous-like swelling of the limbs.

---

### Clinical Pointer

When many pigs within a piggery are lame, examine the coronary region and the interdigital skin specifically for vesicular lesions.

joints, but other lamenesses do not necessarily have typical stances associated with them and are frequently accompanied by voluntary recumbency and an extreme reluctance to rise and stand for examination.

Sows recumbent because of pelvic fractures often lie with their hindlegs abducted, and those with apophysiolysis or epiphysiolysis tend to lie with their legs forward and under the body. However, these are but clinical impressions and, where pigs are recumbent and resist examination, analgesia or light anesthesia may be required for examination and palpation of suspect areas. Examination of the mammary gland is important in breeding females and is dealt with separately below.

## Head and eyes

The eyes are examined at the time of general examination of the head. The examination is usually restricted to an examination of the conjunctivae for color and evidence of inflammation, and a visual examination of the cornea and observable internal structures of the eye. More detailed examinations of the eye and of cranial nerve reflexes and function are restricted to pigs that are showing signs of brain disease. Conjunctivitis is common in young pigs as an accompaniment of upper respiratory disease. Conjunctivitis results in tear staining below the eye, which becomes brown as a result of dust staining.

The nares are examined for nasal discharge. Inclusion-body and atrophic rhinitis are present in most piggeries, and consequently signs of rhinitis, which include sneezing, nasal discharge and, occasionally, epistaxis, are common in young pigs on most farms. Epistaxis may also be observed in growing pigs in the terminal stages of pleuropneumonia.

## Heart and lungs

The lungs and heart are examined by auscultation and palpation. Lung sounds are most audible on auscultation at the area of the bronchial hilus. The caudal boundary for auscultation of lung sounds with deep respirations extends from the costochondral junction of the 7th rib in a gentle curve with a ventral convexity to the top of the 13th rib. Sounds associated with air flow are categorized in terms of intensity, pitch, and character to determine the nature of the lesions in the lung and the possible presence of pleural exudate. The presence of sounds associated with fluid in the airways and with pleuritis is determined.

The heart is most audible at the left 5th intercostal space at the point of the elbow, and is examined using the same criteria as for other domestic species. Careful auscultation for the presence of systolic murmurs associated with endocarditis should be conducted in adult pigs that have exertional dyspnea.

## Mouth

The mouth and tongue are examined with the aid of a gag or speculum, but this is not generally done in routine clinical examination unless there is a specific indication, such as excess salivation, frequent chewing movements, dysphagia, or suspect vesicular disease.

## Abdomen

When acute abdominal accidents are suspected, the presence or absence of intestinal sounds and the presence of a gas-filled viscus are sought by auscultation and auscultation with percussion. Palpation of the abdomen is unrewarding and not usually conducted.

The abdomen may be enlarged where there is ascites, intestinal obstruction such as with rectal stricture, and ill-thriven pigs; pigs with heavy ascarid infestations may appear pot-bellied.

## Feces

The feces should be examined for consistency, color, and the presence of blood and mucus. Determination of the character of the feces, coupled with determination of the epidemiology of the enteric problem, can aid considerably in establishing a list of differential diagnostic possibilities. There may be staining of the perineum in pigs with diarrhea, and baby piglets with

---

### Auscultation in pigs

Auscultation has limited utility in pigs as they are highly vocal animals, especially when restrained. Pigs that are kept stationary by giving access to feed grunt during eating, and the sounds of eating also confound the interpretation of auscultation.

---

### Clinical Pointer

Fluid feces may not be observed easily where pigs are kept on slatted floors or on straw, and they dry rapidly in the warm environment. If enteric disease is suspected defecation can be stimulated by rectal palpation or with a thermometer.

fluid diarrhea may have dried encrustation on the tail and a reddened anus. An examination of the character of the feces should be extended to feces in the environment of the animal, and include observations of others in the group.

## Reproductive tract

### Female

The color of the mucous membrane of the vagina is examined visually by parting the lips of the vulva, and this is a convenient site to assess anemia in sows. Some hemorrhage in the wall is common following farrowing. Partial prolapse of the vagina is not uncommon in recumbent pregnant sows, and presents as a bulging mass protruding from the vulva when they are lying down. The vulva is examined for the presence of abnormal discharge, which may be evident grossly at the vulva or on the floor behind sows in confinement, or suspected from the presence of abnormal staining and encrustation at the vulval lips and on the perineum. A vulval discharge is normal in pigs up to 5 days after farrowing and consists of 30–60 ml of mucus which may contain flecks of thick white or occasionally bloody material. In contrast to the discharge associated with endometritis or retained placenta it does not have an offensive odor and the sow is not sick or pyrexic. The rectal temperature of sows is normally increased (40 °C) for 24 hours after parturition.

Rectal palpation is used for genital tract examination and for pregnancy diagnosis by clinicians with small hands and arms. The examination cannot be performed in gilts and has limited utility in the examination of the abdominal viscera, even in large sows.

### Male

In the boar, the penis is not routinely examined but if there is bleeding from the prepuce, hematuria or hemaspermia, an examination is indicated because these signs frequently reflect injury. The penis can be examined as the boar mounts a sow, the examination being during the stage of erection prior to intromission. Alternatively, tranquilizers can be used to facilitate the examination. There is no distinct glans penis and the free end is covered by the penile integument, which describes a spiral of approximately three and a half twists. Injury is usually to this area.

## Mammary gland and teats

The udder is a focus of examination in sows, especially during lactation. Each gland should be examined both visually and by palpation. The mammary glands of the lactating sow are relatively soft and pliable. Each gland actually has a separate cranial and caudal section, but physical examination does not attempt to localize problems to a section within a gland. There are several lactiferous ducts rather than a single teat canal, as in ruminants. The teats should be examined for patency; the cranial teats can be blind as a result of nipple necrosis occurring in infancy.

Abrasions and cuts are common and the usual causes are trauma from the piglets' teeth or from the flooring. Inverted nipples and blind teats are hereditary defects. Heat, redness, blotchy discoloration, agalactia, palpable firmness in a gland, and edema are usually indications of mastitis. One or more mammary glands may be affected. Milk should be expressed (a large volume is normally not readily expressed) and examined for change in consistency and color. It should be taken for laboratory examination if a gland is suspected as being abnormal, although the sample may largely represent milk from the normal section of the gland. It is difficult to avoid contamination of the sample with environmental organisms because of the nature of the lactiferous ducts. Agalactia can result from mastitis and from systemic disease. Small underdeveloped glands may be due to ergot poisoning. Full glands with no milk letdown in a hyperalert gilt may reflect psychogenic agalactia.

### Cystitis and pyelonephritis

Cystitis and pyelonephritis are common in some piggeries, and the purulent and bloody urine associated with pyelonephritis may be mistaken for a discharge originating from the reproductive tract. Examination of the discharge and of the bladder by rectal palpation is an aid to differentiation.

## FURTHER READING

Blocks GHM, Leengoed LAMG, Verheijden JHM, Van Leengoed LAMG. Integrated quality control project: introduction to a farm visit protocol for growing and finishing pigs. Veterinary Quarterly 1994;16 (2): 120–122.

Done S. Diagnosis of central nervous system disorders in the pig. In Practice 1995;17 (7): 318–327.

Gibson CD. Clinical evaluation of the boar for breeding soundness: physical examination and semen morphology. Compendium on Continuing Education for the Practicing Veterinarian 1983; 5 (5): S244–S249.

Jeppersen LE. Behavioural vices in young pigs. Pig Veterinary Journal 1980;7: 43–53.

Leman AD, Straw BE, Mengeling WL, D-Allaire S, Taylor DJ. Diseases of swine, 7th edn. Ames: Iowa State University Press, 1992.

Martineau GP, Smith BP, Doize B. Pathogenesis, prevention and treatment of lactational insufficiency in sows. Veterinary Clinics of North America, Food Animal Practice 1992; 8 (3): 661–684.

Masters BJ, Hamilton M, Masters PG. Physical examination of swine. Veterinary Clinics of North America, Food Animal Practice 1992; 8 (2): 177–188.

Meredith MJ. Clinical techniques for the examination of infertile sows. Pig Veterinary Society Proceedings 1981; 8: 49–53.

Muirhead MR. The pig advisory visit in preventive medicine. Veterinary Record 1980; 106 (8): 170–173.

Radostits OM, Blood DC, Gay CC. Veterinary medicine, 8th edn. London: Bailliére Tindall, 1994.

Straw BD. Diagnosis of skin disease in swine. Compendium on Continuing Education for the Practicing Veterinarian 1985; 7 (11): S650–S655, S658.

Walton J, Duran O. Pre-purchase examination of boars. In Practice 1993; 15 (4): 162–164.

# Part Three

## Evaluation of Body systems

# 13

# Clinical Examination of the Integumentary System

*D. M. Houston*
*O. M. Radostits*
*I. G. Mayhew*

## CLINICAL MANIFESTATIONS OF DISEASES OF THE SKIN

**Abnormal elasticity, extensibility and thickness**. Abnormal skin may be thin, thick, turgid, or elastic. Loss of elasticity (hypotonia) is manifested by skin that wrinkles excessively and fails to snap back into position when lifted away from the body and released.

**Abscess**. A fluctuant swelling resulting from (dermal or subcutaneous) accumulation of pus. Abscesses are larger and deeper than pustules.

**Acanthosis nigricans**. An area of hyperpigmentation, lichenification and alopecia.

**Acne** is an inflammatory disease of the pilosebaceous unit, the specific type usually being indicated by a modifying term. Clinically it is characterized by comedones which arise from papules and pustules.

**Alopecia**. Loss of hair or wool.

**Anhidrosis**. Failure to sweat appropriately.

**Bulla**. A large well-demarcated elevation of the skin more than 1 cm in diameter.

**Callus**. A thickened, hyperkeratotic plaque.

**Comedo**. An obstructed hair follicle which contains a pigmented impaction of lipid and keratinaceous debris occluding the orifice; also known as comedones (pl.) or blackheads.

**Crust**. A consolidated, desiccated surface mass composed of varying combinations of keratin, serum, cellular debris.

**Cyst**. A fluid-filled cavity within the skin lined by epithelium.

**Epidermal collarette**. A circular patch of alopecia and erythema surrounded by a border of peeling stratum corneum.

**Erosion**. A loss of the viable epidermis although the basal layer is intact.

**Erythema**. Reddening of the skin.

**Excoriation**. An area of epidermal damage as a result of self-trauma. The resulting erosive or ulcerative damage is often linear in appearance.

**Fissure**. A deep crack in the epidermis penetrating to the dermis.

**Fistulous tract**. A tract which connects an area or focus of inflammation to the skin surface.

**Folliculitis** is inflammation of hair follicles characterized by a papule which commonly develop into pustules. Erect hairs are commonly visible over the papule or pustule which may progressively enlarge with the development of a central ulcer which may discharge purulent or serosanguineous material and then become encrusted. When the inflammatory process breaks through the hair follicles and extends into the dermis and subcutis, the process is called furunculosis. When multiple areas of furunculosis coalesce, the resultant focal area of induration and fistulous tracts is called a carbuncle (boil)

**Gangrene**. Severe tissue necrosis and sloughing.

**Hematidiosis**. Blood-stained sweat.

**Hirsutism**. Abnormal hairiness. This is manifested by a long, shaggy, usually curly coat and may extend over the entire body or be limited to specific body regions.

**Hyperhidrosis**. Excessive sweating.

**Hyperkeratosis**. Increased keratin production in the epidermis without normal exfoliation.

**Hyperpigmentation**. An excessive amount of melanin deposited in the epidermis (also known as hypermelanosis).

**Hypertrichosis**. Excessive hair.

**Hypopigmentation**. Decreased amounts of melanin in the epidermis.

**Hypotrichosis**. Less than the normal amount of hair.

**Impetigo** is a staphylococcal infection of the skin characterized by vesicles or bullae that become pustular and rupture, forming yellow crusts.

**Intertrigo.** An erythematous eruption of the skin produced by friction of adjacent parts.

**Lichenification.** A marked thickening of the epidermis, resembling lichen.

**Macule.** A circumscribed area (<1 cm diameter) of change in the normal skin color. The normal contour of the skin is not altered (lesion not palpable).

**Necrosis.** Death of a portion of skin. The affected skin is discolored, cool, may be wrinkled and moist or dry.

**Nodule.** A circumscribed elevation of the skin that is larger than 1 cm.

**Panniculitis.** An inflammation of the subcutaneous fat within the panniculus adiposus (the pad of fat that constitutes the deepest layer of the skin).

**Papule.** A circumscribed, solid elevation of the skin up to 1 cm in diameter.

**Parakeratosis.** Thickening of the skin due to incomplete keratinization of the epithelial cells of the skin.

**Paronychia.** Inflammation of the nail bed.

**Patch.** This is a macule that is over 1 cm in diameter.

**Plaque.** A flat and typically wide (>1 cm) elevation of the skin.

**Pruritus** or **itchiness.** Scratching or rubbing a region of the skin.

**Pustule.** A circumscribed elevation of the superficial layers of the epidermis filled with pus.

**Pyoderma.** A general term to include any purulent skin disease and includes pustules, acne, impetigo, and furunculosis.

**Scab.** A dried crust composed of body fluids and cellular debris covering a skin lesion.

**Scale.** Excessive accumulation of clumps of keratinocytes (superficial cornified epithelial cells).

**Scar.** A mark remaining after the healing of a lesion.

**Seborrhea.** Excessive scale formation and excessive greasiness of the skin and haircoat.

**Sinus tract.** An epithelial-lined channel connecting a deep lesion to the skin surface.

**Slough.** A mass of necrotic tissue which is being expelled from normal tissue.

**Tumor.** A mass of neoplastic tissue, whether benign or malignant.

**Ulceration.** Loss of the epidermis with involvement of the dermis and inflammation and scarring of the dermis.

**Urticaria (hives).** An allergic condition characterized by the appearance of wheals on the skin surface.

**Vesicle.** A well-demarcated elevation of the superficial layers of the skin with underlying fluid, less than 1 cm in diameter.

**Vitiligo.** Absence of melanocytes in small or large circumscribed areas resulting in white skin in affected areas.

**Warts** are fibropapillomas characterized clinically by fleshy masses of the skin which may be sessile (attached to the skin by a broad base) or pedunculated (attached to the skin by a peduncle of stalk).

**Wheal.** A visible dermal plateau or elevation, of irregular outline and diameter.

# INTRODUCTION

The skin is the outer covering and largest organ of the body and is the anatomic and physiologic barrier between the animal and its environment. It provides protection from physical, chemical and pathogen injury, and its sensory components perceive heat, cold, pain, itchiness, touch and pressure. The skin is an integral part of the regulation of body temperature through its support of the haircoat, its regulation of the cutaneous blood supply and sweat gland function. The skin assists in the maintenance of water and electrolyte balance, and is a reservoir for vitamins, fat, carbohydrates, proteins and other materials. Vitamin D is produced in the skin through stimulation by solar radiation. The skin has immunologic, endocrine and antimicrobial properties. Processes in the skin (melanin formation, vascularity and keratinization) help determine the color of the coat and skin. Color and pheromone production assist in animal identification and camouflage when needed. Pigmentation of the skin also helps prevent injury from solar radiation. The flexibility, elasticity and toughness of the skin allow motion and provide shape and form. The skin produces keratinized structures such as hair, claws, and the horny layer of the epidermis.

Skin disease is common in all species of animals, particularly dogs and cats, and is the most common presenting problem for the small animal practitioner.

Diseases of the skin may be primary or secondary in

---

### Primary versus secondary skin disease

To differentiate between primary and secondary skin diseases, it is necessary a complete clinical examination of the patient. If there is no evidence that body systems other than the skin are affected it can be assumed that the disease is primary.

origin. In primary skin disease the lesions are restricted initially to the skin, although they may spread to involve other body systems. On the other hand, cutaneous lesions may be secondary to disease originating in other body systems.

When a careful clinical examination has been made and an accurate history taken it is then necessary to make a careful examination of the skin itself. A knowledge of the normal structure and function of the skin makes it possible to determine the underlying abnormality present.

## STRUCTURE AND FUNCTION OF THE SKIN

There are several features of the structure and function of the skin that are relevant to the clinical examination. These are briefly described here.

### Epidermis and dermis

The thickness of the skin varies in different parts of the body. It is thickest over the dorsal trunk, thinnest on the ventral abdomen and decreases in thickness proximally to distally on the limbs. It is thickest on the forehead, dorsal neck, dorsal thorax, rump and base of the tail, and thinnest on the lateral surfaces of the pinnae and on the axillary, inguinal and perineal areas, and on the undersurface of the tail. The elasticity of the skin is variable, being relatively immobile on the lower limbs but quite mobile on the trunk. The skin of the distal phalanges is modified into claws or hooves; the skin of the planum nasale is thickened and hairless.

At each body orifice the skin is continuous with the mucous membrane of the digestive tract, the respiratory tract, the conjunctiva and the urogenital tract. The skin and haircoat vary in quantity and quality between species, between breeds within a species, and between individuals within a breed. Skin also varies from one area to another on the body, and in accordance with age and gender.

Skin consists of three distinct layers: epidermis, dermis and subcutis. The epidermis is separated from the dermis by the basement membrane, on which rests the stratum germinativum, the layer actively producing the cells above it. The stratum germinativum contains melanocytes – pigment-producing cells which provide melanin. Melanin is synthesized within melanocytes and stored within organelles called melanosomes, which are passed from the melanocyte to the keratinocyte and account for skin pigmentation. The normal color of the skin is also due to erythrocytes in the superficial dermal vessels, which may carry oxygenated or reduced hemoglobin, and other pigments such as carotene. When the skin is inflamed or subjected to prolonged friction or exposure to sunlight, the melanocytes are stimulated to produce more pigment, which darkens the skin. When the hair is closely clipped the skin beneath will darken, because of the increase in melanin production caused by exposure of the epidermis to more light. Above the stratum germinativum is the stratum spinosum that contains Langerhans' cells, cells with an immunological function. As the cells in the stratum spinosum migrate to the surface they become keratinized (keratinocytes), die and become flattened. The keratinocytes enter the stratum corneum, the outer dead layer of the skin, and are exfoliated. Normally this process takes approximately 21 days. Many skin diseases hasten this process, resulting in excess scale and subsequently aroma.

The dermis or corium is part of the body's connective tissue system. It is composed of fibrous connective tissue containing blood and lymph vessels, nerve fibers and cells, sebaceous and sweat glands, hair follicles and piloerector muscles. In areas of thick haired skin the dermis accounts for most of the depth, whereas the epidermis is thin. In very thin-haired skin, the decreased thickness of the skin results from the thinness of the dermis. The dermis accounts for the majority of the tensile strength and elasticity of the skin.

### Cutaneous ecology

The skin forms a protective barrier, without which life would not be possible. There are physical, chemical and microbial barriers to pathogens. Hair provides the first line of physical defense by preventing contact of pathogens with the skin and minimizing external physical or chemical insults to the skin. Hair may also harbor a variety of microorganisms. The strateum corneum provides the basic physical defense barrier. Its thick, tightly packed keratinized cells are permeated by

---

**Structure of the skin**

The skin has three layers:

1. Epidermis – a protective barrier producing cells and pigment
2. Dermis – vascular layer containing nerves, sebaceous and sweat glands and hair follicles
3. Subcutis (hypodermis) – a fibrofatty layer providing energy reserves, heat insulation and protective padding.

an emulsion of sebum and sweat which provides a physical and chemical barrier to potential pathogens.

The normal skin microflora also contributes to defense of the skin. Bacteria, yeasts, and filamentous fungi are located in the superficial epidermis and the infundibulum of hair follicles. The normal flora is a mixture of bacteria which live symbiotically. The flora may change with different cutaneous environments and are affected by factors such as

- pH
- salinity
- hydration
- serum albumin concentration
- serum fatty acid concentration.

The single factor with the greatest influence on the microflora is the degree of hydration of the stratum corneum. If the quantity of water at the skin surface is increased by increased ambient temperature or increased relative humidity, the result is a marked increase in the number of microorganisms. In general, the moist or greasy areas of the skin support the greatest population of microflora.

The close relationship between the host and its cutaneous symbiotic microorganisms enables bacteria to occupy microbial niches and to inhibit colonization by invading pathogens. Those microorganisms permanently present are known as resident microflora. Their numbers can be reduced using germicide techniques but they cannot be totally eliminated. Other microorganisms, known as transients, are occasional contaminants acquired from the environment and can be removed by simple hygienic techniques. In dogs and cats, *Micrococcus* spp., coagulase-negative staphylococci, α-hemolytic streptococci and *Aerobacter* spp. are normal residents of the skin. Certain saprophytic fungi can be cultured from the skin of normal dogs and cats. A large number of bacterial and fungal species can be cultured from the skin of normal farm animals (Scott 1988).

## Sweat and sebaceous glands

Sweat and sebaceous glands are exocrine skin glands and are widely dispersed throughout the general body surface of the skin of mammals. They are not present in all species or in all body areas. In haired species they are located in association with the hair follicles as part of the basic follicular unit.

Sebaceous glands tend to be largest in areas where hair follicle density is lowest. They are largest and most numerous near mucocutaneous junctions, interdigital spaces, on the chin, the dorsal tail, the coronet, and over the dorsal neck and rump. Sebaceous glands are largest in the horse and smallest in intact male goats at the beginning of the rut period. The oily secretion (sebum) produced by the sebaceous glands tends to keep the skin soft and pliable by forming an emulsion that spreads over the surface of the stratum corneum to retain moisture and thus maintain proper hydration. The oil film spreads over the hair shafts and gives them a glossy sheen. During periods of illness or malnutrition the haircoat may become dull and dry as a result of inadequate sebaceous gland function. The sebum–sweat emulsion provides a physical and chemical barrier against potential pathogens.

Sebaceous glands have an abundant blood supply and appear to be innervated. Their secretion is thought to be under hormonal control, with androgens causing hypertrophy and hyperplasia, and estrogens and glucocorticoids causing involution.

Sweat glands are generally coiled and saccular or tubular and are distributed throughout all haired skin. They are localized below the sebaceous glands and usually open through a duct into the piliary canal in the infundibulum, above the sebaceous duct opening. Apocrine sweat glands tend to be largest in areas where hair follicle density is lowest. They are largest and most numerous near mucocutaneous junctions, interdigital spaces, the coronet, and over the dorsal neck and rump.

Specialized glandular structures have been described in the skin of large animals.

- Nasolabial glands occur in the muzzle and lip of cattle, sheep, and goats. These multilocular, tubuloalveolar, seromucoid glands appear to secrete almost constantly in cattle.
- Seromucoid glands are also found in the snout and lip and at the caudomedial aspect of the carpus of swine. These glandular structures occur at the junction of the deep dermis and subcutis, consist of basophilic cuboidal to columnar epithelial cells, and contain large myoepithelial cells.
- The mental, or mandibular organ of swine, a round, raised structure located in the intermandibular space, consists of large sebaceous and apocrine glands and very coarse sinus hairs (vibrissae).
- Eccrine sweat glands are found in the foot pads of small animals.

---

### Defense of the Skin

The skin has three barriers to pathogens:

1. physical defense – the stratum corneum
2. chemical defense – sebum and sweat
3. microbial defense – bacteria, yeasts and filamentous fungi.

---

## Integumentary changes with senility

In some dogs and cats changes may occur in the skin with senility:

- the hair becomes dull and lustreless
- alopecia and calluses appear over pressure points
- white hairs appear on the muzzle and body
- footpads and noses become hyperkeratotic
- claws become malformed and brittle.

## The importance of animal pelage to humans

- fiber from goats and sheep are important economic products
- hair of pet animals is of esthetic importance to owners
- hair (dander) from pets is an important contributor to respiratory disease in humans.

Horses sweat moderately to markedly in response to exercise, high ambient temperatures or fever, pain and stress. They have the ability to produce copious amounts of sweat as a major component of thermoregulation. Sweating is also a significant mechanism for heat loss in cattle. In goats and sheep, both the local application of heat and exposure to a hot environment result in increased sweat production. The skin of cats and dogs does not possess extensive superficial arteriovenous shunts as found in humans and swine that are designated to disseminate heat in hot weather. Carnivores also lack eccrine sweat glands in the hairy skin. Because of the inability to sweat effectively, dogs and cats have developed the ability to vaporize large volumes of water from their respiratory passages and pant to dissipate heat.

## Subcutis (hypodermis)

The subcutis (hypodermis) is the deepest and usually the thickest layer of the skin. It is a fibrofatty structure consisting of lobules of fat cells – lipocytes or adipocytes – interwoven with connective tissue. The subcutis functions as an energy reserve, in heat insulation, as protective padding, and in maintaining surface contours. There is no subcutis in some areas such as the lips, cheeks, eyelids, external ear and anus, where the dermis is in direct contact with musculature and fascia.

## HAIR

Hair is a characteristic feature of mammals; the coat (hair, fur or wool) is also known as the pelage. Most of the body surface is covered by hair, although in some regions, such as around the orifices and in the inguinal and axillary regions, the hair is sparse. Hair is important in thermal insulation, in sensory perception, and as a barrier against chemical, microbial and physical injury to the skin. Hair also harbors many bacteria and fungi, which may contribute to various disease states.

In general, no new hair follicles are formed after birth; except in sheep, wherein new follicle formation can take place for a short time. With growth, hair follicle density decreases and size increases. All hair follicles grow obliquely in relation to the epidermis. The direction of the slope of the hairs, which varies from one region of the body to another, gives rise to the hair tracts. With hair slope that generally runs caudally, benefits would include minimal impediment to forward motion and water flowing off the body on to the ground and not soaking the haircoat, which would reduce its thermal insulating properties. In general, the shape of the hair is determined by the shape of the follicle, with straight follicles producing straight hairs and curly follicles producing curly hairs.

Hairs usually occur in two basic arrangements: simple or compound. In the simple arrangement, characteristic of horses and cattle, hair follicles occur singly and at random, displaying no obvious distribution pattern. Hairs of various colors may occupy the simple follicle. Each hair emerges from a separate follicular opening, and there are no secondary hair follicles. In the compound arrangement, characteristic of cats, dogs, goats and sheep, follicles occur in clusters of variable composition. In general, a cluster consists of 2–5 large primary hairs (guard hair, topcoat hair, outercoat, kemp) surrounded by groups of smaller secondary hairs (down, undercoat). One of the primary hairs is the largest (central primary hair) and the remaining primary hairs are smaller (lateral primary hairs). The primary hairs generally emerge independently through separate pores, whereas the secondary

## Hair follicles of sheep and pigs

- Hair follicles in sheep are twisted so that the hair produced by them grows in a spiral as woolfibers.
- The hair follicle arrangement of the pig is intermediate, between simple and compound, with hairs occurring singly or in clusters of two or three.

hairs emerge through a common pore. Between 5 and 25 secondary hairs may accompany each primary hair. Compound follicles share a common pore into which the sebaceous glands and apocrine glands open.

In all common domestic animal species, with the exception of the goat, primary and secondary hairs are medullated. Hair shafts are divided into a medulla, the cortex, and the cuticle. The medulla is the innermost part of the hair and is composed of cells flattened from top to bottom. The cortex, the middle layer, consists of pigmented cornified cells. The cuticle, the outermost layer of the hair, is made up of flat, cornified, anuclear cells. The large secondary hairs of the goat are medullated, but the small secondary hairs are non-medullated. In sheep and Angora goats there are three main types of hair fibers: true wool fibers are fine, tightly-crimped and usually non-medullated; kemp fibers are very coarse, poorly crimped, fairly short and heavily medullated; hair fibers are intermediate between wool and kemp. Kemp fibers are undesirable in good wool because the large medulla causes brittleness and leaves little solid substance to take up dye. The hairs of the cat have also been divided into three types: guard hairs (thickest, straight, evenly tapered to a fine tip), awn hairs (thinner, with subapical swelling below the tip) and down hairs (thinnest, evenly crimped or undulating).

Adaptive changes in the length and density of the pelage, related to seasonal variation, are an important thermoregulatory device. The ability of the haircoat to regulate body temperature correlates closely with length, thickness, density per unit area and medullation of individual hair fibers. Together, these factors govern the depth of the layer of air trapped within the haircoat. Short-term and relatively minor increases in insulation are brought about by piloerection; this increases the depth of the haircoat.

Glossiness of the haircoat is important in reflecting sunlight, and tropical breeds of animals tend to have glossy coats that reflect sunlight well, whereas breeds with dull, woolly haircoats respond with increased body temperature and respiratory rate when in the tropics.

---

### The hair cycle

Hair growth tends to occur in a three-phase cycle:

- a growing period (*anagen*), during which the hair follicle is actively producing the hair
- a resting period (*telogen*), when the hair is retained in the hair follicle as a dead or 'club' hair that is subsequently lost
- a transitional period (*catogen*), between these two stages.

---

## Hair growth and cycle

Hairs do not grow continuously but rather in cycles. From the time it is first formed, each hair follicle undergoes repeated cycles of growth and rest. The relative duration of the various phases varies with the age of the individual, the region of the body, the breed and gender, and can be modified by a variety of factors, both physiological and pathological.

The replacement of hair is mosaic in pattern (the activity of a hair follicle is independent of that of its neighbors) and responds predominantly to photoperiod and to a lesser extent ambient temperature and nutrition. The photoperiod initiates shedding (molt). Ambient temperature, nutrition and other factors may modify the progress of the molt. Two exceptions to this are the wool follicle of the domestic sheep, in which virtually no cyclic activity occurs (always in anagen), and the coarse permanent hairs of the equine mane, tail and fetlock (horse hairs). In temperate latitudes normal cats, dogs, cattle, goats and horses may shed noticeably in the spring and fall. In general, shedding is a mechanism of adaptation to changing environmental temperatures and conditions. The increasing photoperiod in spring, and the decreasing photoperiod in fall, influence the hair cycle through the eyes, the hypothalamus, the hypophysis,

---

### Hair as a thermoregulator

- Haircoats composed of short, thick, medullated fibers are most efficient at high environmental temperatures.
- Those composed of long, fine, poorly medullated fibers, with coat depth increased by piloerection, are most efficient for thermal insulation at low environmental temperatures.

---

### Control of the hair cycle

The hair cycle, and thus the haircoat, is controlled by:

- photoperiod
- ambient temperature
- nutrition
- other environmental factors
- hormones
- general state of health
- genetics
- intrinsic factors.

### Hormonal influences on hair growth

- Thyroid hormones accelerate hair growth
- Glucocorticoids suppress hair growth.

the pineal gland, the thyroid gland, the adrenal gland and the gonads. Shedding is usually completed in about 5 weeks. Hair follicle activity is usually maximal in spring and early summer, and minimal in winter. In winter, up to 100% of the primary hair follicles and 50% of the secondary hair follicles may be in telogen.

Because hair is predominantly (65–90%) protein, nutrition has a profound effect on its quality and quantity. Poor nutrition may produce a dull, dry, brittle, or thin haircoat, and in cattle and horses may result in retention of the winter coat.

The hair cycle and haircoat are also affected by hormonal changes. Anagen is initiated and advanced, and hair growth is accelerated, by thyroid hormones. Conversely, excessive amounts of glucocorticoids inhibit anagen, suppress hair growth rate, and in sheep produce a tender fleece (wool-break).

Under conditions of stress, ill health or generalized disease, anagen may be considerably shortened. Accordingly, a large percentage of body hair may be in telogen at one time. Telogen hairs tend to be more easily lost, so the animal may shed excessively. Thus, shedding of these hairs (telogen defluxion) occurs simultaneously, often resulting in visible thinning of the haircoat or actual alopecia. This is common in dogs in the postpartum period. Disease states may also lead to faulty formation of hair cuticles, resulting in a dull, lusterless coat. In sheep, excessive amounts of gluco-corticoids, exogenous or endogenous, are associated with tender fleece and wool-break. Androgens significantly change the rate of hair growth on the chin of billygoats after puberty.

The maximum length of hair or wool fibers is genetically determined for each species, and depends on two factors: the rate of hair growth and the duration of anagen.

The rate of hair growth is genetically determined and varies between species, individuals and body regions on the same individual. It also seems to be related to the ultimate length of hair in each site.

### Hair growth rates (mm/d)

- 0.2–0.75 sheep
- 0.3 cats
- 0.04–0.71 dogs.

### Development of wool fibers

Wool is the natural fiber produced by the skin of the domesticated sheep and is characterized by its quality of intertwining, or felting together, by virtue of its imbricated surface. The wool follicle of the domestic sheep is always in anagen and thus there is no cyclic growth activity, as with hair. The duration of anagen is greatly prolonged in domestic sheep, and may last 7 years in merinos, thus eliminating seasonal shedding. The growth of wool fibers varies from 3 to 12 mm/month, with the greatest growth occurring in summer and early autumn.

The primary skin follicles provide the outer haircoat of the wild sheep and the kemps and hairlike fibers of domestic breeds. The secondary follicles provide the undercoat of wild sheep and the true wool fibers of domestic sheep.

The character of continuous growth in the wool fiber is one of the most interesting features in the biology of the sheep. The highly evolved wool sheep is an outstanding example of artificial selection. Its fleece, unlike the pelage of its primitive ancestors, which is shed periodically, grows continuously, and would become an unbearable burden if left unshorn. Its integument is densely populated with follicles that produce wool at a rate which is grossly in excess of the animal's need for heat conservation, and which imposes nutritional demands that are in many ways unique.

## CLINICAL EXAMINATION OF THE SKIN

The skin is the most readily accessible organ for examination. As with other body systems, it is important to examine the skin in a systematic manner to increase the probability of making a definitive diagnosis and providing rational therapy in the most cost-effective manner. There may be a tendency to assess skin lesions too quickly as being trivial and unimportant. Ideally, a thorough examination and appropriate diagnostic procedures should be carried out the first time the patient is examined and before any treatments have been initiated that may change the physical appearance of the skin and haircoat.

### Clinical examination of the skin

The complete clinical examination of the skin includes:

- taking the patient's history
- a physical examination of the skin
- the use of diagnostic aids.

## History taking

The most common complaints made by clients about animals with skin diseases are pruritus, alopecia, the appearance of a variety of lesions (which may be primary or secondary), the development of an abnormal odor or, more frequently, a combination of these signs.

A standard history recording form is helpful to record the history and results of the clinical examination. The use of a standard form or questionnaire can assist the examiner to ensure that most of the common questions are asked. It provides a standard historical database, allowing meaningful and valuable data retrieval and disease surveillance, and becomes an integral part of the patient's medical record, so that clinicians unfamiliar with the case can rapidly familiarize themselves with it. An adequate history should include the following.

### Signalment

The signalment is a description of the characteristics of the patient and includes age, breed, color, gender and use of the animal (e.g. companion, breeding or working).

#### Age

Many skin diseases are age-associated. For example, contagious echthyma of sheep (orf) is a highly contagious disease of lambs less than 6 months of age. The virus persists from year to year in scabs on the mammary glands and is transmitted to the lips of lambs during suckling. The lesions then spread to the muzzle, genitalia and limbs. The disease spreads rapidly and nearly all young animals in a group may be affected. Ehlers–Danlos disease (cutaneous asthenia) is a congenital disease of cats, dogs, cattle, sheep, pigs and horses. There is increased elasticity to the skin and it tears easily. Border disease of sheep is an example of an in utero viral disease causing a hairy coat in lambs at birth. A localized form of demodicosis causing alopecia occurs in young dogs. Middle-aged animals are more likely to be affected by immune-mediated and allergic skin disease. Warts (papillomata) are most common in young animals, and skin tumors are most common in older animals. Genital squamous cell carcinoma is common on the penis and prepuce of aged horses. Alopecia is often a feature of senility.

#### Gender

Certain diseases are gender-related. For example, hyperestrogenism in the dog with cystic ovaries is manifested by symmetrical flank alopecia extending into the perineum and by enlargement of the nipples. A male dog with a Sertoli cell tumor of the testicle may have similar clinical signs of hyperestrogenism. It is not uncommon for postpartum dogs to shed their haircoats (postpartum effluvium). Intact male dogs are predisposed to perianal adenomas.

#### Breed

The incidence of some diseases of the skin is higher in some breeds of animals than others, for example hypotrichosis is an inherited symmetrical alopecia in Friesian (Holstein) cattle and dermatophytosis is common in Persian cats.

#### Color

The color of the animal may also be related to certain problems.

- Color mutant or dilution alopecia is most commonly reported in blue or fawn Doberman pinschers and predisposes these dogs to bacterial folliculitis.
- Yellow-eyed, 'blue smoky' Persian cats are predisposed to Chediak-Higashi syndrome, an autosomal recessive disorder characterized by partial oculocutaneous albinism, a bleeding tendency, an increased susceptibility to infection, and enlarged granules in many blood cell types.
- White-eared cats and cattle with predominately white faces commonly suffer from solar dermatitis and squamous cell carcinoma.

### General history

#### Diet

Nutritional factors can influence hair growth. Hair is about 90% protein with a high percentage of sulfur-containing amino acids, and normal hair growth and skin keratinization requires about 25% of an animal's daily protein requirement. The growth rate and strength of hair and wool fibers are particularly sensitive to the amounts and proportions of amino acids available to the follicle.

---

### The influence of protein deficiency on the haircoat

Protein deficiency, through starvation, low-protein diets, or chronic catabolic disease, can result in

- abnormal texture of the coat
- decreased length and diameter of fibers
- diffuse thinning or alopecia.

---

Nutritional deficiencies or excesses cause a variety of skin conditions in different species.

1. Hypothyroidism in large animals may result from iodine deficiency or from iodine suppression by certain plants fed in excessive quantities. Iodine deficiency produces diffuse alopecia with telogenized, hypoplastic hair follicles.
2. Copper deficiency results in fiber depigmentation, and loss of hair or wool fiber tensile strength and elasticity with resultant breakage in cattle and sheep. In sheep, the crimp of fine wool fibers is lost and the wool becomes straight and 'steely'. Bands of depigmentation in an otherwise black wool fleece are the result of a transitory deficiency of copper in the diet.
3. Cattle on diets containing excess molybdenum and deficient copper show a peculiar speckling of the coat caused by an absence of pigment in a proportion of hair fibers. The speckling is often most marked around the eyes giving the animal the appearance of wearing spectacles. There is also a general loss of density of pigmentation in all coat colors. Hereford cattle, for example, change from normal deep red to a washed-out orange.
4. Herbivores grazing selenium-accumulating plants will develop lesions associated with selenium toxicity including loss of the long hairs of the mane, tail, and fetlock of horses, and occasionally generalized alopecia in horses and pigs.
5. Unbalanced vegetarian diets may lead to canine zinc deficiency. A zinc-responsive dermatosis occurs in Siberian Huskies and Alaskan Malamutes.
6. Some animals require additional fatty acids in the diet to maintain a healthy hair coat. Essential fatty acid deficiency in cats fed largely on human food causes skin changes including generalized scaling, dry skin, dry haircoat and variable alopecia.
7. Mycotoxicoses such as ergot and fescue toxicities can result in skin lesions, characterized by lameness and necrotic skin on the feet, ears and tail.
8. Cobalt deficiency leads to rough, faded and brittle hair and wool fiber, as well as decreased fiber production in sheep and cattle.

Food allergies, although not common in small animals, pose a real challenge to control. Knowing the animal's diet and attempting the elimination of individual food items over a period of time is necessary to establish a diagnosis of food allergy.

*Geographical location*
The geographical location of the animal or where it has been recently may be a risk factor. Dermatophilosis of ruminants is most common in countries with a wet and humid climate. Lumpy skin disease of cattle occurs in Africa.

*Season and environment*
The date when the lesions first appeared is important because some diseases have a seasonal incidence.

1. Seasonal diffuse flank alopecia, beginning in the autumn with hair regrowth occurring the following spring, is seen in a number of breeds including Doberman pinschers, Airedales, and Boxers.
2. Dogs housed on earthen or grass runs where hygiene is poor and temperatures are mild are predisposed to hookworm infestation as conditions are ideal for a large population of the infective third stage larvae to build up in soil.
3. Greasy heel occurs most commonly in cows on pastures that are being constantly irrigated, or in muddy conditions in tropical areas.
4. Greasy heel of horses occurs when horses stand for long periods in wet, unsanitary stables.
5. Horse flies are common in warm, moist weather.
6. Rain scald (dermatophilosis) occurs in horses exposed to heavy rainfall.
7. Squamous cell carcinoma is most common in animals with white ears or faces, exposed to sunlight for long periods.
8. Photosensitization occurs in light-skinned ruminants exposed to prolonged periods of sunshine usually under grazing conditions.
9. Ringworm in cattle is most common in winter when young animals are closely confined; similarly with lice (pediculosis).
10. Atopy due to inhaled pollen hypersensitivity will be seen when plants are in flower.
11. Frost bite of the ears, tails and distal extremities occurs in winter.
12. Staphylococcal eczema of the face of sheep is mainly seen in winter and early spring.
13. A relatively common complaint of dog and cat owners is persistent marked shedding of the hair coat of their animals. This may be associated with the unnatural environment in the modern home with little variation in light and heat throughout the year.
14. Recent changes in a family's life-style may also be important in the initiation of a psychogenic dermatosis.

## Disease history

*Present disease history*
The owner is asked to describe the present complaint in as much detail as possible.

## Clinical Pointer

Ask specific questions such as

- how many times daily does your animal scratch?
- does it scratch in many different sites, or just a few like its ears?
- does it shake its head?
- does it lick its paws?
- does it stamp its feet to the ground?
- does it chew its flank and groin areas?

*Pruritus (itchiness)*

The presence or absence of pruritus is a key aspect of the history that must be determined. The nature of the itching and how the animal behaves during episodes are important facts to determine.

*Previous skin disease*

Any previous skin diseases should be investigated. Where were the lesions? What did they look like? How long did they last? The date and onset of the original lesions, their locations on the body, their initial appearance and changes that have occurred since their first being noticed, and treatments given, along with the response, are important aspects of the history.

*Previous and current therapy*

The precise details of any previous or current therapy are necessary. Many dogs and cats with skin disorders have been bathed, dipped, sprayed or treated with one or more medications prior to presentation to a veterinarian. It is important that all types and dates of treatment are recorded, because a modification of the clinical signs may have resulted.

- Shampoos may remove significant numbers of ectoparasites.
- Anti-inflammatory medications (steroids) will decrease pruritus, removing an important clue.
- Prolonged anti-inflammatory therapy may predispose to bacterial infection, ectoparasitism (Demodex) or iatrogenic Cushing's disease.
- Steroids can markedly alter skin biopsy findings.
- Many drugs, particularly the penicillins and sulphonamides, are capable of producing hypersensitivity reactions.
- The use of certain topical insecticides in farm livestock may be associated with a subsequent mild dermatosis.
- Severe drug eruptions may result from medication given days, weeks, or even months before.

*Other signs of illness*

A number of endocrine diseases have profound systemic effects and result in skin pathology, most often alopecia. Animals with hyperadrenocorticism (Cushing's disease) often present with polydipsia and polyuria. Those with hypothyroidism may be lethargic, heat seeking and overweight. The hepatic–cutaneous syndrome in dogs is characterized by severe dermal ulceration and erythema associated with extensive liver pathology.

*Other animals or people affected.*

In groups of companion animals from a home, or groups or herds of farm animals, more than one animal may be affected.

## Clinical Pointer

Ask if any humans have skin problems similar to those of the animals

Exudative epidermitis of newborn piglets is characterized by most animals in the litter being affected within a few days. Owners must be asked if they themselves have any skin problems, as because of embarrassment they may be unwilling to volunteer this information. Scabies, cheyletiellosis, fleas and dermatophytosis are highly contagious and zoonotic.

## PHYSICAL EXAMINATION OF THE SKIN, HAIR AND APPENDAGES

### Inspection, palpation and smell

It is important to be systematic about the physical examination. Inspection of the animal's behavior, skin and hair, palpation, and smelling of the skin, are the most common physical methods used.

### Distant examination

The body condition is evaluated and the general condition of the haircoat assessed. The haircoat may be glossy and well-groomed or lusterless and unkempt. Dry, brittle, lusterless hair may be seen in many infectious diseases and with malnutrition and cachexia.

The regions of the body that must be examined include:

- Head and face
- Ears (pinna)
- Neck and thorax

- Abdominal wall
- Mane of horses
- Dorsal aspects
- Ventral aspects
- Tail head and tail switch
- Genitalia
- Mammary glands, including teats
- Perineum
- Limbs
- Hooves, including coronary bands
- Mucocutaneous junctions (lips, nares, vulva, prepuce, anus).

---

**Clinical Pointer**

The important prerequisites for the clinical examination of skin are

- adequate restraint and positioning of the animal
- good lighting such as natural light or day-type lamps
- clippers to trim the animal's hair when necessary to visualize lesions
- a hand lens to magnify lesions.

---

**Clinical Pointer**

Observe the entire animal from a distance to get an overall impression and to observe the distribution pattern of the lesions.

---

## Close inspection, palpation and smell

Close inspection, palpation and smelling of the skin and haircoat are necessary to identify and characterize lesions. Magnifying spectacles or an illuminated magnifying glass may prove useful.

All parts of the head, including the nose, muzzle and ears, are examined. The lateral trunk and the extremities are then examined. The feet of large animals need to be picked up to examine the interdigital clefts and parts of the coronary bands. The skin of the udder and teats of cattle, sheep, goats and horses must be inspected. The ventral aspect of the body is carefully examined, using a light source to illuminate the underside of adult cattle and horses. Visual, tactile and olfactory senses are used. Every part of the skin must be examined for the presence of lesions in different stages of development. The presence or absence of some ectoparasites can be determined by visual

---

**Clinical Pointer**

Inspect the dorsal aspect of the body by viewing it from the rear – elevated hairs and patchy alopecia may be more obvious from that angle.

---

inspection: for example, lice and ticks of cattle are usually easily visible. Parting the hairs slowly, and carefully and methodically examining the haircoat will reveal the dark-colored lice moving or burrowing into the skin, but they may be easily missed on a cursory examination. Fleas are the most common cause of skin disease in the dog and cat, and haircoat brushings to detect parasites should be part of every examination of the skin. The foul odor of the skin in some diseases may be offensive. Dermatophilosis in cattle is characterized by a foul and musty odor. The seborrhea in the infected ears of Cocker Spaniels emits a very rancid odor.

It is necessary to part the hairs with the fingers or by gently blowing on them to evaluate the length of the hair shafts. Broken hairs, changes in color and the accumulation of exudative material on the shafts are noted. The texture and elasticity of the skin must be assessed by rolling it between the fingers. Careful digital palpation of haircoat which appears normal on visual inspection may reveal underlying lesions such as pustules. In some cases, tufts of hairs may be seen protruding through an accumulation of exudate. The wool coat of sheep is inspected carefully and systematically by parting the fibers and evaluating their condition and that of the underlying skin.

---

**Clinical Pointer**

The hair coat should not be clipped, groomed or washed before the lesions have been identified and characterized. Palpation can be used to assess the consistency of lesions, the thickness and elasticity of skin, and to determine the presence of pain associated with disease.

---

## CLINICAL MANIFESTATIONS OF DISEASES OF THE SKIN

The skin responds in a limited number of ways to a wide variety of external and internal insults. Clinical manifestations of diseases of the skin include primary and secondary lesions and combinations of both.

Other common manifestations include:

- Abnormal coloration
- Pruritus or itchiness
- Evidence of pain
- Abnormalities of sweat secretion
- Abnormalities of sebaceous gland secretion
- Changes in elasticity, extensibility and thickness
- Abnormalities of hair and wool fibers
- Abnormalities of footpads, nails, hooves, and coronary bands and horns.

There are also secondary effects of diseases of the skin, such as dehydration, toxemia, and loss of body weight or chronic wasting.

The lesions are examined for three major characteristics:

- Distribution pattern
- Configuration
- Morphological appearance.

## Distribution pattern

The distribution pattern is a description of the location of the lesions on the body and tends to be typical for most skin diseases. It may be symmetrical, asymmetrical, localized, generalized or diffuse, or regional.

### Symmetrical

The distribution is bilaterally symmetrical when the occurrence of lesions is relatively the same on both sides of the animal when viewed from the dorsal or ventral aspects.

- In dogs, hyperadrenocorticism causes bilateral symmetrical alopecia of the flanks. The epidermis is thinner than normal, the skin bruises easily and purple macules may be visible.
- Growth hormone deficiency in the Keeshond dog typically causes bilaterally symmetrical alopecia of the caudal thighs and the neck and pinnae; seborrhea and hyperpigmentation may also be present.
- Dermatophilosis in cattle is characterized by symmetrical lesions which extend over the sides and down the legs and the ventral surface of the body.

---

### Clinical Pointer

Symmetrical distribution of alopecia suggests an underlying endocrine disease such as hypothyroidism or hyperadrenocorticism.

---

### Asymmetrical

When the distribution of the lesions is not the same on both sides the pattern is asymmetrical. Skin diseases caused by infectious agents are commonly asymmetrical in distribution. Examples include ringworm, swinepox, and papillomatosis.

### Localized

Lesions may be single, such as the solitary lesion of dermatophytosis or a foreign-body reaction. The areas of skin involved aid in establishing the differential diagnosis, as most skin diseases have a typical distribution pattern.

- In photosensitization, the unpigmented skin is affected, the pigmented parts unaffected, and only the lateral aspects of the teats in cattle are affected.
- Pruritus of the tail head of dogs is highly suggestive of flea allergy.
- Comedones and scales are typical of chin acne in cats.
- An ill-fitting harness or flea collar may cause alopecia or irritation to the affected area.
- Squamous cell carcinoma are common on unpigmented skin regions, noticeably the eyelids of cattle and the ears of white cats.
- Myiasis (fly strike) in sheep affects soiled parts of the body.
- Sarcoptic mange in dogs is typically located over the pressure points (elbows, hocks) and ear margins.

### Generalized or diffuse

Lesions involving a major part or the whole of the body surface may indicate generalized infection or a contact dermatitis following bathing.

- Ringworm in cattle may become generally distributed over the entire body.
- Exudative epidermitis in piglets is characterized by diffuse involvement of the entire body.

### Regional

Lesions may be restricted to certain regional areas.

- Mucocutaneous lesions (ears, lips, foot pads, anus, nasal planum) are typically associated with autoimmune disease (lupus, pemphigus) although pyodermas and zinc-responsive dermatoses can cause similar signs.
- Edema associated with systemic immune reactions in large animals may be most noticeable on the dependent parts of the body where the skin is somewhat loose, and the eyelids, vulva and perineum.
- Zinc deficiency dermatosis results in hyperkeratinization of the muzzle and feet in cattle, horses and dogs.

- In sheep, dermatophytosis causes extensive heaped up pyramidal crusts of the trunk (lumpy wool), severe enough to make the fleece worthless.
- In contagious ecthyma of sheep the lesions are most common on the lips, muzzle, and nostrils.
- Facial alopecia with pruritus and secondary excoriations is seen in cats with food allergies.
- Hookworm infection in dogs commonly affects the feet and lower limbs particularly at the junction between the skin and foot pads.
- Ectoparasitism, in particular, *Chorioptes* spp. of cattle and horses, affects the lower limbs, hind quarters and forelimbs.

## Configuration or spatial arrangement

The configuration of skin lesions refers to their spatial relationship to each other as viewed from above. These characteristics aid in making a differential diagnosis. Skin lesions evolve over time. Primary lesions such as pustules and vesicles may appear quickly and then disappear rapidly. They may leave behind secondary lesions such as focal alopecia, epidermal collarettes, scaling, hyperpigmentation and crusts, which may be more chronic and provide clues as to the presence of previous primary lesions.

*Annular or ring-shaped* configurations occur when the central part of the lesion clears, leaving a ring-like border. This configuration is found in superficial spreading folliculitis, local seborrhea, demodicosis and dermatophytosis, as well as bacterial and fungal infections and healing bullous eruptions.

*Polycyclic* configurations result from the confluence of lesions or a spreading process. Examples are spreading bacterial folliculitis, demodicosis and pyotraumatic dermatitis.

*Grouped* lesions are clusters of lesions, often the result of new foci developing around an old lesion. They occur in folliculitis, insect bites, contact dermatitis and calcinosis cutis.

*Serpiginous* lesions creep from area to area and have a wavy or snake-like border. They develop as a result of spreading, such as in canine scabies or demodicosis.

They may also occur as a result of the confluence and partial resolution of polycyclic lesions.

*Linear* lesions may indicate an exogenous cause, such as trauma from an irritant material, a scratch or a whip, or endogenous disorders such as linear eosinophilic granulomas, which characteristically affect the hindlimbs in cats. In other cases linear lesions may reflect the involvement of blood or lymphatic vessels.

*Arciform* lesions usually result from the partial resolution of polycyclic lesions such as spreading folliculitis, but may also result from spreading, as in canine scabies and demodicosis.

*Iris or central healing* configurations occur when the skin heals behind an advancing front of a disease process. It is typical of certain dermatophytoses, demodicosis and bacterial folliculitis.

*Single* lesions are confined to a single location and are solitary.

## Morphological appearance of primary and secondary lesions

The morphology of skin lesions has been classified into primary and secondary.

### Primary lesion

A primary lesion arises *de novo* in the skin and usually reflects the underlying etiology, and although it may not be pathognomonic it can be attributed to a limited number of diseases. Primary lesions are not always present at the time of examination because they may be very transient. Vesicles, for example, may persist for only a few hours. In other cases the primary lesions may be difficult to identify among the secondary changes that will invariably be present.

Many skin lesions undergo a sequential evolution resulting in a variety of identifiable changes to the skin, and it is the presence of all these lesions, coexisting and often in close proximity, that allows the clinician to deduce the underlying pathology. Thus the recognition of a pustular phase, its precursor the papule,

---

**Clinical Pointer**

Skin lesions evolve over time, the different patterns represent their natural history.

**Clinical Pointer**

Primary lesions are useful diagnostically but must not be considered in isolation.

and a non-scarring, healing phase will allow the conclusion that the lesions are superficial and epidermal in origin.

### Secondary lesion

A secondary lesion is due to changes in the skin caused by factors such as scratching, secondary infection, drug therapy and healing processes. Secondary lesions may not be helpful in making a diagnosis but are commonly the ones that are present. They may be difficult to classify because of the changes that have occurred over time, but it is necessary to describe and interpret them as precisely as possible.

## Evaluation of primary and secondary lesions

Close inspection of the affected skin is necessary. The ability to recognize a lesion and its distribution, to appreciate its development and its evolution, is a crucial first step in making a diagnosis and formulating a differential diagnosis. It is important to look at the lesion, feel it, and determine what changes have occurred in the skin.

The following are morphological descriptions of primary and secondary lesions (see Fig 13.1–13.16). Color atlases of the lesions in horses (Pascoe 1990) and dogs and cats (Wilkinson and Harvey 1994) are available.

### Primary lesions (see Clinical Manifestations for definitions)

**Erythema** may be physiological and associated with heat loss. It is the first sign of inflammation in the skin. By pressing a clear piece of plastic or glass over an erythematous lesion, vascular engorgement can be differentiated from hemorrhage (petechia or ecchymosis). A lesion that blanches on pressure indicates

---

**Clinical Pointer**

Consider these questions when assessing skin lesions.

- Are there any changes in color of the skin?
- Is the surface of the skin normal or thickened, raised or flat, filled with fluid, filled with pus, freely movable, atrophic, excoriated, or ulcerated?
- What is the state of the hair or wool coat?
- Are the hair fibers completely missing or are broken hair shafts protruding through the lesion?
- Are there any crusts, scales, or scabs present?

---

**Clinical Pointer**

Use diascopy to assess erythema:

- vascular engorgement blanches on pressure
- hemorrhage does not.

---

that the reddish color is due to vascular engorgement. This technique is known as diascopy.

**Macules** (Fig. 13.1) may be up to 1 cm in diameter and may be a pronounced feature of canine hyperadrenocorticism.

A **patch** is a macule that is over 1 cm in diameter. The discoloration of macules and patches results from several processes: an increase in melanin pigmentation, depigmentation, and erythema or local hemorrhage. Erythema is the commonest cause and may be seen in localized inflammatory reactions, and in other conditions such as localized demodicosis. Hemorrhage into the skin is less common and suggests clotting defects, poisoning (Warfarin) or defects in vascular integrity, as may occur for example in Rocky Mountain spotted fever or drug eruption.

Changes in pigmentation may be congenital or acquired and may involve both the loss, or the acquisition, of pigment. **Hyperpigmentation** is more common, and may be postinflammatory, as in the healing lesions of superficial pyoderma or a feature of a non-inflammatory disease such as an endocrine dermatosis. In general, endocrine disorders are associated with widespread changes in pigmentation rather than macules or patches, but exceptions do occur.

**Hypopigmentation** may also be postinflammatory, particularly when the damage extends through the basement membrane and results in healing with scar formation. Non-inflammatory, possibly hereditary,

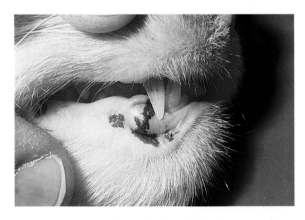

**Fig. 13.1** **Macules** due to lentigo simplex in an orange cat.

acquired loss of pigmentation (**vitiligo**) may be seen in some breeds, notably the Belgian Tervuren or the Rottweiler. Vitiligo frequently begins on the head, particularly the muzzle and lips, and is often symmetrical.

**Wheals** (Fig. 13.2) may be traumatic, allergic or immune mediated in origin. They may be round, oval or plaque-like and adjacent wheals may coalesce, giving irregular shapes. They arise rapidly and frequently disappear within hours. Wheals are a consequence of edema in the superficial dermis and there is no accompanying pathological change to the cells of the epidermis. They may be colorless or pink-tinged and the color blanches on diascopy.

**Urticaria** (**hives**) is most common in horses and occurs occasionally in cattle and dogs. Occasionally edema will cause distension of a region of the body such as an eyelid, the muzzle or a paw, and this is termed **angioedema**.

A **papule** (Fig. 13.3) may be due to an accumulation of cells, fluid, debris or metabolic deposits, and may be follicular or interfollicular in orientation. The cellular infiltrate will vary with the pathological process, but in the commonest cause of papules, i.e. superficial pyoderma, the infiltrate will be neutrophilic in nature.

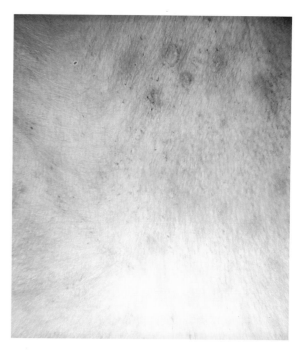

**Fig. 13.3 Papules** due to flea bites in a white cat. (Courtesy of REW Halliwell, University of Edinburgh)

Most papules are erythematous but may be variably colored, for example cream-colored papules are seen in sebaceous adenomatoma. If there is a hair or hairs protruding from the center of a papule this may indicate a bacterial infection of the hair follicles.

Follicular papules may be seen in cases of follicular dystrophy and defects in keratinization, when the accumulation of keratinaceous debris under the occluded follicular orifice produces the swelling. Papules resulting from metabolic deposits may contain calcium, as in calcinosis circumscripta, or other products of metabolic origin, such as mucin or lipid.

Papules often begin as erythematous macules, particularly in superficial pyoderma, when they may outnumber the pustules by 10 or 20:1. They may also evolve into crusted papules, as in miliary dermatitis in the cat or sarcoptic mange in the dog. In allergic contact dermatitis, where the papule is the primary lesion, the progression to pustules does not occur and hence other lesions associated with pustules, such as epidermal collarettes (see below), are also absent.

**Pustules** (Fig. 13.4) are thin, fragile and transient, and rapidly rupture and become crusted. They may be follicular or interfollicular in distribution and originate from the epidermis or the hair follicle. Interfollicular pustules typically begin as macules which become papular and then pustular. Pustules may

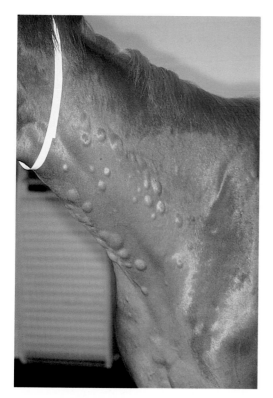

**Fig. 13.2 Wheals** due to a drug reaction in a horse.

---

### Pyoderma versus hives

In short-haired dogs the papules of superficial pyoderma may cause multiple elevations of groups of hairs which mimic wheals and may lead to an erroneous diagnosis of hives. Administration of glucocorticoids to these cases may make subsequent management of the pyoderma difficult. Careful examination and identification of lesions is of paramount importance.

---

be infected (bacteria) or sterile in nature. They may be cream-colored, yellow or green. The typical yellowish color results from the stretching of the upper layer by the gradual accumulation of infiltrate beneath, which then becomes visible. In the most common cause, i.e. bacterial infection, the infiltrate will contain neutrophils, bacteria, debris and perhaps a few free keratinocytes. The latter are unattached owing to the action of bacterial and neutrophil toxins; in consequence they appear rounded in shape and are termed acanthocytes. In follicular infection the toxins may accumulate to sufficiently high levels that large numbers of acanthocytes are present.

Examination of the aspirated pustular contents in these cases may reveal sufficient numbers of acanthocytes to suggest the possibility of pemphigus foliaceus. In addition to pyoderma and pemphigus foliaceus, pustules also may be a feature of

- demodicosis
- dermatophytosis
- sub-corneal pustular dermatosis
- drug eruption.

**Superficial pyoderma** is defined as bacterial skin disease of the superficial portion of hair follicles or the interfollicular epidermis immediately below the stratum corneum (impetigo). Deep pyoderma involves not only the hair follicles but also the dermis or even the subcutis. The follicular wall may rupture to release hair shaft keratin, bacteria and bacterial products into the dermis, resulting in furunculosis.

Occasionally pustules may be unusually colored, hemorrhagic (for example), very large or surrounded by a zone of erythema, and in these situations consideration should be given to staphylococcal hypersensitivity. These florid lesions are often found in cases where long-standing or recurrent bacterial infection is a feature of an underlying disease, particularly a hypersensitivity, such as atopy.

In contrast, very large and flaccid pustules with minimal inflammation suggest immunosuppression, particularly hyperadrenocorticism.

Most cases of superficial pyoderma exhibit only a few frank pustules but many papules and secondary lesions, such as crust and scale (Fig. 13.5). Some cases will also exhibit epidermal collarettes and perhaps postinflammatory hyperpigmentation. In addition, many animals exhibit a patchy alopecia as a consequence of the follicular damage and associated self-trauma.

**Abscesses** can be dermal or subcutaneous and are larger and deeper than pustules.

**Plaques** (Fig. 13.6) may result from edema (wheals), the coalescence of adjacent papules, or may be

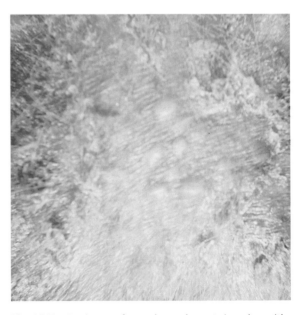

**Fig. 13.5** A mixture of pustules and **crusts** in a dog with pemphigus foliaceous.

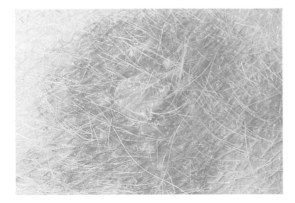

**Fig. 13.4** A **pustule** in a dog with pemphigus foliaceous.

neoplastic in origin. They may result from hyperplasia of the dermis or epidermis or both, and may also result from the deposition of metabolic products in the skin. Plaques are formed by the extension or coalition of papules. Plaque-like accumulations of lipid scales or crust may occur in some of the dermatoses, accompanied by a defect in keratinization, such as vitamin A-responsive dermatosis or *Malassezia pachydermatis* infection.

In addition to being larger than papules, **nodules** (Fig. 13.7) often extend into the dermis rather than remaining confined to the epidermis. As is the case with papules the infiltrate may be infectious, inflammatory, granulomatous, neoplastic or of metabolic origin. **Panniculitis** is manifested by the development of deep-seated, firm and painful nodules anywhere over the body. Nodules need to be distinguished from neoplastic proliferations (**tumors**).

The term **tumor** (Fig. 13.8) is often applied to a large nodule. Tumors may be mobile or locally infiltrative, ulcerated or domed, plaque-like or pedunculated, malignant or benign.

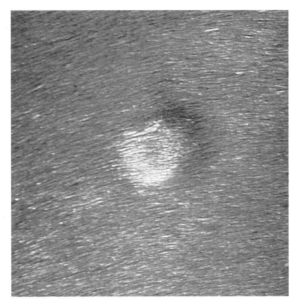

**Fig. 13.7** A singular **nodule** formed as an eosinophilic granuloma with collagen necrosis (nodular necrobiosis) in a horse.

## Clinical Pointer ❋

Take care to distinguish between

- nodules – circumscribed elevations of the skin, more than 1 cm in diameter

*and*

- neoplastic proliferations (tumors) – masses of neoplastic origin, benign or malignant.

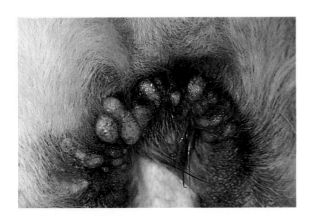

**Fig. 13.6** Inflammatory **plaques** due to urine scalding associated with an ectopic ureter in a dog.

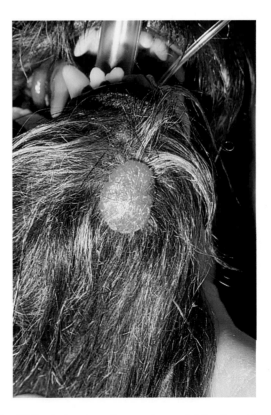

**Fig. 13.8** A singular cutaneous **tumor** (histiocytoma) in a dog.

**Cysts** within the skin are lined by epithelium, usually of adnexal origin rather than epidermal (Fig. 13.9). The contents of the cyst reflect the epithelial lining, i.e. sebaceous cyst derived from the sebaceous gland, or apocrine cyst derived from the epitrichial sweat gland. Cysts may burst or discharge to the surface via a fistula or sinus. They may be congenital or developmental in origin. Developmental cysts, usually located at specific anatomic sites, include branchial cysts in the neck, and false nostril cysts in horses and in the wattles of goats.

**Vesicles** are less than 1 cm in diameter (Fig. 13.10) and are fluid-filled sacs originating in the epidermis or dermis. They protrude above the skin surface, and are very transient in nature. Vesicles are seen in the early stages of viral infections and may also result from irritants, heat and autoimmune skin disease. Viral vesicles may quickly be infiltrated by inflammatory cells and progress to pustules. The elevation of the skin is due to the accumulation of intercellular fluid beneath the roof of the vesicle. The fluid is usually serum or an inflammatory exudate which imparts a pale, almost translucent nature to the vesicle, in contrast to the yellow, opaque nature of pustules.

Compared to vesicles, **bullae** are fluid-filled elevations of the skin more than 1 cm in diameter. The fluid is usually clear and composed of serum, but may be

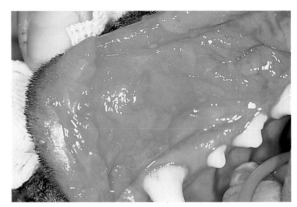

**Fig. 13.10** **Bullae** and **vesicles** on the gum of a dog with bullous pemphigoid.

pink or red if blood is present. Bullae are very transient in animals and are characteristically found in some autoimmune and viral diseases. They may occur as lesions in their own right, perhaps due to cleft formation in the epidermis, or may arise from the coalescence of adjacent pockets of intercellular epidermal edema. The depth of the bulla will affect the appearance of the lesion. In deep lesions, such as occur with bullous pemphigoid (where the cleft is at the basement membrane), the intact bullae may be tense and well defined, whereas with the more superficial, suprabasal clefting of pemphigus vulgaris any intact bullae are rather flaccid, with a tendency to enlarge at the edges.

### Secondary lesions

A **callus** or thickened, hyperkeratotic plaque, usually is alopecic, and develops most commonly over bony prominences (elbows, hocks) as a result of pressure and friction. It is characterized by annular, well-circumscribed plaques of lichenification and hyperkeratosis.

---

### Clinical Pointer ✳

If an autoimmune disorder is suspected

- hospitalize the animal
- examine the animal repeatedly for the presence of vesicles
- take biopsies for a definitive diagnosis.

---

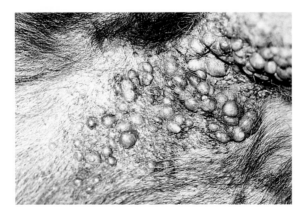

**Fig. 13.9** Multiple epidermal inclusion **cysts** in a German Shepherd dog.

---

### The Nikolsky sign

The Nikolsky sign is a diagnostic test based on the tendency of bullae to underrun and cleft. The Nikolsky sign is produced when the normal-appearing skin peripheral to vesiculobullous and erosive or ulcerative lesions can be dislodged with sliding digital pressure. Lateral pressure or a shearing force applied to the skin adjacent to a lesion in a case of pemphigus vulgaris may result in a vesicle being produced. This is not usually present in cases of bullous pemphigoid.

---

The erythematous eruption of skin due to friction, or **intertrigo** usually occurs at the vulva, the lips, and on lateral aspects of the udder.

The color of superficial, dried **crusts** is determined by their content: yellow-green if formed from pus; dark red or brown if from blood. Unusually thick crusts are found in hairy areas of skin because the dried material tends to adhere more tightly than in glabrous skin. For example, in dermatophilosis of cattle, exudates may be mixed with scales to produce a palisade or layered crust.

**Scales** containing keratinocytes (Fig. 13.11) may be white or gray, and greasy if containing excessive lipid. Scale and dandruff are commonly seen with seborrhea.

Under normal conditions in the dog, the process of keratinization ensures a steady replacement of the epidermis with cells derived from a dividing pool in the basal layer. It takes about 21 days for cells to reach the upper layer of viable epidermis, the stratum granulosum. In Cocker Spaniels with defects of keratinization, this time is reduced to 3 or 4 days; furthermore, there is a larger percentage of the basal cell population involved in the process. As a result there are increased numbers of poorly differentiated cells shed from the surface of the skin, where aggregates of them are visible as scale.

Keratinization is easily altered by numerous other internal factors, and thus scale, oiliness and smell are secondary features of many diseases, particularly those caused by ectoparasites, but also bacterial skin disease, endocrine dermatoses and dermatoses with a hypersensitive etiology.

**Seborrhea** is a defect in keratinization resulting in increased scale formation and excessive greasiness of the skin and haircoat. Although idiopathic or primary seborrhea has been recognized in the horse and dog,

> ### Clinical Pointer ✳
>
> Some crusts may be hidden from view below the hair coat and digital palpation is necessary for detection.

most cases are secondary to an underlying problem such as hypothyroidism, ectoparasitism, pyoderma, fatty acid deficiency or ringworm. Seborrhea occurs in several diseases of animals, including greasy heel of horses and exudative epidermitis of pigs, but its pathogenesis is poorly understood. Seborrhea oleosa denotes greasy skin and hairs with a rancid odor to the coat; seborrhea sicca refers to dryness of the skin and coat with non-adherent scales. Seborrhea sicca causes surface scaling and nit-like keratotic deposits on the hair shafts.

In **hyperkeratosis** the increased keratin production in the epidermis results in the skin being thicker than normal and usually corrugated and hairless. Dryness and scaliness are characteristic. Fissures develop in a grid-like pattern, creating a scaly appearance. Hyperkeratinization is a characteristic finding with zinc deficiency, as in **parakeratosis** where gray thickening of skin due to incomplete keratinization of the epithelial cells occurs.

A **fistulous tract** seen as a draining opening on the skin may be seen in cases of deep pyoderma, anal furunculosis, foreign-body penetration, panniculitis or mycetoma. Fistulous tracts are commonly seen in botryomycosis, and anal furunculosis in dogs, and in bovine actinomycosis.

A **sinus tract** is also seen as a draining opening but this tract is epithelium-lined. This is seen in dermoid cyst and sinus in the Rhodesian Ridgeback. Long-standing foci of deep pyoderma, such as are seen in canine acne or pododermatitis, may also be accompanied by sinus formation.

**Fissures** (Fig. 13.12) are often multiple, occurring in chronic dermatoses where the skin is thick and inelastic and then subjected to sudden swelling from inflammation or trauma. They are typically found in moist, poorly aerated areas. Extensive fissuring is found in anal furunculosis of the German Shepherd dog.

A **comedone, comedo** or **blackhead** (Fig. 13.13) is usually slightly elevated above the skin surface and may be white or black in color. The comedo is the primary lesion of acne in man but is not pathognomonic. Comedones are commonly found in animals suffering from defects of keratinization, both primary and secondary; they are found in cases of demodicosis and are a frequent finding on the abdomen of dogs with hyperadrenocorticism. Comedones are the primary lesion in feline acne and are commonly observed in endocrine disorders and in senile skin.

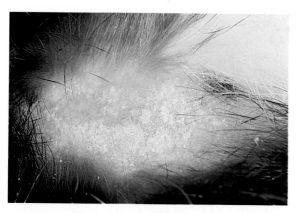

**Fig. 13.11  Scale** due to *Cheyletiella parasitovorax* in a lop-eared rabbit.

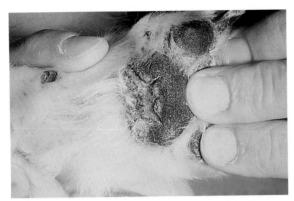

**Fig. 13.12 Fissure** in a footpad of a dog suffering from metabolic epidermal necrolysis.

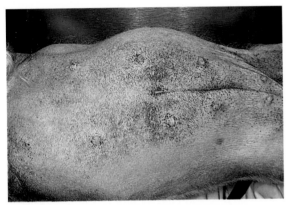

**Fig. 13.13 Comedones** associated with Cushing's disease in a dog.

**Excoriations** are superficial and often linear, and are a result of self-trauma by rubbing, chewing or licking. They are thus a feature of the pruritic dermatoses and in some individuals can be very severe. Excoriations are prone to secondary infection. They may be linear or punctate in appearance, and the associated hair is often broken and saliva stained.

**Erosions** have an intact basal layer and are formed when vesicles or bullae rupture to expose their base.

---

### Clinical Pointer ✳

Ulceration may be a feature of

- deep bacterial or fungal infection
- self-trauma as in feline eosinophilic plaque
- calcinosis cutis in canine hyperadrenocorticism
- irritant contact dermatitis
- neoplasia.

---

They may be found in diseases characterized by vesicles or bullae (such as autoimmune disorders) and in cases due to exposure to physical or chemical agents. Healing occurs without scar formation.

Inflammation and scarring of the dermis results in **ulcer** formation in which healing is often by scar formation (Fig. 13.14).

**Ulcers** may result from ischemia due to pressure, neoplasia, deep mycosis or bacterial infection. Pressure sores or decubital ulcers occur as a result of prolonged pressure on a relatively small area of the body sufficient to compress the capillary circulation, causing tissue damage and necrosis. Decubital ulcers are common when nursing care in recumbent animals is inadequate. Pressure sores are characterized by erythematous to reddish-purplish discoloration which progresses to oozing, necrosis and ulceration. The ulcers are usually deep, undermined at the edges, secondarily infected and slow to heal.

When skin becomes necrotic, the affected area is discolored, cool, may be wrinkled and moist or dry. More severe necrosis results in **gangrene** that may be moist or dry. Moist gangrene is caused by impairment of lymphatic and venous drainage together with infection of the tissues. Moist gangrene is characterized by swollen and discolored tissues with a foul odor. Dry gangrene occurs when the arterial blood supply is occluded but venous and lymphatic drainage is intact, and there is no local infection. Dry gangrene is characterized by a dry, discolored and leathery appearance.

Fourth-degree thermal burns, photosensitization and ischemic necrosis of the skin of the ears, tail and feet can result in a skin slough of necrotic tissue.

**Lichenification** is a response to chronic trauma, particularly friction, but also inflammation. The gross thickening, that often is hyperpigmented, results in exaggeration of the folds and fissures and intertriginous

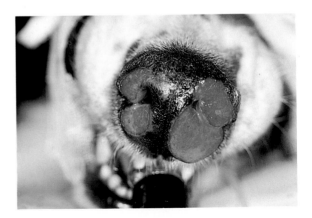

**Fig. 13.14 Ulcers** on the nasal planum of a dog.

maceration with secondary infection common. The skin often appears dry. Lichenification may occur at the sites of pressure points, such as the elbow and hock of large dogs.

A **scar** or healed wound occurs when the basal layers of the epidermis have been breached and the underlying dermis is damaged and involved in an inflammatory reaction. The ensuing healing process involves fibrosis and often contraction. The resultant skin surface is often thin, devoid of hair and hypopigmented. Scars are most common following burns, surgical incisions, bites, traumatic wounds and deep pyoderma.

An **epidermal collarette** (Fig. 13.15) is usually caused by a superficial pyoderma, although rupture of a pustule or bulla can result in a similar lesion. Older lesions may be 2 cm in diameter with a dark pigmented center.

Epidermal collarettes are regarded as secondary lesions by some authorities and as primary lesions by others. Epidermal collarettes are best conceived as decapitated pustules, vesicles or bullae which are spreading peripherally, giving the appearance of a ring of scale. Adjacent lesions may coalesce, giving rise to a large polycyclic ring of scale. There is often a peripherally spreading zone of accompanying erythema. Central healing with postinflammatory hyperpigmentation is common.

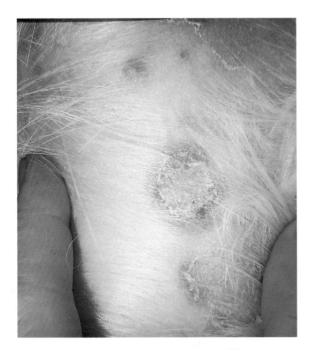

**Fig. 13.15  Epidermal collarette** in a dog. (Figure courtesy of REW Halliwell, University of Edinburgh)

**Clinical Pointer**

Epidermal collarettes look like bull's eyes or targets.

### Abnormal coloration of the hair and skin

Inspection of the hair may reveal evidence of licking which, if prolonged, may cause brown staining. Psoroptic mange in sheep damages the fleece, which hangs in untidy hunks from the body. There is associated extensive yellowish encrustation, and the skin is cool and feels moist.

Abnormal skin colorations, including jaundice, pallor and erythema, may be visible and are best seen in the oral or vaginal mucosae or in the conjunctiva. In animals with light-colored skins they may be visible at first glance. Skin pallor may indicate decreased vascularity or anemia. Erythema may result from inflammation, pruritus or hyperthermia. Early erythema is a common finding where more definite skin lesions are yet to develop, as in early photosensitization. The red to purple discoloration of the skin of white pigs affected by various systemic infectious diseases may be extreme, and no diagnostic significance can be attached to its degree. The same patchy discoloration can be observed in cases of salmonellosis, pasteurellosis, erysipelas and hog cholera. The blue coloration of early gangrene is characterized by coldness and loss of skin elasticity. This is particularly evident on the udder and teat skin of cows in the early stages of acute mastitis caused by *Staphylococcus aureus*. White-yellow deposits in the skin may indicate calcinosis cutis as a result of hyperadrenocorticism.

**Hypopigmentation** may be congenital or acquired. Hypopigmentation of the hair occurs in senility and may follow repeated trauma from ill-fitting harnesses. Hypopigmentation may occur as a postinflammatory phenomenon, for example after a bite wound or an episode of superficial pyoderma. Loss of pigment may also be idiopathic. German Shepherd dogs and Doberman pinschers may frequently be seen with loss of pigment on the planum nasale. Actual depigmentation of the hair occurs in congenital leukotrichia of horses and in vitiligo in several species. Generalized depigmentation of the hair may be seen in severe

**Clinical Pointer**

When assessing abnormal skin color, inspect the oral or vaginal mucosae or the conjunctiva in natural light.

systemic infections and with Johne's disease and malnutrition. Periorbital lightening of the hair occurs in bovine hypocuprosis. Hypopigmentation of the skin may be general, as in albino, pseudoalbino and lethal white animals.

The absence of melanocytes in **vitiligo** results in patches of depigmentation, often with a hyperpigmented border, and often enlarging slowly. The condition is common in horses and cattle, often occurring after surgery. It has been reported in the Belgian Tervuren and the Rottweiler.

Freeze-branding is depigmentation of the haircoat with supercooled instruments: the carefully gauged degree of cold application causes selective destruction of the melanocytes.

In **hyperpigmentation** or hypermelanosis the excessive amount of melanin is deposited in the epidermis and often in dermal melanophages. Excess melanin may be due to increased numbers of melanocytes or an increased amount of melanosomes in the epidermis. Increased numbers of melanocytes are present in lentigo. In contrast, in postinflammatory hyperpigmentation due to chronic inflammation or an endocrine dermatosis, there is increased melaninization and melanin deposition. This usually results from increased production of melanin in the skin (hypermelanosis) which may be seen in

- hypothyroidism
- hyperadrenocorticism
- some chronic inflammatory skin diseases such as generalized demodicosis.

With **acanthosis nigricans** areas of hyperpigmentation, lichenification and alopecia commence in the axillae and often spread to involve the flexural surfaces of all limbs, as well as the ventral body. Dachshunds are particularly predisposed to the disease, often developing the earliest changes at a young age. An endocrine etiology has been postulated. Sporadic cases are secondary to systemic disease, hypersensitivity reactions and friction in body folds.

## Pruritus or itchiness

**Pruritus** or **itchiness** is a common manifestation of skin disease (allergies, ectoparasites, secondary to bacterial and fungal infections) and is almost always caused by abnormalities of the epidermis. Pruritus results from the stimulation of free nerve endings located at the junction between the dermis and the epidermis. A number of mediators, including histamine, serotonin and prostaglandins, are involved in the production of pruritus, which is manifested by scratching, chewing, biting, rubbing or licking. If the

### Clinical Pointer

When assessing the cause of pruritus take care to differentiate between

- abnormalities of the epidermis
- licking and self-excoriation associated with pain or psychosis
- hyperesthesia, increased sensitivity to normal stimuli
- paresthesia or perverted sensation, this is subjective in nature and can hardly be defined in animals.

trunk of a sheep with psoroptic mange is gently scratched by hand, there is characteristic nibbling movement of the jaws and apparent pleasure; the neck may arch and the animal may even topple over.

All sensations that give rise to rubbing or scratching are therefore included with pruritus. The abnormality is more properly defined as scratching.

## Pain

A disease of the skin may cause pain, which is manifested by anxiety, reluctance to move, and a painful response on palpation of the affected skin. Piglets with exudative epidermitis may squeal when the affected skin is palpated. Severe thermal burns of the skin are painful to palpation. Cattle with photosensitization may exhibit uncomfortable behavior because of lesions on the skin of the muzzle and teats, and sloughing of necrotic skin. Vesicles of the coronary bands, interdigital clefts and teats of farm animals, as occur in foot-and-mouth disease and other vesicular diseases, can cause considerable lameness and painful teats. Cracks and fissures of the skin, and vesicles, folliculitis and scabs are accompanied by pain on palpation or when the animal moves and flexes or stretches the skin.

## Abnormalities of sweat secretion

The activity of the sweat glands is controlled by the autonomic nervous system and is, for the most part, a reflection of body temperature. Excitement and pain may cause sweating before the body temperature rises; here the sweating is due to central autonomic activity and increased epinephrine release. Local areas of abnormal sweating may arise from peripheral nerve lesions or the obstruction of sweat gland ducts.

**Hyperhidrosis** is important only in large herbivores (cattle, horses). Noticeable sweating of the head, neck and flanks is seen in horses following hard exercise, after exposure to high ambient temperatures, with severe pain, and occasionally following some drug therapies. A form of hyperhidrosis, apparently inherited, has been recorded in Shorthorn calves. Localized sweating in horses may be seen with local injections of epinephrine, with dourine, and with sympathetic decentralization (denervation) of skin.

**Anhidrosis** with lack of appropriate sweating is seen in horses and occasionally cattle, and is a significant problem in working animals in hot and humid countries. The cause is unknown.

**Hematidiosis** is bloodstained sweat and may be seen in equine infectious anemia, purpura hemorrhagica, and various bleeding diatheses.

## Abnormalities of sebaceous gland secretion

The degree of hydration of the skin is assessed by gently taking a fold of skin between the fingers and then releasing it. Dehydrated skin 'tents' and retracts slowly. The skin may feel damp in normally sweating large animals but will be exaggerated in horses with hyperhidrosis. Animals that have been chewing or licking the skin may feel damp. This may be accompanied by brown pigmentation caused by the action of bacteria on lipids in the hair. Alopecic skin may feel hot and dry to the touch. The skin of the atopic dog may feel hot and moist. The skin in hypothyroidism feels cool and dry, and the senile skin of all animals feels dry.

## Changes in elasticity, extensibility and thickness

The mechanical properties of skin are dependent mainly on the dermis. Skin tone is maintained by elastin, and toughness and tensile strength by collagen. Abnormal skin may be thin, thick, turgid, or elastic. Loss of elasticity (hypotonia) is manifested by excessive wrinkling and skin that fails to snap back into position when lifted away from the body and released and may be seen with

- hyperadrenocorticism
- catabolic states (malnutrition and diabetes mellitus)
- hereditary defects (cutaneous asthenia)
- senility.

Hyperelasticity and hyperextensibility are seen with cutaneous asthenia. Thin skin is usually generalized, associated with cutaneous atrophy (and occasionally cutaneous asthenia), and characterized by excessive fine wrinkling, and/or loss of normal skin markings and increased translucency (underlying vessels and fat more easily visualized). Thin skin may be seen with

> ### Ehlers–Danlos Syndrome
>
> Ehlers–Danlos Syndrome is characterized by marked elasticity of the skin. In young animals, the skin is hyperelastic, fragile and tears easily with slow healing.

hyperadrenocorticism, catabolic states and senility. Localized cutaneous atrophy (as occurs after dermatitis or panniculitis) may also produce actual depressions in the skin. Thick skin may be generalized or localized (sclerosis) and usually indicates inflammation or infiltration.

## Abnormalities of hair and wool (the pelage)

**Primary alopecia** may be due to failure of the hair follicles either to develop or to produce a hair or wool fiber. Follicular dysfunction occurs in endocrine disorders, such as hypothyroidism in dogs. Thyroid hormone is necessary for the initiation of the anagen phase of the hair follicle cycle, and deficiency of the hormone results in failure of hair growth and alopecia. Thyroid hormone also increases the growth rate of hair and hair fiber length. Hyperadrenocorticism is the second most common hormonal cause of alopecia in dogs. Glucocorticoids inhibit follicular activity, decrease hair growth rate, and decrease fiber diameter. Telogen defluxion is commonly recognized in cats, dogs, horses and cattle. Various stressors, such as fever, shock, severe illness, pregnancy, lactation, anesthesia and certain drugs, may cause an abrupt, premature cessation of anagen and sudden synchrony of many hair follicles in telogen. Hairs are then shed profusely 2–3 months later as a new wave of follicle activity begins. Decreased fiber growth rate and increased shedding may be seen during estrus, pregnancy and lactation. The capacity of the follicular epithelium to produce a fiber may be congenitally defective or may be temporarily reduced because of nutritional deficiency or severe systemic disease. Bands of weak fiber through a haircoat or fleece may result in 'breaks' and loss of the major part of the coat.

**Secondary alopecia** is due to loss of preformed fiber. Common causes include dermatophytosis, metabolic

> ### Clinical Pointer
>
> When assessing alopecia check if the hair fiber is completely absent or if it has been broken off along the shaft.

changes associated with malnutrition, and traumatic injury to the fiber from scratching, rubbing or chewing the skin and haircoat.

**Hypertrichosis** or excessive hair growth is rare in animals and is usually due to hormonal or developmental causes. **Hirsutism** is manifested by a long, shaggy, usually curly coat that may extend over the entire body or be limited to specific regions (Fig. 13.16).

Hypertrichosis is seen

- most commonly in aged ponies with adenomas of the pars intermedia of the pituitary gland (Ackerman 1989)
- in association with maternal hyperthermia in sheep
- in utero togavirus infection (Border disease) in sheep
- in horses suffering from chronic disease
- subsequent to virtually any injury or irritation (focal hypertrichosis)
- in cattle following recovery from foot-and-mouth disease
- inherited hypertrichosis has been reported in cattle and pigs.

## Abnormalities of footpads, nails, hooves and coronary bands, and horns

The specialized appendages of the skin must be examined. In dogs, erythema and pruritus in the skin adjacent to the footpads may indicate hookworm dermatitis or autoimmune disease. Hyperkeratosis of

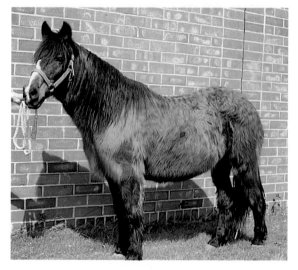

**Fig. 13.16** Hypertrichosis (hirsutism) associated with Cushing's disease in a 21-year-old pony.

the pads is seen in dogs that survive distemper infection, and in dogs with zinc deficiency, and is familial in Irish Terriers. Brittle and/or distorted nails may indicate poor nutrition (including zinc deficiency) or bacterial or fungal infection. **Paronychia** is inflammation of the nailbed. Bacterial paronchyia is characterized by severe painful swelling of the nailbeds in small animals. In racing dogs, corns up to 1 cm in diameter may be observed in the footpads. Feline plasma cell pododermatitis may produce softening and a swelling of one or more footpad and occasionally dermal dehiscence may occur. Nail loss may be due to infection, trauma or autoimmune disease. In dogs, the interdigital skin of all four feet should be examined for interdigital cysts. In cattle, interdigital granulomata may be present, and foot scald (interdigital erythema with erosions) may be observed in sheep grazing lush pastures or abrasive stubble.

In ungulates, hooves, interdigital clefts, and the coronary bands are of major importance in the clinical examination of the skin. Foul in the foot of cattle is an acute and necrotizing infection involving the skin and underlying soft tissues of the interdigital space, and originating in the dermis. Interdigital dermatitis or foot scald is an acute or chronic inflammation of the interdigital skin without extension to the subcutaneous tissues. Verrucose dermatitis is an inflammation of the dorsal or plantar end of the interdigital cleft of cattle. Digital dermatitis of cattle is a specific form of dermatitis of the plantar aspect of the pastern and bulbs of the heels. Interdigital skin hyperplasia is an excess of epidermal and hypodermal tissue occupying most of the interdigital space of cattle, especially bulls.

Foot rot of sheep is a contagious chronic bacterial infection causing inflammation of the epidermal tissues of the hoof, which is characterized by separation of the horn of the hoof progressing from an initial interdigital dermatitis. Several viral infections may produce erythema, vesicles and erosion of the coronary band, and swelling at this site may indicate ergotism or photosensitivity. Dermatophilosis in cattle and horses may be seen here as erythematous areas with scale formation and hair loss. Autoimmune disease also may produce erythema, scaling and ulceration. Equine eosinophilic dermatitis and stomatitis initially produce ulceration of the buccal cavity and coronary bands before becoming more generalized.

## Clinical Pointer

The wall of the hoof is a sensitive indicator of systemic disease or malnutrition.

Distal or proximal cracks in the hoof may be due to trauma or infection. Local heat may result from acute laminitis, and horizontal ridges may result from chronic laminitis, selenium toxicity or molybdenosis (the latter in cattle). Lack of exercise, as for example in stalled cattle, may result in hoof overgrowth and malformation. Some diseases, such as foot-and-mouth, can cause shedding of the cleats in pigs and chronic selenium poisoning in cattle may cause shedding of the hoof.

Examination of the feet of cattle and horses is described in the chapters on clinical examination of the musculoskeletal system.

**Horns** can reflect systemic and nutritional disturbances by becoming brittle or by showing circular ridges. The skin around the base of the horn is a favored site for biting flies in cattle, goats and sheep, with signs such as erythema, edema, local hair loss, papules, crusts and wheals. Other parts of the body may be similarly affected. Signs may be particularly severe in young animals with newly emerging horns.

## Examination of the ears

**Otitis externa** is an inflammation of the epithelial lining of the external auditory canal, which is the portion of the external ear located between the pinna and the tympanic membrane. Physical findings indicative of otitis externa include

- erythema
- swelling
- scaling
- crusting
- alopecia
- broken hairs
- head shyness
- otic discharge
- malodor
- pain on palpation of the auricular cartilage.

Some affected animals attempt to scratch the ear with the ipsilateral hindfoot or shake the head during or after palpation of the ear canal.

On palpation the thickness, firmness and pliability of the vertical and horizontal canal are determined. Thicker, firmer and less pliable canals are associated with proliferative changes. In sarcoptic mange, the lateral aspects of the pinna may be thickened and alopecic because of scratching.

Erythema of the concave surface of the pinna with a normal convex surface is strongly suggestive of atopy or, less likely, food hypersensitivity. Scaling and ulceration of the inner pinna may be seen with some autoimmune skin diseases.

> **Clinical Pointer**
>
> For a thorough examination of the horizontal canal and tympanic membrane almost all animals require some chemical restraint. The ear can be cleaned at the same time.

Purple coloring of the skin of the ears may occur in septicemia in porcine salmonellosis or swine fever. Necrosis of the tips of the ears occurs with frostbite and ergotism.

The standard otoscope is the preferred instrument for the routine examination of the vertical and horizontal ear canals and the tympanic membrane. A halogen light source is desirable and is bright enough to illuminate the depths of the long canine ear canal. Cones for the veterinary otoscope are available in a variety of lengths, diameters and shapes to accommodate the various sizes and shapes of the ears of dogs and cats.

To visualize the ear canal properly with an otoscope the pinna is pulled up and out from the head so that the canal is straight, and the cone is slowly inserted to the necessary depth while the canal is observed through the otoscope. The normal ear canal may contain small amounts of pale yellow or yellow-brown wax. Some breeds of dog, such as poodles, Schnauzer and terriers, normally have hair growing in the canals and this may have to be removed with alligator forceps before a complete examination can be made. Hair, wax, debris, exudate and foreign material must be removed so that a complete examination of the ear canals and tympanic membrane can be made. The use of a bulb syringe or a dental water-propulsion device to flush the ears has been advocated. Pain and palpable abnormalities of the tympanic bulla imply the presence of otitis media.

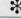

> **Clinical Pointer**
>
> The normal tympanic membrane is
>
> - translucent
> - glistening
> - pearl gray in color
> - slightly concave.
>
> Pathological changes result in
>
> - cloudiness
> - opacity
> - color change
> - bulging.

## Examination of the skin of mammary gland and teats

Several diseases of domestic animals are characterized clinically by lesions of the skin of the mammary glands and teats. Such diseases are most common in cattle and can be of economic importance in the dairy herd because the teat lesions cause pain and discomfort during milking. In swine, necrosis of the teat skin of newborn piglets may occur in outbreak form. The skin of the mammary gland and teats of ewes may be affected by the lesions of contagious ecthyma.

The entire skin of the cranial, lateral and caudal aspects of the udder is examined by inspection and palpation. The skin of the teats must be inspected around their entire circumference and palpated to detect lesions covered by scabs. It may be necessary to superficially irrigate and gently wash the lesions with saline in order to see their morphology and spatial arrangement. Lesions may be restricted to the lateral aspects of the udder and teats, as in photosensitization, or completely surround the teats as occurs in pseudo-cowpox or bovine ulcerative mammillitis.

## Lesions of the skin of udder and teats

Common lesions of the skin of the udder include

- erythematous areas
- papules
- vesicles
- pustules
- scabs
- necrotic sloughing.

In North America the most common viral diseases of the teats of cattle which result in vesicles or erosions are:

- pseudocowpox
- bovine ulcerative mammillitis
- vesicular stomatitis.

The vesicular diseases of the teats are particularly important because they require differentiation from the exotic vesicular diseases such as foot-and-mouth and vesicular stomatitis. The appearances of the lesions of each of these diseases are similar, which makes clinical diagnosis difficult. However, in most cases the morphological and epidemiological differences in the lesions in groups of animals aid the diagnosis.

**Traumatic injuries** to teats vary from superficial lacerations to deep lacerations into the teat cistern, with the release of milk through the wound. Cows which accidentally trample a teat may cause its amputation.

**Thermal burns** of the skin of the udder and teats may occur in mature cattle exposed to grass fires. The hairs of the udder and the base of the teats are singed black. Thermal injury to the skin varies from marked erythema of the teats to blistering and necrosis and weeping of serum.

**Papillomata** (warts) of the teats are caused by the papillomavirus and are characterized clinically by small white slightly elevated nodules 0.3 cm in diameter, or elongated tags 1 cm long which are removable by traction.

**Frostbite** of teats occurs in dairy cows housed outdoors during severely cold weather without adequate bedding. The skin of the teats is cold, necrotic, and oozes serum.

**Thelitis,** or inflammation of the tissues of the teat wall leading to gangrene, is a common complication of gangrenous mastitis, most commonly associated with peracute *Staphylococcus aureus* mastitis. The skin of the teats is cold, edematous, dark-red to purple-black and oozes serum, and the subcutaneous tissues are commonly distended with gas. Sloughing may be evident.

**Chapping and cracking** of the skin of the teats occurs commonly in dairy and beef cattle. The cracks are commonly linear and multiple and are painful when palpated, or when the milking machine cups are applied to the affected teats. Cracks initiated by milking machine action can be aggravated by environmental factors to form chapping. The condition is common when adverse weather conditions follow spring turn-out. Linear lesions appear on the teat wall near the junction with the udder and extend transversely around the teat.

**Udder impetigo** caused by *Staphylococcus aureus* is characterized by pustules 2–4 mm in diameter at the base of the teat which may spread to involve the entire teat and the skin of the udder.

**Flexural seborrhea** of cattle occurs most commonly in young dairy cows which have recently calved. Lesions are present in the groin between the udder and the medial aspect of the thigh, or in the median fissure between the two halves of the udder. There is severe inflammation and a profuse outpouring of serum.

**Photosensitization** of the teats is characterized by erythema followed by edema and subsequently weeping, and finally gangrene of the non-pigmented areas. The lesions are most pronounced over the lateral aspects of the teats. The intense irritation may cause the cow to kick at her abdomen.

**Bovine ulcerative mammillitis** is characterized by the formation of variable-sized vesicles, severe edema and erythema of the teat, with subsequent erosion of the epithelium. The vesicles rupture within 24 hours, and copious serous fluid often exudes from the dermis. Scabs form over the lesions by the fourth day, and the epithelium is re-established under the scab by the third week, although the trauma of milking may delay healing, especially when secondary infection occurs. Scar formation on recovery is uncommon. Lesions may be present on several teats and/or on the udder.

**Pseudocowpox** is characterized clinically by a painful localized edema and erythema with a thin film of exudate over the edematous area. Vesicle formation is uncommon. Within 48 hours of the onset of signs a small orange papule develops, followed shortly by the formation of an elevated, small dark-red scab. The edges of the lesion then extend and the center becomes umbilicated; at 1 week the lesion measures approximately 1 cm in diameter. By 10 days the central scab tends to desquamate, leaving a slightly raised circinate scab commonly termed a ring or horseshoe scab. One teat may have several such lesions, which coalesce to form linear scabs. The majority of lesions desquamate by 6 weeks without leaving scars, although occasionally animals develop chronic infections.

**Teat-end lesions** are common in dairy cattle. These are described as teat canal eversion, teat canal prolapse, prolapse of the meatus, eversion of the meatus, and teat orifice erosion. It is normal to see a 2 mm wide white ring around each teat orifice in machine-milked cows. The first stage of a teat orifice abnormality occurs when this ring undergoes hypertrophy, keratinization and radial cracking. Progression leads to increased hypertrophy, secondary bacterial infection, scab formation, eversion of the distal teat canal, and eventually orifice erosion.

---

## Teat end lesions

Teat end lesions are common in dairy cattle and can be caused by

- excessive or fluctuating vacuum levels
- faulty teat cup liners
- incorrect pulsation ratios
- faults caused by poor maintenance of machines
- careless use of milking machines.

A high milking vacuum combined with a relatively low pulsation chamber vacuum can result in bruising and hemorrhage of the teat end by the slapping action of the liner.

---

# DIAGNOSTIC METHODS

If the diagnosis is not obvious from the history and clinical examination, several diagnostic and laboratory tests can be used to assist in making a probable etiological diagnosis and to provide a rational basis for therapy. The tests selected should be based on the most likely diagnostic possibilities and their cost-effectiveness.

## Special examination and sampling of the skin surface

### Simple magnification

The use of a hand magnifying lens in good natural light, or a combined light and magnifying lens, allows closer examination of lesions and visualization of larger ectoparasites such as fleas, lice and mites. Otoscopic examination is necessary in any animal with clinical manifestations of irritation or inflammation of the ears.

### Examination for parasites

#### Skin scraping

A skin scraping provides a sample of the superficial elements of the skin for laboratory examination for ectoparasites and fungal elements. Skin scrapings are among the most frequently used tests in veterinary dermatology and are recommended when the differential diagnosis includes microscopic ectoparasitic diseases, including demodectic mites, *Cheyletiella* mites, sarcoptic mites, lice, chigger mites, poultry mites, cat fur mites and ear mites. The equipment required is:

- Scalpel blade (no. 10)
- Mineral oil
- Glass microscope slides
- Coverslips
- Microscope.

A drop of mineral oil is placed on the glass slide and scrapings are collected from several lesions and several regions of the body and mixed into the oil. It is beneficial to clip the hair with scissors before scraping because hairs may block the access of the blade to the skin and makes the collection of parasites difficult. The location scraped and the technique used for external parasites varies with the species of parasite and its predilection for certain parts of the body and layers of the skin.

Scrapings must be deep enough to cause capillary bleeding over an area of 1–2 cm$^2$ of an active lesion, and taken from multiple sites to increase the probability of finding the parasites. Once samples have been

- If sarcoptic mange is suspected take scrapings from ear margins, hocks and elbows.
- For demodectic mange take scrapings wherever areas of alopecia are visible.

collected they are examined systematically using light microscopy.

*Acetate tape impression.*
This technique is recommended to find superficial ectoparasites (*Cheyletiella* mites, poultry mites and cat fur mites), and to isolate yeasts such as *Malassezia pachydermatitis* or *Candida albicans* from the skin .

*Hair and skin combing*
Some ectoparasites are small and difficult to see by direct visual examination, and may be seen more easily if a fine-toothed comb is passed through the haircoat, sampling from all representative areas of the body. The debris on the comb is placed on to black paper to discern movement (a magnifying glass may help) or on a slide for microscopic examination. A fine comb will also collect flea feces if present, which will be seen as comparatively large irregular black granules. Placing these granules on a white tissue or cotton wool and wetting them with water allows a brown halo (effect of water on dried blood) to be seen around each one.

*Hair and skin vacuuming*
A battery-operated vacuum cleaner is useful for isolating ectoparasites not visible in the haircoat. A Whatman filter paper is made into a cone and fitted

into the intake nozzle. The coat is then vacuumed over the entire body surface, the cone removed and the debris placed on a slide with mineral oil for microscopic examination.

*Fecal examination*
Animals that chew or lick their skin may have ectoparasites in their feces (*Cheyletiella* spp., *Sarcoptes* spp.). In hookworm-related skin disease helminth ova may be present in the feces.

*Wood's lamp examination*
The Wood's lamp is an ultraviolet (UV) light with a wavelength of 253.7 nm filtered through a cobalt or nickel filter. It is used for the diagnosis of dermatophytosis (ringworm).

The animal is examined in a dark room. Several dermatophytes produce an apple-green fluorescence under UV light, caused by tryptophan metabolites produced by the fungus. These metabolites are produced only by fungi that have invaded actively growing hair. *Microsporum canis* is the most likely dermatophyte to fluoresce. Fluorescence does not occur over scales or crusts or in cultures of dermatophytes. Dandruff and debris may fluoresce with a white-to-yellow shine (not true fluorescence). The Wood's lamp is not as useful for the diagnosis of dermatophytes in large animals, in which most ringworm is caused by *Trichophyton* spp.

*Direct examination for dermatophytes*
Hair, scales and claw material may first be cleared by placing the specimens in several drops of 10–20% potassium hydroxide (KOH) on a microscope slide. A coverslip is added and the slide gently heated for 15–20 seconds, or allowed to stand for 30 minutes at room temperature.

*Fungal culture*
Hairs (8–12 in number) that fluoresce with the Wood's lamp are plucked with a forceps or a hemostat, or brushed out with a sterile toothbrush, and cultured on Sabouraud dextrose agar (SAD) or dermatophyte test medium (DTM) in the dark at 30°C with 30% humidity. The pH indicator phenol red is added to the medium.

To take acetate tape impressions

- press a fresh 3 inch strip of clear (not frosted) adhesive tape onto the skin
- remove gently

and either

- place immediately on a clean glass slide and examine microscopically for mites

or

- apply to the surface of an appropriate media in a petri dish to detect the presence of yeasts.

A Wood's lamp should be turned on and allowed to warm up for several minutes because the stability of the light's wavelength and intensity is temperature dependent.

Dermatophytes first use protein in the medium, with alkaline metabolites turning the medium from yellow to red. When the protein is exhausted the dermatophytes use carbohydrates, giving off acid metabolites, and the medium changes from red to yellow. The cultures are examined daily for 14 days and color changes recorded daily. Any dermatophyte grown on culture should be identified.

## Examination for bacteria and yeasts

*Bacterial culture and antimicrobial sensitivity testing*
Intact pustules are ideal for culturing, although fluid from an abscess, fistulous tract or area of cellulitis can also be cultured. The hair is clipped over the lesion, which is gently wiped with alcohol and allowed to dry. A 22–25 g needle is used to lance the lesion and a culture swab touched to the area. The collected material is placed on appropriate culture medium and incubated. Samples collected from patients with deep pyoderma, fistulous tracts or cellulitis are cultured for aerobic and anerobic bacteria. Culture and antimicrobial sensitivity testing may be performed.

*Skin scrapings or direct impression smears for yeast*
A dry scalpel blade can be used to scrape any lesion. As organisms are usually superficial, scrapings are also superficial. The scale collected is pressed on to a glass slide. Impression smears are obtained by pressing the glass slide directly on to the skin at the site of the lesion.

## Examination for viruses and protozoa

Several viral diseases of the skin occur in hooved farm

animals. Poxvirus infections are diagnosed by skin biopsy and demonstration of the virus by electron microscopy. Isolation of the virus from tissue and fluid samples of the lesions is also possible for several viral diseases. Laboratory diagnosis of viral diseases of teat skin is done by submitting samples for electron microscopic examination. Tissue culture techniques are also used to isolate the virus causing bovine ulcerative mammillitis. Serology can also be a useful diagnostic aid. Protozoal infections that cause skin disease, such as besnoitiosis, are commonly diagnosed by skin biopsy.

## Examination of hairs

Plucking hairs from the skin and examining them microscopically is known as trichography. A small number of hairs are grasped with the fingertips or rubber-covered hemostats and epilated completely. The pulled hairs are placed on a microscope slide, covered with mineral oil and examined with a low-power objective of the microscope. Inactive hair roots (hairs in telogen) have a club shape; active hair roots (hair in anagen) have bulbous ends that glisten. Normal adult animals have an admixture of anagen and telogen hairs, the ratio of which varies with breed, age, season, management factors, and many other influences. A normal hair shaft is uniform in diameter and tapers gently to the tip. Straight-coated animals have straight hair shafts; curly- or wavy-coated animals have twisted hair shafts. Trichography is helpful in the diagnosis of

- self-inflicted alopecia: hairs with a normal shaft are suddenly and cleanly broken
- dermatophytosis: hairs with abnormal shafts are broken
- lice: louse eggs are stuck by their bases to the hair shaft.

## Skin biopsy

A skin biopsy is the removal of a small section of skin for histopathological examination. It can be a valuable aid in making an etiological diagnosis of skin disease.

It is important to select the most representative lesions and to use proper biopsy technique. It is equally important that the pathologist correctly detect the lesions and interpret them according to an accurate clinical history.

Skin biopsies are made for several reasons particularly if

- the lesions appear to be neoplastic
- the lesions are unusual, atypical and the diagnosis is uncertain

- a diagnosis has not been possible with the usual diagnostic aids such as skin scrapings and culture
- a diagnosis is critical, for example if the suspected disease is serious (e.g. cancer), inherited (dermatomyositis) or requires expensive, potentially dangerous or extended therapy (e.g. immune-mediated diseases)
- the lesions are common to several different causes, for example histopathology can usually distinguish between endocrine, inflammatory, and behavioral causes of alopecia
- the lesions fail to respond to therapy after about three weeks or the lesions change in character during therapy
- persistent ulcerations and vesicles are present.

In most cases skin biopsies can be obtained in a conscious animal but occasionally sedation or general anesthesia is required. A general anesthetic may be necessary to obtain biopsies of the pinnae, footpads, planum nasale or extremities of small animals.

In order to preserve the surface features of a lesion, no surgical scrub is used. If needed, the hair is gently clipped. The owner is advised of this as hair regrowth may be slow. A small amount (0.5–0.75 ml) of local anesthetic (1–2% lidocaine) is infiltrated subcutaneously around the area to be biopsied. It is important to avoid intradermal anesthesia as this can distort the histopathology of the tissue. Intradermal inoculation of local anesthetic may simulate dermal edema and hinder evaluation of dermal collagen. A 4 or 6 mm biopsy punch is placed over the area to be sampled and is rotated in one direction with moderate pressure until it cuts through the skin. The entire lesion – or as much of it as possible – is biopsied. For neoplasms and larger inflammatory lesions Tru-cut or excisional biopsy may be best.

The biopsy specimen must be handled with care. Tiny mosquito hemostats, Adson thumb forceps or a 25 g needle are used to grasp the edge of the specimen, which is separated from the underlying fat or connective tissue. Multiple samples are taken, representing all stages of the lesion, and each is placed in a separate container with appropriate labels. It is important to take representative samples and to avoid areas where secondary complications (excoriations, indurations, hyperpigmentation) have occurred. A section of normal tissue is included with this lesion, but this should be only a small portion because the pathologist may rotate the specimen in the wrong direction and fail to section the affected tissue. The biopsies are fixed in an adequate volume of 10% buffered formalin (at least 10 parts per one part tissue). Freezing is avoided by adding 95% ethyl alcohol as 10% of the fixative volume. To prevent sample shrinkage the biopsy can be placed epidermal side down on a piece of wooden tongue depressor. Biopsy sites are sutured with one cruciate or one or two simple interrupted sutures.

The biopsy is submitted to a dermatopathologist along with an adequate history and description of the animal and the lesions. Immunofluorescence and immunohistochemical staining of biopsy specimens may be necessary to confirm autoimmune skin disease.

## Cytologic examination of tissue smears or fluids

Fine-needle aspiration of papules, pustules and nodules, and impression smears of lesions can be placed on to a clean glass slide, dried and stained with Wright's stain (Diff Quik) or new methylene blue for microscopic examination. Cytology is helpful in diagnosing bacterial skin infection, cutaneous neoplasms and yeast and fungal infections.

## Allergy testing

### Food allergy
The only satisfactory test for investigating food allergy is a dietary elimination trial. A number of commercial 'hypoallergenic' diets are available, or the owner can be instructed in the preparation of a home-made diet.

### Intradermal tests
Steroid therapy should be withdrawn for a minimum of 3 weeks prior to intradermal testing; 10 days for antihistamines, and 10 days for essential fatty acids. The skin should not be erythematous or excoriated. In some dogs, sedation is required and xylazine or thiamylal may be used without interfering with test

---

**Clinical Pointer**

1. Take skin biopsies early in the course of the disease before the lesions are modified by therapy.
2. Discontinue antibiotics and anti-inflammatory agents 2–3 weeks before biopsies are taken.

---

**Clinical Pointer**

As pustules and vesicles are fragile and transient it may be necessary to hospitalize the patient for a 'blister watch' and a biopsy taken immediately when a vesicle appears.

results. For intradermal testing the hair over the lateral thorax of small animals or the lateral aspect of the neck in large animals is gently clipped with a no. 40 blade and the sites for challenge are marked with a permanent felt-tipped pen in rows, each about 2.5 cm apart. Twenty to forty allergens are administered. These are available from a number of allergen producers and should be specifically for veterinary use. Only those to which the animal might be exposed are selected.

A small volume (0.05 ml) of an allergen or control is injected intradermally at each site. The needle is inserted with the bevel up and parallel to the skin to produce a visible bleb. Only the bevelled part of the needle is buried at the time the injection is made. A 26–27 gauge, 3/8 inch (0.9 cm) needle attached to a 1 ml disposable tuberculin syringe is used. Two controls are used: a negative one containing vehicle alone and a positive control of 1:100,000 histamine sulfate solution. Positive reactions show as erythematous papules and are at least twice the size of the negative control (which must show no erythema) and are about the same size as the histamine control. It is recommended that the diameter of each wheal be measured in millimeters. The sites are examined at 15 and 30 minutes. Allergens have a short shelf-life and expiry dates should be checked before use. It must be emphasized that positive dermal reactions do not necessarily indicate hyperactivity to that particular allergen: merely that the patient has skin-sensitizing antibody, mast cells that degranulate on antigen exposure, and target tissue that responds to the released mediators. The results of intradermal tests must be taken into consideration along with the clinical history and signs in making specific diagnoses.

*Immunologic tests*

Radioallergosorbent test (RAST), enzyme-linked immunosorbent assay (ELISA), and liquid-phase immunoenzymatic assay are three tests that detect relative levels of allergen-specific IgE in the serum. Some laboratories offer these tests, in which a sample of the patient's serum is subjected to radioimmune assay using a range of allergens. The tests tend to be expensive and more difficult to interpret than intradermal testing.

*Endocrine tests*

Tests of thyroid or adrenal gland function may be undertaken indicated.

## REFERENCES

Ackerman LJ 1989 Practical equine dermatology, 2nd edn. American Veterinary Publications. Goleta, CA.

August JR 1986 Taking a dermatologic history. Compendium on Continuing Education for the Practicing Veterinarian 8: 510–518.

Baker KP, Thomsett LR 1990 Canine and feline dermatology. Blackwell Scientific, Oxford, UK.

Carolotti DN, Pages JN, Sorlin M 1992 Advances in veterinary dermatology. Vol 2. Pergamon Press pp 229–238.

Locke P, Harvey RG, Mason IS 1993 Manual of small animal dermatology. British Small Animal Veterinary Association.

Nesbitt GH, Ackerman LJ, eds. 1991 Dermatology for the small animal practitioner. Exotics. Feline. Canine. Veterinary Learning Systems Company.

Noxon JO 1995 Diagnostic procedures in feline dermatology. Veterinary Clinics of North America. Small Animal Practice 25: 779–799.

Pascoe RR 1990 A color atlas of equine dermatology. Wolfe Publishing, London, UK.

Scott DW 1988 Large animal dermatology. WB Saunders, Philadelphia, PA.

Scott DW, Miller WH, Griffin CE 1995 Muller and Kirk's Small animal dermatology, 5th edn. WB Saunders, Philadelphia, PA.

von Tscharner C, Halliwell REW 1989 Advances in veterinary dermatology. Proceedings of the First World Congress of Veterinary Dermatology, Dijon, France, 27–30 September, Vol 1. Bailliere Tindall, London, UK.

Wilkinson GT, Harvey RG 1994 Color atlas of small animal dermatology. A guide to diagnosis, 2nd edn. Times Mirror International.

Yager JA, Wilcock BP 1988 Skin biopsy: revelations and limitations. Canadian Veterinary Journal 29: 969–972.

### Some common allergens of dogs

Allergens reported to be important in dogs in North America are

- house-dust mites
- house dust
- human dander
- feathers
- kapok
- molds
- weeds
- grasses.

# 14
# Clinical Examination of the Cardiovascular System

*C. C. Gay*
*O. M. Radostits*

## CLINICAL MANIFESTATIONS OF CARDIOVASCULAR DISEASE

**Anemia** is a reduction below normal in the number or volume of erythrocytes or in the quantity of hemoglobin in the blood.

**Arrhythmia** is an irregularity of cardiac rhythm. The term includes changes in heart rate, amplitude, or both.

**Bradycardia** is a decrease in the heart rate below the normal range for that species and age.

**Capillary refill time (CRT)** is the time required for the gingival mucosa to return to its original color after being blanched by digital pressure. Normal is 1 to 2 seconds; prolonged CRT is >2 seconds.

**Cardiac (pericardial) tamponade** is the syndrome caused by distension of the pericardial sac by fluid (e.g. pus or blood) and detected clinically as venous congestion, muffled heart sounds and decreased arterial pulse pressure.

**Congested or injected visible mucous membranes** occur commonly in peripheral circulatory failure, as in shock in the horse with surgical colic.

**Cor pulmonale** is the syndrome of right heart failure resulting from an increase in right heart workload secondary to pulmonary disease and pulmonary hypertension.

**Cough** is a sudden noisy expulsion of air from the lungs.

**Cyanosis** is a bluish discoloration of the visible mucosae and skin owing to excessive concentration of reduced (desaturated) hemoglobin in the blood.

**Dehydration** is a systemic state resulting from inadequate body water.

**Dyspnea** is labored or difficult breathing.

**Edema** is an abnormal accumulation of fluid in intercellular spaces and body cavities. Edematous swellings are soft, painless, and **always** pit on pressure.

- **Anasarca** is extensive subcutaneous edema occurring in the brisket region, under the jaw, and along the ventral midline.
- **Ascites** is the accumulation of transudate in the peritoneal cavity.
- **Hydropericardium** is the accumulation of transudate in the pericardial sac, and is characterized by muffling of the heart sounds.
- **Hydrothorax** is the accumulation of transudate in the pleural cavities, resulting in decreased audibility or absence of lung sounds over the ventral parts of the lungs and dullness on acoustic percussion.
- **Pulmonary edema** is excessive fluid in the interstitial spaces of the lung and in the alveoli; this can be the result of left heart failure. In congestive heart failure the heart is unable to maintain circulatory equilibrium at rest and ventricular output is less than venous return. This results in congestion of the venous circuit, accompanied by dilatation of vessels and edema of the lungs or periphery.

**Fatigue** is a state of increased discomfort and decreased efficiency resulting from prolonged exertion, with loss of power or capacity to respond to stimulation.

- **Exercise intolerance** is cardiovascular and respiratory distress on exercise.

**Gangrene** is death of body tissues generally in considerable mass, usually associated with loss of nutritive supply.

- **Dry gangrene** is due to the death of tissues, usually associated with loss of vascular blood supply to the extremities, such as the feet, tail, and ears.
- **Moist gangrene** occurs when the insult occurs abruptly.

**Heart failure** (congestive heart failure) indicates the heart cannot maintain cardiac output sufficient for the body's requirements. **Right-sided heart failure** results in venous hypertension, peripheral edema, ascites and enlarged abdominal organs. **Left-sided heart failure** is seen as pulmonary hypertension enlargement of the heart and associated increased respiratory rate, cough and pulmonary edema.

**Heart murmur** is any adventitious sound heard in conjunction with the normal heart sounds.

**Jugular vein pulsation** A pronounced jugular vein pulsation which extends up the neck when the head is in the normal position, and which is synchronous with the heart cycle and is systolic in time, indicates insufficiency of the right atrioventricular valve.

**Orthopnea** is dyspnea when recumbent.

**Pallor** is paleness of the visible mucosae or skin.

**Pericardial friction sound** is a scraping or squeaking noise audible with the heartbeat, usually a to-and-fro sound, associated with an inflamed pericardium. Fluid-splashing sounds may also accompany pericardial friction sounds.

**Poor growth or loss of body condition** may be present in some animals with cardiac disease.

**Pulse deficit** is a pulse rate lower than the heart rate, usually associated with cardiac arrhythmias which result in audible heart sounds but failure of the heart to produce an arterial pulse.

**Repeating episodes of fever and shifting lameness** A history with repetitive episodes of fever, ill-defined illness and of lameness that is variable between and with episodes is highly suggestive of periodic bacteremia and endocarditis, and accompanied by polysynovitis.

**Shock** is a systemic state of generalized, acute, and severe reduction in the perfusion and oxygenation of tissues; the failure of the circulation to maintain the perfusion of tissues.

- **Cardiogenic shock** is a primary reduction in cardiac output, usually due to heart failure.
- **Hypovolemic shock** is due to inadequate intravascular volume producing decreased cardiac output (e.g. acute hemorrhage).
- **Vasogenic shock** is due to inadequate vasomotor tone. This can follow severe brain damage (neurogenic), endotoxic shock, systemic toxicity (toxic shock), or bacterial or septic shock.

**Sudden and unexpected death** Cardiac disease may be the cause of sudden death in both large and small animals.

**Syncope** or fainting is loss of consciousness due to transient cerebral ischemia.

**Tachycardia** is an increase in the heart rate above the normal range for that species and age of animal.

**Thrombosis** is the presence of a fixed blood clot in an artery or vein. **Arterial thrombosis** is the presence of a thrombus in an artery resulting in lack of circulation to the part supplied by that artery. **Venous thrombosis** is the presence of a thrombus in a vein, usually associated with phlebitis.

**Venous engorgement** of the large veins, such as the jugular and the subcutaneous abdominal veins, is a manifestation of obstruction of return of the blood to the heart, as in right-side congestive heart failure or a space-occupying lesion in the thoracic inlet.

# INTRODUCTION

The cardiovascular system consists of two main structural units, the heart and the blood vessels, both of which are jointly involved in maintaining the circulation of the blood and thereby ensuring normal exchange of oxygen, carbon dioxide, electrolytes, fluid, nutrients, and waste products between the blood and the tissue fluids and cells.

Physical examination of the cardiovascular system is a routine part of the initial clinical examination, and is an important aspect of monitoring animals during anesthesia and during the clinical course of almost any disease.

The clinical examination of the cardiovascular system consists of a carefully elicited history of the patient and a thorough physical examination. The information obtained from the clinical examination is used to generate a differential diagnosis and to direct the diagnostic approach. This chapter will describe the physical examination of the peripheral circulation (arterial and venous) and the heart. Some of the common abnormalities of the cardiovascular system will be described, but details of specific diseases can be obtained from other specialty textbooks.

### Primary and secondary cardiovascular disease

Cardiovascular disease may be

- the primary cause for the presentation of an animal for clinical examination
- detected secondarily when an animal is presented for evaluation of a different problem.

Some dysrhythmias and murmurs, considered an indication of cardiac abnormality when they occur in companion animals, are considered part of normal physiological variation in horses and cattle, and the clinician should be familiar with their occurrence and characteristics.

## HISTORY AND SIGNALMENT

The history of the case may indicate the possibility of cardiovascular disease with such evidence as

- dyspnea
- fatigue and exercise intolerance
- cough
- edema
- poor growth or loss of body condition
- intermittent fever
- lameness
- syncope
- sudden and unexpected death.

### Dyspnea

In animals, dyspnea is apparent as respiratory distress. When related to cardiac disease it is usually a manifestation of pulmonary edema. Interstitial pulmonary edema reduces pulmonary compliance and is clinically apparent as tachypnea, or an increase in respiratory rate. Severe pulmonary edema floods the alveoli and causes a ventilation/perfusion mismatch. The resultant hypoxemia causes 'air hunger', which is apparent as tachypnea and polypnea. Dyspnea can develop in the absence of pulmonary congestion when cardiac output is low and the delivery of oxygen to peripheral tissues is inadequate. This is sometimes observed in patients with, for example, severe pulmonary stenosis; respiratory distress may be evident following exercise or even at rest because pulmonary blood flow is inadequate. It should be recognized that in any individual the stress required to provoke the development of dyspnea varies, and depends partly upon the severity of cardiac disease. For example,

- exercise intolerance and dyspnea may develop after exercise in a horse with relatively mild heart disease, however
- cats are usually sedentary and cardiac disease commonly progresses unseen until a minimum of stress or exertion provokes severe dyspnea.

The sudden development of dyspnea often suggests pneumothorax, pulmonary embolism, or pulmonary edema. Lower airway disease or obstruction typically

### Clinical Pointer

Dyspnea provoked by exertion can result from either cardiac or respiratory tract disease.

causes an expiratory dyspnea. Inspiratory dyspnea, especially that accompanied by stridor, is indicative of upper airway disease or obstruction. Nocturnal dyspnea and orthopnea are both suggestive of left-sided heart failure. Dyspnea is a feature of the history in sheep that develop myocardial disease from plant or other toxicities. It occurs in goats that develop atrial fibrillation secondary to cor pulmonale. In general dyspnea is not common in cattle and horses with cardiac disease compared with dogs.

### Fatigue and exercise intolerance

Signs of fatigue and exercise intolerance may indicate the presence of either respiratory or cardiovascular disease. In either case, compensatory mechanisms are able to prevent clinical signs at rest but not when the cardiopulmonary system is challenged by exertion. A sudden or chronic decline in expected performance is much more apparent in active animals than in sedentary ones. Regardless of the activity, it is the owner's perception that there is a decline in the animal's ability to participate in normal activities, whether racing or walking up stairs.

### Cough

Cough is a common clinical sign of heart disease in the dog, yet is rarely associated with heart disease in cats. An effort should be made to ensure the owner's assessment is correct, and that coughing has not been mistaken for sneezing or gagging.

The cough is generally characterized according to

- the time of day when it occurs
- its association with exercise or activity
- whether it is productive or non-productive.

These characterizations are occasionally helpful in

### Clinical Pointer

Exercise intolerance may be manifested by a decline in performance, prolonged recovery time from exertion, cough, dyspnea, and syncope.

attempting to determine whether a cough is secondary to heart disease or to respiratory disease. However, the diagnostic importance of these characteristics should not be overemphasized. For example, coughing that is related to heart disease or respiratory tract disease can be provoked by both activity and exercise. During recumbency the intrathoracic blood volume increases; as a consequence, pulmonary venous pressures may rise and favor the development of pulmonary congestion and edema. For this reason, coughing that is heard primarily at night may suggest a cardiac cause. However, it must be recognized that pets are often observed most closely at night. Coughing related to compression of the main-stem bronchi by an enlarged left atrium or tracheobronchial disease is usually non-productive and is often harsh or hacking. In contrast, cough related to diseases of the lower airways is more often soft, and may be productive. When a cough is related to frank pulmonary edema, dyspnea is usually evident on inspection. Determining whether or not a cough is productive presents a further difficulty. Dogs rarely expectorate: often, they swallow sputum that is produced during a cough and it is therefore difficult for owners to recognize when a cough is productive. That a cough can be elicited by tracheal palpation is generally of limited diagnostic value: dogs that cough for any reason may do so following this maneuver. The patient history is of great value and its importance should not be underemphasized. However, in the vast majority of cases the physical examination and diagnostic tests such as thoracic radiographs are the means to determine the cause of coughing in dogs.

## Edema

There are four pathophysiological mechanisms that can explain edema:

1. an increase in the hydrostatic pressure in the capillaries, such as occurs in congestive heart failure
2. a fall in oncotic pressure of the blood, such as occurs in hypoalbuminemia
3. obstruction to lymphatic drainage
4. damage to capillary walls, as occurs with inflammation.

When edema, pleural effusion, and acites are related to the presence of heart disease they are manifestations of right-sided congestive heart failure. Here, the accumulation of fluid is explained by an increase in intracapillary hydrostatic pressure resulting from venous hypertension. Venous engorgement precedes the development of visible fluid accumulation and can usually be detected on physical examination when heart disease explains edema or effusions.

Where edema is due to cardiac failure the liver can be palpated on the right side of the abdomen under the ribs. In horses, the subcutaneous edema associated with heart disease occurs in the limbs or ventrum. It should be noted that in this species the presence of edema more commonly results from extracardiac disease. Dogs and cats seldom develop peripheral or subcutaneous edema as a manifestation of congestive heart failure, but peripheral edema is more commonly associated with hypoalbuminemia, vasculitis, or lymphatic obstruction. Pulmonary edema is common in dogs and cats with congestive heart failure.

## Poor growth or loss of body condition

A history of poor growth and ill thrift may be present in some young animals with congenital cardiac disease, and adults with acquired cardiac disease often present with a history that includes falling body condition.

## Repeating episodes of fever and shifting lameness

A history with repetitive episodes of fever, ill-defined illness, and lameness that is variable between and with episodes is highly suggestive of periodic bacteremia and endocarditis, and accompanied with polysynovitis.

## Syncope

Syncope is uncommon in the history of large animals with cardiac disease but is highly suggestive of heart disease when it does occur. It is usually indicative of arrhythmic heart disease. Syncope occurs with complete heart block, in which case there are other indicators of cardiac disease in the history. It also occurs in horses with long-standing 'benign' atrial fibrillation, where strong vagal tone may result in a sufficient period without a cardiac contraction to result in syncope. These horses may have no other history suggesting heart disease. In acute heart failure there is

- sudden loss of consciousness
- falling with or without convulsions
- pallor of the visible mucosae
- either death or complete recovery from the episode.

Acute heart failure should be a major consideration as a cause of sudden death in large animals, especially when associated with exertion or excitement.

Common causes of syncope in animals include cardiac arrhythmias and structural heart disease. Animals experiencing syncope are usually presented for evaluation because of the dramatic clinical signs and the concern of the owner. Owners may report that their pet has fainted, had a seizure, or a 'heart attack'. In order to plan an appropriate evaluation an effort should be made to differentiate syncope from seizure activity and from sleep attacks (narcolepsy). There are several distinguishing features and it is important to ask owners specific questions regarding the event in order to make the differentiation. In cases where cardiovascular disease is responsible for episodes of syncope there are often additional clinical signs referable to the cardiovascular system, such as cough and exercise intolerance. In addition, syncope in these patients is often precipitated by vigorous activity and/or coughing.

## Sudden and unexpected death

Cardiac disease may be the cause of sudden death in both large and small animals. Subclinical cardiac disease and acute cardiovascular accidents are common causes of sudden death which occurs in association with exertion in horses and other species. Sudden death associated with exertion in previously confined animals is strongly suggestive of cardiac disease, and commonly results from myocardial

> ### Clinical Pointer
>
> Animals experiencing syncope secondary to hypoglycemia usually have a history of episodic weakness.

disease. Some causes of sudden death include

- white muscle disease in calves turned out to pasture in the spring after winter housing
- myocardial necrosis precipitated by excitement at feeding time in young calves
- certain forms of copper deficiency in adult cattle (falling disease)
- heart disease, not manifest in sows while they are confined in stalls, but which results in acute heart failure precipitated by the exertion of breeding or by movement to a different area of the piggery.

Although a history of sudden death is one that is obtained prior to postmortem rather than clinical examination, it is included here because large animals are usually raised in groups and risk factors that lead to sudden death in one member of the group may apply to the group as a whole. This is especially true when death is the result of myocardial disease resulting from toxicoses. A history of sudden death in a member of a group of animals can indicate that examination of the cardiovascular system of other members should be part of the clinical examination.

## Physical traits linked to congenital/inherited abnormalities

These are rare and tend to be limited according to geographic concentration of the genetic defect. Examples include

- the curly haircoat associated with calves with cardiomyopathy
- the long thin limbs, joint and tendon laxity, and ocular abnormalities in cattle with Marfan syndrome
- microphthalmia, commonly accompanied by ventricular septal defect in calves
- eye (cyclopia, anophthalmia, microphthalmia), and other (atresia ani, agnathia) defects with atrioventricular septal defects in lambs.

## Single versus multiple cases

Most diseases of the cardiovascular system are sporadic in occurrence and involve individual animals. Where cardiovascular disease results from a toxic, nutritional, or infectious agent, it may occur in several animals in a group that has been exposed to the same management procedure or noxious insult. There are considerable geographical differences, but some examples include

- plant poisonings from group exposure to canary grass
- exposure to feeds containing ionophores
- exposure to feeds containing blister beetles
- nutritional cardiomyopathy associated with vitamin E/selenium deficiency in newborn lambs
- low dietary levels of selenium, vitamin E, and sulfur-containing amino acids in conjunction with high dietary concentrations of polyunsaturated fats and pro-oxidant compounds in the genesis of outbreaks of mulberry heart disease in growing pigs
- infectious diseases that affect more than one individual in the group, such as *Hemophilus somnus* myocarditis in cattle and *Erysipelothrix rhusiopathiae* endocarditis in pigs.

In some instances the herd history of the problem will be critical in establishing a diagnosis (e.g. canary grass poisoning). In other instances the examination of an individual animal will lead to a diagnosis that suggests other animals in the group are also likely to be affected (e.g. monensin poisoning, *Hemophilus* myocarditis).

## CLOSE EXAMINATION OF THE PERIPHERAL CIRCULATORY SYSTEM

### Visible mucous membranes and skin

#### Visible mucous membranes

The visible mucous membranes include the mucosa of the conjunctivae, the nasal and oral cavities, and the vulva and prepuce. They represent the arteriolar–capillary–venous circulation and, along with the circulatory and hydration state of the skin, represent the important parts of the peripheral circulation which are easily examined.

Inspection of the mucous membranes, especially of the oral cavity, is best done in natural daylight or with the aid of a flashlight for optimal illumination. The lips are retracted to expose the mucosa of the gingiva, which are easiest to examine. The oral mucosa is normally a pale pink, but the color will vary with different sources of light

- direct daylight reveals the true 'salmon pink' color
- tungsten light makes the mucosa appear slightly more red
- fluorescent light makes it appear a blue-gray.

Pale mucous membranes, or pallor, occurs when anemia is present or when there has been cutaneous vasoconstriction, as in hypovolemic shock. When shock or any other impairment of cutaneous circulation is present the lips will also be cool to the touch.

The conjunctivae are examined by depressing and slightly everting the lower eyelid. If digital pressure is applied over the upper eyelid just caudal to the medial canthus the third eyelid or membrana nictitans will protrude, exposing another conjunctival surface for examination. The conjunctivae of both eyes must be examined, so that abnormalities due to local disease are detected and not confused with general clinical findings. The appearance of the normal conjunctiva varies in the different domestic animals. In horses and dogs the color is pale rose; in cattle and sheep it is paler.

The nasal mucosa in the rostral part of the nasal cavity can be inspected with the aid of a light source. In mature horses and cows several centimeters of the nasal mucosa can be seen by direct inspection. It is normally a deep pink to slightly red color and is moist. The presence of an abnormal nasal discharge is significant and reflects disease of the respiratory tract.

The mucosa of the vagina or rectum can be inspected by eversion through the anus and vulva using an appropriate illuminated speculum. The concealed mucous membranes of the nares, pharynx, larynx, trachea, stomach, and bladder may be inspected with the aid of endoscopic or fiberoptic instruments.

The visible mucosae are examined for the presence of

- pallor, indicating the existence of anemia or shock
- hyperemia arising from engorgement of the blood vessels
- petechial hemorrhages
- cyanosis due to defective heart or lung function
- jaundice
- erosions or ulcerations
- swelling of the conjunctivae, as in congestive heart failure
- dryness occurring in dehydrated and febrile states
- discharges.

In mild dehydration the membranes will feel dry and appear pale pink to slightly blanched. Severe

---

**Clinical Pointer**

The color and capillary refill time of the oral mucous membranes is a useful aid in the diagnosis and prognosis of animals with hypovolemic and endotoxemic shock.

## Hyperemia

Hyperemia of the mucous membranes occurs secondary to polycythemia.

- In a young animal it is suggestive of a right-to-left shunting congenital heart defect
- In older animals, it is usually a sign of sepsis.

## Clinical Pointer

The episcleral vessels can easily be seen against the background of the sclera. Note their color: they are normally dark red but in cardiopulmonary disease or peripheral stasis they may be cyanotic.

abdominal pain results in stimulation of the sympathetic nervous system, which results in stimulation of α-receptors and contraction of vascular smooth muscle. These activities cause blanching of the mucous membranes of the oral cavity. With venous congestion or endotoxemia the membranes will appear red to brick-red.

Abnormalities of the erythron may also be detectable by examination of the visible mucosae. These include

- a dark brownish-red color in animals with methemoglobinemia caused, for example, by nitrite toxicity in cattle and acetaminophen toxicity in cats
- a bright red color in animals with either carbon monoxide inhalation or cyanide intoxication
- jaundice associated with hemolysis
- a bluish tinge associated with severe cyanosis.

## Clinical Pointer

Although mucous membrane color is not a sensitive indicator of disease, the diseases causing changes in color can be life-threatening and require a rapid diagnosis.

Abnormalities in hemostasis may also be recognizable by examination of the visible mucosae. Hemostatic functions are maintained by the balanced interaction of platelets, clotting factors, fibrinolytic factors, and blood vessel wall integrity. Petechiae and ecchymotic hemorrhages due to low platelet numbers or platelet dysfunction are often observed on conjunctival, oral,

nasal, and vaginal or preputial mucous membranes. Other commonly observed clinical signs of abnormalities of hemostasis include

- hematomas
- prolonged bleeding of incisions or traumatic injuries
- occult or overt hematuria and fecal blood
- epistaxis
- hyphema
- multiple limb lameness associated with hemarthrosis
- recognition of fluid accumulations in the thorax or abdomen.

**Cyanosis** is a bluish discoloration of the skin and mucous membranes resulting from an increased amount of reduced (desaturated) hemoglobin or of abnormal hemoglobin pigments in the blood perfusing these areas. In most cases the oral mucous membranes are examined for evidence of cyanosis, although the skin of the pinnae and the urogenital mucous membranes will suffice. Artificial lighting and skin pigmentation affect the ability to detect cyanosis.

Cyanosis due to right-to-left cardiac shunts is uncommon in large animals but does occur with tetralogy and pentalogy of Fallot, other less common congenital cardiac defects, and with Eisenmenger's complex and Eisenmenger's syndrome.

Central cyanosis is characterized by decreased arterial oxygen saturation due to right-to-left shunting of blood or impaired pulmonary function. That due to congenital heart disease or pulmonary disease characteristically worsens during exercise. Central cyanosis usually becomes apparent at a mean capillary concentration of 4 g/dl reduced hemoglobin (or 0.5 g/dl methemoglobin). Because it is the *absolute* quantity of reduced hemoglobin in the blood that is responsible for cyanosis, the higher the total hemoglobin content the greater the tendency towards cyanosis. Thus

- cyanosis is detectable in patients with marked polycythemia at higher levels of arterial oxygen saturation than in those with normal hematocrit values
- cyanosis may be absent in patients with anemia despite marked arterial desaturation.

Patients with congenital heart disease often have a history of cyanosis that is intensified during exertion because of the lower saturation of blood returning to the right side of the heart and the augmented right-to-left shunt. The inspiration of pure oxygen (100% $FiO_2$) will not resolve central cyanosis when a right-to-left shunt is present, but may resolve when primary lung disease or polycythemia is causing the problem.

Peripheral cyanosis occurs when there is increased extraction of oxygen from normally saturated blood or decreased blood flow to a peripheral area, as occurs with thromboembolism of the external iliac arteries in the cat with a 'saddle thrombus'. Causes of regional cyanosis include cold exposure, reduced cardiac output or shock, and venous and arteriolar obstruction. Venous obstruction usually results in a congested and cyanotic extremity because of the stagnation of blood.

**Capillary refill time** of the oral mucous membranes is a useful indicator of perfusion of peripheral tissues and the state of the cardiovascular system. The gingiva over the incisor teeth is *lightly* compressed with the ball of the thumb to blanch the tissue. The time required for the blanched area to return to its original color is the capillary refill time. Normally this is between 1 and 2 seconds. The procedure should be repeated at least three times and the seconds should be counted by saying 1000-1-1000-2-1000-3 and so on, to represent actual seconds, rather than simply counting 1, 2, 3, etc.

In the horse with surgical colic the prognosis generally worsens as the oral mucosa becomes cool, congested, then cyanotic and drier as capillary refill time increases. A refill time of 3 seconds or more, accompanied by cyanotic oral mucosae, indicates a poor prognosis, and a refill time of 10 seconds or more indicates potentially fatal peripheral circulatory failure. The color and capillary refill time of the oral mucous membranes are monitored closely and carefully in the horse with suspected acute intestinal obstruction. It is important to remember that this test is not highly sensitive and that a normal capillary refill time may be found in an animal with significant heart disease.

## Skin

Palpation and inspection of the skin is useful for assessment of the peripheral circulation. Feeling the temperature of the skin of various parts of the body, especially the ears, limbs, feet, tail, and over the thorax and abdomen, provides an indication of normal

| Capillary refill times (seconds) | |
|---|---|
| Normal animal | 1–2 |
| Dehydrated animal | 2–4 |
| Severely dehydrated animal | 5–6 |

warmth, increased warmth, or coolness. In animals in shock the skin may be cool and clammy. In white-skinned animals, such as pigs with iron deficiency anemia, the pale, almost white skin is readily obvious. Cyanosis and deep purple blotching of the skin over the ears and abdomen are associated with vascular lesions of the skin caused by septicemias. In the early stages of local gangrene the skin will appear blue and cool and lack elasticity. Cold injury or frostbite of the ears is common in cats and calves, and of the distal extremities in newborn animals exposed to outside cold temperatures during the winter months in temperate climates. In the newborn the feet of the hind limbs are most commonly affected. The skin just above the coronary bands is usually swollen, painful and cool to touch initially. If the animal is brought indoors and the feet gradually warmed, the affected skin becomes moist. Dry gangrene may follow, with ultimate sloughing of the affected tissues, including the claws.

### State of hydration and dehydration

The state of hydration and dehydration is evaluated by inspection and palpation of the skin, and examination of the eyes. Normally, the skin is elastic and, when picked up or tented with the fingers, it returns to its previous position when released. In dehydrated animals the skin will remain tented for varying periods of time (Table 14.1).

The degree of dehydration can also be assessed by examining the amount of space between the eye and the orbit (the sunken eye). As dehydration progresses above approximately 6% of body weight, the eyes are more sunken because of the loss of periorbital and ocular fluid. This is the state of enophthalmos. The depth to which the eyes are sunken and the amount of

---

### Differential cyanosis

Differential cyanosis is cyanosis of the caudal body while the cranial structures (head and neck) receive normally oxygenated blood. It suggests a right-to-left shunting patent ductus arteriosus, a condition in which desaturated blood of the pulmonary artery enters the aorta at a site distal to the origin of the arteries supplying cranial structures, thereby causing cyanosis of caudal structures only.

---

### Clinical Pointer

The urogenital mucous membranes can be used to assess capillary refill time

- in pure-bred Chow or Chow-mix dogs that have pigmented oral mucous membranes
- in aggressive animals.

space around the eye is an approximation of the degree of dehydration. The absolute amount of space visible around the eye varies according to the size of the animal and the species in question.

Obviously, the depth of space around the eyes of a severely dehydrated mature cow will be much greater than that in a severely dehydrated calf under 30 days of age. In the horse the degree of sunken eyes is not as reliable a measure of dehydration as in other species.

## Arterial pulse

The arterial pulse is examined for rate, rhythm, amplitude, and quality. The pulse is felt by placing the ball of one to three fingers transversely on the skin over the artery and applying gentle pressure until the pulse wave can be felt. Only gentle digital pressure is applied to avoid obliterating the pulse wave, and finger pressure is varied until maximal detection is achieved.

- In horses the arterial pulse is taken at the external maxillary artery (facial artery), where it crosses the ramus of the mandible at the rostral border of the masseter muscle. To palpate the pulse, pressure is applied against the artery on the medial aspect of the ventral border of the mandible.
- In cattle the pulse is taken at the ventral coccygeal artery. This is palpable in the ventral midline of the tail at the level of the tip of the vulva in females, or an equivalent distance in males.
- In young calves and in sheep, goats, and pigs the pulse is taken at the femoral artery, high up in the inguinal region on the medial aspect of the thigh.
- In small animals the arterial pulse is usually taken at the femoral arteries. The pulse rate and quality are assessed by palpation of the proximal femoral arteries, close to their origin from the inguinal ring. Both femoral arteries are palpated concurrently because there are occasionally differences in pulse strength and quality between left and right femoral arteries.

While taking the pulse the animal should be held relatively quiet and still to ensure a proper examination.

### Palpation of pulse and simultaneous auscultation of heart

When examining the heart it is often necessary to palpate the pulse at the same time as the heart is being auscultated to

- confirm which sound is the first heart sound by timing its occurrence in relation to the occurrence of the apex beat
- determine what arterial pulsations occur at each phase of the cardiac cycle
- relate changes in pulse amplitude or rhythm to findings on auscultation
- correlate abnormalities of the jugular veins with events of the cardiac cycle.

In large animals, this is done using an artery located more conveniently for the heart than the facial or coccygeal, for example at the median artery at the medial aspect of the proximal forelimb close to the junction of the limb with the thorax and deep to the superficial pectoral muscle. Another convenient site is the medial volar metacarpal artery, which is located on the medial side of the carpus and can be felt by compressing the artery against the palmar part of the radial carpal bone. In small animals, auscultation of the heart and palpation of the femoral artery is possible in most cases.

### Rate

The pulse should be felt for at least a minute as abnormalities in rhythm may not be constant. Usually the rate is counted over 30 seconds and the pulse examined for a longer period during which features such as rhythm and quality are assessed. The rates in normal resting animals are given in Table 14.2, with

| Table 14.1. | Degrees of severity of dehydration and guidelines for assessment | | | | | |
|---|---|---|---|---|---|
| Body weight loss (%) | Sunken eyes, shrunken face, dry membranes | Skinfold test persists for (sec) | PCV (%) | Total serum solids (g/l) | Fluid required to replace volume deficit (ml/kg) BW |
| 4–6 | Barely detectable | <2 | 40–45 | 70–80 | 20–25 |
| 6–8 | ++ | 2–4 | 50 | 80–90 | 30–50 |
| 8–10 | +++ | 6–10 | 55 | 90–100 | 50–80 |
| 10–12 | ++++ | 20–45 | 60 | 120 | 80–120 |

the lower rates in larger animals and in quiet, fit animals. In younger animals and those not used to restraint and a human presence, rates will be faster. In arrhythmic heart disease the arterial pulse should be examined in more detail than during routine clinical examination. The pulse rate should be examined over a period to determine whether there is any sudden change, as can occur with a shift in pacemaker to an irritable myocardial focus. At some stage during the examination of animals with tachyarrhythmias the heart and pulse rates should be taken synchronously to determine the presence of a pulse deficit.

The stress associated with different surroundings and handlers can significantly increase the animal's heart rate from its normal resting level. For example

- the mean heart rate of a population of healthy cats at home was 118 bpm; when recorded electrocardiographically at a veterinary hospital the mean rate increased 54% to 182 bpm
- the heart rate of normal dogs in their familiar surroundings (determined by Holter monitoring) ranges from 30 to 200 bpm, depending on activity level.

Nevertheless, published heart rates are useful when examining pets outside their normal environment.

If either bradycardia or tachycardia is detected an ECG is indicated to document the abnormal rhythm. Bradycardias are associated with several conditions such as hypothyroidism, hypothermia, central nervous system disease, toxicities and third-degree AV block. In addition, many commonly used drugs have the potential to cause bradycardia, including phenothiazine tranquilizers, xylazine, digitalis glycosides, β-adrenergic blockers, calcium channel blockers, quinidine, lidocaine and anesthetics. In dogs the most common cause of bradycardia is high vagal tone, which is usually manifested as a sinus arrhythmia and occasionally as first-degree AV block. As vagal tone increases more serious arrhythmias develop, including second-degree AV block and periods of sinus arrest.

Tachycardia in small animals can be rather benign, such as sinus tachycardia resulting from stress and excitement, or life threatening, such as rapid ventricular tachycardia. Other pathological tachy-

| Table 14.2. Normal heart and pulse rates of domestic animals in beats/minute (bpm) ||
|---|---|
| *Animal* | *Range* |
| Horse, adult | 28–44 |
| Foal 1 week–6 months | 60–100 |
| Cattle, adult | 60–80 |
| Calf under 10 days | 80–100 |
| Sheep, goat | 70–90 |
| Pig, adult | 60–90 |
| Piglet under 10 days | 100–120 |
| Dog, adult, large giant breeds | 60–140 |
| Dog, adult, toy breed | 80–180 |
| Dog, medium breed | 70–160 |
| Puppies | 110–220 |
| Adult cat | 120–240 |
| Kittens | 160–240 |

cardias include atrial fibrillation, atrial or supraventricular tachycardia, and atrial flutter. To reduce the elevation in heart rate associated with stress, the pulse is ideally taken when the animal has had a chance to adjust to the new surroundings, and not when it is agitated or extremely nervous. Owners can be taught how to determine the pulse rate so they can assist in monitoring their pet at home, and provide a pulse rate which is much more representative of the actual heart rate. This is very helpful when titrating the dose of cardiac medication used to increase or decrease heart rate.

## Rhythm

The rhythm of the pulse is noted. A regular rhythm is characterized by equal intervals between successive

---

### Clinical Pointer

The ability to assess pulse quality is affected by body condition – arterial pulses are usually quite prominent in thin animals, whereas they may be difficult to palpate in obese animals.

---

### Bradycardia and Tachycardia

- bradycardia – the heart rate is below normal, it is associated with several physiological conditions and the use of certain drugs
- tachycardia – the heart rate is above normal, it can be benign or life threatening. The most common cause is stress.

pulse waves. This is best determined by mentally tapping the rhythm in conjunction with palpation. Where irregularities are detected, the clinician attempts to determine whether the basic rhythm is regular with an occasional disruption to regularity, or whether there is no underlying rhythm to the pulse. The former suggests that the heart is under the control of a single pacemaker but that there is some temporary disruption in transmission. Examples would be sino-atrial block and second-degree atrioventricular block, where the excitatory impulse is occasionally blocked at the sinus node or of the atrioventricular node, with consequent failure of the ventricles to contract and initiate an arterial pulse. The latter indicates the basic rhythm of the pulse is regular but there is an occasional absence of one or more pulse waves (dropped pulse). Where there is no regular rhythm to the pulse and it cannot be predicted as one attempts to tap it out the heart is not under a single pacemaker influence.

## Amplitude and quality

Evaluation of pulse amplitude and quality is subjective and has the least clinical value for interpreting abnormalities in the heart. Perceived pulse strength is a function of the difference between peak systolic pressure and diastolic pressure, i.e. the pulse pressure. When diastolic pressure is abnormally low and systolic pressure is maintained, the pulse pressure will increase and the perceived strength of the pulse will increase. This is referred to as a hyperkinetic pulse. With significant loss of diastolic pressure, such as occurs in aortic valvular insufficiency or patent ductus arteriosus, pulse pressure becomes very high and pulses become hyperkinetic, or bounding. In cases of mitral valve regurgitation the pulse can have a rapid rate of rise because the left ventricular ejection time is shortened by mitral valve incompetence. When systemic vascular resistance is decreased, as in hyperthyroidism, fever or anemia, pulses are often hyperkinetic. A hypokinetic, or weak, arterial pulse may be present whenever there is decreased left ventricular stroke volume. Common conditions associated with reduced stroke volume include hypovolemia, left ventricular failure and cardiac tamponade. A compensatory tachycardia is also usually present in these cases, contributing further to a loss of pulse pressure. In subaortic stenosis, arterial pulses are hypokinetic and also slow rising (parvus et tardus pulse). Pulses are often hypokinetic in cats with dilated cardiomyopathy. Pulses will be absent when an obstruction to flow is present proximally to the site of palpation. The most notable example is in a cat with thromboembolism of the aortic trifurcation (saddle thrombus). In addition to the absence of femoral pulses, the limbs will be cool and the footpads cyanotic. The tail will also be pulseless. A **pulse deficit** is recorded when the arterial pulse rate is lower than the heart rate as determined by auscultation. This occurs when there are cardiac contractions sufficient to generate one or more heart sounds, but where there is an insufficient stroke volume to generate a palpable pulse. This is common when there is an insufficient diastolic filling time, as can occur with atrial fibrillation that establishes at high heart rates and where there are multiple ventricular extrasystoles. As a general rule, where periodic or beat-to-beat changes in pulse pressure are detected during a single examination period they are likely to reflect underlying heart disease, commonly arrhythmic heart disease.

## Venous circulation

The superficial major veins, such as the jugular, saphenous, and median veins, can be inspected and palpated with the animal standing. The examination should ensure that the free flow of blood is not being impeded by a neck chain or other similar device.

**Jugular vein**
Examination of the jugular veins provides a valuable indication of the functioning of the right side of the heart. There are two components to this examination

- the degree of jugular filling
- jugular pulsation.

In the standing animal the jugular vein is higher than the heart and normally appears empty, making it difficult to see and feel. The veins can be examined without clipping the hair in most horses, cattle, and goats. In small animals, llamas and sheep the overlying hair may have to be clipped in order to observe the jugular veins.

*Jugular filling*
The central venous pressure determines the height of the filling of the jugular vein. In the normal adult horse and cow it will be distended with blood some 5–8 cm above the level of the base of the heart. Thus in the standing animal with its head in a normal position the

> ### DeMussett's sign
>
> DeMussett's sign is the jerking of the head and extremities with each pulse, it is sometimes seen in animals with significant aortic insufficiency causing remarkably hyperkinetic pulses.

jugular vein will be distended in the distal one-quarter to one-fifth of the jugular furrow. Changes in head position will alter this proportion, and when the head is down and below the level of the heart, as when grazing, jugular distension will extend to the ramus of the mandible. In normal animals veins below the level of the heart, such as the subcutaneous abdominal ('milk') vein of lactating cows, are normally full.

*Jugular pulsation*

Several events in the cardiac cycle cause pulsation in the jugular veins. Although this is commonly referred to as pulsation it is actually a variation in the degree of vascular distension. There is a rapid but minor fall in the level of jugular distension associated with the fall of blood into the ventricle during the period of rapid filling in ventricular diastole (y-descent). This is followed by a slower rise in the level of jugular filling to its original point. Superimposed on this and immediately preceding the y-descent is a small wave or retrograde distension associated with atrial contraction (a-wave) and a second smaller retrograde wave associated with bulging of the tricuspid valve into the atrium during ventricular contraction (c-wave).

Cardiac abnormalities that result in right atrial or right ventricular hypertrophy will produce an exaggerated a-wave which commonly obliterates a visible c-wave. Tricuspid insufficiency will produce an exaggerated c-wave because during ventricular contraction blood in the right ventricle is forced through the insufficient tricuspid valve into the right atrium and the jugular vein. Abnormal jugular pulsation may also be present with tetralogy of Fallot and tricuspid valve atresia in foals. The genesis of the pulsation in the jugular vein can be determined by observing its occurrence in relation to the occurrence of the first heart sound, determined by simultaneous observation of the vein and auscultation of the heart.

A jugular pulsation associated with transmission of the pulse from the underlying carotid artery through the jugular vein is occasionally palpable in animals with bilateral jugular distension. This can be easily differen- tiated from true jugular pulsation by occluding the jugular vein with the thumb. If the pulsations continue to be palpable cranial to the occlusion then they are associated with a transmitted carotid pulse.

If the vein is compressed digitally in the middle of the neck it becomes distended above the pressure point because of the accumulation of blood, whereas the section below the pressure point empties at the next heart beat – this is the **negative venous stasis test**. If the jugular vein is visibly distended and feels tense then it is said to be engorged. In cattle and small animals engorged jugular veins are usually due to

- right-sided congestive heart failure – pericarditis, endocarditis, myocarditis, cor pulmonale, or
- space-occupying lesions of the thoracic inlet.

In advanced cases of venous stasis the segment of jugular vein below the compression point cannot empty and it remains just as full of blood as before compression: this is a **positive venous stasis test**.

In vasogenic shock and dehydration the jugular veins are usually collapsed. Compression of such veins results in only slight or no distension of the vein proximal to the point of compression. When attempting venepuncture or the insertion of an intra- venous catheter in such cases, simultaneous compression of both jugular veins or elevation of the animal's hindquarters may be necessary to raise the vein. In some cases it may be necessary to cut down through the skin in order to find the vein.

The subcutaneous abdominal vein of lactating cows is normally engorged because it is below the level of the heart. When it is compressed, that section of the vein nearest the heart does not empty. However, it can be compressed and milked out towards the heart, leaving a relatively empty vein.

**Venous stasis**

The functional state of the venous system can be assessed by observing the large superficial veins such as the jugulars, the smaller cutaneous veins, and others such as the auricular, spermatic, and subcutaneous abdominal veins. In long-coated animals venous distension may not be visible but can be detected by

---

**Engorged jugular veins**

Jugular veins that are fully distended when the animal is standing with its head in a normal position are engorged indicating right-sided congestive heart failure. If the engorged vein is compressed the segment of jugular vein below the compression point does not empty rapidly as it does in animals with normal cardiac function.

---

**Clinical Pointer**

Jugular pulsations can be seen in most horses and cattle by careful observation of the jugular vein at its entrance into the thorax at the base of the neck. The presence or absence of the atrial a-wave helps to identify cardiac dysrhythmia.

## Bilateral engorgement of the jugular veins

Bilateral engorgement of the jugular veins with no visible pulsation is most commonly associated with masses such as lymphosarcoma or an abscess in the cranial thorax, that obstruct the flow of blood from the jugular veins to the heart, and impede the retrograde transmission of pressure changes.

palpation. In thin-skinned horses, such as Thoroughbreds, trotting horses and hunters, when the haircoat is short temporary distension and pulsation of the superficial veins is readily seen after active exertion. Persistent dilatation of superficial veins occurs in diseases in which there is an impediment to blood flow on the venous side of the vascular system. The impediment may involve either the systemic or the pulmonary components, or both concurrently. Venous distension is constantly present when the flow of blood into and through the right ventricle is delayed by incomplete emptying during the preceding systolic contraction. This situation may occur in myocardial dysfunction due to

- myocardial dystrophy
- heart block
- cardiac and mediastinal neoplasia
- endocarditis
- interventricular septal defects
- pericardial disease
- cor pulmonale
- endocardial fibroelastosis.

In the horse with chronic obstructive pulmonary disease the superficial veins may become distended after only a short period of exercise, and remain distended for much longer than in the normal animal, indicating the severity of the dyspnea and its influence on the pulmonary circulation and cardiac reserve. Occasionally, however, engorgement of veins may be the result of a purely local condition, such as compression by a neoplasm or by a superficial inflammatory process.

When venous stasis persists it results in clinical findings attributable to the increased hydrostatic pressure in the veins and to the reduction in stroke volume of the heart. If the right side of the heart is primarily involved there is widespread peripheral edema (anasarca) ascites, hydrothorax, and hydropericardium. The anasarca is limited to the dependent parts, including the ventral surface of the thorax and abdomen, the neck, and the lower jaw. In severe congestion the liver is enlarged to varying degrees, so that the thickened, rounded border can be palpated behind the last rib on the right side, especially in cattle. Further retrograde pressure sufficient to involve the portal system will lead to impairment of digestion, malabsorption, transudation into the intestinal lumen and diarrhea.

## Structural abnormalities of blood vessels

In addition to abnormal pulse waves, certain arteries and veins can be examined directly for the presence of abnormalities. These include

- arterial thrombosis
- arterial embolism
- venous thrombosis
- defects in vessel walls.

In large animals arterial thrombosis frequently results from arteritis, and in cats myocardial disease can predispose to arterial thromboembolism. Parasitic arteritis of the cranial mesenteric artery, the iliac arteries, the base of the aorta, and occasionally the coronary, renal, and cerebral arteries, caused by the migrating larvae of *Strongylus vulgaris*, was relatively common in the horse but has declined in incidence with the use of more effective anthelmintics. Ergotism is characterized by arteritis with vasospasm, producing thrombosis and proceeding to gangrene of the extremities. Frostbite has a similar effect on the skin above the digits. In large animals arterial embolism is in most cases recognized only at necropsy in the form of endarteritis. The lesions are most obvious in the lungs and kidneys, and are found in association with a primary suppurative or other inflammatory process elsewhere, for example vegetative endocarditis or arterial thrombosis at other sites. A thrombus at the aortic trifurcation in the cat is not uncommon in myocardial disease. Ultrasound may be used in the diagnosis of thrombi involving the aorta and iliac arteries.

The clinical manifestations associated with arterial thrombosis and embolism are a reflection of the interference with the function of the part supplied by the affected vessel. In parasitic arteritis the thrombi that

## Vasogenic failure

In vasogenic failure, which occurs in toxemic diseases and shock, the jugular vein is not engorged, although the total blood volume is normal, at least initially, and digital compression slowly produces only a slight distension of any of the superficial veins.

> **Clinical Pointer**
>
> Venous stasis originating from the left side of the heart is manifested by an increase in the rate and depth of respiration in the resting animal, with cough, crackles in the bronchial area, and increased dullness over the ventral third of the thorax because of transudation into the lungs and a degree of hydrothorax. As engorgement of the pulmonary vein intensifies dyspnea occurs and cyanosis becomes obvious.

inevitably develop may partially or completely occlude the artery:

- obstruction of the cranial mesenteric artery causes recurrent colic or, in occasional cases, ischemic necrosis of a segment of the intestine
- occlusion of the coronary artery causes a varying degree of cardiac infarction
- thrombi at the terminal aorta cause pelvic limb paresis, lack of an arterial pulse, pallor, and coolness of the extremities in affected animals
- embolic obstruction of the pulmonary arteries causes hypoxic hypoxia.

Venous thrombosis commonly arises from phlebitis, which may be caused by local extension of infection, by localization of a blood borne infection, by bacterial invasion of the umbilical veins at birth, or by injection of irritant substances in the case of the larger veins. Long-term intravenous catheterization of the jugular veins in horses and cattle or the jugular or cephalic veins in dogs and cats may result in thrombophlebitis characterized by an enlarged and painful swelling of the tissues surrounding the vein. In septicemic diseases of the pig phlebitis and venous thrombosis cause the development of purple discoloration, and later sloughing of the ears, which is a feature in many cases.

Defects in blood vessel walls usually involve the capillaries and smaller arterioles. They occur in septicemic (or viremic) diseases and in purpura hemorrhagica. The end effect is increased permeability leading to hemorrhages, which are either petechial or ecchymotic.

## EXAMINATION OF THE HEART

### Applied anatomy of the heart

The heart, suspended at its base by the large blood vessels which traverse the mediastinum, occupies a considerable part of the middle mediastinal region of the thoracic cavity. The apex of the heart is situated in the midline dorsal to the sternum.

### Dog

In the dog the base of the heart faces dorsocranially, and is level with the middle part of the 3rd rib. The apex is blunt and positioned near the diaphragm on the left of the median plane of the body, opposite the 7th costal cartilage. The area of contact between the heart and left thoracic wall, through the overlying pericardium, extends from the level of the ventral parts of the 3rd to 6th ribs. On the right side the area of contact is limited to that extending between the 4th and 5th ribs.

The **left atrioventricular valve** (mitral valve) is located at the 5th intercostal space just below the costochondral junction; the **aortic valve** is at the left 4th intercostal space at the level of the costochondral junction. The **pulmonic valve** is situated at the level of the left 3rd intercostal space; the **right atrioventricular valve** (tricuspid valve) is at the right 3rd to 5th intercostal spaces.

### Horse

In the horse the heart is asymmetrical in position, slightly more than half of the organ being on the left side of the body. The base, which is directed dorsally, extends from the level of the 2nd to the 6th intercostal space. The apex is positioned centrally about 1 cm dorsal to the caudal sternal segment, and about 2.5 cm cranial to the sternal diaphragm. The caudal border of the heart is nearly vertical and approximates to a position level with the sixth rib or interspace. The left surface of the heart, consisting almost entirely of the wall of the left ventricle, covered by the pericardium, is in contact with the ventral third of the thoracic wall from the 3rd to the 6th ribs. The relationship between the heart and thoracic wall on the right side extends from the 3rd to the 4th intercostal space only, because of the relatively small cardiac notch in the right lung and the degree of cardiac asymmetry. Enlargement of the heart from any cause will proportionally increase the area of contact between the organ and the thoracic wall on the right side.

The **left atrioventricular orifice**, guarded by the mitral valve, is situated level with the 5th intercostal space about 10 cm dorsal to the sternal extremity of the fifth rib. The **aortic orifice**, guarded by its semilunar valve, is level with the 4th intercostal space on a line horizontal with the point of the shoulder. The **pulmonary orifice** of the right ventricle, guarded by the pulmonary semilunar valve, is level with the 3rd intercostal space immediately dorsal to the right atrioventricular orifice. The **right atrioventricular orifice,** guarded by the tricuspid valve, is situated opposite the 4th intercostal space about 7 cm dorsal to the ventral extremity of the fourth rib.

### Cattle

In cattle the degree of cardiac asymmetry is slightly greater than in the horse. The base of the heart extends from the level of the 3rd to about the 6th rib. The cardiac apex, which is median in position and about 2 cm cranial to the diaphragm, is level with the articulation of the 6th costal cartilage with the sternum. The caudal border of the heart, which is almost vertical, is level with the 5th intercostal space, where it is separated from the diaphragm by the pericardium. On the left side the heart and enclosing pericardium are in contact with the thoracic wall from the 3rd rib to the 4th intercostal space. On the right side the extent of the contact is limited to a small area level with the ventral part of the 4th rib, and the adjacent 3rd and 4th intercostal spaces.

The **left atrioventricular orifice** is mainly at the level of the 4th intercostal space; the **aortic orifice** is level with the 4th rib about 12 cm dorsal to the sternal extremity. The **pulmonary orifice,** which is slightly more dorsally situated, is level with the 3rd intercostal space; the **right atrioventricular orifice** is level with the 4th rib, almost 10 cm dorsal to the costochondral junction.

### Pig

The heart of the pig is small in proportion to the body weight. It is short and broad, and the blunt apex, which is situated medially, is about 0.5 cm away from the diaphragm. On the left side the pericardium is in contact with the thoracic wall over an area from the 2nd intercostal space to the 5th rib.

## Physical examination of the heart

The heart is examined by palpation, percussion and auscultation. All of these techniques can provide information, but auscultation is the fundamental component of the examination of the heart.

### Palpation

The animal should be in a standing position and bearing weight on all four limbs. In the case of small animals, the palms of both hands are applied simulta-neously, one on each side, and slight pressure is applied to compress the thoracic wall in the anatomical region of the heart. This requires sliding the fingers and the palm of the hand under the elbow and triceps. Large-breed dogs are best evaluated standing on the floor, small and medium-sized dogs, as well as cats, should be examined standing on the examination table.

The objective of palpation is to determine the location and character of the apex beat (cardiac impulse) and to determine whether adventitious vibrations associated with the cardiac cycle are present.

**Apex beat or cardiac impulse**
The apex beat is the low-frequency vibration produced during the contraction and rotation of the heart in early systole. It is synchronous with the first heart sound and

- in the dog it is best felt on the left side, at the 4th or 5th intercostal space
- in the horse it can be felt from the 3rd to the 6th intercostal spaces and is most intense at the 5th intercostal space
- in the cow, sheep and goat it can be felt in the 3rd to the 5th intercostal spaces and is most intense at the 4th.

The apex beat is less intense on the right side, and in animals with condition scores of 3.5 (out of 5) or more it is normally not palpable on the right. It is usually also visible on the left side in young animals and animals with a condition score of less than 3 particularly when lying in lateral recumbency.

A caudal shifting of the cardiac impulse is suggestive of cardiac enlargement. Other less likely causes include thoracic masses displacing the heart, or lung-lobe collapse allowing the heart to shift. An increase in the intensity of the apex beat occurs where there is an increase in sympathetic tone, but may also be an indication of cardiac hypertrophy. A decrease in intensity may be due to decreased intensity of the cardiac contraction, or to an associated peripheral vascular failure. A decreased intensity also occurs where there is more tissue or fluid between the heart and the skin, such as with pericardial effusion, pleural effusion,

---

**Clinical Pointer**

To palpate the heart of small animals stand behind the animal and palpate both sides of the thorax simultaneously, beginning at the axillary area and moving in a caudal direction.

space-occupying lesions in the plural cavity, or subcutaneous fat.

**Precordial thrill**

This is a palpable vibration of the thoracic wall associated with the kinetic energy of intracardiac or intravascular turbulence. A precordial thrill must be distinguished from the active precordium of an animal with a prominent apical impulse. Precordial thrills are associated with the presence of loud cardiac murmurs, the presence of or absence of a thrill is one characteristic used in the assessment of murmur intensity. The point of maximal intensity of the thrill is the same as the point of maximal intensity of the associated murmur. Determination of the point of maximal intensity provides information that has diagnostic significance in the evaluation of cardiac murmurs.

Rarely, vibrations associated with pericardial friction rubs can be detected by palpation.

## Percussion

Percussion is of limited value in the examination of standing large animals because most of the heart underlies the muscles of the forelimbs and the thoracic wall overlying the heart cannot be resonated. The limb overlying the area of the thoracic wall being percussed must be advanced forward to minimize this constraint. Percussion can be used to delineate the dorsal border of cardiac dullness, and this may be displaced if there is cardiac enlargement or pericardial effusion. Percussion is of greater value in the examination of other structures in the thoracic cavity.

The heart is percussed using the same technique as for the lungs (see pp. 333). It is recommended to percuss from the more resonant areas toward the area of cardiac dullness.

The area of cardiac dullness in the horse elicits obvious dullness on percussion, which is readily demonstrable on the left thoracic wall over an area approximately the size of the palm of the hand, situated caudal to the shoulder, just above the level of the elbow, in the region of the 3rd to the 5th intercostal spaces. On the right side of the thorax the area of cardiac dullness is normally much smaller than that on the left side, being demonstrable only in the 4th intercostal space. Considerable experience is required to outline the area of cardiac dullness, especially that of the right side.

The area of cardiac dullness in normal cattle is distinct and measures about 6–8 cm in diameter between the 3rd and 4th intercostal spaces at the level of the point of the elbow, with the left forelimb placed forward. The area of cardiac dullness is much smaller on the right side of the thorax.

An increase in the area of cardiac dullness occurs in

- enlargement of the heart (cardiac hypertrophy or dilatation)
- pericardial effusion (pericarditis, hydropericardium, hemopericardium)
- lateral displacement of the heart (unilateral pulmonary collapse, unilateral pneumothorax, diaphragmatic hernia)
- neoplasia of the heart, pericardium, thymus, or mediastinum.

In the majority of such cases the area of cardiac dullness may be more distinctly enlarged on the right side, the exceptions being those in which the heart is displaced towards the left side. Because of the anatomical relationships of the heart, any detectable increase in size of the area of cardiac dullness involves the dorsal and caudal borders, both of which are extended to a variable degree.

Reduction in the size of the area of cardiac dullness occurs in over-distension of the lungs (emphysema), when more lung tissue is between the heart and the thoracic wall. If a pleural effusion is present it may be impossible to define the area of cardiac dullness because of the complete lack of variation in the tone of the percussion sound throughout the area.

A pain reaction during percussion of the cardiac area suggests the presence of acute pericarditis or pleurisy.

## Auscultation

Auscultation of the heart is the fundamental component of the examination of the cardiovascular system. Auscultation allows the detection and examination of normal heart sounds which mark the mechanical events in the cardiac cycle, and an evaluation of heart rhythm. It also detects abnormal sounds generated during the cardiac cycle, which include cardiac murmurs, pericardial friction rubs and other less common abnormal sounds.

A high-quality stethoscope is recommended. The end pieces of most stethoscopes are dual, consisting of

---

**Clinical Pointer**

Because of the wide variation in the thickness of the thoracic wall, relative body condition, particularly in dogs, and breed differences in the shape of the thorax, considerable experience is necessary to determine the area of cardiac dullness by percussion.

a flat diaphragm and a concave bell. The bell piece transmits low-frequency sounds better than the diaphragm, but in large animals the coupling across the hair restricts the differential value of the bell head and so the flat diaphragm is most commonly used. In order to transmit high-frequency sound it must be pushed firmly against the skin; light pressure will attenuate high-frequency sounds and accentuate low-frequency ones. The construction of a dual head should not be bulky, so that the stethoscope can be slid under the triceps.

The size of the end piece is also important. Standard-sized chest pieces (3 cm) designed for adult humans are ideal for large dogs and horses. An infant or pediatric stethoscope end piece (2 cm) is approximately 50% smaller and is ideal for cats and small dogs. Transmission of heart sounds is increased and it is possible to localize murmurs better in these small patients. Several additional factors are important when evaluating a stethoscope

- the ear pieces should be soft and fit comfortably within the ear canal; they should be replaced every 1–2 years
- the body frame should place the ear pieces within the ear canals without discomfort, yet with enough pressure to ensure an acoustic seal
- a single casing housing the two tubes is generally superior to the tubes hanging free or joined only by a metallic or plastic band (minimally restrained tubes have a tendency to bump one another causing noise)
- the stethoscope end piece should be constructed of a high-quality alloy, the diaphragm well-seated and durable, and the bell–diaphragm switching mechanism should move without resistance.

### Technique of auscultation

The heart must be examined in a systematic manner for best results. The location of the heart sounds is identified with reference to the base and apex of the heart and the **point of maximal intensity** (PMI) of the four valve regions.

1. Auscultation usually begins on the left side at the point of maximal intensity of the mitral valve.
2. The stethoscope is then moved to the base of the heart to hear the sounds over the areas of maximal intensity of the aortic and pulmonic valves.
3. The examination at the right side is usually started at the area of maximal intensity of the tricuspid valve, and the stethoscope is then moved dorsally and cranially to auscultate over the base of the heart on the right side.

The stethoscope will detect extraneous sounds and the examination should be conducted in a quiet environment. Faint but significant abnormalities can go undetected if the animal is examined in a noisy environment. The animal should be moved to quiet surroundings if possible for a careful examination of the heart. Sounds associated with respiration and intestinal motility may also be heard while auscultating over the cardiac area, and must be recognized and ignored. The rustling sounds caused by movement of the chest piece over the haircoat must also be recognized as extraneous.

Respiratory sounds often occur synchronously with heart sounds and may be mistaken for cardiac murmurs. Occluding the nose for several seconds will stop the animal breathing and allow the heart sounds to be heard in isolation. Panting in dogs can be prevented by having an assistant hold the dog's muzzle.

### Normal heart sounds

The first and second heart sounds are clearly audible in all normal animals unless they are exceptionally fat. A third and fourth heart sound may be heard in normal large animals, particularly horses (Fig. 14.1). The first and second heart sounds are the only sounds normally audible in the dog and cat (Fig 14.2).

*First heart sound (S1)*
The first heart sound is associated with closure of the AV valves. In health, mitral valve closure precedes tricuspid valve closure by an imperceptible period; the two sounds therefore fuse to form a single sound known as S1. The first heart sound is lower in frequency than the second (S2) and sounds like **'lubb'**.

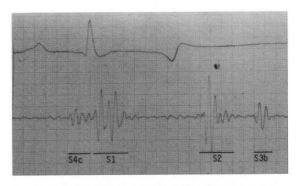

**Fig. 14.1** ECG and phonocardiogram of horse showing the four audible heart sounds. The atrial sound (S4c) is also called the A sound.

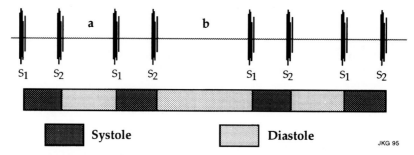

**Fig. 14.2** A phonocardiogram demonstrating the relationship between the first and second heart sounds. The interval between S1 and S2 represents systole (dark gray), while the area from S2 to S1 represents diastole (light gray). Note that the systolic interval remains fairly constant, whereas changes in rate are reflected by a change in the diastolic duration (compare a with b).

*Second heart sound (S2)*

Like the first heart sound the second consists of two components related to closure of the aortic and pulmonary valves. It is shorter and higher pitched than the first, and sounds like '**dupp**'. Pulmonary valve closure follows closure of the aortic valve, and in most healthy animals the two components of S2 are fused to form a single sound. However, right ventricular ejection lengthens during inspiration, and physiological inspiratory splitting of the second heart sound is apparent in some normal animals, particularly horses. The temporal relationship of S1 and S2 varies little over the range of commonly encountered heart rates. Thus when the heart rate is elevated it is the duration of diastole that is noticeably shortened. This is helpful in the identification of the two heart sounds.

*Third heart sound (S3)*

The third heart sound is associated with rapid filling of the ventricle in early diastole and is heard as a dull thud occurring immediately after the second sound. It is usually most audible on the left side just caudal to the area of maximal audibility of the first heart sound. However, it is frequently heard over the base and also over the area of cardiac auscultation on the right side.

---

**Clinical Pointer**

Auscultation of the heart of a purring cat is difficult. The purring can be temporarily stopped by holding of the cat's nose, moving it towards a running faucet, and touching the nose with an alcohol pad. These techniques are variably successful but may provide a period of silence.

---

**The third heart sound**

1. the third heart sound is common in horses and can be detected in the majority of fit racing animals, as well as in cattle
2. the third heart sound is inaudible in normal dogs and cats.

---

*Fourth heart sound (S4)*

The fourth heart sound (also called the atrial contraction sound or 'a' sound) is associated with atrial contraction. It occurs immediately before the first heart sound and is a soft sound most audible over the base of the heart on the left and right. It is common in horses, but its clear separation from the first heart sound depends on the length of the PR interval, which varies between horses. At resting (low) heart rates it is detectable on clinical examination in at least 60% of animals.

The interval between the atrial contraction sound and the first heart sound frequently varies in the same horse at rest, and results in a clear separation in some beats and slurring together of the two sounds in other beats. The fourth heart sound may also be heard in young cattle. The presence of a fourth heart sound in dogs and cats is abnormal.

**Heart rate**

The heart rate is determined by counting the number of beats per unit of time, usually 1 minute, resulting in a measure of beats per minute (bpm). Thus the first and second heart sounds or, in some animals all four heart sounds, constitute one heartbeat. The ranges of heart rates for normal animals are given in Table 14.2.

**Intensity of heart sounds**

The intensity or loudness of the heart sounds depends on the strength of the heartbeat and the thickness of the thoracic wall, or the presence of any factor which interferes with or enhances the transmission of the sounds from the heart to the stethoscope.

---

### Clinical Pointer

Heart sounds are normally more easily detectable by auscultation on the left side in animals of all body condition scores, but may become inaudible on the right side when the body condition score approaches 5/5.

---

Both the absolute and the relative intensity of each heart sound may be increased or decreased. An increase or decrease in intensity suggests that there is either

- a change in the intensity of the generation of sound by the heart, or
- a change in the transmission of the sounds between the heart and the stethoscope.

An increase in the absolute intensity of the heart sounds occurs with cardiac hypertrophy and metabolic diseases such as hypomagnesemia. Increased transmission of normal heart sounds occurs with cranioventral consolidating bronchopneumonia, where there is a reduction in the normal damping of heart sound transmission by normally inflated lung. It also occurs when there is displacement of the heart for any reason (e.g. diaphragmatic hernia) and through reduction of damping tissue in animals that are thin.

Muffling of the heart sounds suggests an increase in tissue and fluid interfaces between the heart and the stethoscope. This can be caused by a shift in the heart due to displacement by a mass, changes in the pericardium (increased fluid or fibrous tissue), changes in the pleural space (pleural effusion or pneumothorax), or increased subcutaneous fat. Perhaps paradoxically, with a pleural effusion the heart sounds are clear and radiate dorsally; this is probably associated with the absence of respiratory sounds in the ventral thorax with such an effusion. Changes in the relative intensity of individual heart sounds result from changes in the end-diastolic volume of the ventricles, pulmonary or aortic hypotension or hypertension, and increased flow volumes.

---

### Decreased intensity of heart sounds

A decrease in the absolute intensity of heart sounds results from decreased strength of cardiac contractility in

- terminal heart failure
- hypocalcemia in cattle
- shock in all species.

---

**Rhythm of heartbeat**

*Normal cardiac rhythm*

Normally the rhythm is in three-time and can be described as lubb–dupp–pause, the first sound being dull, deep, long, and loud, and the second sound sharper and shorter. As the heart rate increases the cycle becomes shortened, mainly at the expense of diastole, and the rhythm assumes a two-time quality. More than two sounds per cycle is called a 'gallop' rhythm, and may be due to reduplication of either the first or the second sounds.

The sequence of occurrence of the four heart sounds in the cardiac cycle is **a–1–2–3**. The intensity of the third and fourth sounds is less than that of the first and second, and the complex can be described as du–lubb–dupp–boo. In some horses the third and/or fourth sound may be inaudible, so that **1–2**, **a–1–2**, and **1–2–3** variations occur. These same variations can occur in cattle, but in sheep, goats, and pigs only two heart sounds are normally heard. The occurrence of a third or fourth heart sound in horses and cattle is not an indication of cardiovascular abnormality.

The relative temporal occurrence and the intensity of the third and fourth heart sounds change with heart rate. At moderately elevated rates the atrial contraction sound may merge with the first heart sound, but the third heart sound usually becomes more audible.

---

### Clinical Pointer

During periods of a rapid change in heart rate (the increase following a sudden noise, for example, and the subsequent decrease in rate)

- the variation in the occurrence and the intensity of the third and fourth sounds, coupled with
- the variation in intensity of the first and second sounds during this change

can give the false impression of an arrhythmia.

---

*Gallop rhythms*

More than two sounds per cycle results in a triple rhythm known as a 'gallop' rhythm. This may be due to doubling or reduplication of either the first or the second sound (split heart sounds, see below) or when the third or fourth heart sounds are audible. A gallop rhythm results when there is accentuation of physiological events in the cardiac cycle and is not an arrhythmia. In small animals the third heart sound is audible when there is rapid deceleration of the blood that enters the ventricle during early diastole. When it reflects disease, an **S3 gallop** is most often associated with

- dilated cardiomyopathy
- restrictive cardiomyopathy
- severe mitral valve incompetence.

An **S4 gallop** resulting from the audibility of S4 is generally associated with diseases that result in decreased ventricular compliance; such is the case in patients with hypertrophic cardiomyopathy.

The finding of gallop rhythm in a dog or cat is usually a specific indicator of cardiac disease; further, the detection of a gallop rhythm in a small animal patient may have grave prognostic implications. As stated, the third and fourth heart sounds are low frequency and usually low intensity. However, the subtlety of this auscultatory finding often belies its clinical significance. In consequence, auscultation of a gallop rhythm justifies further diagnostic evaluation even when clinical signs are absent. The third and fourth heart sounds are often audible in healthy large animals. Other aspects of the physical examination and history must be considered when assessing the clinical importance of a gallop rhythm in large animals.

> ### Summation gallop
>
> In many small animals the heart rate is so rapid that the events of early diastolic filling and atrial contraction fuse – the result is known as a summation gallop.

*Split heart sounds*

A split heart sound is the presence of two components in the first or second heart sound complexes.

*Split first heart sound* (**split S1**)   Because the first heart sound consists of two separate valves closing, a delay in one valve's closure will result in a 'splitting' of this sound. Normally, near-synchronous closure of the right and left atrioventricular valves results in a single first heart sound. Splitting of the first heart sound is not as common as splitting of the second.

Causes of a split S1 include

- structural lesions interfering with valve closure, such as infective endocarditis
- conduction delay of one ventricle, as occurs with a bundle branch block
- premature contraction of one ventricle.

The splitting may not be obvious as there is usually a very short interval between the two components of the first heart sound (Fig. 14.3).

*Split second heart sound* (**split S2**)   The normal second heart sound also comprises the near-synchronous closure of two valves, the aortic and the pulmonic. Splitting of the second heart sound is not uncommon and is usually caused by pulmonary hypertension. This disorder delays emptying of the right ventricle, causing the pulmonic valve to close after the aortic valve. Pulmonary hypertension can be

- primary (idiopathic), or
- secondary to heartworm disease or other causes of cor pulmonale.

Other causes of a split S2 include premature ventricular contraction or delayed conduction (bundle branch block) of a ventricle. A split S2 is usually easier to detect than a split S1, as the splitting is wider (Fig. 14.4).

### Third and fourth sounds in the dog and cat

*Third heart sound* (**S3 gallop**)   In dogs and cats the presence of a third heart sound, S3, is indicative of heart disease. This sound is easily missed.

> ### Clinical Pointer
>
> Take care not to miss an S3 in dogs and cats, it occurs in early to mid-diastole, when a sound is not anticipated, is low pitched and resonant, and resembles the light tapping of a bass drum.

An S3 is of much lower frequency than the first and second heart sounds, is usually of low intensity, or soft, and occurs in diastole, when a sound is not anticipated.

An S3 is produced when there is inadequate ventricular emptying and blood for the next cardiac cycle 'collides' with blood remaining from the previous cycle, or if ventricular compliance is reduced. In large-

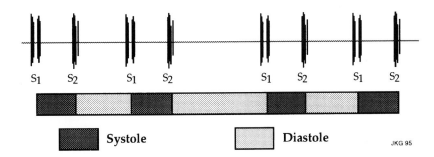

**Fig. 14.3** Splitting of the first heart sound, S1.

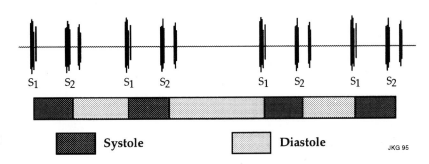

**Fig. 14.4** Splitting of the second heart sound, S2.

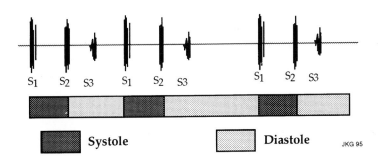

**Fig. 14.5** A third heart sound (S3).

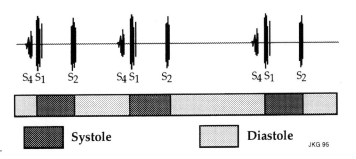

**Fig. 14.6** A fourth heart sound (S4). This sound is associated with atrial contraction and occurs just before the first heart sound.

breed dogs it is almost always indicative of dilated cardiomyopathy. An S3 is differentiated from a split second heart sound by two characteristics

1. the sounds of a split S2 have the same frequency, as opposed to the low frequency of an S3
2. the sounds of a split S2 are much closer together, whereas the S3 occurs later in diastole (Figs 14.4, 14.5).

*Fourth heart sound (S4 gallop)*
An additional sound which is abnormal in the dog and cat is a fourth heart sound, S4 (Fig. 14.6). This sound is produced during atrial contraction and, when heard in the dog or cat, is usually indicative of a non-compliant left ventricle. An S4 is most often heard in cats with hypertrophic cardiomyopathy. It can be difficult to distinguish from a split first heart sound, especially when the heart rate is elevated, and in some cases can only be differentiated phonocardiographically.

---

### Third and fourth heart sounds in cats

An S3 can be difficult to distinguish from an S4 in cats, as both produce a characteristic three-beat gallop-type sound. Since both sounds indicate the presence of heart disease further diagnostics are necessary and the differentiation becomes academic.

---

## PHYSIOLOGICAL AND ABNORMAL ARRHYTHMIAS

Variations in cardiac rate and rhythm include

- tachycardia – increased rate
- bradycardia – decreased rate
- arrhythmia – irregularity in rate and rhythm.

The rate and rhythm of the heart are influenced primarily by the pacemaker, the conduction system and the myocardium, and by the autonomic nervous system. In the normal heart the sinoatrial node is the site of impulse generation and its depolarization is under the influence of the autonomic nervous system. Alterations in autonomic activity, electrolyte imbalance, or structural lesions in the conducting system or myocardium can produce cardiac arrhythmia.

The clinical detection of cardiac arrhythmia is an important skill to learn as there are several arrhythmias in large animals that may occur in the absence of heart disease and which appear to result from excess vagal tone. These occur especially in the horse and include

- sinus arrhythmia
- wandering pacemaker
- sinoatrial block
- first-degree and second-degree atrioventricular block.

---

### Clinical Pointer

Vagal tone can be increased by forceful elevation of the tail in young ruminants.

---

They occur in animals at rest and in horses can frequently be induced by the application of a nose twitch. There is also a diurnal effect, with arrhythmias being more common in horses during the night than the day. There is some debate as to the significance of these disturbances, but it is generally believed that if they are abolished by exercise and if there is no evidence of cardiac insufficiency they are not of pathological significance. All animals with evidence of arrhythmic heart disease should be examined following exercise, as should any animal in which cardiac disease is suspected. The occurrence of cardiac irregularities following exercise is highly indicative of serious cardiac disease. In the examination of the patient with arrhythmic heart disease special attention should be paid to

- the rate, rhythm, and intensity of the individual heart sounds
- the rate, rhythm, and amplitude of the arterial pulse
- the rate, rhythm, and amplitude of the venous pulsations at the jugular inlet. The pulsations in the jugular vein are examined in conjunction with auscultation of the heart.

Transient physiological hypoxemia during birth may result in cardiac arrhythmias in the immediate post-partum period, including sinus arrhythmias and wandering pacemaker, atrial premature contraction, atrial fibrillation, ventricular premature contraction, and partial atrioventricular block. Normal sinus rhythm occurs within 5 minutes of birth.

### Physiological arrhythmias

In the horse the physiological cardiac arrhythmias, that are the result of excessive vagal tone, are more common in trained Standardbreds and Thoroughbred horses and are not commonly encountered in the pony breeds. Sinus arrhythmia can occur in the normal young of all of the large farm animal species. Sinus bradycardia is common in starved cattle.

## Secondary arrhythmias

In cattle, and sometimes in horses

- atrial extrasystole
- second-degree atrioventricular block
- ventricular extrasystole, and
- atrial fibrillation

may occur without evidence of primary cardiac disease. In most cases they are associated with alimentary tract abnormalities and accidents (colic) and also with acid–base and electrolyte abnormalities. If these primary causes are corrected then the heart rhythm returns to normal.

## Sinus tachycardias versus pathological tachycardias

- sinus tachycardias accelerate and decelerate gradually, they are almost always regular
- pathological tachycardias often begin and terminate abruptly, irregular tachycardias are almost always pathological.

### Sinus tachycardia

This is elevation of the heart rate due to increased discharge of the sinoatrial node as a result of excitement, exercise, pain, temporary hypotension, and the administration of adrenergic drugs. The rate returns to normal when the stimulus is removed. Rates above

- 160 bpm in dogs (180 in toy breeds, 220 in puppies, >140 in giant breeds)
- >240 in cats
- 48 bpm in resting adult horses
- 80 bpm in adult cattle

and that are used to being handled are usually classified as tachycardia. Based upon physical examination alone it may not be possible to distinguish sinus tachycardia, which is physiological, from pathological tachycardia.

It is rare for sinus tachycardia to result in heart rates above 120 bpm in either horses or cattle in the usual physical examination situations. Rates well above 120 bpm occur during exercise in the horse, but it is rare for the rate to exceed this at rest in association with pain, fever, or other illness, and rates above 120 in resting cattle and horses are usually indicative of a pathological tachycardia. Excitement producing sinus tachycardia may occur when examining the heart of animals unac-

customed to being handled, and an elevation in rate may occur even in animals used to humans when they are approached by an unfamiliar person. Examination requires patience and quiet, when the rate will usually return to around normal within a few minutes if no further cause of excitement occurs.

### Sinus bradycardia

Sinus bradycardia is a slower than normal heart rate due to a decreased rate of discharge from the sinoatrial node. It is usually defined by a heart rate lower than

- 70 bpm in dogs (<60 in giant breeds)
- <120 bpm in cats
- 28 bpm in the horse, and
- 48 bpm in cattle.

Rates as low as this may occur in well trained, athletic horses at rest, but generally sinus bradycardia suggests cardiac disease. Sinus bradycardia occurs in association with high vagal tone and the rate will become elevated with exercise or the administration of atropine (0.02–0.05 mg/kg SC). In calves and foals vagal tone will be increased, and temporary sinus bradycardia can be induced by firm elevation of the tail dorsally over the back. The application of a nose twitch has the same effect in some adult horses. Low heart rates also occur with space-occupying brain lesions, hypothermia, hypoglycemia, and following the administration of certain pharmaceutical agents. Low rates may also be present in vagus indigestion and diaphragmatic hernia in cattle, and also occur in cattle when the food intake is restricted. Sinus arrhythmia is also observed in cattle deprived of feed. In small animals it occurs with hypothyroidism and hyperkalemia.

## Arrhythmias with normal rates or bradycardia

### Sinus arrhythmia

This is a physiologically normal arrhythmia caused by a variation in the intensity of vagal stimulation to the sinoatrial node. In the common form the arrhythmia is synchronous with respiration. Sinus arrhythmia occurs at slow heart rates, and the rate increases during inspiration and decreases during expiration. Sinus arrhythmia can be detected in young calves and foals and in tame sheep and goats, but is uncommon in adult horses and cattle. Sinus arrhythmia not associated with respiration can occur in horses. Sinus arrhythmia is abolished by exercise or the administration of atropine (10–20 mg/450 kg body weight SC).

On the ECG, sinus arrhythmia is detected by variations in the P–P and P–R intervals and in the horse is frequently associated with a discharge from a **wandering pacemaker**. A wandering pacemaker is associated with differences in the site of discharge from the sinoatrial node, with subsequent minor variations in the vector of atrial depolarization and subsequent minor variations in the configuration of the P wave. In the horse there may be an abrupt change in the contour of the P wave in association with this physiological arrhythmia.

### Sinoatrial block and sinoatrial arrest

This is failure of the sinoatrial node to discharge and consequently there is no atrial contraction or contraction of the ventricle (Fig.14.7). It is characterized by

- the periodic absence of a palpable arterial pulse (dropped pulse), with the interval between the pulse preceding the dropped pulse and that of the following pulse being approximately twice that of the normal pulse interval
- absence of an atrial contraction sound and the absence of sounds associated with ventricular contraction
- absence of an a- and a c-wave and y-descent in the jugular vein
- no third heart sound in small animals
- accentuated first and third sounds in the heartbeat following the block. This is associated with an increased stroke volume and filling pressure in the post-block beat.

This is a relatively common arrhythmia in fit, athletic horses at rest and is considered physiologically normal unless it persists during and immediately after exercise. In normal horses it occurs at slow heart rates. It is not common in cattle. It is easily diagnosed on clinical examination and can be confirmed by electrocardiography. On the ECG there is a complete absence of the P, QRS and T complexes for one beat. In sinoatrial block the distance between the pre- and post-block P waves is twice

the normal P–P interval, or sometimes slightly shorter. Sinoatrial arrest occurs when the P–P interval is greater than twice the P–P interval of the preceding beat.

### Atrioventricular block

In atrioventricular block the depolarization from the atrium is delayed or blocked at the atrioventricular node. The degree of this inhibition leads to a classification of

- first-degree atrioventricular block, in which the impulse is delayed
- second-degree (partial) atrioventricular block, in which the depolarization at the atrioventricular node is periodically inhibited
- complete atrioventricular block (third-degree heart block), where there is no conduction of the depolarization at the atrioventricular node.

---

### Clinical Pointer

Tap out the pulse or heartbeats through the period of sinoatrial block to determine the underlying sinus rhythm.

---

First degree atrioventricular block is an ECG diagnosis. It is common in the horse, where by convention, it is diagnosed when the PQ interval is greater than 400 ms. It may be transient owing to waxing and waning vagal tone. It cannot be diagnosed on physical examination but may be suspected when the interval between the atrial contraction sound and the first heart sound is long. It is commonly accompanied by sinoatrial block of some beats and in most horses is of no pathological significance.

Second-degree atrioventricular block (partial heart block) (Fig. 14.8) occurs when there is atrial depolarization and contraction but depolarization is periodically blocked at the atrioventricular node.

This dysrhythmia is characterized by

- a dropped pulse, with the interval between the preceding pulse and the pulse following the dropped pulse being approximately twice that of the normal pulse interval
- the presence of an atrial contraction sound not followed by the heart sounds associated with ventricular contraction
- the presence of an a-wave in the jugular vein during the period where there is an atrial contraction sound but no sounds associated with ventricular contraction

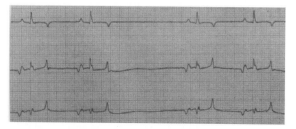

**Fig. 14.7** ECG from horse with sinoatrial block.

- accentuated first and third sounds in the heartbeat following the block. This is associated with an increased stroke volume and filling pressure in the post-block beat (in large animals).

Second-degree atrioventricular block may occur in a random fashion or in a regular pattern: for example, every third or fourth atrial contraction may not be followed by a ventricular contraction. Occasionally two atrial contractions in succession are not followed by ventricular contractions. The underlying rhythm is still sinus in origin and is thus regular. The presence of a fourth heart sound in the horse is a particularly valuable aid to diagnosis. With careful auscultation it can be heard during the block period in the manner of du–LUBB–DUPP–du ... du–LUBB–DUPP. This is diagnostic for this abnormality in the horse.

The ECG shows a P wave associated with atrial depolarization but no QRS complex. Variation of the PQ interval has led to subclassification of types of second-degree heart block, but these do not appear to be important in determining the significance of this conduction defect in horses.

1. With Mobitz type 1 (Wenkebach) second-degree atrioventricular block there is a gradual increase in the PQ interval up to the point of the blocked conduction.
2. With Mobitz type 2 block the PQ interval remains unchanged.

Many second-degree atrioventricular blocks in horses do not fit these categories, and the PQ interval increases until the immediate pre-block complex in which it is decreased. This can often be detected clinically by a gradual increase in the interval between the atrial contraction sound and the first heart sound until the pre-block beat, where the fourth and first sounds are often merged. This can be used to predict the occurrence of a second-degree heart block.

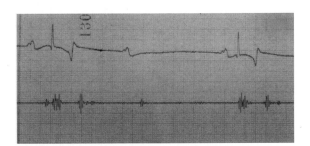

**Fig. 14.8**   ECG and phonocardiogram from horse with second-degree atrioventricular block.

Second-degree atrioventricular block is common in horses and more common in Thoroughbreds and Standardbred horses than in heavy horses and ponies. It is not common in the other large farm species. If associated with excess vagal tone it can be abolished by exercise or the administration of atropine. It has some diurnal variation in occurrence and can often be detected in horses at rest in the evening. This conduction defect is considered abnormal in horses when it persists during exercise. It may be associated in these circumstances with myocarditis and may progress to third-degree block. Second degree heart block occurs

- at fast heart rates in horses with alkalosis in cases of duodenitis and proximal jejunitis
- with electrolyte imbalances in all species
- with overdoses of calcium salts
- with digitalis toxicity, and
- following the administration of α-2 agonist sedative drugs.

It may also reflect cardiomyopathy and myocarditis in infectious and nutritional deficiency diseases.

> ### Clinical Pointer
>
> The application of a twitch to the upper lip of a horse will frequently slow the heart rate and allow the expression of second-degree heart block.

In small animals second-degree heart block is seen most commonly in the dog. It can occur as a normal physiological variation due to variations in vagal tone, and in this instance will be abolished by exercise or the administration of atropine. It has been associated with diseases involving excessive vagal tone (respiratory, gastrointestinal), with drug therapy (digitalis), with hypothyroidism, and with organic disease of the His bundle or bundle branches (ischemic area, scar, infection, neoplasia, or granuloma).

Methods to differentiate clinically between physiological and pathological second-degree heart block have not been established. However, the persistence of the arrhythmia at heart rates above resting normal should be considered to be abnormal.

There is usually no necessity to treat this arrhythmia specifically and treatment is generally directed at the underlying cause. In cases where the block is frequent and syncopal episodes are likely, atropine may alleviate the frequency of the block, but this is only short-term therapy. Second-degree heart block may progress to complete block.

## Abnormal arrhythmias

### Complete heart block (third-degree atrioventricular block)

This is most frequently diagnosed in the dog and occurs only rarely in large animals. In third-degree heart block the depolarization from the atrium is completely blocked at the atrioventricular node or ventricular conduction tissues, and a pacemaker is established in the atrioventricular node or high ventricular conducting tissue. This pacemaker establishes at a low discharge rate, commonly 10–20 bpm in the horse and a similar low rate in cattle. The conduction defect is characterized by

- slow regular pulse rate
- slow regular ventricular contraction rate (first and second heart sounds)
- fast sinoatrial discharge and atrial contraction, this may be detected in both horses and cattle as a faint fast atrial contraction sound superimposed on the ventricular first and second sounds
- atrial contraction (cannon) waves in the jugular vein, these occur when atrial contraction coincides with ventricular contraction and the atrial contraction occurs against closed atrioventricular valves, resulting in a cannon wave in the jugular vein
- variation in the intensity of the first heart sound, this variation occurs with variation in ventricular filling due to temporal variation in atrial and ventricular contraction
- poor exercise tolerance and periodic syncope.

On the ECG, there is complete dissociation between atrial contraction and ventricular contraction. The P waves are of normal configuration and regular, but occur at rates determined by autonomic tone. The QRS complexes occur at slow rates and may be prolonged, with T-wave vectors oriented in the opposite direction. The prognosis using drug therapy in complete heart block is extremely grave unless the block is associated with a correctable electrolyte imbalance. In small animals, placement of a pacemaker is indicated.

### Premature beats

Premature beats or extrasystoles are caused by the discharge of impulses from irritable foci within the myocardium. They are classified according to the site of their origin as

- atrial
- junctional, or
- ventricular.

Premature beats detected at physical examination are characterized by

- heart sounds and arterial pulse occurring earlier than expected from the normal rhythm
- diminished amplitude or absent (dropped) arterial pulse
- variation in the intensity of the first heart sound
- altered amplitude of the first heart sound associated with the premature beat, with increased amplitude of the first heart sound in the complex following the premature systole
- diminished or absent second heart sound in the premature systole
- periods of regular rhythm interrupted by beats with exceptionally short inter-beat periods
- an early ventricular contraction followed by a compensatory pause, following which normal rhythm is continued.

---

### Clinical Pointer

Premature beats may be detected during the physical examination, but electrocardiography is usually necessary to determine their origin in the heart.

---

*Atrial premature beats* These arise from the discharge of an ectopic atrial pacemaker. An atrial premature beat cannot be detected on auscultation unless it has an effect on the ventricular rhythm. This effect can vary. If the stimulus from the premature atrial contraction falls outside the refractory period of the ventricle, it will initiate a ventricular contraction which occurs earlier than expected, and the heart sounds and pulse will occur earlier than expected. If the sinus node becomes reset from the atrial premature beat a regular rhythm is established from this contraction, and in this case atrial premature beats will be detected by the occurrence of periods of regular rhythm interrupted by beats with exceptionally short inter-beat periods. In other instances the sinus node is not reset following the atrial premature contraction, and if its discharge occurs during the refractory period of the atrium then no atrial or subsequent ventricular contraction will occur. This will be detected clinically as an early ventricular contraction followed by a compensatory pause, following which normal rhythm is continued. This character is identical to that produced by many ventricular premature beats. If the stimulus from the atrial premature contraction falls within the refractory period of the ventricle, it will have no effect on ventricular rhythm and may go undetected on physical examination.

At slow heart rates the presence of atrial premature beats is suggested by periodic interruption of an underlying sinus rhythm and by the occurrence of a 'dropped pulse', or a pulse which is markedly decreased in amplitude. The prime differentiations to be made are from sinoatrial block and second-degree atrioventricular block.

On the ECG the P wave of the premature atrial systole is usually abnormal in configuration and occurs early. It may or may not be followed by a QRS complex. When these occur they usually have a normal configuration.

*Junctional premature beats* These arise from the region of the atrioventricular node or perinodal fibers. They produce a premature ventricular contraction which is usually followed by a compensatory pause, owing to the fact that the following normal discharge from the sinus node usually falls upon the ventricle during its refractory period. The P wave may be buried in the QRS-T complex and has a vector opposite to normal. The QRS configurations are normal.

*Ventricular premature beats* These may arise from an irritable focus anywhere within the ventricular myocardium. The normal rhythm is interrupted by a systole that occurs earlier than expected, but in most cases the initial rhythm is established following a compensatory pause (Fig. 14.9). This can be established by tapping through the arrhythmia as described earlier. The amplitude of the heart sounds associated with the premature beat is usually abnormal, whereas the first sound following the compensatory pause is usually accentuated. Occasionally ventricular premature beats may be interpolated in the normal rhythm and not followed by a compensatory pause.

If the diastolic filling period preceding the premature beat is short the pulse associated with it will

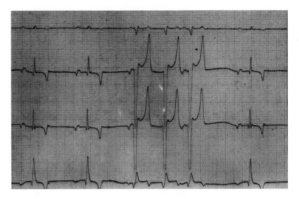
**Fig. 14.9** Ventricular premature systole.

be markedly decreased in amplitude or even absent. Ventricular premature beats are characterized on the ECG by QRS complexes which are bizarre and not preceded by a premature P wave. Conduction over non-specialized pathways results in a complex of greater duration and amplitude than normal, and the complex slurs into a T wave that is also of increased duration and magnitude and with a vector opposite to that of the ectopic QRS complex.

Premature systoles, regardless of their origin in the heart, are usually indicative of myocardial disease. Premature systoles that

- arise from more than one ectopic pacemaker
- are induced by exercise, or
- are associated with paroxysms of tachycardia

indicate severe myocardial disease. A common exception is atrial premature systoles accompanying cases of gastrointestinal diseases in cattle, that can progress to atrial fibrillation. Correction of the underlying cause will result in the return of normal cardiac rhythm.

## Arrhythmias with tachycardia

An ectopic excitable focus or foci within the myocardium may usurp the normal pacemaker in the heart if the discharge rate approaches or exceeds that of the sinoatrial node. Tachycardia may result from an irritant focus within the atria or the ventricles, and these cannot be differentiated on physical examination. Ventricular tachycardia is more common in large animals. Atrial tachycardia and atrial flutter occur rarely, except as transients preceding some cases of atrial fibrillation and in horses being treated for atrial fibrillation with quinidine.

---

### Clinical Pointer

Animals in which premature beats are detected or suspected should be examined after careful exercise, this will usually increase the occurrence and severity of the arrhythmia. Premature beats are most easily detected during the period of slowing of heart rate after exercise.

## Paroxysmal tachycardia

This is an abrupt increase in the heart rate with an equally sudden return to normal. This characteristic usually serves to distinguish this arrhythmia from the transient increases in heart rate that normally follow such factors as excitement. Also the heart rate is elevated to a rate in excess of that which would be normally expected from such stimuli. More commonly the excitable focus discharges repetitively over a long period to produce more continual tachycardia.

## Ventricular tachycardia

Tachycardia from an ectopic focus or foci within the ventricular myocardium may result in a regular or irregular heart rhythm. When the discharge rate of the irritant focus exceeds that of the sinoatrial pacemaker the ectopic focus will establish as the pacemaker, resulting in a rapid but regular heart rate.

The ECG reveals multiple regular QRS complexes that have a bizarre configuration and abnormal amplitude and duration. P waves may be detected but they have no relationship to the QRS-T complex and are frequently lost within them.

> ### Clinical Pointer
>
> - ventricular tachycardia should be considered in the differential diagnosis of tachycardia in any adult horse or cow where the heart rate exceeds 90 bpm at rest
> - it should be strongly suspected with heart rates in excess of 120 bpm
> - it should be suspected where the heart rate is elevated to a level higher than that expected from the animal's clinical condition.

When the discharge rate of the irritant focus within the myocardium is similar to that of the sinoatrial node the ventricular tachycardia can be manifested by a gross irregularity in rhythm. This is common in large animals. Most of the excitatory discharges that originate in the sinus fall on the ventricle during a refractory period from a previous extrasystole, but some reach the ventricle when it is not in a refractory state and are conducted normally. At some periods ventricular contractions may be initiated by the discharges from both sites. The varying influence of each pacemaker on ventricular contraction produces a marked irregularity in cardiac rhythm. Variations in the degree of atrial filling and in the diastolic filling period

result in variations in the intensity of the heart sounds and in the amplitude of the arterial pulse. At fast heart rates there is a pulse deficit. Cannon atrial waves occur in the jugular vein when atrial contraction occurs at the same time as a ventricular extrasystole. The ECG shows runs of ventricular extrasystoles with the characteristics mentioned earlier interspersed with normally conducted complexes, and usually the presence of fusion beats.

Tachycardia produced by ectopic foci in the ventricle is evidence of severe myocardial disease and is usually accompanied by signs of acute heart failure. It occurs with primary myocarditis, secondary to myocardial anoxia, with cardiotoxic plant poisonings in colitis-X in horses, and in severe electrolyte and acid–base disturbance. It is common in the final stages of heart failure and may lead to ventricular fibrillation and death. The severity of ventricular tachycardia is augmented by factors that increase sympathetic tone.

## Ventricular fibrillation

Ventricular fibrillation is the cause of death in most suddenly fatal diseases, including lightning stroke and acute *Phalaris* toxicity, and occurs terminally in the terminal phases of most acquired cardiac diseases. There is complete absence of the pulse and heart sounds, the blood pressure falls precipitously and the animal rapidly becomes unconscious and dies.

## Atrial fibrillation

Atrial fibrillation can occur in all species where there is atrial hypertrophy secondary to other cardiac lesions. It is one of the more common arrhythmias in large animals. In horses it may also be detected unexpectedly during an examination of an animal with no history of cardiac disease. In cattle it occurs most commonly in animals with abnormality of the gastrointestinal tract. In small animals, it occurs most commonly with dilated cardiomyopathy in large breed dogs. There is no synchronous atrial contraction in atrial fibrillation and atrioventricular nodal stimulation occurs in an irregular and random fashion from numerous independent fronts of excitation that course continuously and haphazardly through the atria. The clinical features of this arrhythmia are:

- exercise intolerance
- irregular heart rhythm and arterial pulse rhythm (unpredictable irregularity or irregular irregularity)
- absence of the atrial fourth heart sound
- accentuated third heart sound
- absence of a jugular a-wave

- an irregular variation in the level of jugular distension.

When the heart rate is fast there is also

- variable amplitude of the arterial pulses
- variable intensity of the first heart sound
- pulse deficit.

Atrial fibrillation cannot be detected directly by physical examination and clinical detection occurs through its effects on ventricular function. Random stimulation of the ventricles results in an irregular heart rhythm and arterial pulse rhythm. It is not possible to establish any basic pulse rhythm by tapping out this arrhythmia, and the rate varies in a seemingly chaotic fashion. Because there is no atrial contraction, filling of the ventricles is entirely passive and influenced by the diastolic filling time. Some ventricular contractions occur with little time for diastolic filling, and this produces a marked variation in the intensity of the heart sounds and in the amplitude of the pulse. At fast heart rates there will be a pulse deficit. There is no atrial fourth sound or atrial wave at the jugular inlet. The third heart sound is usually accentuated in the beat that follows a long diastolic interval.

The degree of cardiac insufficiency at rest depends upon the resting heart rate, which is determined primarily by vagal tone and the presence or absence of underlying cardiac disease. Horses with atrial fibrillation fall into two categories

1. those where the arrhythmia is secondary to heart disease
2. those with no evidence of underlying heart disease, sometimes called 'benign fibrillators'.

Benign fibrillators have high vagal tone and conduction through the atrioventricular node is suppressed, resulting in heart rates of approximately 26–48 bpm. At this rate there is no cardiac insufficiency at rest. The heart rate of the benign fibrillator will increase with exercise to allow moderate performance, although it will never perform satisfactorily as a racehorse. This is the most common manifestation in horses and is typified by a complete irregularity in rate, rhythm, and intensity of the heart sounds, and by the occurrence at rest of occasional periods lasting for 3–6 seconds where there is no ventricular activity. At very slow rates periodic syncope may rarely occur.

Where there is underlying heart disease the ventricular rate at rest is much higher and the arrhythmia is accompanied by tachycardia.

There are no P waves discernible on the ECG but the baseline shows multiple waveforms (f-waves) that occur with a frequency of between 300 and 600 bpm. QRS-T complexes are normal in configuration but there is marked temporal variation and no pattern in the QQ intervals.

**Atrial fibrillation in the horse**

The benign form of atrial fibrillation occurs most commonly in the larger breeds of horses, standard breeds, and Thoroughbreds. Racehorses have a history of normality at rest but poor exercise tolerance. There may be a history of sudden loss of performance and stamina, which may occur in the closing stages of a race. Other presenting signs include exercise-induced pulmonary hemorrhage. Once established it is common for the benign form of this arrhythmia to persist for the lifetime of the horse if not converted to normal sinus rhythm by suitable therapy. Occasionally, horses with paroxysmal atrial fibrillation have atrial fibrillation when examined immediately following the race, but convert to normal sinus rhythm shortly afterwards.

Horses with benign atrial fibrillation can be converted to normal sinus rhythm with quinidine sulfate therapy. The necessity for this depends upon the requirement for the horse to perform work, as horses with this arrhythmia can be retired and appear to live a normal life. They may be used successfully as brood mares. There is a greater success with conversion in young horses and when it is attempted shortly following the onset of the arrhythmia. If the arrhythmia has been present for more than 4 months successful conversion is much less common, side effects with therapy are more common, and there is a higher recurrence rate.

Horses may also develop atrial fibrillation in response to underlying cardiovascular disease. Commonly this is mitral valve insufficiency, tricuspid valve insufficiency, or a combination of both, but any acquired or congenital lesion that results in atrial hypertrophy carries this risk. Primary pulmonary hypertension leading to atrial hypertrophy is also a cause. Paroxysmal atrial fibrillation also can occur in newborn foals with respiratory distress and with birth anoxia. Where the arrhythmia is secondary to underlying heart disease it establishes with a high heart rate,

---

### Clinical Pointer

In the resting horse ventricular filling is impaired at heart valve rates above 80/min. At resting heart rates above 100/min the horse will show signs of cardiac insufficiency and cardiac failure.

> ### Clinical Pointer
>
> The treatment of horses with atrial fibrillation at high heart rates is generally unsuccessful as serious cardiac pathology is usually present. Digitalis and quinidine sulfate are used.

and affected horses usually rapidly develop congestive heart failure. In horses with atrial fibrillation a heart rate greater than 60 bpm at rest is suggestive of underlying cardiac disease.

### Atrial fibrillation in cattle

This occurs in association with myocardial disease or endocarditis and in these instances appears to result from the secondary atrial hypertrophy. More commonly it is detected in the absence of structural cardiac disease in association with gastrointestinal disease, with abnormalities causing abdominal pain, and in metabolic disorders such as

- hypocalcemia
- hypochloremia
- hypokalemia
- metabolic alkalosis
- respiratory alkalosis
- metabolic acidosis.

Abnormalities as diverse as left-sided displacement of the abomasum, and torsion of the uterus may be accompanied by this arrhythmia. In these cases heightened excitation of the atria owing to electrolyte and acid–base disturbances or to increased vagal tone lead to atrial premature systoles or atrial fibrillation.

Paroxysmal atrial fibrillation, lasting for a period of a few days and sometimes preceded by atrial premature contractions, also occurs in cows that are otherwise clinically normal. In cattle with atrial fibrillation the heart rate is elevated and grossly irregular and is sufficiently fast to result in a pulse deficit. In cases associated with gastrointestinal disease and in idiopathic cases there are usually no obvious signs of cardiac insufficiency or of congestive heart failure.

The administration of neostigmine to cattle with gastrointestinal disease may precipitate the occurrence of atrial fibrillation. Cattle with atrial fibrillation are not treated with specific antiarrhythmic drugs as the heart will revert to sinus rhythm following the correction of the underlying abdominal disorder.

### Atrial fibrillation in sheep and goats

This can occur where there is atrial hypertrophy secondary to other cardiac lesions. In the goat it is also a complication of interstitial pneumonia and cor pulmonale. The onset of fibrillation is manifest with the development of heart failure, with both severe respiratory distress and signs of right heart failure. The presenting signs are those of respiratory distress and heart failure. Ascites is prominent and there is marked jugular distension, with an irregular jugular pulse.

### Atrial fibrillation in the dog and cat

This is usually caused by abnormalities associated with atrial dilatation, including atrioventricular insufficiency, cardiomyopathy and, less commonly, congenital heart disease. It may occur in the absence of organic heart disease, particularly in giant breeds of dogs. Such individuals usually have slow to normal ventricular rates.

## ABNORMAL HEART SOUNDS

Abnormal heart sounds may originate from the heart and are either audible during a normally silent period of the cardiac cycle or they may overpower normal heart sounds. They include heart murmurs, pericardial friction sounds and, less commonly, other adventitious heart sounds.

### Heart murmurs

Heart murmurs are audible vibrations, caused by turbulent blood flow, that are transmitted to the surface of the thoracic wall. They may occur at any phase of the cardiac cycle. Vibrations of strong intensity may also result in palpable vibrations on the surface of the thoracic wall – a **precordial thrill**. Blood flow is normally laminar and without turbulence. Turbulent flow can be produced by a sudden change in the diameter of the vessel through which the blood is flowing, resulting in the generation of murmurs associated with stenosis or valve incompetence. However, turbulent flow and murmurs are not always due to valve abnormalities. A change from laminar to turbulent flow can occur when the velocity or volume of flow is high or blood viscosity is low. Turbulent flow is most likely when the velocity is high and the vessel large. Blood flow in the aorta of normal horses during the rapid ejection phase is often disturbed, resulting in the relatively common occurrence of ejection murmurs. A large volume of blood flowing with increased velocity through a normal valve orifice may also result in turbulent flow.

When a murmur is heard the diagnosis depends on an accurate determination of its

- location
- intensity
- timing
- duration
- quality
- radiation.

---

### Clinical Pointer

Low blood viscosity contributes to the frequency of murmurs occurring in anemic and hypoproteinemic states.

---

This requires a systematic auscultation of the heart. Other information, such as arterial pulse quality, changes in jugular pulsation, and secondary signs such as the occurrence of peripheral edema, assist in making the diagnosis, and for this reason the examination must include the arterial and venous systems. If the examination is not systematic it is easy to concentrate on listening to the murmur, to the exclusion of the other important diagnostic examinations.

Loud murmurs frequently override auscultatory findings at other periods of the cardiac cycle unless these periods are specifically examined. The systolic component of the murmur associated with a patent ductus arteriosus is loud and audible over a large area of the heart, and may mask the detection of the diastolic component, which can be much less intense and audible over a restricted area. Failure to detect the diastolic component will result in an inappropriate set of probable diagnoses.

Systematic auscultation of the heart requires that the total area of cardiac auscultation on both sides of the thoracic wall is examined. Also, each component of the cardiac cycle should be listened to separately in isolation. This is analogous to having four people all talking at the same time, but by focusing one can listen to and understand what one of them is saying and exclude the others. Thus the first sound is examined and categorized in terms of intensity and quality. The second sound is then examined and categorized by listening over the areas of maximal audibility of the aortic and pulmonic valves, and any temporal differences in closure noted. Then the interval between the first sound and the second sound is examined, followed by the interval between the second and the first sounds.

Heart murmurs are common in horses and physiological and pathological murmurs are frequently found in clinically normal animals. The task of the clinician is to determine the importance of a murmur with respect to the health and performance of the horse and the safety of the rider. In large farm animals the challenge is to determine the importance of the murmur to the health of the animal and to its future production efficiency. This requires a diagnosis as to cause and an assessment of its hemodynamic significance. A knowledge of the relative prevalence of cardiac diseases and murmurs for each species is useful in this assessment.

### Classification of heart murmurs

Murmurs are classified according to

- timing in the cardiac cycle
- intensity
- point of maximal intensity and radiation
- configuration
- quality
- presence of a precordial thrill.

**Timing in the cardiac cycle**

The timing of a cardiac murmur is described relative to the events of the cardiac cycle and may be systolic, diastolic or continuous:

- a systolic murmur occurs during systole in the interval between the first and the second heart sounds
- a diastolic murmur occurs in the interval between the second and the first heart sound
- a continuous murmur begins in systole and continues into diastole.

It is not difficult to distinguish between a systolic and diastolic murmur at slow heart rates because of the temporal difference between the length of the systolic and diastolic periods. However, where a murmur is present at rapid heart rates this distinction is less obvious and it is possible to misclassify the period of the cycle in which the murmur is occurring. For example, with the murmur associated with aortic insufficiency in the horse there is an accentuated third heart sound that may be mistaken for the first heart sound, resulting in misclassification of this diastolic murmur as systolic. This can be avoided by establishing which heart sound is the first and timing the murmur in relation to it. This is most accurately done by timing the occurrence of the heart sounds with the arterial pulse. With an artery close to the heart the arterial pulse occurs in early systole and the sound that immediately precedes it is the first heart sound. Other methods of determining the first heart sound, such as its being the loudest, or its occurrence synchronous with the palpated apex, are not advised. Although these are accurate in the normal heart, with some cardiac abnormalities the third heart sound can be very loud and vibrations associated with the rapid filling of the heart in early diastole can produce a palpable impulse at the thoracic wall.

Having determined the occurrence of the murmur in systole or diastole, systolic murmurs are further classified as early, late, holo- or pansystolic, according to their occurrence and duration in the period between the first and the second heart sounds. Diastolic murmurs are classified as early (occurring between S2 and S3), holodiastolic or presystolic (occurring between the atrial fourth heart sound and S1).

Systolic murmurs are caused by

- turbulent flow and vibrations during the phase of cardiac ejection
- stenosis of the aortic or pulmonic outflow valves, or
- insufficiency of the atrioventricular valves.

Diastolic murmurs are associated with

- turbulent flow or vibrations during the period of filling of the ventricles
- insufficiency of the aortic or pulmonic valves, or
- stenosis of the atrioventricular valves.

A continuous murmur present in both systole and diastole commonly results from the turbulent flow of blood from a high-pressure to a low-pressure system where there is no intervening valve, such as occurs with a patent ductus arteriosus, but it may be associated with

- stenosis and insufficiency of the same valve, or
- multiple valvular lesions.

In general, murmurs that occur throughout systole or diastole are more likely to be associated with problems that compromise cardiac function than those that occur, for example, only in early systole and early diastole.

Insufficiency of the atrioventricular valves (mitral and tricuspid), subaortic stenosis, and pulmonic stenosis all result in systolic murmurs. In Fig. 14.10 note that the second heart sound is present and that the murmur is confined to the systolic phase. This type of systolic murmur is referred to as holosystolic.

Pansystolic murmurs (Fig. 14.11) extend into early diastole and obliterate the second heart sound. This type of murmur is common in small-breed dogs with mitral insufficiency. In this condition the left ventricular pressure remains greater than the left atrial pressure when the aortic valve closes (S2), turbulent regurgitation of blood into the left atrium continues and the murmur extends into diastole.

Diastolic murmurs are uncommon, but their occurrence almost always indicates the presence of significant heart disease (Figure 14.12). Diastolic

## Clinical Pointer

To time the heart sounds with the pulse it is usually easier to detect the arterial pulse by palpation first and then, having found it, to listen simultaneously to the heart sounds.

murmurs are usually soft in intensity and occur between S2 and S1.

The most common causes of diastolic murmurs in small animals are aortic valvular insufficiency (secondary to infective endocarditis) and pulmonic valvular insufficiency (secondary to heartworm disease). Other, more unusual causes include aortic insufficiency due to ventricular septal defect and aortic valvular prolapse and mitral stenosis (congenital or acquired).

Continuous heart murmurs begin in systole and continue into diastole (Fig. 14.13). Such a murmur is strongly indicative of the presence of a patent ductus arteriosus, a defect where there is continuous shunting of blood from the aorta to the main pulmonary artery.

### Intensity

The intensity or loudness of a murmur can be graded subjectively using two systems

- a 6-grade basis, and
- a 5-grade basis.

They differ only in their categorization of moderately loud and loud murmurs (Table 14.3).

## Clinical Pointer

Take care to check all valve areas during cardiac auscultation. In many puppies with a PDA, the characteristic continuous machinery-type murmur is only present at the aortic or pulmonic areas, whereas a prominent systolic murmur is present at the mitral area.

### Point of maximal intensity and radiation

The location of the point of maximal intensity (PMI) of a murmur is related to its area of generation and transmission and may be related to the audibility of the heart valves. The sound of a murmur may radiate from its point of maximal intensity. Commonly this is 'downstream' and occasionally 'upstream' with

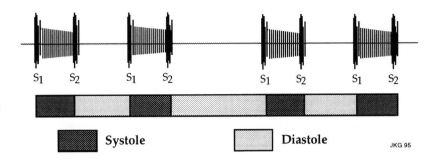

**Fig. 14.10** Phonocardiogram of a holosystolic murmur. In this example, both S1 and S2 as well as the murmur are audible.

Systole    Diastole

JKG 95

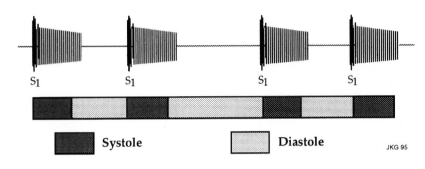

**Fig. 14.11** Phonocardiogram of a pansystolic murmur. In this example, only S1 and the murmur are audible.

Systole    Diastole

JKG 95

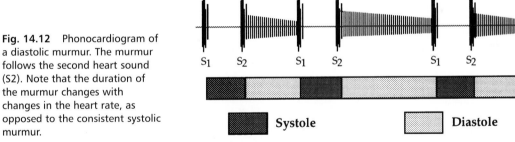

**Fig. 14.12** Phonocardiogram of a diastolic murmur. The murmur follows the second heart sound (S2). Note that the duration of the murmur changes with changes in the heart rate, as opposed to the consistent systolic murmur.

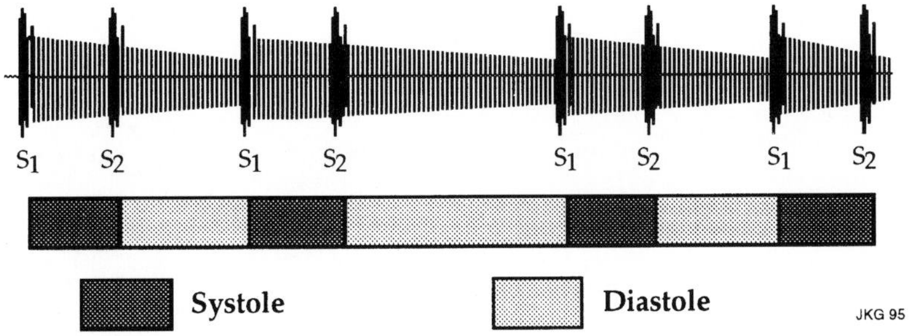

Systole    Diastole

JKG 95

**Fig. 14.13** Phonocardiogram of a continuous murmur. The intensity typically wanes through diastole, as the aortic pressure and shunt magnitude decrease.

Systole    Diastole

JKG 95

| Table 14.3. Gradations of intensity of heart murmurs |
| --- |

*Intensity measured with six gradations*

**Grade 1**  A faint murmur that can be heard only after careful auscultation over a localized area.

**Grade 2**  A quiet murmur that is heard immediately the stethoscope is placed over its localized point of maximal intensity.

**Grade 3**  A moderately loud murmur.

**Grade 4**  A loud murmur heard over a widespread area with no thrill palpable.

**Grade 5**  A loud murmur with an associated precordial thrill.

**Grade 6**  A murmur sufficiently loud that it can be heard with a stethoscope raised just off the chest surface.

*Intensity measured with five gradations*

**Grade I**  The faintest audible murmur. Generally only detected after careful auscultation.

**Grade II**  A faint murmur that is clearly heard after only a few seconds' auscultation.

**Grade III**  A loud murmur which is immediately audible as soon as auscultation begins and is heard over a reasonably large area.

**Grade IV**  An extremely loud murmur accompanied by a thrill. The murmur becomes inaudible if the stethoscope is held with only light pressure on the chest.

**Grade V**  An extremely loud murmur accompanied by a thrill. The murmur can still be heard when the stethoscope is held with only light pressure against the chest.

reference to blood flow occurring at the site and time of the murmur. These characteristics can be of value in further defining the type and cause of the murmur. Low-intensity murmurs are generally restricted to the auscultatory area overlying their area of generation. Murmurs and thrills can be restricted to local areas and it is essential to examine all auscultatory areas of both sides of the heart.

## Configuration

A description of the change in the intensity of a murmur during its production is known as its configuration. The murmur is described as

- crescendo
- crescendo–decrescendo
- decrescendo, or
- plateau.

These patterns are determined by the pathophysiology of the lesion responsible for the murmur. Mitral valve regurgitation (MR), for example, begins early in systole. Except in very severe MR the pressure gradient between the left atrium and left ventricle is maintained throughout systole and the resultant murmur has a plateau shape; it begins coincident with the first heart sound and may obscure the second. Plateau-shaped murmurs are often described as 'regurgitant'. In contrast, the pressure gradient between the left ventricle and aorta that is present in aortic stenosis develops during the course of ventricular systole and peaks at midsystole, resulting in a crescendo–decrescendo or 'ejection' murmur. The terms ejection murmur and regurgitant murmur have the distinct limitation that they lack specificity. A ventricular septal defect, for instance, results in a plateau-shaped murmur similar to the one that arises from AV valve regurgitation. This is because the genesis of these murmurs is similar: both arise because of a pressure gradient that persists throughout systole. The terms holosystolic and pansystolic have been inconsistently defined and applied. Some authors use them as synonyms, whereas others make a distinction between holosystolic murmurs that end before the second heart sound and pansystolic murmurs which obscure S2. As these terms are generally meant to convey information regarding pathophysiology, it is probably preferable to use descriptions of murmur quality and configuration. For example, crescendo–descrescendo midsystolic clearly refers to the type of murmur that results from stenosis of the ventricular outflow tract.

## Quality

Murmurs may also be described according to their frequency characteristics by terms such as blowing, harsh, musical, or sighing, but these interpretations are very subjective and often not repeatable between examiners. Quality types include machinery, regurgitant, and ejection

- a machinery murmur is almost always associated with the continuous murmur of patent ductus arteriosus

- regurgitant murmurs are coarse and do not change much in intensity through systole or diastole (Fig. 14.14a)
- ejection murmurs have a build-up (crescendo) followed by a waning (decrescendo) (Fig. 14.14b).

The murmur of subaortic stenosis is typically ejection in type, whereas that of mitral insufficiency is typically regurgitant.

### Presence of precordial thrill

This is a sensation of vibration felt on palpation over the point of maximal intensity of the murmur and on the thoracic wall over other areas of the heart. The presence of a thrill indicates that there is considerable energy generated by the turbulent flow, and defines the intensity of the murmur in the top two grades in both grading systems.

## Interpretation of murmurs

The defect in function producing the murmur and the valve involved are determined from the characteristics of the point of maximal intensity and radiation, the timing in the cardiac cycle and the intensity and character, and also from any secondary effects that may be present in arterial or venous pulse characteristics. The cause of the lesion cannot be determined from auscultation but may be determined from the results of general clinical and special pathological examinations, and by a consideration of the prevalence of causes of valvular disease that involve the particular valve affected in the animal species being examined.

## Innocent murmurs

Murmurs not associated with a cardiac defect are called innocent. Those caused by turbulence during periods of high-velocity flow are called **functional** or **flow** murmurs; those associated with turbulence due to decreased viscosity and increased flow are called **physiological.** Innocent murmurs occur in all large animal species and particularly in the horse, and must be differ-

---

### The importance of murmurs to health

The importance of a cardiac murmur to health is determined not just by its intensity, but by an assessment of hemodynamic significance and cardiac function. In general the following are all considered pathological

- holodiastolic murmurs
- pansystolic mitral or tricuspid murmurs
- murmurs accompanied by a precordial thrill.

---

entiated from pathological murmurs. The common innocent murmurs in large animals are described below.

### Functional ejection murmurs

These are common in the horse and occur occasionally in cattle, sheep, and pigs. They are detected more commonly in young and fit horses. Functional systolic murmurs are usually low intensity (grade 1–3/6), early to midsystolic and crescendo–decrescendo or decrescendo in character. They are best heard over the base of the heart, usually on the left side and in some horses on the right side, but not on both sides in the same horse. In some horses they are more audible at heart rates slightly elevated above resting. In cattle they are most common at the left base of the heart. Occasionally in horses an ejection murmur is audible over the pulmonary valve. Ejection murmurs are believed to be associated with turbulent blood flow during the rapid ejection phase in early systole. They occur in the absence of any evidence of cardiac insufficiency. Holosystolic murmurs (grade 1–3/6) are heard in some calves in the first 2–3 weeks of life. They are probably associated with minor deformation of the atrioventricular valves by hemacysts at the edge of the valve leaflets. These are common in young calves and resolve with age.

### Early diastolic murmur in horses

This is a soft (grade 1–2/6) high-pitched early diastolic murmur that is usually heard over the mitral valve area and is believed to be due to vibrations associated with

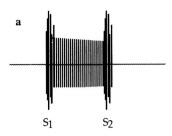

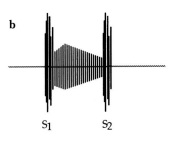

**Figure 14.14** In a, a phonocardiogram of a regurgitant-type murmur; in b, an ejection-type murmur is present. Note the waning intensity of the ejection-type murmur.

the rapid flow of blood into the heart in early diastole. It is heard more commonly in Thoroughbreds and standard breeds than other breeds, and occurs mainly in younger horses. When heard over the apex area it is probably a variation of the S3 sound.

### Presystolic murmur

This is a soft (grade 1–2/6) rumbling murmur that is occasionally heard in horses and is probably a component of the atrial A sound.

### Murmurs in recumbent animals

A low-intensity (grade 1–3/6) crescendo–decrescendo systolic murmur is frequently heard over the right side of the heart in recumbent cattle. It will disappear when the animal stands. A similar murmur occurs where there is ruminal distension and bloat.

### Hemic murmurs

Hemic murmurs occur in animals that are anemic and hypoproteinemic. They are low-intensity (grade 1–3/6), crescendo–decrescendo early to midsystolic murmurs detected at the area of the tricuspid valve. The intensity fluctuates with respiration, increasing with inspiration and decreasing with expiration.

### Murmurs in newborn animals

A continuous or a systolic murmur is frequently audible over the base of the heart in newborn animals owing to a partial temporary patency of the closing ductus arteriosus.

## Valvular disease and heart murmurs

In large animals nearly all valvular lesions are acquired and the murmurs are produced by valvular insufficiency. The common murmurs are those associated with mitral, tricuspid, or aortic valve insufficiency. Pansystolic or holosystolic plateau-type murmurs with the PMI over the atrioventricular valve are typical of mitral or tricuspid regurgitation. Holodiastolic, decrescendo murmurs with the PMI over the heart base are typical of aortic valve regurgitation.

In cattle, sheep and pigs valvular lesions are commonly the result of bacterial endocarditis. In horses bacterial endocarditis is uncommon and the valvular lesions are usually due to myxomatous degeneration of unknown etiology. Murmurs associated with valvular insufficiency can be present in animals that have little evidence of impaired cardiovascular function. In the horse their significance needs to be assessed by performance testing. In small animals, valvular abnormalities may be congenitally (especially aortic and pulmonic stenosis) or acquired (mitral and tricuspid insufficiency).

### Mitral valve insufficiency

This is common in horses, cattle, pigs and dogs. In large animals it tends to result from endocarditis or rupture of the mitral valve chordae. In small animals it tends to be the result of degenerative changes on the valve leaflets. Mitral murmurs are loudest over the left cardiac apex (dog, horse) or the 4th intercostal space (cattle). There is a loud harsh holosystolic or pansystolic plateau-type murmur that is most intense in the mitral area. The murmur radiates dorsally and cranially, and in severe cases may also be heard on the right side. In large animals frequently there is modification of the first and second heart sounds, with marked accentuation of the occurrence of a third heart sound, which may be mistaken for the second. The pulse characters are unchanged until the stage of cardiac failure ensues. Cases of mitral insufficiency may compensate at rest and may only be evident as decreased work tolerance. Failure, if it occurs, will be initially associated with left ventricular volume overload. However, in some cases the retrograde flow of blood through the mitral valve may lead to pulmonary hypertension and the additional occurrence of right-sided heart failure. Acute-onset heart failure is usually associated with rupture of the valve chordae. In the horse mitral insufficiency may predispose to atrial fibrillation.

In all species insufficiency of the mitral valve may result from an inflammatory condition known as endocarditis, or from rupture of the mitral valve chordae.

### Tricuspid valve insufficiency

This is the most common acquired valvular lesion in cattle, pigs, and sheep and is due to endocarditis. Insufficiency may also result from dilatation of the valve annulus associated with chronic anemia, and from cor pulmonale in conditions such as high-altitude disease in cattle. Tricuspid regurgitation can also develop secondary to left-sided cardiac disease and pulmonary hypertension. Because of the association with bacterial endocarditis tricuspid insufficiency in

> ### Assessment of murmurs
>
> - an echocardiogram can give an objective assessment of the hemodynamic significance of a murmur
> - Doppler echocardiography can indicate whether valvular regurgitation is present and semi-quantify its severity
> - Doppler echocardiography can detect clinically silent regurgitation.

---

### Mitral valve insufficiency in dogs

- this is the most common acquired valvular disease in dogs
- it occurs typically in the older, small breeds
- it often follows tricuspid insufficiency
- it is thought to be due to a degenerative or aging phenomenon, with deposition of mucopolysaccharide on valve leaflets, a process known as endocardiosis.
- the valve undergoes non-inflammatory degenerative change, resulting in thickening and shortening of the leaflets, and thickening and shortening of the chordae tendinae.

---

cattle, pigs, and sheep is usually indicative of significant cardiac disease. However, in horses the murmur of tricuspid insufficiency may be present with little evidence of impaired performance. There is a harsh holosystolic or usually pansystolic murmur that is most audible over the tricuspid valve area. In cattle this is low over the costochondral area. Murmurs of high intensity radiate dorsally and to the cranial part of the thoracic cavity on both right and left sides. The valvular insufficiency is usually accompanied by an exaggeration of the v-wave in the jugular vein. Severe lesions are accompanied by congestive heart failure.

In dogs the murmur associated with tricuspid insufficiency is similar to that of mitral insufficiency, and in many instances the development of tricuspid disease is usually followed by the appearance of mitral disease. In such instances the existence of tricuspid insufficiency is difficult to determine because the systolic mitral murmur is often transmitted to the right side of the chest.

### Cor pulmonale

Cor pulmonale is the syndrome of right heart failure resulting from an increase in right heart workload secondary to increased pulmonary vascular resistance and pulmonary hypertension. It is accompanied by tricuspid insufficiency associated with cardiac hypertrophy and dilatation of the tricuspid valve annulus.

Acute alveolar hypoxia results in contraction of the precapillary pulmonary vessels and is a potent cause of pulmonary hypertension, particularly in cattle. Prolonged hypoxia and persistent pulmonary vasoconstriction results in medial muscular hypertrophy of the small pulmonary arteries and arterioles and a further increase in pulmonary vascular resistance. This mechanism by itself may produce cardiac insufficiency in cattle living at high altitudes, usually above 2200 m, and is also known as **high-altitude disease**.

Pulmonary hypertension can also result from partial destruction of the pulmonary vascular bed and a reduction in its total cross-sectional area. Pulmonary thromboembolic disease can produce right heart insufficiency by this mechanism. Chronic interstitial pneumonia and emphysema in cattle and chronic obstructive pulmonary disease in horses can induce cor pulmonale. Heart failure more commonly occurs when additional cardiac stress is superimposed, for example by

- pregnancy
- moderate altitude anoxia in cattle
- the development of atrial fibrillation.

Atrial fibrillation as a sequelae to cor pulmonale and leading to acute-onset heart failure is a sequela of interstitial pneumonia in goats, and cor pulmonale can lead to atrial fibrillation in horses.

### Stenosis of the mitral or tricuspid valve

Stenosis of either atrioventricular valve is uncommon in all species. There is a diastolic murmur caused by the passage of blood through a narrow valve during diastolic filling and audible over the base of the heart on the relevant side. The severity of the lesion will govern the duration of the murmur, but there is likely to be a presystolic accentuation due to atrial contraction. Right atrioventricular valve stenosis may be accompanied by accentuation of the atrial component of the jugular pulse. It is possible that some degree of mitral stenosis may occur in acquired lesions that manifest primarily as an insufficiency.

### Stenosis or insufficiency of the pulmonary valve

Acquired and congenital lesions of this valve are rare in large animals. In dogs, pulmonary valve insufficiency has been noted in *Dirofilaria immitis* infestation. The murmur is maximally audible over the left heart base at the level of the costochondral articulations. The signs are similar to those produced by aortic valve lesions, except that there are no pulse abnormalities. Differentiation may be difficult in such cases.

### Stenosis of the aortic valve

This is a common congenital heart defect in the dog. There is a harsh systolic murmur, most audible dorsally and caudally over the base of the heart on the left side. In the dog it is of maximum intensity in the 4th left intercostal space on a horizontal line through the shoulder joint; in the horse it is most audible midway up the 5th intercostal space on the left side. The murmur replaces or modifies the first heart sound and is often crescendo–decrescendo in character. A systolic thrill may be palpable over the base of the heart and

## Pulmonic stenosis in dogs

- it is the third most common congenital heart defect in dogs
- it causes a systolic murmur which is most intense over the left heart base at or below the level of the costochondral articulations
- pulmonary valve lesions are more audible cranial to the aortic valve area on the left side of the thorax
- heart failure, if it occurs, is right-sided.

the cardiac impulse is increased because of ventricular hypertrophy. Occasionally, the murmur radiates up the carotid arteries to the top of the dog's head. The stenosis has most functional significance when the pulse is abnormal, with a small amplitude rising slowly to a delayed peak, reflecting the diminished left ventricular output. There may be signs of left-sided heart failure and this lesion may also be associated with syncope. In dogs the murmur may be an incidental finding with no clinical signs. In some animals sudden death may occur because of a rhythm disturbance.

**Aortic valve insufficiency**
This is a common acquired valvular defect in the horse. There is a loud holodiastolic murmur, frequently accompanied by a thrill caused by the reflux of blood from the aorta into the left ventricle during diastole. The murmur is generally audible over the left cardiac area, is most intense at the aortic valve area, and radiates to the apex. It may modify the second heart sound but usually starts immediately following it. The intensity varies from case to case and the murmur may be noisy or musical. Frequently it is decrescendo in character, but other variations in intensity occur. The murmur is common in older horses and its significance to cardiovascular function must be assessed by exercise tolerance.

The diastolic murmur arising from aortic insufficiency in dogs is uncommon and most often due to

bacterial endocarditis. It is usually high pitched in type and of maximum intensity in the 4th left intercostal space, just below a horizontal line through the shoulder joint.

**Endocarditis**
Endocarditis can occur as mural or valvular infection. Most frequently it occurs – or is detected – as a valvular endocarditis. It can involve any valve, although each species has its particular predilections. In the horse, and dog, the mitral and aortic valves are more commonly affected than the tricuspid, whereas in cattle, pigs and sheep the tricuspid is most commonly affected and the mitral is second in predilection. Endocarditis is a risk where there is a chronic and prolonged bacteremia with a primary focus from an ongoing septic process, such as

- sole abscess
- mastitis
- metritis
- traumatic reticuloperitonitis
- liver abscess.
- periodontal disease in dogs

Commonly there is a presenting history of ill-thrift and of periodic attacks of malaise, anorexia, listlessness, lameness, pyrexia and, in dairy cattle, transient but dramatic falls in milk yield. Horses have a history of poor exercise tolerance and poor performance.

The clinical findings on physical examination are related to chronic bacteremia, septic emboli, and signs referable to the valve lesion. Thus these can be moderate, fluctuating fever, and secondary involvement of other organs may cause the appearance of signs of

- peripheral lymphadenitis
- embolic pneumonia
- nephritis
- arthritis
- tenosynovitis, or
- myocarditis.

In addition there are changes in the hemogram strongly suggestive of a chronic septic process, with varying degrees of anemia, leukocytosis and left shift, elevated fibrinogen, hypoalbuminemia, and elevated globulins.

## Clinical Pointer

Aortic valve insufficiency of functional significance is accompanied by an arterial pulse of very large amplitude and high systolic and low diastolic blood pressures (water hammer pulse). The pulse wave may be great enough to cause a visible pulse in small peripheral vessels.

## Clinical Pointer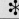

Intermittent and shifting lameness is a common complaint in the history of animals presented with endocarditis.

Blood cultures should be attempted, but a single sampling is frequently negative and repeated samples should be taken. Determination of the sensitivity of the organism to antibacterial drugs may aid in treatment.

The signs referable to damage to individual heart valves and the specific findings on auscultation are detailed above. Some cases of valvular endocarditis and cases of mural endocarditis in cattle can present with a history as above, but on auscultation have an elevated heart rate and a loud pounding heart but no detectable murmurs.

The course in endocarditis may be as long as several weeks or months, or animals may die following a rapid onset of heart failure. Endocarditis may predispose to rupture of the chordae tendinea of the mitral valve or of the medial cusp of the aortic valve, producing acute left heart failure in horses.

### Congenital cardiac abnormalities causing heart murmurs

Congenital cardiac anomalies occur in all animal species but are not common in any one of them. Some are simple and others are complex. The age at manifestation varies between and within the individual defects, depending upon the extent of cardiac insufficiency. Some are clinically manifest at birth, whereas others result in cardiac insufficiency later in life or not at all. Atrial septal defects are common at necropsy in cattle but are rarely clinically manifest. There are apparent differences between species in the prevalence of these defects and, for example, atrial septal defects are more common in calves and pigs than in foals or lambs. Ventricular septal defect and patent ductus arteriosus are among the more common anomalies and have features that allow a tentative diagnosis from physical examination.

#### Ventricular septal defects

Ventricular septal defects are one of the more common congenital cardiac defects in sheep, cattle, and horses. They are usually subaortic and occur high in the membranous portion of the interventricular septum. In the absence of other defects their presence results in the shunting of blood from the left to the right ventricle, under the septal leaflet of the tricuspid valve.

The magnitude of the shunt and the fate of the animal are determined by the size of the defect and the degree of resistance to flow from the right ventricle, as determined by pulmonary vascular resistance and the size of the defect. Animals with large defects and a large shunt may die at birth or show lassitude, growth depression, and dyspnea on moderate exercise at a few weeks to a few months of age. Horses may present with a history of poor performance when they begin athletic work. Less severe shunts may not result in obvious cardiac insufficiency and the defect may be detected incidentally during examination of the animal for other reasons, or incidentally at necropsy. The defect produces a flow load on the left and right ventricles and, depending on the degree of increase in pulmonary vascular resistance, a pressure load on the right ventricle. An increase in pulmonary vascular resistance occurs as the result of increased pulmonary blood flow. In cattle this increase may be sufficient to cause reversal of the shunt, and cyanosis develops. This syndrome, sometimes referred to as an Eisenmenger complex, develops most commonly between 1 and 3 years of age.

On auscultation there is a loud harsh pansystolic murmur audible over a large area on both sides, but most intense at the left 4th and 5th intercostal spaces and on the right side at the sternal border ventral to the tricuspid valve. The murmur is more intense on the right than the left, and is one of the loudest and most obvious murmurs encountered. A pronounced precordial thrill is palpable on the right side at the sternal border, and frequently also on the left thoracic wall over the mitral area.

Turbulence associated with flow across the defect may produce secondary changes in the valves located close to the defect. Cattle are prone to develop endocarditis in the region of the septal cusp of the right atrioventricular valve. Horses may prolapse the medial cusp of the aortic valve into the septal defect, or rupture the medial cusp, with the consequent development of aortic insufficiency and acute left heart failure.

Ventricular septal defects may occur in association with other congenital cardiac or vascular defects.

The signs of heart failure, if present, vary. The defect produces a flow load on the left and right ventricles and, depending on the degree of increase in

---

### Complex congenital cardiac defects

These can rarely be diagnosed accurately by physical examination and require special examination, particularly echocardiography, for differentiation.

---

### Clinical Pointer

A sudden onset of cyanosis and exercise intolerance in an animal between 1 and 3 years of age is highly indicative of ventricular septal defect.

pulmonary vascular resistance, a pressure load on the right ventricle. Signs of acute left-sided failure are usually evident in animals dying with this defect at or shortly following birth, whereas in cattle right-sided congestive heart failure is more common in later life. In cats the murmur may be an incidental finding. If the defect is large the kitten will fail to grow and may develop signs of heart failure at an early age.

### Patent ductus arteriosus

This defect results from failure of the ductus arteriosus to close following birth. There is a loud continuous murmur of variable intensity associated with the shunting of blood from the aorta to the pulmonary artery. The intensity waxes and wanes with each cycle owing to the effects of normal pressure changes on blood flow, giving rise to the term 'machinery murmur'. The systolic component is very loud and usually audible over most of the cardiac auscultatory area. It may be accompanied by a precordial thrill. The diastolic component is much softer and confined to the base of the heart just dorsal to the aortic valve area. Without careful auscultation of the area this component may be missed and the type of murmur misdiagnosed. The pulse is large in amplitude but has a low diastolic pressure.

Patent ductus arteriosus is probably the second most common defect in horses after ventricular septal defect, and is one of the most prevalent cardiac defects in dogs. Predisposed breeds include the Miniature Poodle, Collie, Sheltie and Pomeranian. Surgical ligation of the ductus arteriosus is a recommended option.

### Tetralogy of Fallot

This is almost always lethal. The tetralogy consists of
- a ventricular septal defect
- pulmonary stenosis
- dextral position of the aorta so that it overrides both ventricles
- secondary right ventricular hypertrophy.

---

### Patent ductus arteriosus in normal animals

Murmurs associated with a patent ductus arteriosus can be heard during the first day after birth in normal animals owing to a partial temporary patency of the closing ductus arteriosus. The continuous murmur may persist for periods up to 5 days and the systolic component up to 2 weeks. When these are detected the animal should be re-examined later in the neonatal period to determine whether the ductus has closed and the murmur is no longer present.

---

The marked increase in resistance to outflow into the pulmonary artery results in right-to-left shunting, with the major outflow of blood through the aorta. The condition presents with clinical signs very early in life, frequently results in death at or shortly following birth, and has been reported predominantly in foals, calves, and dogs. The Keeshond is a breed of dog predisposed to this congenital defect. Occasionally affected animals may live for longer periods and a case is recorded in a 3-year-old mare. Affected animals show lassitude and dyspnea after minor exertion such as suckling. Cyanosis may or may not be present, depending upon the degree of pulmonary stenosis, but is usually prominent, especially following exercise. On auscultation a murmur and sometimes a thrill is present, and is most intense in the left 3rd or 4th intercostal spaces. Diagnosis can be confirmed by cardiac catheter pressure measurements, by detecting a shunt by the dye dilution curve, by blood gas analysis and angiocardiography, and by echocardiography.

### Endocardial fibroelastosis

Congenital endocardial fibroelastosis has been observed in calves, pigs, dogs, and cats. The endocardium is converted into a thick fibroelastic coat, and although the wall of the left ventricle is hypertrophied the capacity of the ventricle is reduced. The aortic valves may be thickened and irregular, and obviously stenotic. In all species the cause is unknown. The syndrome is one of congestive heart failure, but there are no signs that indicate the presence of specific lesions of the myocardium, endocardium, or pericardium. On the other hand, the defect may cause no clinical abnormality until the animal is mature.

### Subvalvular aortic stenosis

Subaortic stenosis is one of the most common congenital inherited heart defects in the dog. Breeds predisposed include the Newfoundland, German Shepherd, Boxer, Golden Retriever, Rottweiler, Bull Terrier, Bouvier de Flandres, and Bernese Mountain Dog. The animal may remain asymptomatic or experience syncope and sudden death. Stenosis of the aorta at or just below the point of attachment of the aortic semilunar valves has been recorded as a common, possibly heritable, defect in pigs.

## Friction sounds

### Pericardial friction sounds

These are audible vibrations heard over the thorax produced by friction occurring with movement of the heart in an inflamed pericardial sac. **Pericarditis** is a

Clinical Pointer

### Clinical Pointer

Animals with subvalvular aortic stenosis may die suddenly with asphyxia, dyspnea, and foaming at the mouth and nostrils, or after a long period of ill-health with recurrent attacks of dyspnea. In the acute form death may occur after exercise or be unassociated with exertion.

### Clinical Pointer

The character of pericardial friction sounds varies between cases and daily within a case. Usually it is consistent during any one examination period.

common accompaniment of several systemic infections and may occur by extension from bronchopneumonia. It can be severe or may be clinically silent. It occurs in horses, and in cattle is most commonly associated with foreign-body penetration from the reticulum. In the early stages of pericarditis the loss of the smooth lubricating surface results in pericardial friction sounds.

Pericardial friction sounds generally have a to-and-fro rubbing character (Fig 14.15). They may be restricted to one part of the cardiac cycle but are synchronous with it. If gas is present fluid-splashing ('washing machine') sounds will be heard.

An increase in the volume of pericardial fluid results in muffling of the heart sounds, a decreased intensity of the apex beat and an increase in the area of cardiac dullness. There is general venous congestion, most easily observed by engorgement of the jugular veins. The a-wave of the jugular pulsations is pronounced. The arterial pulse amplitude is poor. Death may occur at this stage, or the animal may survive and the condition progress to that of chronic fibrinous inflammation resulting in chronic constrictive pericarditis. Cardiac insufficiency results from a filling defect, with a decrease in the diastolic reserve volume and the stroke volume. Myocarditis may occur from extension of the primary lesion.

Fever, depression, toxemia, and reluctance to move are evident and cattle may stand with the thoracic wall fixed and the elbows abducted. Evidence of pain may be elicited by percussion over the cardiac region of the sternum.

The following triad is typical of pericardial tamponade.

- venous congestion
- muffling of heart sounds,
- decreased arterial pulse pressure

### Pleural–pericardial friction sounds

These occur in cattle with adhesions between the pleura and the pericardium. They are squeaky sounds of low intensity that occur at the peak of inspiration, usually during systole. They may have a metallic 'click' quality.

## OTHER ADVENTITIOUS HEART SOUNDS

### Systolic clicks

A clicking sound occurring in midsystole is heard during auscultation in some horses. Its genesis is unknown but its occurrence does not appear to be associated with impaired cardiac performance. In small animals brief, sharp, non-resonant sounds occurring during systole are typically heard in middle-aged small-breed dogs with early degenerative valve disease. Such sounds have been attributed to prolapse of the mitral valve leaflets. They are of similar frequency to the first and second heart sounds but lower in intensity

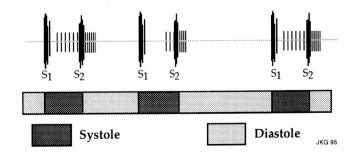

**Fig. 14.15** Pericardial friction sounds. Note the to-and-fro pattern and the slight variation in intensity and character from beat to beat.

(Fig. 14.16). First impressions may cause one to suspect a gallop rhythm, as three heart sounds are heard; however, once the landmark first and second heart sounds are identified the extra sound can be timed to midsystole. A soft systolic murmur of mitral insufficiency often accompanies a systolic click.

Sounds generated in areas of the body other than the heart may be heard over the area of cardiac auscultation. These include

- friction sounds of the skin and hair on the stethoscope head
- sounds associated with respiration
- sounds referred from the abdomen.

The same method of exclusion as mentioned above can be used to exclude these sounds while auscultating the heart.

## SPECIAL EXAMINATION OF THE CARDIOVASCULAR SYSTEM

Evidence of subclinical cardiovascular disease is sometimes detected incidentally during routine veterinary examinations. However, cardiovascular disease becomes clinically apparent when there are signs of diminished cardiac performance. The clinical signs of cardiovascular disease are often associated with the development of congestive heart failure (CHF), although syncope, exercise intolerance, or failure to thrive can certainly be observed in its absence.

Congestive heart failure (CHF) is a syndrome that is a potential consequence of virtually any cardiac disease. When the disease that has resulted in the development of CHF cannot be eliminated or reversed, the syndrome is associated with an inexorable decline in cardiac performance and, ultimately, death. Thus the prognosis in CHF is typically unfavorable. This holds true for all species

- if pulmonary edema develops in a dog with mitral valve endocardiosis, death is likely within 6–12 months even with palliative medical therapy

- horses that develop pulmonary edema as a consequence of aortic valve incompetence have a survival that is generally measured in months.

Also, it is important to recognize that CHF is simply a syndrome of cardiac dysfunction and associated neuroendocrine abnormalities. It is not a specific disease, but rather the potential outcome of cardiac disease. Of the cardiac diseases that result in CHF, most have a chronic and progressive course associated with the development of myocardial hypertrophy and activation of other compensatory mechanisms that temporarily preserve cardiac performance. Because of this, enlargement of the cardiac chambers generally precedes the development of CHF.

Although CHF is a potential outcome of many cardiac diseases, there are some disorders that cause morbidity through different avenues. For example, when arrhythmias develop in the absence of structural cardiac disease, clinical manifestations may include syncope, exercise intolerance and sudden death.

Evaluation of the patient's history and undertaking a thorough physical examination form the basis for the clinical investigation of cardiovascular disease. Special diagnostic studies, such as electrocardiography, thoracic radiography, and echocardiography, are chosen depending on the nature of the clinical problems identified. The components of the non-

---

### Objective of the cardiovascular examination

In the most general sense it is the objective of the cardiovascular examination to answer the following questions.

- What is the cardiac rate and rhythm?
- Is the heart enlarged?
- Is congestive heart failure present?
- If congestive heart failure is present, what is the disease that has caused it?

---

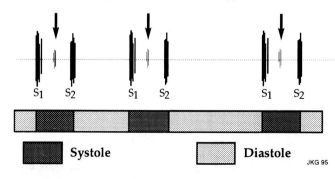

**Fig. 14.16** Systolic clicks arrows are brief, high-frequency sounds occurring in early to mid-systole.

invasive cardiovascular examination provide information that is distinct but complementary. Each diagnostic test has not only a specific utility, but also limitations. An appraisal of the clinically available means to evaluate the cardiovascular system follows. The utility of each diagnostic modality is assessed with respect to the basic objectives of the cardiovascular examination.

Electrocardiography, radiography, echocardiography, and methods for indirect determination of blood pressure are available in some general practices, specialist clinics, and teaching hospitals.

The prevalence and economic importance of cardiovascular disease in large animals that requires examination by these methods is generally not significant enough to warrant their use in a general practice. Furthermore, spurious and misleading readings can be obtained with such equipment if the principles underlying its use are not appreciated. Examination of the cardiovascular system of large animals using these techniques has been limited and generally confined to teaching hospitals and investigative units.

## Electrocardiography

Many cardiac arrhythmias in large domestic animals can be diagnosed with reasonable certainty on physical examination when they occur at slow heart rates. However, diagnosis by physical examination is extremely difficult when the heart rate is fast, and the ECG is the major method of diagnosis. Because of the importance of electrocardiography in the diagnosis of arrhythmias the salient features are presented here.

The ECG provides a graphic record of the varying potential difference occurring over the surface of the body as a result of electrical activity within the heart associated with depolarization and repolarization of the myocardium. The potential difference at the surface of the body is the sum of this activity, and at any one instant the electrical activity in the heart registers as a single dipole vector that has polarity, magnitude, and direction. The polarity is determined by the charge on the surface of the cells, whereas the magnitude and direction are determined by the mass of muscle being depolarized or repolarized. The process of ventricular activation differs between domestic animals. In **category A** animals, including dogs and cats, there are

- three broad fronts of depolarization of the ventricle which occur in sequence
- in the second of these fronts there is depolarization of both ventricular free walls towards the epicardium from the termination of the Purkinje fibers.

In these species this enables the ECG to be used to give an approximation of changes in regional ventricular muscle mass. In the horse, cow, sheep, goat, and pig there is much more extensive ramification and penetration of the Purkinje fibers into the ventricular muscle mass, and the major depolarization of the ventricle occurs in multiple areas which cancel and are silent to the surface ECG. Consequently, with these **category B** animals there are only two fronts of sequential depolarization detected by the surface ECG. These are

- the initial depolarization of an endocardial shell in the apex of the left ventricle
- a simultaneous excitation of the interventricular septum from the right ventricular endocardium towards the left, as occurs in category A animals.

The second front is associated with terminal depolarization of the middle and base of the interventricular septum in a general apicobasilar direction. As a consequence the depolarization of a large proportion of the myocardial mass is not recognized by the surface ECG, and the detection of cardiac hypertrophy and myocardial abnormality by vector analysis of the ECG is, in general, not possible in these large animal species.

The ECG may be taken with the traditional limb lead system or with a single bipolar lead placement. The traditional lead system consists of standard bipolar limb leads (I, II, and III), the augmented unipolar limb leads (aVR, aVL, aVF), and an exploring unipolar chest lead. This is the lead system in common use in small animals. In large animals the routine diagnosis of

---

### Clinical Pointer

The prevalence of cardiovascular disease in dogs and cats is high and warrants the routine use of electrocardiography and radiography.

---

### ECGs in large animals

The major use of the ECG in large animals is in the detection and diagnosis of conduction abnormalities and arrhythmic heart disease. These are detected by measurement of the various waveforms and intervals in the ECG that represent conduction and depolarization in the heart, and by observation of their absence or abnormality.

abnormalities of conduction can be achieved by a single bipolar limb system, and this is the lead system most commonly used in clinical work. The bipolar lead system and its placement is the one least affected by movement of the animal. The most commonly used lead placement in horses and cattle consists of two electrodes, one positive and one negative, the Y lead system attaches

- the left arm lead (positive electrode) at the xiphoid about 8–10 cm behind the girth, and
- the right arm lead (negative electrode) at the thoracic inlet.

Lead I on the standard electrocardiograph is used for recording. An alternate and common lead system is the base–apex monitor lead. The right arm electrode is attached two-thirds of the way down the neck in the right jugular furrow and the left arm electrode is placed over the apex of the heart just behind the left elbow. Again, lead I is used for recording. With both systems the ground electrode is placed remote from the heart, usually over the withers. With sheep, where the wool interferes with placement on the neck, the negative electrode can be placed on the midline of the poll. The electrodes can be placed using alligator clips and a gel contact, or disposable human stick-on type electrodes. In order to ensure good adherence the skin should be shaved and cleansed with alcohol prior to application of the gel.

Either of these lead systems can be used to record a simple ECG and this can be done in field situations:

- the recording is made distant from areas of electrical interference
- the animal stands square on dry ground or a rubber mat
- the electrocardiograph is calibrated so that an input of 1 mV produces a 1 cm deflection of the recording pen.

Recording speeds are generally 25 or 50 mm/s.

Discharge of the sinoatrial node results in a wave of depolarization over the atria to produce a P wave in the ECG. The delay in conduction at the AV node is registered by no electrical activity at the body surface and an isoelectric PR interval on the ECG. Depolarization of the ventricles occurs with several sequential fronts to produce the QRS complex, which is followed by another isoelectric period before repolarization, represented by the T wave.

Electrocardiography has become an important diagnostic tool in many small animal practices. An ECG is indicated in any dog or cat with heart failure, a history of a heart murmur, or indication of cardiac arrhythmia or auscultation. Electrocardiography is also of potential benefit in animals with syncope, cyanosis, suspected electrolyte or acid/base abnormalities (e.g. hyperkalemia in a cat with urinary obstruction or a dog with hypoadrenocorticism), and as part of a preanesthetic screening procedure in geriatric dogs and cats. The ECG provides valuable information on heart and rhythm, state of the myocardium (looking for evidence of premature ventricular contractions or microscopic myocardial infarcts) and, in dogs and cats, also provides information on cardiac chamber enlargement.

To perform an ECG in a dog or cat, the animal is ideally placed in right lateral recumbency and the labelled electrodes are placed on the corresponding elbow and stifle regions. Alcohol or contact gel is applied at the electrode contact points and the ECG machine is turned on. Usually the paper speed is set at 50 mm/sec and the voltage is at 1 cm = 1 mV (sensitivity). There are 6 commonly used ECG limb leads. Leads, 1, 11 and 111 are termed standard bipolar limb leads, and compare the voltage between two sites. For example, lead 1 compares the electrical potential at the left arm (+) to that at the right arm (–), a left to right axis. Lead 11 compares the electrical potential at the right arm (–) compared with the left leg (+) and lead 111, the left arm (–) compared with the left leg (+). The other standard limb leads (aVR, aVL, aVF) are the augmented unipolar limb leads and they compare the voltage at one limb to a standard, internally calculated reference point at the center of the heart. For further information on obtaining and reading an ECG, the reader is referred to the references found at the end of this chapter.

## Continuous ambulatory electrocardiography

Considering the transient nature of many cardiac arrhythmias, and the observation that daily events often trigger arrhythmias, a technique has been developed to overcome the limitations of routine electrocardiography in detecting arrhythmias. With continuous ambulatory electrocardiography (Holter monitoring) the cardiac rhythm is recorded for 24 hours, preferably when the animal is in its natural surroundings. Transient arrhythmias are easily detected and those with a circadian pattern are documented. Holter monitoring is indicated:

- in the evaluation of dogs with syncope that have a normal routine ECG
- as a method of determining antiarrhythmic drug efficacy
- in screening asymptomatic dogs for arrhythmogenic cardiomyopathy.

## Radiography and angiocardiography

Obtaining high-quality thoracic radiographs is essential in the evaluation of small animals with suspected heart disease.

---

### Radiography and heart failure

Radiography is a sensitive diagnostic test used to detect left heart failure. This is indicated by the presence of increased interstitial densities and/or air bronchograms.

---

If it is deemed that a dyspneic animal can tolerate radiography, the DV (dorsoventral) view is less stressful than the VD (ventrodorsal) view. For stable animals the conventional views are VD and right lateral. Others prefer the left lateral view, but there is no real advantage to either. More importantly, positioning needs to be consistent from case to case. Radiography is also important in determining the progression of heart disease in a particular case (serial radiographs) and the response to therapy. Radiographs should be interpreted systematically to avoid missing abnormalities. The superficial structures, bony thorax, cardiac silhouette, lungs, and airways must be evaluated.

---

### Clinical Pointer

Never restrain an overly dyspneic animal for radiography as the stress can be fatal. In this situation it is necessary to alleviate the cause of respiratory distress (thoracocentesis or diuresis) prior to obtaining radiographs.

---

In small animals radiography is the most readily available means to identify pulmonary edema and pulmonary venous congestion. It can also assist in the diagnosis of

- chamber enlargement
- great vessel enlargement
- heartworm disease
- pericardial effusion
- pleural effusion.

Lateral and DV or VD radiographs should be obtained at end inspiration.

Because of the size of horses and cattle these methods of examination are largely confined to neonates of these species.

Angiocardiography can be a diagnostic method of examination in congenital cardiac defects where the passage of contrast media through abnormal routes can be detected.

## Phonocardiography

Phonocardiography allows the recording and measurement of heart sounds. A special microphone is placed over the various auscultatory areas of the heart and the sounds are recorded graphically on moving paper or on an oscilloscope. Prior to recording they are usually passed through high-pass, low-pass, or bandpass filters to allow better discrimination of the individual sounds and to allow a crude frequency examination. Phonocardiograms are usually recorded in conjunction with an ECG, which permits their occurrence in relationship to the electrical activity within the heart to be timed.

Phonocardiograms can provide considerable information on heart sounds in addition to that acquired by stethoscopic examination. In cardiovascular disease they are used primarily for the characterization and timing of murmurs, especially at fast heart rates, where simple stethoscopic examination may not allow this.

## Echocardiography

In echocardiography, high-frequency sound waves are pulsed through tissues at known velocities. When the waves encounter an acoustic tissue interface echoes are reflected back to the transducer. In M (motion) mode echocardiography a unidimensional view of the heart provides excellent temporal resolution, which is displayed on an oscilloscope in conjunction with an ECG. Determinations of ventricular wall thickness, luminal dimensions, and valve motion can be made. Alternatively, two-dimensional (real-time) echocardiograms can be obtained that have depth and width. Doppler echocardiography can be used to investigate the flow of blood within the cardiovascular system. The echocardiograph is capable of determining spatial orientation and the distance of the returning echo from the transducer. Regurgitant jets associated with valvular insufficiency can be observed using color Doppler echo. Measurements of cardiac and individual chamber dimensions can be of value in assessing the effects of cardiac lesions on cardiac structure and function, and can also be used to predict the type of lesion likely to result in these changes. Valvular defects and endocarditis may be diagnosed by imaging

- abnormal valve motion
- incompetent valve orifices, or
- vegetative masses associated with the valves.

Similarly, echocardiography can be of value in the diagnosis of congenital cardiovascular defects, and the injection of echogenic materials, such as microbubble-laden saline, may aid in the detection of shunts. Echocardiography can also be used to determine

- indices of contractility
- the presence of tumor masses within the thorax
- the presence and extent of pleural and pericardial effusion.

In the examination of the vascular system ultrasound is capable of the early detection of iliac thrombosis in horses and cats, and is more sensitive than manual palpation per rectum.

## Central venous pressure

Central venous pressure (CVP) measurement is the determination of the venous blood pressure in a central vein, such as the cranial vena cava. The CVP closely reflects the right atrial pressure and changes in response to dehydration and parenteral fluid administration. To avoid excessive fluid administration and to monitor the patient, the CVP can be followed. A large-bore catheter placed within the cranial vena cava is attached to a manometer.

## Blood pressure measurement

Blood pressure measurement is indicated when

- evaluating a patient for hypertension
- monitoring a critically ill animal with cardiovascular disease, and
- to determine the response to therapy when vasodilators are used.

There are two general methods: direct and indirect. Direct blood pressure measurement involves catheterization of a peripheral artery and the use of a pressure transducer and manometer. This technique is invasive and sedation is usually required. Indirect blood pressure measurement is done by applying a cuff to a limb or the tail, and determining blood flow by oscillometric or Doppler transducers.

## Pericardiocentesis

Pericardiocentesis is the technique of removing fluid from the pericardial space. In most cases this is done to relieve the life-threatening pressure caused by a progressive pericardial effusion (cardiac tamponade). Fluid removed should be examined cytologically,

although there is a significant potential for false negatives and false positives for neoplasia when examining serosanguinous effusions. A large over-the-needle catheter is preferred.

## Exercise testing in large animals

Dyspnea, fatigue, and a prolonged elevation in heart rate following exercise are signs suggestive of cardiac insufficiency. Frequently animals with suspected cardiac disease are exercised in an attempt to elicit these signs and to obtain an estimate of exercise tolerance. In most practice situations the assessment of exercise tolerance is subjective.

Exercise followed by electrocardiography allows the detection of abnormalities associated with underlying heart disease. These include changes in the ST segment (elevation or depression) and the occurrence of arrhythmias. After a vigorous run a multilead ECG is recorded and compared to a pre-exercise ECG. This test is capable of revealing transient arrhythmias which may have gone undetected by routine electrocardiography.

---

**Clinical Pointer**

Although unlikely, there is a risk of sudden death during exercise tolerance testing in patients with undiagnosed transient arrhythmias.

---

## ACKNOWLEDGEMENT

The Authors would like to thank Dr. John-Karl Goodwin for supplying the phonocardiograms used in this chapter.

## FURTHER READING

Bernard W, Reef VB, Clark ES, Vaala W, Ehnen SJ. Pericarditis in horses: six cases (1982–1986). Journal of the American Veterinary Medical Association 1990; 196: 468–471.

Bonagura JD. Echocardiography. Journal of the American Veterinary Medical Association 1994; 204: 516–522.

Claxton MS. Electrocardiographic evaluation of arrhythmias in six cattle. Journal of the American Veterinary Medical Association 1988; 192: 516–521.

Constable PD, Muir WW, Freeman L, Hoffsis GF, St. Jean G, Welker FH. Atrial fibrillation associated with neostigmine administration in three cows. Journal of the American Veterinary Medical Association 1990; 196: 329–332.

Constable PD, Muir WW, Bonagura JD, Rings DM, St-Jean G. Clinical and electrocardiographic characterization of cattle with atrial premature complexes. Journal of the American Veterinary Medical Association 1990; 197:1163–1169.

Cornick JL, Seahorn TL. Cardiac arrhythmias identified in horses with duodenitis/proximal jejunitis: six cases (1985–1988). Journal of the American Veterinary Medical Association 1990; 197: 1054–1059.

Deem DA, Fregin GF. Atrial fibrillation in horses: a review of 106 clinical cases, with consideration of prevalence, clinical signs, and prognosis. Journal of the American Veterinary Medical Association 1982; 180:261–265.

Dowling PM, Tyler J W. Diagnosis and treatment of bacterial endocarditis in cattle. Journal of the American Veterinary Medical Association 1994; 204: 1013–1016.

Elwood CM, Cobb MA, Stepien RL. Clinical and echocardiographic findings in 10 dogs with vegetative bacterial endocarditis. Journal of Small Animal Practice 1993; 34: 420–427.

Gay CC. Diseases of the cardiovascular system. In: Radostits OM, Gay CC, Blood DC, Hinchcliffe DC (eds) Veterinary Medicine. 9th edn. London: W B Saunders 2000; 361-398

Goodwin JK, Lombard CW, Ginex DD. Continuous ambulatory electrocardiography (Holter monitoring) in a cat with hypertrophic cardiomyopathy. Journal of the American Veterinary Medical Association 1992; 200: 1352–1354.

Machida N, Nakamura T, Kiryu K, Kagota K. Electrocardiographic features and incidence of atrial fibrillation in apparently healthy dairy cows. Journal of Veterinary Medicine Series A 1993; 40:233–239.

Manohar M, Smetzer DL. Atrial fibrillation. The Compendium on Continuing Education for the Practicing Veterinarian. 1992; 14:1327–1333.

McGuirk SM, Bednarski RM, Clayton MK. Bradycardia in cattle deprived of food. Journal of the American Veterinary Medical Association 1990; 196: 894–896.

Miiten LA. Cardiovascular causes of exercise intolerance. Veterinary Clinics of North America Equine Practice 1996; 12:729–746.

Parry BW, Anderson GA. Importance of uniform cuff application for equine blood pressure measurement. Equine Veterinary Journal 1984; 16: 529–531.

Patterson MW, Blissitt K. Evaluation of cardiac murmurs in horses: clinical examination. In Practice 1996, 18:367–376.

Patterson MW, Cripps PJ. A survey of cardiac auscultatory findings in horses. Equine Veterinary Journal 1993; 25: 409–415.

Reef VB. Evaluation of the equine cardiovascular system. Veterinary Clinics of North America Equine Practice 1985; Vol.1, No.2, 275–288.

Reef VB. The significance of cardiac auscultatory findings in horses: insight into the age-old dilemma. Equine Veterinary Journal 1993; 25:393–394.

Reimer JM, Reef VB, Sweeney RW. Ventricular arrhythmias in horses: 21 cases (1984–1989). Journal of the American Veterinary Medical Association 1992; 201:1237–1243.

Tilley LP. Essentials of canine and feline electrocardiography, 3rd edn. Philadelphia: Lea and Febiger, 1992.

West HJ. Congenital anomalies of the bovine heart. British Veterinary Journal 1988; 144: 123–130.

Yamamoto K, Yasuda J, Too K. Arrhythmias in newborn Thoroughbred foals. Equine Veterinary Journal 1992; 24: 169–173.

# 15
# Clinical Examination of the Lymphatic System

*J. W. Tyler*

## CLINICAL MANIFESTATIONS OF DISEASE OF THE LYMPHATIC SYSTEM

**Lymphadeniaopathy** is hypertrophy of the lymph nodes.

**Lymphadenitis** inflammation of the lymph nodes. The lymph nodes are usually enlarged and painful.

**Lymphangiectasia**, is dilatation of lymphatic vessels. Intestinal lymphangiectasia is a common cause of protein-losing enteropathy.

## EXAMINATION OF LYMPH NODES

Examination of the lymphatic system consists of inspection and palpation of the accessible lymph nodes, and if possible the course of the lymphatics. A fine needle aspirate or biopsy may also be taken.

A number of superficial lymph nodes are readily identified in domestic animals. Lymph nodes are palpable in the loose subcutaneous tissues. Their size will vary with location and the species under examination. Lymph nodes are bean-shaped and have a smooth contour. Ruminants have additional lymphoid organs – hemal lymph nodes – which are most readily identified in the subcutaneous tissues of the paralumbar fossa. Hemal lymph nodes are usually about 1 cm in diameter and roughly spherical. In normal animals the thymus is typically not palpable. Thymic enlargement may be identifiable as a mass which extends from the thorax, through the thoracic inlet and cranially along the ventral surface of the neck. Gross enlargement of the thymus is strongly suggestive of lymphoproliferative disease.

The proportional distribution of lymph nodes varies depending on the species of animal. Lymph nodes that are normally palpable in small animals include the

- mandibular
- prescapular
- superficial inguinal, and
- popliteal.

If the cervical, retropharyngeal, axillary, accessory axillary, or femoral nodes are palpable, disease is likely. Occasionally the superficial cervical, superficial inguinal, and facial lymph nodes are palpable. A number of different lymph nodes are palpable in other species.

## LOCATIONS OF PALPABLE LYMPH NODES

*Submandibular* In the horse these nodes are situated beneath the skin towards the caudal part of the

---

### Clinical Pointer ✳

In cattle and horses several abdominal lymph nodes are palpable by rectal examination.

### Clinical Pointer

Refer to a textbook of veterinary anatomy for the exact size, shape, position, and area drained by the individual nodes in each species.

intermandibular space; they are as thick as a finger and converge anteriorly. In cattle the corresponding lymph nodes lie further caudal near the angle of the mandible.

In small animals, the mandibular lymph nodes form a group of two or three and lie ventral to the angle of the jaw.

*Pharyngeal* These consist of two groups.

1. The subparotid (parapharyngeal in the horse) lymph nodes are situated on the caudal part of the masseter muscle beneath the parotid salivary gland. In the horse the nodes lie on the dorso-lateral surface of the pharynx, just ventral to the guttural pouch, where they are not directly palpable. They are readily palpable in cattle.
2. The retropharyngeal (or subpharyngeal) lymph nodes in horses and cattle are situated on the caudal aspect of the pharynx. In the horse they are comparatively small and because of their situation are sometimes known as the guttural pouch lymph nodes.

*Cranial, middle, and caudal cervical (prepectoral)* These are situated respectively in the vicinity of the thyroid gland (under cover of the caudal part of the parotid salivary gland in the horse), in the middle of the neck on the trachea, and near the entrance to the thorax, ventral to the trachea.

*Prescapular* These are situated in front and slightly dorsal to the point of the shoulder. In the horse they lie on the cranial border of the cranial deep pectoral muscle; in cattle they are located at the cranial border of the supraspinatus muscle.

*Cubital* These are situated on the medial aspect of the humerus between the elbow and the wall of the thorax (regularly present only in the horse); they are covered by muscle and are palpable only in a lean animal.

*Axillary* Situated deep in the axilla beneath muscle masses which prohibit effective palpation in horses and cattle.

*Prefemoral (precrural)* Located above the fold of the flank on the cranial border of the tensor fasciae latae, dorsal to the stifle.

*Popliteal* Located between the biceps femoris and semitendinosus muscles caudal to the gastrocnemius muscle.

*Supramammary* These are located in the perineum dorsal to the mammary gland. In the cow there are

---

> ### Clinical Pointer
>
> To palpate the supramammary lymph nodes in the cow stand behind the animal, using both hands begin in the upper third of the hindquarters of the udder and work towards the perineum.
>
> - If the caudal nodes are situated near the skin, or the udder is to any degree pendulous, the glands are usually palpable.
> - When the mammary gland is closely attached to the abdominal wall, or the lymph nodes are deeply situated, palpation is not possible.

usually two nodes on each side, and sometimes more; the larger nodes of the group, which are caudal, resemble sheep kidneys set on edge, flattened from side to side and approximately 4 cm in height. They are often fused caudally, giving the impression of a single mass when palpated.

*Superficial inguinal* In the stallion these form an elongated group on either side of the penis. In the bull and ram they are situated in fatty tissue caudal to the spermatic cord at the neck of the scrotum.

*External iliac* Located in the caudal part of the flank medial to the ilium and not palpable from the exterior. They are occasionally found to be enlarged on rectal palpation in dogs with disorders such as prostatic carcinoma.

## OTHER LYMPH NODES

Certain other lymph nodes are clinically important but in general they can only be identified when they are enlarged. In cattle, enlargement of the caudal mediastinal lymph nodes may occur with

- lymphosarcoma
- actinobacillosis, and
- tuberculosis

which may cause compression of the esophagus and so reduce its lumen; this can sometimes be recognized by passing a stomach tube. The condition is suggested by encountering a sudden increase in resistance well before the instrument enters the cardia. During withdrawal the sequence of events is reversed. Occasionally enlarged lymph nodes can be palpated at other sites, such as the subcutaneous tissues at the base of the ear or on the wall of the thorax and abdomen.

## Internal lymph nodes

In large animals the iliofemoral nodes are accessible by rectal examination in the retroperitoneal space, cranial and medial to the body of the ilium. When palpable, they are the size of a large walnut. They collect lymph from the subiliac, popliteal, mammary, and scrotal lymph nodes. They may be felt with the extended arm and hand on each side of the pelvic inlet just in front of the upper part of the body of the ilium; internal iliac nodes sometimes are palpable at the bifurcation of the aorta.

## PHYSICAL EXAMINATION OF THE LYMPH NODES AND LYMPHATIC VESSELS

Physical examination of the palpable lymph nodes involves inspection and palpation. Inspection reveals changes in normal contours caused by enlargement. Palpation provides more critical evaluation of any changes. Lymph node enlargement should be assessed according to physical characteristics, distribution, and the signalment. Physical characteristics to assess include

- size
- response to palpation
- lobulation
- consistency
- temperature of the overlying skin
- abscess formation, maturation, and discharge
- adhesions between the lymph node and the skin or surrounding tissues.

The number of palpable lymph nodes involved is noted, and whether the involvement is unilateral or bilateral.

The lymph nodes are normally flaccid or tensely elastic, easily displaced, and in one piece.

---

### Lymph node size

Consider the age and condition of an animal with lymphadenopathy:

- young animals are exposed to a variety of new antigenic stimuli, increased lymph node size is a normal immunological response
- as an animal ages lymph node size often decreases, and the nodes become difficult to palpate
- in cachectic patients loss of fat surrounding the nodes makes them seem more prominent.

---

Lymph node enlargement may be due to

- benign proliferation of lymphocytes and macrophages in response to antigenic stimulation
- infiltration with inflammatory cells
- in situ proliferation of hematopoietic neoplasia
- infiltration by metastatic neoplastic cells.

When assessing the significance of an increase in the size of a lymph node it should be remembered that the enlargement may represent any of the following.

1. An acute local inflammatory reaction which may either resolve completely (non-specific wound infection) or lead to suppuration (equine and puppy strangles).
2. Part of a systemic reaction to a major specific disease (malignant catarrhal fever).
3. A chronic inflammatory reaction (chronic suppuration of the sinuses or guttural pouch).
4. Neoplasia, which may be primary (lymphosarcoma) or metastasis as the result of spread from neighboring tissues (carcinoma).
5. Part of a generalized neoplasia of lymphatic tissue (myeloid leukemia).

The physical characteristics of enlarged lymph nodes, as determined by palpation, may aid in differentiation between reactive and neoplastic lymphadenopathy: reactive lymph nodes tend to be painful and less firm.

Fixation of nodes to surrounding tissues suggests metastatic neoplasia, marked inflammatory reactions, fungal disease, or extracapsular lymphoma. The enlarged lymph nodes in individuals with lymphoma are firm, freely moveable, and non-painful. If lymph nodes are extremely firm, nodal fibrosis (as occurs with coccidioidomycosis) or metastatic neoplasia are likely.

In pyogenic involvement of lymph nodes fluctuation may be demonstrated and the overlying skin may be hot and the surrounding tissues painful and swollen (collateral inflammatory edema and lymph stasis).

The distribution of lymphadenopathy may provide clues to the etiology of lymph node enlargement. If one or a localized set of lymph nodes is involved, the sites drained by these lymphatics are carefully examined for infection, inflammation, or neoplasia. If

---

### Clinical Pointer

Reactive lymph nodes tend to be painful and less firm than neoplastic nodes. An exception is the painful axillary lymph node enlargement secondary to mammary carcinoma metastasis.

---

**Lymph node changes in acute versus chronic diseases**

- in acute inflammatory conditions the swollen lymph node is warm and painful and the lobulation is indistinct
- in chronic diseases, the lymph node when enlarged is painless, firm, normal in temperature and sometimes adherent to the skin or the contiguous tissues, lobulation may still be perceptible.

---

**Bovine lymphoma (BL)**

This may be suspected based on the age of the animal and the distribution of lymphadenopathy

- juvenile BL (calves, less than 6 months of age) and 50% of adult BL (cattle more than 18 months of age) cases present with generalized lymphadenopathy
- adolescent BL (cattle 6–18 months of age) affects the thymus.

---

several peripheral lymph nodes are involved, systemic antigenic stimulation or primary lymphoid neoplasia should be considered. Grossly distended lymphatic vessels may be palpable and visible in the subcutaneous tissues distal to a regional lymphatic obstruction. This finding is more readily apparent in large animal species.

The signalment and clinical circumstances in which lymph node enlargement is observed may determine its significance. Young healthy animals routinely develop lymph node enlargement after routine vaccinations or exposure to new antigenic stimuli. Cats may be asymptomatic yet develop transient generalized lymphadenopathy during the initial viremic stages of feline immunodeficiency virus and feline leukemia virus infections. Cachectic animals may have lost sufficient perinodal fat to produce a false impression of lymphadenopathy. History and other physical examination findings (cutaneous lesions, splenomegaly, signs of systemic illness) should be considered when developing a diagnostic plan.

Lymphoid hypoplasia is less common and usually associated with developmental or inherited defects of lymphoid differentiation and proliferation. Examples include lethal trait A46 of cattle, severe combined immunodeficiency of Arabian horses, and juvenile immunodeficiency of llamas.

Animals may be presented with clinical signs directly resulting from lymphadenopathy, including coughing due to tracheal compression by enlarged hilar lymph nodes and difficulty in defecating owing to sublumbar lymphadenopathy.

When grossly enlarged, lymph nodes may exert pressure on important structures in their vicinity and so produce secondary clinical findings, such as

- dysphagia or recurrent ruminal tympany as a result of enlargement of the caudal mediastinal lymph nodes
- dyspnea from swellings of the retropharyngeal or bronchial lymph nodes

- obstructive edema of the head and neck through pressure on the jugular vein by enlarged caudal cervical lymph nodes.

The peripheral lymphatic vessels may be grossly distended as a result of inflammation (lymphangitis) forming tortuous branching cords as in streptococcal lymphangitis in foals. If suppuration develops the abscesses and resultant nodular swellings occur at approximately equal distances apart, owing to the presence of valves in the vessels, at which invading bacteria tend to be arrested. This produces the 'pearl necklace' arrangement of nodular swellings, noted in glanders, and so-called 'skin tuberculosis'.

## THE SPLEEN

The shape and size of the spleen may vary between normal animals of different species. In the simple stomached species it is situated in close relationship to the greater curvature of the stomach on the left of the median plane, but does not normally extend beyond the costal arch sufficiently to be recognizable by external abdominal palpation. The position of the spleen is influenced in simple stomached animals by the degree of fullness of the stomach itself. In the dog, when the stomach is full of food the spleen is situated medial to the last rib on the left side. However, even in this location recognition of the spleen by palpation is dubious. In cattle, sheep and goats the spleen is related intimately on its medial surface to the dorsal curvature of the rumen, just below the left pillar of the diaphragm. Although the dorsal border extends just beyond the last rib, the normal spleen is not usually palpable in these species.

### Clinical examination of the spleen

This is limited mainly to palpation and percussion, which may reveal the presence of pain or gross enlargement.

External palpation of the cranial abdomen in the dog will, in the majority of instances, suggest when there is significant enlargement of the spleen by reason of detecting a vague, indeterminate mass in this position. The dorsal and caudal margins of the spleen usually are palpable rectally in horses, lateral to the left kidney and apposed with the left body wall. Rectal palpation of the spleen can be useful in certain cases of equine colic, such as nephrosplenic entrapment of the colon.

Splenic enlargement is often identified on abdominal palpation in companion animals. Palpation of the spleen is especially indicated in small animals with lymph node enlargement, to assess for evidence of

- splenic neoplasia such as lymphoma (dog and cat)
- mast cell tumor (cat), and
- malignant histiocytosis (dog).

Other causes of splenic enlargement include torsion, hematoma, extramedullary hematopoiesis, hypersplenism, and anesthetic drugs, particularly barbiturates. Recognition of splenic enlargement is usually followed by ultrasound examinations and either exploratory celiotomy or cytological examination of paracentesis samples.

# FURTHER READING

Casley-Smith JR. The fine structure and functioning of tissue channels and lymphatics. Lymphology 1980; 12: 177–183.

Faller DV. Diseases of the lymph nodes and spleen. In: Wyngaarden JB, Smith LH, Bennet JC (eds) Cecil textbook of internal medicine, 19th edn. Philadelphia: WB Saunders,1992; 978.

Haynes BF. Enlargement of lymph nodes and spleen. In: Wilson JD (ed) Harrison's principles of internal medicine, 13th edn. New York: McGraw-Hill, 1994; 323.

McGuire TC, Banks KL, Poppie MJ. Combined immunodeficiency in horses: characterization of the lymphocyte defect. Clinical Immunology and Immunopathology 1975; 3: 555–556.

Rogers KS, Barton CL, Landis M. Canine and feline lymph nodes. Part I. Anatomy and function. Comp Cont Educ Pract Vet 1993; 15: 397–408.

Rogers KS, Barton CL, Landis M. Canine and feline lymph nodes. Part II. Diagnostic evaluation of lymphadenopathy. Comp Cont Educ Pract Vet 1993; 15: 1493–1503.

Theilen GH, Madewell BR. Hematopoietic neoplasms, sarcomas and related conditions. Part V Bovine. In: Theilen GH, Madewell BR (eds) Veterinary cancer medicine, 2nd edn. Philadelphia: Lea & Febiger, 1987; 408.

# 16

# Clinical Examination of the Respiratory Tract

*B. C. McGorum*
*P. M. Dixon*
*O. M. Radostits*
*J. A. Abbott*

## CLINICAL MANIFESTATIONS OF RESPIRATORY TRACT DISEASE

**Abduction of the elbows** may occur with thoracic pain.

**Absent or reduced breath sounds** A decreased intensity or audibility or absence of breath sounds audible over the lung fields, usually associated with a space-occupying lesion of the lung or the pleural cavity, or obesity.

**Breath sounds** The normal sounds clearly audible by auscultation over the larynx, trachea, and the hilus and parenchyma of the lungs.

**Cough** An explosive expiration of air from the lungs following brief closure of the glottis.

**Crackles** Short-duration discontinuous sounds detectable on auscultation of the thorax and trachea and characterized by clicking, popping, or bubbling sounds. Formerly known as moist rales.

**Cyanosis** A bluish discoloration of the skin and mucous membranes caused by excessive concentration of reduced hemoglobin in the blood, which usually indicates profound ($PaO_2$ < 5.33 kPa) arterial hypoxemia. Cyanosis is most noticeable when the mucous membranes are examined, although it can also be detected by examining unpigmented nailbeds or unpigmented non-haired skin.

**Diaphragmatic flutter** or **'thumps'** is a contraction of the diaphragm (hiccup) which is both audible and visible over the thorax and flanks in horses. It is probable that acid–base or electrolyte disturbances make the phrenic nerve sensitive to the depolarizing electrical activity of the adjacent myocardium. The 'thump' is synchronous with the heartbeat.

**Dyspnea** Difficult or labored breathing. The head and neck may be extended, the movements of both the thoracic and abdominal walls may be excessive, the body may rock back and forth with each respiration, the facial expression may be anxious, and respiratory noises such as stertor, stridor, or grunting may be present with each respiration. Dyspnea may be primarily inspiratory or expiratory in nature.

**Epistaxis** Hemorrhage visible at the external nares; can be unilateral or bilateral.

**Excercise induced pulmonary hemorrhage** Bleeding from the lungs as a consequence of exercise; occurs in the racehorse and is diagnosed by endoscopic observations of blood in the tracheobronchial airways.

**Expiratory dyspnea** Prolonged and forceful expiration, usually associated with diffuse or advanced obstructive lower airway disease.

**Expiratory grunt** An audible grunt during expiration, produced by sudden laryngeal opening after a period of breath-holding against a closed larynx. Common in cattle with severe pneumonia, pleuritis, and pulmonary emphysema. May also occur in painful conditions.

**False nostril flutter or high blowing** A loud expiratory sound in horses caused by a snoring-like vibration of the nasal structures, including the true nostrils.

**Halitosis** Offensive odor of the breath.

**Heave line** Linear depression which develops ventral to the external abdominal oblique muscles when these muscles hypertrophy in horses with chronic and severe expiratory dyspnea, as in chronic obstructive pulmonary disease (COPD) (Fig. 16.1). The muscular hypertrophy renders the costal arch prominent. Heave lines must be distinguished from the hypertrophied external abdominal oblique muscles in fit performance horses.

**Hemoptysis** Coughing up blood from the lower respiratory tract indicates pulmonary hemorrhage. The blood is usually bright red and frothy with air bubbles.

**Hyperpnea** Abnormal increase in the depth of breathing.

**Inspiratory dyspnea** Prolonged and forceful inspiration, usually due to obstruction of the extrathoracic airways, such as with laryngeal obstruction or collapse of the cervical trachea, or by abnormalities restricting thoracic expansion, such as restrictive lung diseases and space-occupying lesions of the thorax.

**Loud breath sounds** Increased intensity or loudness of breath sounds audible over the lung fields, usually associated with increased rate and depth of respirations or consolidation of the lungs.

**Nasal discharge** Increase in the amount or change in the character of the respiratory secretions normally visible at the external nares.

**Open-mouthed breathing** Labored breathing with the mouth held open. Occurs commonly in advanced pulmonary disease and obstruction of the nasal cavities. Does not occur in horses.

**Panting** Rapid shallow breaths, characteristic of a heat-losing mechanism in dogs; represents an increase in dead-space ventilation, resulting in heat loss without necessarily increasing oxygen uptake or carbon dioxide loss.

**Pleuritic friction source** Loud coarse rubbing sound audible on auscultation of the thorax during both inspiration and expiration, indicating pleural disease.

**Reduced exercise tolerance** Reduced ability to perform physical activity. Characterized by rapid onset of an unusual degree of dyspnea and tachycardia following physical activity.

**Reverse sneezing** This is a brief, rapid inspiratory effort seen in dogs. The reflex is protective and intended to clear the nasopharynx.

**Roaring** A stertor in respiration caused by air passing through a stenosed larynx; the commonest cause is laryngeal hemiplegia in the horse.

**Sneezing** A characteristic forceful exhalation of air from the respiratory tract, initiated by stimulation of the nasal mucosa. Occasional sneezing occurs in normal animals.

**Snorting** A voluntary, short, explosive expiration through the nasal cavities; common in cattle and horses.

**Stertor** Low-pitched 'snoring' sound that occurs during breathing owing to vibration of the soft palate, pharynx, or nasopharynx. Stertor can be a 'normal' finding in brachycephalic dogs such as the English Bulldog, Boston Terrier, and Pug.

**Stridor** High-pitched inspiratory sound indicating upper airway obstruction; the sound is usually audible without the aid of a stethoscope at a distance from the patient.

**Subcutaneous crepitus** Air or gas in the subcutaneous tissues characterized by a soft, mobile swelling which crackles like bubble-wrap when palpated.

**Syncope** or fainting is a transient loss of consciousness most commonly due to reduced cerebral perfusion. Syncope is occasionally precipitated by bouts of coughing and is then known as tussive syncope, or the 'coughdrop' syndrome.

**Tachypnea and polypnea** Very rapid breathing, often due to hypoxemia and/or hypercapnia. Tachypnea may also be a response to anxiety or pain. It must be differentiated from panting, which is a thermoregulatory mechanism noted in normal dogs and sometimes in cats.

**Thoracic pain** Pain originating from the thoracic wall or thoracic viscera, including the pleura and pericardium, causing an audible grunt or groan when the animal moves or when digital pressure is applied to the thorax.

**Wheezes** Continuous musical sounds detectable on auscultation of the thorax and trachea. Formerly known as dry rales or rhonchi.

**Whistling** A high-pitched inspiratory respiratory sound made by force breathing through a very narrow opening of the larynx.

## INTRODUCTION

The upper respiratory tract includes the nasal cavities, nasopharynx, the larynx, and the trachea to the thoracic inlet. The lower respiratory tract includes the intrathoracic trachea, bronchi, lungs, pleura and pleural space, diaphragm, and thoracic wall. This chapter will describe the clinical examination of the respiratory tract according to anatomical location and species differences.

## CLINICAL EXAMINATION OF THE RESPIRATORY TRACT

### History

Factors such as age and breed of the animal, the duration of clinical findings, the environment and management, recent travel or transportation, vaccination history, and previous and current medications may provide clues to the cause and nature of respiratory disease.

## Age

In general, congenital abnormalities or their sequelae are most often detected in young animals. Congenitally stenotic nares are occasionally observed in brachycephalic breeds of dogs and cats; severe stenosis may result in clinical signs of upper respiratory tract obstruction. In brachycephalic dogs stenotic nares may be only one element of a spectrum of structural upper respiratory abnormalities that include

- tortuous compressed turbinates
- redundant soft palate
- everted laryngeal saccules
- tracheal hypoplasia.

Cleft palate also occurs as a congenital abnormality in all species and predisposes the neonate to dysphagia and aspiration pneumonia. Recently weaned beef calves with toxemia, anorexia, fever and rapid shallow breathing are likely to be affected with pneumonic pasteurellosis. Unthriftiness in foals with respiratory disease suggests pneumonia due to *Rhodococcus equi*. Housed dairy calves with a history of coughing and unthriftiness suggests enzootic pneumonia. A mature stabled horse with a history of coughing and poor exercise tolerance is suggestive of chronic obstructive pulmonary disease (COPD). A 12-year-old cow with chronic worsening respiratory disease is more likely to be affected with a pulmonary neoplasm than with pneumonic pasteurellosis.

## Breed

Brachycephalic dogs are predisposed to congenital structural abnormalities of the upper respiratory tract. Nasal neoplasia occurs most commonly in dolichocephalic (long-nosed) dogs. Small-breed, middle-aged, and geriatric dogs, such as miniature poodles, are commonly presented for evaluation of persistent coughing due to chronic bronchitis and a collapsing trachea. These diseases may occur concurrently and the presence of left atrial enlargement resulting from chronic mitral regurgitation may complicate the clinical presentation. Feline bronchitis is diverse in its clinical manifestations, but Siamese cats may be particularly predisposed. Laryngeal paralysis occurs most commonly in older large-breed dogs.

## Nature and duration of clinical signs

A history of cough of several years' duration in a dog would suggest a primary respiratory tract disease such as chronic bronchitis; cardiac disease or congestive heart failure are unlikely to be the cause. However, geriatric animals may suffer from several concurrent cardiorespiratory diseases. In addition, subclinical diseases may progress and complicate pre-existing chronic diseases. Evidence that a disease has progressed, and the rate of progression, is an important aspect of the history. A history of spontaneous improvement might suggest infectious diseases that are typically self-limiting, such as uncomplicated viral tracheobronchitis. A seasonal exacerbation of clinical signs suggests allergic disease. An acute onset of severe respiratory distress in pastured beef cattle in the autumn suggests acute interstitial pneumonia.

**Syncope** is occasionally the clinical sign that first causes the owner of a pet with cardiorespiratory disease to seek veterinary attention. Hypoxia associated with diseases such as collapsing trachea can also cause syncope. Some patients with pulmonary hypertension associated with cor pulmonale experience syncope on exercise or excitement.

## Environment and management

The patient's environment may be a risk factor for respiratory disease.

> **Clinical Pointer**
>
> In the stabled horse a history of coughing of over 2 months' duration is highly suggestive of COPD.

Infectious and immune-associated diseases of the respiratory tract in large animals are common in groups of animals raised indoors with inadequate ventilation. Examples include

- pleuropneumonia of pigs
- enzootic pneumonia of pigs and calves
- chronic interstitial pneumonia of cattle exposed to dusty feed
- COPD in the mature horse exposed to moldy hay or straw.

## Travel

The stress of transportation has been associated with diseases of the respiratory tract. Acute pneumonic pasteurellosis is common in weaned beef calves transported to the feedlot. Transportation of racehorses over long distances is a major risk factor for acute bacterial pleuropneumonia.

### Environmental influences in dogs and cats

**Outside** – dogs that roam free are at greater risk of exposure to parasites such as heartworm, toxicoses, infectious diseases, and trauma.
**Indoors** – indoor animals are subject to poor ventilation and allergenic factors such as tobacco smoke, dusty bedding, and cat litter.
**Boarding kennels** – exposure to unfamiliar animals transmits diseases such as infectious tracheo-bronchitis (kennel cough) or infectious feline upper respiratory tract disease.

## Vaccination status

The incidence and severity of many infectious diseases of the respiratory tract may be greater in unvaccinated animals or those which have no naturally acquired immunity than in those vaccinated at strategic times before being exposed to natural infection.

## Previous and current medications

Previous and current medications may alter the clinical findings on presentation of the animal

- for example, corticosteroids may cause temporary remission of signs resulting from inflammatory airway disease
- antibiotic therapy can decrease or eliminate the purulent component of a nasal discharge that results from foreign-body, neoplastic, or mycotic nasal disease, but the purulent component will generally recur after the cessation of therapy.

### Geographical distribution of respiratory disease

Always note the animal's geographical home and travel history when infectious and parasitic diseases are considered. A distinct geographical distribution is noted for

- mycotic diseases such as *Blastomomyces* or *Histoplasma* pneumonia
- complications of the plant awns of foxtail Hordeum spp inhalation or porcupine quill migration.

## PHYSICAL EXAMINATION OF THE RESPIRATORY TRACT

### Audiovisual inspection of breathing

To minimize any changes in the rate and depth of breathing which may occur because of handling the animal, the audiovisual inspection of breathing is usually performed first, followed by examination of the lower respiratory tract and the upper respiratory tract, and finally by any special diagnostic tests.

The examination is best done in a quiet location, by distant observation, without disturbing the animal. When animals are examined out of their normal environments, such as in an outpatient clinic, they are invariably anxious and an altered breathing rate and pattern may be observed. The audiovisual inspection of breathing includes evaluation of the rate, rhythm, type, depth, and symmetry of breathing, and any respiratory noises associated with breathing.

**Rate**
The rate of breathing is best observed from behind and to one side of the animal, by watching the movements of the costal arch and the abdominal wall at the flank. In normal resting horses breathing movements may be so subtle that determination of the rate can prove very difficult. In such instances the rate may be determined by placing a hand near the nostrils and feeling the expiratory air flow. On cold days the breathing rate in horses may be determined by observing the condensed water vapor as it is exhaled from the nostrils. One inspiration, one expiration, and a pause between inspiration and expiration, is one breath or respiratory cycle. The number of breaths per minute is counted.

Inspiration and expiration are approximately equal in duration. Panting occurs in normal dogs and cats as a thermoregulatory mechanism.

**Rhythm**
The normal rhythm of breathing is inspiration, expiration, pause. In diseases of the respiratory tract, the pause may be considerably shortened and either the inspiratory or expiratory phase or both may be prolonged.

**Type**
Breathing may be of the thoracic (costal) or the abdominal type. In thoracic breathing the excursions are mostly done by the thoracic wall. In abdominal breathing inspiration and expiration are accomplished mainly by the abdominal muscles and diaphragm. The breathing pattern is assessed by observing how the movements are shared between the thoracic and

abdominal walls. If they are equal in extent the respiration is classified as costoabdominal. In cattle, sheep, and goats the movement of the abdominal wall is greater than that of the thoracic wall.

The breathing pattern of the horse differs from that of other mammals, which have a passive expiration and thus only require activity of the breathing muscles during inspiration. In the normal resting horse, both expiration and inspiration are biphasic. The horse inhales

1. initially by passive relaxation of the abdominal muscles
2. then by active contraction of the intercostal muscles and diaphragm.

Exhalation comprises

1. an initial passive relaxation of the intercostal muscles and diaphragm
2. followed by an active contraction of the abdominal muscles, creating an end-expiratory abdominal 'lift'.

This 'lift' can often be observed in the normal resting horse. The biphasic pattern, and in particular the end-expiratory abdominal 'lift', may be exaggerated in horses with dyspnea. Neonatal animals with severe dyspnea may have *paradoxical* breathing: on inspiration their highly compliant thoracic wall may collapse while the abdomen expands.

### Depth

Variations from the normal excursions of the thoracic and abdominal wall may be shallow or deep. During relaxed breathing normal horses have relatively subtle movements of the nostrils, costal arch, and intercostal and abdominal muscles.

### Symmetry of thoracic wall movements

Normally both thoracic walls move symmetrically. In pneumothorax or painful conditions of one thoracic wall the movements of one hemithorax may be more obvious than those of the other.

### Dyspnea

Dyspnea is difficult or labored breathing, characterized by excessive and obvious movements or

| Normal respiratory rates (breaths/min) | |
|---|---|
| Dogs and cats | 15 to 50 |
| Cattle | 12 to 36 |
| Horses | 8 to 12 |
| Ponies | 15 to 20 |
| Foals | 30 to 60 |

---

> ### Clinical Pointer
>
> - prolonged inspiratory phase suggests a lesion of the upper respiratory tract, usually the larynx or trachea, restrictive lung disease or space-occupying lesions of the pleural cavity
> - prolonged expiratory phase suggests obstructive lower respiratory tract disease such as COPD.

excursions of the thoracic and abdominal walls with each breath.

*Inspiratory dyspnea*

Inspiratory dyspnea is characterized by a prolonged and labored inspiratory phase with exaggerated intercostal activity and, if due to an upper respiratory tract obstruction, will be accompanied by stridor. Inspiratory dyspnea may arise from an upper respiratory obstruction, from a restrictive lung disease or from a space-occupying lesion of the thorax.

*Expiratory dyspnea*

Expiratory dyspnea is characterized by a prolonged and labored expiratory phase, with exaggerated abdominal effort or 'heave'. The latter may give rise to pumping of the anus and, if chronic, to a 'heave line' in horses (see Fig. 16.1). Expiratory dyspnea usually arises from obstructive lower airway disease such as COPD in the horse.

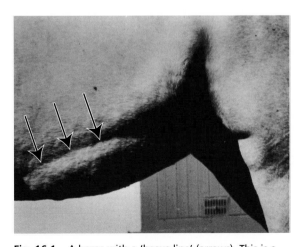

**Fig. 16.1** A horse with a 'heave line' (arrows). This is a linear depression which develops ventral to the external abdominal oblique muscles, when these muscles hypertrophy in horses with long-standing severe expiratory dyspnea.

## Characteristics of dyspneic patients

- anxious facial expression
- they prefer to remain standing or to lie in sternal recumbency
- when standing, the elbows may be abducted from the thorax
- the head and neck are usually held horizontal to the ground, possibly to reduce airflow resistance through the upper airway.

## Interpretation of abnormal breathing patterns

Abnormal breathing patterns may be divided into five broad categories

1. rapid deep breathing – this may be associated with
   - physiological causes such as anxiety and exercise
   - pathological causes, including lung disease, pyrexia, endotoxemia, anemia, and acidosis
2. slow deep breathing – this is occasionally seen in animals with severe airway obstruction, when inspiratory or expiratory air flow is restricted to such an extent that the duration of inspiration or expiration is prolonged and the breathing rate cannot be increased
3. fast shallow breathing – this may occur with
   - anxiety
   - conditions that make breathing painful, such as fractured ribs or pleuropneumonia
   - restrictive lung diseases, such as interstitial pneumonia and pulmonary fibrosis, which restrict lung inflation; affected animals often adopt a fast shallow breathing pattern, which is energy efficient
   - space-occupying lesions that reduce thoracic volume and limit lung expansion, such as pleural effusion, pneumothorax, and diaphragmatic herniation
4. slow shallow breathing – may occur in animals with central nervous system depression, or as a compensatory response to metabolic alkalosis
5. Cheyne–Stokes breathing – this rare finding is characterized by a cyclical waxing and waning of the respiratory rate and depth; it has been associated with central nervous system disease.

### Abnormal breathing sounds

Certain respiratory sounds or noises may be audible during breathing without the aid of a stethoscope. When they occur at rest they usually indicate respiratory tract disease. They include expiratory grunting, coughing, snorting, stridor, stertor, sneezing, and reverse sneezing.

### Clinical Pointer

Respiratory sounds that are audible at rest without a stethoscope usually indicate respiratory tract disease.

### Coughing

Coughing is a reflex initiated by stimulation of the cough center in the medulla oblongata which results from irritation of sensory receptors in the respiratory tract. The cough receptors are located mainly in the larger airways. The stimulus may originate in the pharynx, larynx, trachea, and bronchi. The act of coughing consists of several stages

- deep inspiration followed by closure of the glottis
- a vigorous and forced expiration
- compression of the air in the lungs
- sudden opening of the glottis permitting an explosive expiration during which linear velocities of several hundred meters per second are attained.

The purpose of coughing is to remove excess mucus, inflammatory products, or foreign material from the respiratory tract distal to the larynx. Coughing usually indicates pulmonary disease. A paroxysm of coughing (numerous coughing bouts one after another) suggests the presence of marked irritation of the respiratory tract mucosa.

Coughing is usually painless, but in acute laryngitis, bronchitis, and pleuritis it can be accompanied by pain and attempts at cough suppression. A cough is productive if there is obvious expulsion of mucus, inflammatory debris, or blood through the nasal or oral cavities. A productive cough indicates the presence of exudative lesions, which results in the production of large quantities of inflammatory debris and mucus. A non-productive cough is usually known as a dry cough and indicates inflammation with minimal exudation.

When the cough is infrequent and does not occur spontaneously during the clinical examination it may

### Clinical Pointer

Coughing in the horse is a reliable overt or clinical indicator of pulmonary disease, although it is inexplicably absent in some horses with significant pulmonary disease and excessive respiratory secretions.

be necessary to induce it. In animals with airway inflammation a cough may be provoked by inducing forced breathing, either by temporary (30–60 seconds) occlusion of the external nares and mouth, or by using a rebreathing bag. In the presence of laryngitis and tracheitis external manipulation and slight compression of the larynx or trachea may induce a cough. In the horse coughing is often heard at the beginning of exercise as the animal clears accumulations of mucus, or the airways react to changes in air flow, humidity, and temperature.

In small animals a harsh, dry cough is usually due to irritation of the airways, such as with chronic bronchitis, collapsing trachea, and compression of the main-stem bronchi by an enlarged left atrium. Pulmonary venous congestion can result in stimulation of the juxtapulmonary receptors, resulting in bronchoconstriction and an increase in bronchial mucus production, which may contribute to the genesis of the 'hacking' cough noted in some dogs with cardiac disease.

**With pulmonary edema**

If pulmonary edema is present

- the cough tends to be soft and sometimes productive, resulting in a pink frothy sputum
- dyspnea is usually evident.

**Clinical Pointer**

Coughing in cats is usually the result of primary respiratory disease are rarely cardiac disease.

The cough of pneumonia tends to be soft. In dogs laryngeal or pharyngeal disease (such as an elongated soft palate) may be associated with a soft cough or a gag; sometimes there is a noticeable voice change with laryngeal disease.

**Sneezing**
This is a characteristic forceful exhalation of air from the respiratory tract, mediated by a central reflex, intended to clear the nasopharynx, and initiated by stimulation of the nasal mucosa. Occasional sneezing occurs in normal animals. Persistent sneezing indicates a local disease process, such as the presence of a nasal foreign body, inflammation, or neoplasia. Sneezing does not occur in large animals.

**Reverse sneezing**

1. this is a spastic inspiratory effort in dogs. It is a protective reflex intended to clear the nasopharynx of irritants
2. reverse sneezing is unfamiliar to many pet owners and thus the episode may be misinterpreted as a 'fit'
3. repetitive reverse sneezing suggests nasopharyngeal or paranasal sinus disease
4. it is not seen in horses.

## DETAILED EXAMINATION OF UPPER RESPIRATORY TRACT

### Nose and muzzle

The nose and muzzle are inspected and palpated for the presence of masses, symmetry, and depressions.

### Dog and cat

In dogs and cats the muzzle is the more rostral portion of the head and includes the upper and lower jaws. The length of the muzzle varies between species and between individual breeds. It is covered with haired skin except for the apical portion of the nose, the nasal planum, which is hairless and variably pigmented. In dogs the normal planum is moist. Senile hyperkeratosis can result in the appearance of a dry and hard nose in otherwise normal elderly dogs. The nose of the healthy dog or cat is free of discharge. If a discharge is present it should be quantified and characterized. Chronic nasal discharges, as occur with nasal aspergillosis or neoplasia, can result in ulceration of the hairless area of the nose.

### Cattle

The muzzle of cattle is devoid of hair and is normally moist and cool because of the continuous secretion of serous fluid (beads of sweat). A small amount of serous nasal discharge may be pooled on the ventral aspects of the nostrils in healthy cattle, which regularly lick off nasal discharges. When cattle are anorexic, depressed, toxemic, or pyrexic, the muzzle becomes dry

- any abnormal nasal discharge accumulates, dries, and adheres to the surface
- large amounts of discharge mixed with feed particles accumulate on the muzzle
- the surface of the muzzle appears dirty and may be painful
- the accumulated material on the muzzle may extend to occlude the external nares, resulting in varying degrees of nasal stridor.

Lesions associated with specific diseases, such as infectious bovine rhinotracheitis, bovine virus diarrhea, malignant catarrhal fever and bovine papular stomatitis, may occur on the muzzle.

### Horse

The muzzle is fully covered with hair and is very mobile and tactile. The nasal area is normally dry, except for a few drops of serous (clear and water-like) fluid, which consists mainly of tears that drain via the nasolacrimal duct into the rostral nasal cavity and may flow down the lateral aspect of the muzzle. Unlike the dog the horse rarely develops a streak of excoriation and depigmentation of the ventral nostril along the course of chronic nasal discharge. Some normal horses have areas of white hair ('snips') on their external nares, which should not be confused with pathological secondary depigmentation.

## Nares (nostrils) and nasal cavities

Examination of the nares and nasal cavities includes inspection of the nares and examination of breath from the nostrils, nasal discharge, nasal mucous membranes, and patency of the nasal cavities.

### Nares

The nares and the rostral part of the mucous membranes of the nasal cavities are examined by inspection with the aid of a good light source and by endoscopy. The nares should be symmetrical. In cattle the nares are relatively small and thick and are less dilatable than those of the horse.

In the horse the nostrils are semilunar in outline during normal breathing, but when the tidal volume increases they dilate and become circular. The alar fold projects laterally into the dorsal part of the nostril and divides the nostril into dorsal and ventral passages.

The dorsal passage leads into a blind cutaneous pouch, the nasal diverticulum (false nostril). The ventral passage leads into the nasal cavity.

During dilation of the true nostrils, such as during exercise, the lumina of the equine false nostrils become reduced in size. These latter structures are about 6–8 cm deep and are lined with epithelium, most of which contains dark pigmented skin. Particles of dark sebaceous secretions normally lie on their surface. Soft, oval-shaped fluctuant swellings of the lateral aspect of the false nostril are caused by cysts (atheromas) of its epithelial lining. Because of the mobility of the horse's nostrils it is possible, unlike in other domesticated species, to readily examine a significant area of nasal mucosa and the rostral aspect of the nasal conchae (turbinates). The nasolacrimal orifice is readily identifiable in the ventrolateral aspect of the nostril, adjacent to the boundary between the nasal mucosa and the pigmented nostril epithelium. Most of the nasal cavity can only be visually examined by endoscopy.

### Breath from nostrils

The stream of expired air is examined by holding the back of the hand or some cotton wool in front of the nostrils. By manually occluding both nostrils (and mouth) for about 30 seconds, air flow subsequently can be temporarily increased, making it easier to assess. In small animals the patency of the nares is assessed by holding a mirror or microscopic slide in front of the patient's nose and evaluating the pattern of condensation produced by exhalation. In the normal animal the flow of air from both nostrils is approximately equal. If there is an obstruction in a nasal cavity, as in neoplasia, or fracture, the airflow will be reduced or absent. Variations in the volume of expired air can be further assessed by occluding each nostril individually.

The expired air may have an offensive odor detectable from a distance. This is usually produced by putrefaction of the tissues, as in

- gangrenous pneumonia
- necrosis of the turbinate bones,
- suppurative inflammation of the larynx.

If the origin of the odor is unilateral it can be detected on one side only when the exhaled air is smelled; if it

---

### Clinical Pointer

The nostrils of cattle and horses with dyspnea will dilate fully during inspiration, and may remain fixed in permanent dilation with severe dyspnea.

originates caudal to the pharynx it can be detected at both nostrils. In ketosis in cattle there may be a sweet sickly acetone odor from the expired air, which cannot be detected by some clinicians.

## Nasal discharge

Nasal discharges can be characterized as

- unilateral or bilateral
- continuous or intermittent
- scanty or copious
- serous
- malodorous
- mucoid
- mucopurulent
- serosanguinous
- hemorrhagic
- containing feed/gastrointestinal contents.

> ### Clinical Pointer
>
> Differentiate malodor from the respiratory tract from malodor of the oral cavity (halitosis) by smelling nasal air flow and the oral cavity separately.

Inflammation of the nasal mucosa elicits increased mucus production and, if large numbers of leukocytes are not present, the discharge will remain mucoid (clear or slightly opaque in appearance and viscous in nature). Serous and mucoid nasal discharges thus represent non-specific responses of the nasal mucosa to irritation. A purulent discharge suggests bacterial infection of the respiratory tract. Unilateral nasal discharge occurs in unilateral disease of the nasal cavity and adjacent structures, such as the paranasal sinuses and teeth. In large animals the presence of bilateral nasal discharge is usually indicative of pulmonary lesions, with the respiratory secretions being transported up to the pharynx by the mucociliary escalator, or by gravity when the head is lowered below the level of the thoracic trachea, and also by coughing. Once transported to the pharynx these secretions are usually swallowed, but if large volumes arrive the discharge may flow down the nostrils and has an equal chance of traveling down either side. Some diseases, such as viral respiratory infections, will have concurrent upper and lower respiratory tract inflammation. In such cases the nasal discharge may therefore also be of upper respiratory tract origin.

Although primary bacterial rhinitis is rare in all species, bacterial infections often complicate neoplastic or mycotic disease as well as intranasal foreign bodies.

> ### Clinical Pointer
>
> The presence of a bilateral nasal discharge containing fresh food, immediately after eating, is indicative of pharyngeal or esophageal dysphagia or cleft palate.

### Dog and cat

The presence of nasal discharge in small animals is most often associated with upper respiratory tract disease but is occasionally noted in patients with bacterial pneumonia. A serous or mucopurulent nasal discharge in young cats can be related to infectious upper respiratory tract (URT) disease. Causative agents include herpesvirus, calicivirus and chlamydia; infectious URT disease is an important cause of morbidity, particularly in young cats. Mucopurulent nasal discharge can also be explained by the presence of an intranasal foreign body, neoplasia, or mycotic infection. Primary bacterial rhinitis is uncommon. However, mention should be made of chronic bacterial rhinosinusitis, which can be observed in cats and results in a chronic mucopurulent nasal discharge. It is presumably a sequel to previous viral infection.

### Cattle

Cattle normally lick and swallow their nasal discharges and keep their external nares clean. A persistent nasal discharge may cause an area of dermatitis of the muzzle and external nares. A purulent nasal discharge indicates the presence of varying degrees of suppurative inflammation at any location in the respiratory tract. In pneumonic pasteurellosis in cattle a mucopurulent nasal discharge is common but does not necessarily originate from the pulmonary lesion. Secondary bacterial infection of the nasal cavities may account for much of the discharge in these cases. However, cattle with chronic suppurative pneumonia may have a copious purulent nasal discharge of pulmonary origin.

In pharyngitis, pharyngeal dysphagia, esophageal obstruction and esophagitis the nasal discharge may contain masticated feed particles mixed with saliva, which may impart a green color. The presence of rumen contents in the nasal discharge suggests regurgitation of ingesta into the nasal cavities, as may occur in cattle with advanced milk fever.

### Horse

Nasal discharge in horses commonly accumulates in the external nares and is readily evident. A few drops of watery (serous) discharge (which is probably mainly composed of tears from the nasolacrimal duct) are commonly present at the nostrils of normal horses.

In the horse the presence of chronic unilateral nasal discharge is usually due to disorders rostral to the caudal border of the nasal septum (Fig.16.2), for example

- a purulent discharge originating from the drainage ostium of an infected caudal maxillary sinus will flow down the nasal cavity on the affected side
- the presence of ipsilateral (on the same side) submandibular lymphadenopathy along with unilateral nasal discharge is confirmatory evidence of a unilateral URT disorder.

### Clinical Pointer

A nasal discharge containing pus and blood often suggests a destructive disease process such as neoplasia or mycotic infection.

### Clinical Pointer

Unilateral nasal discharge usually indicates disease of the ipsilateral nasal cavity, rostral to the nasopharynx or ipsilateral sinus.

The submandibular lymph node group, which in the horse contains 70–150 small nodes, is usually not palpable or barely palpable. Even when these lymph nodes are enlarged they may not be detected unless the dorsomedial aspect of the mandible is specifically examined for their presence. Very rarely in horses these lymph nodes are swollen by secondary neoplasms. Nearly all cases of unilateral nasal discharge have some underlying disorder, such as dental abscessation or poor sinus drainage, underlying a secondary bacterial infection. Consequently, identification and treatment of the cultured bacteria will simply result in delaying the establishment of a specific diagnosis and institution of appropriate treatment (which is usually surgical) to allow permanent resolution of the problem.

The association of pulmonary disease with bilateral nasal discharge is not absolute and a small percentage of horses with pulmonary disease will inexplicably have unilateral nasal discharge.

The presence of bilateral submandibular lymphadenopathy will occasionally be due to bilateral upper respiratory disorders, such as bilateral sinusitis or guttural pouch disorders, but is most commonly due to generalized viral respiratory infections, such as equine influenza, herpesvirus 1 and 4 infections, or strangles.

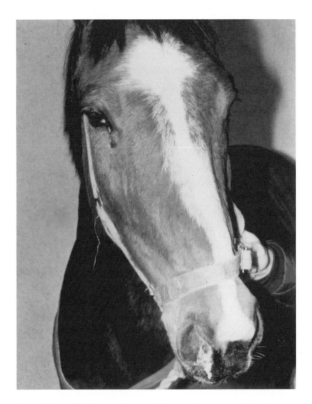

**Fig. 16.2** This horse has a right purulent nasal discharge and also right maxillary swelling and epiphora due to empyema of the right maxillary sinus.

With lesions of the upper respiratory tract caudal to the nasal septum, such as pharyngitis associated with strangles, nasal discharge will be bilateral. With unilateral pharyngeal and guttural pouch disorders where large ( >50 ml) volumes of discharge are suddenly released, the discharge will flow into the nasopharynx and then down both nostrils. Thus with unilateral guttural pouch mycosis massive hemorrhage from the internal carotid artery will cause bilateral epistaxis.

In the horse the most common causes of respiratory mucosal inflammation are viral infections such as influenza or herpes 1 or 4 infections, or pulmonary

### Clinical Pointer

The horse has few cough receptors in its upper respiratory tract, thus coughing together with bilateral nasal discharge confirms the pulmonary origin of nasal discharge and indicates pulmonary disease.

allergies such as COPD. In these conditions increased mucus production is accompanied by transmucosal migration of large numbers of leukocytes, primarily neutrophils, into the mucus. Owing to the presence of these neutrophils the respiratory secretions, whether of upper or lower respiratory tract origin, will be mucopurulent in nature and will be viscous and pale. Mucopurulent respiratory secretions are characteristic of most equine pulmonary diseases. With primary bacterial respiratory mucosal infections, such as strangles, pharyngitis, or bacterial pneumonia, the respiratory secretions will contain so many leukocytes, predominantly neutrophils, that they will have a purulent nature. These then will be of very high viscosity, and intensely white, yellow, or green, the color being partially dependent on bacterial pigments. With the involvement of anaerobic bacteria the purulent respiratory secretions will frequently be malodorous. Such bacteria are common pathogens in equine sinusitis and also in pulmonary abscessation.

*Nasal discharge containing food*
In the horse with pharyngeal or esophageal dysphagia some masticated feed will become displaced dorsal to the soft palate during attempts at swallowing. This feed material and saliva will flow down both nasal cavities, especially when the head is lowered, usually within a minute or so after the ingestion of food or liquids. During breathing some of this food will also flow caudally over the soft palate into the open larynx, and will enter the trachea. Inhalation of food or liquid is termed aspiration. Inhaled food will stimulate cough receptors, which are mainly present in the distal trachea of the horse, resulting in some of the aspirated food being expelled by coughing via the nasal and oral routes. The horse has a large 'sump-like' dependent area at the rostral intrathoracic trachea which traps most aspirated material until it is cleared by either coughing, mucociliary transport or gravity when the horse lowers its head below the thoracic tracheal level. The tracheal contents then flow out through the nasopharynx and nasal cavities. Consequently, aspiration (inhalation, foreign body) pneumonia does not usually occur with aspiration in the horse.

Unlike ruminants the horse does not normally regurgitate food. However, food material from the gastrointestinal tract can be discharged from the nostrils if a build-up in pressure occurs in the stomach and small intestine. This process is termed gastric or gastrointestinal reflux. It is most commonly caused by stomach and small intestine obstruction, with subsequent fluid distension of the intestine proximal to the obstruction. Reflux of the gastrointestinal contents up the esophagus into the pharynx may then occur.

Because of the normal subepiglottic position of the equine soft palate, most gastric reflux will flow down the nasal cavities. This watery discharge containing partially digested food usually has a foul smell.

In contrast to pharyngeal or esophageal dysphagia, gastrointestinal reflux with nasal food discharge is not usually be associated with food ingestion, as the refluxed material may have been ingested many hours previously. Also, horses with marked ileus will show no inclination to eat and have gastrointestinal distension and abdominal pain (colic).

> ## Clinical Pointer
> - true gastric fluid is acidic
> - fluid from the small intestine is yellow/green and alkaline.

### Epistaxis and hemoptysis

Epistaxis or bleeding from the nose may be due to

- traumatic injury to the nasal mucosa
- hemorrhage elsewhere in the respiratory tract.
- increased fragility of capillaries
- systemic hypertension
- bleeding disorders such as thrombocytopenia.

Injury may be due to erosion or ulceration of the mucosa by a systemic disease or by a local disease of the nasal mucosa, such as trauma to the head, or a foreign body in the nasal cavities. Blood originating from sites other than the nasal mucosa is a potentially serious occurrence in all species. The sudden passage of large amounts of blood is usually associated with pulmonary hemorrhage, and in horses and cattle may be fatal.

Unilateral epistaxis suggests a lesion rostral to the nasopharynx. Bilateral epistaxis indicates a lesion caudal to the nasopharynx, such as occurs in exercise-induced pulmonary hemorrhage in the horse or pulmonary thromboembolism in cattle.

In some cases the origin of the blood in epistaxis and hemoptysis may be obvious, but usually other diagnostic procedures are required, including careful auscultation of the lungs to detect abnormal sounds indicative of pulmonary disease. A thorough examination of the nasal cavities, nasopharynx, larynx, trachea and large bronchi using a flexible fiberoptic endoscope may be necessary. Clotting defects can be identified by means of suitable hematological techniques. Radiography of the head may be necessary in some cases to detect lesions of the nasal cavities and surrounding structures which may be the source of the hemorrhage.

Hemoptysis, or coughing up blood through the oral or nasal cavity, is usually associated with disease of the lower respiratory tract.

---

### Clinical Pointer

Sudden bleeding from the nose in the horse at rest is commonly from the guttural pouch and is due to mycotic erosion of the blood vessels in the pouch.

---

**Dog and cat**

In dogs and cats epistaxis can result from

- local disease processes, including trauma, neoplasia, and fungal infection
- systemic disorders, including thrombocytopenia and systemic hypertension.

Some dogs with heartworm disease develop severe hemoptysis associated with thromboembolic events that follow the administration of heartworm adulticide.

**Cattle**

Epistaxis in cattle may result from trauma to the nasal cavities caused by

- the passage of a stomach tube
- injury to the facial or nasal bones
- entry of a foreign body into the nostril.

In acute pulmonary congestion associated with anaphylaxis small amounts of rust-colored serous fluid may be observed in the nostrils. In acute pulmonary edema the nasal discharge consists of grayish-white or bright-red froth containing small bubbles; the quantity of the escaping material is often considerable and its passage often accompanied by coughing and severe dyspnea. Epistaxis may also be caused by dicoumarol poisoning, purpura hemorrhagica, and other bleeding disorders of cattle in which there are no physical lesions.

Hemoptysis in cattle results in blood being coughed up from the lungs and expelled through the oral cavity and both nostrils. Some blood is swallowed. Hemorrhage from the lungs, with prominent hemoptysis, occurs in pulmonary arterial aneurysm and thromboembolism from caudal vena caval thrombosis, which usually originates from a ruptured hepatic abscess.

**Horse**

Epistaxis in the horse may result from

- injury to the nasal mucosa
- disease of the guttural pouch
- pulmonary hemorrhage
- bleeding diseases such as thrombocytopenia.

Traumatic injury of the nasal mucosa by the passage of a nasogastric tube or endoscope usually results in a transient episode of unilateral epistaxis. Lesions of the nasal mucosa usually result in intermittent episodes of mild epistaxis. Mycosis of the guttural pouch involving the internal carotid artery, or with early cases of the disorder termed progressive ethmoid hematoma, the nasal discharge will be largely or wholly composed of blood. In the former instance it will usually be a large volume (many liters) of pure blood. Exercise-induced pulmonary hemorrhage (EIPH) is bleeding from the lungs as a consequence of exercise. Most affected horses do not exhibit clinical epistaxis. Definitive diagnosis is established by endoscopic observations of blood in the tracheobronchial airways. The blood may be mixed with mucoid or mucopurulent respiratory secretions. If after a few days they will become brown colored owing to the breakdown of hemoglobin pigments to hemosiderin.

### Nasal mucosa

The nasal mucosa is normally salmon pink in color and moist. With the aid of a light source it is possible to view from 5 to 8 cm of the rostral aspects of the nasal mucosae in the mature cow and horse; proportionately less in calves and foals. The more caudal parts of the nasal mucosae of cattle are bluish-red in color because of the greater vascularization.

With primary disease of the nasal mucosa, such as with generalized respiratory infections, the nasal mucosa will become

- inflamed
- edematous
- erythematous (reddened)
- ulcerated, and
- covered with mucopurulent secretions.

In some diseases, such as infectious bovine rhinotracheitis, lesions of the nasal mucosa are readily visible and characteristic.

With the localized disorder of nasal mycotic infection that is usually caused by *Aspergillis fumigatus*, gray or black fungal plaques may be apparent, but endoscopy is usually required for their detection.

---

### Ulceration of the nasal mucosa

Marked ulceration of the nasal mucosa is characteristic of diseases such as glanders and epizootic lymphadenitis in horses, and malignant catarrhal fever in cattle.

---

## Obstruction of the nasal cavities

### Dog and cat

Obstruction of the opening of the nasal cavity (the naris or nostril) or one or both nasal cavities may occur in the dog and cat. Common causes include traumatic injury, presence of a foreign body or tumor, or congenital anatomical defects. The external naris (plural nares) should be examined for movement during inspiration, patency, and the presence of discharge. Collapse of an external naris can occur following traumatic injury or destruction of nasal carti-lages. Bilateral collapse of the narrowed external naris resulting in complete loss of patency is a congenital characteristic of brachycephalic breeds of dogs. Bilateral stenosis and inspiratory collapse of the external nares are characteristic of the brachycephalic airway obstruction syndrome. The dyspnea common in these breeds is due to the combined effect of

- the abnormal nares
- reduced nasal and pharyngeal air space
- an excess of soft palate, and
- possible distortion and collapse of the larynx.

At rest the airway through the external naris is extremely narrow but patent. During inspiration the naris does not dilate, but the wing of the nostril is sucked medially against the philtrum, thus closing down the air space. Total closure necessitates mouth breathing, but in the presence of partial occlusion, nasal breathing is possible if the inspiratory effort is increased to overcome the obstruction. When the size of the external naris permits, anterior rhinoscopy is easily achieved in the dog by use of a long auroscope cone or small-diameter flexible endoscope. Evaluation of the vestibule, the common, dorsal, and ventral nasal meatus, and the dorsal and ventral conchae is possible.

### Horse

The horse is an obligate nasal breather, as the caudal border of the long soft palate lies beneath the epiglottis during breathing, forming an effective seal between oropharynx and nasopharynx. The caudolateral extensions of the soft palate (the palatopharyngeal arch) form a seal around the larynx which partially protrudes into the nasopharynx during breathing. Thus the rostral larynx (the corniculate processes of the arytenoids, the aryepiglottic folds and the epiglottis) are in an intranarial (intranasopha-ryngeal) position during respiration.

Obstructions of the nasal airways are therefore of much greater significance in horses than in other domestic species that can also breathe via the oral cavity.

---

> ### Nasal paralysis in horses
>
> Nasal paralysis, caused by damage to the dorsal buccal nerves (from a kick to the side of the head, or from iatrogenic facial nerve damage during dental extraction by the lateral buccotomy technique) is of major significance in the equine athlete
>
> - because the horse is an obligate nasal breather
> - because of the great mobility of its nostrils compared to those of most other domestic species.

---

Unilateral nasal obstruction is most commonly due to swellings of the paranasal sinuses, in particular by a pus-filled maxillary sinus (maxillary empyema) or a maxillary cyst.

A common loud expiratory sound in horses caused by a snorting-like vibration of the nasal structures, including the true nostrils, is termed 'false nostril flutter' or 'high blowing'. These normal sounds often occur at the beginning of exercise, and are also common in aggressive animals at rest or work.

During exercise increases in tidal volume and respi-ratory rate can increase air flow sixtyfold in horses. Respiratory sounds can then become audible from a distance of over 25 meters in normal animals. In very unfit horses increased levels of normal respiratory noises, or coarse low-pitched noises, may occur during fast work, and horses making such noises are referred to as being 'thick winded'. These noises normally disappear when the animal becomes fitter. After prolonged and fast exercise, such as racing, even normal fit horses will exhibit post-exercise dyspnea, in which they will continue to breathe fast and deep and make loud but normal respiratory sounds for a period of 5–15 minutes.

In horses with upper airflow obstructions, no abnormal respiratory sounds will be present at rest but increased volumes of respiratory sounds and abnormal sounds may be produced during cantering or galloping. These exercise-induced **inspiratory** sounds are often termed 'noises' by owners and may be audible at more than 50 m from the exercising horse. Some horses make repetitive abnormal rattling or snoring-type noises (like a brachycephalic dog) during inspiration and expiration while performing very fast work, as a result of dorsal displacement of the soft palate (DDSP) above the epiglottis.

Because of the absence of an exercise area, inclement weather, or intercurrent problems such as lameness, it may not always be possible to have a horse exercised and thus the importance of obtaining a complete and accurate history cannot be overemphasized.

> ### Clinical Pointer
>
> During fast exercise normal expiratory sounds are about twice as loud as inspiratory sounds.

### Determining expiration and inspiration during fast exercise

It is highly diagnostic in horses with suspected upper airway obstruction, to determine whether any abnormal noises made during fast exercise occur during inspiration or expiration. This can be done by observing

- the moist air being expelled from the nostrils in cold weather
- the relationship of the horse's gait to the respiratory cycle; at the canter and gallop locomotion and respiration become fully synchronized, expiration occurring when the forefeet hit the ground, inspiration occurring when the forefeet are being elevated.

> ### Clinical Pointer
>
> If the horse cannot be exercised during the examination, the owner can make a video or audio recording of the horse exercising while producing the noise.

### Cattle

Obstruction of the nasal cavities is uncommon in cattle but may occur as a result of the presence of foreign bodies such as plant materials and inflammatory exudate associated with nasal infections.

> ### Clinical Pointer
>
> Hold a strand of cotton wool in front of each external naris to assess patency of the nares and the nasal cavity airways.

There is nasal stridor on inspiration and occasional episodes of snorting. Nasal obstruction may occur without any nasal discharge, but there is reduction or complete absence of expired breath from the nostrils.

Most obstructions of the nasal cavities cannot be visualized by direct inspection through the external nares. Percussion of the nasal cavities which are obstructed with exudate may yield a dull sound.

When an endoscope is not available a simple field test to determine the location of an obstructive lesion and the patency of the nasal cavities is to attempt the passage of nasogastric tubes of varying diameters through each, beginning with a small tube and gradually using larger ones. Inability to pass a tube of an appropriate diameter for the size of the animal may indicate the presence of an obstruction. Depending on the nature of the lesion, the attempted passage of tubes will often cause episodes of snorting and may cause epistaxis and the release of abnormal nasal discharges, which should be collected for laboratory analysis. When available, endoscopy of the nasal cavity using a flexible fiberoptic endoscope is much more effective. Radiography can also assist in assessing the size and nature of any lesion and the tissues involved.

### Paranasal sinuses

Diseases of the paranasal sinuses occur frequently in the horse. The most common is an accumulation of pus in the maxillary sinuses due to excessive production of exudate combined with an impairment of drainage, which is naturally very poor in the horse. Other domestic species with more freely draining maxillary sinuses (dog, cat, cow) suffer infrequently from maxillary sinusitis.

#### Dog and cat

Primary disease of the paranasal sinuses is uncommon in small animals. However, the paranasal sinuses may be involved secondarily when diseases such as aspergillosis or neoplasia affect the nasal cavities. Examination of the paranasal sinuses requires general anesthesia and radiographic studies.

#### Horse

The paired paranasal sinuses in the horse include the rostral and caudal maxillary sinuses (Fig. 16.3). The rostral maxillary sinuses communicate freely on their medial aspects (dorsal to the infraorbital canal and dental alveoli) with the ventral conchal sinuses (formerly called the medial aspect of the maxillary sinus). The caudal maxillary sinus communicates freely via a large circular opening with the frontal sinus. The portion of the frontal sinus formerly known as the turbinate part of the frontal sinus is now termed the dorsal conchal sinus, and both parts are now termed the conchofrontal sinus. The smaller and paired ethmoidal and sphenopalatine sinuses also communicate with the nasal cavity via the caudal maxillary sinus into the caudal aspect of the middle meatus. The smaller paired rostral maxillary sinuses drain separately at a more rostral point into the middle meatus (Fig. 16.3).

Inflammatory conditions that cause maxillary sinusitis in the horses include

- respiratory viral and bacterial infections
- cysts and neoplasms
- local mycotic infections
- abscessation of the apices of the caudal cheek teeth.

Bacterial sinusitis may be secondary to cysts or neoplasms.

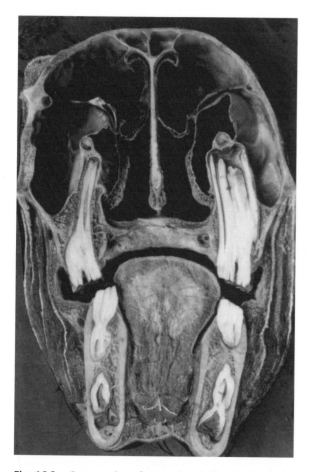

**Fig. 16.3** Cross-section of an equine skull at the level of the fifth cheek tooth. The length of reserve crown indicates that it is a young horse. Note the relationship between cheek teeth and maxillary sinus.

The thick lateral (external) maxillary wall is usually not distorted unless gross sinus distension and bone softening occurs, but the thin medial walls readily become compressed medially towards the nasal septum, causing unilateral nasal airflow disruption. The naso-lacrimal duct runs on the dorsolateral aspect of the maxillary sinuses and compression of this structure during sinus disease may lead to unilateral epiphora. With sinus disease unilateral epiphora and nasal airflow obstruction will often be accompanied by ipsilateral purulent nasal discharge and submandibular lymph node enlargement.

With empyema of the maxillary or frontal sinuses (Fig. 16.2) percussion of the sinus may be of value to assess the density of the tissues directly beneath the site. An exudate-filled sinus, which in chronic cases may develop thinning and demineralization of its walls, may lose the resonance of a normal air-filled sinus. However, affected horses frequently resent percussion of a painful sinus and occasionally the rapid closure of the eyelids during percussion produces a noise that may be mistaken for a dull percussion sound. In general, percussion is unreliable unless advanced sinus disease is present.

With low-grade sinusitis all clinical examinations are unreliable. Therefore, if sinusitis is suspected the diagnosis should be confirmed by radiography to detect the presence of characteristic fluid lines in these normally air-filled structures (Fig. 16.4). The radiographic anatomy of this area is complex and it is useful to have normal sinus radiographs of a similarly aged horse for comparison.

Malodorous breath is usually indicative of a necrotizing upper airway disease associated with anaerobic bacterial infection, especially of the paranasal sinuses, but can also be due to necrotizing pulmonary conditions, such as inhalation (gangerous) pneumonia. A unilateral (or markedly asymmetric) nasal malodor indicates that its source is somewhere in the ipsilateral (same) side of the head. Malodorous oral disorders, in horses such as dental, and in particular periodontal, disease will be detected from the mouth, but not usually from the (nasal) breath.

---

**Clinical Pointer**

To assess sinusitis in the horse, place a hand over the maxillary sinuses on both sides and assess for increased heat and, by local compression, for softening of the bones and evidence of pain.

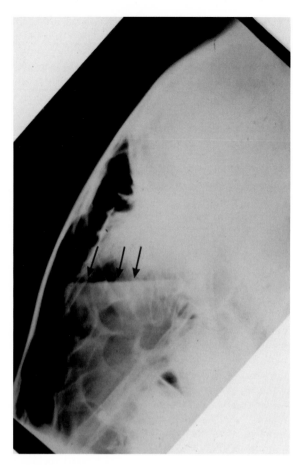

**Fig. 16.4** Lateral radiograph of a standing horse which clearly shows fluid accumulation in the maxillary sinus (arrows). In this instance the maxillary sinus was filled with pus.

### Cattle

Anatomically the paranasal sinuses connect either directly or indirectly with the nasal cavity, of which they are diverticula. There are four pairs

- the frontal – these are very large
- the maxillary
- the sphenopalatine
- the ethmoidal.

The first part of the examination consists of observing whether there is any abnormal prominence or depression in the area overlying any of the sinuses and then, by palpation, determining whether there is any rarefaction or fracture of bone, or heat. Percussing with the fingers or with a plexor determines the state of the sinus by the character of the sound elicited. The paranasal sinuses can also be assessed by auscultation with the stethoscope over the middle of the frontal sinus. Sound is generated by flicking the finger or a plexor against the frontal and maxillary sinus walls. Dullness or, more reliably, asymmetry of sound conduction between the two sides of the face is listened for. In normal animals the acoustic sound is clear and loud, but if the sinus contains

- exudate
- neoplastic tissues
- a dental retention cyst

the percussion sound may be dull. These evaluations should always be done by comparing findings on each side of the head with only distinctive differences being considered of diagnostic value.

In cattle, apart from occasional cases of actinomycosis or neoplasia of the maxillary sinus, frontal sinusitis is most commonly a sequel to dehorning.

### Cranial cervical region

The cranial cervical region is immediately caudal to the vertical ramus of the mandible and includes the

- parotid salivary gland
- larynx
- thyroid gland
- parotid and pharyngeal lymph nodes.

The region is examined by inspection and palpation and, in the case of the larynx and trachea, by auscultation. Both sides should be examined. Enlargement of the thyroid gland may cause swelling in the cranioventral part of the neck overlying the caudal region of the larynx. Local or general enlargement of the esophagus, which may indicate an esophageal obstruction, diverticulum, stenosis or paralysis, may be associated with a swelling of variable extent in the left jugular groove.

External palpation of the cranial cervical region in all species is usually performed with both hands, one on either side, stroking lightly at first and gradually increasing the pressure, because otherwise the animal may show resentment even though there is no pain in the area. Palpation may reveal heat, swelling, and pain, indicating inflammatory diseases, and deep-seated swelling which may be caused by esophageal foreign bodies or neoplasia.

External inspection of the pharyngeal region reveals whether there is any swelling associated with inflammation of the parotid salivary gland, lymphadenitis, enlargement of the thyroid gland or neoplasia.

## Pharynx

### Dog and cat

A brief examination of the pharynx and soft palate of some small animal patients can be accomplished without chemical restraint. The upper jaw is held by the examiner's dominant hand and the lower jaw is abducted with the other. Gently forcing the fingers of the dominant hand between the premolars and molars may encourage a dog to open the mouth. The oral mucosa is carefully examined for lesions such as ulcers or foreign bodies. Calicivirus infection in cats, can cause oral mucosal ulceration. The teeth are also carefully examined. Tooth root abscessation is an important cause of purulent nasal discharge. Detailed examination of the pharynx usually requires general anesthesia. The complete oropharynx, the tonsils, and soft palate should be inspected. Retraction of the soft palate using a spay hook can allow visualization of the nasopharynx with a dental mirror, but the use of a flexible endoscope may be required. The normal mucosa is a healthy pink color. The nature and location of lesions should be recorded. The presence of pharyngeal foreign bodies can explain clinical signs such as dyspnea or gagging.

### Nasopharyngeal polyps

These can be detected when the nasopharynx is visualized. They are common in young cats and can cause

- nasal discharge
- dyspnea
- loud breath sounds.

### Horse

The pharynx is a rectangular musculomembranous cavity which serves as a common conduit for both the respiratory and alimentary tracts. The oropharynx is the part of the pharynx between the soft palate, the tongue, and the epiglottis. The large vertical ramus of the equine mandible covers most of the lateral aspect of the pharynx, with the large parotid salivary glands covering the pharynx caudal to the mandible. Ventrally, the omohyoid muscles, the cricothyroid ligament and the hyoid apparatus fully cover the ventral aspect of the oropharynx. Therefore, little information can be gained from external examination of the equine pharynx.

Internal pharyngeal inspection and palpation can be performed with difficulty only in larger horses. Without general anesthesia it is advisable to

- have adequate assistance
- have the horse well sedated
- use a full mouth speculum.

The base of the tongue, the large midline glosso-epiglottic fold, the oropharyngeal walls and floor, the overlying caudal aspect of the soft palate and the base of the epiglottis are palpable when the soft palate and epiglottis are in the normal breathing position. This examination will often cause the soft palate to become dorsally displaced, and all of the epiglottis and the rostral aspect of the larynx will then be palpable.

Pharyngeal dysphagia can be due to neuromuscular dysfunction, caused by lesions affecting its sensory or motor nerves (cranial nerves IX, X, and XI) or the pharyngeal muscles. Neuromuscular dysfunction may be part of a generalized neural disorder, such as botulism, or can be the result of a local disorder such as guttural pouch mycosis, with damage to cranial nerves IX, X, or XI. Mechanical causes of pharyngeal dysphagia include

- cleft palate
- excessive surgical resection of the soft palate (staphylectomy)
- subepiglottic cyst
- pharyngeal foreign body (usually at the piriform recesses), and occasionally
- epiglottic entrapment associated with marked local ulceration.

Acute pharyngitis as occurs with strangles will occasionally cause a transient pharyngeal dysphagia due to pain and retropharyngeal lymphadenitis, but the other clinical signs, such as bilateral purulent nasal discharge, lymphadenitis and febrile response, will aid diagnosis.

In contrast to the dog, foreign bodies are only rarely encountered in the equine oropharynx, but occasionally will be found in the piriform recess (lateral to the arytenoid cartilages) or oropharynx.

Viral respiratory infections are often mistermed 'upper respiratory infections' when in fact they usually

---

**Pharyngeal dysphagia in the horse**

This is manifested by

- food and saliva flowing down the nasal cavity during or immediately after eating
- coughing owing to food inhalation
- evidence in the water bucket of froth and masticated food that has been discharged down the nasal cavities during attempts at swallowing.

---

cause their most significant pathology in the lungs. However, signs of inflammation of the upper respiratory tract epithelium, including the nasopharyngeal epithelium (the oropharyngeal mucosa does not become infected), the mucosa of the larynx, the guttural pouches, nasal cavities and sinuses, can be manifested as a bilateral mucopurulent nasal discharge and bilateral swelling of the submandibular lymph nodes. Swelling of the parotid lymph nodes frequently occurs with strangles, but may not be readily detectable because of the presence of the large overlying parotid salivary gland. However, deep palpation of this area may reveal increased heat and pain, especially with inflammation of the parotid lymph nodes.

The entrance to the esophagus, which is surrounded by the palatopharyngeal arch, lies immediately dorsal to the larynx. This area cannot be palpated and is normally occluded from endoscopic view by the caudodorsal nasopharyngeal roof. If a horse has been sedated a mucosal fold of the palatopharyngeal arch, or occasionally of the dorsal pharyngeal mucosa, will bulge down over the dorsal larynx. This is due to a sedative-induced loss of tone of the caudal pharyngeal constrictor muscles (thyropharyngeus and cricopharyngeus). This must be differentiated from a more marked and permanent prolapse of the palatopharyngeal arch caused by a congenital absence of the cricopharyngeus muscle in the disorder termed cricopharyngeal–laryngeal dysplasia.

---

**Disorders of the equine epiglottis**

Two well described disorders of the equine epiglottis that can be palpated orally in adult horses but more accurately diagnosed by transnasal endoscopy are

- entrapment of the epiglottis by a fold of the subepiglottic mucosa
- the presence of subepiglottic cysts.

---

**Clinical Pointer**

Care is required to differentiate between

- the mucosal fold of the palatopharyngeal arch in a sedated horse, and
- prolapse of the palatopharyngeal arch in the disorder cricopharyngeal–laryngeal dysplasia.

---

*Soft palate in the horse*

Because of its anatomical position it is not possible to visualize the equine soft palate directly on oral examination without the use of general anesthesia and an instrument to depress the base of the tongue. Even then, only a very restricted view of the ventrorostral aspect of the soft palate will be achieved. Depending on the relative sizes of the horse's oral cavity and pharynx and the examiner's arm, digital examination of the ventral aspect of the soft palate is possible in the well sedated horse. Consequently, examination of the soft palate is usually performed by nasopharyngeal endoscopy, and to a lesser extent by lateral nasopharyngeal radiography.

In foals, cleft palate most commonly involves the caudal aspect of the soft palate only. A cleft palate is an incomplete separation of the oral and nasal cavities which results in the passage of food or liquids into the nasopharynx during swallowing. This material will flow down the nose within seconds of sucking (Fig. 16.5) and, more significantly, will also flow into the trachea, commonly inducing coughing immediately after swallowing. In some cases this can lead to aspiration pneumonia. During exercise a horse may occasionally have to swallow saliva, or excessive lower respiratory secretions transported up the trachea and accumulating on the soft palate. The act of swallowing necessitates transient dislocation of the larynx from the palatopharyngeal arch. This can be commonly observed during endoscopy in resting normal horses, when the soft palate is seen to move dorsal to the epiglottis. However, if the soft palate becomes dislocated dorsally during very fast work, the free end will become repeatedly sucked into the glottis during inspiration and blown out during expiration, causing the acute respiratory obstruction known as dorsal displacement of the soft palate (DDSP). This usually occurs only during maximal exercise and the soft palate appears endoscopically normal prior to and after exercise. However it is now possible to examine such functional changes by performing endoscopy during high-speed treadmill exercise. In horses suspected of suffering from DDSP it is useful to assess whether previous corrective surgery has been performed and the animal should be examined for the presence of a laryngotomy scar. Also, the rostral sternothyrohyoideus area should be assessed for myectomy scars and muscle absence.

## Guttural pouches (eustachian tube diverticulae)

The guttural pouches of the horse are air-filled diverticulae of the eustachian tubes whose function is unknown: they are unique to equidae. They are positioned medial to the mandible and parotid salivary glands and in the normal horse cannot be visualized or palpated.

In foals a congenital (possibly neuromuscular) defect of the nasopharyngeal ostium of one or both guttural pouches may result in a unilateral or bilateral accumulation of air within the affected pouch. This will present as a unilateral or bilateral marked swelling, caudal to and sometimes below the mandible. Palpation will reveal a gas-filled drum-like painless swelling, which on percussion will be tympanitic.

With marked unilateral or bilateral accumulation of pus (empyema) within the guttural pouches, the overlying parotid salivary gland may become displaced laterally. Occasionally this pus will become inspissated into many egg-like concretions, known as chondroids. A greatly distended guttural pouch may protrude

caudolaterally between the angle of the mandible and the larynx, with the floor of the guttural pouch lying subcutaneously lateral to the larynx, causing a painless doughy swelling.

Guttural pouch mycosis is a more common disorder of this structure and usually involves the dorsal aspect of the medial compartment. This condition can cause a wide and dramatic array of clinical signs due to damage to the large number of major nerves and blood vessels of the medial compartment. It is often the *combination* of these clinical signs that makes the clinical diagnosis of guttural pouch disease possible. Massive and even fatal bilateral epistaxis can occur as a result of erosion of the wall of the large internal carotid artery, which runs in the medial compartment of the guttural pouch. Although the hemorrhage occurs from just one pouch, such large quantities of blood flow into the nasopharynx and drain down **both** nostrils. Damage to cranial nerves IX, X and XI can lead to pharyngeal dysphagia, and damage to the cranial nerve X can also lead to a sudden onset of laryngeal paralysis on the ipsilateral side. Damage to the cranial sympathetic trunk as it passes through the guttural pouch will cause Horner's syndrome. Unilateral facial sweating is often not present in horses in cooler climates, but ptosis and pupil constriction (miosis) are more constant features of Horner's syndrome in horses.

> ### Clinical Pointer
>
> All severe (>1 liter blood) episodes of epistaxis that occur at rest and are unassociated with head trauma should be considered as being of guttural pouch origin.

Endoscopy is the technique of choice for examining the guttural pouches, and is described later.

## Cattle

With the use of a Drinkwater mouth gag in adult cattle, most of the pharynx, the glottis and epiglottis of the larynx, and the proximal esophagus can be palpated through the oral cavity. Most of the pharynx can also be visualized directly or with the aid of a simple rigid plexiglass speculum measuring 4 cm in diameter and 45 cm in length for adult cattle, and smaller sizes for calves. The mouth is held open with the gag and the speculum is placed over the base of the tongue and advanced to the pharynx. Using the tongue as a fulcrum, and with a light source directed down the speculum, the pharynx and the glottis and epiglottis

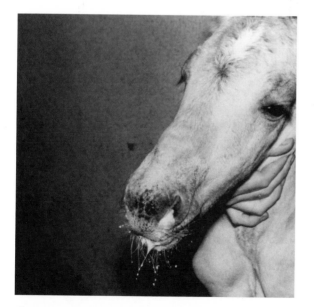

**Fig. 16.5** This 3-day-old foal has just suckled its dam and milk is now flowing down both nostrils and the foal is coughing. These signs indicate the presence of dysphagia with aspiration of milk into the trachea.

are easily visible. If the animal vocalizes during the examination the vocal cords will abduct and the proximal part of the trachea may also be visible. Inflammatory lesions of the larynx are usually easily visible. This method of examination is useful for the identification of

- foreign bodies
- enlargement of the pharyngeal lymph nodes
- traumatic injuries to the pharynx.

It is also possible in adult cattle to palpate the laryngeal rima glottidis to assess suspected lesions such as abscesses and tumors. When the hand is introduced into the isthmus of the fauces (constricted aperture between the oral cavity and the pharynx) in cattle, the pharyngeal reflex is initiated, so that constriction of the pharynx is followed by swallowing movements and mild retching.

The clinical findings of pharyngitis include: anorexia, drooling of blood and feed-stained saliva, dropping of feed from the mouth and coughing. Water is usually swallowed but at a slower rate than normal. Inspiration is prolonged and accompanied by a loud snoring sound.

## Larynx

The larynx has three main functions, namely

- prevention of food aspiration
- regulation of air flow
- phonation.

Five paired muscles (cricoarytenoideus lateralis, ventricularis, vocalis, interarytenoideus and cricothyroid) are present for adduction, compared to only one pair (cricoarytenoideus dorsalis) for abduction.

### Dog and cat

The larynx is carefully assessed by palpation. The normal larynx is symmetrical and gentle manipulation causes no obvious discomfort. Direct examination of the larynx is indicated when functional or structural abnormalities are suspected based on historical and physical findings, and requires sedation or anesthesia. Laryngeal function is assessed as the patient recovers from a light plane of anesthesia. As laryngeal function returns active abduction of the vocal folds is noted during inspiration, but not in patients with laryngeal paralysis (Fig. 16.6). Often this lesion affects the larynx asymmetrically, aiding in diagnosis.

### Horse

The most significant equine laryngeal disorder is caused by a neuropathy of the recurrent laryngeal nerve, causing a unilateral paralysis (hemiplegia) of the larynx. As this is usually a unilateral **partial** paralysis the condition is more correctly termed **laryngeal hemiparesis**. As the etiology is unknown the term idiopathic laryngeal hemiparesis or hemiplegia is widely utilized. However, the term hemiparesis technically does not include total laryngeal paralysis or

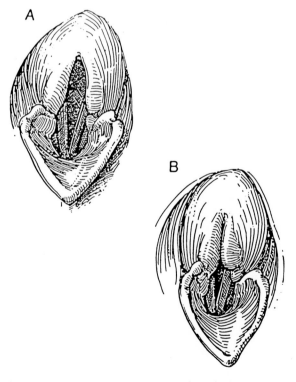

**Fig. 16.6** The laryngoscopic appearance of a normal canine larynx (A) can be compared with the appearance of laryngeal paralysis (B).

subclinical disease, and so many authors prefer the term recurrent laryngeal neuropathy (RLN), which includes all grades of laryngeal muscle dysfunction, from subclinical to total paralysis. The primary clinical sign is caused by inadequate laryngeal abduction during strenuous exercise. This is manifested by the production of abnormal breathing noises, and possibly by reduced exercise performance. Abnormalities of phonation, as in the presence of an abnormal whinny *may* also be present in some badly affected cases, but aspiration is very rarely present.

The dorsorostral aspects of the larynx should be bilaterally palpated to determine the prominence of the muscular process of the arytenoids. If there is significant atrophy of the surrounding abductor (cricoarytenoid dorsalis) muscle the ipsilateral muscular processes will become more prominent. The degree of laryngeal muscling on each side should be compared. A useful way to do this is to

- facing the horse, the mandible is rested on the observer's left shoulder
- the fingers of both hands are advanced beneath the rostral aspect of each sternocephalicus tendon
- the fingers are moved rostromedially along the dorsum of the larynx to the muscular processes of the arytenoids on each side.

Some degree of laryngeal muscle atrophy is present in most large horses, but clinical signs may not appear until it is very marked. A slap test (Chapter 19) has also been used to assess the function of the recurrent laryngeal nerve and cricoarytenoideus muscle. A further assessment of laryngeal muscle function is the 'arytenoid depression maneuver', which consists of stabilizing the right side of the larynx with three to four fingers while pressing the left arytenoid muscular process in a rostromedial direction with the right index finger. Horses with severe RLN usually make stridorous inspiratory noises during this procedure.

The laryngeal adductor muscles (except the cricothyroid) are also innervated by the recurrent laryngeal nerve, and are usually more severely atrophied in RLN than are the abductor muscles. However, this is not usually clinically significant. Most of the affected adductor muscles are deep to the thyroid cartilage and are not palpable. Nevertheless, adductor muscle function was previously commonly used to assess laryngeal function. If a normal horse is suddenly frightened, such as by quickly waving a stick in front of its head, it will usually make a sudden and short grunt. The ability to grunt normally (i.e. quickly) depends on rapid laryngeal adduction. In RLN, adductor muscle damage causes the production of a prolonged, low-pitched grunt during this procedure. Some authors, without objective evidence, have alleged that horses with a wide intermandibular space are less likely to develop RLN and that the converse is also true.

The most common and effective clinical technique to assess laryngeal function is to exercise the horse fast, and during the high airflow rates of exercise to listen for abnormal breathing noises indicative of upper airflow turbulence

- initially during exercise horses with RLN make an abnormal 'whistling-type' inspiratory noise
- with further or faster exercise these whistling sounds change to coarse inspiratory noises resembling 'wood sawing' (termed 'roaring' by owners)
- with severe RLN these sounds become very loud and will become biphasic, occurring during both inspiration and expiration.

Palpation of the larynx, immediately after exercise, may transiently reveal fremitus due to turbulent air flow, if marked laryngeal paralysis is present. A horse may have abnormal breathing sounds for a few seconds after hard exercise and occlusion of one nostril will reduce these sounds, presumably by decreasing air flow and hence turbulence.

Endoscopy before and after exercise is the ancillary technique of choice to examine laryngeal muscle function in the horse. In the normal resting horse the

---

### Some features of recurrent laryngeal neuropathy (RLN)

- it includes all grades of laryngeal muscle dysfunction – subclinical to total paralysis
- it is common in larger horses – up to 85% of those over 16 hands high
- it is rarely seen in smaller breeds of horses
- it can affect adduction, abduction, and phonation
- the inadequate laryngeal abduction during strenuous exercise causes abnormal breathing noises and poor performance.

---

### Clinical Pointer

If laryngeal paralysis is suspected there may be palpable evidence of surgical scars from

- subcutaneous laryngotomy (midline, ventral to the cricothyroid ligament)
- laryngoplasty (ventral to the left external maxillary vein), although these are difficult to detect.

glottis is diamond shaped, with the two corniculate processes of the arytenoid cartilages forming the dorsal sides and the two vocal folds forming the base (Fig. 16.7). With marked left-sided RLN the left arytenoid and vocal fold are displaced medially (laryngeal asymmetry) even in the resting horse (Fig. 16.8). This is usually a sign of clinically significant laryngeal muscle dysfunction. With deeper breathing, which can be induced by temporarily occluding the nostrils (for approximately 30 seconds), the speed of abduction of the arytenoids can be assessed and compared for evidence of delayed opening of one side (asynchrony). Many horses that are clinically normal will endoscopically display trembling of the left arytenoid during abduction, but after nostril occlusion, or during treadmill endoscopy, most can abduct the left arytenoid fully and, more importantly, maintain full abduction.

The epiglottis is a small leaf-shaped cartilage that is the rostral aspect of the larynx. As previously noted, in the horse the soft palate normally lies beneath the epiglottis during breathing. Dysfunction of the soft palate or the epiglottis, or incoordination between these two structures, can cause dorsal displacement of the soft palate (DDSP). In some horses, particularly standard breeds, hypoplasia or flaccidity of the epiglottis is believed to predispose to DDSP. Epiglottic

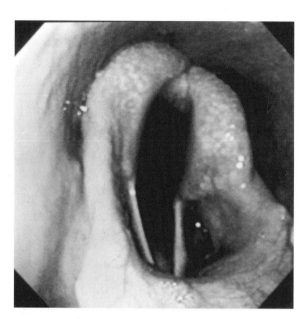

**Fig. 16.8** Endoscopic view of the larynx of a horse after exercise, during which it made loud abnormal inspiratory noises and had exercise intolerance. This demonstrates absence of any abduction of the left side of the larynx due to total left-sided laryngeal paralysis.

size can best be assessed by lateral radiography or endoscopy. The latter will also allow detection of an entrapped epiglottis (when a fold of the loose ventral epiglottic mucosa becomes folded dorsally over the apex of the epiglottis). Depending on the degree of inflammation induced in the entrapped epiglottis and on the entrapping mucosal fold, signs can vary from dysphagia to exercise-related airflow obstruction, or affected cases can be asymptomatic.

### Cattle

The larynx is examined by external palpation for evidence of pain, enlargement, and whether a cough can be induced by mild pressure. Auscultation over the larynx of normal cattle reveals clear breath sounds synchronous with inspiration and expiration. Diseases of the larynx include

- laryngitis
- edema
- stenosis
- foreign bodies
- traumatic injuries
- fractures.

Diseases causing constriction of the larynx may result in abnormal respiratory sounds, consisting of inspi-

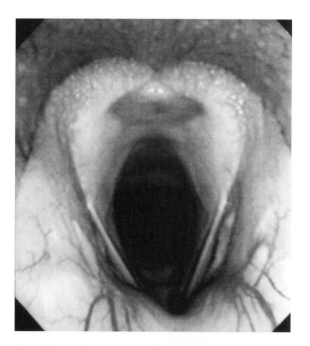

**Fig. 16.7** Endoscopic view of the larynx of a horse immediately after fast exercise. This demonstrates full and bilateral abduction of both sides of this normal larynx.

ratory dyspnea, inspiratory stridor which is commonly audible from a few steps away, and pain and coughing on external palpation. Upper respiratory tract infections causing pharyngitis, laryngitis, and tracheitis are a prominent feature in several common diseases of cattle, including infectious bovine rhinotracheitis and calf diphtheria. In laryngitis, when exudation is present rattling sounds or stridor are audible. When the glottis is constricted, as with laryngitis, allergic edema, or tumor, the laryngeal sounds are stridorous in character. In such cases a vibration or thrill (laryngeal fremitus) may be detected when the hand is placed firmly on the overlying skin. Inflammation and edema of the larynx is visible by nasal endoscopy or examination through the oral cavity, which is made easy by using a simple cylindrical plexiglass speculum.

## Trachea

The trachea extends from the larynx to the main bronchi and consists of a tube-like structure which is kept open by a series of incomplete cartilaginous rings. The cervical trachea is related

- dorsally to the proximal part of the esophagus, but mainly to the longus colli muscles
- laterally to the thyroid gland, the carotid artery, the jugular vein, the vagus, sympathetic and recurrent laryngeal nerves, the tracheal and cervical lymphatic ducts, and the cervical lymph nodes.

The esophagus deviates to the left side of the trachea from the third cervical vertebra caudally.

The cervical portion of the trachea is examined by inspection of the overlying skin and coat, to identify changes in shape or position, scars, or tracheotomy wounds. Palpation will detect pain, local swellings, and deformities. Developmental defects include

- constriction at one or more points
- dorsoventral or lateral collapse
- overlapping or incurving of the ends of some of the tracheal rings.

Mild digital pressure and massage of the trachea in animals with varying degrees of tracheitis will commonly elicit coughing.

Localized painful swellings of the ventral aspect of the neck can be due to trauma, such as a kick injury.

### Dog and cat

In dogs the trachea is almost circular in cross-section at both ends, but the midsection is slightly flattened dorsoventrally. The cartilaginous segments do not meet on the dorsal aspect. The bifurcation, which is level with the 5th rib, forms a very wide angle.

The trachea is carefully assessed by palpation and an attempt is made to elicit a cough. One hand is used to apply gentle compressive force to the proximal trachea and the patient is then observed for evidence of coughing.

In dogs the presence of tracheal collapse often produces a honking coughing and inspiratory dyspnea, which is exaggerated with **slight** digital pressure of the trachea at the level of the thoracic inlet.

In the cat the trachea is comparatively shorter than in the dog but in cross-section is similar anatomically.

### Horse

The space between the caudal aspect of the cricoid cartilage and the first tracheal ring – the cricotracheal ligament – can be readily identified by palpation, both by the large size of the cricoid cartilage and because this ligament is wider than the spaces between the tracheal rings (interannular ligaments). In some horses, even with their heads in the normal flexed position the cricotracheal space can be very large and the ligament may appear to be slack: with digital pressure it can be readily pushed into the airway lumen. This anatomical feature has been considered by some authors to cause inspiratory airflow obstruction during fast work. In many horses, particularly Thoroughbreds, the first five to eight tracheal rings have a degree of flattening, particularly of the ventral aspect. A prominent protrusion on the ventral aspect of these tracheal rings may be palpable in the cranial neck, where they are covered by the relatively thin sternothyrohyoideus muscles. In virtually all cases this deformity is of no clinical significance and endoscopy

---

### Tracheal rupture

This is indicated by

- localized painful swellings on the ventral aspect of the neck
- subcutaneous emphysema (manifested by crepitus on palpation)
- leakage of air and possibly gas-forming bacteria through the ruptured tracheal mucosa.

Weeks or months later affected animals may develop stridor, as a result of tracheal stricture caused by damage to tracheal cartilages. In all species the trachea can be easily examined using a fiberoptic endoscope.

> ### Clinical Pointer
>
> Small animals with many different diseases of the respiratory tract may cough in response to tracheal palpation. However, it is helpful because it assists the owner to reaffirm that the clinical problem is indeed a cough and not a gag, retch or other clinical sign.

of the tracheal lumen at such sites will show a very adequately sized and stable airway.

In small ponies, especially Shetlands, stridor is generally caused by a congenital dorsoventral flattening of the tracheal cartilages. Often there is also separation of the tracheal mucosa from the dorsal cartilage into the tracheal lumen. This deformity usually involves the caudal cervical and intrathoracic trachea. Palpation of the caudal cervical trachea may be very difficult because of the

- thick skin
- greater muscle covering over the distal cervical trachea
- frequently overweight nature of these ponies.

However, deep lateral palpation in the jugular groove may reveal an abnormal sharp lateral edge to the trachea. In addition, with lateral pressure, a flattened trachea will not roll away as will a normal rounded one. In such cases deep midline pressure over the caudal cervical trachea may induce stridor. However this procedure should be performed with care to avoid inducing asphyxia.

### Cattle

The trachea is relatively small in diameter (about 4 cm) in cattle, compared to that of the horse. In cattle laryngotracheitis is characterized by spontaneous coughing, pain, and coughing on palpation and compression of the larynx and cervical trachea, and varying degrees of inspiratory dyspnea.

## EXAMINATION OF THE LOWER RESPIRATORY TRACT

The lower respiratory tract is examined by palpation, auscultation, and percussion of the thorax; several ancillary aids are also available.

## Palpation of the thorax

The thoracic wall is palpated to detect

- fractured ribs
- wounds
- subcutaneous emphysema
- thoracic pain.

Palpation of the entire length of each rib may reveal evidence of a recent fracture or a callus of a healing fracture, especially in young foals. If pneumothorax is suspected the entire thoracic cage should be carefully palpated for evidence of trauma. Firm palpation of the intercostal spaces may elicit a painful response in animals with pleuropneumonia or pericarditis.

Animals with thoracic pain may

- have an anxious facial expression
- be reluctant to move or to lie down
- persistently point one forelimb
- stand with the elbows abducted
- have shallow breathing
- have a soft suppressed cough.

Palpation of the thoracic wall can be used to assess body condition. In a normal individual the ribs may be palpable but not readily visible, as in a well-conditioned and fit racehorse. The precordium is palpated and the point of maximal intensity of the apex

> ### Clinical Pointer
>
> Exercise caution when interpreting the response to thoracic palpation in the horse, as many normal animals resent this procedure.

heartbeat identified.

In cats an attempt is made to gently squeeze the cranial thorax between the thumb and fingers of one hand

- a compliance of the thoracic cage can be detected in normal young cats
- this compressibility is lost in patients with space-occupying lesions of the cranial thorax (e.g. mediastinal lymphosarcoma), and in some elderly cats.

### Subcutaneous emphysema

Air or gas in the subcutaneous tissues is characterized by a soft, mobile swelling which crackles like bubble-wrap when palpated and is known as crepitus. There is no pain, no heat, and no ill effects. It commonly occurs secondary to

- severe airway obstruction which may cause intrapulmonary rupture of the alveoli, with tracking of air into the peribronchial tissues, mediastinum, and subcutaneous tissues of the back
- acute pulmonary emphysema in cattle
- upper respiratory tract surgery or trauma
- postsurgical laparotomy pneumoperitoneum without penetration into the respiratory tract in all species, particularly cattle.

### Subcutaneous edema

An accumulation of fluid within the subcutaneous tissues of the ventral thorax is common with pleuropneumonia. Edema of the head and neck may occur in patients with cranial thoracic masses, as a result of impaired venous and lymphatic drainage from the head.

## Auscultation of the respiratory tract

Auscultation, especially of the lungs, is the most commonly used technique for pulmonary examination in animals. It is cost-effective, fast, and usually provides some diagnostic information. Auscultation may occasionally indicate the nature and location of lesions and the changes occurring in the affected lung over time. A good-quality stethoscope is essential, along with clinical experience. Ideally, auscultation should be done in a quiet area with no background noises. Such circumstances may be possible in small animal practice, but in farm animal practice the circumstances are often noisy because of windy weather, the handling of other animals or the presence of mechanical noises in the background. With practice and experience, and negative adaptation to environmental noises, auscultation of the respiratory tract can yield worthwhile results.

Understanding of the mechanisms of sound production in the respiratory tract, and the transmission and attenuation of sounds in the normal and abnormal lung, has advanced markedly in the last few decades, accompanied by the adoption of new terminology which clearly relates to the acoustic properties of various lung sounds.

### Physics of sound waves

Sound consists of audible vibrations created by alternating regions of compression and rarefaction of air. A sound wave can be depicted as an S-shape described by a sine function, the peaks and valleys in the wave corresponding to the alternating regions of compression and rarefaction. If the waves are in the audible frequency range of 20–20 000 cycles per second Hz, are of sufficient intensity and are transmitted to the ear, the vibrations are transduced, processed, and experienced as sound.

Sound has three principal characteristics:

- frequency
- intensity
- duration.

Frequency is a measure of the number of vibrations per unit of time, in cycles per second or hertz (Hz). A high-frequency vibration results in a high-pitched sound; low frequency in a low-pitched sound. Intensity is governed by four factors:

- amplitude of the vibrations
- source producing the energy
- distance the vibrations must travel
- medium through which they travel.

The duration of the vibrations may be long or short. The quality of a sound is a result of the component frequencies that make up that sound. A violin and a guitar playing the same note will have a different quality owing to the higher frequency harmonics, or overtones, associated with each. Quality also refers to the duration and repetitive nature of a sound. What is referred to as a musical quality, for instance, means that the ear recognizes the periodic nature of the sound waves and distinguishes them from noise, or random sound.

Depending on the damping effect of the surrounding medium, sound waves are transmitted with variable attenuation. That is, the amplitude of the waves decreases with distance from the source of production and the medium through which they move. Reflection occurs at interfaces between media with different physical properties, such as that between visceral pleura and altered pulmonary parenchyma. The proportion of sound energy transmitted depends on the degree of matching of the acoustic properties of the two media, termed acoustic impedance, and is primarily determined by their respective densities.

1. At interfaces of tissues with closely matched acoustic properties little or no reflection occurs and most of the sound energy is transmitted.
2. At interfaces of tissues with markedly different properties, such as air-filled lung and the muscular thoracic wall (Fig. 16.9) a large proportion of sound is reflected.

### Types of air flow and sounds produced

#### Laminar flow of air in tubes

The streamlines in gases flowing slowly along a straight smooth pipe are arranged in a laminar pattern where

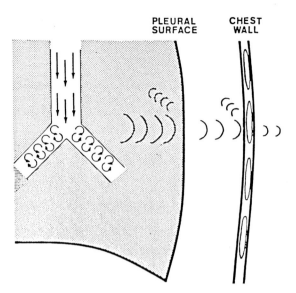

**Fig. 16.9** Schematic representation of sound production in the large airways, and reflection at the pleural surface at the lung and at the thoracic wall.

the path of each layer of gas follows a course parallel with the walls of the pipe. The driving pressure is gradually dissipated by shearing forces between neighboring streamlines, and between the gas and the walls. There are no sudden changes or oscillations of pressure capable of generating sound waves. The sluggish gas flow in the terminal airways and alveoli is laminar and silent (Fig. 16.10a).

**Turbulent flow of air in tubes**

Above a critical flow velocity the orderly arrangement of the streamlines breaks up and small parcels of gas begin to move at random across or against the general direction of flow. In turbulent flow the transfer of energy between these colliding parcels of gas is associated with transient pressure variations. The sound generated by

these fluctuations of gas pressure is a noise varying at random in amplitude, with an even frequency distribution between 200 and 2000 Hz (Fig. 16.10b).

Air passing through the trachea is rapid and turbulent, thereby creating more audible sounds as the molecules of air bounce against the airway wall and against each other. As the volume of air inhaled passes through the ever-branching airways to the alveoli the air flow becomes more laminar, as the sum total of the diameters of each generation increases exponentially. Peripherally in the lung the volume of inhaled gas is 'spread out' over many airways and air flow is slower, laminar, and quiet (Fig. 16.10a).

**Vortices**

When a stream of air in a pipe is forced to change direction abruptly, vortices are produced. In airways, these produce noises with a wide frequency spectrum because flow velocity decreases at each bronchial division as air moves down the bronchial tree (Fig. 16.10c).

## Origin of normal breath sounds

The normal breath sounds are produced by turbulent air flow in the trachea and bronchi (Fig. 16.10b). Because the peripheral airways – the bronchioles – normally maintain laminar air flow they are not believed to be responsible for significant breath sound production, but may play a role in the transmission of the turbulent sounds of the larger airways to the peripheral parts of the thorax.

Breathing (inspiration and expiration) is necessary for the production of breath sounds. The examiner thus relies on the natural breathing of the animal or the hyperventilation which can be stimulated using a rebreathing bag.

## Transmission of breath sounds

The normal air-filled lung acts as a filter for the transmission of sound. It alters the tracheobronchial sounds of the major airways to a softer version heard primarily during inspiration. Changes in lung tissue will alter the sound transmission characteristics of the lung. Diseases that increase the tissue density of the lung will usually increase the sound transmission qualities and result in a significant loss in the filtering effect. As a result, tracheobronchial breath sounds may be heard over areas of consolidation, or atelectasis, provided a patent bronchus is present.

Diminished intensity of breath sounds may result from decreases in sound generation (less turbulent flow) with shallow breathing patterns. This may occur

> ### Selective filtration
>
> This is the reflection of sound, as well as its attenuation during transmission
>
> - certain frequencies may be transmitted through the media with little reflection or attenuation
> - other frequencies may not pass at all.
>
> This concept is important in the understanding of respiratory sounds heard over the thoracic wall and over the trachea.

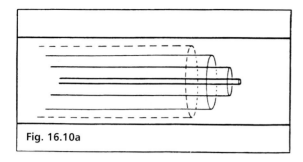

Fig. 16.10a

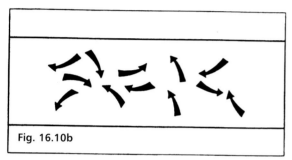

Fig. 16.10b

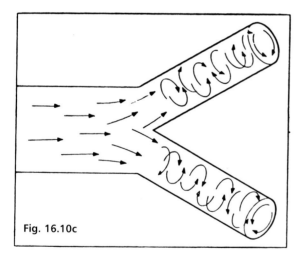

Fig. 16.10c

**Fig. 16.10** Types of air flow. In smooth, straight tubes turbulent flow occurs only at high velocity; this usually occurs only in large tubes such as the main bronchi and trachea, especially when there is hyperpnea. The flow rate in the fine tubes is very low because the total air flow is divided among hundreds of thousands of tubes. However, eddy formation may occur at each branching of the tracheobronchial tree, and the pressure required for eddy flow is approximately the same as for turbulent flow. Turbulence (at low flow rates) or eddy formation is particularly apt to occur where there are irregularities in the tubes, such as those caused by mucus, exudate, tumor or foreign bodies, or partial closure of the glottis. Sometimes air flow is the combination of laminar and turbulent flow with eddy formation. (a) Laminar flow. (b) Turbulent flow. (c) Vortices.

with restrictive lung diseases as a result of inadequate lung inflation. A diminished intensity will also occur when the sound transmission capacity of the lung or thoracic wall is reduced and results in more filtering of the turbulent flow sounds. This can occur

- with muscular and fat-filled thoracic walls
- when the lung becomes hyperinflated (as with emphysema)
- with pleural disease (effusion or pneumothorax).

A muffling or complete absence of lung breath sounds occurs when there are space-occupying masses in the lung or pleural cavity, pleural effusions, and when portions of the distal bronchial tree are occluded with exudate.

### Anatomic landmarks for auscultation and percussion

**Dog and cat**
The dorsal limit of the area of auscultation is the lateral margin of the paravertebral muscles. The basal border of the lung extends in a curve from the costochondral junction of the 6th rib to the margin of the para-vertebral muscles in the 11th intercostal space. The cranial lobes of the lungs are covered by the pectoral limb, and auscultation as far cranial and dorsal as possible is necessary to evaluate the cranial aspects of the lungs.

**Horse**
The dorsal limit of the area of lung auscultation and percussion is the lateral margin of the large paravertebral muscles, the most lateral of which terminates on the angles of the ribs. The cranial border is formed by the triceps muscle and varies with the position of the pectoral limb. In the usual standing position the olecranon is in the transverse plane of the 5th costo-

---

**Normal breath sounds**

It is thought that normal breath sounds are produced regionally within each lung, and probably within each lobe, implying that the breath sounds heard over a specific lobe are predominantly the result of air entry into that lobe. Normal breath sounds differ according to the

- thickness of the thoracic wall
- age of the animal
- respiratory movement patterns
- site of auscultation.

chondral junction. The basal border of the lung extends from the costochondral junction of the 6th rib, through the middle of the 11th and 12th ribs to the margin of the paravertebral muscles in the 16th intercostal space. Approximately one-quarter of both cranial regions is covered by the pectoral limb, which means the stethoscope must be pushed high up into the axilla in order to auscultate the cranial aspects of the lungs.

### Cattle

The dorsal limit of the area of auscultation and percussion is the lateral margin of the paravertebral muscles. In the standing adult animal the olecranon is paravertebral near the sternal end of the 5th rib. The basal border of the lung extends from the costochondral junction of the 6th rib to the margin of the spinal muscles in the 11th intercostal space. The cranial lobes of the lungs are covered by the pectoral limbs, and auscultation as forward and high up as possible in the axilla is necessary to evaluate the cranial aspects of the lung (Fig. 16.11). This is especially important when auscultating the lungs of young calves with suspected enzootic pneumonia, in which the lesions are most pronounced in the cranioventral aspects of the lungs in the early stages of the disease.

**Fig 16.11a**

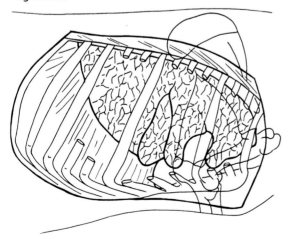

**Fig 16.11b**

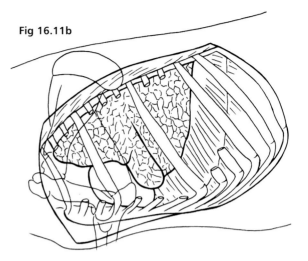

**Fig 16.11** Topographical anatomy of the lungs of an adult cow **(a)** Right side. **(b)** Left side. Note how the pectoral limb covers about one-third of the lung, necessitating auscultation in the axillary region cranial to the triceps musculature.

### *Technique of auscultation of lungs, trachea, and larynx*

The entire aspects of both lung fields and the trachea and larynx should be auscultated in a systematic manner. The breath sounds are evaluated for their

- acoustic characteristics
- timing in the respiratory cycle (inspiration or expiration)
- anatomical location of adventitious sounds
- areas of absence of sounds.

Interpretation of these variables is necessary to evaluate the nature of the lesions present. The acoustic characteristics of breath sounds and their significance are summarized in Table 16.1.

### Cattle

The following description of the auscultation of the lungs of cattle can be applied to other species with some minor modifications.

It is preferable to begin by auscultating the larynx, the trachea, and the thorax over the area of the tracheal bifurcation to assess the intensity of sound heard over the lungs. The diaphragm of the stethoscope is held over the external aspects of the larynx, and then the cervical trachea, to listen for the sounds of inspiration and expiration.

For auscultation of the lungs the thoracic wall can be divided topographically into dorsal, middle and ventral thirds.

**Table 16.1. Identification and clinical significance of breath sounds and extraneous sounds heard on auscultation of respiratory tract**

| Sounds | Acoustic characteristics | Significance and examples |
|---|---|---|
| Normal breath sounds | Soft blowing sounds; longer and louder on inspiration than on expiration; audible over the trachea and lungs | Normal respiratory tract |
| Increased audibility of breath sounds | Mild to moderate increase in loudness of breath sounds; audible on inspiration and expiration over the trachea and lungs | Any factor which increases respiratory rate or depth of respirations, including fever, excitement, exercise, high environmental temperatures, lung disease. Harsh loud breath sounds are audible over the lungs with any disease resulting in collapse or filling of alveoli and leaving bronchial lumina open; e.g. pulmonary consolidation and atelectasis. |
| Decreased audibility of breath sounds | Decreased audibility of breath sounds on inspiration and/or expiration over the lungs. Generalized or localized | Obese animal, pleural effusion, space-occupying mass of lung or pleural cavity, pneumothorax, diaphragmatic hernia, occlusive (lung) airway disease as in bronchial lumina filled with exudate |
| Crackles | Short duration, interrupted, non-musical breath sounds. Coarse crackles are loud and most commonly heard over large airways in animals with pulmonary disease and may be heard during inspiration and expiration. Fine crackles are of short duration, less intense and higher pitched | Coarse crackles are probably caused by air bubbling through, and causing vibrations within, secretions in large airways. Fine crackles caused by sudden explosive popping open of a series of airways closed during expiration. May be detected in early or late inspiration. |
| Wheezes | Continuous musical-type squeaking and whistling sounds audible over the lungs | Narrowing of large airways; expiratory polyphonic wheezing common in equine COPD; bronchopneumonia, any species |
| Pleuritic friction rubs | 'Sandpapery' sound; grating; sound close to the surface; on inspiration and expiration; tend to be jerky and not influenced by coughing | Pleuritis; diminish or disappear with pleural effusion |
| Stridor | A high-pitched sound on inspiration, audible with or without stethoscope over the larynx and trachea | Obstruction of extrathoracic airways, especially the larynx (due to edema) prime example is calf diphtheria or tracheal collapse in horses and dogs |
| Stertor | Snoring sound (low pitched, coarse and raspy) audible without a stethoscope on inspiration and expiration over the pharyngeal and laryngeal areas | Partial obstruction of the upper respiratory tract, commonly due to abnormalities of soft palate and nasopharynx |
| Expiratory grunting | Loud grunting on expiration; audible on auscultation of the thorax, over the trachea and often without the aid of a stethoscope | Due to pain resulting from severe diffuse pulmonary emphysema; extensive consolidation; acute pleurisy and peritonitis |

| Table 16.1. Identification and clinical significance of breath sounds | | |
|---|---|---|
| *Sounds* | *Acoustic characteristics* | *Significance and examples* |
| Transmitted upper respiratory tract breath sounds | Abnormal upper respiratory tract breath sounds audible by auscultation over the extrathoracic trachea during inspiration | Indicates the presence of abnormalities of the upper respiratory tract (larynx, nasopharynx, nasal cavities and upper trachea) resulting in accumulation of respiratory secretions causing constriction of airways. Laryngitis is an excellent example |
| *Extraneous sounds heard on auscultation of respiratory tract* | | |
| Crepitating sounds in subcutaneous tissues | Loud superficial crackling sounds induced by movement of stethoscope over the skin | Subcutaneous emphysema |
| Peristaltic sounds | Gurgling, grating, rumbling, squishing sounds audible over the lungs | Gastrointestinal sounds transmitted from the abdomen. Does not indicate diaphragmatic hernia unless other evidence such as an absence of breath sounds is present. |

It is also critical to auscultate in the axillary region as far cranially and dorsally as possible to ensure that the cranioventral aspects of the lungs are examined.

## A recommended method for auscultating the lungs of cattle

- auscultation commences over the middle third of the thorax at the level of the base of the heart
- the movements of the thoracic and abdominal walls are observed while simultaneously listening to the breath sounds of several breathing cycles (inspiration, expiration, pause)
- the stethoscope is moved caudally along the thoracic wall until the lung sounds are no longer audible at their most caudal border
- the stethoscope is moved systematically in horizontal and vertical directions, like the pattern of a checkerboard, until all lung areas have been examined
- at each site at least two breathing cycles are listened to for any change in the characteristics of the breath sounds and the presence of any adventitious sounds
- areas of abnormality are auscultated again to ensure that the same abnormalities can be heard repeatedly when compared with normal areas.

Increased loudness of breath sounds and adventitious sounds indicative of disease may be clearly audible by auscultation in the axilla, whereas the sounds over the upper third of the lungs may be within the normal range in an animal with pneumonia. Comparison of the lung sounds of the dorsal, middle, and ventral thirds of the lung is helpful in detecting the presence of abnormalities. For example, with a pleural effusion the lung sounds may be diminished or absent over the ventral third of the thorax and within normal range in the middle and dorsal thirds. Only by critically comparing the intensity of the sounds at various anatomical levels can subtle abnormalities be detected. It is also necessary to auscultate both sides of the thorax for comparison.

When lung sounds are just barely audible, it may be necessary to make the animal hyperventilate. Occluding the nostrils with one hand or, in the case of large animals, holding a plastic rebreathing bag over the rostral face for 1–2 minutes (Fig. 16.12), will cause hyperventilation and accentuate both normal and abnormal respiratory sounds, which may not be clearly audible if the animal is breathing with less depth.

The following questions should be considered:

- Is the audibility of breath sounds heard on auscultation of the cervical trachea and thorax normal?
- Are there regional differences in the audibility of breath sounds?

secretions accumulate in horses with respiratory disease, coarse crackles may be most readily detected at this site. During auscultation the clinician should observe the costal arch and abdominal wall to

- determine the stage of the breath cycle at which the sounds occur
- assess the relative intensity of the inspiratory and expiratory sounds.

Auscultation should also be performed while the horse is hyperventilating: this considerably improves the audibility of the breath sounds and hence increases the sensitivity of the examination. Hyperventilation is easily induced using a rebreathing bag or by occluding the external nares for 30 to 60 seconds (Fig. 16.12). Although the latter technique is better tolerated, it often initiates swallowing and chewing, resulting in referred noise which can mask the breath sounds. The clinician should strongly suspect respiratory tract disease if forced hyperventilation induces adventitious breath sounds or coughing, or if the time for the breathing rate to return to normal is excessively long.

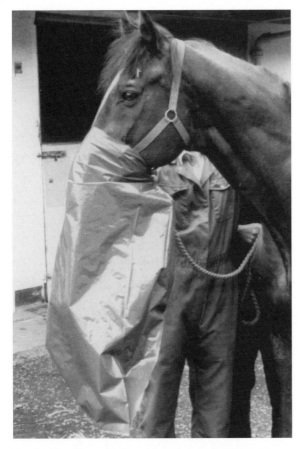

**Fig. 16.12** The audibility of breath sounds detected by auscultation may be increased by using a rebreathing bag. This induces hyperventilation and considerably improves the sensitivity of thoracic auscultation.

- Are abnormal breath sounds present? If so, what are they, what is their location, and at what stage of the breath cycle do they occur?

Learning to recognize breath sounds requires regular and systematic clinical practice on normal animals. Students should begin auscultating the respiratory tract of the different domestic animals early in their careers to become familiar with the respiratory sounds of normal animals.

### Horse

The major limitation of auscultation is the relative inaudibility of breath sounds detectable over the thorax, especially when examining obese horses under noisy field or clinic circumstances. The distal cervical trachea and both lung fields should be auscultated, as breath sounds are usually louder here than at the thoracic wall, and also, as this is where respiratory

**Clinical Pointer**

Forced hyperventilation is contraindicated in animals with thoracic pain or severe dyspnea.

### Dog and cat

Auscultation is performed in a quiet room free of distractions. Except in large-breed dogs or the critically ill, auscultation is best performed with the patient standing on an examination table. Purring in cats and panting in dogs are impediments to reliable auscultation. Sometimes the sound of running water or a mild noxious stimulus such as the odor of rubbing alcohol will stop a cat purring. Briefly occluding the nares is also effective. Holding a dog's mouth closed with one hand while performing thoracic auscultation prevents panting.

Brachycephalic dogs may have very loud stertorous sounds on inspiration which may obscure the normal breath sounds.

## Classification and interpretation of breath sounds

### Normal breath sounds

Normal breath sounds are produced in normal animals as a consequence of the movement of air within airways. This causes oscillations of solid respiratory tissues (tissue vibration) and rapid fluctuations of gas pressure (aerodynamic sound generation). The sounds are generated by turbulent air flow in the large ( >2 mm) airways and transmitted along the tracheobronchial lumen as airborne sound, and peripherally through the lung tissues and to the thoracic wall, where auscultation is commonly performed. The sound is normally filtered or damped as it travels within the lung outward towards the thoracic wall, this probably accounts for the differences in sounds heard over various portions of the thorax. Thus, normal lung sounds heard at the thoracic wall are a composite of individual noises generated by multicentric sources in underlying lung and from elsewhere in the respiratory tract. Nasal, laryngeal, and tracheal sounds can be heard over the thorax, as well as lung sounds. Small airways ( <2 mm) transmit sound waves poorly and probably do not contribute to the generation or transmission of breath sounds.

Normal breath sounds are clearly audible by auscultation over the larnyx, trachea, and lung. Their characteristics vary according to the age of the animal, breathing patterns, thickness of the thoracic wall, and the site of auscultation. The clear breath sounds audible over the cervical trachea and over the bifurcation of the trachea were previously known as tracheal and bronchial breath sounds, respectively. The breath sounds audible over the periphery of the lungs are attenuated and were previously known as vesicular breath sounds. The terms bronchial and vesicular have been replaced by the term **breath sounds.**

The normal breath sounds audible over the different levels of the respiratory tract are as follows.

- Nasal cavity breath sounds – breath sounds audible by auscultation over the nasal cavities or at the external nares.
- Normal breath sounds audible at the larynx – breath sounds audible by auscultation over the ventral aspects of the larynx.
- Normal breath sounds audible at the cervical trachea – the normal breath sounds produced in the large airways are transmitted efficiently through the thin peritracheal tissues and are clearly audible on auscultation of the distal cervical trachea. Normally they are soft blowing sounds which should be neither harsh nor accompanied by adventitious sounds. They are heard predominantly during early inspiration and early expiration, with the audibility of the inspiratory and expiratory noise being approximately equal.
- Normal breath sounds audible over the thorax – only a fraction of the breath sounds produced in the large airways reaches the thoracic wall, the remainder being lost owing to attenuation and reflection (Fig. 16.13). Consequently, the breath

sounds detected over the thorax during normal resting breathing are often barely inaudible and are difficult to interpret. This loss is normally greater for high-frequency than for low-frequency sounds. Normally, breath sounds are louder during inspiration and in the horse louder over the right lung field than over the left.

In adult horses, and probably other large animals, pulsatile inspiratory and expiratory breath sounds can be heard over the cervical trachea and cranial lung fields. These pulsations are synchronous with the heartbeat and are best detected when the beat is very strong and breathing deep and slow. This probably is due to movement of the heart causing fluctuations in the velocity of air in the large airways.

**Variations in audibility of breath sounds**

The amplitude or loudness and the duration of normal breath sounds may be increased or decreased, which in turn increases or decreases their audibility.

*Increased amplitude or audibility*

An increase in amplitude or audibility is usually the first and the most common abnormality of breath sounds that occurs in animals with respiratory disease.

Increased audibility of normal breath sounds over the entire lung field is most commonly due to hyperventilation. This increases breath sound production by increasing the velocity of air flow in the large airways. There are numerous causes of hyperventilation, including

- exercise
- respiratory tract disease
- anxiety
- high ambient temperature
- acidosis
- fever
- severe anemia
- cardiac failure.

The breath sounds are usually louder than normal in the presence of any lung disease that increases airflow velocity. This includes consolidation, pulmonary edema, and atelectasis. The acoustic properties of these abnormal states favor the efficient transmission of high-

---

**Clinical Pointer**

Consider size and condition of the animal when interpreting breath sounds, the sounds may be more audible in thin animals.

frequency breath sounds from the surrounding healthy airways to the overlying thoracic wall (Fig. 16.13). The breath sounds of the conducting airways will usually be transmitted through consolidated lung (i.e. not air-filled) much more effectively than when the lung contains air. Only when the conducting airways to an affected lobe are also occluded with exudate, or when there is a pleural effusion, will the sounds be diminished.

*Decreased amplitude or audibility*
The amplitude of breath sounds may be diminished, barely audible, or absent. Decreased audibility, commonly referred to as muffled lung sounds, usually results from an increase in the loss of sound as it is transmitted from the large airways to the stethoscope. A generalized reduction in the audibility of breath sounds over the entire thorax is common in obese animals, as the thick chest wall considerably reduces sound transmission. Rarely, a generalized reduction in breath sounds may be due to reduced airflow velocity, as occurs with hypoventilation. Regional loss of breath sounds occurs when

- air
- free fluid, or
- intestines

are present within the pleural cavity (Fig. 16.13). In these conditions breath sounds are lost largely by reflection at the tissue/air or tissue/fluid interfaces, which act as near-complete acoustic barriers. Although the accumulation of air within the pulmonary parenchyma, caused by emphysema or lung hyper-inflation, will also increase sound loss due to reflection, this is rarely detectable clinically. Some normal animals, especially horses, will have such quiet breathing at rest that normal breath sounds may be inaudible.

**Abnormal breath sounds (crackles and wheezes)**
Adventitious breath sounds are additional to normal breath sounds and are classified into two major groups

- discontinuous sounds – crackles
- continuous sounds – wheezes.

The identification and clinical significance of respi-ratory sounds are summarized in Table 16.1.

Although adventitious breath sounds are usually present only in animals with respiratory tract disease, the clinician should be cautious when attributing a particular adventitious sound to a specific disease process or etiology. The converse is also true: the absence of adventitious breath sounds does not preclude the presence of lung disease, especially in animals during the recovery stages of pneumonia.

Adventitious breath sounds usually occur at the same stage of the breath cycle, over consecutive breaths. The

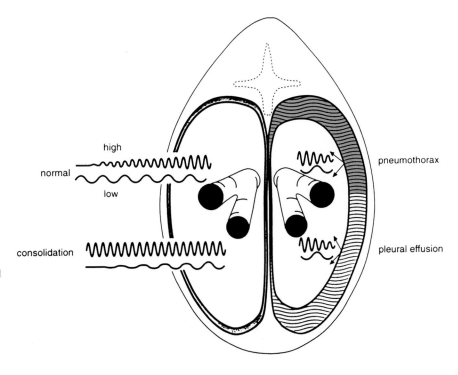

**Fig. 16.13** Schematic diagram showing the effects of pulmonary consolidation, pneumothorax and pleural effusion on the transmission of high and low frequency breath sounds from their source in the large airways to the stethoscope.

stage at which they occur should be determined as it can provide information regarding the nature and location of the underlying airway dysfunction. The location of maximal intensity of adventitious breath sounds should also be determined, as this usually indicates the location of dysfunction. The nature, anatomical location, and audibility of adventitious breath sounds may vary with time, owing to alterations in the underlying airway dysfunction or clearance of airway secretions by coughing.

*Crackles*
These are abnormal sounds of short duration, non-musical, and interrupted or discontinuous in time. Two types may be recognized.

*Coarse* These are loud, short duration (typically 10–30 ms), non-musical, bubbling sounds. They are probably the most common adventitious breath sound heard. They are loudest over the distal cervical trachea, especially during induced hyperventilation, and may be heard during inspiration and expiration. They are probably caused by air bubbling through, and causing vibrations within, secretions in the large airways.

*Fine* Compared to coarse crackles, fine crackles are shorter (typically 1–10 ms), less intense and higher pitched. They can be simulated by rolling a lock of one's hair between the fingers, close to the ear. Most fine crackles are probably caused by the sudden explosive popping open of a series of airways which have become abnormally closed during expiration (Fig. 16.14). The audible sounds are due to sudden equalization of the downstream and upstream airway pressures, or the sudden alteration in the tensions of the airway walls. In some animals fine crackles may be caused by air bubbling through secretions in the large airways. Fine

crackles are detectable mainly in peripheral and dependent lung areas. They are commonly associated with interstitial pulmonary disease.

It is important to note that the presence of crackles does not necessarily imply the presence of fluid within the lung. This is relevant in the elderly canine patient with a cough and an acquired murmur of mitral valve regurgitation. The presence of crackles suggests only that the patient has pulmonary disease, which may be cardiogenic pulmonary edema or perhaps bronchitis and airway collapse. Information gained from the remainder of the clinical examination must be used to make the distinction.

*Wheezes*
These are continuous (>250 ms) whistling, musical, squeaking sounds. They occur when air flows through

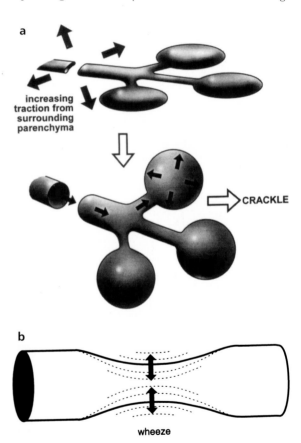

**Fig. 16.14** Schematic representation of mechanisms underlying the production of crackles and wheezes. (**a**) Crackles are caused by a series of collapsed airways suddenly popping open due to increasing traction from surrounding parenchyma. (**b**) Wheezes are produced by air flowing through narrowed airways, causing their walls to vibrate between the closed and barely open positions.

---

**Late inspiratory crackles**

occur in restrictive lung diseases, which reduce the compliance or distensibility of the lung and cause airway closure at low lung volumes. Late-inspiratory crackles over the dependent region of the lung may also be due to atelectasis associated with prolonged lateral recumbency or immobility.

**Early inspiratory crackles**

occur in animals with obstructive pulmonary diseases, which cause expiratory airway collapse as a result of intrathoracic airway narrowing, rather than reduced compliance as occurs in restrictive lung diseases.

narrowed airways, causing the walls to vibrate between the closed and barely open positions (Fig. 16.14). When an airway lumen narrows the airway wall flutters between open and nearly closed states, producing a continuous sound. The loudness, pitch, and duration of the wheeze depend on the velocity of air flow and the mechanical properties of the airway involved. Wheezes can be simulated by most normal humans and all human asthmatics simply by performing a violent forced expiration, which induces a dynamic collapse of the central airways at low lung volumes.

Wheezes may be heard throughout the breath cycle or, if exacerbated by dynamic airway collapse, may be inspiratory or expiratory (Fig. 16.15). Expiratory wheezing is most common

- expiratory wheezes and expiratory dyspnea indicate partial obstruction of the intrathoracic airways, as occurs in equine COPD, in contrast
- inspiratory wheezes and inspiratory dyspnea indicate partial obstruction of the extrathoracic airways, such as occurs in bilateral laryngeal paralysis and cervical tracheal collapse.

Severe obstruction of the extrathoracic airways often produces a particularly loud inspiratory wheeze, termed a stridor, which is usually audible without a stethoscope. Less commonly, late inspiratory wheezes are audible in animals with atelectasis, pulmonary consolidation or restrictive lung diseases. In these conditions wheezes are produced by air entering previously collapsed airways as the lung expands and the airways dilate during late inspiration.

Wheezes are characterized as high-pitched/musical or low-pitched/sonorous, and monophonic (single tone) or polyphonic (multiple tones), and by the timing of their occurrence in the respiratory cycle. A fixed monophonic wheeze is a single note of constant pitch, site, and timing. It indicates partial obstruction of a single airway, usually by a solitary space-occupying lesion. This is relatively uncommon distal to the tracheal bifurcation.

Wheezes are frequently audible at the thoracic wall, cervical trachea, and external nares, as they are transmitted throughout the large airways and through the thoracic wall with very little sound attenuation.

The pitch of a wheeze is determined by the mass and elasticity of the solid structures set oscillating, as well as the linear velocity of the air through the stenosed airway. It is therefore incorrect to attribute high-pitched wheezes to short peripheral airways and low-pitched wheezes to large central airways.

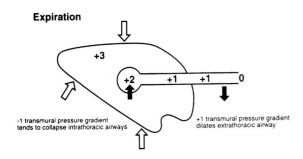

**Inspiration**

+1 transmural pressure gradient dilates intrathoracic airways

−1 transmural pressure gradient tends to collapse extrathoracic airway

**Expiration**

−1 transmural pressure gradient tends to collapse intrathoracic airways

+1 transmural pressure gradient dilates extrathoracic airway

**Fig. 16.15** Schematic diagram showing the pathogenesis of dynamic airway collapse. During inspiration the pressure outside the extrathoracic airways exceeds that within the airway. If this transmural pressure gradient overcomes the rigidity of the airway, dynamic extrathoracic airway collapse will result. Conditions that compromise the rigidity of the extrathoracic airways, including laryngeal paralysis and cervical tracheal collapse, may induce airway collapse and cause inspiratory dyspnea. Conversely, during expiration the transmural pressure gradient favors dynamic collapse of the intrathoracic airways. Conditions that lead to narrowing of these airways, such as chronic obstructive pulmonary disease, exacerbate airway closure and cause expiratory dyspnea.

> ### Polyphonic wheezes
>
> These comprise several different notes of different pitch and timing, starting and ending simultaneously like a chord. They indicate multiple airway obstruction and are commonly heard in
>
> - cats with acute asthmatic bronchoconstriction
> - horses with COPD
> - cattle with bronchitis, as in viral interstitial pneumonia due to bovine respiratory syncytial virus.

*Pleural friction sounds*
Movement of the pleural membranes during breathing is normally silent owing to the lubricant properties of

the pleural fluid. When the visceral and parietal pleurae are inflamed and rub together, frictional resistance may produce pleural friction sounds. These sounds vary considerably, from the classic harsh sounds, which may be simulated by rubbing two sheets of sandpaper together, to sounds similar to crackles. They have also been likened to the creaking of new leather. This variability complicates recognition of these sounds and makes them difficult to differentiate from crackles produced by pulmonary disease. In general they are a combination of continuous and discontinuous sounds, easily audible, and they appear to be very close to the diaphragm of the stethoscope. The crackles of pleural disease are usually louder, lower pitched, and more focal than those associated with deep lung disease. Pleural friction sounds are usually heard during both inspiration and expiration, and tend to recur consistently at similar stages in the breath cycle, features which are diagnostically useful.

Most pleural friction sounds are transient phenomena, disappearing when the pleurae are separated by large volumes of pleural effusion. Thus the absence of pleural friction sounds does not rule out the presence of pleuritis. In chronic pleuritis the pleurae may be adherent, which will not be associated with a friction sound.

*Transmitted abnormal upper respiratory tract breath sounds*
Abnormal breath sounds may be transmitted from the upper respiratory tract to the lungs and misinterpreted as abnormal lung sounds. Partial obstruction of the larynx or trachea, such as due to disease or mechanical constriction of the neck by a restraining rope, or to the presence of excessive respiratory secretions in the upper airway, can result in varying degrees of stertor and stridor which will be transmitted to the lungs and be audible primarily on inspiration. The presence of these sounds on inspiration when auscultating the lower trachea will confirm that they are transmitted from the upper part of the tract.

## Extraneous sounds audible while auscultating the respiratory tract

During auscultation of the respiratory tract some extraneous sounds may be superimposed over normal and abnormal lung sounds. With practice and careful technique it is possible to concentrate on the breath sounds and ignore these. Extraneous sounds include skin and hair noises, heart sounds, muscular contractions, gastrointestinal sounds, and feline purring.

Skin and hair sounds are superficial scratching sounds which occur if the stethoscope is not held firmly against hair-covered skin. They may be mistaken for crackles. Hair noises are diminished if the stethoscope is pressed firmly against the thoracic wall. Subcutaneous emphysema causes crackling and crepitating sounds when the stethoscope is applied to the affected part of the skin.

Heart sounds are commonly heard during auscultation of the lungs. Normal lung sounds are difficult to hear in the region of maximum intensity of heart sounds, but adventitious sounds may be detected. Adventitious respiratory sounds may be mistaken for heart murmurs. The clinician may differentiate cardiac and breath sounds by determining whether the sounds coincide consistently with the cardiac or the breath cycle. Forced cessation of respirations by occluding the external nares for up to 30 seconds will allow auscultation of the heart without interference by lung sounds.

Muscular contractions, especially tremors of the triceps muscle, cause a low-pitched rumbling sound which can interfere with auscultation.

Gastrointestinal sounds are frequently audible when listening to the thorax of normal animals. They include the sounds of

- swallowing
- eructation
- reticulorumen contraction
- gastrointestinal motility.

These must be differentiated from breath sounds as they are sporadic, variable in intensity and duration, and unassociated with the breath cycle. Their presence does not indicate diaphragmatic herniation, unless other signs are suggestive.

### Feline purring

This is a characteristic sound that overshadows all breath sounds. It results from the highly regular intermittent activation (25–30 times/s) of intrinsic laryngeal muscles and the diaphragm. Each laryngeal muscle activation causes glottal closure and the development of high transglottal pressure. The sound is generated when this high pressure is dissipated by glottal opening.

## Acoustic percussion of the thorax

### Indications

Acoustic percussion is a non-invasive technique for detecting pleural and superficial parenchymal lesions

(Fig. 16.16). It is indicated when auscultation of the lungs reveals a decreased audibility of breath sounds. The most common abnormality to prompt acoustic percussion is muffling of the lung sounds by a pleural effusion or a space-occupying lesion of the lungs or pleural cavity (Fig. 16.17).

The objective is to determine whether there are areas of increased resonance or dullness that may indicate the presence of lesions. The technique is done without the aid of the stethoscope. In general auscultation provides more information.

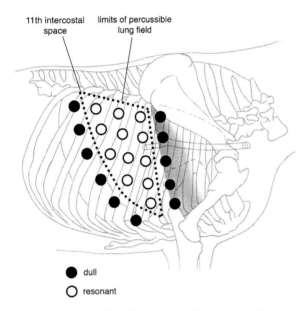

**Fig. 16.16** Normal border for thoracic percussion in cattle. Notice the steep straight caudoventral border (c.f. Fig 16.19.)

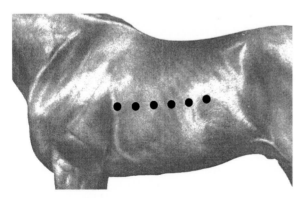

**Fig. 16.17** Acoustic percussion of thorax of this horse revealed dullness of the ventral aspect of the thorax due to pleural effusion. Dotted line indicates ventral limits of lung field in this case.

## Limitations of percussion

- considerable practice is required to attain diagnostic proficiency
- only relatively large space-occupying lesions of the lungs can be detected
- the percussion sound waves penetrate to a depth of several centimeters, and so only pleural and superficial parenchymal lesions can be detected.

### Anatomical landmarks

Clinically normal thoracic fields identified by acoustic percussion have reproducible and readily identifiable boundaries. In both large and small animals the mass of the triceps brachii muscle forms the cranial border of the area of percussion of the lung, precluding meaningful percussion in this area although the lungs extend further forward. The dorsal extent of the area of percussion is defined by a line immediately ventral to the paravertebral muscles. The caudal border varies between species, but extends from a point just caudal to the olecranon to the dorsal aspect of the 11th intercostal space in ruminants and small animals, and to the dorsal aspect of the 16th intercostal space in the horse. In cattle the caudal border is almost a straight line from the olecranon, passing through the middle of the 9th rib and extending to the 11th intercostal space. In the horse the caudal border is a crescent-shaped line extending from just caudal to the olecranon to the 16th intercostal space, and the presence of gas in the underlying large intestine may make delineation of caudoventral limits difficult.

### Technique of percussion

As percussion over the ribs and the intercostal spaces yields slightly different tones the clinician should attempt to restrict it to the intercostal spaces. However, this may not be possible in obese animals, when the ribs and intercostal spaces cannot be palpated.

Percussion should be done in a systematic pattern, usually commencing at the craniodorsal aspect of the thorax and moving dorsal to ventral within each intercostal space, before repeating the examination over the caudally adjacent rib. It is essential to percuss and compare both sides of the thorax.

Various techniques for acoustic percussion are described. The preferred techniques use a manual method and an instrument-based method as depicted in Fig. 16.18. The fingers may be used as both plexor and pleximeter. A right-handed person hyperextends the middle finger of the left hand and presses the distal phalanges firmly against the thoracic wall. The other parts of the hand should not contact the thorax as this will damp the vibrations. The distal interphalangeal joint is then abruptly struck with the tips – not the pads – of the middle three fingers of the right hand, keeping them semiflexed, rigid, and aligned. The right hand is immediately withdrawn to avoid damping the resultant noise.

The indirect method of percussion of the thorax may be used in large animals. A plexor and pleximeter are required (Fig. 16.18C). The plexor is a small hammer with a rubber head; the pleximeter is a metal plate which fits into the intercostal space (a tablespoon can also be used). The pleximeter is held firmly into an intercostal

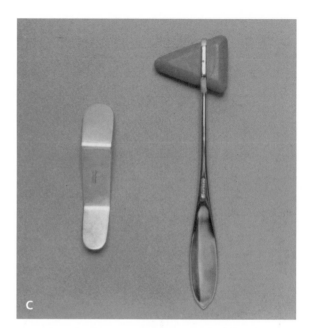

**Fig. 16.18** (C) Plexor (hammer) and pleximeter (plate) used for acoustic percussion in cattle and horses.

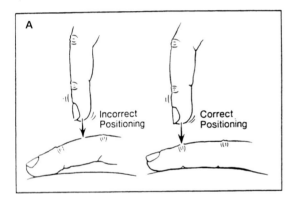

**Fig. 16.18** (A) The most common percussion technique in small animals is an indirect one in which the distal phalanx serves as a pleximeter. The phalanx should maintain close contact with the thoracic wall.

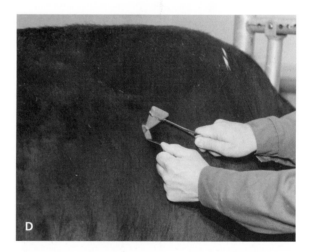

**Fig. 16.18** (D) Acoustic percussion of thorax of cow using plexor and pleximeter instruments.

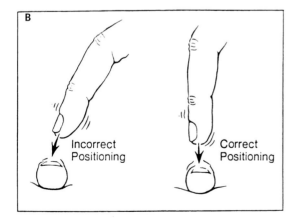

**Fig. 16.18** (B) The plexor finger should be kept at right-angles to the finger serving as a pleximeter.

space while two quick uniform taps with the plexor, using wrist action, are delivered to it (Fig 16. 18D). The pleximeter is then moved to a different location, the percussion is repeated and the resulting sounds are compared. Delivering the percussion blows rapidly and moving the pleximeter briskly to a new location often aids the detection of different resonances. In the normal animal the area of percussion outlined above will yield variable degrees of resonance except over the heart, where the area of cardiac dullness or cardiac silhouette is encountered. When an area of abnormality is detected it should be examined repeatedly to confirm the results.

### *Interpretation of acoustic percussion sounds*

Normally, percussion over the lung fields (Fig. 16.19) results in a low-pitched hollow sound that is termed resonant, whereas percussion outside this area produces a damped, higher-pitched tone described as dull. In normal horses, increased and decreased resonances are occasionally detected at the end of inspiration and expiration, respectively. Percussion yields a more resonant tone in individuals with thin thoracic walls, such as neonates and thin adults. Although many texts describe the use of percussion to

detect enlargement of the lung fields in horses with chronic obstructive pulmonary disease, this is in fact rarely detectable.

The most common abnormal finding during percussion of the thorax in large animals is dullness of the ventral aspect, often delineated by a horizontal line commonly referred to as a **fluid line** (see Fig. 16.17). The cranio-ventral dullness is most often caused by

- a pleural effusion
- widespread consolidation of lungs due to bronchopneumonia, or
- a pericardial effusion.

A hyperresonant sound is a more vibrant, lower-pitched, louder, and longer sound associated with increased air density. The hyperresonant sound is found normally in younger animals and during deep inspiration. The differential diagnosis for an enlarged area of resonance and the presence of tympany over the thorax includes

- pneumothorax,
- tympany associated with herniation of parts of the gastrointestinal tract into the thorax,
- pulmonary emphysema (especially bullous emphysema).

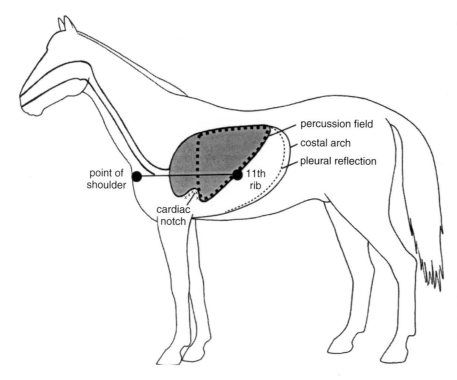

**Fig. 16.19** Schematic diagram showing the line of costodiaphragmatic pleural reflection (.....), the cardiac notch and the outline of the equine lung field as determined by percussion (-----). On percussion the ventral limit of the lung field at the 11th rib is level with the point of the shoulder. The actual anatomical outline of the lung, however, varies during the breath cycle (c.f. Fig 16.16).

## Clinical Pointer

The composite normal resonant note can only be learned from personal experience gained by percussion of the thorax of many clinically normal animals.

## Abnormal findings on acoustic percussion of the equine and bovine thorax

- dull area ventrally – pleural effusion (see Fig. 16.17), diaphragmatic hernia, marked cardiomegaly, marked pericardial effusion
- dull area at any site – pleural or pulmonary abscess or neoplasm
- increased resonance dorsally – pneumothorax
- increased resonance at any site – emphysematous bullae, although these are rarely of sufficient magnitude to be detectable by percussion
- coughing – percussion induces coughing only if there is disease of the underlying lung parenchyma
- pain – percussion is painful only if there is disease of the underlying thoracic wall, pleura or lung parenchyma.

## Endoscopy of the respiratory tract

The respiratory tract can be examined visually with an endoscope. The equipment consists of a light source which transmits cold light through a fiberglass cable to a flexible endoscope. Light transmission is by bundles of non-coherent glass fibers. Image transmission is by bundles of coherent glass fibers, or by a small camera on the endoscope tip. An air and water pump provides the mechanism for demisting and cleaning the objective lens. Various instruments, such as

- catheters
- biopsy forceps
- cytology brushes
- probes
- swabs, and
- guidewires

can be passed down a channel of the endoscope for special diagnostic purposes. Photographs and videos can also be taken. The cone of forward vision is about 60° and the end of the scope can be rotated at least 180° in either direction to view the walls of a hollow tube.

## Endoscopic techniques

Because it is used extensively in the horse, this technique will be described in the horse and can be used and modified in other species.

**Horse**
A 1 m long flexible fiberoptic endoscope allows direct examination of the

- nasal passages
- ethmoturbinates
- nasomaxillary openings of the sinuses
- pharynx
- guttural pouch openings
- larynx, and
- trachea.

Gastroscopes (1 m long) and colonoscopes (2 m long) designed for use in human patients have routinely been used for endoscopy in horses.

## Clinical Pointer

- endoscopy is normally done on the resting horse
- using endoscopy optimal detection of exercise-induced pulmonary hemorrhage is achieved about 30 minutes after fast exercise
- endoscopy can be carried out while a horse is exercising on a high-speed treadmill.

Diagnostic endoscopy of the upper respiratory tract in horses is usually performed in the conscious standing animal, and is thus easily performed in the field. The horse is restrained with a halter and lead rope, and a twitch is usually necessary. The endoscope is a little stiff in cold weather and prior to endoscopy may be warmed and the tip lubricated in warm water. It is introduced into the ventral meatus of the nasal cavities in the same way as a nasogastric tube, and once in the ventral meatus can be advanced further under direct vision into the nasopharynx or trachea.

## Clinical Pointer

Any discomfort usually diminishes after the endoscope has been inserted about 15 cm into the nasal cavity.

The view in the ventral meatus is limited to the

- mucosae of the floor of the nasal cavity
- conchae
- nasal septum.

Exudate may be visible but this often arises further caudally. Towards the dorsocaudal limit of the nasal passage the ethmoid turbinates can be seen as finger-like projections.

---

### Clinical Pointer

Ethmoid hematomas are one cause of chronic low-volume unilateral epistaxis in horses.

---

Despite the fact that an endoscope cannot be inserted through the very small nasal orifices of any equine paranasal sinus, nasal endoscopy is of great value to confirm the presence of sinusitis. With disorders of the frontal, dorsal conchal, caudal maxillary, caudal ventral conchal, ethmoidal and sphenopalatine sinuses, discharge most often will flow from the drainage ostium of the caudal maxillary sinus, and this will be seen at the caudal aspect of the middle meatus, below the ethmo-turbinates. With disorders of the very small rostral maxillary and ventral conchal sinuses discharge will be seen entering the nasal cavity midway along the middle meatus. There is usually also local swelling and reddening of the adjacent conchal mucosa.

A technique also used to investigate sinusitis, in particular chronic cases of unknown etiology, is direct sinusoscopy (sinoscopy), with insertion of a fiberoptic endoscope or arthroscope directly into the maxillary or frontal sinus (Fig. 16.20). This is readily achieved with sedation and local anesthesia of the overlying skin, prior to drilling a small hole wide enough to permit the endoscope to be introduced into the sinus.

As the endoscope is passed caudally through the nasal cavity it will enter the nasopharynx, which dorsally extends into the dorsal pharyngeal recess. Only a thin area of tissue separates the caudal wall of the recess from the guttural pouches. Looking dorso-caudally, the two openings of the guttural pouches should be visible in the lateral wall of the pharynx, completely covered by a shell-like flap of mucosa. Only when the horse swallows do the ostia open.

If indicated, the guttural pouches can be visualized. The endoscope is passed through the guttural pouch opening by following a guidewire. Usually a closed biopsy punch is passed through the biopsy port (arranging the endoscope tip so that the guide is against the pharyngeal mucosa) and into the guttural pouch opening. The endoscope can then follow the probe. The guttural pouch is divided into two compart-ments by the stylohyoid bone. Arteries, veins and nerves are visible in the wall of the pouch, particularly on the dorsocaudal aspect.

As the endoscope is moved further caudally down the nasopharynx the epiglottis will come into view. The normal epiglottis has a scalloped edge, with two small blood vessels visible running parallel to each edge.

---

### Clinical Pointer

If the epiglottis appears to have a smooth edge and the blood vessels are not visible, the area should be examined carefully for epiglottic entrapment.

---

The larynx is carefully evaluated for hemiplegia or hemiparesis, which was described earlier under exami-nation of the larynx.

The trachea can be inspected for evidence of abnormal respiratory secretions. If a long (>2 m in the adult horse) endoscope is available the site of discharge may be localized by following it down the main-stem bronchus into a secondary or tertiary bronchus. However, this is inexact as discharges are often intermittent and sites can be missed.

On endoscopy, the trachea of normal horses is circular in cross-section and should contain no (or only a few) flecks of respiratory secretions. The trachea normally curves towards the right of the median plane as it passes around the heart base, and bifurcates at the level of the 5th to 6th intercostal spaces. The normally asymmetric bronchial anatomy has been described. A summary of abnormal findings on endoscopic exami-nation of the lower respiratory tract is as follows:

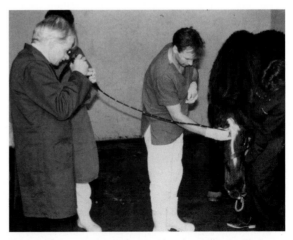

**Fig. 16.20** Under sedation and local anesthesia this horse has had an endoscope inserted through a small surgical opening (sinusoscopy) in its right frontal sinus to allow examination of the sinus lumen.

1. Excessive respiratory secretions within the cranial thoracic trachea (graded 1–5 according to volume)
   - mucopurulent secretions – present in most equine pulmonary diseases
   - purulent secretions – bacterial bronchopneumonia, pleuropnuemonia, or abscessation
   - blood – pulmonary hemorrhage
   - foamy liquid – pulmonary hypertension, cardiac failure, or alveolitis.
2. Mucosal inflammation – hyperemia and edema. Mucosal swelling may blunt the normally sharp carina and bronchial bifurcations.
3. Tracheal collapse (not uncommon in small ponies and miniature horses).
4. Foreign bodies (rare).
5. Airway neoplasia (rare).
6. Airway occlusion due to space-occupying lesion (rare).
7. Adult lungworms (*Dictyocaulus arnfieldi*) (rarely visible).

**Cattle**

Endoscopic examination of the respiratory tract is not performed routinely in cattle. It is recommended without sedation. The nasal septum tapers caudo-dorsally, allowing both ethmoturbinates to be observed from one side. The pharyngeal septum is contiguous with the nasal septum and merges with the caudodorsal wall of the pharynx. The appearance of the vocal cords is similar to those observed in the horse. Cattle lack a laryngeal saccule, and a laryngeal ventricle is not observed rostral to the vocal cords. The more rounded arytenoid cartilages are commonly maintained fully abducted and can be adducted by tactile stimulation of the larynx with the tip of the endoscope. The corniculate process of the arytenoid cartilage in cattle is more obvious and may project more rostrally than in the horse.

---

### Some uses of bronchoscopy

- to assess dynamic changes in airway diameter
- to aid the extraction of foreign bodies with grasping forceps
- to aid the biopsy of mass lesions using biopsy forceps
- for visual inspection of the respiratory tract before taking selective diagnostic samples
- to obtain swabs for bacterial culture or cytology using sterile sheathed brushes.

---

**Dog and cat**

Fiberoptic bronchoscopy can be performed in the anesthetized patient as previously noted. If inhalant anesthesia is used the bronchoscope is passed through the endotracheal tube. The need for anesthesia is a disadvantage in certain cases but does allow direct visual inspection of the airways.

## ANCILLARY DIAGNOSTIC TESTS

### Laboratory evaluation of respiratory secretions and exudates

When an inflammatory process is suspected in the respiratory tract, samples of secretions and exudate can be collected for microbiological and cytological examination. The objective is to obtain a sample which is uncontaminated with environmental or commensal flora (which are common in the upper respiratory tract), and in cases of respiratory infection to isolate the pathogen responsible for the lesion. This can be done by swabbing the nasal cavities or the pharynx, or taking

- a transtracheal aspirate
- a tracheal lavage
- a bronchoalveolar lavage, or
- a sample of pleural effusion
- a tissue biopsy.

### Nasal and nasopharyngeal swabs

For isolation of viruses associated with disease of the upper respiratory tract nasopharyngeal swabs are satisfactory, provided a copious amount of nasal discharge is collected and the swabs are kept in virus transport medium during transport because certain viral pathogens rapidly become inactivated in transit.

When investigating nasal disease in small animals, rhinoscopy is performed following radiographic examination of the nasal cavity. An otoscope, arthroscope, or pediatric flexible endoscope can be used to visualize the nasal cavities. The flexible endoscope can also be introduced into the oropharynx and retroflexed, permitting inspection of the nasopharynx and choanae (see below). This area can also be viewed per os using a dental mirror and penlight. Following rhinoscopy, cytological or histopathological samples of nasal tissue can be obtained from patients with clinical evidence of nasal disease. A nasal wash can be performed by

- introducing a flexible catheter such as a urinary catheter, into the nasal meatus
- injecting then reaspirating saline
- examining the wash cytologically.

## Clinical Pointer ✳

Owing to the large population of commensal organisms in the upper respiratory tract, bacteriological culture of nasal or nasopharyngeal swabs is rarely of value. The exception is in the diagnosis of strangles in the horse, when *Streptococcus equi* is readily cultured.

Most often histological study is required for definitive diagnosis. Biopsy forceps can be used to obtain tissue samples. When possible, a representative tissue sample is obtained under rhinoscopic guidance. When biopsies are obtained without the benefit of rhinoscopic guidance, the distance from the nares to the medial canthus of the eye is carefully measured beforehand and compared with the length of the biopsy instrument to avoid the potential complication of cribiform plate rupture.

### Transtracheal aspirate

The collection and evaluation of tracheobronchial secretions is useful for assessing lower airway disease. Most horses with pulmonary disease have large volumes of respiratory secretions pooling in the most dependent aspect of the trachea, near the thoracic inlet (Fig. 16.21A,B). Although detection of these secretions is a very sensitive indicator of pulmonary disease, cytological and bacteriological analysis is usually required to determine its etiology. Bacteriological evaluation of a transtracheal aspirate may provide useful information on antimicrobial sensitivity and aid in the selection of appropriate drugs.

### Large animals

Percutaneous transtracheal aspiration is a practical method which has been used extensively in the horse and is adaptable to cattle, sheep, and goats. Adequate restraint is necessary. Adult cattle should be in a stanchion or head-restraining device. The head is secured in a slightly elevated position with a halter, and the following procedure used.

1. The skin over the selected site is prepared aseptically and anesthetized locally. The optimum site for penetration is the most distal part of the external trachea not covered by other tissue, and where the trachea can be grasped and the rings easily palpated.
2. A trocar and cannula of suitable size is pushed firmly between two tracheal rings perpendicular to the long axis of the trachea. Once the tracheal

mucosa is perforated and the trocar is in the lumen, air can be heard flowing through the cannula when the trocar is withdrawn.

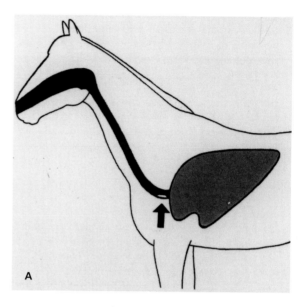

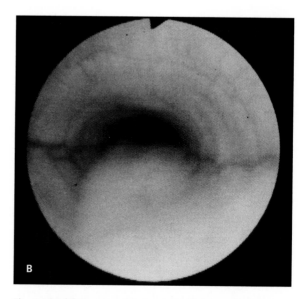

Fig. 16.21 (A) Excess respiratory secretions tend to accumulate at the most ventral part of the trachea, close to the thoracic inlet. At this location they may be detected on auscultation as coarse crackles. Secretions may be collected from this site using transendoscopic or percutaneous aspiration. (B) Endoscopic view of the distal cervical trachea of a horse with pulmonary disease, showing a large pool of respiratory secretions.

3. The cannula is then pushed down the trachea and the catheter threaded through it. A 30 cm long polyethylene catheter in a 14 gauge x 6 cm cannula or a sterile 14 g over-the-needle catheter can be used.
4. The trocar is removed and 20 ml sterile saline instilled. In mature horses and cattle it may be necessary to introduce an additional 30 to 50 ml saline in order to recover sufficient fluid by aspiration.
5. A syringe is then used to aspirate the saline and respiratory secretions from the lowest point of the trachea, which is just distal to the thoracic inlet.
6. The sample is placed in a sterile transport tube for microbiological evaluation, and other plain tubes for cytological evaluation.

Although coughing always occurs, other complications such as subcutaneous emphysema, pneumomediastinum and cellulitis can also occur.

Normal equine tracheal secretions contain mainly macrophages and ciliated columnar epithelial cells, a few cuboidal epithelial cells, and lymphocytes. Percentages of neutrophils appear to be variable, with less than 20% in apparently normal housed horses and less than 5% in most normal pastured horses.

**Dog and cat**

If possible, transtracheal aspiration is done without sedation, which inhibits the cough reflex, using the procedure outlined above for large animals with appropriate modifications for size.

Complications as for large animals are infrequent A tracheal wash can also be obtained through a sterile endotracheal tube while the patient is anesthetized. The risk of sample contamination is perhaps greater than with transtracheal aspiration; however, this technique has advantages for smaller animals, particularly cats, as there is less risk of laryngeal trauma.

## Bronchoalveolar lavage

Bronchoalveolar lavage (BAL) is a safe and relatively simple technique for harvesting cells from the distal airways and alveoli. Examination of BAL fluid (BALF) cytology has proved to be invaluable in the investigation of equine pulmonary disease, particularly chronic pulmonary disease, and is considered the most sensitive method for diagnosis of COPD. BALF cytology is easier to examine and interpret than tracheal RS cytology and also correlates well with pulmonary histopathology. Although there is a good correlation between BALF cytology and lung histopathology for generalized pulmonary diseases, with localized pulmonary diseases such as abscesses inadvertent lavage of a normal area may yield misleading information.

### Technique

Details of the technique are described elsewhere. Briefly, a BAL is performed using a long (>2 m) endoscope or a proprietary BAL catheter. To minimize the marked coughing elicited by passage of the endoscope or catheter beyond the tracheal carina the horse must be sedated. The horse is restrained with a nose twitch and the endoscope or catheter passed distally until it wedges, usually in a third- or fourth-generation bronchus. Isotonic sterile saline, 200–300 ml warmed to 37 °C to minimize coughing, is instilled and immediately aspirated gently using 50–60 ml syringes. On average, 50% of the instilled fluid is recovered. Complications of BAL are very rare.

### Interpretation

BALF from normal animals contain predominantly macrophages and lymphocytes, with few

- ciliated columnar epithelial cells
- neutrophils
- eosinophils, and
- mast cells.

In suppurative pneumonia and in equine COPD the cells are more numerous and are predominantly neutrophils, and there is abundant mucus. The presence of large numbers of eosinophils is abnormal and is consistent with transpulmonary parasite migration or idiopathic pulmonary eosinophilias. The presence of hemosiderin-laden macrophages is evidence of prior pulmonary hemorrhage. Owing to

---

### Bacteriological analysis of tracheal aspirates

- Both aerobic and anaerobic bacterial cultures should be performed.
- Because the trachea is not normally sterile, semiquantitative techniques should be employed.
- Normal secretions usually contain low numbers ($<10^4$ colony-forming units/ml) of a mixed bacterial flora.
- Secretions from animals with bacterial infections of the lower respiratory tract usually contain larger numbers ($>10^6$ colony-forming units/ml), a single pathogenic bacterial species usually predominates.

the unavoidable contamination of lavage fluid with upper respiratory tract bacteria, bacterial culture of lavage fluid is rarely of value in the horse.

## Pleuroscopy

An endoscope may be inserted into the pleural space to enable direct visualization and sampling of lesions affecting the pleurae, mediastinum, pericardium, and diaphragm. Complications of pleuroscopy include exacerbation of respiratory dysfunction due to pneumothorax, infection, and pulmonary laceration.

---

### Clinical Pointer

Pleuroscopy is indicated only when lesions cannot be adequately evaluated using less invasive techniques such as ultrasonography and radiography.

---

## Pleurocentesis (thoracocentesis)

Paracentesis of the pleural cavity is of value when the presence of fluid or air in the pleural sac is suspected. The withdrawal of pleural fluid can provide symptomatic relief in an animal with large quantities of a pleural effusion. Also, the pleural fluid should be examined for the presence of abnormal numbers and types of cells, and infectious agents.

### Dog and cat

Thoracocentesis is indicated when the cause of a pleural effusion is unclear despite radiographic evaluation. The procedure can be performed with an over-the-needle or a butterfly catheter with the patient in sternal or lateral recumbency. Prior to needle puncture the skin is prepared aseptically and locally anesthetized. Usually, the right hemithorax at the 7th or 8th intercostal space is chosen, although the appearance of thoracic radiographs may be helpful in guiding centesis of local effusions. A sample is obtained by gentle aspiration and submitted for cytological and bacteriological analysis.

---

### Clinical Pointer

Pleurocentesis is indicated when a pleural effusion is the cause of dyspnea.

---

### Complications of thoracocentesis

These are rare but include

- collapse of the animal
- pneumothorax
- puncture of the lung or heart.

---

### Large animals

The most common site for needle insertion is either the 6th or the 7th intercostal space below the level of the fluid line, which has been determined by percussion. Ultrasonography may be used to identify the optimal site of aspiration. The skin over the site is prepared aseptically and local anesthesia applied. In a mature horse or cow a 12–14 gauge needle, 8–10 cm in length, or a pleural catheter, is inserted carefully into the caudal aspect of the intercostal space. Immediately upon entering the pleural cavity the pleural fluid will usually drain out of the needle; occasionally it may be necessary to apply suction with a syringe or suction pump.

Normal animals have small volumes of clear to slightly turbid yellowish, non-clotting pleural fluid. It should be bacteriologically sterile and contain less than $10 \times 10^9$/liter nucleated cells, mainly

- neutrophils
- mononuclear/mesothelial-type cells, and
- lymphocytes.

## Lung biopsy

Percutaneous lung biopsy is warranted **only** when a histological diagnosis is essential for management of the case, and when such a diagnosis cannot be obtained using other less invasive techniques such as bronchoalveolar lavage. The technique is potentially hazardous and is contraindicated in animals with bullous or cavitating lesions or coagulopathies.

---

### Potential complications of lung biopsy

These include

- lung collapse
- pneumothorax
- hemothorax
- hemoptysis
- dissemination of infection
- neoplasia.

---

# MEDICAL IMAGING

## Radiography of the upper respiratory tract

Studies of the nasal cavity and frontal sinuses are important in the diagnostic evaluation of patients with chronic nasal discharge. This is particularly so when sinusitis and tooth root disease is suspected in horses. In small animals only, the open-mouth views of the nasal cavity tend to be most informative, although a complete radiographic nasal series is recommended for all small animal patients with clinical evidence of nasal disease. Destructive processes and, mass lesions can be identified

- lytic bony lesions of the nasal structures or loss of turbinate detail suggest neoplastic or advanced fungal disease
- involvement of the paranasal sinuses may be radiographically apparent with fungal disease
- aggressive neoplasms may invade the sinuses but generally arise from within the nasal cavity in dogs, the reverse is true in horses.

The information gained by radiographic examination is sometimes helpful in guiding biopsy attempts. The trachea and larynx can also be studied radiographically. Examination of inspiratory and expiratory views of the thorax and upper airway may increase the sensitivity for detection of airway collapse.

### Thoracic radiography

**Dog and cat**
Despite advances in other technologies, thoracic radiography remains a cornerstone of non-invasive evaluation of the respiratory tract in dogs and cats. Attention to technical factors is essential to gain the optimal amount of information. Radiographic technique, patient positioning and the phase of respiration must be taken into account before information provided by the thoracic radiograph can be considered reliable and useful.

An end-inspiratory radiograph provides the most useful information regarding the pulmonary parenchyma. A systematic approach to interpretation is recommended. After careful examination of the bony structures, the size of the cardiac silhouette is assessed. Examination of the great vessels is followed by careful assessment of the peripheral pulmonary vessels. Chronic respiratory disease is sometimes complicated by pulmonary vascular disease, which results in pulmonary hypertension and cor pulmonale. Distal attenuation and tortuosity of the pulmonary arteries may also be a part of the radiographic appearance of cor pulmonale. The pulmonary veins are generally small, reflecting reduced pulmonary perfusion.

A system of pattern recognition has been applied to the radiographic examination of the pulmonary parenchyma.

1. A bronchial pulmonary pattern is characterized by accentuation of the bronchial structures, resulting in the appearance of 'doughnuts and tramlines'. This pattern usually signifies the presence of inflammatory cells or structural elements (fibrosis) in the walls of the bronchi, and is generally associated with primary respiratory diseases such as chronic bronchitis.
2. An interstitial pulmonary pattern results when cellular infiltrates or edema obscure vascular detail. The causes of an interstitial pulmonary pattern are varied and its presence can suggest

- pulmonary edema
- inflammatory disease, or sometimes
- neoplastic disease.

3. The air bronchogram is the hallmark of the alveolar pulmonary pattern. The presence of fluid or cells within pulmonary parenchyma provides contrast with the air-filled bronchi.
4. Vascular patterns characterized by proximal pulmonary artery enlargement and distal attenuation occur in patients with cor pulmonale as well as some congenital cardiac malformations, such as the right–left shunting occurring with patent ductus arteriosus.
5. An appearance of hyperperfusion is noted in patients with left to right systemic to pulmonary shunts. Pulmonary venous distension suggests elevated left ventricular filling pressures, as might complicate myocardial disease as well as mitral and aortic valve disease.

**Large animals**
Thoracic radiography is not routinely used in the diagnosis of diseases of the respiratory tract of large animals. The large size of mature horses and cattle limits the use of radiography to hospitals where powerful X-ray machines are available for such purposes. Only lateral projections are possible. The large mass of tissue of the

---

## Clinical Pointer ✳

Examination of at least two orthogonal (lateral and ventrodorsal or lateral and dorsoventral) radiographic views of the chest is essential.

thorax in mature cattle and horses creates unique and often insurmountable imaging difficulties. Also, the radiographic image varies considerably with the stage of the breath cycle at which it is taken and with the position of the animal relative to the machine and screen. Radiography may detect

- large space-occupying lesions
- pneumothorax
- fractured ribs
- diaphragmatic herniation
- pleural effusion, and
- severe exercise-induced pulmonary hemorrhage lesions.

The technique and interpretation of equine thoracic radiography have been well described. The thorax of calves and foals up to about 6 months of age can be radiographed with many portable machines and can provide useful diagnostic information almost as precise as for small animals.

## Thoracic ultrasonography

Ultrasonography is a valuable non-invasive technique for imaging lesions of the

- superficial pulmonary parenchyma
- cranial mediastinum
- pleural cavity and thoracic wall

in both small and large animals, and is considerably more sensitive than percussion or auscultation. It is particularly useful for detecting and investigating pleural effusion and for selecting the optimal site for thoracocentesis or lung biopsy. Because ultrasound is totally reflected at a tissue–air interface, images cannot be obtained deep to normal aerated lung parenchyma. The relative diagnostic merits of thoracic ultrasound and radiography in large animal practice are listed below. Both may be required for a complete evaluation of any disease process. The technique of thoracic ultrasonography is well described.

Sonographic examination of the cranial mediastinum can be rewarding in small animals. Thoracic sonography, including echocardiography, provides useful information in the presence of pleural effusion.

## A comparison of the advantages of ultrasonography and radiography

### Advantages of ultrasonography

- more useful for imaging lesions of the cranial mediastinum, chest wall, pleurae, and superficial lung parenchyma
- useful for imaging lesions of the ventral thoracic cavity, which cannot be imaged radiographically as they are obscured by the cardiac and abdominal silhouettes
- enables ultrasound-guided biopsy of lesions
- very useful for determining the optimal site for thoracocentesis
- equipment is relatively inexpensive, portable, safe to use and more commonly available than radiographic equipment.

### Advantages of radiography

- useful for imaging deep parenchymal and caudal mediastinal lesions
- more useful for imaging interstitial lung disease
- more useful for imaging a pneumothorax.

## Fluoroscopy (image intensifier)

Fluoroscopy is similarly helpful in identifying collapse of the large airways, particularly the trachea. The patient is usually studied in lateral recumbency. Stimulation of the cough reflex through tracheal palpation may provoke airway collapse.

## Magnetic resonance imaging and computed tomography

Recent advances in technology allow three-dimensional image construction of the thoracic cavity and upper respiratory tract. Computed tomography (CT) utilizes narrowly collimated conventional X-rays; magnetic resonance imaging (MRI) provides images generated by energy detected when the body is subject to magnetic fields.

## Clinical Pointer

A commercially available device that continually monitors arterial oxygenation is invaluable in the critical care setting.

## Pulmonary function tests

Pulmonary function testing is used in the horse where it can on occasions detect low-grade subclinical respiratory disease. Determination of arterial $O_2$ and $CO_2$ levels, intrathoracic pressure measurements and pulmonary mechanic measurements, especially during treadmill exercise, are also effective but their use is likely to be restricted to research centers.

Pulse oximetry is a technique whereby light is transmitted through a non-pigmented skin fold and the light absorption characteristics of the tissue are analyzed. Practically, this is accomplished by attaching a small clip that is equipped with a light source and sensor to a skin fold. Light absorption during arterial pulsation is compared with the degree of background absorption. Venous blood, tissue, and bone are presumed to be responsible for the latter. The relationship of the absorption characteristics allows instantaneous estimation of oxyhemoglobin saturation. Clinically this parameter can be used to estimate the partial pressure of arterial oxygen. Although the accuracy of the saturation determination is affected by factors that include tissue perfusion, skin pigmentation and anatomical clip placement, the commercially available devices provide a means to continually monitor a parameter of arterial oxygenation.

## Arterial blood gas analysis

Measurement of arterial $CO_2$ concentration provides an assessment of alveolar ventilation, and measurement of arterial $CO_2$ and $O_2$ can provide information regarding pulmonary gas exchange. In large animals, arterial blood is usually collected from the carotid artery using a 21g 3.5 cm needle which is inserted through the caudal cervical jugular groove and directed towards the lateral aspect of the trachea. Other useful sites are

- the transverse facial artery
- the brachial artery
- the lateral metatarsal artery.

In small animals arterial blood is usually collected from the femoral or pedal artery using a 25g needle. Arterial blood will usually spurt or drip from the needle hub. Samples should be collected anaerobically, maintained on ice, and analyzed within 4 hours of collection. The major limitation of this technique is the requirement for expensive equipment and for rapid analysis. Misleading results may be due to inadvertent contamination of the sample with air or with venous blood, delayed analysis, or alterations in the breathing pattern induced by anxiety.

## IMMUNOLOGY

### Allergy testing

Occasionally, to confirm a diagnosis of allergic pulmonary disease it may be necessary to demonstrate that

- exposure of an affected animal to the causal allergens exacerbates the disease
- elimination of the allergen from the animal's environment induces disease remission.

This technique is particularly useful for confirming a diagnosis of COPD in horses, when it is very low grade or when other examinations are inconclusive. Within several hours of exposure to environments containing moldy hay and straw, horses with COPD have an exacerbation in pulmonary inflammation and dysfunction; exclusion of these agents results in a complete disease remission within a few weeks.

### Intradermal antigen testing

Intradermal testing with mold antigens appears not to be of value in the diagnosis of equine COPD. Many normal horses have positive intradermal reactions to mold antigens and there is no significant correlation between the dermal and pulmonary reactivities to mold antigens.

### Serology

Serology is used in the laboratory diagnosis of infectious diseases of the respiratory tract. More recently, proprietary virus antigen detection kits have become available that can allow detection of viral antigens in nasal secretions within 24 hours.

## FURTHER READING

Allen DG. Chronic cough. In: Allen DG (ed) Small animal medicine. Philadelphia: JB Lippincott, 1991; 123–130.
Amis TC, Kurpershoek C. Tidal breathing flow–volume loop analysis for clinical assessment of airway obstruction in conscious dogs. American Journal of Veterinary Research 1986;47: 1002–1006.

Anderson DE, DeBowes RM, Gaughan EM, Yoorchuk KE, St. Jean G. Endoscopic evaluation of the nasopharynx, pharynx, and larynx of Jersey cows. American Journal of Veterinary Research 1994; 55: 901–904.

Anderson DE, Gaughan EM, DeBowes RM, Lowry SR, Yoorchuk KE, St. Jean G. Effects of chemical restraint on the endoscopic appearance of laryngeal and pharyngeal anatomy and sensation in adult cattle. American Journal of Veterinary Research 1994; 55: 1196–1200.

Bauer TG, Woodfield JA. Mediastinal, pleural and extrapleural diseases. In: Ettinger SJ, Feldman E (eds) Textbook of veterinary internal medicine, 3rd edn. Philadelphia: WB Saunders, 1995; 812–842.

Beech J. Tracheobronchial aspirates. In: Beech J (ed) Equine respiratory disorders. Philadelphia: Lea & Febiger, 1991; 41–53.

Bennett DG. Evaluation of pleural fluid in the diagnosis of thoracic disease in the horse. Journal of the American Veterinary Medical Association 1986;188: 814–815.

Bjorling DE. Laryngeal paralysis. In: Bonagura JD, Kirk RW (eds) Kirk's current veterinary therapy – XII – small animal practice. Philadelphia: WB Saunders, 1995; 901–904.

Curtis RA, Viel L, McGuirk SM, Radostits OM, Harris FW. Lung sounds in cattle, horses, sheep and goats. Canadian Veterinary Journal 1986;27: 170–172.

Dixon PM. Collection of tracheal respiratory secretions in the horse. In Practice 1995;17:66–69.

Epstein DM, Gefter WB, Fishman AP. Computed tomography and magnetic resonance of the chest. In: Fishman AP (ed) Pulmonary disease and disorders, 2nd edn. New York: McGraw-Hill, 1988; 529–565.

Farrow CS. Radiographic examination and interpretation. In: Beech J (ed) Equine respiratory disorders. Philadelphia: Lea & Febiger, 1991; 89–119.

Hawkins EC. Tracheal wash and bronchoalveolar lavage in the management of respiratory disease. In: Bonagura JD, Kirk RW (eds) Current veterinary therapy– XI – small animal practice. Philadelphia: WB Saunders, 1992; 795–800.

Hendricks JC. Pulse oximetry. In: Bonagura JD, Kirk RW (eds) Kirk's current veterinary therapy – XII – small animal practice. Philadelphia: WB Saunders, 1995; 117–118.

King LG, Hendricks JC. Clinical pulmonary function tests. In: Ettinger SJ, Feldman EC (eds) Textbook of veterinary internal medicine, 3rd edn. Philadelphia: WB Saunders, 1995; 738–753.

Kotlikoff MI, Gillespie JR. Lung sounds in veterinary medicine. Part I: Terminology and mechanisms of sound production. Compendium of Continuing Education for the Practicing Veterinarian 1983;5:634–639.

Kotlikoff MI, Gillespie JR. Lung sounds in veterinary medicine. Part II: Deriving clinical information from lung sounds. Compendium of Continuing Education for the Practicing Veterinarian 1984;6:462–467.

Kuehn NF. Diagnostic methods for upper airway disease. Seminars in Veterinary Medicine and Surgery (Small Animal) 1995;10:70–76.

Kuehn NF, Roudebush P. Dyspnea. In: Allen DG (ed) Small animal medicine. Philadelphia: JB Lippincott, 1991; 123–130.

Mackey VS, Wheat JD. Endoscopic examination of the equine thorax. Equine Veterinary Journal 1985;17:140–142.

Mair TS, Gibbs C. The radiographic evaluation of pulmonary disease in the horse. Veterinary Annual 1990a; 30:181–189.

Mair TS, Gibbs C. Thoracic radiography in the horse. In Practice 1990;12:8–10.

McCarthy PH. Anatomy of the larynx and adjacent regions as perceived by palpation of clinically normal standing horses. American Journal of Veterinary Research 1990;51: 611–618.

McGorum BC, Dixon PM. The analysis and interpretation of equine bronchoalveolar lavage fluid (BALF) cytology. Equine Veterinary Education 1994;6:203–209.

McKiernan BC. Bronchoscopy in the small animal patient. In: Kirk RW (ed) Current veterinary therapy –X – small animal practice. Philadelphia: WB Saunders, 1989; 219–224.

McKiernan BC. Bronchoscopy revisited – is it worth it? Proceedings American College Veterinary Internal Medicine Forum. 1995; 385–387.

Nickel R, Schummer A, Seiferle. The viscera of the domestic mammals. Second revised edition by Schummer A, Nickel R, Sack WO, 1979. Verlag Paul Parey. Berlin, Hamburg.

Padrid P. Diagnosis and therapy of canine chronic bronchitis. In: Bonagura JD, Kirk RW (eds) Kirk's current veterinary therapy – II – small animal practice. Philadelphia: WB Saunders, 1995; 908–914.

Pringle JK. Assessment of the ruminant respiratory system. Veterinary Clinics of North America (Food Animal Practice) 1992; 8: 233–242.

Pringle JK. Ancillary testing for the ruminant respiratory system. Veterinary Clinics of North America (Food Animal Practice) 1992; 8: 243–256.

Rantanen NW. Diseases of the thorax. Veterinary Clinics of North America (Equine Practice) 1986; 2:49–66.

Raphel CF, Gunson DE. Percutaneous lung biopsy in the horse. Cornell Veterinarian 1981;71:439–448.

Reimer JM. Diagnostic ultrasonography of the equine thorax. Compendium of Continuing Education for the Practicing Veterinarian 1990;12:1321–1327.

Roudebush P. Lung sounds. Journal of the American Veterinary Medical Association 1982; 181: 122–126.

Roudebush P, Ryan J. Breath sound terminology in the veterinary literature. Journal of the American Veterinary Medical Association 1989;194: 1415–1417.

Roudebush P, Sweeney CP. Thoracic percussion. Journal of the American Veterinary Medical Association 1990; 197: 714–718.

Schaer M, Ackerman N, King RR. Clinical approach to the patient with respiratory disease. In: Ettinger SJ (ed) Textbook of veterinary internal medicine. Philadelphia: WB Saunders, 1989; 747–767.

Sweeney CR, Weiher J, Baez, JL, Lindborg SR. Bronchoscopy of the horse. American Journal of Veterinary Research 1992;53: 1953–1956.

Traub-Dargatz JL, Brown CM. Equine endoscopy. CV Mosby, 1997.

Tyler J. Something old, something new: thoracic acoustic percussion in cattle. Journal of the American Veterinary Medical Association 1990;197: 52–57.

Willoughby RA, McDonnell WN. Pulmonary function testing in horses. Veterinary Clinics of North America (Large Animal Practice) 1979;1:171–196.

# 17

# Clinical Examination of the Alimentary System

*Dogs and Cats – D.M. Houston*
*Horses – T.J. Phillips, P.M. Dixon*
*Ruminants – O.M. Radostits*

## CLINICAL MANIFESTATIONS OF DISEASES OF THE ALIMENTARY SYSTEM

**Abdominal distension** An enlarged or distended abdomen usually caused by the accumulation of excessive quantities of gas, ingesta, fluid or tissue (eg. pregnancy) in the abdomen. The distension may also be due to organomegaly of a mass in the abdomen. The distension may be unilateral, bilateral, symmetrical, or asymmetrical. It may also be more prominent over the upper or the lower aspect of the abdomen.

**Abdominal tympany** The accumulation of gas in the lumen of the stomach or intestines; it may result in distension of the abdomen and the possible presence of a ping on simultaneous percussion and auscultation of the abdominal wall. The accumulation of excessive quantities of gas in the rumen, abomasum, or intestines is the most common cause of abdominal tympany in cattle; in the horse, tympany of the large colon is the most common cause. Gastric dilatation and volvulus of the stomach is a common cause of abdominal tympany in the dog. Pneumoperitoneum is a less common cause and is usually associated with intestinal rupture or it occurs postsurgically following a laparotomy.

**Abdominal pain or colic** The various behavioral and systemic manifestations of pain in the gastrointestinal tract or other organs of the abdomen, including the reproductive tract, liver, and urinary tract. Characteristic signs include pawing with the forelimbs, looking at the flank, lying down, rolling, getting up restlessly, sweating, kicking at the abdomen, and prolonged recumbency. Cattle may depress their back

and paddle with their hindlegs, arch their back, or be immobile and reluctant to move. An audible grunt is commonly associated with acute localized peritonitis in cattle. The grunt may occur spontaneously or may have to be elicited by deep palpation of the affected area. Pinching the animal over the withers may also elicit a grunt in cattle with peritonitis. The grunt may be clearly audible with the unaided ear or it may be necessary to auscultate over the trachea to hear it. A grunt may also occur in cattle with pleuritis or pericarditis. Dogs with acute abdominal pain may assume a saw horse stance or praying position in which the forelimbs rest on the ground and the back is arched upwards.

**Abnormal gastrointestinal sounds** These are associated with the presence of excessive gas and fluid in the lumen of the intestines, and increased and decreased intestinal motility. In the presence of distension due to intestinal tympany, the sounds are hyperresonant and can be heard over the entire abdomen.

- A decrease in the audibility of the frequency, intensity, and duration of borborygmi over the right abdominal wall indicates the presence of ileus or varying degrees of hypomotility, as occurs in most cases of acute intestinal obstruction. There may be a complete absence of intestinal sounds indicating an advanced state of ileus.
- An increase in the audibility of the frequency, intensity, and duration of borborygmi over the right abdominal wall in the horse indicates the presence of hypermotility and intestinal tympany.
- **Fluid-rushing sounds**, either continuous or interrupted, are audible over the right abdominal wall in the presence of fluid-filled intestines, as in acute enteritis.

- **Fluid-tinkling sounds** are audible on auscultation of the right abdominal wall in the presence of hypomotile intestines which are filled with fluid and gas.
- **Fluid-splashing sounds** are audible on simultaneous auscultation and ballottement of the right abdominal wall in the presence of intestines filled with fluid and gas.
- **'Ping' or high-pitched metallic sound** audible on simultaneous auscultation and percussion over either the left or the right abdominal wall, or both, indicates the presence of stomach and/or intestines filled with gas.

**Abnormal masses on palpation of abdomen** Abnormal masses may be palpable through the abdominal wall. These include abomasal and omasal impaction, hepatomegaly, splenomegaly and retroperitoneal abscesses of the right abdominal wall.

**Abnormal rumen on palpation** The rumen feels abnormal on palpation through the abdominal wall of the left paralumbar fossa. It may feel more doughy than normal; it may be grossly distended with an excessive quantity of ingesta, gas or fluid; or it may not be palpable through the abdominal wall.

**Abnormal ruminal motility** Ruminal atony or hypermotility observed visually, by palpation and on auscultation.

**Abnormalities of prehension, mastication and swallowing**

- **Inability to prehend food** may be associated with lesions of the lips or the oral mucosa, abnormal teeth, an absence of teeth or loss of function of the tongue.
- **Painful mastication** is characterized by slow chewing movements, interrupted by pauses and expression of pain if due to abnormal or painful teeth.
- **Quidding** or dropping accumulations of masticated or partly masticated feed from the mouth during eating is usually an indication of oral pain caused by dental or gingival disease.
- **Dysphagia** is difficulty in swallowing. A history of gagging, choking, frequent swallowing attempts, and excessive drooling of saliva is suggestive of dysphagia.

**Anorexia** Total lack of food intake.

**Ascites** The abnormal accumulation of fluid in the peritoneal cavity, characterized by distension of the abdomen with fluid.

**Belching (eructation)** The oral ejection of gas or air from the stomach; a normal activity for ruminants but not for monogastric animals.

**Borborygmi** The rumbling, squashing, gurgling sounds audible on auscultation of the abdomen caused by intestinal peristalsis and the propulsion of ingesta and gas through the lumina of the intestines. They are characterized by their intensity, frequency, duration, and pitch.

**Bruxism** Grinding of the teeth is a manifestation of abdominal thoracic, esophageal or oral pain. It also occurs in diseases of the brain.

**Cecal-rush** Periodic, loud rushing and gurgling sounds that propagate in a crescendo-decrescendo pattern most prominently over the cecal base in the right paralumbar fossa of horses.

**Constipation** A reduction in the frequency of defecation and the amount of feces passed, which are usually drier than normal. The most common cause is intestinal hypomotility due to physical or functional obstruction of the intestinal lumen, or as a secondary effect of dehydration, fever or pain from unrelated causes.

**Crib-biting** An acquired habit in stabled horses characterized by stereotypic behavior. The horse grasps a solid object with its incisor teeth, arches the neck pulls upward and backwards and swallows air. The consequences are eroded teeth, occasionally gastric distension and body weight loss. Also called windsucking or cribbing.

**Cud dropping** A temporary condition in which cattle reject a regurgitated bolus to the exterior.

**Dog-sitting posture** Sitting on the haunches like a dog. When the posture is adopted for short periods by horses and associated with other signs of abdominal pain it is usually associated with intestinal colic.

**Diarrhea** An increase in the frequency of defecation, or an increase in the concentration of water and a decrease in the dry matter content in the feces. It reflects a decreased transit time through the large intestine, a loss of the absorptive capacity of the large intestine mucosa, or overload of water in large intestinal contents. Diarrhea may be associated with increased or decreased intestinal motility.

**Drooling saliva** The discharge of saliva from the mouth: it may be an indication of painful oral lesions, diseased teeth, abnormalities of swallowing, or disorders of salivary glands with hypersialosis. As rabies is a possibility protective gloves should be worn.

**Dropping regurgitated 'cuds'** The dropping of regurgitated cuds in ruminants is associated with abnormalities of the cardia of the reticulorumen or the esophagus.

**Dyschezia** Difficult or painful defecation.

**Dysentery** Blood in the feces together with diarrhea. The blood may be uniformly mixed with the feces, indicating hemorrhage in the distal part of the small intestine or the large intestine, resulting in dark red-colored feces. Hemorrhage in the distal colon or rectum results in the presence of frank blood not uniformly mixed with the feces.

**Failure to ruminate** Failure to regurgitate and chew cud.

**Flatulence** Excessive formation of gas in the stomach and intestine, released through the anus.

**Fluid wave** An impulse which can be felt with the hand (fingers) or a visible undulation of the abdominal wall following tactile percussion of one side of the abdomen and simultaneous observation and feeling on the opposite side. A fluid wave indicates the presence of excessive amounts of fluid in the peritoneal cavity, as in ascites. A fluid wave can also be elicited by tactile percussion of the abdomen containing a fluid-filled viscus.

**Gagging** The swallowing-vomiting activity of the gag reflex.

**Gaunt abdomen** A hollow and empty abdomen, usually associated with prolonged anorexia, inappetence, or starvation.

**Halitosis** An offensive oral breath.

**Hematemesis** The vomiting of blood implies gastric or proximal duodenal mucosal damage. The blood may appear as small red flecks, large clots, or, if digested by gastric acid, as 'coffee-ground-like' material.

**Hematochezia** Blood in the feces not necessarily with diarrhea, this is commonly due to trauma in the rectum.

**Inappetence** Failure to eat normal quantities of food or partial appetite.

**Jaundice or icterus** A syndrome characterized by hyperbilirubinemia and the deposition of bile pigment in the skin and mucous membranes, with resulting yellow appearance of the patient.

**Loss of body weight or cachexia** Marked loss of body weight and generalized weakness due to the effects of chronic disease. It includes pathological loss of body condition and muscular weakness.

**Melena** Black, tar-like feces, it is a manifestation of hemorrhage in the upper gastrointestinal tract (stomach, abomasum, or duodenum).

**Nasal discharge** A discharge from the nostrils which may be unilateral, bilateral, serous, purulent, hemorrhagic, or contain feed material which may have originated from regurgitation or vomition.

**Nasogastric regurgitation (gastric reflux)** Stomach contents flowing into the esophagus, and usually into the nasopharynx and nasal cavities, owing to distension of the stomach with fluid, which usually originates in the small intestine. This involuntary process is usually slow and gradual, unlike true vomiting.

In horses the presence of sequestrated gastric fluids can be confirmed only by the creation of a siphon using a nasogastric tube to infuse a volume of fluid and then disconnecting its supply in order to retrieve the **nasogastric reflux**.

**Obstipation** Intractable constipation with resulting fecal impaction throughout the rectum and colon.

**Odontoprisis (baurism)** Grinding the teeth; most common in cattle.

**Periodontitis** Inflammation of the tissues around the tooth or the periodontium, frequently seen with dental disease.

**Polyphagia** Excessive or voracious eating.

**Ptyalism** Excessive production of saliva.

**Putrid breath** Smell of rotting flesh, evidence for a necrotic process in the respiratory tract, mouth, nasal passages, pharynx, larynx or esophagus.

**Quidding** Dropping feed from the mouth while in the process of chewing it; usually due to stomatitis or bad teeth.

**Regurgitation** The expulsion through the oral cavity of food, saliva, or water from the esophagus that has not been swallowed into the stomach.

**Retching** An unproductive effort to vomit or regurgitate.

**Scant feces** Small amounts of feces which are usually pasty.

**Scooting** A behavior in which the animal sits and drags the perineum on the ground or carpet. It is a common manifestation of anal sac disease in dogs.

**Shock** is characterized by varying degrees of failure of the peripheral circulation, manifested by changes in the visible mucosae and the arterial and venous pulse, tachycardia, muscle weakness, cool extremities, and depressed mentation. Changes in the state of the oral mucous membranes include pallor to marked congestion and cyanosis, petechiation, and increased capillary refill time. **Dehydration** is manifested by loss of skin elasticity, sunken eyes and dry mucous membranes.

**Sialosis** The flow of saliva.

**Sweet smelling breath** The sweet aroma of the breath, consistent with ketosis, not smelt by some clinicians.

**Tenesmus** Straining as if to defecate or urinate, it is a common manifestation of disease of the rectum. Persistent tenesmus may result in rectal prolapse.

**Vomiting** The forcible expulsion of stomach (and possibly duodenal) contents through the mouth. This is an active act and is associated with prodromal signs such as nausea, drooling of saliva, and abdominal muscular contractions (heaving motions).

# Dogs and Cats

## SIGNALMENT

The signalment of the patient may suggest certain diagnostic possibilities. Young animals with vomiting and diarrhea more frequently have endoparasites, dietary indiscretion, and gastrointestinal foreign bodies than do older animals with a similar history. A history of vomiting, diarrhea, and weight loss in a 17-year-old dog suggests the presence of a tumor within the intestinal tract or systemic disease such as renal failure. A history of regurgitation in a young dog suggests a vascular ring anomaly, whereas in a mature dog it may suggest the possibility of acquired esophageal weakness due to myasthenia gravis. Vomiting in a mature overweight female dog may be due to acute pancreatitis. Examples of breed susceptibility to disease include

- exocrine pancreatic insufficiency in young German Shepherd dogs
- parvoviral gastroenteritis in the Rottweiler and Doberman Pinscher
- early onset hyperplastic gingivitis in Abyssinian and Persian cats
- gastric dilatation and volvulus in large, deep-chested breeds of dogs such as the Great Dane and Doberman Pinscher.

## HISTORY

In the patient with oral disease the owner may have noticed halitosis, drooling, reluctance to eat, or difficulty in prehension, mastication, or swallowing.

A history of regurgitation, dysphagia and ptyalism is typical with esophageal disorders. Vomiting, melena, anorexia, and abdominal pain are clinical signs suggestive of stomach and small intestinal disorders. Animals with maldigestive/malabsorptive disorders due to disease of the pancreas and small intestine typically manifest signs of weight loss and small intestinal diarrhea. A history of hematochezia, tenesmus, mucoid feces, dyschezia, constipation, fecal incontinence, or flatulence is suggestive of colorectal disease. Icterus is a clinical sign of liver disease.

Whenever possible the clinician should personally observe the signs reported by the owner. For example, the owner may say the animal is vomiting but it actually may be regurgitating. Observing the act will assist in establishing a proper diagnostic course of action.

---

### Some indications of abdominal pain in dogs

A dog with abdominal pain may refuse to move and assume a 'sawhorse' stance, or a 'praying posture' in which the head rests on the forelimbs while the rear end is elevated. If the pain is due to gastric dilatation and volvulus the dog may be extremely restless, lie down and get up frequently, and extend its head and neck.

---

## PHYSICAL EXAMINATION

A reasonable sequence of examination of the digestive tract and abdomen of small animals is recommended. Beginning at the head and moving caudally to the tail is a reliable method. Most dogs and cats enjoy having the dorsum of the head touched and scratched, and this allows the clinician time to socialize with the animal and gain its trust. Examination of the perineum and rectum is left to the end of the physical examination, as most animals resent any manipulation of this area.

### Oral cavity

The oral cavity is examined by inspection, palpation, and smelling. Sedation or general anesthesia may be necessary if the patient is intractable or appears to be painful on handling. If the animal is drooling, protective gloves are recommended.

The oral mucous membranes are examined for

- color
- capillary refill time, and
- hydration status.

Icterus, cyanosis, and anemia may be reflected in the color of the mucous membranes. Bullae, vesicles, erosions, ulcers, gingival hyperplasia or recession, petechiae, and abnormal masses are usually obvious. In the cat, plasma cell gingivitis and lymphocytic–plasmacytic gingivitis are common problems.

The buccal or labial surface of the teeth and gingival tissues can be examined as the upper lip is raised.

---

### Clinical Pointer

Visual observation of the act of defecation and gross examination of the feces will assist in distinguishing between diarrhea due a lesion of the small or the large intestine.

---

Proceeding from rostral to caudal, the mandibular and maxillary teeth and cheek tissues are examined on each side of the mouth. Dental tartar and associated gingivitis, periodontitis, and halitosis are common in small animals and frequently involve the canine teeth and molars.

The occlusion of the mandible and maxilla is assessed. In normal dogs and cats the occlusion pattern is known as a 'scissor bite', in which when the jaw is closed the lower incisors strike immediately caudal to the surface of the upper incisors (Fig. 17.1a). The lower canine occludes between the lateral upper incisor and the upper canine tooth (Fig. 17.1b). The lower third premolar is rostral to its upper counterpart, the third premolar, and the upper fourth premolar covers the lower first molar buccally. Malocclusion is any variation or deviation from normal. Categories of occlusion include

- Class I – occlusion is normal with one or more teeth out of alignment or rotated
- Class II – commonly referred to as brachygnathism or an overshot jaw, the lower premolars and molars are positioned behind or distal to the normal relationship
- Class III – prognathism or an undershot jaw in which the lower premolars and molars are positioned ahead of the normal relationship.

When the animal is relaxed its mouth can be opened. The cat's mouth can be opened by placing one hand around its head with the thumb on one side of the maxilla and the fingers on the opposite side. Extending the head gently backwards allows the mandible to fall open (Fig. 17.2). The dog's mouth can be opened by placing one hand over the top of the muzzle and elevating the nose to a vertical position (Fig. 17.3). In this position the dog is less able to close the jaw. The index finger and thumb should be pressed into the interdental space, just behind the canine teeth, on either side of the maxilla. The index finger of the second hand can be used to lower the bottom jaw, or alternatively the thumb can be placed on one side of the mandible and the fingers on the opposite side (Fig. 17.3).

Any odor from the mouth is noted. Abnormal odors include

- the ammoniacal smell of uremia
- the acetone or sweet smell of diabetic ketoacidosis
- the putrid odor of suppurative respiratory conditions
- the halitosis of periodontal disease and gingivitis.

With the mouth open, the hard and soft palate, the tonsillar region, the tongue, and the teeth are examined (Fig. 17.4).

### Palate

The hard palate makes up most of the roof of the mouth. It extends from the incisor teeth to the level of the last molars. A cleft palate (defect in the integrity of the palate) results in

- regurgitation of milk through the nose
- nasal discharge
- aspiration pneumonia, and
- poor growth in a neonatal puppy or kitten.

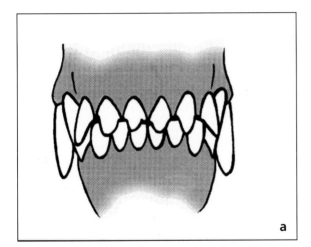

a

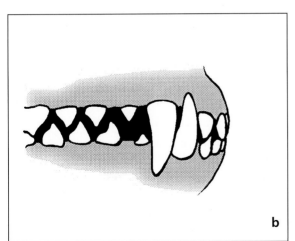

b

**Fig. 17.1** Normal dental occlusion pattern of the mandible and maxilla in a dog. (a) Scissor bite, in which the lower incisor teeth strike immediately caudal to the surface of the upper incisors. (b) The normal relationship of the upper canine and premolar teeth to the lower canines and premolars.

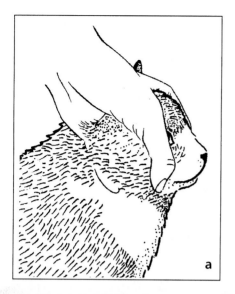

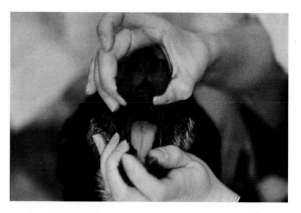

**Fig. 17.3** Technique to open a dog's mouth for oral examination. Note the position of the thumb and fingers on each side of the maxilla pushing in the interdental space just behind the canine teeth.

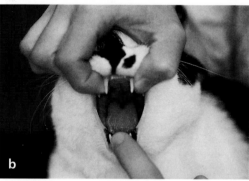

**Fig. 17.2** Technique of opening a cat's mouth for oral examination (a) Note the thumb and forefinger grasping the cheek on each side of the face and the little finger stabilizing the base of the cat's neck. (b) With the head tilted gently backwards, the lower jaw is pressed down with the right hand.

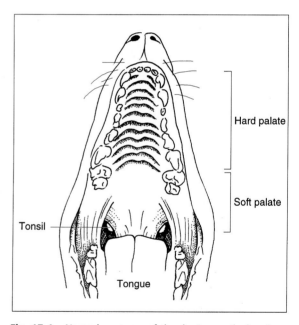

**Fig. 17.4** Normal anatomy of the dog's mouth showing the location of the hard palate, soft palate and tonsillar tissue.

The soft palate extends from the caudal edge of the hard palate to the level of the epiglottis. Elongation of the soft palate leads to inspiratory stridor, a common problem in brachycephalic breeds. The extent of the soft palate is difficult to assess in the average dog or cat and requires general anesthesia for total assessment. The palate should be examined for the presence of ulcers, fissures, fistulae, and foreign bodies.

## Tonsils

The palatine tonsils are located on the oral surface of the soft palate, just caudal to the palatoglossal arch. They are situated in the tonsillar crypts and, unless enlarged, are not usually visible on physical examination. With sedation or anesthesia the tonsils of the dog can be everted from their crypts and examined for the presence of foreign bodies, inflammation, or infection.

## Tongue

The tongue should be examined for symmetry, color, and the presence of foreign bodies or ulcers in the conscious dog and cat. It is important, especially in the cat with a history of vomiting, inappetence, or drooling, to examine under the tongue, as string, thread, or wool may be embedded into the lingual frenulum and may not be visible.

The hypoglossal nerve (CN XII) is the motor nerve to the intrinsic and extrinsic muscles of the tongue. Its function can be assessed by looking at the symmetry of the tongue and gently grasping the tongue and watching for retraction.

---

### Clinical Pointer

Applying gentle pressure to the base of the tongue with the index finger may allow visualization of the tonsils in some dogs.

---

### Teeth

With the mouth open, the buccal and lingual surfaces of the teeth can be examined. The dental formulae of the adult dog and cat and the puppy and kitten are as follows:

| | |
|---|---|
| Adult dog | 3I 1C 4P 2M |
| | 3I 1C 4P 3M |
| Adult cat | 3I 1C 3P 1M |
| | 3I 1C 2P 1M |
| Puppy | 3I 1C 3M |
| | 3I 1C 3M |
| Kitten | 3I 1C 3M |
| | 3I 1C 2M |

Cats and dogs have diphyodont dentition, meaning deciduous teeth that are replaced by permanent teeth. Normally the deciduous incisor and canine teeth erupt at 3–4 weeks of age and the premolar and molar teeth erupt at 5–6 weeks. Permanent incisors appear at 2–5 months and permanent canine teeth at 5–6 months. Premolars and molars appear at 4–6 and 5–7 months, respectively. The presence of retained deciduous teeth should be noted and removal recommended.

---

### Clinical Pointer

The undersurface of the cat's tongue is made visible by pressing upward on the intermandibular tissues.

---

The teeth are examined for the presence of

- tartar
- abnormal wear
- faulty enamel
- root exposure
- malocclusions
- fractures and discharges
- hair around the base of any tooth.

Using a dental instrument, each tooth can be lightly tapped and any sensitivity noted.

### Salivary glands

The anatomical locations of the zygomatic, parotid, mandibular, and sublingual salivary glands are illustrated in Figure 17.5. The zygomatic gland is located medial to the zygomatic arch in the ventral orbital area; its duct opens in the mouth just distal to the first upper molar tooth. The parotid gland lies ventral to the ear; its duct opens in the mouth adjacent to the upper fourth premolar tooth. The mandibular salivary gland is located caudal to the ramus of the mandible and lies ventral to the parotid gland. Its duct opens just lateral to the rostral aspect of the lingual frenulum in the floor of the oral cavity. The sublingual salivary gland lies close to the rostral aspect of the mandibular gland and its duct courses with the mandibular duct, opening on the medial side of the sublingual papilla. The salivary glands are not usually visible or palpable on physical examination. Occasionally the mandibular salivary glands are palpated as firm, unmovable structures at the ventromedial aspect of the angle of each mandible. The submandibular lymph nodes lie directly beneath these glands.

Problems related to the salivary glands that may be apparent on physical examination include

- pain on palpation (seen with sialadenitis), or
- swelling below the mandible (mucocele or sialocele), below the tongue (ranula) or in the pharyngeal space.

Ranulae, mucoceles, or sialoceles are seen when a tear occurs in a salivary duct, with subsequent accumulation of saliva. The sublingual salivary gland is the most commonly affected.

---

### Dental abscesses

- a swelling under the eye may be indicative of an abscess of the upper fourth premolar tooth
- a unilateral nasal discharge may be due to an abscess of the upper canine tooth.

---

A more complete examination of the oropharyngeal area requires sedation or anesthesia.

## Esophagus

The normal esophagus cannot be visualized or palpated on physical examination. Observation of swallowing can provide an indication of the state of the esophagus. Regurgitation is a common clinical manifestation in animals with esophageal disease. Occasionally in an animal with megaesophagus, the esophagus is found to be distended with fluid or gas.

## Abdomen

The abdomen is examined by inspection, palpation, and rectal examination. Auscultation, ballottement, and percussion are occasionally helpful. Ancillary tests, including radiography, ultrasonography, abdomino-paracentesis, endoscopy, laparoscopy, and exploratory laparotomy, may be indicated depending on the results of the clinical examination.

### Inspection

The contour of the abdomen is examined visually for

> **Clinical Pointer**
>
> It may be possible to inflate the dilated cervical esophagus of a dog with generalized megaesophagus by
>
> - holding the mouth closed,
> - occluding the nares and
> - simultaneously compressing the chest.

evidence of an increase or decrease in size, which may be symmetrical or asymmetrical. Enlargement of the abdomen may occur

- in advanced pregnancy
- in gastric dilatation
- in volvulus syndrome
- with large tumors of the liver, spleen, or other abdominal structures
- with ascites.

Decreases in the circumference of the abdomen, resulting in a tucked-up or gaunt appearance, may occur as a result of

- prolonged malnutrition from starvation
- chronic malabsorption syndromes
- other chronic disease states.

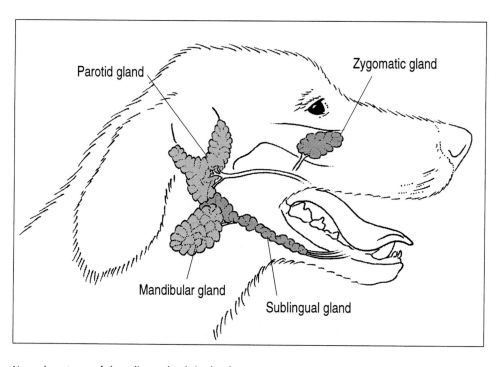

**Fig. 17.5**  Normal anatomy of the salivary glands in the dog.

The perineum, especially the anus and its mucocutaneous junction, are examined visually for the presence of vesicles, ulcers, fistulous tracts, masses, fecal staining, or other abnormalities. Perianal fistulae (anal furunculosis) appear as ulcerating sinus tracts in the perianal tissues (Fig. 17.6). They are painful and often foul-smelling. A purulent discharge may be evident. Perianal fistulae are more common in German Shepherds, Irish Setters, and Cocker Spaniels than in other breeds. If perineal examination, including the lifting of the tail, results in considerable discomfort to the animal a thorough examination of this region is indicated and may require sedation of the animal and clipping of the region. A perineal hernia results from a weakness of the muscles of the pelvic diaphragm and may include rectal, abdominal (bladder, prostate gland, intestine) or pelvic contents. It appears as a soft tissue swelling lateral to the anus (Fig. 17.7). Rectal prolapses and intussusceptions are uncommon. They appear as a tube-like mass of varying length protruding from the anus.

## Palpation

Palpation of the abdomen is diagnostically useful in small animals. Palpation, by definition, is the 'application of the fingers with light pressure to the surface of the body for the purpose of determining the consistency of the parts beneath'. Deep palpation is often needed to localize an area of abdominal pain. The purpose of palpation of the abdomen is to locate all normally palpable structures and abnormalities.

A prerequisite for becoming skilled in palpation of the abdomen is a thorough knowledge of its anatomy and structures. The use of an abdominal radiograph

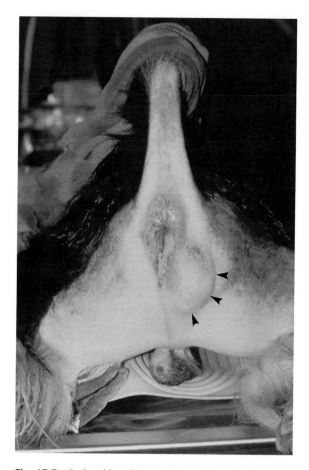

**Fig. 17.7** Perineal hernia in an intact older male dog. The hair has been clipped in preparation for surgery. The arrows are directed at the swelling on the right ventrolateral side of the perineum.

will help to visualize the location of the structures. For descriptive purposes, the abdomen is divided by imaginary lines into sections – cranial, middle, and caudal – and then further subdivided into dorsal and ventral regions (Fig. 17.8).

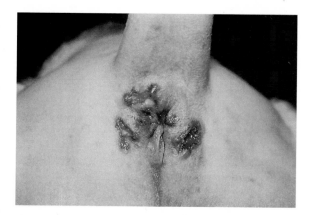

**Fig. 17.6** Perianal fistula in a dog. The tail is elevated showing almost 360° involvement of the perianal tissue.

---

### Palpation of the abdomen in dogs and cats

- in most dogs and cats, loops of the small intestine, the large intestine, and the bladder are easily felt
- in cats, both kidneys can be felt
- in dogs and cats the liver, stomach, spleen, and pancreas are not usually felt.

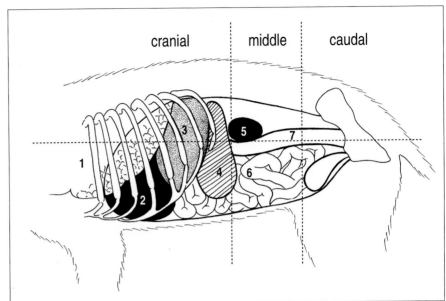

**Fig. 17.8** Abdomen divided into cranial, middle, and caudal regions for ease of identifying abdominal organs by palpation. The horizontal dotted line separates the abdomen into dorsal and ventral regions, (1) thorax, (2) liver, (3) stomach, (4) spleen, (5) kidney, (6) loops of small intestine, (7) colon.

### Cranial abdomen

The cranial section of the abdomen contains the liver, the stomach, the cranial duodenal flexure, and the initial third of the descending duodenum, transverse colon, and pancreas. The spleen occupies a variable portion of this region.

**Liver**

The liver is composed of six lobes grouped into three major divisions

- the left lateral and medial lobes form the left division and contribute about 40% of the liver mass
- the quadrate and right medial lobes are considered the central division and contribute about 30% of the liver mass
- the right division consists of the right lateral and caudate lobes and contribute about 30% of the liver mass.

In most dogs and cats the liver is not palpable because of the thoracic wall (Figs 17.8, 17.9a, b). When the liver extends slightly beyond the costal arch it may be palpable by placing one hand on each side of the cranial abdomen, just behind the costal arch, and applying gentle pressure with the fingers under the ribs. If normal, the edges should be firm, smooth and even (sharp edges). In neonates the liver occupies a large portion of the abdominal cavity and is usually palpable.

Hepatomegaly may be due to several causes, including:

- acute or chronic disorders impairing outflow from the hepatic veins
- extramedullary hematopoiesis
- hyperplasia of the reticuloendothelial system
- infiltrative disorders, such as hepatic lipidosis, lymphocytic–plasmacytic hepatitis, or neoplasia.

When enlarged, the liver extends beyond the end of the costal arch and may be palpable in the right and left portions of the cranial abdomen just caudal to the costal arch (Fig. 17.10a, b). The edges of an enlarged liver are often rounded and thickened. Variable-sized nodules may be palpated on an asymmetrically enlarged liver.

**Stomach**

In the dog the fundus of the stomach lies to the left of the midline, the body lies on the midline, and the pylorus extends to the right of the midline. The liver and small intestines separate the empty stomach from the abdominal floor. When moderately full the stomach expands to the left, touching the diaphragm caudal to the liver but not reaching the ventral abdominal wall. In cats the entire stomach is to the left of the midline. In adult dogs and cats the empty stomach is not normally palpable as it lies within the costal arch caudal to the liver, between the planes of the ninth thoracic and first lumbar vertebrae (Figs 17.8, 17.9a, b). It may

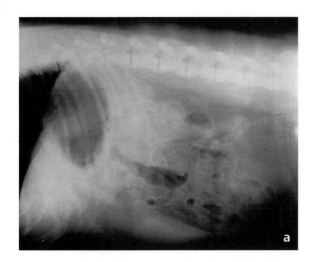

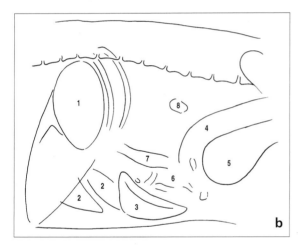

**Fig. 17.9** (a) Lateral radiograph of a normal canine abdomen. (b) Schematic of the lateral radiograph showing (1) stomach, (2) liver, (3) spleen, (4) colon, (5) bladder (6) loops of small intestine, (7) gas within the ascending colon and small intestine, and (8) kidney.

be palpable in puppies who have just eaten a meal. If full, the greater curvature of the stomach bulges beyond the left costal arch, displacing the intestines caudally. The stomach may occasionally be palpated in

---

**Clinical Pointer**

Palpation of the stomach may be assisted by pushing the fingers under the ribcage or by elevating the forelimbs, allowing the abdominal contents to fall caudally.

---

a narrow-chested breed of dog that has just eaten a big meal or, more commonly, in the gastric dilatation volvulus patient, when the stomach is grossly distended with air.

**Pancreas**

The pancreas, consisting of a body and right and left lobes, is anatomically associated with the stomach, liver, and duodenum. The body is located at the pyloroduodenal junction; the right lobe lies next to the descending duodenum, and the left lobe extends along the greater curvature of the stomach, where it is in contact with the liver, the transverse colon, and sometimes the left kidney and spleen.

---

**Palpation of the pancreas**

- it is not palpable in the normal animal
- it is rarely palpable in the diseased state
- it may be palpable in individuals with pancreatic masses (phlegmon, abscess, pseudocyst, tumor), particularly following an acute episode of pancreatitis.

---

**Spleen**

The spleen is the single largest reticuloendothelial organ in the body and is positioned in the left cranial portion of the abdomen (Fig. 17.8). It is loosely attached to the greater curvature of the stomach by the gastrosplenic ligament and varies in location with stomach volume. It is not palpable in normal animals. Temporary generalized splenomegaly is commonly palpated in dogs anesthetized with thiobarbiturates.

Splenomegaly may be

- focal owing to a mass (nodular hyperplasia, neoplasia, hematoma, abscess), or
- diffuse owing to congestion or infiltration with inflammatory or neoplastic cells.

Hemangiosarcoma is the most common neoplasm affecting the spleen, and the German Shepherd dog is a breed at risk. In generalized splenomegaly the spleen may be palpable as a firm, semisolid mass extending backwards caudal to the left costal arch at the cranioventral region of the abdomen. It is sometimes difficult to distinguish the liver from the spleen when the latter is situated in the cranial abdomen.

When enlarged, the spleen may extend into the middle and even the caudal abdominal region (Fig. 17.10a, b). Alterations in the size, shape, or position of

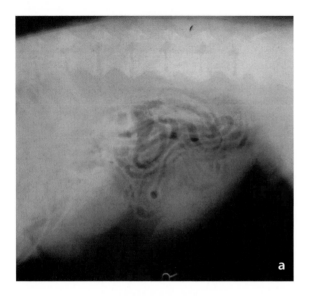

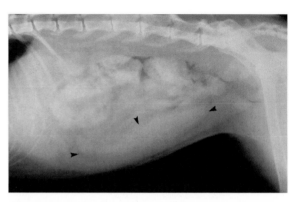

**Fig. 17.11**  Lateral radiograph showing feline splenomegaly. The arrows are directed at the enlarged spleen.

**Intestines**

The duodenum, the shortest and most proximal portion of the small intestine, lies largely to the right of the midline. It receives the openings of the stomach, common bile duct, and pancreatic ducts. The duodenum is the most fixed part of the small intestine. Near the pelvic inlet it forms a flexure by turning medially and then cranially along the medial aspect of the colon and left kidney. At this point it dips ventrally and continues as the jejunum, the largest portion of the small intestine. Loops of small intestine are palpable in normal dogs and cats (Figs 17.8, 17.9a, b).

The transverse colon lies in contact with the greater curvature of the stomach and travels across the midline from right to left.

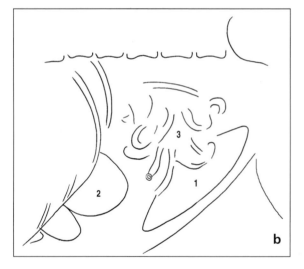

**Fig. 17.10**  (a) Lateral radiograph showing hepatomegaly, splenomegaly, and displaced spleen. (b) Schematic of the lateral radiograph showing (1) large, caudally positioned spleen, (2) hepatomegaly, and (3) loops of small intestine.

the spleen can result in characteristic displacement of other abdominal organs, such as the intestines, the direction and severity of which depends on the magnitude of the splenomegaly and the portion of the spleen involved.

Splenomegaly in the cat differs from that in the dog in that the enlarged organ may lie entirely along the left flank, rather than extending diagonally across the abdomen (Fig. 17.11).

---

### Clinical Pointer

The transverse colon may be palpated if filled with feces or distended with gas.

---

### *Middle abdomen*

The middle abdomen extends from the second to the fifth lumbar vertebrae and contains the middle third of the descending duodenum with its associated portion of pancreas, and the jejunum and ileum. The jejunum, the longest portion of the small intestine, consists of up to eight loops of intestine that occupy most of the middle abdomen and are covered by the omentum (Figs 17.8, 17.9a, b).On the right side the ileum, the shortest section of the small intestine, extends forward in the right sublumbar region and communicates with the proximal part of the colon at the ileocecocolic junction. The colon begins as a short segment termed the ascending colon. This is connected to the descending colon by the transverse colon, the most cranial portion of the large intestine, located at the level of the twelfth thoracic vertebra. The transverse colon passes cranial to and around the root of the mesentery. The descending colon blends into the rectum at the pelvic inlet.

The intestines are palpated for masses such as foreign bodies, tumors, and granulomas. Inflammation and neoplastic infiltration may cause the intestines to become thickened and more prominent on palpation. An intussusception, defined as a prolapse or invagination of one portion of the gastrointestinal tract into the lumen of an adjoining segment may be palpable as a firm tubular, cylindrical, or sausage-shaped structure. Most intussusceptions in small animals are enterocolic in location and are usually palpable in the cranial to middle abdomen regions (Fig. 17.12). Pain may or may not be present.

The cecum is not normally palpable, but may be if impacted with feces (Fig. 17.13).

The ascending colon and proximal part of the descending colon, when filled with feces, are often palpable as a tube-like structure. In most cases of large intestinal disease palpation of the abdomen is normal. Distension of the colon with feces or foreign material, certain neoplasms and intussusceptions may be palpable.

The mesenteric lymph nodes lie within the mesentery along the vessels in the middle abdomen. They are not palpable unless enlarged. Lymphadenopathy may be due to inflammation, infection or neoplasia. Occasionally mesenteric lymphadenopathy occurs in association with inflammatory bowel disease. Neoplasia of the mesenteric lymph nodes is recognizable as an indeterminate mass in the caudal middle abdomen.

### Caudal abdomen

This region contains the distal descending colon, rectum, parts of the small intestine, and the external iliac lymph nodes. The colon is about one-fifth the length of the small intestine. The rectum – the terminal part of the descending colon that lies within the pelvic canal – may be palpable if filled with feces, fluid, or gas, or if the wall is thickened as a result of inflammatory or infiltrative disease.

The external iliac lymph nodes lie under the fifth and sixth lumbar vertebrae. They are not palpable in the normal dog and cat.

## Palpation of the abdomen

### Palpation technique

Palpation is best learned on a calm, non-obese patient. The examination should be made with the animal standing on a table with a non-slip surface; large dogs are best left standing on the floor.

For a two-handed palpation the examiner

- stands to one side of the animal and places one hand on each side of the abdomen
- extends the fingers of each hand keeping them firmly together, with the thumb of each hand pointing outwards
- applies gentle pressure medially using the fingertips of both hands, until they almost touch one another
- moves the hands ventrally, feeling the various internal structures slipping between the fingertips.

At the beginning of the examination most animals will be tense and the tone of the abdominal musculature will intensify, hindering palpation. To help overcome this, gentle but consistent pressure is applied until the tone of the abdominal wall is relaxed and the underlying organs can be identified. The entire abdomen is palpated systematically. When the ventral part is palpated, a double fold of the abdominal wall can often be felt as a cord-like structure. This is a normal finding. Palpation of the abdomen can be difficult in animals which are well-muscled, obese, excitable, or experiencing abdominal pain.

Palpation in the cat is rewarding because the abdominal wall is less tense and the internal organs, including the kidneys, are easily palpable. A one-handed technique is recommended (Fig. 17.14a, b). For restraint, the left hand may be used to encircle the upper left hind limb with the left thumb pressed

---

## Clinical Pointer ✳

Clumping of the intestines can be caused by

- linear foreign bodies (string, tinsel, wool, thread)
- intestinal adhesions.

---

## Clinical Pointer ✳

A two-handed technique is recommended for palpation of most dogs; in the cat and some small dogs, a one-handed technique is adequate.

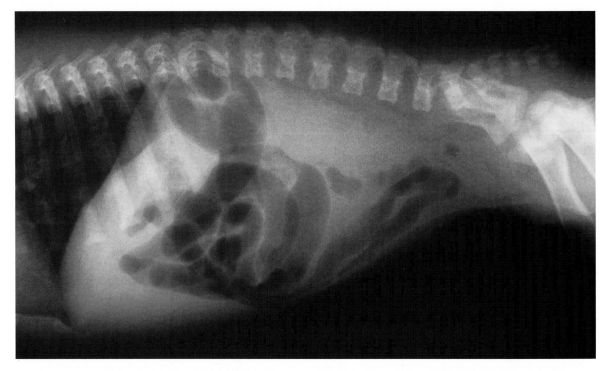

**Fig. 17.12** Radiograph showing intussusception in a young puppy. Note the prominent gas-distended loops of small bowel in the cranial and midabdominal regions.

against the femur and the four fingers grasping the medial thigh. This leaves the right hand free for palpation. An alternative method is to place the left hand on the cat's back. For palpation, the thumb of the

right hand is placed on one side of the body and the four fingers on the other. Gentle pressure is applied medially on the abdomen until the fingers meet the thumb. The hand moves ventrally, feeling the internal structures slipping between the thumb and fingers.

*Positional palpation*

In some cases, elevating the forelimbs or placing the animal in left or right lateral recumbency or in dorsal recumbency may allow mobile abdominal viscera to move with the effect of gravity and assist in palpation. In large dogs, a chair is used to assist in elevation of the forelimbs (Fig. 17.15). In small dogs and cats one hand is used to elevate the forelimbs while the other is used to palpate. The spleen and small intestines float caudally and the liver, stomach, kidneys, and the region of the pancreas are then within reach. The spleen may be distinguishable from the liver and, although the pancreas is not specifically palpable, evidence of pancreatic disease, such as localized pain or masses, may be detectable. In right lateral recumbency the

- left kidney
- left lateral lobe of the liver, and
- dorsal extremity of the spleen

**Fig. 17.13** Radiograph showing cecal impaction in the midabdominal region. The arrows are directed at the stool-filled cecum.

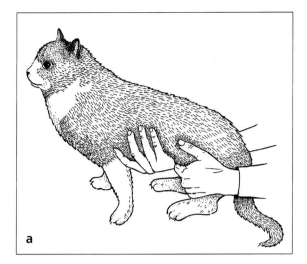

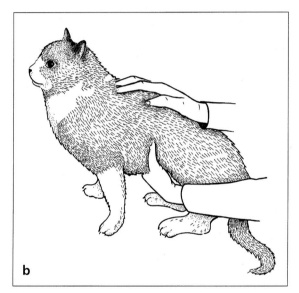

**Fig. 17.14** (a) One-handed abdominal palpation in the cat showing left hand restraining cat by encircling left medial thigh. (b) One-handed palpation in the cat showing left hand supporting cat's back leaving right hand free for palpation.

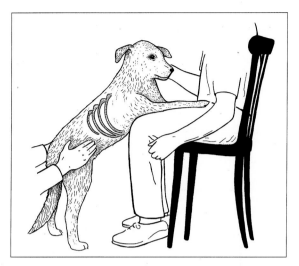

**Fig. 17.15** Positional palpation technique in the dog. With the forequarters elevated the cranial abdominal contents fall caudally and may be palpated.

- the presence of tumors
- enlargement of abdominal organs and visceral structures, such as the liver and spleen
- pain.

Abdominal pain in small animals is characterized by increased tension of the abdominal musculature, arching of the back, crying out, or attempting to bite the examiner when the affected region is palpated.

---

**Abdominal pain**

- pain in the cranial abdomen suggests gastric, pancreatic, hepatic, or splenic origin
- pain in the middle abdomen suggests a small intestinal origin
- pain in the caudal abdomen suggests a colonic origin.

---

**Clinical Pointer**

The presence of fluid in the peritoneal cavity impairs the ability to assess the size, shape, and texture of abdominal structures.

---

may be palpable. The right kidney and pancreatic region become more accessible to palpation when the animal is placed in left lateral recumbency. In dorsal recumbency the ventral and lateral surfaces of the liver, the body and ventral extremity of the spleen, and the kidneys may be palpable.

### Abnormalities detected on palpation

Common abnormalities detected on abdominal palpation include

Displacement of abdominal viscera or organs from their normal location is also detectable by palpation. For example, the stomach in gastric dilatation and volvulus syndrome may be displaced into the right cranial and middle abdominal regions.

Palpation is not the most sensitive method of detecting peritoneal fluid, but small amounts are suspected when the serosal surfaces of abdominal structures slip away from the examiner's fingers.

## Auscultation, ballottement, and percussion of abdomen

### Auscultation

Although auscultation is not used routinely in the examination of the alimentary tract in small animals it is useful in assessing intestinal motility. Intestinal sounds are generated by the movement of fluid and air, with air increasing the amplitude of stomach sounds and fluid increasing the amplitude of the small intestinal sounds. Most normal abdominal sounds originate from the stomach and are best heard with the diaphragm of the stethoscope placed over the cranial and middle abdominal regions; small and large intestinal sounds are too brief in duration to be audible. The rate of sound production varies in the normal animal depending on the phase of the digestive cycle. Intestinal sounds may be decreased or absent in animals with

- ileus (total lack of intestinal movement)
- hypomotility due to chronic intestinal distension or chronic enteritis
- generalized peritonitis.

Intestinal sounds increase in frequency with increased intestinal motility. Borborygmi may be heard in cases of intestinal obstruction and fluid accumulation in the intestine, and with hypersegmentation from acute enteritis.

Auscultation should precede percussion and palpation, as the latter maneuvers may alter the frequency of intestinal sounds.

### Ballottement

Ballottement of the abdomen is of greatest value in detecting peritoneal fluid. With one hand on each side of the abdomen the abdominal wall is lightly tapped with the fingertips of one hand while the other hand is gently held against the opposite side. If a large amount of fluid is present a sensation of fluid movement – the fluid wave – can be felt with the opposite hand (Fig. 17.16). In some cases an undulation of the abdominal wall may be visible after ballottement. Small volumes of peritoneal fluid may not be noticed.

To identify an organ or a mass in a fluid-filled abdomen, one hand is placed on each side and, with

the fingers of one hand straightened and stiff on the abdominal surface, the other hand makes a brief jabbing movement directly toward the suspected structure (Fig. 17.16).

Ballottement may also be used to help identify

- a gravid uterus
- large abdominal tumors
- gastric dilatation and volvulus in the dog.

In gastric dilatation volvulus (GDV) the stomach can be ballotted and auscultated as an air-filled density with a characteristic high-pitched tympanic sound heard in the right cranial abdominal region. Excessive fluid and gas in the intestine will elicit fluid-splashing sounds on ballottement and auscultation.

### Percussion

Like auscultation and ballottement, percussion by itself is of limited value in the examination of the gastrointestinal tract, but may be combined with auscultation, palpation, and ballottement to provide information on gastrointestinal structures. Percussion is the act of

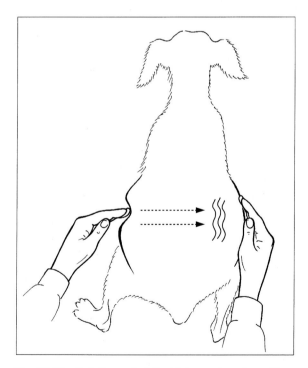

**Fig. 17.16** Ballottement of the abdomen in a dog with ascites. Note the position of the fingers on the left hand. A brief jabbing movement is directed toward the distended abdomen. A fluid wave is created (dotted arrows) and an undulation is felt on the right hand.

striking a part of the body with short, sharp blows in an attempt to set the underlying tissues into motion, producing audible sounds and palpable vibrations. Percussion can help to determine the physical state of underlying tissues. The sounds produced can distinguish between normal and abnormal states

- resonant (tympanic or drum-like) sounds indicate air-filled structures such as the lungs or gas-filled abdominal viscera
- dull sounds indicate the presence of solid tissue or fluid-filled cavities.

In small animals the hand acts as a pleximeter using a recommended technique:

1. hyperextend the middle finger of the left hand – the pleximeter finger – and place its distal interphalangeal joint firmly on the surface to be percussed
2. do not allow any other part of the hand to contact the pleximeter finger as this damps the vibrations
3. using the right middle finger, the plexor, strike the pleximeter finger at the distal interphalangeal joint or between the distal interphalangeal joint and the fingernail with a sharp, but relaxed wrist motion – the action transmits vibrations through the bones of this joint to the underlying organ being percussed
4. withdraw the striking finger quickly to avoid damping the vibrations
5. repeat the percussion twice in the same location
6. percuss all sections of the abdomen to assess the distribution of tympany and dullness.

Several abnormalities may be detected with simultaneous percussion and auscultation. In GDV, the stomach can be percussed and auscultated as an air-filled structure with a characteristic high-pitched tympanic sound heard in the right cranial abdominal region. Enlargement of the liver or spleen, and large superficially located tumors, elicit a dull sound on percussion. When splenic torsion or splenic displacement occurs, the normal tympany of the stomach and colon may be replaced with the dullness of the spleen.

---

### Percussion and auscultation of the peritoneal cavity

- fluid free in the peritoneal cavity gravitates ventrally → dull notes
- gas-filled loops of intestine float dorsally → tympanic notes.

---

## Rectal examination

A digital rectal examination is an important part of the examination of the most caudal part of the alimentary tract in small animals. The pelvic cavity, containing the

- rectum
- descending colon
- pelvic bones
- urethra
- anal sacs, and
- prostate gland (in the male dog)

can be palpated. A fresh fecal sample is usually obtainable for examination during this procedure.

Because most animals resent rectal palpation and find it somewhat uncomfortable, it is best left to the end of the physical examination. Most cats and dogs that are aggressive, too apprehensive, or have evidence of perianal fistula or anal sac abscessation will require sedation for proper rectal examination.

Dogs should be allowed an opportunity to walk and defecate prior to the procedure, during which they should be standing and adequately restrained.

Examination gloves are worn. The index finger of the dominant hand should be lubricated with a petroleum jelly product or commercial lubricant, the tail slightly elevated and the rectum gently entered. If extreme pain is manifested at this point sedation is recommended.

---

### Clinical Pointer

Tone of the anal sphincter is assessed as soon as the finger is inserted – the normal anal sphincter constricts – the finger is not advanced until the sphincter relaxes.

---

Gentle rotary movement of the finger usually aids insertion. Once the finger is beyond the anal sphincter relaxation occurs and non-painful manipulations are tolerated. If there are feces within the rectum a sample is collected for analysis.

The finger is slowly advanced cranially and any resistance or pain noted. If the animal strains, the examination should stop temporarily, allowing the finger to be pushed backwards toward the anus by the intra-abdominal pressure. Once the finger is totally inserted, a 360° palpation is performed around the rectum, moving caudally toward the anus. The walls of the rectum should be smooth and devoid of irregularities. Abnormalities that may be detected on palpation include

- polyps

- tumors
- foreign bodies (e.g. pieces of bone)
- diverticula
- strictures
- roughening of the rectal wall.

Pain may indicate colitis, neoplasia or, in the male dog, prostatitis. A perineal hernia causing a sac-like outpouching of the rectum to one or both sides of the anus is easily palpable. The external iliac lymph nodes, commonly referred to as the sublumbar lymph nodes, are not normally palpable unless enlarged (Fig. 17.17). Occasionally pulsations of the rectal artery can be palpated on the dorsal wall of the rectum, and the urethra can be palpated on the ventral floor of the rectum.

In male dogs the dorsal aspect of the prostate gland can be palpated during rectal examination. It should be a symmetric, bilobed structure immediately in front of the pubis.

---

**Clinical Pointer** ✳

If the anal sphincter fails to constrict when the finger is first inserted, a lesion of the pudendal nerve or sacral spinal cord is suspected, warranting further examination.

---

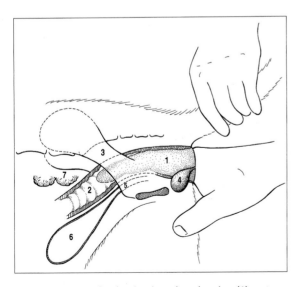

**Fig. 17.17** Rectal palpation in a dog showing (1) rectum, (2) descending colon, (3) pelvic bones, (4) anal sac, (5) urethra, (6) bladder, and (7) external iliac lymph nodes.

## Anal sacs

Animals with anal sac disease are often presented with a history of scooting, dragging, or rubbing the perineum on the ground or carpet, licking or biting at the perineal region, tail chasing, sudden darting across the room, or an usual body odor.

The anal sacs are palpated at the end of the rectal examination. They are located between the internal and external anal sphincters on either side of the anus ventrolaterally, at approximately the 4 and 8 o'clock positions (Fig. 17.17). Their duct openings are located just inside the anus. Anal sacs are variable in size (pea-sized in most cats and dogs, but can expand to 15 mm in diameter in some dogs). The lining of the anal sacs and their associated ducts consists of stratified squamous epithelium. Numerous apocrine and sebaceous glands lie beneath the anal sacs and ducts and the secretion of these glands collect in the sacs. Normal anal sac material is composed of these glandular secretions, desquamated epithelium, and bacteria. The secretion varies in color from light gray to brown, and in consistency from fluid to granular or a putty- or paste-like material. It has a foul, putrid odor reputed to result from bacterial fermentation of cholesterol and its conversion into butyric acid, indole, and skatol. The anal sacs generally empty at the time of defecation.

Anal sac disease is common in dogs, uncommon in cats. Any change in character of the secretion can cause the ducts to become plugged impaction, fermentation, inflammation, and infection of the anal sac can then result.

---

**Emptying the anal sacs**

- to empty the sacs internally, the index finger of the right hand is placed on the gland internally and the thumb of the right hand is placed over the gland externally so that the secretions can be gently 'milked' dorsomedially toward the duct opening and the expressed material is collected in a paper tissue
- to empty the sacs externally, fingers and thumbs are used to gently squeeze the sacs forward against the perineum.

---

### Neurological examination

A neurological examination is indicated

- in any animal with a history of constipation or failure to defecate normally
- in animals in which the anal sphincter appears weak on rectal examination.

Perineal sensitivity can be assessed via the perineal reflex, which is elicited by light stimulation of the perineum with a forceps. A normal response is contraction of the anal sphincter muscle and flexion of the tail. A similar response can be obtained by squeezing the penis or the vulva (bulbocavernosus reflex). Sensory innervation for the perineum is via the pudendal nerve and spinal cord segments (S1–S2, sometimes S3); motor innervation is through the pudendal nerve; and tail flexion is mediated through caudal nerves. The perineal reflex is the best indication of the functional integrity of the sacral spinal cord segments and the sacral nerve roots. Absence or depression of the reflex indicates a sacral spinal cord lesion or a pudendal nerve lesion.

## Ancillary testing

### Clinical pathology

#### Hematology and serum biochemistry

Changes in the hemogram can aid in the diagnosis of inflammatory and infectious disorders. The biochemical profile provides information on liver function, hepatocellular damage, cholestasis, and albumin and globulin levels, both of which are lost in diseases producing protein-losing enteropathy.

Several tests are now available to aid in the diagnosis of specific gastrointestinal diseases

- serum bile acids are commonly used to evaluate liver function
- serum trypsin-like immunoreactivity (TLI) is a sensitive and specific test for the diagnosis of exocrine pancreatic insufficiency
- the D-xylose absorption test is recommended for assessment of intestinal absorption
- hydrogen breath tests are used to assess monosaccharide or disaccharide malabsorption, bacterial colonization of the small intestine, and transit time
- the intravenous administration of $^{51}$Cr-labeled albumin is used to document protein-losing enteropathy.

#### Feces

Fecal examination should be routine in any patient with signs of gastrointestinal disease. A sample can be collected at the time of rectal palpation and should be examined grossly for the presence of blood (frank blood or melena), mucus and foreign material such as bone chips. Laboratory evaluation is done to detect inflammatory cells or infectious agents (parasites, bacteria, viruses).

### Medical imaging

Survey radiographs are routinely used in the examination of the gastrointestinal tract of small animals. Radiographs of the thorax are indicated if

- megaesophagus
- aspiration pneumonia, or
- metastatic disease

are suspected. Radiographs of the abdomen may assist in the diagnosis of

- masses
- radio-opaque foreign bodies
- gastric dilatation and volvulus
- hepatomegaly, and
- peritonitis.

In general, survey radiographs of the colon provide little information.

Contrast radiography is important for the detection of radiolucent foreign bodies, masses, strictures, gastrointestinal wall infiltration, mucosal ulceration, motility problems, and filling defects suggestive of neoplastic or ulcerative disease.

---

### Clinical Pointer

Giardiasis is an important cause of diarrhea in dogs and cats, zinc sulfate centrifugation–flotation of feces for identifying *Giardia* cysts is recommended.

---

A barium enema may detect mural masses, extramural colonic compression, intussusceptions, strictures, and severe mucosal irregularities associated with inflammatory bowel disease.

Abdominal ultrasound is useful for evaluating portosystemic shunts as liver size, consistency, and vasculature can all be assessed. It also aids in the diagnosis of intestinal thickness, intestinal luminal contents, and peristaltic function, and is helpful in detecting neoplasia and intussusception (Fig. 17.18). With an intussusception the ultrasound may actually show one loop of intestine within another (Fig. 17.18).

Fluoroscopy is useful in assessing motility disorders of the esophagus.

### Endoscopy and proctoscopy

Endoscopy of the esophagus, stomach, proximal duodenum, and colon has revolutionized the diagnosis and treatment of patients with gastrointestinal disease.

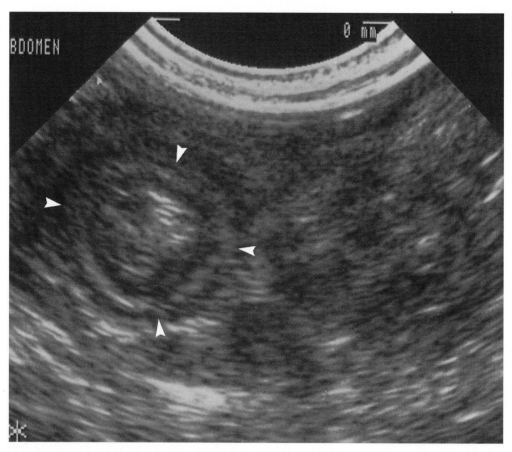

**Fig. 17.18** Abdominal ultrasound in a puppy showing one loop of bowel within another (intussusception). The arrows are pointing at the intussusception. Same puppy as shown in Fig. 17.12.

>
> ### Clinical Pointer
>
> With inflammatory gastric or intestinal disease the endoscopic appearance of the mucosa may be normal but multiple biopsy samples should always be taken.

Proctoscopy is used to evaluate the rectum and distal colon. Endoscopic examination of the luminal surfaces of the esophagus, stomach, duodenum, and colon allows the identification and possible removal of foreign bodies, the identification of certain parasites, and identification and biopsy of areas of inflammation, ulceration or suspected neoplasia.

### Laparoscopy and laparotomy

Laparoscopic surgery or exploratory laparotomy is indicated when

- full-thickness biopsies of the intestinal tract are needed
- the biliary system needs to be examined for patency and culture
- endoscopy is not available for examination of the vomiting patient.

Findings on physical examination, such as a splenic mass, and the results of blood work and radiography may lead the examiner to recommend an exploratory laparotomy.

Cytological evaluation of gastric or duodenal fluid is seldom performed except when *Ollulanus tricuspis* in the cat, giardiasis in the cat or dog, or evidence of bacterial overgrowth in the dog or cat is suspected. The intestinal fluid can be obtained through an aspiration tube during endoscopy or by aspiration with a wide-bore needle and syringe at laparotomy.

### Abdominocentesis

Abdominocentesis, or the collection of fluid from the

peritoneal cavity, is useful for the diagnosis of an acute abdomen, peritoneal effusion and peritonitis.

1. The animal should have an empty bladder and be sedated if necessary.
2. The periumbilical area is shaved and surgically prepared. Alternatively, the abdomen can be divided into four quadrants by bisecting a line drawn through the umbilicus and a small area shaved and prepared for aspiration in each quadrant.
3. A 16–18 gauge intravenous catheter, or a commercial peritoneal catheter with a trocar and stylet, can be used.
4. The animal is left standing or, if sedated, placed in right or left lateral recumbency.
5. The catheter is directed through the linea alba and into the abdominal cavity 1–3 cm caudal to the umbilicus or into each prepared quadrant.
6. Following abdominal puncture the stylet is removed and the catheter connected to a syringe for aspiration.
7. If the aspiration is negative for fluid (which is likely if the volume present is less than 5.2 ml/kg) peritoneal lavage is recommended. For this the animal is placed in dorsal recumbency, the site is aseptically prepared and the catheter inserted. Approximately 20–50 ml/kg of warmed physiological saline is then infused into the abdomen and the animal gently rocked from side to side to mix the peritoneal cavity contents. The abdomen is then drained by gravity flow and about 30–50% of the infusate is recovered and submitted for cytology and culture.

# Horses

## REGIONAL ANATOMY

### Mouth

The oral cavity and its accessory organs the tongue, teeth, and salivary glands, are concerned with the prehension, selection, mastication, and insalivation of feed, and with the conversion of feed to a bolus that can be swallowed. The oral cavity extends from the lips to the entrance into the pharynx, and in the horse is unusually long and relatively narrow. Its osseous support is provided by

- the incisive bone (premazilla)
- the palatine and alveolar processes of the maxilla
- the horizontal lamina of the palatine bone, and
- the mandible.

The oral cavity is bounded rostrally by the lips and laterally by the cheeks. Its dorsal limit, or roof, is the hard palate. Ventrally is the tongue and under its apex and lateral margins there is a crescent-shaped space which is the actual floor of the oral cavity (Fig. 17.19). Caudally the oral cavity communicates with the oropharynx, which is a narrow isthmus formed by the root of the tongue and the soft palate and is usually closed. When the jaws are closed the oral cavity is divided by the teeth and the alveolar processes into the vestibule and the oral cavity proper. In horses the two cavities communicate via the large interdental space between the incisors and the cheek teeth, and the

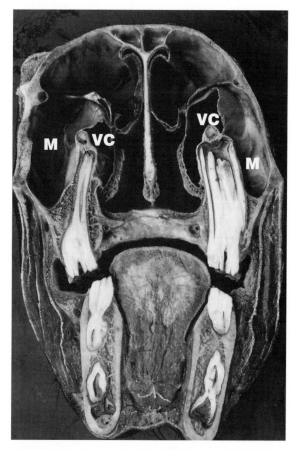

**Fig. 17.19** Cross-section of an equine skull at the level of the fifth cheek tooth. The length of reserve crown indicates that it is a young horse. Note the relationship between the maxillary cheek teeth and maxillary (M) and ventral chouchal (VC) sinus.

space behind the last molars. The mucous membrane of the oral cavity is usually pink, but may be pigmented in certain places. It is well supplied with blood vessels and in its submucosa contains serous or mucous glands known as labial, buccal, and lingual glands, depending on their location.

## Lips

The large upper lip and the smaller lower lip of the horse are highly mobile musculo-membranous folds and are very sensitive tactile and prehensile organs. Both are covered externally with fine hair; on the free borders of the lips the hair is short, stiff, and bristly. Numerous tactile hairs surround the oral cleft. The hairs on each side of the middle of the upper lip are often long. Below the lower lip is the chin, consisting of the poorly developed mentalis muscle and of adipose and connective tissue. The oral cleft extends to the level of the first cheek teeth and is relatively small compared to the length of the oral cavity. This makes examination of the caudal parts of the oral cavity and oral surgery difficult.

## Hard palate

The hard palate extends from the incisors to the level of the last cheek teeth and is of almost equal width throughout. Immediately caudal to the incisors the mucosa covering the hard palate bulges ventrally and may be level with the occlusal surface of the upper incisors, particularly in the foal. This bulge was formerly mistakenly thought to be a pathological swelling ('lampas').

## Tongue

The tongue is long and narrow and occupies the inter-mandibular space. It has tall lateral surfaces. Its apex is highly mobile, long and spatula-like rostrally, has rounded borders and is connected with the floor of the mouth by a well developed frenulum. The filiform papillae are soft and thin and give a velvety texture to the dorsum of the tongue. The fungiform papillae are scattered over the dorsal surface of the apex and the lateral surfaces of the tongue. There is usually only one pair of large vallate papillae at the junction of the body and root of the tongue which are about 7 mm in diameter and have an uneven surface. The foliate papillae are located on the lateral borders of the tongue just rostral to the palatoglossal arches, forming rounded eminences about 20–25 mm long.

## Pharynx

The pharynx of a 500 kg horse is about 20 cm long, but its caudal limit does not extend beyond the caudal limit of the skull. Only the rostral third of the pharyngeal roof is attached to the base of the cranium. The caudal two-thirds are related to the guttural pouches, as are the dorsolateral walls.

The soft palate is long, and from its rostrally arched border to its attachment on the osseous palate it measures 10–13 cm. The mucous membrane on the ventral surface of the soft palate is wrinkled and presents numerous small openings of the large palatine glands. Rostrally there is the median tonsil of the soft palate. Diffuse lymphatic tissue and lymph nodules are also present in the mucosa of the dorsal surface.

---

### The soft palate during normal breathing

During normal breathing the free border of the soft palate lies against the base of the epiglottis, with the epiglottis and part of the arytenoid cartilages protruding through the intrapharyngeal opening into the nasopharynx. Horses are unable to elevate the soft palate sufficiently for effective mouth breathing (regurgitation also flows down the nasal cavity).

---

The palatopharyngeal arches continue the free border of the soft palate along the lateral walls of the pharynx. They measure as much as 1 cm in height and meet dorsal to the arytenoid cartilages. Together with the free border of the soft palate they form the slightly oval intrapharyngeal opening (about 5.5 cm long and 5 cm wide) enclosing the rostral larynx.

The oropharynx, like the soft palate, is relatively long. Except during swallowing it is no more than a narrow elongated cleft between the root of the tongue and the soft palate, being slightly wider caudally than rostrally. The laryngopharynx is relatively short and extends from the base of the epiglottis to the front of the cricoid lamina. The piriform recesses on each side of the entrance to the larynx are 3 cm deep, measured from the edge of the aryepiglottic folds.

## Tonsils

The lingual tonsil is comprised of follicles at the root of the tongue and near the glossoepiglottic fold. The tonsil of the soft palate is an oval, slightly elevated follicular structure located rostrally on the ventral surface of the soft palate.

The palatine tonsils comprise elongated, flat follicular tissue, 10–12 cm long and 2 cm wide located on the floor of the oropharynx, lateral to the glosso-epiglottic fold and extending caudally to the base of the epiglottis.

## Teeth

The formula for the permanent dentition of the horse is:

2[I 3/3, C 1/1, P 3 (4)/3, M3/3] = 40 (42).

Equine teeth are hypsodont (high crowned) and slowly erupt over the life of the animal to compensate for the high occlusal wear that occurs in herbivorous animals which can spend up to 18 hours per day chewing tough forage containing silicate particles.

The incisors (I) of the horse are designated I1, I2, and I3, and are also known as the central, interme-diate, and corner incisors, respectively. Their lengths (permanent incisors) range from 5.5 to 7 cm, most of which is reserve (unerupted) crown. They are embedded in the incisive (premaxilla) bone and the rostral aspect of the mandible, with their reserve crowns and apices converging slightly towards the median plane. Each tooth is curved, the concavity being toward the tongue, and the curvature of the upper incisors is generally more marked than that of the lower. In young animals the clinical crowns (exposed parts) are close together, and when the jaws are in apposition they form a semicircle on both dorsoventral and lateral inspection.

The clinical crowns of the incisors are curved more strongly than the reserve crowns. Because of this the clinical crowns of the young horse meet their antago-nists almost vertically, that is, the angle between the upper and the lower incisors when viewed in profile is nearly 180°. As the horse ages the less curved reserve crown comes into wear and the angle between the upper and lower incisors becomes progressively more acute. At the same time, the arch formed by the occlusal surfaces as seen on dorsoventral inspection becomes progressively flatter.

Each incisor has a centrally placed **infundibulum** (**cup**) that is partially filled with cement; the remaining lumen becomes filled with food, giving it a black appearance. As the tooth wears (at a rate of about 2 mm per year) the cup gradually narrows and disap-pears. The bottom of the infundibulum, however, remains as a small raised **enamel spot** close to the lingual surface of the tooth for some years. The pulp cavity beneath the occlusal surface progressively fills with secondary dentine. When this secondary dentine is eventually exposed through occlusal wear, usually

after 5–6 years, it is termed the **dental star** and lies between the infundibulum and the labial aspect of the tooth.

The canine (C) teeth develop fully only in the male, but vestigial canines are encountered occasionally in the mare. When fully developed the canines have a total length of 4–5 cm, with a 1–3 cm long cone-shaped clinical crown. The canines are closer to the corner incisors than to the first cheek teeth, the upper being located at the junction of the incisive bone and the maxilla. Signs of wear on the canines are present only in old subjects. Between the canines and the cheek teeth is the extensive diastema ('bars of the mouth').

The horse has six upper and six lower cheek teeth on each side, three premolars (P) and three molars (M) (premolars 2, 3 and 4, and molars 1, 2 and 3). They form two slightly curved rows which extend from the diastema to beneath the eye in the upper jaw and to the vertical ramus of the mandible in the lower. The external enamel of these teeth is extensively folded and covered in cement. They complete true longitu-dinal growth when the horse is 6–7 years old, and at that time they are about 8–10.5 cm long (Fig. 17.20) with clinical crowns projecting about 1.5–2 cm above the gums. Only as longitudinal growth ceases do roots develop. The upper cheek teeth are nearly square on cross-section, whereas those of the lower jaw are rectangular. The upper cheek teeth each have two infundibula, the lower cheek teeth have none. With wear all three dental calcified tissues (enamel, dentine, and cement) are exposed on the occlusal surface, and because of their different hardnesses differential wear will occur. This results in the deeply folded hard enamel ridges becoming raised between depressions of dentine and cement. On the buccal (lateral) surface of the upper cheek teeth are three longitudinal ridges of differing heights separated by two longitudinal grooves. There is a centrally placed longitudinal ridge on their palatal (medial) surface which is accompanied on either side by two longitudinal grooves. The lower cheek teeth contain two deep enamel infoldings on their lingual (medial) aspect and one on their buccal

---

### Cross section of the occlusal surfaces

The shape of the occlusal surface of the incisors, on cross section, is of value in estimating a horse's age

- in the young animal they are rectangular to oval
- they become rounder then somewhat triangular, and finally
- oval in the old horse.

aspect. The lower cheek teeth have two roots, except the sixth which has three. Occasionally, a rudimentary upper P1 (wolf tooth) is present. The reserve crowns of the cheek teeth diverge as shown in Figure 17.21. In the upper jaw the clinical crowns of the first two cheek teeth incline caudally, the third and fourth are more or less vertical to the masticatory surface, and those of the fifth and sixth incline rostrally.

## Occlusion

Because the horse has a narrower mandible than maxilla (i.e. is anisognathic) only the lingual third of the occlusal surface of the upper cheek teeth is in contact with the buccal half of the lower cheek teeth at centric occlusion (Fig. 17.20). As the mandible moves to one side during

mastication all contact between the upper and lower cheek teeth on the opposite side is lost.

The lingual (medial) aspect of the occlusal surface of the lower cheek teeth is higher than the buccal aspect, with the occlusal surface at a 10–15° angle in this direction. Conversely, the palatal surface of the upper cheek teeth is lower than the buccal. As a result, the occlusal surface of the lower cheek teeth slopes towards the cheeks and the occlusal surface of the upper cheek teeth slopes toward the hard palate. Occasionally, owing to incomplete lateral movement of the mandible during mastication (probably associated with high-concentrate diets and less time spent eating forage), the lingual aspects of the lower cheek teeth and the buccal aspects of the upper cheek teeth become very sharp and damage the buccal and lingual mucosa. This is known as enamel points or, in its extreme form, 'shear mouth' (Fig. 17.21).

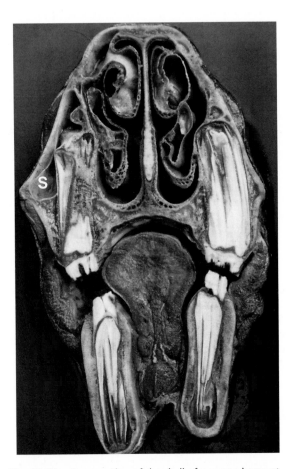

**Fig. 17.20**  Cross-section of the skull of a young horse at the level of the third cheek teeth. This shows remnants of the deciduous teeth ('caps') lying on the crowns of the permanent teeth. The nasal conchae and rostral aspect of the right rostral maxillary sinus (S) are also visible.

> **Clinical Pointer**
>
> The angulation of the cheek teeth crowns is essential to keep the teeth in tight contact at the occlusal surface throughout the horse's life.

The formula for the deciduous dentition of the horse is:

2[Di 3/3 Dc 1/1 Dp 3/3] = 28.

The deciduous incisors (Di) are smaller and whiter than the permanent incisors. Their crowns are shovel-shaped and there is a distinct neck and a relatively short root. An infundibulum is present, but it is only about 4 mm deep. Short vestiges of the deciduous canines (Dc) develop in both sexes but never erupt. The three deciduous premolars (Dp) of both upper and lower jaws are smaller than the permanent premolars, but resemble them in shape and structure.

## Dental assessment of age

The central, middle, and corner permanent incisors usually erupt at 2.5, 3.5 and 4.5 years of age, respectively, and come into full wear over the following 12 months or so (Table 17.1). Aging horses up to 6–7 years old by dental examination has been shown to be relatively acccurate. Beyond this age, and despite much anecdotal literature, horses cannot be accurately aged by dental examination. Nevertheless, some general principles can be of value.

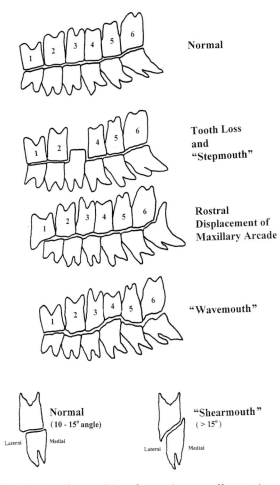

**Fig. 17.21** Abnormalities of wear that can affect equine cheek teeth.

| Table 17.1. Eruption and replacement of teeth in the horse | | | |
|---|---|---|---|
| Teeth | Time of eruption | Teeth | Time of eruption (in wear) years |
| Di 1/1 | Before or shortly after birth | I 1/1 | 2½ – (3) |
| Di 2/2 | 3–4 weeks and, rarely, up to 8 weeks | I 2/2 | 3½ – (4) |
| Di 3/3 | 5–9 months | I 3/3 | 4½ – (5) |
| Dc 1/1 | Rarely erupt | C 1/1 | 4–5 |
| Dp 2/2 | Before birth or | P 2/2 | 2½ |
| Dp 3/3 | during first week | P 3/3 | 2½ |
| Dp 4/4 | after birth | P 4/4 | 3½ |
| M 1/1 | 6–9 months, and rarely, up to 14 months | | |
| M 2/2 | 2–2½ years | | |
| M 3/3 | 3½ –4½ years | | |

caudally on the dorsal surface of the trachea. In the middle third of the neck it deviates to the left and comes to lie lateral to the trachea from about the 5th cervical vertebra caudally, occasionally reaching the

1. Recently erupted incisors have deep enamel infoldings (infundibulae) on their occlusal surface that usually wear away between 2 and 5 years after eruption.
2. With increasing wear, areas of secondary dentine laid down at the site of the former pulp cavity appear: these are termed 'dental stars'.
3. With age the incisor teeth also lose the rectangular cross-sectional shape and large curvature towards the occlusal surface of the young horse and become triangular on cross-section and project rostrally with little curvature (Figs 17.22, 17.23).

## Esophagus

The esophagus follows the short laryngopharynx dorsal to the cricoid cartilage of the larynx and passes

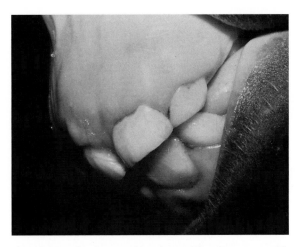

**Fig. 17.22** The degree of brachygnathism (parrot mouth) present in this young horse is clinically insignificant.

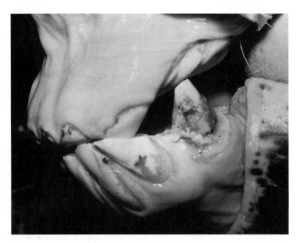

**Fig. 17.23** This 43-year-old pony has gross wear of its remaining incisors, which protrude at a very rostral angle. Note the calculus on its canine teeth.

median plane ventral to the trachea. It passes through the thoracic inlet between the trachea and the left 1st rib, and soon regains the dorsal surface of the trachea. It continues caudally in the mediastinum dorsal to the base of the heart and tracheal bifurcation, crossing the aorta on the right. At the level of the 14th thoracic vertebra and about 12 cm ventral to the vertebral column it passes through the esophageal hiatus of the diaphragm, slightly to the left of the median plane. As it enters the abdominal cavity it joins the stomach at an acute angle. At its cranial end the esophagus receives the two lateral longitudinal esophageal muscles, which originate from the pharyngeal raphe and are covered by cricopharyngeus and thyropharyngeus muscles that are the caudal constriction of the pharynx and act as the rostral valve of the esophagus.

---

### Esophageal muscle

The muscular coat of the esophagus

- consists of striated muscle to the level of the tracheal bifurcation and of smooth muscle from there to the cardiac part of the stomach
- is 4–5 mm thick proximally, increasing gradually toward the cardia, where it reaches an extraordinary thickness of 1.2–1.5 cm.

---

## Stomach

The stomach of the horse is unusually small relative to body size and has a normal capacity of only 8–15 liters. It is bent sharply so that the cardia and pylorus lie close to each other, and it has a very pronounced fundus which projects as a true blind sac, well above the level of the cardia. The stomach lies under cover of the ribs, for the most part on the left side of the median plane, only the pyloric part being on the right. Even when greatly distended it never reaches the ventral abdominal wall. The greater curvature, traced from the cardiac part over the summit of the blind sac to the pylorus, faces at first to the right, then dorsally, then to the left, and then ventrally, and over the pyloric part again to the right. The lesser curvature is short and faces dorsally and to the right. The parietal surface faces craniodorsally and slightly to the left, and is applied dorsally against the diaphragm and ventrally against the left lobe of the liver, on which it produces the distinct gastric impression. Laterally the parietal surface lies against the gastric surface of the spleen. The visceral surface of the stomach, facing caudoventrally, is in contact with jejunum, descending colon, the diaphragmatic flexure and right dorsal segment of the ascending colon, and the left lobe of the pancreas. The blind sac is the most dorsal and also the most caudal part of the stomach, and lies at the level of the 14th or 15th intercostal spaces. The body of the stomach lies cranioventral to the blind sac and is opposite the 9th to the 12th intercostal spaces. When the stomach is distended it expands principally to the left and caudally, but it may also advance cranially to the level of the 8th or 7th intercostal spaces.

The shape and structure of the equine stomach fits the description of a simple stomach. The **cardiac loop**, which is formed by the internal oblique fibers and which continues along the inside of the lesser curvature, is especially well developed. Thick bundles of the circular muscle layer cross the internal oblique fibers externally and provide the floor of the gastric groove. In the vicinity of the cardia these fibers combine with the cardiac loop to form the strong **cardiac sphincter**, which keeps the cardia tightly closed even after death. This strong sphincter and the very oblique angle at which the esophagus joins the stomach make it practically impossible for stomach contents and gases to enter the esophagus. Also, being entirely within the bony thorax, the stomach is not directly influenced by extra-abdominal pressure. Thus the horse – with rare exceptions – is unable to relieve even a greatly distended stomach by vomiting, and if acute gastric distension is left untreated the stomach will rupture. The circular muscle layers form the **pyloric sphincter**, in the region of which the longitudinal muscle layer is also unusually thick. Proximal to the sphincter is a muscular ring, causing a constriction at which the pyloric part is divided into the pyloric antrum and the pyloric canal.

## Abdomen and abdominal cavity

The abdomen is that part of the body trunk between the 18th rib and costal arch cranially and the level of the pelvic inlet caudally. The abdominal cavity is contained within the abdomen, but a significant volume of it lies deep to the ribcage because of the cranial convexity of the dome-like diaphragm. The dorsal wall of the abdominal cavity comprises the subvertebral (hypaxial) muscles and the lateral walls are formed by abdominal muscles and fasciae that attach to

- the transverse processes of the lumbar vertebrae dorsally
- the ribs and sternum cranially, and
- the pelvic girdle caudally (as the linea terminalis).

Ventrally the aponeuroses of these muscles form the sheaths of the rectus abdominis muscle, the two bellies of which extend from the sternum to the prepubic tendon, joined in the midline by the thick fascial linea alba. The walls of the abdominal cavity are lined by the parietal peritoneum, a thin serous membrane which extends beyond abdominal boundaries via outpouches around structures within the pelvic cavity and, in males, through the inguinal canals as the tunica vaginalis of the spermatic cords and testes. Visceral peritoneum is closely applied to the surfaces of intra-abdominal organs, except for the kidneys and adrenal glands, which lie in a retroperitoneal position. Visceral and parietal layers of peritoneum are continuous with each other through reflections of the latter to form intra-abdominal connective structures such as

- the intestinal mesentery
- the omenta, and
- certain ligaments (e.g. the suspensory ligament of the spleen).

The gastrointestinal tract constitutes the bulk of the abdominal viscera (Fig. 17.24). The horse's cecum and large colon are especially capacious, with the result that they necessarily dominate descriptions of the topo-graphical anatomy of the abdomen. The cecum occupies a large part of the right side of the abdominal cavity. The bulbous cecal base lies against the right paralumbar fossa and the caudal four ribs. The body of the cecum arcs cranioventrally from the base and tapers into the apex, which sits on the floor of the abdominal cavity at approximately the level of the midpoint of the ventral abdomen. The large colon is arranged in a folded double-barrelled shape which has along its length three flexures giving rise to four segments. The right ventral colon arises at the ceco-colic orifice on the lesser curvature of the cecal base and passes cranioventrally, roughly along the line of the right costal arch. At the level of the xiphoid, the colon passes from right to left as the sternal flexure and continues caudally on the left side of the floor of the abdominal cavity towards the pelvis. At this point the left ventral colon becomes the left dorsal colon via the pelvic flexure, passing from ventral to dorsal. Depending on how full it is, this region of colon may occupy most of the area deep to the left paralumbar fossa. The left dorsal colon passes cranially, dorsal to the left ventral colon along the left abdominal wall and axial to diaphragmatic attachments on the left ribcage, and medial to the spleen to reach the most cranial aspect of the abdominal cavity. The colon then passes from left to right as the diaphragmatic flexure and becomes the right dorsal colon, passing caudally, dorsal to the right ventral colon, and then merges into the transverse colon medial to the cecocolic junction.

The pylorus of the stomach is just to the right of the midline and the short duodenum is relatively fixed in position by its dorsal hepatoduodenal ligament and the mesoduodenum. The ileum is also relatively short (approximately 1.5 m) and is similarly restricted in mobility by the antimesenteric ileocecal fold which attaches the ileum to the dorsal cecal tenia. It follows, then, that the vast majority of the length of the small intestine comprises loops of jejunum. These are suspended by a mesentery whose root arises ventral to the first and second lumbar vertebrae but which, in an average horse, fans out to some 25 m in length along its intestinal attachment. At its midpoint the mesentery may be 50 cm or more deep, so that the jejunal coils have great mobility and tend to fill spaces between the more fixed structures. As a general guide small intestine occupies

- the midcranial abdomen, and
- the dorsal and left caudal abdomen.

However, intestinal loops may lie ventrally between the large colons or against the right flank, depending on the state of filling of the large intestinal segments and individual variations. The small colon is a continuation

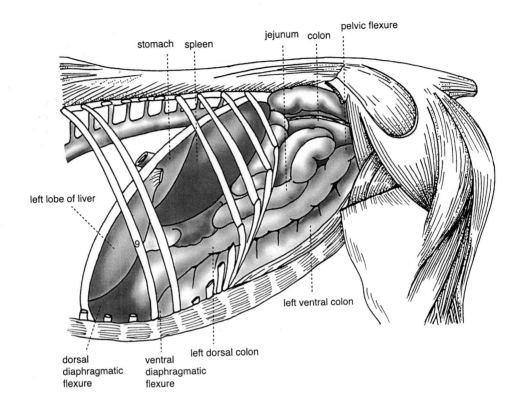

**Fig. 17.24** Topographical abdominal anatomy of the horse from (A) left and (B) right lateral aspects.

of the transverse colon and, although shorter than the small intestine, also has considerable mobility afforded by an extensive mesentery. Small colon loops therefore mingle with those of the small intestine. Terminally the small colon occupies the midline as it becomes the rectum and leaves the abdominal cavity.

## Liver

The liver of the horse is indistinctly lobated, partly because of the absence of a gallbladder. It lies against the diaphragm, traversing the midline in an oblique, right/dorsal to left/ventral orientation. The right abaxial surface of the liver lies against the abdominal surface of the dorsal half of the diaphragm between the 6th and 15th ribs, with pleural cavity interposed over much of this area. The left surface of the liver has a still less direct relationship with the lateral abdominal wall, and ventrally the liver is protected by the sternum.

## Kidneys

The right kidney is almost completely covered by the dorsal limits of the 18th, 17th, and 16th ribs. The craniolateral pole juxtaposes against the renal impression on the caudal aspect of the right liver lobe. The left kidney is longer and narrower and is situated further caudally than the right, extending from beneath the dorsal limits of the 16th, 17th, or 18th rib to beneath the transverse processes of the first three lumbar vertebrae. The ventrolateral border of the left kidney is related to the dorsal pole of the spleen and the two are connected by the renal part of the suspensory ligament of the spleen (nephrosplenic ligament).

## Spleen

The spleen lies flat against the left abdominal wall and is usually covered by ribs, but sometimes extends further caudal than the costal arch. The wide dorsal margin is related to the left kidney in the region of the 16th and 17th intercostal spaces. The body tapers cranioventrally toward the ventral half of the 9th to 11th intercostal spaces, but the exact position is variable depending on

- the state of filling of the stomach and large colon (to which the spleen is attached)
- the type of horse (fitter, athletic types have larger spleens)
- the state of sympathetic drive (the equine spleen is highly contractile).

# PHYSICAL EXAMINATION OF THE DIGESTIVE TRACT AND ABDOMEN

## Sequence of clinical examination

The sequence of the different parts of the clinical examination will vary according to the history and the clinical findings of the initial general examination. If abdominal pain is obvious then careful examination of the abdomen is indicated. If dysphagia is obvious then a detailed examination of the oral cavity, pharynx, and esophagus, including nasogastric intubation, may be necessary in the early part of the examination. The sequence of the clinical examination recommended here can be modified to meet individual circumstances.

## History taking

Factors such as the body condition, the presence or absence of feces and their nature, a normal or dull, erect haircoat, the type of bedding material in use, disruption of the bedding, recent changes in diet or management, concurrent medications and skin abrasions might suggest the type or course of the disease encountered. Any changes in the severity of the case in the previous several hours should be determined.

Colonic impactions, such as confinement and the opportunity to ingest poorly digestible roughage, are typically associated with stressful events. A well-conditioned horse that is abruptly confined on a straw bed because of an injury is at particular risk of developing colonic impaction. A higher incidence of particular abnormalities is associated with certain age, gender or breed groups

- entrapment of intestine in the epiploic foramen and obstruction by mesenteric pedunculated lipomata are more likely to occur with advancing age
- stallions are almost exclusively associated with scrotal herniation
- large-framed horses and brood mares are shown to be at higher risk of colonic displacement than other types of horse.

## Clinical Pointer

Horses with major gastric or colonic distension may progress from violent colic to relative calm following the rupture of a viscus, a subdued patient, with signs of a previous struggle is consistent with this event.

## Distant examination

A general distant examination includes evaluation of demeanor, behavior, mentation, appetite and eating, postural changes, and ease of handling. The amount and character of feces passed within the previous few hours is valuable information. Observing the animal for 10–15 minutes may reveal important clinical findings that provide diagnostic clues.

Examination for abdominal distension is best made from behind the horse, standing alternately just to one side then the other to compare right and left sides of the abdomen. Normally there are visible depressions in the body walls at the sublumbar fossae and concavities cranial to the tuber coxae. Subtle losses of this abdominal contour are physiologically normal. This can be caused by such factors as

- high-volume feed intake and greater body fat
- lack of fitness
- advancing age
- mid- to late pregnancy
- thick haircoat.

Pathological distension tends to be rapid in onset and usually reflects tympany of the large intestine. The relative rigidity of the ribcage means that abdominal distension is most obvious in the regions of the muscular flanks. In general, right- or left-sided abdominal distension will be caused by cecal or left colonic tympany, respectively, although the changes in contour are not as pathognomonic as they can be with forestomach distension in cattle. The relatively smaller dimensions of the small intestine and its more internal positioning within the abdomen mean that abdominal distension is an infrequent sign of small intestinal obstruction. However, particularly in cases of the more aborally located obstructions, "full flanks" may be recognized in some cases. Distension occurs only rarely in diseases of other abdominal organs, hydroallantois being one exception.

The muzzle, lips and nares are visually inspected for evidence of swellings, drooling saliva, nasogastric reflux in the nasal discharge, and any evidence of malodorous breath on oral membranes.

Horses spend a large part of their time chewing feed, and the normal sound of coarse forage being chewed between the irregular occlusal surfaces of the cheek teeth is a vigorous coarse grinding sound. With dental disease, especially the very common painful condition of enamel overgrowths of the edges of the cheek teeth, a less vigorous and often slurping type of chewing noise will be detected.

The horse cannot readily breathe through its oral cavity and consequently malodorous oral disorders, such as dental peridontal disease, will be detected on oral mucous membranes but not usually from the (nasal) breath.

Prehension, chewing, and swallowing are complex activities that depend on the coordinated functioning of many neural, muscular, skeletal, and dental structures of the mouth, pharynx, and esophagus. Dysfunction of any of these can adversely affect or even prevent normal eating and drinking. Thus dysphagia, the inability to swallow, can be oral, pharyngeal, or esophageal in origin.

---

### Clinical Pointer

If dysphagia is suspected it is useful to see the horse eat and drink, therefore the owner should be asked to starve the animal for a short time before the examination.

---

### Belching

Belching may indicate certain pharyngeal disorders, e.g. cricopharyngeal–laryngeal dysplasia.

---

### Evaluation of abdominal pain

This is an important aspect of the distant examination. The behavioral manifestations of abdominal pain include

- pawing the ground with the forefeet
- turning the head and neck and looking at the flanks
- assuming the dog-sitting position (Fig. 17.25A) or a sawhorse stance
- a tendency to lie down and roll (Fig. 17.25B)
- prolonged periods of dorsal or lateral recumbency with minimal other activity.

The horse with unrelenting abdominal pain may exhibit these behavioral changes over several hours. A horse manifesting abdominal pain can usually be allowed to behave instinctively and unrestrained for a short period so that the behavior can be evaluated and interpreted. The client can be assured that allowing a horse with abdominal pain to lie down and roll does not predispose to a volvulus or torsion. As a general rule the severity of abdominal pain reflects the severity of the abnormality. Gastrointestinal pain arises through different mechanisms which can be broadly categorized under four headings

1. hyperperistalsis
2. intestinal distension causing mural stretching

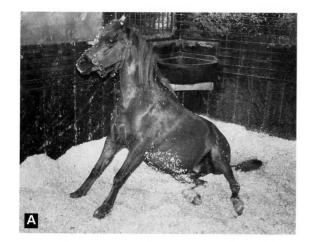

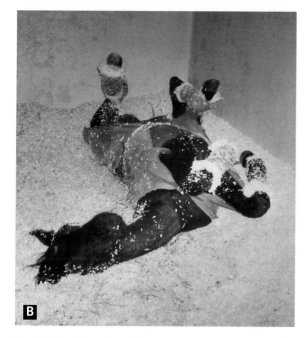

**Fig. 17.25** (A) A 'dog sitting' posture is an unusual sign of colic, sometimes seen in grass sickness. Note also the patchy sweating, which is another feature of this syndrome. (B) Increasingly severe pain causes increasingly violent colic, such as continuous rolling.

3. tension on the mesentery
4. inflammation and ischemia of the intestinal wall.

Thus an impaction of the large colon which, at least in the early stages, will involve primarily distension of the intestine, might be expected to be less painful than a large colon displacement, in which a greater degree of distension may be compounded by mesenteric tension. Strangulating volvuli have the additional noxious

pathogenic factor of ischemia. These lesions tend to be the most painful of all intestinal obstructions and the most likely to be associated with a horse that rolls violently and incessantly. Certain behavioral characteristics suggest the mechanism of pain involved in a given case and hence the root cause. For instance

- compulsive and strenuous pawing at the ground with a forelimb suggests marked gastric distension and, by extrapolation, raises the index of suspicion of small intestinal obstruction
- a dog-sitting posture has also been related to gastric distension but is rarely seen
- prolonged periods of lateral or dorsal recumbency suggest an attempt by the animal to relieve mesenteric tension and would be typical of the type of pain experienced by a horse with a non-strangulating colonic displacement
- occasionally horses will be seen to press their haunches against the wall of the stall, or to 'sit' on a drinking bowl or manger, this tends to occur in cases of caudal colonic impaction, presumably as a response to pressure at the pelvic inlet
- many horses with moderate chronic colic adopt a stretched stance (frequently misinterpreted by owners as an inability to urinate normally).

If the duration and pattern of painful episodes are known or can be deduced circumstantially, such evidence also adds to the pool of diagnostic information. Because most bouts of colic resolve spontaneously, it is self-evident that the more protracted the period the more likely it is that a significant problem exists. Non-strangulating lesions might cause pain that persists for days without marked cardiovascular or metabolic deterioration, thus presenting a clinical challenge. Furthermore, the pattern of pain manifestations within one abdominal event varies with the nature of the obstruction. Generally, continuous pain, even if relatively low grade, represents the presence of a more severe lesion than do intermittent bouts.

The classic 'spasmodic' colic, associated with loud borborygmi, flatulence, and soft feces, can lead to episodes of intense pain punctuated by periods of apparent normality. The pain of impactions is also characteristically intermittent, probably associated with waves of peristaltic activity against the obstruction.

---

**Clinical Pointer**

- moderate chronic colic pain → stretched stance
- lower urinary tract problems → overt signs of dysuria with full posturing and tenesmus.

The assessment of how well a horse with colic responds to analgesic drugs is an essential part of the examination. It is a useful rule of thumb that abdominal pain that is fully responsive to non-steroidal anti-inflammatory drugs (NSAIDs) is unlikely to be due to a lesion requiring surgical intervention, and vice versa. NSAIDs are more discriminating than $\alpha_2$-adrenergic agents, the sedative action of which is capable of suppressing signs of colic due to more sinister lesions, at least in the short term. Similarly, opioid drugs will mask most abdominal pain and should be used judiciously. There is some evidence that within the group of NSAIDs, flunixin is a more potent inhibitor of pain than, for example, phenylbutazone. However, this is controversial. A greater disadvantage of flunixin may be its apparent ability to obscure signs of advancing circulatory shock, thereby possibly delaying a decision for surgery to be made.

# CLOSE PHYSICAL EXAMINATION

## Palpation and ballottement

Following the distant examination both the right and left sides of the abdomen are palpated for evidence of distension and abdominal pain, and are ballotted with concurrent auscultation to detect the presence of fluid-splashing sounds. However, the large size of most horses renders techniques of external abdominal palpation of little value compared with smaller species. Other than the late-pregnancy uterus and the fetal prominences, it is not possible to reliably identify any viscus by palpation through the abdominal wall of the horse. When inflammation of the parietal peritoneum is present, steady compression of the flanks with a clenched fist may be resented. In more advanced cases ballottement may also cause pain when a displaced viscus rebounds against the abdominal wall. In severe peritonitis the abdominal musculature may be tense and palpation resisted.

---

### Palpation of the scrotum

The scrotum of a male horse with abdominal pain should always be inspected and palpated for evidence of scrotal herniation. Signs of strangulation in the affected testis include

- swelling
- hardness
- coolness.

Torsion of the spermatic cord is a differential diagnosis for this condition.

---

## Auscultation and percussion

The abdomen is auscultated to determine the functional status of the gastrointestinal tract. However, the correlation between

- audible intestinal sounds (borborygmi)
- the intestinal segment or abdominal area from which they emanate, and
- the presence of propulsive motility

is not clear. Furthermore, there is no objective means by which the sounds can be quantified and compared with a 'normal' model. Even in a healthy horse the pattern of audible intestinal sounds varies between individuals, with feeding practices and with other prevailing circumstances. Thus, sounds need to be interpreted critically with due regard to complementary diagnostic procedures and, where possible, using changes in the clinical findings detectable over repeated examinations, rather than depending on a single examination.

A methodical and careful auscultation of the entire abdomen takes several minutes and involves a systematic placing of the stethoscope so as to cover right and left ventral abdominal walls. The abdomen can be divided into four quadrants: dorsal and ventral left, and dorsal and ventral right, viewed from the rear of the animal. Beginning in the dorsal quadrant in the paralumbar area the stethoscope should be moved cranioventrally in an arc cranial to the border of the costal arch on both the left and right sides of the abdomen.

There is a general consensus that small intestinal motility is not reliably reflected by audible intestinal sounds. Ileus of the small intestines does appear to be associated with a persistently quiet abdomen that may reflect widespread hypomotility. It has been suggested that most of the left-sided sounds are due to gastric contractions, and that small intestinal borborygmi are audible over the lower abdomen. However, the consensus of opinion generally attributes intestinal sounds to large intestinal activity. The sounds are the result of mixing of intestinal contents caused by peristaltic contractions. In the normal abdomen it should be possible to detect arrhythmic background noises of intermittent short-duration low-pitched gurgles and squelches, accompanied by occasional high-pitched squeaks and tinkling over the entire abdomen. Superimposed on this are the periodic, louder 'cecal rush' sounds that propagate in a crescendo–decrescendo pattern. The latter are most prominent on the right side and have been associated with the coordinated cecal contractions that empty its contents into the right ventral colon.

The audible intestinal sounds are interpreted by comparing their characteristics with those of a subjective impression of normality. The characteristics of audible intestinal sounds to be noted are

- intensity
- duration, and
- frequency.

In the normal horse the intestinal sounds are clearly audible (intensity), there are periods of quiescence (frequency), and the sounds have a certain detectable duration. The intensity, frequency, and duration commonly increase during and following normal eating. A reduction in intensity is generally more significant than an increase. In spasmodic colic the borborygmi may be so loud that a stethoscope is barely necessary. This indicates that there is no intrinsic functional impairment and reflects a state of hyper-peristalsis. Similar increases in activity after a period of quiescence sometimes indicate the commencement of an impaction breaking up, and may be associated with more intense bouts of pain.

An absence of borborygmi or a quiet abdomen is less reliably indicative of hypoperistalsis at the first examination. If such a finding persists through repeated examinations, or is progressive, the probability of an acute physical intestinal obstruction increases. An absence of cecal sounds does not necessarily imply that the underlying abnormality is of cecal origin, as there is a reflex cecal hypomotility secondary to most abdominal crises. However, specific cecal atony may occur as a complication in the treatment of unrelated abnormalities, particularly musculoskeletal injury, or subsequent to general anesthesia.

Tinkling or high-pitched resonant sounds may be audible over the abdomen. These are caused by a gas–fluid interface where there is a larger than normal accumulation of gas under pressure. Resonance can be detected best by percussion using finger-flicking, or with a plexor, against the abdominal wall and simultaneous auscultation over the regions of suspected tympany (Fig. 17.26). The areas of increased resonance, or pings, can be delineated by moving the stethoscope to multiple sites, and it is possible to map out the approximate dimensions of the tympanitic viscus. Frequently the

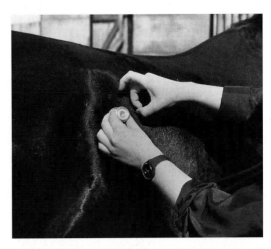

**Fig. 17.26** Flicking the abdominal wall close to where the stethoscope has been placed causes a resonant 'ping' to be heard if there is an underlying tympanitic viscus present.

affected viscus is the cecum, high in the right flank. When this feature is recognized it either indicates a primary tympany or, more likely, is secondary to colonic obstruction. Tympanitic areas on the left side will involve the left colon and again suggest colonic obstruction. In general, simple intraluminal impactions of the colon do not completely obstruct the passage of gas, so that intestinal tympany represents a relatively high index of suspicion for displacement of the colon.

Along with examination of the abdomen the thorax is also auscultated. Referral of loud intestinal sounds into the thorax is common in the horse because of the overlap of the abdominal and thoracic cavities.

---

### Intestinal sounds audible over the thorax

These can be differentiated into

- referred abdominal sounds, or, extremely rarely
- a diaphragmatic hernia – only the presence of colic in association with tachypnea accompanied by intestinal sounds overlying the lung fields and displacement of heart sounds craniad might indicate displacement of intestines through the diaphragm.

---

### Rectal examination

Rectal examination of a horse with a history and clinical findings of colic or other manifestations of

---

### Clinical Pointer

In cases of sand impaction, gravity causes the dense material to accumulate ventrally, and movements of the semifluid mass can create a noise that mimics sounds of the seashore.

abdominal disease is an extremely valuable diagnostic aid and should be considered routine. There are some limitations and precautions to consider.

1. Only the caudal third of the abdominal cavity is within reach.
2. Foals and miniature ponies are too small even to attempt rectal examination.
3. Fractious patients represent a risk to the safety of both themselves (rectal tear) and the examiner (kick), and adequate restraint must be used. The intravenous administration of a smooth muscle relaxant (e.g. hyoscine 0.2 mg/kg body weight) prior to examination is effective in reducing rectal tone and straining, reducing the risk of iatrogenic damage, and improving diagnostic accuracy.
4. Exploration around the abdomen should be slow, smooth and deliberate. Temptation to push the arm through a region of resistance or to use the fingertips excessively must be avoided.

Depending on the size of the horse, fat depositions, hydration status, and the presence or absence of distended viscera, the ease of examination is highly variable. Care should be taken to prevent the introduction of tail hairs into the rectum. Lubricant should be used liberally and topical local anesthetic added when necessary.

## Normal findings (Figs 17.27A, B)

The rectal mucosa should be moist. Formed or semi-formed feces are encountered at about the level of the rectal ampulla and must usually be evacuated before deeper penetration can be achieved. Approximately spherical fecal balls are distributed throughout the length of the small colon and can be palpated scattered around the midregion of the palpable caudal abdomen. The small intestine is normally not palpable. The caudal border of the spleen is palpable as a firm, rubbery edge lying close against the left abdominal wall, although in a variable position both craniocaudally and dorsoventrally. Tracing the line of the splenic base dorsocranially leads to the caudal pole of the left kidney, which is fixed to the dorsal abdominal wall. Between the caudal pole of the left kidney and the dorsal, axial surface of the spleen is the nephrosplenic

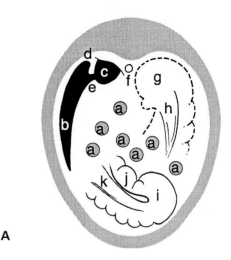

**A**

**Fig. 17.27** **(A)** Diagram representing the cross-section of the caudal abdomen indicating the approximate positions of structures that might normally be palpable during examination per rectum.

| | |
|---|---|
| a = small intestine | g = base of cecum |
| b = spleen | h = cecal teniae |
| c = left kidney | i = pelvic flexure |
| d = nephro-splenic space | j = left dorsal colon |
| e = nephro-splenic ligament | k = left ventral colon |
| f = aorta | |

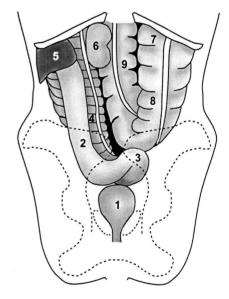

**B**

**Fig. 17.27** **(B)** The spatial relationships between caudal abdominal structures, viewed dorsally.

| | |
|---|---|
| 1 = bladder | 6 = left kidney |
| 2 = left dorsal colon | 7 = base of cecum |
| 3 = pelvic flexure | 8 = body of cecum |
| 4 = left ventral colon | 9 = apex of cecum |
| 5 = spleen | |

## Clinical Pointer ✳

Fecal balls can be distinguished from ovaries or abnormal masses by their mobility and the ability to disperse them by gentle digital compression.

space, bordered ventrally by the nephrosplenic ligament. This is palpable as a short, tight band and usually two or three fingers can be inserted over it into the space. This is more difficult in large horses. In male horses the two slit-like vaginal rings lining the deep inguinal rings can be felt on either side of the ventral midline, just beyond the pelvic brim. In relaxed or smaller horses the root of the mesentery, centered on the cranial mesenteric artery, can be identified at the cranial extent of reach. This is like a firm band of tissue suspended from the dorsal body wall in the midline. Moving to the right of the midline the hand encounters the base of the cecum, the semifluid contents of which can be appreciated by ballottement with the hand. The base of the cecum is attached to the dorsal body wall and the body and apex run ventrally, medially, and cranially. This can be delineated by palpating the ventral and/or medial cecal band (tenia) running in that direction. Cupping the fingers around these bands (left to right) allows a caudal traction to be applied on the cecum (Fig. 17.27C). This is normally

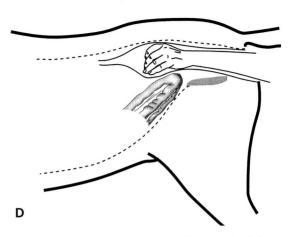

**D**

**Fig. 17.27 (D)** Gentle pressure applied by trapping left colon wall against the pelvic brim assists in determining the textures of colonic wall and contents.

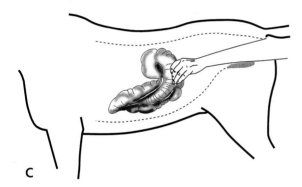

**C**

**Fig. 17.27 (C)** Caudal traction on the ventral/medial cecal tenia might elicit a pain response, particularly in horses with an ileal or cecal lesion.

not resented. The terminal part of the left ventral colon, the pelvic flexure, and the proximal part of the left dorsal colon may or may not be palpable, depending on the amount of ingesta contained therein. Pressing ventrally may allow intestinal wall or teniae to be detected between fingers and body wall, or may allow ingesta to be palpated (Fig. 17.27D). In the former case the intestinal wall should feel relatively thin and roll easily beneath the finger without pain. Normal ingesta has a semifluid consistency without the intestinal wall being stretched around it or contracted down on it. The pelvic flexure varies somewhat in position and may be quite far cranial on the left side, or

the left colons may be transverse inside the pelvic brim with the pelvic flexure situated to the right of the midline. In general, rectal examination in a normal horse should allow identification of the above landmarks; exploration usually should be comfortable for the horse and be unobstructed by distended viscera, tight bands, or abnormal masses (Fig. 17.57a,b).

The identification of abnormal findings on rectal examination might lead to a specific diagnosis or merely to a conclusion about the nature of the disease process, on which further investigative or therapeutic approaches can be based. These non-specific abnormalities are often indicative of the need for an exploratory laparotomy and might thus be fundamental to the successful outcome of the case.

There are several major general features to be considered

1. The amount, nature, and consistency of the feces and the state of the rectal mucosa.
2. Firm enlargements of intestine in the form of long columns, caused by impaction of feces in the large or small colon, or ingesta in the terminal ileum at the ileocecal valve. These commonly pit on digital pressure and indicate impaction.
3. Distension of segments of intestine with fluid or gas. These are tense, resilient, and fluctuate with digital pressure. Loops of small intestine can be distinguished from large colon by their smaller diameter (4–6 cm maximum) and from the small colon by the absence of an antimesentric band. Large intestinal segments can become abnormally much larger, such that their full contents cannot be palpated.

4. Tight bands indicating stretching of mesentery, due to either a heavy intestinal segment at the end of it or a folding together of mesentery when the intestine is twisted on itself (volvulus torsion) or telescoped into itself (intussusception).

5. The absence of certain intestinal segments which are normally palpable suggests displacement; cranial retroflexion of the pelvic flexure is, however, a normal variant.

6. The position of the spleen depends to some extent on the fullness of the stomach. If the caudal edge of the spleen appears too far caudal, it could be due to gastric distension.

### Rectal mucosa

A dry, tacky rectal mucosa and small, hard fecal balls are indicative of dehydration and a relative absence of feces suggests an obstruction. However, in the early stages, after the onset of an acute physical intestinal obstruction, dehydration might not have had time to develop and the ingesta caudal to the obstructed site may still be passed, this can be erroneously interpreted as a patent intestinal tract.

### Feces

The nature and consistency of the feces are important clues. A mucoid covering over the feces suggests a delay in intestinal transit time. Liquid feces are not generally associated with acute gastrointestinal disease but are most commonly encountered with hypermotile 'spasmodic' colic. However, colic is sometimes the prodromal sign of acute diarrheic disease, and horses sometimes pass liquid feces in the presence of a cecal impaction. The presence of frank blood in the feces suggests the possibility of a rectal tear, but can occur with strangulation of the small colon.

### Distended viscera

Tympany almost invariably involves the large intestine, especially the cecum (Fig. 17.27E). Massive accumula-

tions of large intestinal gas might obstruct the rectal examination. Involvement of the cecum can usually be identified because it remains possible to pass the arm medial to the base of the cecum, which is immobile. On occasions it is helpful to decompress a tympanitic cecum in order to complete the rectal examination. This is performed aseptically through the right sublumbar fossa under local analgesia

- a 14 gauge 12 cm catheter and stilette, or other suitable trocarized cannula, is passed through a skin stab incision and directed towards the point of the left elbow
- removal of the stilette then allows the release of trapped gas
- blockage of the cannula can be cleared by the injection of a soluble antibiotic solution.

Primary tympanitic colic does not occur as frequently as is sometimes suggested, and the presence of space-occupying gas-distended intestines should be assumed to be the result of a large intestinal displacement unless there is a compelling reason to think otherwise.

### Tight bands

Tight bands, usually orientated approximately horizontally across the abdomen, are another marker of large intestine malpositioning, as they are created by a combination of distension and flexion of the viscus. They should be distinguished from the medial and/or ventral cecal band(s), which can be palpated normally but which can also feel tense if the cecum is distended. Traction on these bands may elicit a pain reaction (Figs 17.27C,E).

Secondary impactions of large intestinal segments develop as a sequel to dehydration, whatever its cause. These can be recognized by dry ingesta being palpable through a corrugated, contracted intestinal wall, highlighting the sacculations. Sometimes it is possible to feel changes in the intestinal wall or mesentery that suggest vascular compromise. Intestinal wall (mural) edema feels like a soft thickening of a visceral surface. Often the easiest place to detect this is the pelvic flexure, which can be compressed against the abdominal wall (Fig. 17.27D). Ischemic intestine may be painful to this manipulation. Occlusion of mesenteric vessels leads to congestion and hemorrhages, which feel like gelatinous swellings unassociated with the intestinal wall. This usually represents a taut and engorged mesocolon which has become more palpable by some sort of intestinal malpositioning.

### Palpable loops of small intestine

If small intestinal segments can be picked up and the walls palpated between thumb and finger without there being any distension, then the wall is abnormally

---

## Texture of serosal surfaces

The texture of the serosal surfaces indicates the animal's condition

- normal viscera are well lubricated
- more resistance is felt on palpation as the abdomen becomes drier
- peritonitis results in a fibrinous roughening of the serosae
- frank ingesta or fecal contamination lead to a grating, crepitant feeling.

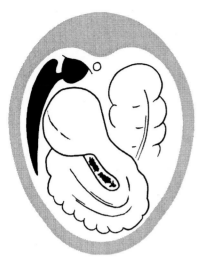

**Fig. 17.27** (E) Tympany of the large intestine is often a non-specific sign of large colon malpositioning and might involve the cecal base (rightt) and/or left colons (left). If taeniae of the ventral colon can be palpated ventral to the dorsal colon which has no taeniae the displacement either does not involve a volvulus or the degree of rotation is greater than 180°. These two possibilities can usually be differentiated by the degree of pain that the animal is showing. The dimension of the distended viscera varies and is sometimes so great as to preclude viscus identification. Flexure of loops and/or mesentery results in tight bands. Jelly-like palpable masses suggest mesenteric edema or hemorrhage and indicate vascular obstruction.

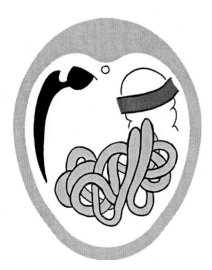

**Fig. 17.27** (F) Small intestinal distension usually presents as a stack of turgid loops of bowel with smooth, thin walls occupying the mid abdomen.

thickened. This may be due to infiltrative intestinal disease or to chronic, partial obstruction with muscular hypertrophy, usually associated with a history of chronic intermittent colic and perhaps weight loss. Fluid and gas distension in the small intestine can be identified by the presence of stacked, turgid loops of thin-walled intestine ('garden hosepipe' appearance) occupying the midregion of the palpable abdomen (Fig. 17.27F). The type, site, and duration of obstruction dictate the degree of distension.

### Specific abnormalities

Several specific abnormalities may be palpable by rectal examination. The accuracy varies with the experience of the clinician and with factors affecting the ease of examination. One report states that a definitive diagnosis by rectal examination alone was possible in 50% of colic patients.

---

**Clinical Pointer**

On rectal examination

- strangulating obstructions of the distal small intestine result in loops, measuring about 6 cm in diameter, which may obscure all other abdominal structures
- functional obstructions (e.g. ileus, grass sickness) tend to cause less tense intestinal distension.

---

**Impactions**

Impactions of the intestinal tract tend to occur at sites of abrupt changes in the diameter of the lumen or its direction. Impaction at the pelvic flexure and left ventral colon is one of the most common and can usually be palpated on rectal examination. The left ventral colon fills with dry ingesta and may become so large that it occupies a part of the pelvic cavity, making it difficult to advance the examiner's arm beyond the pelvic inlet. The pelvic flexure may fill excessively and become a blunt bulbous end in the pelvic cavity. The distension results in stretching and turgidity of the intestinal wall, which obliterates the sacculations of the left colon. This feature can be used to distinguish primary colonic impactions from those that result in dehydration of ingesta or partial impaction secondary to other abnormalities.

Impactions at other sites are less consistently palpable. The right dorsal colon is not uncommonly involved, but this segment can be reached only in smaller animals or those that have received a smooth muscle relaxant. Impaction of the ileum at the ileocecal valve may be recognizable as a vertically orientated, firm cylindrical structure palpable through the dorsal body of the cecum. Impaction of the small colon is recognizable as a convoluted 'sausage-like' structure occupying the caudal and midregion of the palpable abdomen. The wide tenial band is identifiable by palpation and will differentiate this from small intestinal distension. Cecal impactions are also infrequent causes of colic. Two syndromes have been described

- one is a primary impaction of firm ingesta
- the other is secondary to disturbance of cecal motility, in which the contents are fluid but do not move through the cecocolic orifice.

It is usually possible to define cecal involvement by reference to its landmarks: fixation of the base of the cecum to the dorsal body wall and the medial/ventral cecal band on the greater curvature which faces caudally.

---

### Clinical Pointer

To detect ileocecal intussusception a doughy mass palpable in the region of the cecal base is felt for. This can be difficult to distinguish from a cecal impaction, but tends to move with a separate inertia when ballotted per rectum.

---

Displacements of the large colon can sometimes be detected if the orientation of the tenia on the left colons can be felt and interpreted. If these appear to be dorsal to a segment of left dorsal colon (which has no free tenia) then there must be a volvulus. Entrapment of the left colon in the nephrosplenic space (left dorsal displacement of the colon) can be conclusively diagnosed if the colon is directly palpable draped over the nephrosplenic ligament. More often, gas accumulations in the colon and cecum obstruct detailed palpation of this area, but the orientation of the loops of distended intestines and teniae towards the space raises a high index of suspicion. However, the use of these indirect criteria may result in overdiagnosis of the condition.

Obstructions involving the small intestine tend not to lend themselves to specific diagnosis, with the exception of inguinal/scrotal herniation, in which case loops of distended small intestine will be palpable fixed in the region of the right or left deep inguinal ring on the ventral body wall just cranial to the pelvic inlet.

### Rectal tears
Lacerations of the rectal wall as a result of intraluminal trauma are potentially fatal. Occasionally injuries occur

---

### Right dorsal displacement of the colon

- if the colon can be palpated to the right of the cecum against the right body wall it is reasonable to make this diagnosis
- it often coexists with a non-strangulating volvulus of the colon.

---

following accidental penetration (usually during attempted breeding) or as unexplainable spontaneous ruptures, but the majority occur during rectal examinations. Rectal tearing is commonly a result of lack of caution or overzealous palpation. However, this is not invariably the case, and it appears that some animals are prone to rectal tears either intrinsically or perhaps because of inherent weakness of the dorsal rectum or scarring created at previous examinations.

Rupture of the rectal wall may be evident at the time it occurs

- if there is a sudden loss of resistance from the rectal wall around the hand, tearing should be suspected
- if extraluminal structures can be palpated directly a full-thickness tear must have occurred.

However, shallow tears and even some deeper ones can occur without being recognized.

Small amounts of blood on a rectal sleeve often reflect mucosal injury only, which is of minor consequence. More substantial tears often bleed profusely, sometimes to the extent that clots have already formed by the time the arm is withdrawn. On other occasions the hand will be withdrawn without any evidence of blood, thus leaving no suspicion of the injury. Horses with rectal tears involving more than mucosal layers usually exhibit evidence of discomfort soon after the occurrence. Clinical findings include

- restlessness and anxiety
- tail elevation
- tenesmus, and possibly
- sweating

are common. If a rectal tear is suspected it is desirable to be able to assess the degree of damage as soon as

---

### Clinical Pointer

As a routine, immediately after every rectal palpation the gloved hand and arm are inspected for streaks of fresh blood.

possible. However, further palpation runs the risk of worsening the injury and should not be performed until the patient has received sedation and smooth muscle relaxation. The latter can be achieved by the use of epidural anesthesia or hyoscine (0.2 mg/kg body weight). Thereafter, a careful evacuation of the rectum and palpation of the defect, perhaps performed most accurately with ungloved fingers, can proceed. Most tears occur perpendicular to the luminal axis across the dorsal aspect of the rectum. Rectal tears have been classified according to the tissue layers involved. Referral to an equine hospital is indicated.

1. **Grade 1 Mucosa-only tears** These are usually within the pelvic rectum and can be felt to occur when a peristaltic wave passes over the clinician's knuckles. Infection of the deeper layers of the wall results, but provided antibiotic therapy is given, the feces are kept soft, and the diet is reduced in bulk, systemic signs or long-term complications are unlikely.
2. **Grade 2 Disruption of the mucosal and muscular layers of the rectal wall** The outer layers of the rectal wall are left intact. These will probably not be recognized immediately, but rather as incidental findings or when a resulting diverticulum causes impactive colic.
3. **Grade 3 Tears of the wall into the pelvic fascia (retroperitoneal)** These are likely to bleed heavily and cause discomfort fairly rapidly. Immediate action is required to save the patient.
4. **Grade 4 Rupture of layers of the rectal wall extending into the peritoneal cavity** These also cause discomfort but, paradoxically, bleeding may appear to be minimal if it occurs intraperitoneally. Fairly heroic treatment is required immediately.

Tears that occur distal to the level of the peritoneal reflection around the rectum (approximately 30 cm from the anus in the average horse) may develop into impactions in diverticuli some time after the injury, or may lead to pararectal cellulitis or abscessation. Tears occurring within the region of the peritoneal part of the rectum are liable to develop peritonitis. Grade 4 tears result in frank contamination of the abdominal cavity and the onset of endotoxic shock is rapid. Grade 3 tears cause peritonitis by diapedesis of bacteria through the serosal wall, and the onset of signs of peritonitis is less acute. If doubt persists, analysis of peritoneal fluid cytology is a good indicator of the presence of a grade 3 lesion. Grade 4 tears that occur dorsally may be protected from the abdominal cavity by the mesocolon. In such cases the signs mimic those of a grade 3 tear.

# EXAMINATION OF ORAL CAVITY, PHARYNX, ESOPHAGUS, AND STOMACH

Some horses resent their head and neck region being touched, particularly around the ears and nose, but with patience and gentle handling the animal's confidence will usually be gained. With more difficult horses some restraint such as a nose twitch or restraint stocks may be required, both for personal safety and for completeness of the examination. The oral cavity, pharynx, esophagus, and stomach are examined using visual inspection, palpation, and the use of the nasogastric tube to evaluate the esophagus and stomach. Endoscopy is also frequently used.

## Regurgitation, nasogastric reflux, and vomiting

Regurgitation in monogastric animals means the return of swallowed but undigested feed, usually from the esophagus. Gastric or gastroesophageal reflux is the return of stomach contents into the esophagus which may then move to the nasal cavities and be known as nasogastric reflux. The term gastric reflux is also in common use when the stomach is distended with fluid which has refluxed from the small intestine. This fluid can be released with a nasogastric tube. Vomiting is the projectile return of swallowed, partially digested food which has reached the stomach or small intestine.

In pharyngeal or esophageal dysphagia some masticated feed will become displaced dorsal to the soft palate during attempts at swallowing. This feed material and saliva will flow down both nasal cavities and appear at the external nares, especially when the head is lowered, usually within a minute or so after ingestion. During breathing some of it will also flow caudally over the soft palate into the open larynx and enter the trachea. Inhalation of feed or liquid is termed **aspiration**. Aspirated particles of feed will stimulate cough receptors, which are present mainly in the distal trachea of the horse, resulting in some of the aspirated feed being expelled by coughing via the nasal and oral routes. The horse has a large 'sump-like' dependent area at the cranial intrathoracic trachea which traps

> ### Clinical Pointer
>
> Vomiting, the projectile return of swallowed food from the stomach, probably never occurs in horses.

most aspirated material until it is cleared either by coughing, mucociliary transport, or gravity when the horse lowers its head below the thoracic tracheal level. The tracheal contents then flow out through the nasopharynx and nasal cavities. Consequently, aspiration (inhalation, foreign-body) pneumonia does not usually occur with aspiration in the horse.

Unlike pharyngeal or esophageal dysphagia, gastrointestinal reflux with nasal feed discharge will **not** usually be associated with feed ingestion, as any particulate material refluxed may have been ingested many hours previously and the reflux consists mostly of stomach and intestinal secretions that are unable to move aborally. Also, horses with marked ileus will show no inclination to eat. Gastrointestinal distension causes severe continuous abdominal pain (colic) in the horse, the distress being manifested by signs such as looking at the flank, restlessness, pawing and adopting a dog-sitting posture. However, horses with total gastro- intestinal ileus due to grass sickness may show no signs of colic.

---

### Gastric or gastrointestinal reflux

- this occurs most commonly with small intestinal obstruction and subsequent distension of intestine with fluid proximal to the obstruction
- the fluid later causes gastric distension and reflux of gastrointestinal contents up the esophagus and possibly into the pharynx
- because of the normal subepiglottic position of the equine soft palate, most gastric reflux will flow down the nasal cavities
- the liquid discharge, containing partially digested food, usually has a foul smell and a very low pH owing to the presence of gastric acid
- it is not associated with feed ingestion.

---

## Oral cavity

### Prehension activity

The very mobile and tactile equine lips direct the forage between the incisors and, once grasped, the forage is torn away using a quick head movement. Many horses have a slight degree of mandibular brachygnathism (parrot mouth). This hereditary defect is mainly cosmetic and will not significantly affect prehension. When severe it prevents contact between the upper and lower incisors, with resultant overgrowth of the incisors. Trauma, most commonly from kicks, is the most frequent cause of incisor teeth damage. In some young horses the broken incisors may have the

pulp exposed and yet the pulp and thus the tooth remains vital. These teeth survive by laying down secondary dentine and sealing off the exposed pulp. They will continue to erupt and will eventually develop contact with their opposite tooth, which erupts more quickly than normal because of the lack of occlusal pressure; in addition it will undergo no natural wear because of the absence of occlusal contact.

Retention of the deciduous incisors adjacent to their permanent counterparts that have erupted may occur and, less commonly, supernumerary permanent incisors develop. Neither of these abnormalities usually affects prehension. Even in very old horses with grossly worn incisors, prehension is usually not a major problem, and such horses can maintain their body weight.

### Mastication

The constant grinding of fibrous food containing biological abrasives, especially silicates, for up to 18 hours a day causes much wear on the occlusal surface of the teeth. This is compensated for by continuous eruption of the reserve crown of these long-crowned (hypsodont) teeth until they are fully worn, usually at 25–30 years of age. Uneven wear of the occlusal surfaces of the cheek teeth will result in the development of sharp prominences that may cause mechanical obstruction to feed grinding. In addition, these sharp edges on the lingual aspect of the lower (mandibular) and the buccal aspect of the upper (maxillary) arcades will lacerate the mucosa of the tongue and cheeks respectively during chewing. Pain from these soft tissue lesions then causes an additional hindrance to normal mastication.

Normal horses have a vigorous side-to-side masticatory effort. Because equine teeth are composed of layers of constituents of different hardness (enamel is harder than dentine or cementum) differing rates of wear normally lead to the development of an irregular and self-sharpening occlusal surface that is very effective at grinding fibrous plant material. Normal mastication of fibrous food produces a loud grinding sound. In the presence of mechanical and/or painful hindrances mastication is much less vigorous, producing more 'slurping-type' sounds. Restricted lateral movement of the mandible may also be apparent in such cases. This

---

### Cheilitis

Inflammatory nodules of the mucosal aspect of both upper and lower lips due to plant awns results in cheilitis (inflammation of the lips), making prehension painful and difficult.

---

may be detected by stabilizing the proximal aspect of the maxilla with one hand and assessing the range of lateral mandibular movement with the other.

With painful oral lesions propulsion of a chewed bolus of feed back to the oropharynx is often ineffective, and feed falls out of the mouth. This is termed quidding, which is an oral dysphagia. Examination of the ground in front of the feeding area, or outside a half-doored box of a horse with such dental lesions, usually reveals masticated boluses of feed about 5 cm in diameter. Abnormal mastication may also lead to a 'hamster-like' pocketing of feed in the cheeks, and also at the gum margins. The latter may eventually lead to secondary periodontal disease and may also occur with facial (cranial nerve VII) paralysis. Non-dental causes of oral dysphagia include

- fracture of the mandible, premaxilla (incisive), maxilla, or hyoid bones
- bilateral paralysis of the tongue (cranial nerve XII) or masticatory muscles (cranial nerve V)
- glossitis, and
- stomatitis.

## Clinical Pointer

By palpating through the cheeks the presence of sharp edges on the lateral aspects of the rostral maxillary cheek teeth can be detected. Resentment of this procedure indicates pain.

## Swallowing

Swallowing is a complex act involving the sensory and motor nerves and muscles of the tongue, pharynx, hyoid, larynx, and esophagus. It can be divided into oral, pharyngeal, and esophageal phases. In the horse

- the free edge of the very long soft palate becomes elevated into the nasopharynx during swallowing
- simultaneously, contractions of the lingual and hyoid muscles compress the epiglottis against the base of the tongue, tilting it dorsocaudally and occluding the laryngeal opening
- contractions of the laryngeal adductor muscles then fully adduct the arytenoid cartilages (both of these latter mechanisms prevent aspiration)
- the feed bolus is then squeezed towards the esophagus, whose entrance is opened by the coordinated relaxation of the caudal pharyngeal constrictor muscles (thyropharyngeus and cricopharyngeus) and thus of the palatopharyngeal arch.

## Examination of the oral cavity

Like all herbivores, the horse has a very limited angle of opening of the jaws. In addition, the commissures of the lips are very rostral and the dental arcades long. These three factors make clinical examination of the equine oral cavity, especially its caudal aspects, difficult. In a quiet horse a partial clinical examination of the rostral oral cavity is possible with the animal unsedated. The horse is restrained by a halter with a loose noseband that permits full jaw opening. A bridle will provide better restraint but the bit greatly obstructs the examination. The examiner's hand is introduced into the space between the incisor and cheek teeth (interdental space, or bars of the mouth) and the tongue is grasped and drawn out of the mouth to one side, ensuring that the operator's hand does not come between the horse's incisors. The tongue can be grasped with the thumb and 2–3 fingers and the noseband grasped with the small and ring fingers, thus ensuring that if the horse moves its head the examiner's hand will move with it and not get bitten, and also that the horse's tongue will not be injured. The tongue should not be pulled vigorously and should not be used to control a fractious horse. The mouth may also be opened further by pressing the thumb of the free hand against the hard palate. Using a headlight or mobile light source the rostral aspect of one side of the cheek teeth arcades may now be examined. The tongue is then drawn out of the opposite side of the mouth and the opposite arcade similarly examined. Withdrawal of the tongue will often be resented, and if painful oral lesions are present or the animal is unbroken or fractious it may not be possible to perform even this superficial examination. Preferably, a speculum is used.

With many equine dental abnormalities feed will be retained in the oral cavity, particularly on the lateral aspects of the cheek teeth, and its presence will prevent a full clinical examination of the teeth. Starving the horse for a few hours beforehand is effective in some cases, but gross impaction of feed in the cheeks will not

## Esophageal obstruction (choke)

- this results in an inability to swallow, characterized by a bilateral intermittent nasal discharge consisting of feed and saliva
- attempts by the horse to drink and eat are followed by a profuse bilateral nasal discharge consisting of a mixture of water, saliva, and feed particles; accompanied by arching and lowering of the neck and coughing.

be cleared by starvation. In such cases flushing the oral cavity with a very large syringe of warm water is useful, but when feed impaction is gross careful manual removal is required; this is best performed with use of a speculum and with a gloved hand, because of the foul odor of impacted feed.

Even when visual examination of the oral cavity is possible, the medial aspects of the cheeks and the lateral aspect of the tongue lie close against and prevent complete visualization of the caudal 2–3 cheek teeth. This problem can be partially overcome by use of a thin metal rod to displace the tongue or cheeks away from the dental arcade, and thus attempting to expose all the teeth. The use of a headlamp greatly assists visual examination.

Manual examination of the caudal arcades is needed to allow a more complete examination and may reveal periodontal pocketing of feed and displaced, fractured, cariotic or missing teeth. This procedure can only be performed using a speculum (gag) (Fig. 17.28). A variety of gags can be used to keep the jaws open, but should only be used in quiet or sedated horses as sudden movement of the animal's head can injure the examiner and any assistant. The current availability of a variety of safe and effective short-acting sedatives (usually $\alpha_2$-adrenergic agonists) greatly facilitates safe oral examination in horses with a gag. It is best to have at least two assistants for such examinations

- one to hold and to elevate the horse's head
- the second to withdraw the tongue to the side opposite to that being examined.

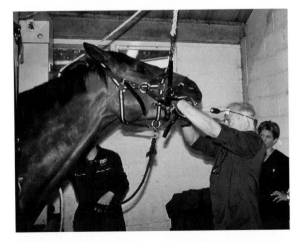

**Fig. 17.28** This sedated horse is restrained in stocks, has its head elevated using a dental head halter, and is wearing a Hausmann gag (speculum). The examiner is performing an oral examination by palpation and by visual inspection with the aid of a strong head light.

This allows the examiner's hands to be free to hold a light source and a metal rod to move the tongue and cheeks and for oral examination as necessary.

Care should be taken that the sharp enamel ridges that are commonly present on the medial aspect of the equine mandibular cheek teeth do not cut the operator's hand or arm during manual examination of the oral cavity. If these ridges are very prominent they should be rasped in advance of the examination. Some horses resent manual examination of the caudal aspect of their oral cavity, even when sedated. Consequently, during this part of the examination sudden movements of the horse's head can result in the metal gag severely injuring the head of the examiner and any assistant. During caudal oral or oropharyngeal examinations horses will also constantly make vigorous chewing movements which can rostrally dislodge a gag that is not tightly retracted by a tight headband or held in position on the incisors. This can also potentially injure the operator's hand or arm. It has been suggested that the effects of sedation make horses more prone to chew the operator's arm or their own tongue.

### Clinical Pointer

In advanced periodontal disease bacterial growth, particularly of anaerobic bacteria, results in a foul smell in the oral cavity. It is useful to smell one's hand for such odors after performing an oral examination. However, sick, anorexic horses also develop foul-smelling oral cavities.

### Oral mucous membranes

Examination of the oral mucous membranes to assess the peripheral circulation is an important part of the general clinical examination of the horse. Eversion of the lips (Fig. 17.29) allows visual and digital inspection of the mucous membranes. Most changes to the oral mucosa are caused by systemic abnormalities (see Chapter 14).

The capillary refill time, determined by timing (by slowly counting ... pause/one second/pause/two seconds/pause ...) the return of color to the gum following blanching by minimal digital pressure of the mucous membranes above the upper incisor teeth is usually less than 2 seconds in the normal horse. In advanced shock the capillary refill time will increase and terminally might be more than 4 seconds.

## Color of the mucous membranes

- normal mucous membranes are pink, moist, and warm
- in the earlier vasoconstrictive stage of shock and dehydration the mucous membranes may be pale, dry, and cool
- in advanced shock they become congested, brick-red, and eventually cyanotic

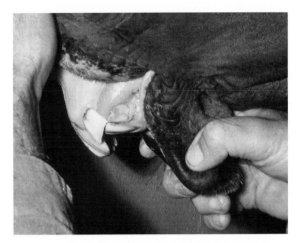

**Fig. 17.30** This horse has gross brachygnathism. There is partial occlusal contact between the caudal aspect of the upper corner incisor and the middle lower incisor and gross overgrowth of the remaining teeth.

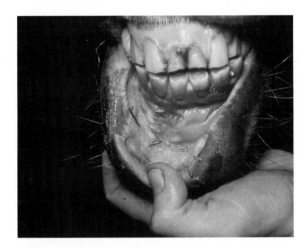

**Fig. 17.29** Gross ulceration of the oral mucosa secondary to chronic renal disease. The dental wear pattern indicates that this is an aged horse and also that it is a crib biter (excessive wear on the rostral aspect of incisors, especially centrals).

## Teeth

### Dental disease

*Incisor teeth*

Horses that 'crib-bite' (biting on stable objects) will eventually develop abnormal wear on the rostral angles of their central incisors. Palpation of the neck of such horses also commonly reveals hypertrophy of the sternocephalicus (sternomandibularis) muscles.

Abnormalities of the incisors include mandibular brachygnathism (undershot lower jaw, parrot mouth) which may not be clinically significant unless gross (Fig. 17.30). Prognathism (overshot lower jaw, sow mouth) is less common in the horse. An increased number of incisors (> 6 teeth per arcade) is most commonly the result of deciduous incisors being retained in younger animals: some of the incisors (deciduous) will be smaller and whiter than the permanent ones. A developmental disorder of supernumerary permanent incisors can also occur, where all (>

6) incisors will be of similar appearance. Fractures of the incisors are obvious and have been previously discussed (page 388).

*Canine and wolf teeth*

The vestigial first maxillary premolar (wolf tooth) is sometimes present, either erupted or unerupted, and can be seen or palpated at the rostral border of the first cheek tooth. Despite its traditional alleged role as a cause of many oral problems, it is difficult to rationalize how this structure causes any such problems.

*Cheek teeth*

Because of the sloping occlusive surfaces of the cheek teeth, sharp edges ('enamel points') commonly develop on the lateral aspect of the maxillary arcade and on the medial aspect of the mandibular arcade. These can cause buccal and lingual lacerations, respectively, which can be detected on oral examination. A more extreme form of this disorder occurs when the mandibular arcade is excessively narrow in relation to the maxilla. The full occlusal surfaces of upper and lower cheek teeth now become triangular in shape in the condition termed shear (scissor) mouth (see Fig. 17.21).

Some horses have a rostral displacement of the whole maxillary arcade in relation to the mandibular arcade. This results in the development of a large overgrowth (hook) on the rostral aspect of the first maxillary cheek tooth (P2), which is readily identified. The corresponding hook on the caudal aspect of the sixth mandibular cheek tooth (M3) will not be apparent without a full examination of the caudal oral cavity (see Fig. 17.21). With some dental disorders unevenness in wear or in eruption of the cheek teeth can cause the cheek teeth arcades, which are normally level (or slightly curved) in the sagittal plane, to assume an irregular undulating appearance. This is termed wave mouth (see Fig. 17.21).

Equine teeth, including the erupted clinical crown, have an external layer of cementum, although this is often worn off the rostral aspect of the incisors. This peripheral cementum gives teeth an irregular, cream to brown colored, chalky appearance, very different from the white shiny enamel surfaces of brachydont (short-crowned) teeth such as is present in humans. This normal peripheral cementum should not be mistaken as calculus.

---

### Calculi

True calculi, often very large (> 30 mm diameter), sometimes develop on the lower canine teeth (usually only in male horses) and may be accompanied by localized and usually non-significant inflammation of the adjacent gum. Such large irregular calculi may cause mechanical ulceration of the overlying buccal mucosa.

---

Localized periodontal disease is a common finding in horses during eruption of the permanent cheek teeth and is manifested as a narrow (5–10 mm) band of redness at the gingival margin of recently erupted teeth. With further eruption of these hypsodont teeth and exposure of new periodontal membranes, this usually resolves within months. This is in contrast to its chronic nature in species with brachydont dentition, such as the dog, where periodontal disease is irreversible.

During eruption of the first three permanent cheek teeth (between 2.5 and 4 years of age), the remnants of the overlying deciduous teeth, termed 'caps' (see Fig. 17.50) may become trapped between the adjacent teeth or by some remnants of gingiva, and may cause oral discomfort and even temporary oral dysphagia. Deciduous and permanent cheek teeth can be differentiated by palpation as the occlusal surfaces of deciduous teeth are smooth in contrast to the rough occlusal surface of recently erupted permanent teeth.

Cheek tooth disease is commonly caused by abscessation of the periapical region. In some horses with advanced periapical infection, evidence of caries (dental necrosis) may be obvious on the occlusal surface, with secondary sagittal fractures even occurring in some advanced cases. In older horses

(> 20 years) cheek tooth loss may occur as the result of normal wear or be secondary to disease, especially periodontal disease. Subsequent overgrowth of the opposing cheek tooth will cause an irregularity known as 'step mouth' (see Fig. 17.21).

Periapical abscessation of the cheek teeth may result in detectable changes on the erupted (clinical) tooth crown and also formation of an external sinus tract from the mandible or maxilla. In the absence of these changes, radiography (lateral-oblique projections) is necessary to confirm the presence of periapical dental disease. Great changes occur in the radiographic appearance of equine teeth with age, and care must be taken when comparing differences between adjacent cheek teeth that can vary in age by up to 3 years. Where sinus tracts are present, additional radiographs with probes or contrast medium in these tracts can be of great diagnostic help, especially in cases without clear-cut radiographic changes.

### Salivary glands

Like all herbivores, horses have large and well developed salivary glands. These are the large, paired parotid and smaller mandibular (positioned deep to the mandible) and sublingual (positioned between the rostral aspect of the tongue and medial aspect of mandible) glands. The parotid salivary glands lie relatively superficially in the retromandibular fossa beneath the base of the ear, caudal to the vertical ramus of the mandible and extend ventrocaudally for nearly the full length of the mandible. In normal horses the lateral aspect of the parotid salivary gland lies about a finger's depth medial to the mandible. The parotid salivary glands can be freely elevated on their caudoventral aspect, where their caudal lobulated border is about 2–3 cm thick, depending on the size of the horse and the type of diet it is currently on. The lateral aspect of this gland does not normally feel lobulated owing to the overlying parotidoauricularis muscle and dense fascia. In other domestic species, such as cattle and sheep, large well defined parotid lymph nodes are present within or beneath the parotid salivary glands, but in horses a much smaller, less well defined group of 6–10 lymph nodes (the parotid lymphocenter) lies within or beneath the mid-dorsal aspect of this salivary gland.

Because of their small size and deep position it is not usually possible to clinically detect inflammation in the equine parotid lymph nodes, even when marked inflammation exists in areas they would be expected to drain, such as the maxillary sinus. However, with certain local infections such as strangles, gross inflammation of these parotid lymph nodes will occur, causing hot and painful and usually bilateral diffuse swelling of the parotid area. A purulent sinus tract to the exterior will occasionally develop owing to abscessation and rupture of the nodes.

Bilateral parotid salivary gland swelling of unknown origin does occur in grazing horses and this enigmatic condition is termed idiopathic parotiditis. Such swellings may be due to gross overproduction of saliva on lush pasture and will bring the parotid salivary gland level with, or even protruding beyond, the lateral mandibular surface. The swellings are sometimes accompanied by local subcutaneous edema and slight pain and stiffness of the area. After withdrawal of the animal from pasture the swellings usually resolve within 12–24 hours. Such swellings may also be due to dependent edema in horses sick for many reasons, when the head remains constantly low.

A less common but more serious type of parotid salivary gland swelling is a firm irregular, nodular swelling caused by infiltration of the salivary gland and the associated lymph nodes by melanoma (melanotic carcinoma) in gray horses (Fig. 17.31). The biology of

---

**Clinical Pointer**

The parotid salivary glands are the second most common site of melanoma in gray horses, the ventral base of the tail and perianal area are the areas most frequently involved.

---

these tumors at this site is variable, with most growing slowly over many years, sometimes developing into massive swellings; metastasis seldom occurs.

The parotid salivary gland or duct is occasionally damaged by trauma, and this may result in a chronic salivary–cutaneous fistula which may secrete increased volumes of saliva in response to the presence of food in the mouth.

### Soft palate

Because of its anatomical position it is not possible to visualize much of the equine soft palate on oral examination without the use of general anesthesia and an

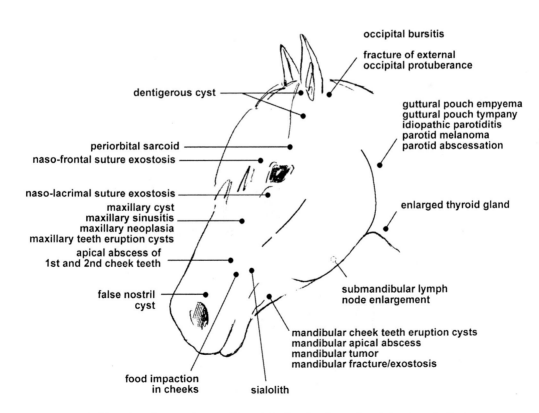

**Fig. 17.31**  Anatomical location of some abnormalities of the head and associated structures in the horse.

instrument to depress the base of the tongue. Even then, only a very restricted view of the ventrorostral aspect will be achieved. Depending on the relative sizes of the horse's head and the examiner's arm, a digital examination of the ventral aspect of the soft palate is possible orally but requires the use of sedation and a speculum. The soft palate can also be examined by nasopharyngeal endoscopy and by lateral nasopharyngeal radiography.

In foals, cleft palate most commonly involves the distal aspect of the soft palate. A cleft palate causes an incomplete separation of the oral and nasal cavities, resulting in the passage of food or liquids into the nasopharynx during swallowing. This material will flow down the nose within seconds of sucking and, more significantly, will also flow into the trachea, commonly inducing coughing immediately after swallowing. In some cases such aspiration will lead to a foreign-body pneumonia.

## Pharynx

This rectangular mucosa-lined cavity serves as a common pathway for both the respiratory and the alimentary tracts. The large vertical ramus of the equine mandible covers most of the lateral aspect of the pharynx, with the large parotid salivary glands covering the pharynx caudal to the mandible. Ventrally

- the omohyoid muscles
- the cricothyroid ligament, and
- the hyoid apparatus

fully cover the ventral aspect of the oropharynx. Little information can therefore be obtained from external examination of the equine pharynx.

Internal pharyngeal palpation can be performed only in larger horses. To do this without general anesthesia it is advisable

- to have adequate assistance
- to have the horse well sedated, and
- to use a gag.

The base of the tongue, the large midline glossoepiglottic fold, the oropharyngeal walls and floor, the overlying caudal aspect of the soft palate and the base of the epiglottis are palpable when the soft palate and epiglottis are in the normal breathing position. This examination will often cause the soft palate to become dorsally displaced, and all of the epiglottis and the rostral aspect of the larynx will then be palpable. However, the equine pharynx is relatively small and constant swallowing and head movements further restrict the usefulness of this examination in the unanesthetized subject.

Foreign bodies are only rarely encountered in the equine oropharynx, but will occasionally be found in the piriform recess or lateral nasopharynx.

The entrance to the esophagus, surrounded by the palatopharyngeal arch, lies immediately dorsal to the larynx. This area cannot be palpated and is normally occluded from endoscopic view by the caudodorsal nasopharyngeal roof. If the horse has been sedated a mucosal fold of the palatopharyngeal arch, or occasionally of the dorsal pharyngeal mucosa, will bulge down over the dorsal larynx. This is caused by a sedative-induced loss of tone of the caudal pharyngeal constrictor muscles (thyropharyngeus and cricopharyngeus). This must be differentiated from a more marked and permanent prolapse of the palatopharyngeal arch caused by a congenital absence of the cricopharyngeus muscle in the disorder termed cricopharyngeal–laryngeal dysplasia. In some such cases, and also with acquired damage to these muscles, such as occasionally happens after laryngeal surgery, the esophageal opening may be permanently open.

---

### Disorders of the equine epiglottis

The two well described disorders of the equine epiglottis that can be palpated orally, but are more accurately diagnosed by endoscopy, are

- entrapment by a fold of the subepiglottic mucosa
- the presence of a subepiglottic cyst.

---

## Esophagus

As previously noted, gastric (gastrointestinal) reflux via an inserted nasogastric tube is a very common and significant finding in horses suffering from gastrointestinal ileus and foals with advanced gastroduodenal ulceration. Some gas may also be released from the stomach during passage of a nasogastric tube to remove gastric contents in horses suffering from ileus.

Eructation is very rare in horses and this may also be due to the presence of strong caudal esophageal musculature and sphincters. Another type of 'eructation' in the horse is caused by a congenital disorder (cricopharyngeal–laryngeal dysplasia) that includes unilateral or bilateral absence of the cricopharyngeus muscle (one of the caudal pharyngeal constrictor muscles). Absence of this muscle disrupts the rostral esophageal sphincter and allows the entry and accumulation of air into the esophagus and proximal gastrointestinal tract. Intraesophageal air will occasionally be released with an eructation-type sound.

The esophagus is not normally palpable in the horse, but during passage of a nasogastric tube the esophageal wall will be seen to distend dorsal to the left jugular groove during transit.

In equine esophageal obstruction (choke), commonly caused by impaction of a large segment of the esophagus with particulate matter, such as sugar beet pulp or pelleted feed, a firm to doughy distended esophagus may be palpable in the left jugular groove.

---

### Clinical Pointer

The presence of subcutaneous crepitus in the left jugular groove is a grave prognostic sign, usually indicating either

- esophageal rupture with periesophageal air leakage, or
- infection of the damaged periesophageal tissues by gas-forming bacteria.

---

Assessment of possible esophageal choke is usually done by gentle passage (swallowing) of a suitably sized lubricated nasogastric tube to assess the presence and possible site of obstruction. Pharyngeal dysphagia prevents a nasogastric tube from being passed beyond the nasopharynx, and such cases may resemble esophageal choke where the obstruction extends to its pharyngeal opening. However, in most cases the nasogastric tube can be swallowed and will pass freely through the esophagus until it encounters the proximal aspect of the obstruction, which is often in the cervical region. By marking the tube at the level of the nostrils before withdrawing it, the rostral limit of the obstruction can be determined by placing the tube along the side of the head and the path of the esophagus. The presence of blood on the nasogastric tube after withdrawal indicates that the tough esophageal mucosa has been lacerated. This may be due to previous misguided attempts to dislodge esophageal obstructions by force. The clinical examination of a case of equine esophageal choke should also include evaluation of the horse's hydration status. A horse with esophageal choke initially will often attempt to drink and eat, which is followed by regurgitation of ingesta with saliva through the nose. The trachea and lungs should be examined for evidence of aspiration.

The esophagus can also be examined radiographically and ultrasonographically. The normal equine esophagus may not be detectable on radiographs or may just contain thin longitudinal streaks of air. The presence of large volumes of intraesophageal air indicates dysfunction of the rostral esophageal valve. Choke may be detected by the presence of feed (homogeneous, granular appearance radiologically), which is most obvious if the obstruction is in the cervical esophagus. The additional use of a contrast medium such as barium is also of value in assessing

- esophageal patency
- shape, and
- motility

with certain esophageal disorders, but should not be used per os in suspected cases of esophageal choke to avoid aspiration.

Endoscopic examination of the esophagus is done by advancing a long (approximately 2 m) endoscope into the caudal nasopharynx and then directing it dorsal to the larynx and advancing it slowly until it touches the nasopharyngeal mucosa, using the procedure described below.

1. The endoscope is passed in the same way as a nasogastric tube. It should be pressed gently against the nasopharyngeal wall until the horse swallows it into the esophagus.
2. It should then be slowly advanced down the esophagus, holding both vertical and horizontal controls relatively fixed, to prevent the endoscope tip from becoming stuck in the mucosa and doubling back on itself, which can seriously damage both the esophagus and the instrument.
3. By insufflating with air, the esophagus can be examined during descent of the endoscope, but it is easier to examine the esophageal mucosa during endoscope withdrawal, as it collapses closed over the tip of the instrument.

Esophageal obstructions such as choke, strictures, dilatations, mucosal erythema, ulceration, and rupture can be detected endoscopically.

## Nasogastric intubation and siphonage, and examination of the stomach

The technique of gastric decompression is partly therapeutic but the results of attempts to release fluid or

---

### Clinical Pointer

The nasogastric tube is used primarily as a diagnostic tool in esophageal choke in the horse which usually develops choke from particulate objects.

Attempts to dislodge particulate obstructions by pressure from a nasogastric tube may result in a fatal esophageal rupture.

---

gas from the stomach are also diagnostically useful. Gastric distension is a highly distressing feature of some colic cases and the mere pain relief of gastric decompression facilitates the clinical examination. The retrieval of significant volumes (2 liters or more) of sequestrated gastric fluid is also a highly specific indicator of intestinal obstruction, especially of the small intestine, and a reasonably specific indicator that surgical intervention may be necessary.

## Technique

The largest-diameter tube possible for the patient should be chosen (16–20 mm outside diameter for adult horses). A transparent tube is preferable so that the liquid being refluxed within the lumen can be seen. Gastric contents are particulate and the bore of the tubing needs to be as wide as possible to prevent blockage. Some clinicians prefer the distal end of the tube to have additional side holes. Plastic tubing stiffens in cold temperatures, so it is best to optimize malleability by immersing it in hot water immediately prior to use. The application of lubricating gel to the first few inches of the tube wall eases its passage. A minimum of three people are usually required, one to handle the horse, one to pass the tube and one to operate the pumping system. Restraint of the patient depends on the individual circumstances. A confident handler using a bridle is usually sufficient. Nose twitches or even sedation may be required but tend to suppress the swallow reflex, thereby increasing the difficulty of intubation. Before the procedure begins the tube should be marked at the approximate insertion lengths expected to encounter first the larynx and then the cardia of the stomach.

The position from which to perform intubation is a matter of personal preference. One method is to stand to one side (usually the left) of the horse's head facing in the same direction. The hand nearest to the horse is passed beneath its jaw and wraps around the right side of the face, so that backward restraint can be applied over the bridge of the nose; this tends to flex the horse's head, which is the optimal position for the tube to enter the esophagus. The tube should be directed into the ventral meatus and advanced slowly and smoothly into the pharynx. If resistance is encountered the ethmoturbinates may have been impacted and the tube should be withdrawn a little then readvanced. The presence of the tube in the nasopharynx will commonly stimulate the swallowing reflex. This should be anticipated, so that a gentle thrust of the tube can be synchronized with it. If unsuccessful initially, the tube is withdrawn slightly and the process repeated. Sometimes it can take several minutes to accomplish

this part of the intubation, and care is needed not to allow frustration to lead to increasing force being applied while maneuvering the tube, which would predispose to trauma. Clearly it is vital to distinguish between esophageal and tracheal intubation and there are a number of factors to consider in this regard, most of which depend on the differences in mechanical properties between the cartilaginous rigidity of the trachea and the muscular elasticity of the esophagus.

1. The implosion of the esophageal wall around the tube end offers a resistance to its onward movement that is not evident when the trachea is entered.
2. Blowing and sucking through the tube will be easy when the tube is in the trachea, but not when it is in the esophagus. This is less true when the tube has reached the stomach, as the movement of gastric gases can mimic the air flow of breathing. The acidic aroma of stomach contents is usually reliably distinctive.
3. As the tube passes down the cervical esophagus a ripple in the region of the left side of the trachea can be detected by sight and touch as the esophageal wall distends. This does not occur if the trachea has been entered.
4. Blowing sharply and briefly through the tube immediately after it has passed the level of the larynx results in a bubble of air distending the esophagus, seen just to the left of the trachea if the tube is in the esophagus.

In general the cough reflex indicates tracheal intubation, although some horses cough simply because of the pharyngeal stimulation. In some horses, particularly those with gastric distension, considerable resistance will be met at the cardia. This can be overcome either by

- gentle pressure
- blowing through the tube
- instilling a small volume of water to stimulate relaxation, or
- instilling 25–30 ml of local analgesic solution.

On entering the stomach there is usually an emission of pungent gases. If there is gaseous gastric distension

---

### Clinical Pointer

The most sensitive part of nasogastric intubation is the passage of the tube through the nostril and into the nasal cavity. This should be completed as quickly as possible, avoiding finger contact with the skin or mucosa.

this emission will be prolonged. If no gas flows it may be necessary to blow down the tube to clear its distal end of any blockage and wait for a possible reflux of gas. In cases of extreme gastric distension with fluid, spontaneous efflux might occur. Such a finding tends to suggest that the site of intestinal obstruction is relatively craniad. Abnormalities inducing intestinal ileus, such as grass sickness or duodenitis/proximal jejunitis, would be included in this category. More frequently it is necessary to create a siphon in order to obtain stomach contents by reflux. This is done by infusing a controlled volume of water (1–2 liters) by dose syringe or pump and then disconnecting the tube while the end of it is held below the level of the patient's stomach. If the nozzle of the tube is within a fluid pocket in the stomach a siphon will be created and flow will continue while the nozzle remains immersed. Periodically the flow may be temporarily obstructed by particles clogging the tube end, or by the stomach wall being sucked into it. On these occasions short, outward jerking movements of the tube can establish or resume flow. It is useful to collect the fluid obtained so that, after subtracting the volume of water infused, the retrieved sequestrated fluid can be measured. This entire procedure must be repeated several times to ensure that all possible material is removed from the stomach. In spite of this the stomach can be impacted with a large volume of ingesta with little or no liquid reflux being obtained.

Finding that the stomach contains excessive secretions is both specific and sensitive in predicting that a small intestinal obstruction exists. This in turn increases the probability that surgical intervention will be necessary, although not inevitable. Neurogenic obstructions that occur with grass sickness, secondary to prolonged mural stretching or as a sequel to inflammatory conditions, might also result in gastric distension. In addition, it is not necessarily true that stomach distension is synonymous with primary small intestinal obstruction. Protracted cecal or colonic obstructions may eventually lead to reduced ileocecal outflow and certain non-strangulating (particularly right dorsal) colonic displacements will passively obstruct the small intestine, resulting in reflux.

## CLINICAL PATHOLOGY

The extent to which laboratory data are used in the examination and diagnosis of equine abdominal disease will vary according to the nature of the abnormality under investigation. There is a temptation to gather laboratory test results indiscriminately, carrying the danger of placing inappropriate emphasis on a laboratory 'screen', which should always be subordinate to the findings of the physical examination. It follows that those cases most likely to have markedly abnormal hematological or biochemical values are also those in which the tests may be diagnostically superfluous, as the abnormalities could have been reliably predicted from the clinical picture anyway. Before embarking upon a given test it is prudent to first consider its cost–benefit analysis in the context of the individual case. None the less, there remain occasions when laboratory data are valuable in the diagnosis of abdominal disorders, and perhaps even more so in guiding therapy, developing a prognosis, and in monitoring progress.

### Peritoneal fluid collection and analysis

Abdominal paracentesis is the technique used to collect a sample of fluid from the peritoneal cavity for laboratory evaluation. This can be a valuable diagnostic aid in the clinical examination of the horse with a suspected abdominal disorder, as the changes that occur in the peritoneal fluid reflect abnormalities of the visceral or parietal peritoneum, or both. However a number of caveats should be considered before the test is performed and the results interpreted. Normal peritoneal fluid is not synonymous with a normal abdomen. Lesions that do not affect mesothelial surfaces do not cause changes in the peritoneal fluid.

---

**Peritoneal fluid analysis**

- in principle, acute or chronic diseases of any body system in which the peritoneum is affected have the potential to cause changes in the peritoneal fluid
- in practice the diagnosis and monitoring of septic peritonitis and the investigation of gastrointestinal tract diseases are the most common indications for collecting and analyzing peritoneal fluid.

---

These are exemplified by impaction of the large colon and other types of simple intestinal obstruction, although in more advanced cases serosal damage may occur secondary to protracted stretching of the intestinal wall. Further, there are certain instances when strangulated intestine can exist with its surfaces effectively sealed from the peritoneal cavity, thus preventing the cellular changes in the peritoneal fluid compartment that might otherwise be expected. Intussusceptions, scrotal herniae, and some cases of herniation through the epiploic foramen are the most common examples. Historically, sanguinous peritoneal fluid was considered to be the most important criterion in deciding whether or not to opt for exploratory laparotomy and abdominal paracentesis became a routine procedure in the clinical examination of horses with acute abdominal pain. However, this clinical reasoning requires reappraisal. There is inevitably a lag phase between the onset of tissue damage and the appearance in the peritoneal fluid of the products of that damage. In cases of strangulating intestinal obstruction it may take several hours before diagnostic changes are detectable. It is also possible to aspirate from pockets of normal fluid before pathological changes have become homogeneous within the full peritoneal compartment. Thus, waiting for erythrocytes to appear in the peritoneal fluid as the marker that surgery is indicated is a highly insensitive test which imparts a potentially fatal delay into the decision-making process.

Where doubt remains about a diagnosis or an appropriate course of treatment, or where it would be useful to record cell counts (e.g. for serial monitoring of a case) the benefits of abdominal paracentesis outweigh the disadvantages and the test is justified. Conversely, if the clinical signs are decisive regardless of the findings of peritoneal fluid analysis, then the test is not indicated.

## Complications of abdominal paracentesis

Complications, rare in practice, include

- iatrogenic puncture of the intestine – if it involves a normal loop of intestine there are generally no major clinical consequences
- puncture of distended, atonic intestine situated against the ventral abdominal wall – this can cause leakage of intestinal contents and hence peritonitis, or possibly cellulitis of the abdominal wall caused by contamination during withdrawal of the needle
- puncture of the spleen or a mesenteric vessel – this occurs fairly easily and the consequent hemorrhage then obscures the true cytological picture of the fluid.

### Technique

The purpose of the procedure is to penetrate the parietal peritoneum with a cannulated instrument to establish a spontaneous, gravitational fluid flow (Fig. 17.32). Slight variations in technique include the use of a blunt bovine teat infusion cannula placed through a stab incision into (not through) the linea alba in

order to minimize the risks of intestine penetration; the use of a bitch urinary catheter to penetrate deep retroperitoneal fat; and the use of paramedian puncture sites. The following protocol is safe, uncomplicated and reliable

1. Adequate restraint is essential; stocks are ideal.
2. A 10 cm band of skin of the midline ventral abdomen is close-clipped from the sternum to the umbilicus.
3. The skin and the operator are prepared for an aseptic procedure.
4. An 18-gauge x 1.5″ needle (or 18-g x 2″ for fat animals) is used.
5. A site is identified on the midline a few centimeters cranial to the umbilicus on the caudodorsally inclined contour of the belly, some way caudal to the most dependent point (Fig. 17.32).
6. The needle is advanced in one confident movement, penetrating the skin only (this may cause a reaction from the animal).
7. The needle is advanced through the insensitive linea alba slowly, pausing at intervals to see whether fluid flows.
8. If the hub of the needle begins to move when left unheld, this suggests that it is against intestine. If no fluid flows the needle is rotated to redirect the bevel away from the intestinal wall. If this is unsuccessful the lower flanks are ballotted to try to shift fluid pockets toward the needle.
9. If still no fluid flows a second needle is inserted, usually closer to the xiphisternum, leaving the first in place. The second needle may release the subatmospheric pressure and allow a free flow of fluid. Three or four different puncture sites can be tried, but it is necessary to accept that on occasions it will prove impossible to obtain fluid, even in normal horses.

Fluid should be collected into a sterile tube with anticoagulant added. It is worth watching the fluid as it flows. Blood contamination might occur through puncture of vessels in the skin, the abdominal wall, the intestinal mesentery or the spleen.

### Analysis of peritoneal fluid

#### Volume and rate of flow

Assessment of the volume of fluid collected is purely subjective, based on the assumption that the easier it is to obtain a sample and the faster the fluid flows then the more fluid there is likely to be present in the abdomen or the greater the pressure it is under. Usually fluid will tend to flow in spurts of a few milliliters, stimulated by subtle changes in needle depth or

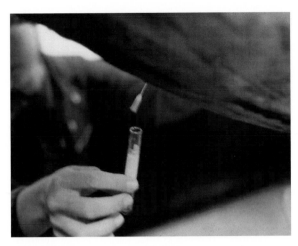

**Fig. 17.32** Collection of peritoneal fluid. The needle is placed aseptically through the linea alba, starting at a site between the most dependent point of the ventral body wall and the umbilicus.

rotation. Both intra- and extra-abdominal abnormalities can lead to an increased net production of fluid. Peritoneal effusions may reflect systemic hemodynamic disorders arising from increased capillary hydrostatic pressure or hypoalbuminemia. Thus, primary disease might originate in the heart, liver, kidney, or gut. Intra-abdominal lesions usually cause discolored effusions, depending on whether hemorrhagic or exudative conditions are present. However, space-occupying intestinal distensions will increase the fluid pressure; large colon impactions or non-strangulating displacements characteristically yield high volumes of fluid which appears grossly normal. Retroperitoneal fat may

### Blood contamination in peritoneal fluid

- transient streaks of blood in the fluid indicate puncture of blood vessels
- a serosanguinous sample indicates an intra-abdominal lesion
- the appearance of dark, tarry blood suggests splenic puncture, this can be confirmed by recording a packed cell volume (PCV) higher than that of peripheral blood
- fluid resembling whole blood may be caused by puncture of a mesenteric vessel or by intra-abdominal hemorrhage
- the loss of erythrocytes from strangulated intestine can be so great as to cause fluid resembling whole blood also.

prevent access to the fluid, and in severe dehydration, as in grass sickness, there may be insufficient fluid present. It is also possible that ventral colonic distension may be severe enough to exclude fluid pockets from the ventral abdomen.

**Gross appearance**

The appearance of peritoneal fluid is highly indicative of certain conditions.

- Normal peritoneal fluid is virtually translucent, ranging from almost clear to straw colored.
- Opacity develops with increasing cellularity or rising protein content (usually the two go together).
- Erythrocytes give a red tint to the fluid and a reddish discoloration of the sediment. Both become more intense the greater the number of cells, through to overt red discoloration.
- An amber to orange tint to the supernatant fluid suggests that erythrocytes have hemolysed.
- A sanguinous aspirate can arise following bleeding from a previous tap or from peritoneal inflammation. However, the usual source is diapedesis of erythrocytes from an ischemic intestinal wall.
- Leukocytes indicate an inflammatory response and result in a milky to gray opaque change to the fluid and sediment.
- Fluid with a dirty brown or greenish hue suggests that intestinal contents have been aspirated, and the presence of particulate plant debris confirms this. It may also be possible to detect the acidic odor of gut contents. Two possibilities have then to be considered: either the sample was obtained by inadvertent enterocentesis, or there has been a rupture of the gastric or intestinal wall. When intestinal contents are encountered the needle should be rapidly withdrawn and discarded. Intestinal punctures generally seal spontaneously without adverse consequences, although fatal lacerations of the intestinal wall and cellulitic reactions do rarely occur. If the same result is obtained with the next sample the index of suspicion for intestinal rupture rises. However, it is relatively easy to repeatedly puncture a distended viscus and it can be surprisingly difficult to decide between the two possibilities in some cases. Reference to other signs is important. It is worth noting that small intestinal contents can appear misleadingly clear, and may be recognized only microscopically by a complete lack of cells.

**Protein content**

This can readily be estimated by refractometry, which provides adequate accuracy for clinical purposes. The protein concentration in peritoneal fluid is a function of the endothelial permeability at the interface between the peritoneal surface and the subperitoneal vasculature. Increased permeability leads to increased protein concentrations and is the result of inflammatory processes, although neoplasia and liver disease have also been associated with elevated levels. There are small variations between quoted normal range values, but in general up to 15 g/l is considered normal and anything above 25 g/l abnormal. An increased protein content tends not to occur in the absence of other changes – notably a raised leukocyte count – and it is therefore a rather non-specific marker of intra-abdominal pathology.

## Clinical Pointer

Ideally perform cytological and biochemical analyses on peritoneal fluid and peripheral blood and serum concurrently. A comparison of the two can differentiate between

- changes that originate within the peritoneum or its related organs
- changes that are secondary to systemic disease.

### Cytology

A full cytological analysis includes total erythrocyte and leukocyte counts, a differential leukoctye count and a morphological examination. It is worth noting that cell counting machines do not give very accurate results for samples of low cellularity, such as normal peritoneal fluid. Thus, despite the ease and speed of automation, hand counting using a hemocytometer slide is in many instances more appropriate. Differential cell counts and cell morphology are best assessed from a stained, direct smear of the collected fluid. If cell density is low then the fluid can first be spun in a centrifuge to condense the cells into a sediment.

Erythrocytes are not present in normal peritoneal fluid. However, it is almost inevitable that some contamination will occur during sampling, and even fluid that appears grossly normal usually has low erythrocyte counts – up to $0.005 \times 10^{12}$/liter. Significant blood contamination can obscure the cytological evaluation, although Malark et al (1992) suggested that up to 17% v/v blood contamination does not affect clinical interpretation in normal horses. As an approximation, $1 \times 10^{12}$/liter contaminating erythrocytes will falsely raise a sample's leukocyte count by $1 \times 10^9$/liter and the protein content by 10 g/l. Erythrocytes will appear in the peritoneal fluid under various pathological circum-

stances. True hemoperitoneum is uncommon but may arise following

- trauma
- spontaneous rupture of a major vessel, or
- in certain cases of neoplasia, such as gastric carcinoma.

It may be possible to distinguish hemorrhage which occurred prior to the paracentesis procedure if there is evidence of erythrophagocytosis on a stained smear. Also, true hemorrhage of any source will result in platelets being present in the peritoneal fluid. More commonly in inflammatory and ischemic states erythrocytes appear by diapedesis. Advanced intestinal strangulation or fulminating peritonitis may be associated with erythrocyte counts of up to $1 \times 10^{12}$/liter.

Nucleated leukocytes are a normal constituent of peritoneal fluid but there is variation in reported normal values, particularly for the differential counts. Most sources cite $0.5 \times 10^9$/liter as the upper limit for a total leukocyte count (McGrath 1976, Wendell Nelson 1979). Between 50% and 70% of the leukocytes in normal peritoneal fluid are neutrophils, the remainder comprising mostly macrophages and mesothelial cells, a few lymphocytes and the occasional eosinophil, basophil or mast cell. Neutrophils in peritoneal fluid do not return to the bloodstream and therefore degenerative changes such as apoptotic and toxic neutrophils are a common finding. Macrophagocytosis of neutrophils may also be observed.

## Clinical Pointer

In most cases, changes in the leukocyte profile of peritoneal fluid provide non-specific evidence of intra-abdominal lesions, rather than pointing to specific disease entities

- inflammatory processes, ischemic or infectious in nature, lead to an influx of neutrophils
- with increasing chronicity of an inflammatory process the proportion of large mononuclear cells rises, particularly those engaged in phagocytosis.

### Other features of the stained smear

During the examination of a stained smear bacteria may be encountered. Given adequate aseptic technique there should be negligible or no contamination of samples, but occasional clusters of cocci will occur iatrogenically. Primary septic peritonitis is likely to lead to a high bacterial density, with a marked toxic peritoneal neutrophilia. Organic plant fibers and/or ciliated protozoa suggest enterocentesis or intestinal rupture. In the former there will be a lack of cells and in the latter an abundance, unless contamination has occurred only very recently.

## Hematology

Changes in the circulating blood cell profile can only give indirect information regarding pathological processes originating within the abdomen. Essentially the relevant tests are those to measure red cell and leukocyte responses.

### Packed cell volume

The relative volume occupied within a blood sample by the erythrocytes is quantified as the packed cell volume (PCV %) or hematocrit (in liters/liter). In the horse the contribution of the intestinal tract to the body's fluid balance is profound. The large intestine must recover each day a volume of water equivalent to the total extra-cellular volume. Thus most types of intestinal obstruction tend to result in hypovolemia and hemo-concentration. The added propensity for the development of endotoxic shock means that assessment of hemoconcentration is a mandatory part of the investigation of horses with suspected intestinal problems.

The PCV of a horse may rise by approximately 50% above normal values quoted (28%–42%) because of sympathetic stimulation of the highly contractile spleen. Further, PCV values are variable with

- breed (higher in Thoroughbred types)
- age (higher in individuals up to 2 years old), and
- state of training (higher in fit horses).

Thus a value of 38% might represent significant dehydration in an unexcited Shire horse yet be normal in a racehorse. Some sort of validation can be afforded by the concurrent analysis of total serum protein, which have less physiological variability.

### Total serum protein concentration

Plasma or serum protein concentrations offer the most readily available alternatives and can easily be estimated by measuring total solids by refractometry. Normal values range from 58 to 64 g/l, but dehydration may cause this figure to approach 80 g/l. It should be noted that where *plasma* levels have been measured the antico-agulant in the sample tube maintains fibrinogen and other coagulable proteins in solution, and thus hyperfib-rinogenemia resulting from any extreme inflammatory processes could account for up to 10 g/l protein in the sample, irrespective of dehydration. Hypoproteinemia

and hypoalbuminemia tend not to occur with liver disease in horses, compared to other species.

### Leukocyte count

Leukocyte evaluations can aid in the detection and monitoring of inflammatory processes. A full assessment requires total and differential counts as well as cell morphological examination. It is popular to express differential cell fractions as percentages, but this results in misinterpretation and is emphatically discouraged in equine medicine. For instance, 90% neutrophils in a total count of $5 \times 10^9$/l is reflective of primary lymphopenia rather than neutrophilia. A single circulating leukocyte profile is necessarily a static representation of the highly dynamic processes involved in leukocyte kinetics.

> ### Clinical Pointer
>
> Although sequential leukocyte counts offer more diagnostic help, the nature of the condition may demand action on the basis of the first clinical tests. It is therefore essential to interpret results in the context of other clinical parameters.

Sequestration of neutrophils at sites such as the peritoneal cavity might account for circulating leukopenia, particularly if endotoxemia (which causes margination of neutrophils in small vessels) is also present. Persistent neutropenia (beyond 3 days) has been associated with a poor prognosis, particularly in foals.

### Serum biochemistry

The use of assays of various serum (or plasma) biochemical constituents is routine, for both diagnosis and monitoring of abdominal disease processes. There is a danger of misinterpretation by oversimplification, and the profile of tests chosen should be driven by the preceding clinical evaluations rather than vice versa.

### Fecal examination

The clinical findings that indicate the need for a fecal examination are diarrhea, weight loss, or chronic or recurrent colic. Fecal examination might be used to detect direct evidence of

- infectious agents (metazoa, bacteria, viruses, and protozoa)

- indirect evidence of enteric infection (e.g. leukocytes)
- dental disease (long fiber length)
- sand impaction, and
- occult blood as evidence of gastrointestinal tract hemorrhage.

Immunological techniques exist for detecting certain viral and protozoal pathogens (e.g. rotavirus and *Giardia* sp.), and similar applications plus DNA diagnostic testing are likely to become available for the more common enteric disease-producing agents.

Modern anthelmintics appear to have been associated with a decrease in the prevalence of the *large* strongyle species in the equine population.

---

### Clinical Pointer

- a negative fecal worm egg count does not rule out prepatent parasitic disease as many of the pathogenic effects of large strongyle and cyathostome (small strongyle) infestations are mediated by the early larval stages which do not produce eggs
- a positive worm egg count is not necessarily indicative of clinically significant adult worm burdens.

---

As a generalization, individuals with a count of 1000 or more eggs per gram (epg) of feces can reasonably be expected to be adversely affected by adult strongyles, and a herd mean of at least 400 epg can be taken as supportive evidence that strongylosis could be involved in any individual showing clinical signs consistent with such a diagnosis.

Bacteriological examination of equine feces is inevitably clouded by the huge number of organisms that normally populate the large intestine. In addition, primary bacterial enteritis is rare in adult horses, *Salmonella* and *Clostridia* spp. being the only organisms generally associated with recognized clinical syndromes. To some extent the isolation of causative bacteria in enteritis is immaterial and the treatment of such cases rests more on supportive therapy than on specific antibacterial medication.

## Biopsies

For acute diseases the inevitable time requirements often preclude the use of biopsy techniques. One exception to this is grass sickness which can cause signs of an acute small intestinal obstruction or, in its subacute form, signs that clinically resemble protracted impaction colic. In these situations examination of frozen or formalin-fixed ileal biopsy tissue sections for characteristic histological changes can provide a rapid diagnosis of grass sickness to be made during, or soon after, surgery. Such samples may be obtained by routine exploratory laparotomy or by minimally invasive, standing, flank laparotomy.

For the investigation of more chronic abnormalities, biopsy might be the definitive diagnostic test once other procedures have indicated the organ of interest, such as the small bowel.

The liver is the organ most commonly subjected to percutaneous biopsy. Renal biopsy is regarded to be less safe and the potential for obtaining specific diagnostic information more limited. The use of ultrasound imaging increases confidence with regard to the position of organs, and will occasionally provide guidance to specific lesions within organs. The use of laparoscopy and exploratory laparotomy enables greater accuracy of biopsy sampling for tissues that are visible by this technique, such as the

- liver
- spleen
- accessible mesothelial surfaces, and
- extramural intestinal lesions

but full-thickness biopsy of the bowel wall still requires a laparotomy.

### Liver biopsy

The approach is made through the right 13th or 14th intercostal space on an imaginary line drawn from the point of the shoulder to the tuber coxa using the following procedure.

1. The presence and location of hepatic tissue is defined ultrasonographically.
2. An area of skin around this point is aseptically prepared and local analgesic solution infiltrated into the subcutis and intercostal muscles.
3. A stab incision is made through the skin with a small scalpel blade. If excessive and continuous bleeding is seen the procedure is terminated because of the risk of uncontrollable bleeding.
4. A biopsy instrument at least 15 cm long is then advanced slowly in a slightly cranial and ventral direction through lung tissue until the diaphragm is engaged, as evidenced by movements of the needle synchronous with breathing when the instrument is left free.

5. Advancing deeper than this should cause the instrument to enter hepatic tissue, and the intention should be to embed the full depth of the cutting blade of the needle within the liver.
6. Close inspection of the tissue withdrawn will usually confirm whether liver, lung, diaphragm, or other tissue has been obtained.
7. Samples should be preserved in 10% formalin.

Ultrasound planning and/or guidance for this procedure is paramount.

# IMAGING TECHNIQUES

## Radiography

Younger horses commonly develop infections of the apices of the long reserve crowns of their cheek teeth that also cause infection and swelling of the supporting (maxillary and mandibular) bones. Radiography is the ancillary technique of choice to investigate such cases and, for example, to differentiate such infections from the traumatic fractures of these bones that are also common in this age group. Radiography of such maxillary cheek teeth suspected to be associated with secondary dental sinusitis is also essential and is discussed in Chapter 16.

---

### Computed tomography (CT)

CT gives very good imaging of the cheek teeth, jaws, and soft tissues without the superimposition of the many other head structures, including the opposite teeth, that often makes radiographic interpretation difficult. Consequently, much additional information can be obtained using CT.

---

Following barium swallow or feeding barium mixed with food, radiography of the pharynx and esophagus can be of value in cases with dysphagia. In addition to obtaining still (plain) radiographs, the use of an image intensifier allows dynamic radiographs of these areas to be evaluated and consequently allows functional problems such as megaesophagus to be detected. However, endoscopy is a simpler technique that is often equally as effective in arriving at a diagnosis.

Although it is practical and effective to incorporate radiography into the investigation of foals with colic (Fig.17.33), for adult horses the technique is at best crude and often futile. The hazards of scattered radiation should be considered at all times. If diaphragmatic herniation is suspected then a lateral standing caudal thoracic radiograph may provide diagnostic information. Radio-opaque enteroliths can sometimes be detected, as can sand accumulations in ventral colonic segments.

## Ultrasonography

Most soft tissue lesions of the oral cavity and oropharynx of adult horses can be detected by clinical examination. Likewise, most such lesions of the nasopharynx and esophagus can be evaluated well endoscopically. However, soft tissue lesions such as abscesses and tumors lying deep between the mandibular bones or on the lateral aspect of the pharynx (in the region of the parotid gland) are best be evaluated by ultrasonography, or CT/MRI if available.

Ultrasonography has become a valuable diagnostic aid in the clinical examination of abdominal diseases. All organs that lie adjacent to the abdominal wall are accessible to transcutaneous ultrasound and the use of rectal probes allows imaging of parts of the deep caudal abdominal viscera. The great depth of penetration required through an adult horse's abdominal wall dictates that low-frequency (3.0 or 2.5 MHz) transducers be used. For foals or for transrectal imaging 5.0 MHz is probably adequate. Sector scanners are preferable to linear array scanners because of the extra ease of contact between the scanner head and the skin and of imaging between the ribs.

Parenchymal organs that can reliably be examined ultrasonographically include the liver, kidneys, and spleen. In addition, the walls of the stomach and various parts of the intestinal tract, the bladder, uterus, and ovaries can also be imaged. Pockets of peritoneal fluid can also be seen, sometimes aiding sample collection. Peritoneal effusions are usually of low echogenicity. Echogenic particles visible within fluid suggest fibrinous peritonitis or the presence of extraluminal particles of gut contents.

In the right cranial abdomen the liver is scanned ventral to the right lung lobe. Deep to the liver at this site it is possible to image the wall of the right dorsal colon and the duodenum. Further caudally on the right the right kidney is detectable dorsally, the remainder of the surface area being occupied by the cecum (with the duodenum dorsomedial to it, just ventral to the kidney) and large colon. On the left side the liver shadow is less extensive and the spleen and left kidney can be scanned. The spleen has fewer vascular channels than the liver and is more echogenic. Sometimes the left kidney is obscured by the dorsal pole of the spleen, which lies lateral to it. Deep to these structures there are normally intestinal loops in which peristaltic movements can be seen. Ventrally the large

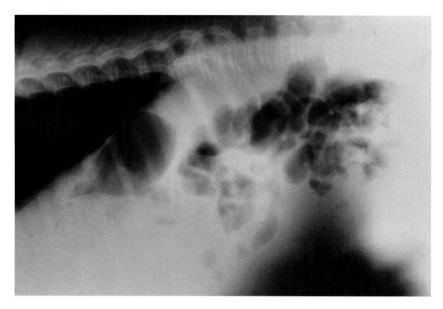

**Fig. 17.33** A standing lateral abdominal radiograph of a foal with colic. Dorsal gas accumulations are visible in the stomach, small intestine and large intestine. However, none of these structures appears to be extremely enlarged and the radiography was helpful in deciding to persist with conservative treatment.

colon sits close against the abdominal wall, although caudally the bladder may be within view. In foals (see page 411) the umbilical remnants are identifiable.

### Clinical Pointer

As the ultrasonographic examination is made in real-time dynamic functions such as gut peristalsis can also be evaluated.

Identification of changes in parenchymal architecture, such as

- focal or diffuse cellular infiltrates
- fibrosis, and
- cystic conditions (e.g. hydronephrosis or hepatic hydatidosis)

can be a useful adjunct in the investigation of liver, kidney, and splenic disease. Renal calculi or cholelithiasis may also be detected by the presence of high-amplitude echoes in the respective organs. Normal peritoneal fluid appears as areas of hypoechogenicity between the shadows of other structures. Acoustic interfaces within them suggest particulate deposits such as fibrin. Small intestinal distension can be detected by the presence of multiple, usually hypomotile, loops in cross-section or longitudinal section, with relatively hypoechoic centers.

Santschi and colleagues (1991) reported the use of transcutaneous ultrasonography to accurately diagnose the presence of left dorsal displacement of the colon by the presence of gas-filled intestinal segments between the dorsal spleen and the left kidney. In practice this can be difficult owing to the presence of bowel lateral to the kidney in some normal horses. Neoplastic conditions of the gastrointestinal tract can sometimes be detected by ultrasound. In fact, it is one of the more definitive means of identifying gastric tumors (squamous cell carcinomas), many of which can be detected from the left body wall as an interposition of low-echogenic tissue between the spleen and stomach wall–gas interface.

### Clinical Pointer

The 'bull's-eye target' appearance of a double-ringed loop in cross-section is classically diagnostic of an intussusception (Fig. 17.34), this is relatively common in foals.

The use of a transducer rectally allows imaging of the left kidney, bladder, uterus, and ovaries, and of intestinal structures that are within reach of a rectal examination. Directing the probe dorsally enables the walls of and blood flow within the caudal aorta and origins of the iliac arteries to be assessed. Thrombotic occlusion at this site, apparent as echogenic shadows impinging into the vascular lumen, is an unusual cause of low-grade abdominal discomfort.

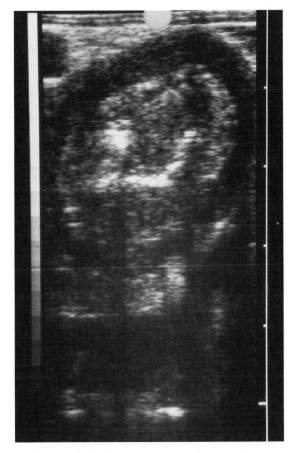

**Fig. 17.34** A sonogram, obtained in this case per rectum, of a part of the gastrointestinal tract. The typical 'target' lesion is shown with a central core of echodense material surrounded by a halo of relatively hypoechoic tissue (gut lumen) and further echodense tissue outside. This appearance of 'gut within gut' is usually created by an intussusception, but in this case was due to a swollen ileocecal valve protruding into the lumen of the distal ileum. The ultimate diagnosis was eosinophilic enteritis. (Courtesy of RS Pirie, Royal (Dick) School of Veterinary Studies, Edinburgh.)

## Diagnostic endoscopy

Endoscopy of the caudal oral cavity should only be performed in sedated horses that have a full mouth speculum in place. Endoscopic evaluation of the nasopharynx is readily performed per nasum in the unsedated horse and the presence of food in this area is a most sensitive indication of dysphagia. Less severe cases of dysphagia without foodstained nasal discharge will often have such endoscopic abnormalities. Lesions such as cleft palate or cricopharyngeal–laryngeal dysplasia also should be obvious on endoscopic examination.

The presence of esophageal obstruction (choke) can be confirmed endoscopically, usually without sedation, and this technique will also allow the detection of other esophageal abnormalities, such as ulceration, stricture, and dilatation.

Flexible fiberoptic endoscopes or, preferably, videoendoscopes can be used to inspect

- the lumen of the esophagus
- the stomach, and
- the most oral part of the duodenum.

The length of endoscope required for gastroscopy means that custom-built instruments are necessary in most cases. Although the stomachs of small foals may be little over 1 m from the nostrils, that of a larger adult horse might approach 2.5 m. Generally the procedure is best carried out under standing sedation. Some foals need to be examined in recumbency. A minimum of three people are required for adult horses and four for foals, which usually require greater manual restraint. Except for suckling foals, patients should be starved for 12–24 hours prior to gastroscopy. The lubricated end of the endoscope is

- passed routinely along the ventral meatus of one of the nasal chambers
- directed dorsal to the larynx to elicit a swallow reflex, and thence
- passed into the esophagus and on to the stomach.

Insufflation with air aids this passage. The esophageal side of the cardiac sphincter is recognizable as an oblique cleft, which should normally be closed, effectively sealing the esophagus from gastric fluid, and therefore it is normally free of mucosal inflammation. Some knowledge of the orientation of the internal features of the stomach wall is vital if perspective is to be maintained.

The endoscopic anatomy of the equine stomach has been well illustrated and described by Adamson and Murray (1990). With experience it is possible to consistently locate the saccus cecus and non-glandular squamous fundus, the margo plicatus and glandular fundus, the lesser curvature and the pyloric antrum. The visibility of the latter landmarks depends on the volume of gastric fluid present. Squamous mucosal surfaces normally appear with a pale, furry film

**Clinical Pointer**

Air insufflation to distend the stomach helps to obtain a panoramic view.

covering them. Glandular mucosal surfaces are deep pink in color and smooth in texture. The margo plicatus appears as an obvious sharp demarcation between the two. By a combination of bending the tip of the endoscope to the horse's left and deflecting it off the greater curvature it is sometimes possible to inspect the duodenal ampulla and pyloric sphincter.

Most young foals undergo desquamation of the non-glandular fundus. Lesions of the glandular portions are more subtle but more significant. These appear as roughening, reddening, and ulceration of the mucosal surface. In older foals and adults lesions of the squamous epithelium might be of greater significance, although interpretation is somewhat empirical. Generally, the deeper, the more extensive and the more hemorrhagic the lesions, the greater the likelihood of their being related to clinical disease syndromes. *Gasterophilus* larvae attached to the stomach wall and papular lesions attributed to *Habronema* and *Draschia* spp. are relatively common findings. Squamous cell carcinoma causes a marked distortion of the nature of the mucosal surface, and lesions often start close to the margo plicatus. Such lesions are relatively easy to biopsy using instruments designed to pass down the biopsy channel of the endoscope.

Lesions within the rectal or small colon lumina are relatively uncommon but on occasions it is useful to inspect these regions endoscopically. In particular, the site, extent, and progress of rectal tears can be assessed. The view is enhanced by air insufflation and care should be exercised in advancing the endoscope for fear of converting partial-thickness defects into full peritoneal penetrations.

---

### Endoscopy of the duodenum

Once the pylorus is in view, in some animals it is possible to advance the endoscope into the duodenum

- 5–6 cm beyond the pylorus the hepatic and pancreatic duct openings can be seen
- duodenal ulceration may be detected in foals
- *Gasterophilus* spp. may be seen attached to the mucosal surface of the duodenum.

---

### Laparoscopy

In recent years laparoscopy has successfully been applied to the horse and has provided another dimension in diagnostic procedures for investigating abnormalities within the abdomen. The procedure is well tolerated by standing, sedated animals. The instrumentation required is basically that available for human surgery, although there may be some advantage in acquiring specially made laparoscopes with extra length or different viewing angles.

Laparoscopy enables the direct visualization of intra-abdominal regions that are out of sight at laparotomy. It is a valuable diagnostic aid when clinical examinations have indicated the existence of an abdominal abnormality without precision as to its cause. The diagnostic potential is further enhanced by the ability to take biopsies of grossly abnormal tissues, although for intestinal samples there is too great a risk of contamination. Laparoscopy has so far been reported to yield diagnoses in the following conditions:

- abdominal cryporchidism
- ovarian tumors
- extraluminal lymphosarcoma and other neoplasms
- adhesions
- fibrinous peritonitis
- abdominal abscessation
- diaphragmatic hernia
- colonic displacement.

### Exploratory laparotomy

An exploratory laparotomy is the most invasive diagnostic procedure available for the evaluation of intra-abdominal abnormalities. Sometimes it is indicated as an emergency procedure in order to detect a life-threatening condition (usually an intestinal crisis) with a view to its immediate surgical correction. On other occasions the procedure might be elective, for the purpose of obtaining intestinal biopsies or for the investigation of the cause of chronic or recurrent colic. In the latter instance consideration should be given to the respective advantages and disadvantages of laparoscopy and laparotomy. Indeed there might in some cases be a justification for both. Current equine surgery texts should be consulted for the laparotomy procedure.

---

### Laparotomy versus laparoscopy

- Disadvantages of laparotomy – it requires general anesthesia, carries higher mortality and morbidity rates, involves protracted convalescence, and is more expensive than laparoscopy. Some regions of the abdomen that are visible on laparoscopy remain examinable only by palpation at laparotomy.
- Advantages of laparotomy – it offers a fuller examination and currently it allows more scope for undertaking corrective procedures than laparoscopy.

---

# EXAMINATION OF THE DIGESTIVE TRACT AND ABDOMEN OF THE FOAL

In addition to the fundamental size difference there are certain differences in the physiology and behavioral characteristics of foals that require different emphases in the tests performed and their interpretation when evaluating a foal with a suspected abdominal disorder.

## History and distant examination

Colic within the first 24 hours of life with a history of absence of feces could be consistent with

- functional impaction (meconium retention), or
- congenital atresia

of part of the hindgut. **Atresia ani** can be diagnosed by direct inspection of the perineal region. Male foals are more prone to retention of meconium because of their narrower pelvic canal. Colostrum has laxative properties and a history of late or inadequate intake might raise the suspicion of meconium retention. Rupture of the bladder at or before parturition tends to result in a depressed attitude a little later than that resulting from meconium retention, depending on the extent of the tear and the rate of build-up of uroperitoneum. Male foals have a higher relative risk for the condition than do females. Failure of passive transfer of maternal antibodies is an important factor in the development of a range of infections in foals, many of which might arise in or localize to abdominal organs. Also, a history of prepartum lactation or vulval discharge, dystocia, or signs of placentitis in the mare and/or deficiency of foal maturity should alert the clinician to the possibility of neonatal infections, which might take a variety of forms, including enteritis or peritonitis. Diarrhea is common in foals and may result from bacterial, protozoal, viral, parasitic, or nutritional causes. Almost all suckling foals will experience a transient bout of diarrhea coinciding with the time of the mare's first postpartum estrus (usually during the second week).

Gastroduodenal ulceration can be a clinically significant syndrome in foals. It probably has a multifactorial etiology but stress, concurrent disease and the administration of non-steroidal anti-inflammatory drugs are thought to be the main predisposing factors. In older foals ulceration might be associated with a pattern of ill-thrift and intermittent colic (possibly associated with duodenal strictures), but parasitism with *Parascaris equorum* or cyathostomes and chronic intussusception are both relatively common diseases that could cause a similar clinical presentation. The enteric form of *Rhodococcus equi* infection is another differential diagnosis, although less probable.

## Inspection and palpation of abdomen

Abdominal distension is probably more easily detected in the foal than in the adult horse, but is also less specific as distension of either the small or the large intestine, as well as uroperitoneum, results in a visibly distended abdomen. The fluid accumulation of uroperitoneum pools ventrally in the standing patient, giving a pendulous appearance compared to that created by gas accumulations within intestinal loops. Percussion can also help to discriminate between the two. Fluid in the abdomen (intraluminal and intraperitoneal) will not cause resonant pings on auscultation but does transmit vibrations, so that fluid thrills can be palpable by percussion and transabdominal palpation. The smaller size of the foal makes palpation of the abdomen a more realistic proposition in general, although the instances when significant information is yielded by the technique remain few.

The umbilicus is a common site of problems in young foals. Urine leakage from a patent urachus and marked swelling or purulent discharge due to septic omphalophlebitis usually are visible. The swelling and discomfort caused by infection of the umbilicus are also readily detected by palpation. Scrotal and umbilical congenital herniae occur quite frequently in the horse. Heavy and miniature breeds are particularly susceptible to the former. Large herniae are apparent at gross inspection. Palpation allows the detection of smaller herniae or might help to establish the nature of the contents of any hernial sac. Unless herniated intestine becomes obstructed there will be no other clinical signs.

---

**Clinical Pointer**

Occasionally in cooperative foals abdominal masses such as colonic impactions are palpable.

---

**Clinical Pointer**

- foals with retained meconium adopt a lordotic stance (depressed back)
- foals with bladder rupture appear kyphotic (hunched-up).

---

The critical evaluation of abdominal pain in foals is more problematic than that described for adults. Foals appear in marked discomfort whatever the cause, often adopting contorted positions in recumbency. None the less, relentless intractable intense colic carries a high index of suspicion for a lesion requiring surgical attention. Persistent straining, an elevated tailhead and tail swishing are all consistent with retained meconium. Foals with ruptured bladders may show similar signs, and the voiding of urine does not preclude this diagnosis.

Signs typical of gastroduodenal ulceration in foals include

- bruxism (grinding teeth)
- ptyalism (drooling saliva)
- inappetence
- postprandial colic
- prolonged dorsal recumbency
- pain elicited by pressure exerted through the xiphisternum.

However, overreliance on the presence of any of these for diagnosis is unwise. As with adults, the response (or lack of it) to analgesic medication is an important discriminant in determining the severity of a condition and the need for an exploratory laparotomy.

## Rectal examination

A rectal examination of the caudal abdomen is not possible in foals. Although a digital rectal examination can be performed it allows extremely limited access – perhaps enough to reach the caudal limit of a meconium impaction. However, injury to the anus and perineum, manifested by edema and soreness, occurs rapidly with apparently minimal trauma and the procedure should be performed

- only with care
- never repeatedly.

## Abdominocentesis

The collection of peritoneal fluid for laboratory evaluation is potentially more important in foals because of the unavailability of results of rectal examinations. However, there is also a greater risk of puncturing the intestine, partly because the intestinal wall of young foals has a mechanically lower resistance and partly because patient compliance is less reliable. These factors might favor the use of blunt-ended cannulae instead of sharp needles. The use of ultrasound guidance to detect fluid pockets is also helpful. Broadly speaking, the constituents of peritoneal fluid show no significant age-related differences, although the upper limit for a normal nucleated cell count might be lower in foals. Uroperitoneum can be diagnosed by estimating the ratio of creatinine concentration in peritoneal fluid and

serum, with a value greater than 2:1 being abnormally high. In addition, the instillation of a dye (e.g. methylene blue) into the bladder via a urinary catheter and its subsequent identification in a peritoneal aspirate will establish a bladder wall disruption. However, bladder defects that intermittently seal and ureteral defects may not be detected by this means.

## Clinical pathology

Hematological and biochemical profiles tend to be used more in examinations of foals than with adults. In part this is another reflection of the relative difficulty of arriving at a diagnosis, but it is also true that foals are susceptible to a wider range of systemic illnesses in which abdominal abnormalities play a part, and they are probably more rapidly vulnerable to the effects of metabolic compromise. For these reasons, whenever facilities and budget allow, it is advisable to incorporate serum IgG and blood glucose concentration estimation, blood culture, and blood acid–base status analysis as routine procedures for sick neonatal foals unless the clinical signs lead to an immediate diagnosis that renders them unnecessary. The principles of interpretation of hematological and biochemical values are the same for foals and adults, but it is necessary to be aware of age-related differences in normal ranges.

The prevalence of diarrhea in foals, especially between 1 week and 2 months of age, perhaps presents more opportunities to perform fecal examinations in foals than in adults. However, the inclination to perform fecal analysis is tempered by the facts that

- the recovery of pathogenic agents is not consistent
- most potential pathogens can also be found in the feces of asymptomatic foals
- the majority of cases are self-limiting
- knowledge of the causative agent rarely dictates specific therapy.

Tests are more important in the face of outbreaks of a diarrheic syndrome in one establishment. Agents that are generally accepted as being potentially pathogenic include

- *Salmonella* spp.
- Rotavirus
- *Aeromonas hydrophila* has been found to be significantly associated with diarrhea
- Older foals are susceptible to cyathostomiasis (although infection in animals older than yearlings is more typical)
- *Strongyloides westeri* infection is common in young foals and can be associated with diarrhea. Standard flotation techniques allow detection of the parasite in feces

- *Parascaris equorum* infection is prevalent in foals and yearlings, fecal detection of the eggs is straightforward, although the shedding of ova is intermittent. Clinical signs relate mostly to the migration of larvae through the respiratory tract, but the presence of large numbers of adult worms in the intestines may lead to unthriftiness. Sporadically a syndrome of acute colic caused by simple obstruction of the ileum by a mass of worms arises, sometimes following the use of anthelmintics.

## IMAGING TECHNIQUES

### Radiography

In contrast to its limitations in larger animals, radiography is a valuable and perhaps underused diagnostic aid in the investigation of foal abdominal (principally gastrointestinal) disorders. Lateral projections can be obtained with the patient standing or in lateral recumbency using kV and mAs settings within the capability of many portable X-ray units. Rare-earth screens are preferable and grids assist image quality if the power of the machine is suitable for their use. Normal radiological features have been described by Campbell and colleagues (1984). These include

- the identification of the stomach with a gas cap overlying ingesta in the cranial abdomen
- gas collections in small intestinal loops in the mid-abdomen
- gas caps over ingesta in the cecum and large colon caudodorsally
- gas accumulations in small colon loops caudally near the pelvic inlet.

Knowledge of these features allows the segment(s) of bowel distended to be predicted reasonably accurately. Gastric distension can be associated with ulcerative disease. Multiple tubular distensions indicate small intestinal obstruction.

### Clinical Pointer

Small intestinal distension is considered to be present when the width of a loop of intestine exceeds the length of the first lumbar vertebra.

The distinction between mechanical and functional obstructions of the small intestine remains problematic, particularly given the propensity for foals to develop ileus from dietary upset or enteritis, whose signs mimic those caused by lesions requiring surgical intervention. Large intestinal distension in foals is more likely to be associated with functional obstructions or to be secondary to small colon impactions, which can usually be readily diagnosed radiologically. None the less, displacements of the large colon do occur in foals and reference to other clinical findings is important. Free peritoneal gas is an indicator of intestinal rupture and visualization of the cranial margin of the renal silhouette is regarded as a reliable indicator of free gas. Radiography after the administration of barium sulfate, by mouth or as a rectal enema, further enables the identification of sites of obstruction. Retrograde contrast radiography in particular has been found to significantly enhance diagnostic accuracy for colon obstructions.

### Ultrasonography

The use of abdominal ultrasonography in foals has all the benefits described for its use in adults, with the added ability to penetrate to a greater relative depth transcutaneously but without the possibility of positioning the scanner head rectally. Ultrasonography can be diagnostic of certain conditions such as intestinal intussusception, bladder rupture and ascending infection in umbilical remnants. It is also of use in determining indirect evidence of disease, such as bowel thickness, contents, motility, and distension, as well as locating pockets of peritoneal fluid prior to aspiration. However, some sonographic findings describe the state of a segment of bowel without defining the cause, i.e. an amotile length of distended, thickened small intestine could arise through enteritis or strangulating obstruction, and Reimer (1993b) warns against misdiagnosis through overinterpretation.

# Ruminants

The clinical examination of the alimentary system of cattle can also in general be applied to sheep and goats.

## REGIONAL ANATOMY AND PHYSIOLOGY

The digestive system includes the alimentary canal and several accessory glands. The alimentary canal consists of the

- mouth
- pharynx

- esophagus
- compartments of the forestomach (rumen, reticulum, omasum)
- true stomach (abomasum)
- small intestines
- large intestines
- anal canal.

## Forestomach and abomasum

The stomach of ruminants is divided into a forestomach and a true stomach. The forestomach is composed of the reticulum, rumen, and omasum; the abomasum is homologous to the stomach of non-ruminants.

### Rumen

The rumen is a large, laterally compressed sac which occupies a major portion of the abdominal cavity. It extends from the diaphragm to the pelvic inlet and fills the left half of the abdominal cavity. Its caudoventral part may extend well over the median plane into the right half of the abdominal cavity.

The parietal surface of the rumen faces mainly to the left and is related to the diaphragm, the left abdominal wall, and the floor of the abdomen. The visceral surface faces to the right and is related chiefly to the intestines, the liver, the omasum, and the abomasum. The dorsal curvature lies against the diaphragm and the roof of the abdominal cavity; the ventral curvature follows the contour of the abdominal floor.

The rumen is divided into several parts by a number of grooves of varying depth. Shallow left and right longitudinal grooves on the parietal and visceral surfaces respectively are connected cranially and caudally by two deep transverse grooves, the cranial and caudal grooves. These four grooves form a nearly horizontal constriction which divides the rumen into dorsal and ventral sacs. The dorsal sac lies to the left of the median plane and the ventral sac extends often into the right half of the abdominal cavity. The left longitudinal groove begins at the cranial groove and, passing at first dorsocaudally, extends along the left side of the rumen to the caudal groove, giving off an accessory groove that extends for a short distance along the surface of the dorsal sac. The right longitudinal groove splits into two limbs which enclose an elongated area of the wall of the rumen. Although the dorsal limb is more prominent, the deep wall of the greater omentum attaches to the ventral limb. The dorsal and ventral coronary grooves extend in opposite directions from the caudal end of the longitudinal grooves and

mark off the caudodorsal and caudoventral blind sacs. The ventral coronary groove extends completely around the base of the caudoventral blind sac, but the dorsal groove is deficient dorsally:

- in cattle the two blind sacs are of about equal length
- in small ruminants the caudoventral blind sac extends farther caudally than the caudodorsal sac.

### Reticulum

The reticulum is the most cranial compartment of the ruminant stomach. It is spherical but slightly flattened craniocaudally, and lies between the diaphragm and the rumen at the level of the 6th to the 9th intercostal spaces, about equally to the right and left of the median plane. Dorsally it is continued without demarcation by the cranial sac of the rumen, whereas ventrally and to the sides it is sharply separated from the rumen by the deep ruminoreticular groove. Its diaphragmatic surface is convex, following the curvature of the diaphragm; its visceral surface is applied against the rumen. On the right the reticulum is related to the left lobe of the liver, the omasum, and the abomasum; on the left it lies against the costal part of the diaphragm and occasionally is in contact with the ventral end of the spleen. Its ventral relations are the sternal part of the diaphragm, the caudal end of the sternum, and the xiphoid cartilage.

### Omasum

The omasum of cattle is a spherical organ which is somewhat compressed laterally between its visceral and parietal surfaces. It has a curvature facing dorso-caudally and to the right, and opposite the curvature is the flat base which faces in the opposite direction. The omasum is separated from the reticulum by a neck-like constriction and from the abomasum by a similar, but wider, constriction.

The bovine omasum lies ventrally in the intra-thoracic part of the abdominal cavity, to the right of the median plane, between the ventral sac of the rumen on the left and the abdominal wall on the right. Craniodorsally it is related to the liver. Its visceral surface faces mainly to the left, but also slightly caudally, and is applied against the ventral sac of the rumen. Its parietal surface faces in the opposite direction and is related to the diaphragm, liver, and gallbladder. Between the 6th and 11th intercostal spaces the omasum is in contact with the right abdominal wall, protruding ventrally by about 10 cm from the costal arch. Ventrally it is related to the reticulum and abomasum, and caudally to the jejunum. The omasum of the sheep and goat lies more medially, at about the level of the 8th to 10th ribs, and is not in contact with the right abdominal wall, although its other relations are similar to the ones described for the ox.

## Abomasum

The abomasum is the most distal compartment, after the three compartments of the forestomach. It is a bent, pear-shaped sac which is set off from the omasum by a deep annular constriction. It looks much like a simple stomach and consequently has been divided into a fundus, a body, and a pyloric part. It has a greater curvature facing ventrally and to the left, and a lesser curvature facing dorsally and to the right. The fundus and body lie on the abdominal floor caudal to the reticulum; the longitudinal axis of this portion crosses the midline somewhat obliquely from left cranial to right caudal, overlying the region caudal to the xiphoid cartilage between the ventral ends of the costal arches. The pyloric part of the abomasum is directed dorsolaterally behind the omasum and is followed at the pylorus by the duodenum. The abomasum is closely related on the left to the recessis ruminis and may, when distended with fluid and gas, extend to the left and come to lie ventral to the cranial sac of the rumen, making contact with the left abdominal wall.

## Intestines

### Small intestine

The small intestine is situated almost entirely to the right of the midline and in the dorsal part of the abdomen. Its capacity is relatively less than that of the small intestine of other species and it lies in a 'sling-like' suspension of the greater omentum, the supraomental recess.

### Duodenum

The duodenum of adult cattle is approximately 1 m long. It arises at the pylorus of the abomasum approximately at the level of the ventral end of the right 9th intercostal space or 10th rib, and extends to the visceral surface of the liver, where it takes the form of an S-shape curve, the ansa sigmoidea, which with the cranial duodenal flexure forms the cranial part of the duodenum. It then passes caudally high in the sublumbar region as the descending duodenum, and

### Hepatoduodenal ligament

This ligament is a part of the lesser omentum

- it is not as ligamentous in appearance in the bovine species as it is in other domestic species
- it anchors the cranial portion of the duodenum to the liver, making it invulnerable to torsion
- it continues as the mesoduodenum, a portion of the common dorsal mesentery, carrying vessels and nerve fibers to and from the duodenum
- the mesoduodenum attaches the duodenum to portions of the liver, pancreas, right kidney, and cecum.

near the pelvic inlet it turns cranially at the caudal duodenal flexure as the jejunum.

### Jejunum and ileum

As in other domestic species there is no clear boundary between the jejunum and ileum, which together form many short coils within the free margin of the mesentery. The position of these coils depends upon the fullness of the rumen and the size of the uterus, but usually most of the jejunum lies within the recess bounded by the rumen and greater omentum. However, some small intestine may be found behind the rumen and thus against the left flank.

## Large intestine

The **cecum**, a tubular organ with a rounded, blind tip which projects caudally from the intestinal mass, is the first portion of the large intestine and is separated from the colon by the entrance of the ileum.

The tip of the cecum, when filled with gas, is located high in the abdomen but sinks to the abdominal floor when its contents are heavier. The length of the cecum in cattle is about 75 cm and its diameter is approximately 12 cm.

The **colon** is divided into the ascending, transverse, and descending parts. The ascending colon is unusually long and is divided into proximal, spiral, and distal loops. The proximal loop is a direct continuation from the cecum. It is continued ventrally as the centripetal gyri, which makes two full turns toward the center of the intestinal mass; the intestine then reverses its direction and at this point it is called the central flexure. From here the intestinal coil turns toward the outside and is termed the centrifugal gyri, continuing as the distal loop of the colon, which passes dorsally and caudally on the surface of the proximal loop to be continued on the transverse body just in front of the cranial mesenteric artery; from here it is continued as the descending colon.

The descending colon courses caudally high in the abdomen, bound by mesentery to the ascending duodenum. At about the level of the sixth lumbar vertebra the descending (sigmoid) colon makes a bend and is more movable than the rest of the colon owing to its longer mesentery.

The **rectum** is the intrapelvic portion of the colon. Most of the rectum has a mesorectum, with only its caudal part being retroperitoneal and relatively immovable. The muscular layers are thick, with intermittent transverse folds produced by circular smooth muscle. The anal canal is the short terminal segment of the bowel which ends at the exterior as the anus. Rectal columns – longitudinal mucosal folds – are found for a distance of approximately 10 cm at the junction of the rectum and anal canal.

### Clinical Pointer

Unlike the large intestine of the horse and the pig, the ruminant large intestine does not possess teniae coli.

## Liver and gallbladder

In ruminants, the liver lies to the right of and parallel to the median plane and is directed obliquely ventral and cranial toward the right portion of the diaphragm. The liver has a diaphragmatic surface located next to the diaphragm and a visceral surface which is in contact chiefly with the omasum and reticulum.

Ruminants possess a gallbladder, a pear-shaped structure approximately 10–13 cm long, lying partly against and attached to the visceral surface of the liver at approximately the level of the 10th or 11th intercostal space.

## The spleen

In ruminants, the parietal surface of the spleen lies against the diaphragm, to which it is attached, and its visceral surface lies firmly against the rumen, thus allowing little opportunity for the spleen to rotate upon itself and produce constriction of its vessels as seen in torsion of other organs.

The spleen in adult cattle measures approximately 60 cm in length, 2 cm thick, and 15 cm wide, and weighs about 0.9 kg. It extends downward and forward on the left side of the body from the 12th and 13th ribs

(its dorsal extremity) to approximately the junction of the middle and lower thirds of the 7th rib. Thus under normal conditions the spleen is protected by the thoracic cage and does not extend caudally as far as the paralumbar fossa.

## Abdomen and abdominal cavity

In cattle, the abdominal cavity is both absolutely and relatively more capacious than that of the horse (Figs 17.35, 17.36). The larger capacity arises from the greater transverse and longitudinal diameters.

### Clinical Pointer

The compound stomach, consisting of the rumen, reticulum, omasum, and abomasum, occupies almost three-quarters of the abdominal cavity.

The compound stomach fills the left half of the abdomen – the spleen and a few coils of small intestine are situated in this part – and extends considerably over to the right of the median plane. The total volume of the stomach compartments varies according to the age and size of the animal, the total capacity is

- 136–180 liters in average-sized adult cattle
- 180–270 liters in large cattle
- 115–160 liters in small cattle.

In the neonatal calf the reticulum is very small and the capacity of the rumen is less than half that of the abomasum; when the calf is 10–12 weeks old the rumen has become twice as large as the abomasum, the latter remaining functionless during this period. In the 4-month-old calf the capacity of the rumen and reticulum together is four times that of the omasum and abomasum together. At around 18 months the four compartments each have attained their final relative capacities.

The ruminant stomach occupies most of the abdominal cavity and leaves little room for the intestinal tract. The ruminoreticulum occupies the left half of the abdominal cavity and, with the ventral sac of the rumen, at times also a considerable portion of the right half. The omasum lies under cover of the ribs to the right of the median plane, and dorsocranial to it is the liver. The abomasum occupies the floor of the abdominal cavity in the xiphoid region. The remaining space, essentially the caudal part of the right half, contains the intestines, which form a disc-shaped mass, roughly sagittal in position, reaching from the liver to the pelvic cavity, and often into it. The intestinal mass is suspended from the roof of the abdominal cavity and,

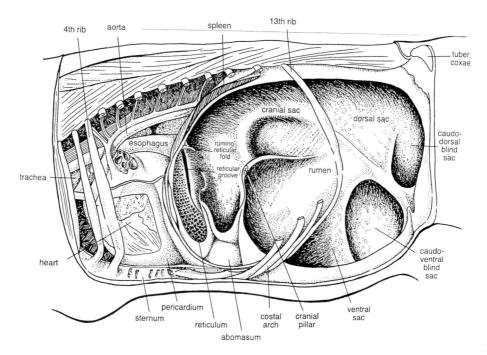

**Fig. 17.35**   Topographical anatomy of abdomen of cattle, left side.

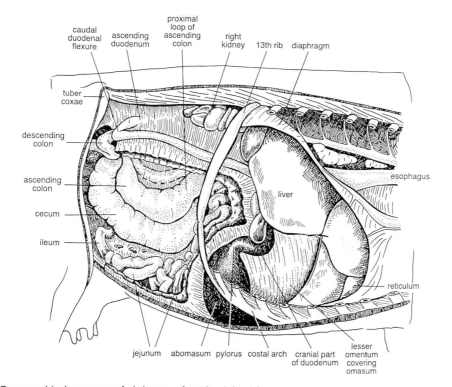

**Fig. 17.36**   Topographical anatomy of abdomen of cattle, right side.

with the exception of the cecum and a few caudal jejunal coils, is contained in the supraomental recess. The left surface of the intestinal mass lies against the dorsal sac of the rumen and the deep wall of the greater omentum covering the ventral sac. On the right side the intestinal mass is related to the right abdominal wall, but is separated from it by the two walls of the greater omentum. Cranially, the intestines extend deeply into the intrathoracic part of the abdominal cavity and are in contact here through the deep wall of the greater omentum with the omasum, the abomasum and the visceral surface of the liver; dorsally they are related to the kidneys and the pancreas. Obviously, stomach contractions – those of the ruminoreticulum in particular – and variations in the fullness of the stomach or the intestines change the position and the relations of the intestinal tract.

During pregnancy the uterus expands mainly cranioventrally and to the right, displacing the rumen and the intestinal mass craniodorsally and to the left. In the latter part of pregnancy the soft abdominal wall caudal to the costal arch and last rib becomes distended so as to prevent undue pressure from the greatly enlarged uterus on the other abdominal organs.

## APPLIED PHYSIOLOGY

### Rumination

Rumination is the complex process of

- regurgitation
- remastication
- ensalivation, and
- reswallowing

of reticulorumen contents. It is also called chewing the cud, or cudding. Rumination requires a positive approach by the animal and is easily stopped by fright or the offering of feed. Determining the causes of failure to ruminate is a major diagnostic challenge.

The stomach compartments occupy almost 75% of the abdominal cavity. Because of its comparative size and its situation in relation to the left abdominal wall, the rumen compartment is the one most readily examined by routine clinical methods. An assessment of its functional state obtained in this manner may reflect the condition of the other stomach compartments, which are intimately interdependent and consist of microbial degradation and synthesis and physical maceration. The latter involves motility, the periodicity and vigor of which are readily ascertained in respect of the rumen. The contractions of the stomach compartments are organized and controlled

through the vagus nerve and the ruminoreticular motor center in the medulla oblongata.

The cyclical movements, which ensure thorough mixing of the contents of the rumen and reticulum, occur at the rate of 1–3 per minute, the greater frequency being related to recent ingestion of feed. The cycle of motility commences with a double contraction of the reticulum, the second phase being associated with a simultaneous strong contraction of the anterior dorsal sac of the rumen. As a result of these movements the fluid contents of the reticulum are spilled over the reticuloruminal fold on to the surface of the dry ingesta in the rumen. A sequential contraction of the ventral sac of the rumen then returns the fluid to the reticulum.

---

> ### Clinical Pointer
>
> The interdependency between the stomach compartments, means that disease of one compartment will modify the activity of the others.

---

Eructation contractions, which are independent of the mixing contractions, mainly occur following the mixing cycle, their frequency being related to the gas pressure in the rumen. The contraction is initiated in the dorsal sacs of the rumen, from where it passes cranially to the esophageal groove. Relaxation of the reticulum and cardia follows, depressing the level of the fluid so that the gas enters the esophagus and is freely expelled. Frothiness of the fluid will prevent clearing of the cardia so that eructation is impossible.

Regurgitation movements are an essential prelude to rumination; the associated ruminal contractions occur immediately prior to the normal mixing movements of the rumen. The function of the specific movements is to flood the esophageal cardia with fluid. The next stage in rumination necessitates voluntary action by the animal, consisting of an inspiratory effort with the glottis closed, whereby the intrathoracic negative pressure is greatly increased. This action is associated with a visible lifting movement of the abdomen. As a result, some of the reticular fluid, containing solid material, enters the esophagus and, after initiating antiperistalsis, is carried up to the pharynx. At this point a movement of the tongue directs the solid material between the tables of the molar teeth on one side of the mouth, the jaws are brought together and the base of the tongue is retracted into the pharynx, so that the regurgitated fluid is reswallowed. The mastication of the bolus then commences and is continued on the same side of the mouth.

In healthy cattle the periods of rumination vary in length from a few minutes to more than an hour, and may occur at any time of the day. Although the animal usually lies down to ensure greater comfort, rumination in the standing position is not abnormal. When ruminating, cattle present an appearance of comfort and placid contentment. Each bolus is methodically chewed some 50–80 times (the number of masticatory movements depending on the character of the food) before being reswallowed; the next bolus is regurgitated into the mouth within a few seconds. Generally, in any given period of rumination the number of masticatory movements per bolus varies very little in healthy animals. Normally there are about 60 jaw movements per minute, which is slower than that for ordinary mastication during initial feeding. The total time devoted to rumination on a daily basis is related to the character of the feed, for example sheep spend

- up to 9 hours ruminating when fed poor-quality rough hay
- 5 hours ruminating on a diet of ground grass meal
- 2.5 hours ruminating when fed concentrates alone.

The healthy calf usually commences to ruminate for short and irregular periods on about the 10th day of life if it has access to forage. By the time it is 6 weeks old the calf is ruminating regularly, but at the comparatively rapid rate of 80 jaw movements per minute. The adult rate of mastication is not established until the animal is about 1 year old.

When reticulorumen dysfunction is present, particularly hypomotility, the problem is to decide whether the cause is directly associated with the stomachs and/or the other parts of the alimentary tract, or is due to an abnormality of another system. Differentiation requires a careful clinical examination, including simple laboratory evaluation of the rumen contents.

When the animal is influenced by excitement or fear rumination ceases abruptly. The absence of coarse fiber in the rumen when cattle are fed on a diet of finely ground or pelleted feeds will cause diminished rumination. There are many reasons why rumination may be infrequent, irregular, or completely suppressed, or be performed slowly, with a reduced number of jaw movements per bolus

- febrile disease
- ruminal atony
- acute impaction of the rumen
- traumatic reticulitis
- vagus indigestion
- actinobacillosis of the rumen and/or reticulum

- rumenitis
- impaction of the omasum
- displacement and torsion of the abomasum.

In painful diseases affecting the mouth structures or abdominal or other organs, including those associated with erosive and ulcerative lesions of the oral mucosa, dental defects, traumatic reticulitis, ulceration of the abomasum, and acute hepatitis, rumination is irregular.

The abomasum in its normal position in mature cattle cannot be examined by the standard techniques of physical examination, with perhaps the exception of auscultation and paracentesis. Some gurgling and peristalsis-like sounds may be audible on auscultation but they are not usually diagnostic.

---

### Clinical Pointer

Irregular rumination associated with grunting often indicates abdominal disease.

---

## CLINICAL EXAMINATION OF THE DIGESTIVE TRACT AND ABDOMEN

A routine general clinical examination of the animal is performed prior to a close examination of the gastrointestinal tract and abdomen. When gastrointestinal dysfunction is suspected a thorough clinical examination is necessary to determine the location and nature of the lesion. The methods used include inspection, external palpation, ballottement, tactile percussion, succussion, auscultation, percussion and simultaneous auscultation and rectal palpation. Passage of the stomach tube, abdominocentesis, ultrasonography, laparoscopy, and exploratory laparotomy may also be implicated. The sequence of clinical examination recommended here can be modified to meet individual circumstances.

### History taking and examination of the environment

Details of the recent disease history and management of the animal are necessary. The events of the illness should be obtained in chronological order, and

- stage of the pregnancy/lactation cycle
- days since parturition
- nature of the diet
- speed of onset
- duration of illness

will often suggest diagnostic possibilities. An accurate description of the appetite will suggest whether the disease is acute or chronic. In lactating dairy cattle an indication of the precise decline in milk production over what period of time can provide useful information for formulating diagnostic hypotheses. Any previous treatments used and the response obtained should be determined. Any history of abdominal pain and its characteristics should be determined. The nature and the volume of the feces may suggest enteritis or alimentary tract stasis. The state of the immediate environment and any evidence of unusual animal activity, such as disturbed ground surfaces or bedding, should be noted. Inspection of the feed and water supplies may offer clues to diagnostic hypotheses.

## Distant examination

The habitus, appetite, feces and rumination are evaluated from the history, the distant examination and the initial part of the clinical examination.

### Habitus

Changes from normal behavior are much less obvious in cattle affected with painful conditions than they are in horses in similar circumstances. Behavioral manifestations of abdominal pain in cattle include kicking at the abdomen, and lowering the back and stretching the forelegs forward and the hind legs backward while in a standing position. Spontaneous grunting or groaning suggests abdominal pain associated with distension of a viscus or acute diffuse peritonitis. Sudden onset of acute abdominal pain in calves is characterized by recumbency, with stretching of the legs, bellowing, and repeatedly lying down and getting up. Marked changes in the contour of the abdomen occur in cattle with diseases of the digestive tract and should be noted. The significance of grunting in cattle is not always related to disease of the alimentary system. After a full feed of highly palatable food cattle may grunt intermittently when they move or lie down because of the slight respiratory embarrassment caused by the distended rumen restricting movement of the diaphragm.

Grinding of the teeth or bruxism may occur with abdominal pain in cattle but is not specific.

### Appetite

The degree of appetite and the presence or absence of rumination are reliable indicators of the state of the alimentary tract, including the liver. Complete anorexia persisting for more than 3 days is unfavorable. The return of appetite and ruminating following medical or surgical treatment for alimentary tract disease is a favorable prognostic sign. Persistent inappetence and failure of rumination suggests a chronic lesion, usually with an unfavorable prognosis.

### Feces

It is vital to determine the amount and character of feces being passed (or not passed) in the previous several hours. A complete absence of feces for more than 24 hours suggests an intestinal obstruction, which could be functional or physical.

### Inspection of the abdomen

**Contour**
The contour or silhouette of the abdomen is inspected at a few steps from the rear of the animal, and each lateral region viewed from an oblique angle. This will assist in determining the presence and possible causes of abdominal distension, which may be unilateral, bilaterally symmetrical or asymmetrical, or more prominent in the dorsal or ventral half of one side or the other. Inspection may reveal evidence of distension of the left paralumbar fossa, as in frothy bloat.

Figure 17.37 illustrates the various silhouettes of the contour of the abdomen of cattle, viewed from the rear, representing different diseases of the abdominal viscera.

The differential diagnosis of abdominal distension in cattle is summarized in Table 17.2.

The cause of distension is determined by a combination of

- inspection of the contour or silhouette of the abdomen to determine the site of maximum distension
- auscultation and percussion of the abdomen to detect the presence and location of gas-filled viscera
- relief of rumen contents with a stomach tube to determine whether the distension is due to an enlarged rumen (the ruminal contents can also be examined grossly at the same time)
- rectal examination to determine the presence and location of distended viscera
- paracentesis to examine the amount and nature of the peritoneal fluid, this may indicate the presence of ischemic necrosis of intestines or peritonitis

---

**Clinical Pointer**

Mature cattle are stoic and do not exhibit the postural changes with abdominal pain that are so common in the horse.

- trocarization of severe gas-filled swellings, such as an abomasal torsion in a calf.

Distension of the abdomen may be due to excessive quantities of feed, late pregnancy and multiple fetuses, excessive abdominal fat, or abnormal amounts of fluid in the peritoneal cavity (urine, ascites, peritoneal exudate). An excessive amount of fluid in the peritoneal cavity usually causes distension of the lower part of the abdomen – the pear-shaped abdomen. Gastrointestinal gas (tympany) usually distends the flank upwards, distending the hollows of the paralumbar fossae. Distension of the left abdomen in cattle suggests ruminal tympany. Distension of the right abdomen suggests dilatation of the abomasum, cecum, intestines, or a gravid uterus.

A reduction in the size of the abdomen may be due to starvation, reduced feed intake, after parturition, especially following multiple births, chronic illness causing anorexia, or following prolonged diarrhea. Increased tenderness (splinting) of the abdominal wall due to peritonitis may make the contour of the abdomen appear smaller than normal.

**Umbilical region**
Hemorrhage from the umbilical vessels may occur in newborn calves. Inspection of the umbilical region of

> ### Vagus indigestion
>
> This is characterized by distension of the left upper and lower abdomen and right lower abdomen in a mature cow (known as a 'papple-shaped' abdomen). The rumen is grossly enlarged with distension of the
>
> - dorsal sac → left upper and lower abdominal distension
> - ventral sac → right lower abdominal distension.

the ventral abdomen of calves under a few weeks of age may reveal the presence of enlargements, which may be due to herniation or painful swellings associated with navel-ill or omphalophlebitis. Dribbling of urine from the umbilicus suggests a patent urachus in the newborn. Skin lesions of the ventral midline of the abdominal wall of mature cattle may suggest stephanofilariasis.

**Anal region**
The anal region is examined for evidence of swellings, fecal staining, rectal prolapse, fissures or swellings, or the absence of an anus.

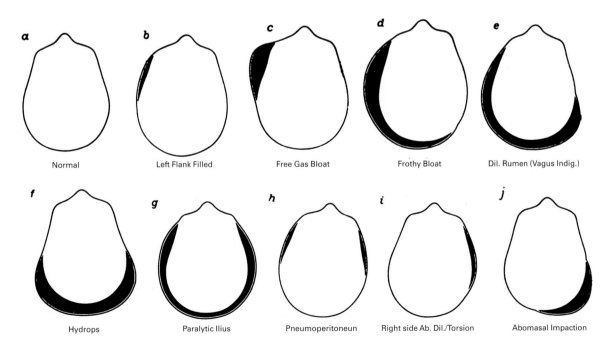

**Fig. 17.37**  (a–j) Silhouettes of the contour of the abdomen of cattle, viewed from the rear, with different diseases of the abdominal viscera.

**Table 17.2. The differential diagnosis of abdominal distension of cattle**

| Cause | Major clinical findings and methods of diagnosis |
|---|---|
| **Distension of rumen:** | |
| Acute ruminal tympany | Marked distension of left abdomen, less of right. Very tense distended left paralumbar fossa, dull resonance on percussion. Pass stomach tube and attempt to relieve gas or froth |
| Vagus indigestion | Marked distension of left abdomen, less of right. Fluctuating rumen on palpation. Excessive rumen activity or complete atony. Large L-shaped rumen on rectal examination. Pass large-bore stomach tube |
| Grain overload | Moderate distension of left flank, less of right. Rumen contents are doughy or fluctuate. Fluid-splashing sounds may be audible on ballottement. Rumen static and systemic acidosis. Rumen pH below 6.5 |
| Simple indigestion | Moderate distension of left flank; rumen pack easily palpable and doughy. Contractions may be present or absent depending on severity. Systemically normal. May be dropping cuds |
| **Distension of abomasum:** | |
| Right-side dilatation, displacement and torsion | Right flank and paralumbar fossa over right flank normal to severely distended. Ping on percussion. Rectal palpation of fluctuating or tense viscus in right lower quadrant |
| Impaction | Right lower flank normal to moderately distended. Doughy viscus palpable caudal to costal arch. Rectal palpation feel doughy viscus in right lower quadrant |
| Left-side displacement | Abdomen usually gaunt. Occasionally left paralumbar fossa distended due to displaced abomasum. Ping on percussion over upper aspects of 9–12 ribs |
| Abomasal trichobezoars | Older calves (2–4 months of age). Right lower flank distended. Fluid-splashing sounds. Painful grunt on deep palpation. Confirm by laparotomy and abomasotomy |
| **Distension of intestines:** | |
| Enteritis | Slight to moderate distension of right abdomen. Fluid-rushing and splashing sounds on auscultation and ballottement. Diarrhea and dehydration |
| Intestinal obstruction | Slight to moderate distension of right abdomen. Fluid tinkling, percolating and splashing sounds on auscultation and ballottement. May palpate distended loops of intestine or intussusception rectally. Scant dark feces. Paracentesis abdominis |
| Paralytic ileus | Slight to moderate distension of right abdomen. Tinkling sounds on auscultation. Tympanitic ping on percussion. Loops of distended intestine palpable per rectum. Scant feces that return to normal if no physical obstruction |
| Cecal dilatation and torsion | Right flank may be normal or moderately distended. Ping present in right paralumbar fossa. Palpate movable blind end cecum on rectal examination. Confirm by laparotomy |
| **Enlargement of uterus:** | |
| Physiological | Gross distension of both flanks, especially right. Normal pregnancy with more than one fetus. May palpate fetus rectally |
| Pathological | |
|   Hydrops amnion | Gradual enlargement of lower half of abdomen in late gestation. Flaccid uterus, fetus and placentomes are easily palpable per rectum |
|   Hydrops allantosis | Gradual distension of lower half of abdomen in late gestation. Palpable uterus rectally, cannot palpate placentomes or fetus |
|   Fetal emphysema | History of dystocia or recent birth of one calf, twin in uterus and emphysematous. Diagnosis obvious on vaginal and rectal examination |
| **Fluid and gas accumulation in peritoneal cavity:** | |
| Ascites | |
|   Congestive heart failure, peritonitis, ruptured bladder | Bilateral distension of lower abdomen. Positive fluid waves. Abdominocentesis. May feel enlarged liver behind right costal arch |
| Pneumoperitoneum | Perforated abomasal ulcer, postsurgical laparotomy. Bilateral distension of both paralumbar fossae with a ping over each fossa |

### Defecation

The act of defecation is observed for any evidence of inability to posture or any pain associated with the passage of feces.

### Movements of abdominal wall

Movements of the abdominal wall may be associated with contractions of the rumen and movements of the fetus in late pregnancy.

## Systemic state (temperature, peripheral circulation, state of hydration, heart and respirations)

The body temperature, peripheral circulation including the arterial pulse and venous circulation, and the state of hydration are examined, as well as the heart and respiratory tract.

The vital signs will indicate the severity of the disease and suggest whether it is acute, subacute, or chronic. In acute intestinal obstruction, abomasal torsion, acute diffuse peritonitis and acute carbohydrate engorgement the heart rate may be 100–120 per minute and dehydration is usually obvious. If cattle with any of the above diseases are recumbent and unable to rise the prognosis is usually unfavorable. A marked increase in the rate and depth of respirations associated with alimentary tract disease usually indicates the presence of fluid or electrolyte disturbances, and possibly subacute pain. Fever is an indication of an inflammatory lesion such as peritonitis.

---

### Clinical Pointer ✳

Pallor of the mucous membranes is an important indicator of alimentary tract hemorrhage, especially if there is concurrent melena.

---

## Examination of left abdomen

### Inspection

Contractions of the rumen are visible by inspection of the left paralumbar fossa and the left lateral abdominal region. The alternate rising and sinking of the left paralumbar fossa on normal mature ruminant cattle is associated with the concurrent contraction and relaxation of the dorsal and ventral sacs of the rumen. It occurs more frequently and is seen more easily in mature cattle during and after eating and during rumination, and is visible in both the standing and the recumbent animal.

Coincidental with each rising of the paralumbar fossa, a ripple can be seen moving slowly in a dorsal direction over the surface of the left lateral abdominal region toward the fossa. With each sinking of the fossa, there is a less distinct and slightly more complex ventral regression of the ripple.

During contractions of the rumen there is an alternate rising and sinking of the left paralumbar fossa in conjunction with abdominal surface ripples. The ripples reflect ruminal motility and occur during both the primary (or mixing) cycle and the secondary (or eructation) cycle. As the left paralumbar fossa rises during the first part of the primary cycle there are two horizontal ripples which move from the lower left abdominal region up to the paralumbar fossa. When the paralumbar fossa sinks, during the second part of the primary cycle, the ripple moves ventrally and fades out at the lower part of the left abdominal region. Similar ripples follow up and down after the rising and sinking of the paralumbar fossa, associated with the secondary cycle movements. In vagus indigestion there may be three to seven vigorous incomplete contractions of the rumen per minute. They may not be audible because the rumen contents are porridge-like and do not cause the normal crackling sounds. However, they are visible and palpable as waves of undulations of the left flank.

### Palpation of rumen

After observation of its movements, the rumen is palpated in the left paralumbar fossa and left lower flank to determine the nature of its contents. The left paralumbar fossa is normally slightly concave. Palpation of the rumen is done with the extended fingers, the palm of the hand, or the back of the closed fist applied to the abdominal wall on the left side (Fig. 17.38). A systematic procedure should be adopted, starting at the dorsal part of the abdominal wall beneath the extremities of the lumbar transverse processes and continuing down towards the ventral aspect of the abdomen. The mass of rumen contents palpable indirectly through the abdominal wall of the left paralumbar fossa is commonly known as the 'rumen pack'. It normally feels doughy and pits on digital pressure. Palpation above the rumen pack will reveal the normal gas cap, which is resilient and tympanic. If the gas cap is enlarged the left paralumbar fossa may be convex and the rumen pack not readily palpable. If moderately firm pressure is applied at this location the abdominal and ruminal walls move inwards for a short distance before the rumen contents are felt. Palpation of the normal rumen enables assessment of the frequency, strength, and cyclical pattern of the movements. In the more ventral areas of the left paralumbar fossa and flank the abdominal wall is more resistant to pressure because of the weight of the rumen contents, and the motility contractions are much less obvious.

If the rumen pack cannot be felt in the left paralumbar fossa it may be because of displacement of the rumen medially, most commonly by a left-sided displacement of the abomasum, a decrease in the amount of rumen contents, or a collapsed rumen, which occurs in cattle anorexic for several days.

In bloat or ruminal tympany the left paralumbar fossa will be distended to varying degrees of prominence and the distension will be resilient to very tense, depending on the amount of intraruminal pressure. Pneumoperitoneum or intraperitoneal gas will cause distension of both paralumbar fossae.

### Clinical Pointer

The severity of ruminal tympany and distention of the abdomen of cattle can be evaluated by the amount of skin which can be grasped over the left paralumbar fossa. In the normal animal, a 'tent' of skin can be easily grasped (Figure 17.38B). In severe ruminal tympany, it may be impossible to grasp and tent the skin which is an indication of severe distention and an unfavourable prognosis which necessitates emergency relief of the ruminal tympany.

The diet influences the consistency of the 'rumen pack'

- in roughage-fed cattle the rumen contents are usually doughy and pit on pressure
- in cattle fed long cereal-grain straw the rumen may be large with firm contents
- in dehydrated animals the contents may feel firm
- in grain-fed cattle the contents are usually soft and porridge-like.

When the rumen contains excessive quantities of fluid the left flank will fluctuate on deep palpation. In the atonic rumen distended with excess gas the left flank will be tense, resilient and tympanitic on percussion and the 'rumen pack' cannot be felt.

In mature cattle anorexic for several days the rumen may be smaller than normal and the dorsal sac will be collapsed (rumen collapse); palpation of the left paralumbar fossa fails to identify a rumen pack but rather a sense of emptiness, in which nothing but the abdominal wall can be felt.

### Clinical Pointer

An excessively dry and firm rumen pack indicates primary or secondary dehydration.

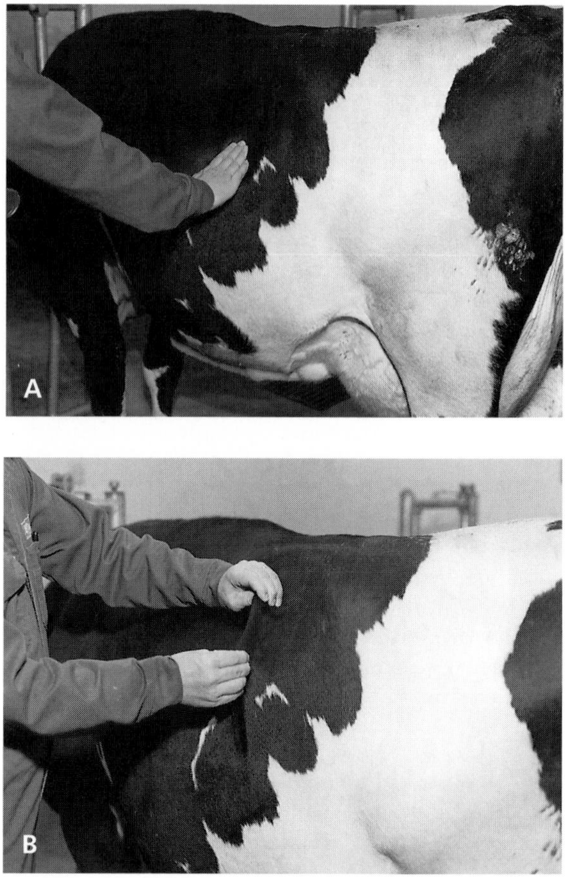


**Fig. 17.38** (A) Palpation of rumen with open hand. (B) Picking up skin over the left flank as a measure of the degree of abdominal distension.

### *Auscultation of the rumen and left abdomen*

Auscultation of the rumen allows evaluation of its functional status, and to a varying degree that of the other stomach compartments can be assessed. Rumen contractions are audible with the stethoscope placed in the left paralumbar fossa and extending cranially over an area from the dorsal third of the 10th to the 13th ribs (Fig. 17.39).

The rumen contraction sounds should be evaluated for **intensity**, **duration**, and **frequency**. The sounds are influenced by

- time after feeding
- recent excitement

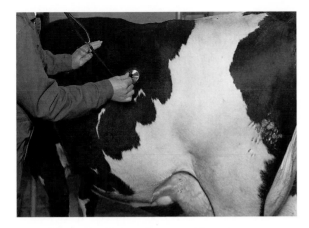

**Fig. 17.39** Auscultation of rumen with stethoscope.

- composition of the diet, and
- access to water supply.

In the normal animal on a roughage diet there are two independent contraction sequences of the reticulo-rumen.

1. The **primary cycle contraction** occurs approximately every minute and consists of a biphasic contraction of the reticulum followed by a monophasic contraction of the dorsal sac of the rumen, and then by a monophasic contraction of the ventral sac. These contractions occur with the alternate rising and sinking of the left paralumbar fossa. They are the mixing contractions of the rumen and assist the passage of rumen contents into the omasum.
2. The **secondary cycle contractions**, which occur at intervals of about 2 minutes, are confined to the rumen and consist of a contraction of the dorsal sac followed by a contraction of the ventral sac. The former causes the fluid contents of the dorsal sac to be forced ventrally and the gas layer to be forced cranially to the region of the cardia, where eructation takes place. Contractions of the dorsal and ventral sacs cause undulations of the left paralumbar fossa and lower flanks which are readily visible and palpable.

A decrease in the intensity or the absence of ruminal sounds over the left paralumbar fossa and the area cranial to it suggests the presence of a viscus or mass between the rumen and the abdominal wall. The most common cause is left-side displacement of the abomasum.

Rumen contractions are reduced in frequency, duration, and amplitude, or entirely absent, in

- hypocalcemia

### Normal rumen contraction sounds

The sounds of rumen contractions in an animal consuming roughage are similar to a series of exploding/crackling/grating sounds. When the rumen contains less coarse roughage or primarily grain, the sounds may be less distinct but still possess a crackling/grating characteristic.

- endotoxemia
- simple indigestion
- acute carbohydrate engorgement
- traumatic reticulopertonitis

and in other diseases of the ruminant stomachs that inhibit primary contractions.

In traumatic reticuloperitonitis, rumen contractions are absent or reduced to a frequency of one every several minutes, with decreased amplitude. The rumen is also mildly tympanitic, resulting in a moderate degree of distension in the left paralumbar fossa. Palpation in the dorsal aspect of the fossa reveals the presence of a larger than normal gas cap overlying the firm doughy mass of solid rumen contents.

The presence of **fluid-tinkling** or **splashing sounds**, along with a static rumen, suggests that the rumen contains an excessive quantity of fluid. Fluid-splashing sounds suggest diseases, such as grain overload, or an atonic rumen associated with prolonged anorexia, as in chronic diffuse peritonitis or abomasal or omasal impaction. The sounds are similar to those present in left-side displacement of the abomasum. To assist in the differential diagnosis, the outline of the rumen can be percussed to observe a much wider area of metallic sound than would normally be expected in left-side displacement of the abomasum.

In vagus indigestion with an enlarged hypermotile rumen the contractions are

- obvious and frequent (3–6 per minute)
- visible and palpable as prominent undulations of the wall of the left flank
- not usually audible because the rumen contents are homogeneous and porridge-like owing to prolonged maceration in the rumen.

Complete atony of the rumen may also occur in vagus indigestion. Achalasia of the reticulo-omasal and pyloric sphincters is the pathogenetic mechanism that results in failure of outflow of contents from the reticulorumen through to the omasum and abomasum. Large quantities of fluid and rumen contents accumulate in the rumen, resulting in marked ruminal distension often accompanied by pyloric dysfunction and impaction of the abomasum.

The effects of achalasia of the reticulo-omasal sphincter occur as one or other of two syndromes

- ruminal distension with hypermotility
- ruminal distension with atony.

The former is characterized by moderate to severe tympany with almost continuous, forceful rumen contractions, which are readily detected by palpation although the sounds are barely audible or absent. The latter affects cows in late pregnancy and comprises a syndrome in which there is distension of the abdomen, reduction in or complete absence of ruminal movements, a mild degree of tympany, anorexia, and the passage of small amounts of soft, pasty feces. The type in which pyloric obstruction occurs also affects cows in late pregnancy. In this form rumen motility is usually completely absent and pasty feces are passed in reduced quantity.

The clinical recognition of the presence or absence of either the primary cycle or secondary cycle contractions or both may aid in determining the cause and severity of the disease and the prognosis.

### Auscultation of the reticulum

Auscultation of the reticulum requires considerable experience to be able to detect those sounds which are specifically related to its functional activity, as well as the ability to interpret the significance of any departure from normal. The cycle of mixing movements commences with a biphasic contraction of the reticulum, which pours the liquid contents of the reticulum over the reticuloruminal fold, producing a soft fluid sound, adequately described as having a swishing character; it persists for several seconds. A somewhat similar sound is heard when fluid is returned to the reticulum by the succeeding contraction of the ventral sac of the rumen. Fluid sounds are also detectable at the same location in association with eructation contractions and those for rumination, the former occurring immediately after, and the latter just prior to, the mixing sounds. The usual readily observable signs associated with both these actions will indicate that the origin of the sounds is distinct from that of the mixing cycle.

> ### Site for auscultation of the reticulum
>
> The most informative point is over the costochondral junction of the 7th left rib, which is approximately 10 cm caudal to the point of the elbow.

### Percussion and simultaneous auscultation

Percussion and simultaneous auscultation is used to detect the presence of gas-filled viscera in the abdomen (Fig. 17.40A, B).

Percussion and simultaneous auscultation over both sides of the abdomen is a useful diagnostic technique to elicit 'pings' or 'pungs' – resonant sounds indicating the presence of excessive quantities of gas in the lumen of the gastrointestinal tract or in the peritoneal cavity, a ping is a high-pitched resonant musical sound, a pung is a low-pitched resonant musical sound.

The area being examined is percussed with a flick of the finger, flexed fingers, or a plexor (a percussion hammer). The stethoscope is placed immediately adjacent to the area being percussed and the examiner listens for a tympanitic sound, which may vary from a high-pitched bell-like sound to a low-pitched bass drum sound. The most commonly known ping is that associated with left-side displacement of the abomasum. Percussion over distended loops of intestine containing fluid and gas will also result in a ping. A pung is a low-pitched sound commonly heard by percussion and auscultation over an atonic rumen containing some gas.

> ### Clinical Pointer
>
> gas-filled viscera → pings (distended abomasum, cecum, or intestines)
> gas-filled rumen → pungs

The factors that dictate whether or not a resonant sound can be elicited include

- the size of the gas-filled viscus
- the location of the viscus and its proximity to the abdominal wall
- the amplitude of the percussion applied.

The most reliable method of eliciting these resonant sounds is to use a plexor or percussion hammer rather than the flicking fingers, which may not provide sufficient percussion and consistency, both of which can be achieved with a plexor.

The presence of a ping denotes three basic characteristics about the structure from which the sound originates.

1. It must be a hollow viscus with a significant free gas component. This may either largely fill the viscus, as in most cases of abomasal or cecal dilatation, or it may be accompanied by a sizeable fluid component, as in volvulus of the abomasum.

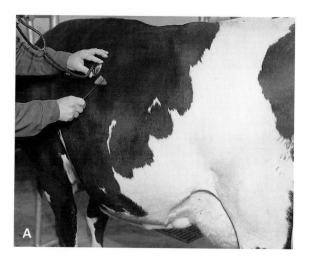

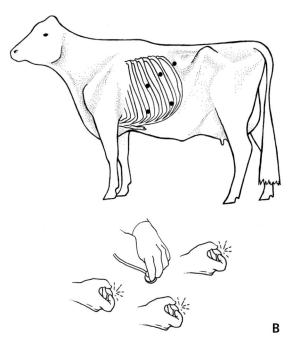

**Fig. 17.24** (A) Percussion and simultaneous auscultation of left abdomen for pings and pungs using the plexor. (B) Percussion and simultaneous auscultation of left abdomen for pings and pungs using the flick of a finger as plexor. Location of pings which may be audible by percussion and simultaneous auscultation over left abdomen. (C) Left lateral aspect of abdominal viscera of a cow with left-side displacement of abomasum (Sack 1968).

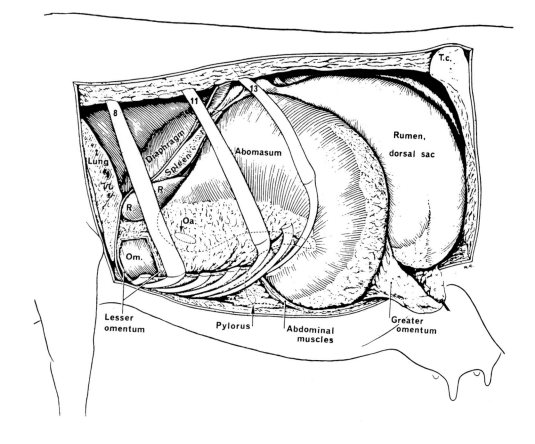

2. The viscus must lie next to or against the parietal peritoneal surface; the ping is heard over the area of abdominal wall that contacts the viscus.

3. The area of abdominal wall being percussed must be sufficiently thin to transmit the energy generated by the plexor from the skin surface to the viscus, and the resulting ping sound from the viscus to the skin, where it can be picked up by the stethoscope bell. For example, a gas-distended cecum in the dorsal portion of the abdomen caudal to the right tuber coxae would not yield a ping because the thick gluteal musculature and associated bony structures would prevent the transmission of the audible sound.

It is important to appreciate that a variety of abdominal viscera other than the abomasum can be associated with right-side pings. It is possible for the correct structure to be identified through careful, thorough simultaneous auscultation and percussion combined with rectal palpation. Knowledge of the particular viscus involved will allow appropriate clinical management of the patient and may help to avoid unnecessary surgery.

### Percussion and simultaneous auscultation of the left abdomen

Percussion and simultaneous auscultation of the left abdomen, including the left paralumbar fossa and an area extending from the midpoint of the 9th to the 13th ribs, is used to detect the presence of a ping associated with left displacement of the abomasum. Percussion is done with a flick of the finger or, most reliably, with a plexor (Fig. 17.40). In left-side displacement of the abomasum, percussion and auscultation elicits a ping over the area. The area of the pings may extend from the center of the left paralumbar fossa to the ventral parts of the 9th to the 13th left ribs. In pneumoperitoneum, a ping can be elicited on both sides of the abdomen over the paralumbar fossae. Other causes of pings on percussion of the left abdomen in mature cattle are an atonic rumen and pneumoperitoneum.

In the normal state, the upper part of the dorsal sac of the rumen contains rumen gases in the gas cap. This is reflected in the slightly tympanic note obtained from percussion of the gas cap in the dorsal aspects of the rumen in mild gaseous distension which, if the tympany is severe, becomes ringing in character.

#### Pings and pungs in the left abdomen
*Left displacement of the abomasum (LDA)*
The physical displacement of the atonic, moderately distended abomasum to the left side of the abdomen

> **Clinical Pointer**
>
> In frothy bloat the gas in the rumen is finely dispersed throughout the ingesta, causing a tympanic sound that is
>
> - more resonant
> - much lower down on the abdominal wall than in the normal animal.

involves

- the fundus and greater curvature
- displacement of the pylorus and duodenum
- a degree of rotation of the omasum, reticulum, and liver.

The greater curvature of the abomasum passes beneath the rumen and is retained between it and the left abdominal wall, sometimes reaching beyond the costal arch in the midflank region (Fig. 17.40C). The displaced abomasum contains fluid and gas, which results in a ping on percussion and auscultation. Percussion and simultaneous auscultation of the left abdominal wall over an area extending from the middle of the 9th to the 13th rib, above and below an imaginary line drawn between the point of the elbow and the tuber coxae, is used to elicit a ping associated with left-sided displacement of the abomasum (Fig. 17.41A). The area of concern should be examined carefully and methodically to ensure that the presence of a ping is not missed. The presence of fluid in the abomasum can be determined by eliciting fluid-splashing sounds on ballottement and auscultation of the left lower flank. In a proportion of cases displacement is in a cranial direction, the abomasum being trapped between the reticulum and diaphragm; this requires careful percussion and auscultation over a wide area.

In left displacement of the abomasum, the ruminal movements are reduced in frequency and amplitude and often can only be recognized – at least in the upper part of the left paralumbar fossa – when the abdominal wall is manually depressed inwards into contact with the rumen, which is displaced slightly medially. This often results in the animal appearing to be slab-sided. In unusual cases the gas-filled abomasum may extend up to the left lower paralumbar fossa, where it may be possible to palpate the bulging, cylindrical mass of the viscus just caudal to the costal arch, with the rumen pack just caudal to the distended abomasum (Fig. 17.40C).

*Rumen atony and collapse*
Diseases of cattle that cause anorexia and rumen stasis may result in the rumen collapse syndrome and a pung

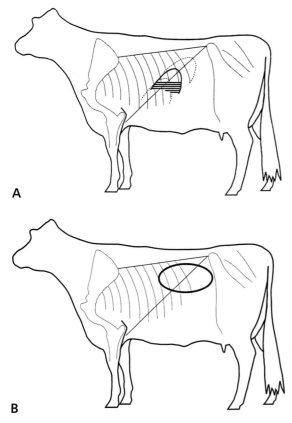

**A**

**B**

**Fig. 17.41** (A) Location of ping in left-side displacement of abomasum (clear zone). (The dotted lines represent the various locations of the left-displaced abomasum. The horizontal solid lines represent fluid levels in the displaced abomasum.) (B) Location of pings or pungs which may be audible by percussion and simultaneous auscultation over left paralumbar fossa in ruminal atony (rumen collapse).

(lower pitched than a ping) over the left abdomen in an area similar to where the ping is audible in left-side displacement of the abomasum (LDA) (Fig. 17.41A). It could therefore be misdiagnosed as LDA. The resonant sound is lower pitched – a pung – and its area is rectangular in shape, including the left paralumbar fossa but extending anteriorly and dorsally, resulting in a resonant sound over a much larger area than in LDA. The resonant sound is not associated with abdominal distension and the rumen pack cannot be palpated in the left paralumbar fossa. Rectal examination reveals the dorsal sac of the rumen to be collapsed in the left quadrant of the abdomen.

*Ruminal distension*
Distension of the rumen with foamy contents as in frothy bloat will result in a low-pitched tympanitic

sound. Distension with free gas will result in a medium-pitched ping or pung.

*Pneumoperitoneum*
The accumulation of air in the peritoneal cavity of cattle occurs following laparotomy. Both paralumbar fossae may be slightly enlarged and a dull ping may be detectable on percussion and auscultation of the upper third of both right and left abdomen.

### Ballottement of left abdomen

The left abdomen can be ballotted with the closed fist over the lower one-third of the left paralumbar fossa. Auscultation at the same time may reveal fluid-spashing sounds, which indicates the presence of fluid-filled viscera such as left displacement of the abomasum or an atonic rumen (Fig. 17.42).

### Tactile percussion of the abdomen

Tactile percussion of the abdomen is used to detect a fluid wave – an undulation of the abdominal wall created by a sharp percussion of the abdominal wall on the opposite side. It may be present when the abdominal cavity contains an excessive quantity of fluid. The tactile impulse of the percussion of one abdominal wall is transmitted across the fluid medium to the other side of the abdominal cavity, and the

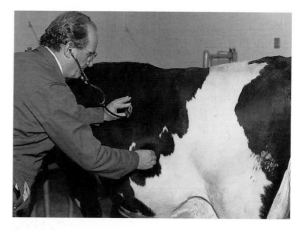

**Fig. 17.42** Ballottement and simultaneous auscultation of left abdomen.

### Clinical Pointer

At least the ventral one-third of the abdominal cavity must contain fluid before a fluid wave is detectable.

undulation can be seen and felt. The magnitude of the fluid wave depends on the presence of a certain amount of fluid in the peritoneal cavity.

A fluid wave can occur in any disease resulting in an excessive amount of fluid in the abdominal cavity, for example

- uroperitoneum
- ruptured bladder
- ascites associated with hepatic disease or congestive heart failure
- diffuse peritonitis.

## Examination of the right abdomen

The right abdomen is examined by inspection of the contour, palpation, ballottement, simultaneous percussion and auscultation, and succussion (shaking or rocking the animal from side to side). The primary objective is to detect the presence of viscera which are distended with gas, fluid, or ingesta.

### Inspection

The contour of the right abdomen is inspected for evidence of distension, which may be due to a viscus filled with fluid, gas or ingesta, ascites, or a gravid uterus. The common causes of abnormal distension of the right abdomen are

- dilatation and volvulus of the abomasum
- cecal dilatation and torsion
- acute intestinal obstruction, usually of the spiral colon
- abomasal impaction
- ascites.

In severe distension of the rumen the ventral sac may be markedly enlarged and may distend the lower half of the right abdomen. A marked gauntness of the right abdomen is present in chronic unthriftiness and prolonged inappetence.

### Palpation and ballottement

**External palpation**
Using the palms of both hands or the closed fist, the abdominal wall caudal to the right costal arch from the dorsal to ventral aspects is palpated for evidence of distension or heaviness, which may suggest an enlarged viscus or a gravid uterus, and for evidence of a grunt indicating pain (Fig. 17.27A).

The pregnant uterus after 7 months' gestation is easily detectable by ballottement. Deep palpation in the normal animal with both extended hands will reveal a resilient abdomen. The normal abomasum cannot be felt by external palpation. Palpation of a distended viscus in the right flank caudal or ventral to the right costal arch may be due to

- abomasal volvulus or impaction
- omasal impaction
- cecal dilatation and volvulus, and sometimes
- an enlarged ventral sac of the rumen extending over to the right abdominal wall, or
- enlargement of the liver.

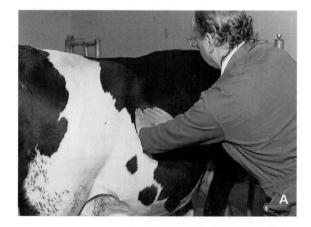

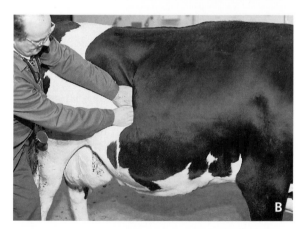

**Fig. 17.43** (A) Palpation of right abdomen. (B) Deep palpation of the right abdomen in cranial direction to feel enlarged liver.

---

**Clinical Pointer**

In the normal calf and in non-pregnant adult cattle, no organs or viscera can be palpated distinctly through the abdominal wall of the upper or lower right flank.

Impaction of the abomasum or omasum is characterized by a firm and doughy mass palpable behind the right costal arch from the middle third to the ventral third of the flank. An enlarged liver may be palpable immediately caudal to the middle third of the costal arch at the lower limits of the right paralumbar fossa (Fig. 17.43B). A rectal examination is necessary to identify the distended viscus and a laparotomy may be necessary to positively identify the lesion.

## Ballottement and succussion

Ballottement of the right abdomen is a variation of palpation and is useful for the detection of firm or solid masses situated near the abdominal wall (Fig. 17.44).

Using the extended fingers or the clenched fist, the examiner gives the abdominal wall a short jab. This causes any firm or tense mass to move away from the abdominal wall and then rebound, when it can be felt by the examiner. The best example is ballottement of the fetus in the right flank of cattle in late pregnancy (after 7–8 months). An impacted abomasum or omasum may also be palpable by simple deep palpation or ballottement of the abdominal wall.

Succussion is the shaking or moving of an animal from side to side while auscultating the abdomen for evidence of fluid-splashing sounds caused by fluid- and gas-filled intestines or viscera.

Fluid-splashing sounds audible on ballottement or succussion may be due to

- fluid-filled intestines in enteritis
- fluid-filled distended abomasum
- fluid- and gas-filled intestines in acute intestinal obstruction or diffuse peritonitis.

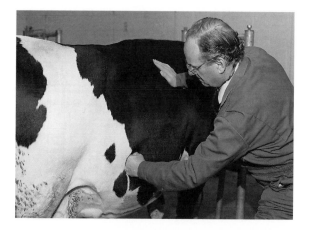

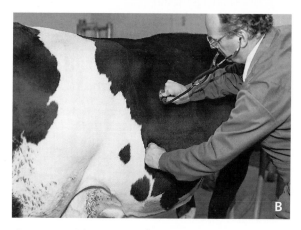

**Fig. 17.44**  (A) Ballottement of right abdomen. (B) Ballottement and auscultation of right abdomen.

---

### Clinical Pointer ✳

Free fluid in the peritoneal cavity will not usually cause fluid-splashing sounds on succussion or ballottement.

---

## Auscultation

In normal mature ruminating cattle, auscultation over the right flank will reveal the squishing peristaltic sounds of the small and large intestines about every 15–20 seconds. Auscultation over the right lower flank over the anatomical location of the abomasum, will reveal the squishing sounds of the contraction of the pyloric part of the abomasum. The intensity and frequency of these abomasal and intestinal sounds vary

widely from one animal to another and their presence or absence is not diagnostic. Fluid-rushing sounds audible over the right flank usually indicate the presence of an excessive quantity of intestinal contents, such as occurs in enteritis or grain overload.

When the intestines are distended with gas and fluid, it is often possible to elicit a ping by simultaneous percussion and auscultation of the abdominal wall directly over the abnormal intestine. Ballottement and

---

### Obstruction of the small and large intestine

This causes a decrease in frequency and intensity of normal peristaltic sounds. Eventually these sounds are completely absent and are replaced by fluid-tinkling sounds due to the movement of fluid and gas within distended loops of intestine.

---

succussion and simultaneous auscultation may reveal fluid-splashing sounds, which indicate that fluid and gas are in distended loops of intestine in acute intestinal obstruction, paralytic ileus and distension of the abomasum.

Fluid-rushing sounds audible on auscultation may be due to enteritis or acute intestinal obstruction.

### Percussion and simultaneous auscultation

The identification of structures and conditions responsible for pings over the right abdomen of adult cattle are depicted in Figures 17.45–17.55. The stippled areas represent the anatomical location and approximate relative size of the pings for each of the abnormalities. The causes of pings include

- right-side dilatation and volvulus of the abomasum
- cecal dilatation and torsion
- torsion of the coiled colon
- descending colon and rectum filled with gas associated with tenesmus
- intestinal tympany of uncertain etiology
- torsion of the root of the mesentery in young calves
- intussusception
- pneumoperitoneum
- intestinal tympany in the postparturient cow (postpartum pings).

---

### Clinical Pointer

Failure to release gas with a stomach tube in frothy bloat requires alternative techniques such as

- trocarization of the rumen
- administration of surface tension-reducing agents.

---

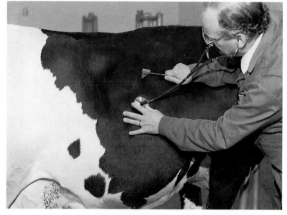

**Fig. 17.45** Percussion and simultaneous auscultation of right abdomen.

### Rumen contents

Examination of the rumen contents is often essential to help determine the state of the ruminal environment. Passage of a stomach tube into the rumen will determine the patency of the esophagus and whether there is increased intraruminal pressure associated with a frothy or free-gas bloat. In a free-gas bloat large quantities of gas are usually released within a minute. In a frothy bloat the ruminal end of the tube may become occluded by the froth and very little if any gas is released. Moving the tube back and forth within the rumen and blowing air into it to clear the ruminal end may result in the release of some gas.

When the tube is in the rumen some rumen juice can be siphoned or pumped out and collected for field and laboratory analysis. The color, depending to a limited extent on the feed, will be a green, olive green, or brown-green. In cattle on pasture or being fed good-quality hay the color is dark green. When silage or straw is the diet the color is yellow-brown. In grain overload the color of the rumen contents will be a milky-gray, and greenish-black in cases where rumen stasis is of long duration and where putrefaction is occurring. The consistency of the rumen contents is normally slightly viscid, and watery contents are indicative of inactive bacteria and protozoa. Excess froth is associated with frothy bloat, as in primary ruminal tympany or vagus indigestion. The odor of the rumen contents is normally aromatic and, although somewhat pungent, not objectionable. A moldy, rotting odor usually indicates protein putrefaction, and an intensely sour odor indicates an excess of lactic acid formation due to grain or carbohydrate engorgement. The pH of the rumen juice varies according to the type of feed and the time interval between the last feed and taking a sample for pH examination. The normal range, however, is between 6.2 and 7.2. The pH should be examined immediately after the sample is obtained, using a wide-range pH (1–11) paper.

| Rumen pH | |
|---|---|
| Normal | 6.2–7.2 |
| High | 8.0–10.0 |
| Low | 4.0–5.0 |

High pH values (8–10) will be observed when putrefaction of protein is occurring or if the sample is mixed with saliva. Low pH values (4–5) are found after the feeding of carbohydrates. In general, a value below 5 indicates carbohydrate engorgement and this level will be maintained for between 6 and

**Figs 17.46–17.55** Location of pings detectable on percussion and simultaneous auscultation of right abdomen of cattle.

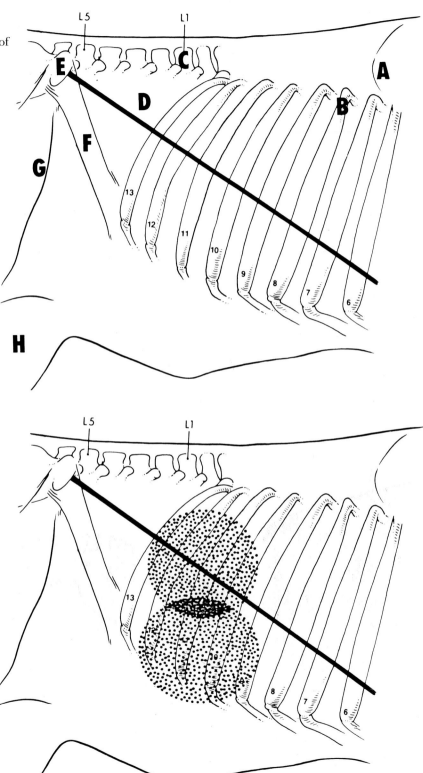

**Fig. 17.46** Right side of the bovine abdominal wall with reference points. A=caudal border of scapular cartilage; B=rib 8 (exposed ribs 6–13 are shown); C=first lumber vertebra (L1 and L5 are labeled; D=paralumbar fossa; E=tuber coxae; F=prominence caused by internal abdominal oblique muscle (caudovertebral border of paralumbar fossa); G=cranial border of tensor fasciae latae muscle; H=mammary gland. The straight line extends from the tuber coxae to the tuber olecrani (not shown). Smith et al. 1982).

**Fig. 17.47** Stippled regions represent typical areas of tympanitic resonance (ping) heard over the right side of the abdominal wall of adult cattle with conditions causing gas distension of intra-abdominal viscera. Right side displacement of the abomasum. Two commonly heard areas are indicated.

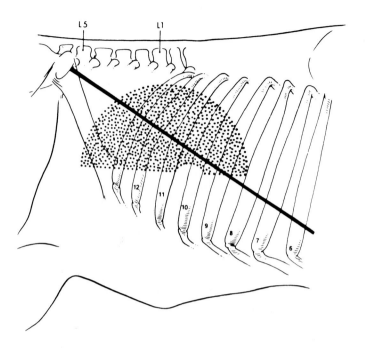

**Fig. 17.48** Volvulus of the abomasum (and omasum).

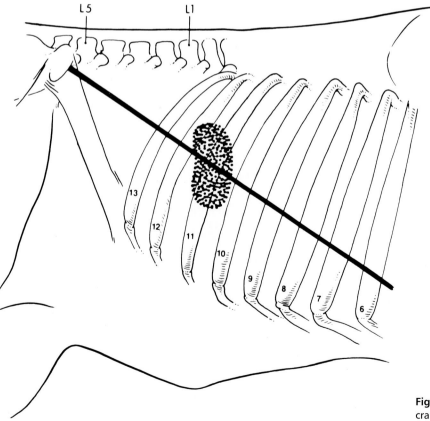

**Fig. 17.49** Dilatation of the cranial duodenum.

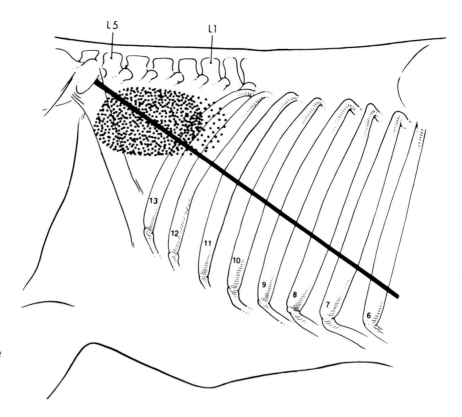

**Fig. 17.50** Dilatation of the cecum. The light stipple indicates the area where the ping is less commonly heard.

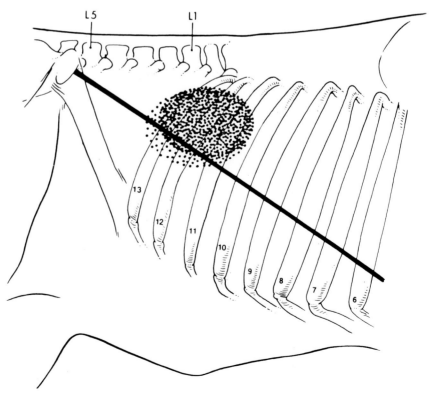

**Fig. 17.51** Dilatation of the ascending colon.

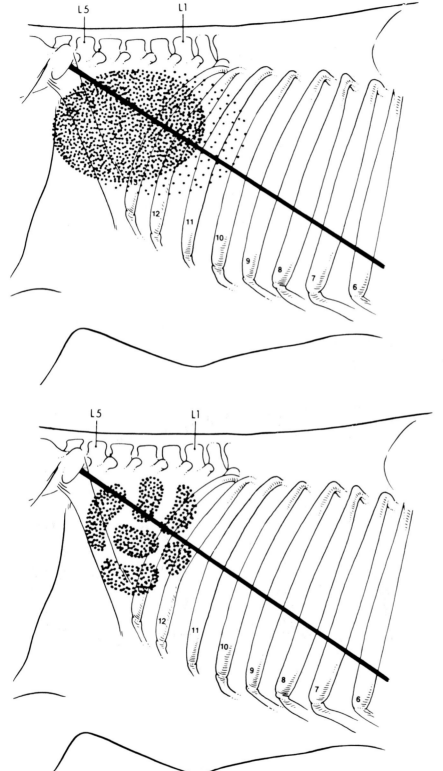

**Fig. 17.52** Dilatation and volvulus (rotation) of the cecum and ascending colon.

**Fig. 17.53** Dilatation of the jejunoileum.

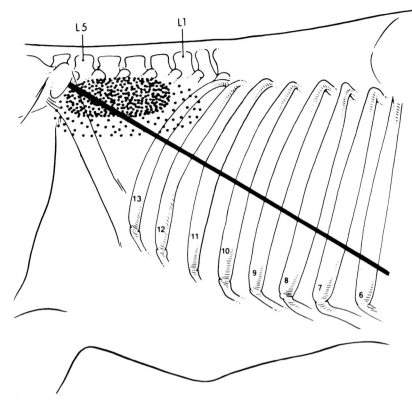

**Fig. 17.54** Dilatation of the descending colon and rectum.

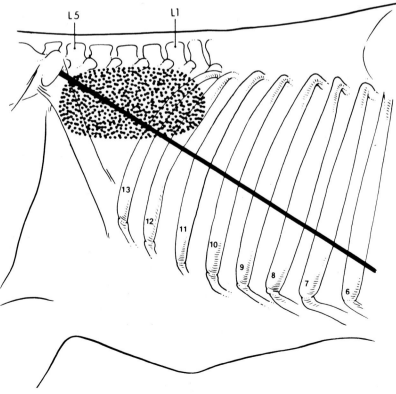

**Fig. 17.55** Pneumoperitoneum.

24 hours after the animal has actually consumed the carbohydrate diet. Microscopic examination of a few drops of rumen fluid on a glass slide with a low-power field will reveal the level of protozoan activity. Normally five to seven protozoans are active per low power field.

In adult cattle with severe abdominal distension due to gross distension of the rumen it is difficult, if not impossible, to assess the status of the abdomen. To determine whether the rumen is distended and/or to relieve the pressure, a large-bore stomach tube should be passed (Colorado Kingman Tube, 2 m long and 3 cm inside diameter). In vagus indigestion the rumen may be grossly distended with fluid contents, which will gush out through a large-bore tube: in some cases 100–150 liters may be released. If no contents are released it may be because the contents are frothy or mushy, and the rumen end of the tube will plug almost instantly. Rumen lavage may then be attempted using a water hose to deliver 20–40 liters of water at a time, followed by back drainage by gravity flow. After the rumen is partially emptied it is usually possible to assess both it and the abdomen more accurately.

The rumen contents of calves from about 1 week to 2 months of age affected with gastrointestinal disease may be abnormal. Affected calves are often presented with abdominal pain, a distended abdomen, fluid-splashing sounds in the rumen and over the right abdomen, diarrhea, and dehydration. The passage of a stomach tube will release significant quantities of abnormal odoriferous ruminal fluid.

---

### Clinical Pointer ✳

In lactic acidosis usually no active protozoa are seen in the rumen fluid, or only a few dead ones are visible.

---

## Examination of the abomasum

### Dilatation

Dilatation of the abomasum, which is usually right abomasal displacement, results in a syndrome of subacute pain suggestive of alimentary tract obstruction. There is distension of the right abdomen and the presence of fluid can be detected by palpation and combined percussion and auscultation, which induces a high-pitched ping when the abomasum contains fluid and gas (Fig. 17.47). Rectal examination will reveal the distended abomasum almost completely filling the lower right side of the abdomen, being almost comparable in size to the rumen; the wall is usually under considerable tension.

### Volvulus

Volvulus of the abomasum is a much more severe disease than right-side dilatation and displacement. Distension of the abdomen occurs as the result of distension of the abomasum with fluid and gas. In some instances there may be a bulge in the lower right paralumbar region. External palpation of the abdominal wall on the right side, below the costal arch, will reveal the existence of the distended tense viscus, and fluid-splashing sounds can be elicited. Auscultation with simultaneous percussion reveals a high-pitched ping (Fig. 17.48). The distended abomasum is usually palpable on rectal examination in the right side of the abdomen.

### Ulceration

The clinical findings in mature cattle depend on whether the ulcer

- erodes an artery of sufficient size to cause severe hemorrhage, or
- perforates the wall of the abomasum.

If perforation occurs local or diffuse peritonitis also occurs. With localized peritonitis omental adhesions develop. External palpation over the region of the right lower abdomen may elicit a painful response and the distended fluid-filled abomasum may be felt. Fluid-splashing sounds may be heard on ballottement and auscultation similar to those occurring in right-side displacement of the abomasum. Ulceration of the abomasum may also occur in left abomasal displacement, and perforation may occur resulting in localized peritonitis. Rupture of the abomasum results in diffuse peritonitis and shock and death within a few hours.

### Impaction

Impaction of the abomasum may be due to

- vagal nerve injury, as in vagus indigestion
- the ingestion of large quantities of poor-quality roughage, or
- the ingestion of sand or dirt along with certain diets.

---

### Acute and subacute hemorrhage from abomasal ulceration

- acute hemorrhage may cause death within 24 hours
- subacute hemorrhage causes sudden loss of appetite, mild abdominal pain, teeth grinding, heart rate up to 100 bpm, marked reduction in milk yield, melena, and the development of hemorrhagic anemia and scanty feces which are black and tarry in consistency, with occasional periods of diarrhea.

---

The enlarged abomasum will be situated in the right lower quadrant of the abdomen and will be palpable as a full and firm mass behind the right costal arch, extending from the middle to the ventral third. The impacted abomasum can usually be palpated on rectal examination in the right lower quadrant unless the animal is in advanced pregnancy. Commonly the omasum is also impacted and enlarged and can be palpated in the lower midline of the abdomen.

## Summary

Clinical examination of the right side of the abdomen is performed to detect the presence of enlarged organs such as the liver, or viscera distended with gas, fluid, or ingesta. A rectal examination will often assist in the identification of the distended viscus. A laparotomy may be necessary to accurately identify it, the extent of the distension or displacement, and the viability of its tissue and circulation. It is not possible on rectal palpation to determine the severity of the ischemic necrosis that may be present, which is important for the prognosis.

---

### Clinical Pointer

- gas-filled viscera are usually situated in the upper half of the right flank
- impacted viscera are usually in the lower half of the right flank.

---

# CLINICAL EXAMINATION OF THE INTESTINES

The intestines and their activity can be examined only to a limited extent using clinical examination techniques. The intestines are in the right side of the abdomen, but examination of the right abdomen is of limited value for the assessment of intestinal activity. The character of the feces, and other clinical findings such as hydration status and body condition, are indicators of the functional activity of the small and large intestines.

Clinical examination of the small and large intestines includes the detection of distension, abdominal pain, absence of feces, diarrhea and dysentery, and abnormal feces.

1. Distension of intestines with fluid and gas can result in distension of the abdomen, pings on percussion over the abdomen, and fluid-spashing sounds on ballottement and auscultation. Distended loops of intestine may be palpable on rectal examination.
2. Abdominal pain may be the result of distension of intestines with fluid and gas in acute intestinal obstruction or peritonitis. Abdominal pain may also be elicited on rectal examination of distended loops of intestine in acute intestinal obstruction.
3. A decrease in the amount or complete absence of feces for an extended period of time suggests intestinal obstruction, which may be due to a functional (adynamic ileus) or physical obstruction (dynamic ileus).
4. A profuse diarrhea with or without dysentery is characteristic of acute or chronic enteritis.
5. Abnormal feces indicate an enteropathy, either acute or chronic.

## Intestinal obstruction

Obstruction of the intestine is caused by torsion of the mesentery, intussusception and strangulation, in all of which there is virtually a complete absence of defecation for more than several hours, except for the passage of bloodstained mucus accompanied by severe shock and acute abdominal pain. In calves, torsion of the root of the mesentery is the most common form of intestinal obstruction.

An important clinical finding of intestinal obstruction is fluid-splashing sounds audible on ballottement and simultaneous auscultation of the right abdomen. The obstruction results in distended loops of intestine anterior to the obstruction which are filled with excessive fluid and gas, and are in a state of ileus. Auscultation over the distal part of the 13th rib and deep ballottement of the right flank will commonly elicit clear fluid-splashing sounds which are highly reproducible between observers and over a period of time.

In intestinal obstruction which develops suddenly with complete occlusion there is usually an episode of acute abdominal pain during which the animal

- is restless
- depresses its back
- kicks at the abdomen, and
- grunts or groans

all signs indicating severe pain. These behavioral changes are most pronounced in the young calf with acute intestinal obstruction. This and even more dramatic behavior, including rolling, continues spasmodically for between 6 and 12 hours in conjunction with complete anorexia and retention of feces. During this period the temperature and respiratory rate are not significantly altered and the heart rate increases moderately, compared to a similar abnormality in the horse.

When the period of acute pain is past, the signs of shock become more evident and the animal is more depressed, with complete absence of ruminal and intestinal motility. Careful rectal examination is important in order to identify distended loops of intestine.

When intestinal obstruction develops over a period of time, or is incomplete, as in dilatation and torsion of the cecum, the signs indicating pain are not so acute, also

- the appetite is suppressed to a variable degree
- lactating cattle show a decline in milk production over a period of days
- feces are passed more frequently but in small amounts, are soft in consistency, and may contain bloodstained mucus.

In the absence of strangulation and necrosis the animal survives for about 7 days, by which time moderate abdominal enlargement, somewhat pendulous in character, is apparent, along with signs of severe toxemia. Dilatation and torsion of the cecum may result in a distended right paralumbar fossa, with a tympanic or fluid sound on percussion and simultaneous auscultation. The temperature, pulse, and respirations may remain within normal ranges in the terminal stages. In the last phase a moderate degree of dehydration is clinically apparent, and hypochloremia and hypokalemia have a significant effect on the animal.

### Cecal dilatation and volvulus in cattle

In cecal dilatation without volvulus there are varying degrees of anorexia, mild abdominal discomfort, and a decreased amount of feces. In some cases there are no clinical signs and the dilated cecum is found coincidentally on rectal examination. A distinct ping may be elicited on percussion and simultaneous auscultation over the right paralumbar fossa, extending forward to the 10th intercostal space (Fig. 17.52). Simultaneous ballottement and auscultation of the right flank may elicit fluid-splashing sounds. There may be slight distension of the upper right flank, but in some cases the contour of the flank is normal. On rectal exami-

nation the distended cecum can usually be palpated as a long cylindrical movable organ measuring up to 20 cm in diameter and 90 cm in length. Palpation and identification of the blind end of the cecum directed towards the pelvic cavity is diagnostic. In simple dilatation the cecum is enlarged and easily compressible on rectal palpation.

In cecal volvulus

- anorexia
- ruminal stasis
- reduced amounts or the complete absence of feces
- distension of the right flank
- dehydration and tachycardia

are evident, depending on the severity of the volvulus and the degree of ischemic necrosis. There may be some evidence of mild abdominal pain, characterized by treading of the pelvic limbs and kicking at the abdomen. The area of tympanitic resonance is centered over the right paralumbar fossa and may extend to the 10th and 12th intercostal spaces. Fluid-splashing sounds are usually audible on ballottement and auscultation of the right flank. The cecum is usually distended with ingesta and feels enlarged and tense on rectal palpation. The blind end of the cecum may be displaced cranially and laterally or medially, and the body of the cecum is then felt in the pelvic cavity. Varying degrees of distension of the colon and ileum may occur, depending on the degree of displacement or volvulus present.

### Congenital atresia of intestine

Congenital atresia of the intestine and anus is a cause of intestinal obstruction in newborn calves. The abdomen may be grossly distended before birth when the defect is in the small intestine, and the distension may interfere with normal parturition.

In defects of the large intestine distension usually occurs after birth. In these the anus is normal and the part of the intestine caudal to the obstructed section may be normal or absent. The passage of a rectal tube or a barium infusion and radiography may assist in the detection of atresia of the intestine. There are usually large quantities of thick tenacious mucus in the rectum, with no evidence of meconium or feces. In the latter case only exploratory laparotomy can reveal the extent and nature of the defect. The principal clinical findings are depression, anorexia and abdominal distension. Frequently the owner has not seen the calf pass meconium or feces. In many cases the animal has not suckled since the first day and 5–6-day-old animals are very weak and recumbent. The intestine may rupture and acute diffuse peritonitis develop.

### Clinical Pointer

If cecal volvulus is suspected the animal must be handled with care, rectal palpation or transportation may cause rupture of the distended cecum. This is followed by shock and death within a few hours.

## Intestinal hypermotility

With an increase in the frequency of intestinal peristalsis the decreased transit time results in reduced intestinal absorption and a profuse diarrhea. Functional diarrhea occurs in excitement and is also an expression of disturbed motor nerve control. The passage of soft feces persists for a variable period in cattle when they are turned out to graze lush pasture in the spring season. The high water and protein content of the herbage is probably the important factor in producing this effect.

## Enteritis

The clinical manifestations of enteritis include

- diarrhea
- variable abdominal pain
- sometimes dysentery
- dehydration
- toxemia with fever in certain cases.

The signs vary considerably in severity according to the specific nature of the causal agent. In some acute systemic diseases enteritis is less obvious than in others in which it is a prominent feature initially. Chronic diarrhea is characterized by persistently abnormal feces, frequent defecation, unthriftiness, and inappetence.

## RECTAL EXAMINATION

In general, the procedure can be easily done on animals over 1 year of age. Depending on the breed it is usually not possible to do a rectal examination of the abdomen in cattle under 6–8 months of age.

The purpose of a rectal examination is to determine the presence or absence of abnormalities of the gastrointestinal tract which are not detectable with the general clinical examination, or abnormalities that might explain certain clinical findings. The presence of a ping over the right abdomen in a cow may suggest the presence of a dilated cecum, dilated abomasum, or intestinal tympany. A rectal examination may reveal the presence of a gas-filled viscus, which accounts for the ping, and the location of the viscus may provide clues to its identity. In other situations the general clinical examination may reveal no evidence of a specific abnormality in an animal with gastrointestinal dysfunction, but a rectal examination may reveal the presence of peritoneal adhesions, distended viscera, or multiple intra-abdominal masses. The general rule is, when the general examination reveals the presence of an uncertain abdominal abnormality a rectal examination should be performed.

## Restraint and equipment

The animal must be suitably restrained, ideally in a stanchion or stocks device which prevents movement from side to side. With most cattle kicking backwards is not a problem as it is in the horse, and anti-kicking hobbles or devices are not necessary.

A protective rubber or plastic glove and sleeve, thoroughly lubricated with liberal quantities of lubricant, is used and the prepared, glove-covered hand is introduced through the anal sphincter by extending the fingers in the form of a cone with the thumb pointing towards the base of the middle finger. The tone of the anal sphincter is reduced by gentle insertion of the fingers, and the hand is then inserted with a rotatory movement into the anal canal and then the rectum. Unnecessary force must be avoided and forward pressure applied with gentle caution.

Palpation is performed with the open hand, the extended fingers being maintained in close apposition. If, on introducing the hand, the rectum is found to be filled with feces, these should be removed before proceeding further. They can be removed manually or by stimulation of defecation by raking of the rectal wall with the fingers. If the animal arches its back during a rectal examination, patiently waiting for a minute or two will usually relax it. If the rectum is ballooned, peristaltic contractions and expulsion of the air, followed by collapse of the rectum, can be achieved by gently stroking its dorsal wall.

Rectal examination is best done in the standing animal. In the recumbent animal the gastrointestinal viscera, and the uterus of the cow in late pregnancy or within a few days after calving, will be displaced caudally towards the pelvic inlet, making it difficult to adequately palpate the structures which are normally palpable in the standing animal. The recumbent cow may have to be rolled from one side to the other in order to examine the caudal abdomen as much as possible.

A systematic method of palpating all accessible parts of the caudal abdominal cavity is used. For reference purposes, the abdomen is divided into four quadrants

- upper left
- lower left
- upper right
- lower right

as viewed from the animal's rear.

## Normal findings

Only the caudal part of the abdomen can be palpated. In the normal mature cow or bull the rectum usually contains several handfuls of feces of variable consistency, depending on the diet being fed. In cattle grazing on lush pasture the feces may be voluminous and soft. In animals fed large quantities of roughage the feces are well formed. In the normal animal the rectal mucosa feels smooth and the lubricant enables the slow introduction of the hand and arm into the rectum, which is the intrapelvic part of the descending colon. Within the pelvic cavity, the hand is moved in a systematic sequence to feel the different structures.

1. The bony pelvis can be felt ventrally, laterally, and dorsally.
2. Move the hand and arm forward along the floor of the pelvic cavity to feel the brim of the pelvis – a reliable landmark.
3. Beyond the pelvic brim the hand is in the descending colon, which has a longer mesentery than the rectum and is thus freely movable in all directions.
4. Move the hand and arm slowly forward until the caudal border of the left kidney is palpable, this represents another reliable landmark for rectal exploration of the abdomen of cattle.
5. By moving the hand from the kidney to the left upper quadrant the caudal part of the dorsal sac of the rumen can be felt and palpated with the extended fingers.
6. Slide the hand down the right lateral aspects of the dorsal sac of the rumen to feel the right longitudinal groove of the rumen, this marks the approximate junction of the dorsal and ventral sacs of the rumen.

Palpation of the right upper and lower quadrants of the caudal abdomen in normal cattle reveals a feeling of emptiness. The small and large intestines, including the cecum, cannot usually be felt because the intestines are displaced by the palpating hand. Occasionally a contracting segment of intestine can be grasped momentarily during peristalsis or segmentation. In the normal animal, ingesta in the spiral colon or in the cecum cannot be palpated. Feces may be present in the rectum and descending colon as far as can be reached within the lumen.

In large mature cattle, particularly large cows and bulls of the large breeds, it may not be possible to palpate the fullest extent of the caudal abdomen because of the long abdomen. It may be necessary to ask an experienced clinician with a longer arm to palpate the animal in order to identify certain abnormalities which may be difficult to reach.

## Non-specific abnormalities

Identification of abnormal findings in the gastrointestinal tract might lead to a specific diagnosis or merely to a conclusion about the nature of the disease process, from which further investigative or therapeutic approaches can be formulated. Non-specific abnormalities may indicate the need for an exploratory laparotomy or, if remarkable enough, may warrant a recommendation for euthanasia or slaughter for salvage.

Several different non-specific abnormalities may be found on palpation

- in diarrheic states the feces may be excessive in quantity and liquid in consistency
- alimentary tract hemorrhage is characterized by the presence of a variable amount of blood, which may be bright red, dark red, or black, depending on the location of the hemorrhage
- the feces may be scant and tenacious, or almost completely absent all the way up to the descending colon
- the rectal mucosa may be dry and feel roughened
- the animal may exhibit pain during the rectal palpation, which indicates the presence of inflammation or stretching of a serous membrane
- the palpable parts of the rumen may be grossly distended and extend dorsally to the sublumbar region, or the ventral sac may be enlarged and extend to the right lower quadrant
- the rumen may be smaller than normal and feel as though the dorsal sac is collapsed
- other viscera which may be palpable because of enlargement and/or distension include the cecum, abomasum, omasum, and intestines.

Gas- and fluid-filled viscera fluctuate on palpation;

viscera which are impacted will pit on digital pressure. Grasping and palpating a portion of a distended viscus may cause pain, which is manifested as grunting and tenesmus. Often it is only possible to just barely touch a distended viscus (volvulus of the abomasum) with the extended fingers, but its presence is a major diagnostic aid. Masses of varying shapes and sizes, including tumors, abscesses, and fat deposits, may be palpable anywhere in the caudal abdomen or pelvic cavity. Peritoneal adhesions feel like roughened surfaces and it may be possible to separate adherent viscera with the palpating hand.

The behavior of the animal during insertion of the hand into the rectum, and when the various organs are handled, is noted. In intestinal obstruction vigorous straining and pain result from the intestinal contractions that are induced. The rectum is also usually empty, except for a small quantity of bloodstained mucus which adheres to the hand and arm. Intestinal incarceration due to a tear in the mesentery, or through the development of peritoneal adhesions following injury or hemorrhage, may be palpable if the affected segment is within reach. Gaseous distension of the small intestine is not a marked feature in obstruction because fermentative digestion is of minor significance at this point in the digestive tract in cattle.

> ### Intussusception
>
> In intussusception of the small intestine the affected segment is sometimes palpable as a firm sausage-shaped mass, which when handled initiates a sharp painful reaction.

In torsion of the coiled portion of the colon distension of loops of small intestine does occur and is readily palpable. Dilatation and volvulus of the cecum is characterized by a grossly distended viscus extending into the pelvic inlet.

The strength and frequency of ruminal contractions, as well as the nature of the contents, which may be fluid, solid or gaseous, can be determined, as well as any reduction or increase in size. Reduction in size, in conjunction with displacement towards the median plane, occurs when the abomasum is displaced to the left. An increase in the size, so that the dorsal blind sac projects into the pelvis, occurs when the rumen is distended with contents or is tympanitic.

The cranial parts of the rumen, the reticulum, and the omasum, are inaccessible during rectal examination which is therefore of no direct value in assisting the diagnosis of traumatic reticuloperitonitis. When the abomasum has been displaced to the left there may be a feeling of emptiness in the right dorsal abdomen, with a reduction in the size of the rumen, and only rarely the distended abomasum may be palpable to the left of the rumen.

Extensive masses of fat necrosis and lipomas, which may surround the rectum, are readily palpable because of their mobility and firm consistency. Enlarged iliac and sublumbar lymph nodes, when recognized, suggest the presence of lymphomatosis.

## Specific abnormalities

Some of the common specific abnormalities of the gastrointestinal tract which may be palpable on rectal examination of cattle are described briefly. Some of the specific abnormalities of the digestive tract, which are commonly palpable on rectal examination are illustrated in Figure 17.56.

> ### Clinical Pointer
>
> The abomasum, normally out of reach during rectal examination, occasionally becomes so distended in dilatation and volvulus that it fills the right half of the abdomen and can be differentiated from the rumen on the left by the tense condition of its wall.

### L-shaped rumen (Fig. 17.56b)

This occurs commonly in vagus indigestion and chronic bloat, or any diseases of the reticulorumen characterized by gradual distension of the rumen. The caudal part of the dorsal sac of the rumen is grossly enlarged and commonly extends to the pelvic inlet. The ventral sac is easily palpable and extends to the right abdomen. The enlarged ventral sac may be mistaken for an enlarged abomasum, but can be distinguished from it by being continuous with the dorsal sac. Identification of the right longitudinal groove of the rumen will assist in determining that the enlarged ventral sac and dorsal sac are part of the same viscus. An impacted abomasum is separate from the rumen even though it may feel close to it.

### Cecal dilatation and volvulus (Fig. 17.56c)

Cecal dilatation is characterized by a long cylindrical dilated viscus with a blind end, commonly near the pelvic inlet. The dilated cecum may contain only gas, or it may contain soft ingesta and be tense and feel full of contents. In most cases, characteristically the enlarged cecum can be gently displaced. In some cases the blind end of the enlarged and twisted cecum has moved forward either medially or laterally, and the tense rounded body is palpable near the pelvic inlet.

## Right-side distension, displacement, and volvulus of the abomasum (Fig. 17.56d)

The tense fluid- and gas-filled viscus can be palpated in the upper right quadrant of the abdomen. In large cattle it may be possible to feel the presence of a tense viscus only with the fingertips; in other cases it may be possible to extend the fingers over part of the distended abomasum. In early dilatation the abomasum feels slightly tense; at volvulus stage it feels tense.

## Abomasal impaction (Fig. 17.56e)

The abomasum is palpable as a doughy mass in the right lower quadrant of the abdomen. It may require several minutes to move the palpating hands slowly toward the impacted abomasum. It is usually not palpable in late pregnancy because of the gravid uterus.

## Left-side displacement of the abomasum (Fig. 17.56f)

It is not usually possible to palpate a left-side displacement of the abomasum because it is out of reach by rectal examination. Rare cases of severe displacements are sometimes palpable as a gas-filled viscus lateral to the left aspect of the rumen, which is usually smaller than normal and may feel slightly displaced to the right by the displaced abomasum.

## Intussusception (Fig. 17.56g)

An intussusception may be palpable as a firm cylindrical tubular structure in the right side of the abdomen. In most cases of acute intestinal obstruction the intussusceptum is not palpable, but gas- and fluid-filled distended loops of intestine cranial to the obstruction may be palpable in the right abdomen. In intestinal incarceration a distended loop of intestine may be felt passing through a portion of the mesentery.

## Mesenteric torsion (Fig. 17.56h,i)

Torsion of the root of the mesentery of the intestine is uncommon in adult cattle. Distended loops of intestine are palpable over a large part of the right abdomen.

## Peritonitis (Fig. 17.56j)

Fibrinous adhesions may be palpable in acute local or diffuse peritonitis involving the caudal abdomen. The affected surfaces are roughened and palpation between loops of intestine, which are adhered together or to the abdominal wall, elicits a feeling of separating two pieces of buttered bread.

## Lipomatosis (Fig. 17.56k)

These are commonly palpable as 'lumps' or floating corks in the abdomen and pelvic cavity. They are usually freely movable.

## Omental bursitis (Fig. 17.56l)

This abnormality is characterized by a large firm to soft mass palpable in the midline below the left kidney, far forward in the caudal abdomen.

As part of the differential diagnosis of digestive tract disease in the postparturient cow the uterus should be examined for evidence of retained placenta and metritis. Both vaginal and rectal examinations should be done. The toxemia caused by retained fetal membranes and postpartum metritis may cause anorexia, rumen stasis, paralytic ileus, scant feces, and sometimes a 'ping' in the right flank, all of which may be misinterpreted as primary digestive tract diseases.

## Defecation and feces

Cattle defecate 10–18 times a day, usually just after standing up and during feeding. Defecation is accompanied by slight arching of the back and raising of the tail. Tenesmus, or straining as if to pass feces, may occur if the feces are firm and dry or if there is inflammation in the rectum or in the soft tissues of the pelvic cavity. Acute or chronic peritonitis may also cause painful defecation because of the pain caused by the posturing for defecation. In tenesmus, the tail is often held up continuously. The passage of small quantities of feces (scant feces) or the complete absence of feces in cattle indicates failure of movement of ingesta caudally in the digestive tract. The most common causes are

- acute intestinal obstruction
- failure of outflow from the forestomach and abomasum
- ileus due to peritonitis or acid–base imbalances.

Rarely there is paralysis of the rectum, which becomes

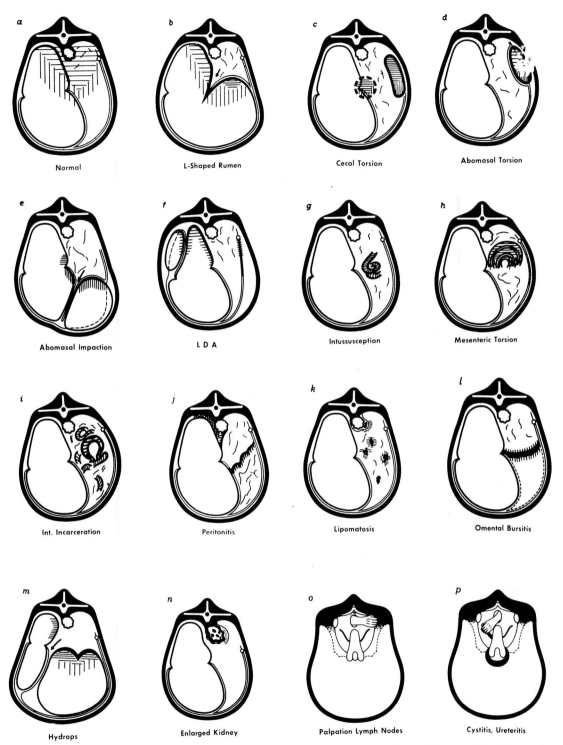

**Fig. 17.56** (a–p) Schematic illustrations of the rectal findings in cattle affected with different diseases of the abdominal viscera. (From Stober and Dirksen, 1977) courtesy of the authors and the editor of *Bovine Practitioner*. (Fig. 17.40a–l illustrates the abnormalities through a transverse section of the abdomen; Fig. 17.40m–p are included for the differential diagnosis of the diseases each represents)

impacted with firm feces. Diarrhea is the frequent passage of liquid feces and indicates abnormality of gastrointestinal function, usually enteritis or dietary indigestion.

## Gross examination of feces

The gross appearance of the feces is not only an indicator of disease of the digestive tract but can provide valuable clues for the differential diagnosis of disease elsewhere.

### Amount

A reduction in the bulk of feces can be due to a decrease in feed or water intake or a retardation of the passage through the alimentary tract. In diarrhea the feces are passed more frequently and in greater amounts than normal, and contain a higher water content (over 90%).

Diseases causing disturbances of motility of the reticulorumen and abomasum often result in a relative absence of feces. Ileus due to peritonitis or idiopathic intestinal tympany also results in a marked reduction in feces – sometimes a complete absence – for up to 3 days. The marked reduction of feces that occurs in functional obstruction is a major source of diagnostic confusion because it resembles physical obstruction of the intestines. The causes of physical and functional obstruction of the alimentary tract of cattle are summarized in Figure 17.57.

> ### Clinical Pointer
>
> Failure to pass any feces for 24 hours or more is abnormal, and may be due to physical or functional intestinal obstruction.

### Color

The color of the feces is influenced by the

- nature of the feed
- concentration of bile in the feces
- passage rate through the digestive tract.

Calves reared on cow's milk normally produce gold-yellow feces, which become pale brown when hay or straw is eaten. The feeding of milk substitutes adds a variable gray component.

The feces of adult cattle eating green forage are dark olive-green; on a hay ration they are more brown-olive;

and the ingestion of large amounts of grain produces olive-gray feces. A retardation of the ingesta causes the color to darken. The feces become ball-shaped and dark brown, with a shining surface due to the mucus coating. Diarrheic feces tend to be paler than normal because of their higher water content and lower concentration of bile.

The presence of large amounts of bile produces a dark olive-green to black-green color, as in cattle with hemolytic anemia. In cattle with obstruction of the common bile duct the feces are pale olive-green because of the absence of bile pigments.

### Blood

Blood in the feces may originate in the following ways.

- The swallowing of blood coughed up from pulmonary hemorrhage (uncommon, usually detected as occult blood with Hemetest tablets).
- Hemorrhage into the abomasum: acute hemorrhage usually appears as tarry black feces (melena); chronic hemorrhage as occult blood. The degree of darkness or the presence of melena depends primarily on the degree of hemorrhage and the amount of blood entering the lumen of the stomach or the intestines.
- Hemorrhagic enteritis of the small intestines; the feces are uniformly dark red.
- Hemorrhagic enteritis of the large intestines. Blood originating in the cecum or colon appears as frank blood evenly distributed throughout the feces. Blood originating in the rectum appears as streaks or chunks of frank blood unevenly distributed throughout the feces (hematochezia).

If the feces are dark-colored and alimentary tract hemorrhage is suspected, the occult blood test can be used to detect the presence of the heme ion (from the blood).

### Odor

Fresh bovine feces are not normally malodorous. Objectionable odors are usually due to putrefaction or fermentation of ingesta, which are usually associated with inflammation. The feces of cattle with salmonellosis may be fetid, and in advanced pericarditis with visceral edema due to passive congestion, the feces are profuse but do not have a grossly abnormal odor.

### Consistency

The consistency of the feces depends on the water content, the type of feed, and the length of time the ingesta have remained in the digestive tract. Normally, milk-fed calves excrete feces of a medium to firm porridge-like consistency. After transition to a plant

# SOME COMMON CAUSES OF PHYSICAL AND FUNCTIONAL OBSTRUCTION OF THE ALIMENTARY TRACT OF CATTLE

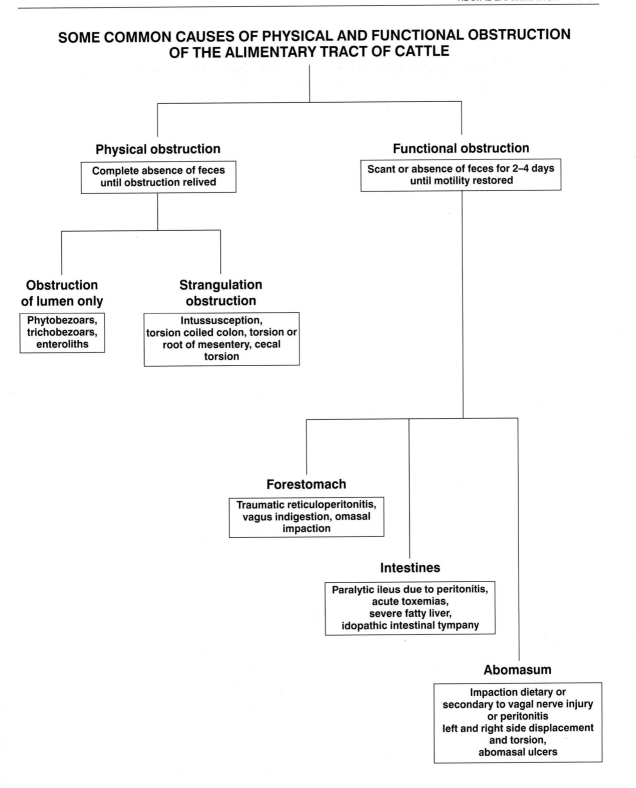

**Physical obstruction**

Complete absence of feces until obstruction relived

**Functional obstruction**

Scant or absence of feces for 2–4 days until motility restored

**Obstruction of lumen only**

Phytobezoars, trichobezoars, enteroliths

**Strangulation obstruction**

Intussusception, torsion coiled colon, torsion or root of mesentery, cecal torsion

**Forestomach**

Traumatic reticuloperitonitis, vagus indigestion, omasal impaction

**Intestines**

Paralytic ileus due to peritonitis, acute toxemias, severe fatty liver, idopathic intestinal tympany

**Abomasum**

Impaction dietary or secondary to vagal nerve injury or peritonitis left and right side displacement and torsion, abomasal ulcers

**Fig. 17.57**  Some common causes of physical and functional obstruction of the alimentary tract of cattle.

diet the first solid particles begin to appear. Normal bovine feces are of a medium porridge-like consistency. A moderate thickening leads to the passage of fecal disks of a more solid consistency, and severe dehydration causes the formation of firm balls arranged in facets inside the rectum, the surfaces of which are dark and coated with mucus.

### Degree of digestion

The proportion of poorly digested plant particles in the feces depends on the duration and thoroughness of rumination and the rate of passage of ingesta through the forestomach. The length of time the ingesta are in the postruminal digestive tract seems to have no appreciable influence on digestion. Poor comminution of feces indicates failure in rumination and/or the accelerated passage of ingesta through the forestomachs. Thus in some cattle with acute traumatic reticuloperitonitis the feces may contain small walnut-sized chunks of undigested plant fibers which have escaped the cellulose digestive processes of the forestomachs. The presence of large numbers of grain kernels in the feces is associated with the ingestion of large quantities of unprocessed grain, such as whole wheat or barley.

---

### Abnormal feces

- left displacement of the abomasum → pasty feces
- obstruction of the forestomachs (vagus indigestion, chronic peritonitis) → sticky and tenacious feces.

---

## Other substances in feces

### Mucus

The presence of mucus on the surface of fecal balls suggests increased transit time of the ingesta in the large intestine. The presence of a plug of mucus in the rectum is suggestive of a functional obstruction (ileus). In enteritis, large quantities of clear watery mucus may be passed which sometimes clot to form gelatinous masses.

### Fibrin

In fibrinous enteritis, as occurs commonly in enteric salmonellosis, fibrin may be excreted in the form of long strands which may mold into a print of the intestinal lumen (intestinal fibrinous casts).

### Laboratory examination of feces

The kind of laboratory examination carried out on fecal samples will depend on the suspected diagnosis. Because of the cost, it is desirable to select only those examinations that are likely to yield diagnostically useful results.

Feces can be examined in the laboratory for many pathogens and substances, including

- chemicals, heavy metals such as arsenic, lead, and many other toxic agents
- intestinal helminth ova
- protozoal oocysts
- bacteria and viruses.

---

### Techniques to detect enteropathogenic bacteria and viruses

- cultural isolation techniques
- indirectly by immunofluorescence
- the newer DNA probe techniques.

---

## DETECTION AND LOCALIZATION OF ABDOMINAL PAIN

The manifestations of abdominal pain in cattle and calves varies widely. Acute abdominal pain in mature cattle with acute intestinal obstruction may be manifested by stretching of the body with depression of the back, kicking at the abdomen and restlessness. In calves, acute abdominal pain is usually more dramatic and is characterized by bellowing, repeatedly lying down and standing up, compulsive walking and restlessness, and pain on palpation. However, some mature cattle with intestinal obstruction may not exhibit outward signs of abdominal pain and its presence must be determined by close clinical examination.

A grunt is a guttural sound caused by a forced expiration against a closed glottis. In cattle, a grunt is best elicited using deep palpation with the closed fist or the examiner's knee applied to the abdomen at the end of inspiration and the beginning of expiration. The inspiratory and expiratory breath sounds are auscultated over the trachea with a stethoscope for a few respirations and then, without warning, deep palpation pressure is applied. The presence of a grunt indicates the presence of a lesion of a serous membrane, including the peritoneum, pleura, and pericardium (stretching, inflammation, edema). The absence of a grunt does not, however, exclude the presence of a peritoneal lesion. In acute traumatic reticuloperitonitis the grunt may be absent or barely audible and inconclusive 3–5 days after the initial penetration of the reticulum.

A rigid bar or wooden pole may be necessary to apply sufficient pressure to the abdomen in large cattle (large mature cows and bulls)

- with the aid of two assistants the bar is held in a horizontal position just behind the xiphoid sternum
- a third person auscultates over the trachea when the bar is lifted quickly up into the abdomen
- several attempts to elicit a grunt are made before concluding its absence
- the ventral and both sides of the abdomen are examined, beginning at the level of the xiphoid sternum and moving caudally to a point caudal to the umbilicus, thus the anterior and caudal aspects of the abdomen will be examined for evidence of painful points.

---

### Grunting as an indication of pain

A grunt or groan is characteristic of abdominal and thoracic pain in cattle

- animals with acute local or diffuse peritonitis may grunt spontaneously with almost every respiration
- the grunt is exaggerated in the recumbent position
- grunting may also be caused by severe pneumonia, pleurisy, and severe pulmonary emphysema
- careful auscultation and percussion of the thorax are necessary to exclude the presence of pulmonary disease
- not all grunts occur spontaneously, deep palpation of the abdomen using the closed hand or knee may be necessary to elicit a grunt
- simultaneous auscultation over the trachea is often necessary to hear the grunt.

---

Manual pinching of the withers in the average-sized cow to depress the animal's back is also used to elicit a grunt. In an animal with an inflammatory lesion of the peritoneum a grunt elicited in this way may be audible without auscultation over the trachea, but auscultation will usually be necessary.

The term **cranial abdominal pain** refers to abdominal pain associated with several diseases of the cranial abdomen of cattle, which would include traumatic reticuloperitonitis, hepatic abscesses, abomasal ulcers and intestinal obstruction. The differential diagnosis includes diseases that cause thoracic pain, such as pleuritis, pericarditis, and severe pulmonary disease (Fig. 17.58).

## CLINICAL EXAMINATION OF THE LIVER

In cattle, the liver is situated entirely in the right half of the abdominal cavity. Topographically it is covered by the right ribcage and cannot be palpated in its normal state. The liver extends from its most cranial point at the level of the 6th intercostal space, with its long axis extending caudodorsally to the 12th intercostal space or the dorsal end of the 13th rib, with its caudoventral border extending ventrally to about the ventral aspect of the 10th intercostal space. The normal area of liver dullness and any increase in size can be outlined using acoustic percussion.

If the liver in cattle is grossly enlarged its edge can be felt on deep palpation caudal to the costal arch, usually at the middle third. The edge of the enlarged liver is usually rounded and thickened, compared to the more defined edge of its normal counterpart. The liver may be enlarged and palpable in cases of

- advanced right-sided congestive heart failure
- multiple liver abscesses
- diffuse hepatitis.

---

### Clinical Pointer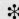

An enlarged liver may be felt by

- deep palpation caudal to the costal arch, at the middle third
- rectal examination in the right upper and lower quadrant in a very cranial direction.

---

## EXAMINATION OF THE ORAL CAVITY, PHARYNX, AND ESOPHAGUS

### Oral cavity

When there are obvious clinical manifestations of disease of the oral cavity it can be examined before any other part of the alimentary tract. Such clinical manifestations include

- drooling saliva because of painful conditions of the oral cavity and inability to swallow
- protrusion of the tongue associated with inflammation or paralysis of the tongue
- inability to prehend because of painful lesions of the tongue
- difficulty or painful mastication
- difficulty swallowing
- regurgitation following difficult swallowing, with resultant dropping of cuds out of the mouth
- smacking of the lips owing to painful conditions of the lips and oral cavity
- foul-smelling odor due to necrotic lesions of the oral cavity
- swellings of the cheeks associated with impaction of feed between the cheek teeth and cheek mucosa.

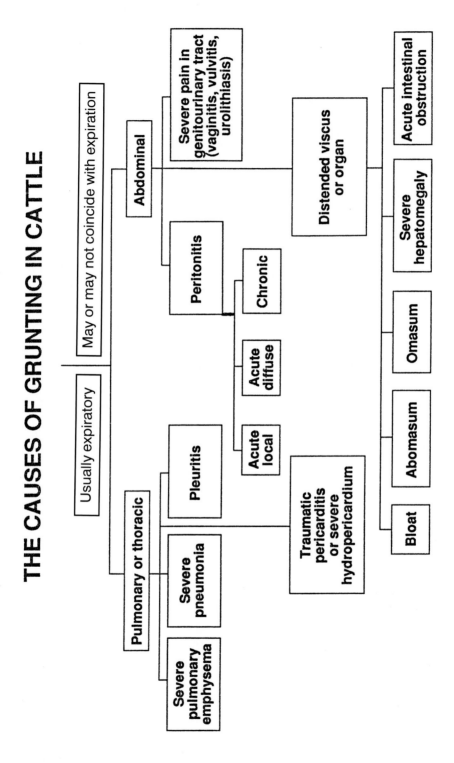

Fig. 17.58 Causes of grunting in cattle.

Suitable restraint is required for a detailed examination of the oral cavity. Protective gloves are recommended, especially if rabies is a possibility. It may be necessary to use a pair of nose tongs for additional restraint. The oral cavity of the newborn calf is easy to open and examine (Figs 17.59A, B, 17.60, 17.61).

Examination of the oral cavity should begin with inspection of the mucosa and mucocutaneous junctions of the lips.

The upper lip of cattle is thick, firm, and not very mobile. Its central portion is hairless and takes part in the formation of the nasolabial plate. The upper lip is covered with hair laterally, including tactile hairs. Relative to the large oral cavity, the lips are short. The lower lip, being shorter, is slightly covered by the margin of the upper lip. The external surface of the lower lip is covered with hair and also has tactile hairs.

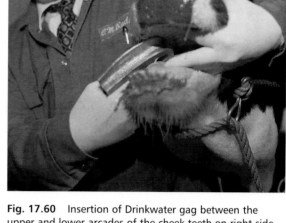

**Fig. 17.60** Insertion of Drinkwater gag between the upper and lower arcades of the cheek teeth on right side.

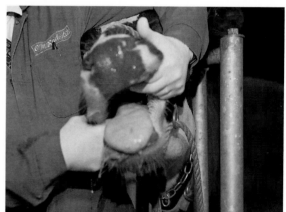

**Fig. 17.61** Gag held securely in place with hand.

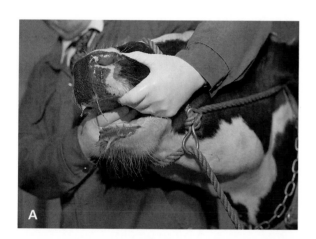

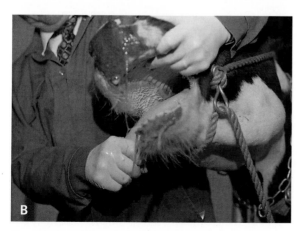

**Fig. 17.59** (A) Opening the mouth using two hands, (B) grasping tongue with one hand.

At the free margin the hair-covered skin gives way to a narrow hairless zone with small rounded papillae along the edge of the lip. The chin is well developed and consists mainly of adipose tissue. Numerous cornified labial papillae are present on the inside of the lips near the angle of the mouth. They are caudally directed conical outgrowths of the mucous membrane and are continued on the inside of the cheeks. The labial glands are concentrated in the vicinity of the angle of the mouth, and are often imbedded between bundles of the labial muscles. The short lips and oral cleft make both inspection of the caudal parts of the oral cavity and oral surgery difficult, even when the animal's mouth is fully opened.

The lateral aspects of the upper lips are retracted dorsally to view the mucosae and the papillae of the upper and lower lips. The lower lip adjacent to the

### Clinical Pointer

In stomatitis, accumulations of viscid and foamy saliva are common in the mucosae of the commissures of the mouth.

incisor teeth is also everted for inspection. The mucosae of the commissures of the mouth are examined at the same time for evidence of pallor, icterus, hemorrhages, and mucosal lesions such as erosions, vesicles, ulcers, traumatic injuries and proliferative lesions.

The oral cavity of cattle is capacious and distensible. Its mucosa carries the large conical buccal papillae, which are directed toward the pharynx and are covered with a cornified epithelium. They are longest and most numerous around the angle of the mouth and decrease in size and number caudally.

The hard palate is wide rostrally and caudally, with a narrow part in the middle. In ruminants the upper incisors are absent and are replaced by a dental pad. This is a thick semilunar plate of dense connective tissue attached to the underlying body of the incisive bone. The tough mucous membrane covering the pad has a thick, heavily cornified epithelium. A narrow caudal zone of the dental pad carries short conical papillae and, centrally, the incisive papilla. The latter is surrounded by a circular groove, into the bottom of which the incisive ducts open on each side of the papilla. The mucous membrane of the hard palate overlies a layer of venous plexuses and may either be partly or completely pigmented. The palatine ridges number 15–19 in cattle, are set with caudally directed horny papillae and gradually diminish in size, so that caudal to the level of the second cheek teeth the hard palate is smooth.

In mature cattle, with suitable restraint of the head and neck and with the examiner standing beside the animal's head and neck and facing in the same direction as the animal, the oral cavity is opened by

- placing one hand over the head and into the side of the mouth while the opposite hand is available to assist
- the hand over the head of the animal is inserted into the mouth and moved towards the hard palate of the upper jaw
- the oral cavity can usually be held open with ease by maintaining slight hand contact with the hard palate
- the other hand is free to illuminate the mouth with a flashlight and to grasp the tongue.

The tongue of cattle is firm and plump, highly mobile and protusile, and has an important function in the prehension of feed. The rounded borders of its pointed apex blend caudally with the high lateral surfaces of the body. The lingual frenulum is wide. The caudal part of the dorsum of the tongue is raised and forms the characteristic oval torus linguae, rostral to which is the transverse fossa linguae of varying depths. The mucous membrane of the dorsum of the tongue is thick, firm, often pigmented, and adheres intimately to the subjacent tissues.

- The filiform papillae are directed caudally, pointed and threadlike, and are found on the dorsum rostral to the fossa.
- The papillae on the torus are either blunt and conical or round and flat, and decrease in number toward the root of the tongue.
- The fungiform papillae are numerous, especially along the edges of the apex, but are also found in smaller numbers on the dorsum and along the lateral surfaces of the tongue.
- The vallate papillae number 8–17 on each side. They vary in size, and form irregular rows on each side of the caudal part of the torus.

### Clinical Pointer

Occasionally barbed awns or husks of grain lodge in the fossa of cattle and cause infection of the tongue.

### Ingestion of foreign bodies

The rasp-like tongue and the caudally directed papillae make it difficult for ruminants to discharge foreign bodies from the mouth. Domestic ruminants, particularly cattle that eat fast with poor mastication, swallow many foreign bodies, such as nails and pieces of wire, these settle in the reticulum of the stomach causing traumatic reticuloperitonitis.

The rasp-like roughness of the tongue, the papillae on the palatine ridges and the large caudally directed papillae on the lips and cheeks facilitate the prehension and swallowing of coarse feed.

A cloth towel will assist in grasping the tongue if it is slippery from excess saliva. The tongue is retracted from the mouth and pulled to one side and then the other, so that it can be examined for evidence of lesions. During this process a large part of the oral cavity can be inspected.

A lack of tone in the tongue is characterized by the tongue being pulled out of the mouth with little effort and the animal unable to retract it. This suggests glossoplegia due to a defect in the hypoglossal nerve.

The mucosa of the oral cavity is normally warm to touch, salmon pink in color, glistening, and (slightly) slippery with saliva. It is examined visually for discoloration, such as pallor, icterus and cyanosis, and by palpation for the hypothermia and dryness of dehydration and shock, and mucosal lesions. Erosions, vesicles, ulcers, traumatic injuries, and proliferative lesions are distinct and must be recognized in order to make a definitive diagnosis.

The tone of jaw muscles can be assessed by the force needed to open the mouth and keep it open manually. Some cattle resist having their mouths opened but this is usually due to fractious behavior. Trismus, or lockjaw as occurs in tetanus, is characterized by the inability to open the mouth even with excessive manual force. Lack of tone in the jaw muscles and the dropped jaw syndrome are usually associated with cranial nerve deficits or fracture of the mandible.

## Clinical Pointer

Using a strong light source the oral cavity is examined carefully, the erosions of mucosal disease may occur on any aspect of the tongue and throughout the oral cavity, including the lower lips.

Abnormal odors may be noted when the mouth is opened and can provide some indication of the lesions present or of systemic illness

- cattle with acetonemia have an acetone breath
- cattle with advanced azotemia associated with pyelonephritis may have a uremic breath
- a foul necrotic odor is associated with oral necrobacillosis in calves.

Cattle which have been eating normally may have a bolus of partially masticated feed in the mouth.

## Clinical Pointer

The capillary refill time of the gingiva in cattle is not as reliable a test for peripheral perfusion as it is in the horse.

Regurgitated rumen contents may be present in the oral and nasal cavities of cattle which have had third-stage milk fever. Foreign bodies, such as small pieces of wood, wire, and other objects that cattle may attempt to swallow, can often be found in the oral cavity.

Calves with oral necrobacillosis may have large necrotic ulcers almost anywhere in the oral cavity, but commonly on the dorsum of the tongue and in the cheek mucosa. The ulcers are painful, covered with foul-smelling necrotic material, and may be impacted with feed. A newborn calf with a history of difficulty in sucking but a desire to suck may have a cleft palate, which is very obvious when the mouth is opened and the hard palate examined.

## Actinobacillosis

An enlarged firm and lumpy tongue which may be protruding slightly from the oral cavity is characteristic of actinobacillosis of the tongue (wooden tongue). There may be no clinical evidence of the lesion except anorexia, and failure to examine the oral cavity would result in the diagnosis being missed.

## Teeth

The teeth of cattle, sheep, and goats consist of the lower incisors, and the upper and lower premolars and molars. Evaluation of the teeth requires knowledge of the formulae of dentition, including the age at which the deciduous teeth are replaced and eruption of the permanent teeth. The age of domestic ruminants can be determined from the

- eruption and replacement of teeth
- size and shape of the occlusal surfaces of the incisors
- loss of teeth in advanced age.

All the deciduous incisor teeth may be present at birth or erupt within a few days, and are functional by 2–4 weeks of age.

The formula for deciduous dentition in ruminants is

$$2[Di0/4, Dc0/0, Dp3/3, Dm0/0] = 20$$
where Di  = deciduous incisors
     Dc  = deciduous canines
     Dp  = deciduous premolars
     Dm  = deciduous molars

The incisor teeth can be used to determine the age of cattle, sheep, and goats. In addition to their numerical designation, I1 to I4, the incisors are also known, respectively, as central, first intermediate, second intermediate, and corner incisors. Each of them has a shovel-shaped asymmetrical crown which is slightly more drawn out laterally. The eruption and replacement of teeth in cattle, sheep and goats are summarized in Tables 17.3, 17.4, and 17.5.

The formula for the permanent dentition of cattle, sheep and goats is:

$$2[I0/4, C0/0, P3/3, M3/3] = 32$$

where D is deciduous, I is incisor, C is canine, P is premolar and M is molar. The incisor teeth are used for gripping and cutting forage and their periodontium is modified to accept rotating or turning forces encountered during grazing. These anatomical modifications allow the normal incisors to move up anteroposteriorly under gentle pressure. The periodontium of the cheek teeth is designed to hold the teeth in place against the downward and lateral forces of cudding.

Dental disease is an economically important problem in sheep flocks and requires knowledge of the normal dentition and the clinical manifestations of dentition. Scoring systems for the clinical examination of the incisors of sheep for evidence of broken mouth have been described. The teeth of sheep can be examined by straddling and restraining the animal and retracting the lips. Examination of the lingual aspect of the

**Table 17.4.  Eruption and replacement of teeth in sheep**

| Teeth | Time of * eruption | Teeth | Time of replacement* |
|-------|--------------------|-------|----------------------|
| Di /1 | Before birth to up to 8 days | I /1 | 12–18 months |
| Di /2 | Before birth | I /2 | 21–24 months |
| Di /3 | Before birth | I /3 | 27–36 months |
| Di /4 | Birth to up to 8 days | I /4 | 36–48 months |
| Dp 2/2 | Before birth to up to 4 weeks | P 2/2 | 21–24 months |
| Dp 3/3 | Before birth to up to 4 weeks | P 3/3 | 21–24 months |
| Dp 4/4 | Before birth to up to 4 weeks | P 4/4 | 21–24 months |
| M 1/1 | 3 months | | |
| M 2/2 | 9 months | | |
| M 3/3 | 18 months | | |

* The lower figures are for early-maturing breeds, the higher figures for late-maturing breeds.

**Table 17.3.  Eruption and replacement of teeth in cattle**

| Teeth | Time of * eruption | Teeth | Time of replacement* |
|-------|--------------------|-------|----------------------|
| Di /1 | Before birth | I /1 | 14–25 months |
| Di /2 | Before birth | I /2 | 17–33 months |
| Di /3 | Before birth to up to 2–6 days | I /3 | 22–40 months |
| Di /4 | Before birth to up to 2–14 days | I /4 | 32–42 months |
| Dp 2/2 | Before birth to up to 14–21 days | P 2/2 | 24–28 months |
| Dp 3/3 | Before birth to up to 14–21 days | P 3/3 | 24–30 months |
| Dp 4/4 | Before birth to up to 14–21 days | P 4/4 | 28–34 months |
| M 1/1 | 5–6 months | | |
| M 2/2 | 15–18 months | | |
| M 3/3 | 24–28 months | | |

* The lower figures are for early-maturing breeds, the higher figures for late-maturing breeds.

**Table 17.5.  Eruption and replacement of teeth in goats**

| Teeth | Time of eruption | Teeth | Time of replacement |
|-------|------------------|-------|---------------------|
| Di /1 | At birth | I /1 | 15 months |
| Di /2 | At birth | I /2 | 21 months |
| Di /3 | At birth | I /3 | 27 months |
| Di /4 | 1–3 weeks | I /4 | 36 months |
| Dp 2/2 | 3 months | P 2/2 | 17–20 months |
| Dp 3/3 | 3 months | P 3/3 | 17–20 months |
| Dp 4/4 | 3 months | P 4/4 | 17–20 months |
| M 1/1 | 5–6 months | | |
| M 2/2 | 8–10 months | | |
| M 3/3 | 18–24 months | | |

incisors and lower dental pad is possible by further retraction of the lips until the mouth opens. Clinical examination of the cheek teeth requires the use of a mouth gag and light source. This will allow evaluation of the alignment and angle of the tables and the spaces left by missing teeth. Changes in periodontium and teeth occur in all sheep with advancing age. Some changes are clinically significant, whereas others are not yet well understood. Some common abnormalities are

- broken mouth
- dentigerous cysts
- dental caries
- incisor wear
- wavy mouth
- fluorosis.

The loss of permanent incisor teeth in sheep is known as 'broken mouth', and the premature loss of incisors of animals in a flock results in decreased production. The shape of the incisor teeth can change with age. Healthy aged ewes should have closely packed, short, spade-shaped incisors. Peg-like incisor teeth are common in flocks where dental disease is not a problem, but long peg-like incisors may indicate developing broken mouth. Excessive wear of the incisor teeth can reduce them to pebble-like structures in 1 or 2 years and reduce grazing efficiency. Irregular cheek teeth wear occurs sporadically in sheep, resulting in decreased feed intake and diseases such as pregnancy toxemia and loss of body weight, and incomplete mastication leading to severe halitosis because of impaction of feed between the teeth and cheek mucosa. Irregular wear is seen as 'steps' between the cheek teeth and may result from tooth loss, loosening or maleruption. The opposing teeth passively erupt into the gap left by the missing or moved tooth, abrading the mucous membrane of the cheek and surrounding gums. Abnormal molar wear is often present in association with developing broken mouth. Wavy or shear mouth is seen as

- angulation and peaking of the tables
- exceedingly sharp cutting edges
- injury to the surrounding soft tissues.

Tooth surface deposits consist of supragingival bacterial plaques attached to all teeth at the entrance to the gingival sulcus. Supragingival plaque must be differentiated from subgingival plaque, which is important in the initiation and development of gingivitis, periodontitis and tooth loss. Brown staining of teeth is common and variable. It is presumably caused by feed staining the porous cementum that covers the enamel. Thicker mineralized deposits, or calculus, commonly accumulate on cheek teeth and, less often, on incisors. The amount, color, and consistency vary widely, from flaky coal-black deposits to mirror-like, hard metallic silver or bronze encrustations. Feed impaction between the cheek teeth of sheep is common, particularly where teeth have been lost and the incisors are peg-like and long.

The teeth are also examined for occlusion. In animals with normal dentition the incisors meet the upper dental pad within 5 mm of its rostral edge, the position depending upon

- the relative lengths of the mandible and maxilla
- the angles of the cranial incisors within their sockets
- the length of the clinical crown.

All three change with age, and the incisors also drift forward on the upper dental pad with age. The most common clinical abnormality of the bite which reduces grazing ability is the malpositioning of the incisors on the front of the dental pad. Although severe congenital prognathism (abnormal protrusion of one or both jaws) does occur, this type of bite is most often caused by the abnormal proclination of incisors. Teeth meeting far back on the pad are less common and are more likely to be a result of congenital brachygnathia (abnormal shortness of the mandible, resulting in protrusion of the maxilla; also called overshot or parrot mouth) rather than retroclination.

---

### Tooth enamel

- normal tooth enamel has a polished translucent white surface
- chalky irregular surfaces are possibly caused by the use of fluorine-rich phosphate fertilizers
- localized hypoamelogenesis (enamel pitting) is an incidental finding during dental examination of sheep teeth
- caries causes deep circumscribed holes in the enamel near the gum margins, weakening the crowns which fracture leaving irregular stumps.

---

### Drinkwater gag

The Drinkwater gag, left and right types, is a simple and excellent device for use in mature-sized cattle. The gag fits between the upper and lower arcades of the cheek teeth and because of its wedge-like structure can be held in place with slight digital pressure. With the gag in place it is possible to palpate the entire oral cavity, including the pharynx, the nasopharyngeal openings, and the rostral aspects of the larynx (Fig. 17.60).

> ### Actinomycosis (lumpy jaw)
>
> This causes an osteomyelitis of the mandible resulting in malocclusion of the upper and lower molar teeth.

## Gingivitis

Gingivitis is inflammation of the gums and may be found in almost all sheep. It is characterized by localized redness of the gingival margin close to one or more teeth. Severe gingivitis, with reddening, swelling, and edema of the gingival margins, occurs in flocks that develop broken mouth, and may be present for up to 2–3 years before teeth are actually lost.

Traumatic injury to the gums and either the maxillary or mandibular dental pad is common and is associated with the sheep's grazing habits. Common sites affected are the gums and the gingival margin below the two central pairs of incisors.

A gingival pocket is a deepening of the gingival sulcus following injury to the tooth supports. In broken mouth, pocketing occurs around the incisors in the year before tooth loss.

Gingival recession is the relative movement of the incisor upwards out of the gum or the downward contraction of the gingiva following periodontal tissue injury. It is recognized clinically by the presence of pale crescents of newly exposed cementum close to the gingival margin.

In cattle, with the mouth held open the incisor teeth and the cheek teeth can be inspected. Pulling the tongue to one side and then the other allows the observer to see the teeth of the opposite side. The use of a left- or right-side Drinkwater gag allows for palpation of the maxillary and mandibular cheek teeth of one side and then the other. Abnormalities of the cheek teeth are uncommon in cattle. The teeth are visually inspected for

- evidence of excessive wear
- malalignment

> ### Clinical Pointer
>
> The incisor pocket can be gently examined by inserting a periodontal pocket probe down the sulcus parallel to the tooth. The probe will penetrate easily to the bottom of the pocket, except on the lingual aspect of the incisors where the curvature of the tooth traps the probe.

- malocclusion
- discoloration
- fractures
- missing teeth
- foreign bodies wedged between teeth.

The incisor teeth of cattle may be excessively worn if the animals are grazing on pastures or rangelands on sandy soils. Occasionally premolar and molar teeth become fractured and the loose portion of the tooth is visible on examination. In actinomycosis (lumpy jaw), on visual inspection and palpation of the affected area the gingiva of the teeth involved in the lesion of the mandible is usually prominently enlarged and the teeth may be grossly malaligned.

## Pharynx

The pharynx of cattle is relatively short and does not extend caudally beyond the base of the skull.

The soft palate varies from 8 to 12 cm in length, it reaches the base of the epiglottis and is held in this position during normal breathing. Elevation of the soft palate occurs during regurgitation. This dilates the oropharynx and the regurgitated bolus is directed into the mouth, where it can be remasticated. Eructated gas from the rumen may also pass through the oral cavity. Most of the gas, however, is forced into the lungs. This is accomplished by closing the intrapharyngeal opening and the mouth, and by opening the glottis. The intrapharyngeal opening is closed by the elevation of the soft palate and the rostral pharyngeal constrictors. If eructation is inhibited for some reason, gas rapidly accumulates in the rumen.

The submucosa of the ventral surface of the soft palate contains a thick layer of glands which produce mucus and make up approximately one-third to half of the thickness of the soft palate. They extend dorsally between the palatine muscles and laterally into the wall of the pharynx. Diffuse lymphoid tissue and lymph nodules are also present on the ventral surface of the soft palate. The delicate mucous membrane on the dorsal surface of the soft palate is covered with ciliated pseudostratified epithelium.

The oropharynx is wide and dilatable. The rostral part of the larynx projects upward from the floor of the laryngopharynx through the intrapharyngeal opening. The piriform recesses are deep in cattle. The laryngopharynx is relatively short and extends to about the rostral third of the cricoid lamina.

The nasal septum is continued into the nasopharynx as the pharyngeal septum, which divides the dorsal part of the nasopharynx into right and left recesses. The pharyngeal septum is high in the calf and somewhat lower in adult cattle. The pharyngeal openings of the auditory tubes are small slits in the caudal part of the nasopharynx.

Because of the bulge of the dorsum of the tongue, the pharynx cannot be viewed directly unless the tongue is depressed with a flat instrument or a cylindrical speculum. In mature cattle a cylindrical speculum 40 cm in length and 3–4 cm in diameter placed over the dorsum of the tongue, which is also used as a fulcrum, and with the use of a flashlight, makes viewing the pharynx and opening of the larynx easy. The pharynx, glottis, larynx and tonsillar crypts can also be palpated with the hand. Pharyngeal lesions associated with traumatic injury from balling guns used for the oral administration of boluses may be visible and palpable.

The lingual tonsil of cattle consists of many follicles and extends to the base of the epiglottis on either side of the glossoepiglottic fold.

## Esophagus

The esophagus begins at the laryngopharynx and lies with its initial portion on the lamina of the cricoid cartilage. The length of the bovine esophagus is 90–95 cm, the cervical part being 42–45 cm and the thoracic part 48–50 cm. In the cranial third of the neck it lies between the longus colli and the trachea; in the caudal half of the neck it deviates to the left and lies against the lateral surface of the trachea for the remainder of its cervical course. The thoracic part of the esophagus extends caudally in the mediastinum, and soon after passing through the thoracic inlet it returns to its original position between the longus colli and the trachea, until it reaches the end of the muscle at the level of the sixth thoracic vertebra. The esophagus passes dorsal to the tracheal bifurcation and the base of the heart, crosses the right surface of the aorta opposite the 4th to the 7th intercostal spaces, and passes through the esophageal hiatus of the diaphragm at the level of the 8th intercostal space. Before reaching the diaphragm it is related dorsally to the long caudal mediastinal lymph node. Enlargement of this node may affect the esophagus and the accompanying dorsal vagal trunk.

The muscular wall of the esophagus consists of striated muscle, which varies in thickness in the different segments of the tube. The lumen of the esophagus varies in the different segments. At the

**Clinical Pointer**

To assess the functional condition of the esophagus (provided the animal is eating) it first needs to be determined whether swallowing occurs at all.

**Clinical Pointer**

- Rumen contents dropped on the ground indicates dysfunctional regurgitation
- 'Quidding' indicates a painful condition of the mouth.

junction of the middle and caudal thirds of the neck the lumen narrows, but caudal to this constriction steadily widens again. In the cervical part it is rosette-shaped in cross-section. Caudal to the heart the lumen is large and oval in cross-section, measuring 7–8 cm dorsoventrally and 4–5 cm from side to side.

The cervical portion of the esophagus is examined in the depth of the jugular furrow; in rare cases it is situated on the right side of the neck. Difficulty in swallowing (dysphagia) usually results from physical obstruction by a foreign body or neoplasm in the pharynx or esophagus, although occasionally it is caused by local pain or inflammatory swelling. Esophageal diverticulum, or segmental paralysis, invariably contributes to functional obstruction, which is manifested by dysphagia. The signs of dysphagia are forceful attempts to swallow, initially accompanied by extension and then flexion of the head, with contractions of the cervical and abdominal musculature. These can be detected by observation during and immediately after the ingestion of food or water. When swallowing, the bolus can be seen as a mobile swelling in the esophagus moving downwards, along the left jugular furrow.

If dysphagia exists the animal takes an unusually long time to consume its feed. Slow eating may, however, be caused by diseases of the nervous system. When the difficulty in swallowing is less severe liquids can still be swallowed fairly readily, but not solids.

Abnormalities of the cervical portion of the esophagus which cause changes in shape or contour, e.g. impacted foreign bodies or tumors, are detectable by inspection or palpation. In dilatation of a part or the whole length of the esophagus, or in constriction (stenosis), a swelling develops at the site of or anterior to the lesion while the animal is feeding. This is reducible on pressure and disappears spontaneously after a variable time, but recurs whenever the animal eats. In certain conditions firm pressure at almost any point along the left jugular furrow may cause eructation, regurgitation and vomiting (esophagitis, dilatation, spasm). Primary esophagitis may follow the ingestion of chemical or physical irritants and is usually accompanied by stomatitis and pharyngitis. Inflammation of the esophagus is a concomitant, but usually unrecognized, feature of many specific diseases, particularly those causing stomatitis.

By introducing a suitably sized stomach tube or probang, i.e. a sufficiently flexible, firm rubber or plastic tube, through the nasal cavity and into the esophagus it is possible to determine whether the esophagus is patent and whether

- constrictions
- foreign bodies
- masses of feed, or
- neoplasms

are present. Enlargement of the posterior mediastinal lymph nodes in cattle, which may be caused by actinobacillosis or leukosis, may be detected by this method because the compression stenosis produced by the enlarged node offers some resistance to the passage of the instrument. The tube must be lubricated before use and should be introduced only when the head and neck are fully extended and the patient is adequately restrained.

## SPECIAL DIAGNOSTIC TECHNIQUES

### Abdominocentesis

Collection of a sample of peritoneal fluid can be a useful aid in the diagnosis of diseases of the peritoneum and intestines.

In mature cattle the choice of sites for abdominocentesis (paracentesis) is a problem because the rumen occupies a large portion of the ventral abdominal wall, and avoiding its penetration is difficult. One recommended site is 8–10 cm caudal from the xiphoid sternum and 8–10 cm lateral from the midline. A teat cannula is recommended, but with care and caution a 16 gauge 5 cm hypodermic needle may also be used. The skin is prepared aseptically, local anesthetic applied and the skin incised with a stab scalpel blade. The cannula is pushed carefully and slowly through the abdominal wall, which will twitch when the peritoneum is punctured. Fluid may drip from the cannula or it may be necessary to connect a syringe to apply vacuum. It may be necessary to move the cannula back and forth

in a few different directions before fluid is obtained. Failure to obtain a sample does not preclude the presence of peritonitis. The exudate may be thick, large masses of fibrin may be present, or the peritonitis may be localized with a minimal amount of fluid.

Examples of four different samples of peritoneal fluid from cattle are shown in Figure 17.62

- normal fluid is amber colored
- cloudy fluid suggests an increased concentration of protein
- serosanguineous fluid contains blood suggesting ischemic necrosis of intestine as in intussusception
- turbid fluid containing particulate material occurs in cattle with a perforated abomasum.

Normal cattle may yield 1–5 ml of clear serum-like fluid containing mesothelial cells, lymphocytes, neutrophils, a few red blood cells and occasional monocytes and eosinophils:

- in normal cattle lymphocytes and segmented neutrophils are found in a ratio of approximately 1:1
- in acute peritonitis there is an increase in the total number and percentage of neutrophils
- in chronic peritonitis the number of neutrophils decreases whereas the number of monocytes increases (Table 17.6).

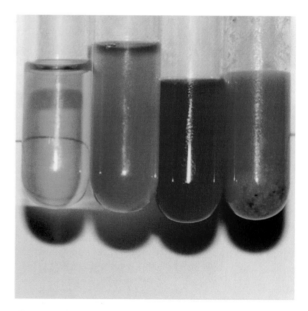

**Fig. 17.62** Peritoneal fluid from mature cattle. From left to right: normal amber-colored fluid; cloudy fluid with increased concentration of protein (peritonitis); serosanguineous fluid from cow with intussusception; turbid fluid containing particulate matter from calf with perforated abomasal ulcer.

---

### Peritoneal fluid samples

Using abdominocentesis to collect peritoneal fluid:

- in acute diffuse peritonitis a sample is usually readily obtainable
- in local peritonitis or in long-standing cases it may be necessary to attempt as many as four different sites.

**Table 17.6.** Guidelines for the classification and interpretation of bovine peritoneal fluid

| Classification | Physical Appearance | Total protein g/dL | Specific gravity | Total RBC x 10⁶/ul | Total WBC x 10³/ul | Differential WBC count | Bacteria | particulate matter (plant fibers) | Interpretation |
|---|---|---|---|---|---|---|---|---|---|
| Normal | Amber, crystal clear 1–5 ml per sample | 0.1–3.1 (1.6) does not clot | 1.005– 1.015 | Few from puncture of capillaries during sampling | 0.3–5.3 | Polymorpho-nuclear and mononuclear cells, ratio 1:1 | None | None | Increased amounts in late gestation, congestive heart failure |
| Moderate inflammation | Amber to pink, slightly turbid | 2.8–7.3 (1.6) | 1.016– 1.025 | 0.1–0.2 | 2.7–40.7 (8.7) | Non-toxic neutrophils, 50-90% macrophages may predominate in chronic peritonitis | None | None | Early stages of strangulation destruction of intestine; traumatic reticuloperiton-itis; obstruction; acute diffuse peritonitis; abomasal ulcer; rupture of uterus, stomachs or intestine; ruptured bladder; chronic peritonitis |
| Severe Inflammation | Serosanguin-eous, turbid, viscous commonly clots,10–20 ml per sample | 3.1–5.8 (4.2) | 1.026 - 1.040 | 0.3–0.5 | 2.0–31.1 (8.0) | Segmented neutrophils, 70–90%. Presence of (toxic) degenerate neutrophils containing bacteria | Usually present | May be present | Advanced stages of strangulation |

## Exploratory laparotomy (celiotomy)

An exploratory laparotomy may assist in the diagnosis and treatment of diseases of the digestive tract or abdomen. When a significant lesion is found at laparotomy, surgery is usually justifiable whether or not the outcome is favorable.

The diagnostic challenge is to decide whether surgery should be performed and whether a left- or a right-side laparotomy should be done. However, because a properly done laparotomy is time-consuming and expensive, the number of laparotomies in which no significant lesions are present must be minimized.

There are some well recognized diseases in which, if a clinical diagnosis can be made, a laparotomy is indicated. In some cases slaughter for salvage may be indicated.

Other than rumenotomy for the treatment of traumatic reticuloperitonitis, grain overload, and cesarean section, the most common indications for a laparotomy in cattle are for the surgical correction of displacements or obstructions of viscera, such as

- left-side displacement of the abomasum
- right-side displacement and volvulus of the abomasum
- torsion of the root of the mesentery
- torsion of the spiral colon
- cecal dilatation and volvulus, and
- intussusception.

---

### Clinical Pointer

The accuracy of diagnosis should be maximized before an unnecessary laparotomy is done.

---

In other cases the diagnosis may be suspected but not obvious, and the indications for laparotomy, slaughter, euthanasia, or conservative medical treatment are unclear.

The major question is, 'under what conditions is a laparotomy indicated if the history and clinical and laparotomy findings suggest an obstruction but the obstruction cannot be located on clinical examination?' The following criteria are useful indicators of the need for laparotomy (Table 17.7).

- The most important clinical indicator is gastro-intestinal hypomotility with the accumulation of gas, fluid, and ingesta in the ruminant stomachs or intestines; a reduction in the amount of feces or complete absence of feces; anorexia, along with varying degrees of abdominal pain; and progressively worsening shock and dehydration.
- Sudden onset of abdominal pain along with tachycardia, shock and dehydration, anorexia, ruminal atony, failure to drink, and absence of feces for several hours.
- Distension of the abdomen which cannot be relieved by passage of a stomach tube (owing to distension of the cecum, abomasum, intestines); shock and dehydration; ruminal atony.
- Absence of feces over several hours and/or bloodstained scant feces along with distended viscera, ruminal atony, and shock and dehydration.
- Fluid-spashing sounds on ballottement of the right flank, along with distended viscera palpable on rectal examination, ruminal atony, anorexia, shock, and dehydration.
- Presence of a ping over a large area of the right abdomen, along with tachycardia, ruminal atony, shock and dehydration, anorexia, and a palpable tense viscus on rectal palpation suggesting dilated cecum, dilated abomasum, intussusception.

- Presence of a grunt on deep palpation of the abdomen, along with anorexia, ruminal atony, and reduced or absent feces.
- Peritoneal fluid containing evidence of inflammation or vascular congestion, along with evidence of anorexia, ruminal atony, reduced amount of feces, and distended viscera palpable on rectal examination.
- Hemogram indicating inflammation; serum biochemistry indicating metabolic hypochloremic, hypokalemic alkalosis, along with anorexia, reduced feces, gas-filled and fluid-filled viscera, and shock and dehydration.

### *Making a decision about a laparotomy*

How long can the clinician delay doing a laparotomy in a cow in which the history and clinical findings suggest the possibility of a surgically correctable obstruction of the digestive tract but in which the clinical evidence is not sufficiently definitive? For example

- initial bouts of abdominal pain which have now subsided
- complete anorexia
- absence of feces
- no palpable distended loops of intestine or viscera
- obvious clinical dehydration.

Is this an intussusception located in the anterior abdomen or a case of idiopathic paralytic ileus which will resolve spontaneously in 12–24 hours? How long can the clinician delay before doing a laparotomy in a cow with an intussusception and still be early enough to correct the obstruction successfully?

Deciding to recommend a laparotomy or delaying monitoring the animal for several hours while awaiting evidence of improvement or progressive worsening depends on the value of the animal to the client, the practicability of examining the animal every few hours, and the availability of laboratory services. Clinical evidence of improvement or worsening is usually detectable within several hours of the initial examination (Table 17.7).

### Laparoscopy

Laparoscopy can be readily performed through the

- right paralumbar fossa
- left paralumbar fossa, and
- cranioventral midline.

A 32 cm rigid laparoscope with a direct-viewing lens has been used to view the abdomen and viscera. The laparoscope is introduced through the right and left

**Table 17.7.  The use of guidelines and criteria to decide when to do a laparotomy in cattle with disease of the digestive tract and abdomen**

| Parameter/Criteria | Significance and Interpretation of Criteria |
| --- | --- |
| History | Does the history suggest a surgically correctable condition? |
| Systemic state, habitus | Heart rate over 100 per minute suggests impending shock but rates below 100 do not preclude existence of an obstructive lesion. Progressive dehydration, progressive weakness, persistent recumbency indicates worsening situation and laparotomy unless can detect incurable lesions. Temperature unreliable. Complete anorexia suggests a severe lesion. |
| Abdominal distension | Laparotomy indicated if distension of abdomen caused by distension of rumen, abomasum, cecum, intestines. |
| Nature and amount of feces | Scant or absence of feces for more than 36 to 48 hours indicates a functional or physical obstruction. In functional obstruction (i.e. peritonitis) some dark feces usually present. In physical obstruction (intussusception) feces are very scant and dark red due to leakage of blood into intussusceptus. Laparotomy indicated unless can determine that cause of absence of feces is not surgically correctable (diffuse peritonitis or impaction of abomasum or omasum). |
| Rectal findings | Distended viscera other than rumen (abomasum, cecum, small and large intestines) warrants laparotomy. Palpable 'bread and butter' fibrinous inflammation in caudal part of abdomen suggests acute, diffuse peritonitis and laparotomy would not be rewarding. |
| Peritoneal tap | Peritoneal fluid which is blood-stained, turbid, and clots in few minutes suggests leakage of the intestinal wall and warrants laparotomy if history and clinical findings suggest a strangulation obstruction. |
| Hemogram | A degenerative left shift in the leukogram indicates inflammation. Laparotomy indicated if the history and clinical findings suggest the possibility of strangulation obstruction. Persistent hyperfibrinogen indicates chronic inflammation. |
| State of the rumen | The fullness of the rumen, the nature of the rumen contents and the regularity and intensity of the contractions are reliable indicators of the state of the digestive tract beyond the rumen. Complete rumen stasis suggests a significant lesion of the rumen itself or of the abomasum, intestines or peritoneum. |
| Abdominal pain (colic) and grunting | Behavioral and postural signs of acute abdominal pain (colic) such as kicking at the belly, stretching the body, suggest acute distension of the stomach or intestines with fluid and gas. A laparotomy is indicated if the clinical evidence suggests that obstruction is the cause of the distension. Spontaneous grunting with each respiration, which usually becomes pronounced in sternal recumbency, or the presence of a grunt on deep palpation of the abdomen suggests inflammation of the peritoneum. |

paralumbar fossae and $CO_2$ gas used to insufflate the abdominal cavity, after the introduction of a trocar and cannula and prior to introduction of the laparoscope. The laparoscope is directed cranially then moved counterclockwise to examine the caudal portion of the abdomen. With right paralumbar laparoscopy, cranially the descending part of the duodenum, caudate and right lobes of the liver, and right kidney can be viewed. The costal part, the lateral part of the right crus and the central tendinous portions of the diaphragm are identifiable. Multiple peristaltic movements are also visible. The body and right lobe of the pancreas can also be identified. Caudally the free edge of the greater omentum and the cranial border of the broad ligament create a space through which the laparoscope can be advanced into the caudal portion of the abdominal cavity. Caudally, from the right side the following structures can be identified

- ovary
- descending colon
- mesocolon
- uterus
- segments of small intestine
- vascular arcades of the mesenteric border
- cecum
- spiral colon
- parts of the urinary bladder.

With left paralumbar fossa laparoscopy, cranially the dorsal sac of the rumen and spleen are visible. The reticulum cannot be observed. Caudally the dorsal sac and caudodorsal blind sac of the rumen are visible. The left kidney is visible medial to the rumen in the mid-dorsal portion of the abdomen. Portions of the small intestine may be visible caudomedial to the rumen. Cranioventral laparoscopy over the ventral midline allows viewing of the sternal and tendinous center of the diaphragm. To the right of the midline the body of the abomasum is identifiable, with its smooth serosal surface without an overlying omentum and large fundus tapering caudally into its pyloric part. The omasum may be obscured by the greater omentum. The reticulum may be difficult to distinguish from the adjacent rumen, unless it is distended with gas. When it is distended with gas it may have an irregular serosal surface with multiple indentations similar to its honeycombed interior. The caudal portion of the abdominal cavity is obscured by the greater omentum.

---

### Clinical Pointer

- a flexible fiberoptic colonoscope, 14 mm diameter and 1120 mm working length, may be useful as an aid for the diagnosis of traumatic reticuloperitonitis
- this instrument did not help the detection of left-side displacement of the abomasum when used through the right flank in cattle.

---

## MEDICAL IMAGING

The large size of mature cattle restricts the use of radiography of the abdomen to veterinary teaching hospitals.

### Radiography of cranial abdomen and reticulum

Radiological examination of the reticulum with the animal in dorsal recumbency (dorsal reticulography) is

an accurate diagnostic method for the evaluation of cattle with suspected traumatic reticuloperitonitis. However, the technical difficulties of positioning the animal and the increased potential of personnel exposure associated with manual restraint suggests that it may not be practical.

The cranioventral abdomen of cattle can be evaluated using two cranial abdominal and one caudal thoracic radiographs. An X-ray machine with a capacity of 1000–1250 mA and 150 kV is necessary, which is usually only available in veterinary teaching hospitals. However, such techniques may be appropriate in valuable animals in which an accurate diagnosis and prognosis for surgical treatment may be desirable.

### Ultrasonography of reticulum

Ultrasonography is a suitable method for the investigation of reticular contractions in healthy ruminants and in cattle for the diagnosis of traumatic reticuloperitonitis. The reticulum and adjacent organs of cows can be examined with ultrasonography using a 3.5 MHz linear transducer applied to the ventral midline of the thorax over the 6th and 7th intercostal spaces, and from the left and right sides of the midline. It may not be possible to image the reticulum in large good-body-condition cows because of the high proportion of fat in the muscle layers. In older cows calcification of the xiphisternum may interfere with imaging. The most common reason for being unable to visualize the reticulum in sick animals is the displacement of the reticulum by a markedly distended rumen or by space-occupying lesions, such as abscesses and fibrin-containing effusions. It is possible to visualize the

- pattern
- number
- amplitude, and
- duration

of the intervals between contractions. The contour of the reticulum, reticular contractions, and the organs adjacent to the reticulum can be imaged. The biphasic reticular contractions can be visualized at the rate of 4 per 4-minute period. During the first incomplete contraction the reticulum contracts by a mean of about 7.2 cm, and during the second contraction it disappears from the screen.

### Ultrasonography for traumatic reticuloperitonitis

The reticulum can be visualized in more than 90% of cows, in spite of interference by the ribs and sternum. In cows with disturbed reticular motility biphasic contractions are slower than normal or indistinct, and the number of contractions is reduced. Fibrinous material appears as echogenic deposits, sometimes accompanied by hypoechogenic fluid. Reticular abscesses have an echogenic capsule with a hypoechogenic center. Involvement of the spleen, omasum, liver, and abomasum may also be imaged.

Reticular abscesses associated with traumatic reticuloperitonitis can be visualized by ultrasonography. The amplitude of reticular contractions is reduced, the reticulum is displaced from the ventral body wall, and the abscesses have hypoechogenic centers and echogenic capsules.

# CLINICAL PATHOLOGY

## Hematology

Hematology can assist in the diagnosis of inflammatory diseases of the digestive tract. The total and differential leukocyte counts provide good diagnostic and prognostic information. The differential leukocyte count is usually considerably more indicative of the acute peritonitis than is the total count. In acute local peritonitis there is commonly a neutrophilia (mature neutrophils above $400/\mu l$) and a left shift (immature neutrophils above $200/\mu l$). This is a regenerative left shift. Both the neutrophilia and the left shift will be increased on the first day and will last for up to 3 days when, in uncomplicated cases, the count begins to return to normal. In chronic cases the levels do not return completely to normal for several days or longer, and there is usually a moderate leukocytosis, neutrophilia, and a monocytosis.

In acute diffuse peritonitis there is often a leukopenia (total count below $4000/\mu l$) with a greater absolute number of immature neutrophils than mature neutrophils (degenerative left shift), which if severe suggests an unfavorable prognosis. The degree of lymphopenia (lymphocyte count below $2500-3000/\mu l$) is an indication of the stress reaction to the infection. In cases of severe diffuse peritonitis the fibrinogen levels may be increased up to $10-20$ g/l.

There are varying degrees of hemoconcentration (increased PCV and total serum proteins). The determination of total plasma protein has been used as an aid to the diagnosis of traumatic reticuloperitonitis. There is a significant difference in total plasma protein levels between cattle with traumatic reticuloperitonitis and those with other diseases of the gastrointestinal tract that might be confused with the former. The mean plasma protein concentrations, measured before surgery, were

- $88 \pm 13$ g/l for traumatic reticuloperitonitis, and
- $77 \pm 12$ g/l for controls.

Serum fibrinogen levels are commonly elevated in acute traumatic reticuloperitonitis, and continue to increase in chronic cases unresponsive to treatment.

## Serum biochemistry and urinalysis

Diseases of the digestive tract can result in marked changes in serum electrolyte concentrations, metabolic alkalosis, hypochloremia and hypokalemia. Paradoxic aciduria may also be present.

## Laboratory tests for hepatic disease and function

Hepatic disease is difficult to diagnose based on clinical findings alone and the use of laboratory tests is necessary. The results and interpretation of such tests, however, depend on the

- nature of the lesion
- duration and severity of the disease
- species variations.

Specific tests which specify the exact nature of the lesion are not available, and a combination of tests is usually necessary to make a diagnosis. In cattle it is suggested that the serum activities of SDH, GGT and GOT, and the concentration of bile acids provide sensitive indicators of hepatocellular dysfunction.

The laboratory tests for the diagnosis of hepatic disease and to evaluate hepatic function in farm animals can be divided into

- those that measure the ability of the liver to remove substances from the serum and detoxify them
- those that measure the serum levels of liver enzymes which increase following hepatic injury
- the non-specific tests which provide some indirect assessment of hepatic function, such as blood glucose, serum proteins, clotting factors and urinalysis.

## Liver biopsy

Liver biopsy can be informative and useful in confirming the presence of liver disease and, in many cases, for determining its etiology. Diffuse and zonal lesions occurring in most of the toxic, infectious, and metabolic liver diseases can usually be diagnosed on biopsy. Some veterinarians have been reluctant to perform liver biopsy because of the risk to the animal and the time involved; however, with the methods described here, using the disposable 'Tru-Cut' needle, liver biopsy is a relatively safe and simple procedure

- cattle should be suitably confined for the procedure; a squeeze chute may be preferable for beef cattle, but a stanchion and nose lead should suffice for the dairy cow
- the puncture site can be located by extending a horizontal line craniad from the middle of the paralumbar fossa
- the site can be confirmed by ultrasound examination
- the needle is inserted where this line crosses the 11th intercostal space on the right side (Fig. 17.63)
- the needle is directed slightly craniad and ventrad, in the direction of the opposite elbow joint
- the length of the needle required will vary with the size and condition of the animal.

The major deficiency of the method lies in the small sample obtained: unless the liver change is diffuse the sample may not be representative. The procedure has been repeated many times on one animal without injury.

---

**Some risks of liver biopsy**

- if the direction of the needle is incorrect it may approach the hilus and damage the large blood vessels or bile ducts
- if the liver is shrunken or the approach too caudal no sample will be obtained
- fatal hemoperitoneum may result if a hemorrhagic tendency is present
- peritonitis may occur if the liver lesion is an abscess containing viable bacteria
- biliary peritonitis results if a large bile duct is perforated
- always confirm site with ultrasonographic examination.

---

## CLINICAL EXAMINATION OF THE CALF

Clinical examination of the digestive tract and abdomen of the calf and the interpretation of the clinical findings may be more difficult than in the adult animal. The rumen of the preruminant calf is not yet

functional and is thus not a reliable indicator of the state of the alimentary tract. Rectal examination of the abdomen is not usually possible until the animal is about 10–12 months old, depending on the breed. A digital examination of the rectum of young calves is useful to determine the nature and amount of feces present or the absence of feces and may indicate the presence of diarrhea which may not yet have begun. A complete absence of feces may suggest

- the presence of an acute intestinal obstruction
- acute diffuse peritonitis, or
- atresia coli.

In addition to a routine systematic clinical examination the important parts of the digestive tract and the abdomen which should be examined are the oral cavity, the left and right sides of the abdomen, the rumen and rumen contents, the abomasum and intestines, a rectal examination, feces, and the umbilicus.

### Oral cavity

The oral cavity is easily examined. The oral mucous membranes are examined for

- evidence of discoloration
- lesions such as erosions or ulcers
- changes in temperature
- the degree of moistness.

The suck reflex is easily examined by inserting one's finger deep into the oral cavity and assessing the vigor of the suck.

### Abdomen

Abdominal distension is common in calves under 3 months of age. It usually appears symmetrical and it is often difficult to determine whether it originates in the rumen, the abomasum, the intestines, or is due to fluid accumulation in the peritoneal cavity. The differential diagnosis of the common causes of abdominal distension and abdominal pain in the calf are set out in Table 17.8.

Examination of the abdomen of the young calf includes inspection of the contour to determine the site of maximum distension, deep palpation and ballottement of each flank to determine the presence of fluid-splashing sounds indicating a fluid-filled viscus, and percussion and auscultation to determine the presence of a gas-filled viscus.

### Rumen

Distension of the left abdomen occurs in calves of any age. In the preruminant calf it is commonly associated

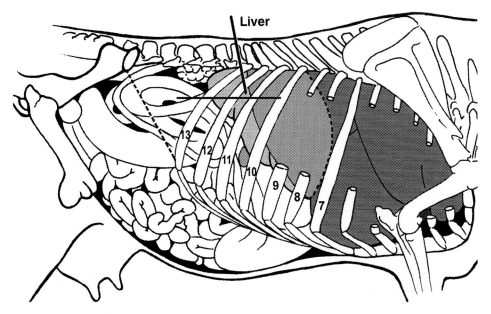

**Liver**

13 12 11 10 9 8 7

**Fig. 17.63**   The liver biopsy site in cattle illustrating the anatomical locations of liver, lungs and ribs.

with excessive putrefaction and fermentation of milk in the rumen. This results in the accumulation of foul and putrid-smelling liquid contents in the rumen, with gas formation and distension. Rumen contractions are not present but ballottement and auscultation over the left paralumbar fossa elicits fluid-splashing sounds indicating the presence of excessive quantities of fluid. Passage of a stomach tube into the rumen will relieve any pressure and commonly release odorous gray fluid containing milk clots. Obstruction of the reticulo-omasal orifice by a foreign body, such as baling string, will cause ruminal distension with the accumulation of excessive quantities of dark fluid. In ruminant calves, the rumen may contract 3–5 times per minute, as evidenced by abdominal ripples, but the typical sounds of rumen contractions may be absent. The fluid-splashing sounds are obvious on ballottement and auscultation.

### Abomasum and intestines

Distension of the abomasum or the intestines, or both, can result in distension of the right side of the abdomen caudal to the costal arch and over the right paralumbar fossa. Palpation of both the left and right sides may reveal a distended and tense abdomen. Percussion and ballottement with simultaneous auscultation may reveal a high-pitched ping and fluid-splashing sounds, indicating a fluid-filled viscus or intestines.

Positioning the calf on its hindquarters allows the viscera to move to the caudal abdomen and may allow inspection and palpation of a distended abomasum

below the xiphoid sternum. Palpation of the abdomen in this position may elicit a painful site. With the calf in left lateral recumbency, careful palpation and ballottement with simultaneous auscultation may reveal the approximate location of the distended viscus.

With severe distension of the right abdomen accompanied by severe abdominal pain (kicking, bellowing, rolling, getting up and lying down) it may be necessary to relieve pressure with a large-gauge needle (12–14 gauge, 7–10 cm). The most common cause of severe right-side abdominal distension in a young calf which can be relieved by **trocarization** is abomasal dilatation. The diagnosis of perforation of an abomasal ulcer with diffuse peritonitis, and torsion of the root of the mesentery requires abdominocentesis, which is easily done in the calf, and at least three taps should be done before concluding a negative tap. In some cases it may be necessary to do an exploratory laparotomy to determine the cause of the distension.

---

### Some common causes of abdominal distension in young calves

- early cases of severe enteritis
- abomasal dilatation associated with the ingestion of excessive quantities of milk
- abomasal volvulus
- torsion of the root of the mesentery
- perforated abomasal ulceration with peritonitis

**Table 17.8. Differential diagnosis of diseases of the digestive tract of young calves with abdominal pain and distension**

| Disease | History, clinical and laboratory findings, treatment |
|---|---|
| Dietary gastrointestinal tympany | Nursing calves 2 to 6 weeks of age sucking high-producing cows. May be due to ingestion of excessive quantities of milk and abnormal gas formation in the abomasum and large intestine. Abdominal pain (kicking of the belly, stretching) and fluid-splashing sounds and pings over right abdomen. Will not suck or eat. Feces are absent or scant and foul-smelling. At laparotomy, gaseous distension of the abomasum and intestines. Spontaneous recovery in 12–24 hours. |
| Abomasal torsion (volvulus) | Acute to peracute, one week to six months of age, acute abdominal pain, bellowing, up and down, severe tight distension of abdomen, loud and large ping with fluid-splashing sounds over right abdomen. Emergency surgery necessary; recovery about 50% if recognize and correct early. |
| Abomasal dilatation (fluid, milk, hairballs and often abomasal ulcers) | Chronic or acute onset, calves one to six months of age, history of abnormal feces, may be unthrifty, mild to moderate abdominal distension and pain, fluid-splashing sounds over right flank, mild dehydration, no peritoneal fluid. Laparotomy and abomasotomy are required. |
| Perforated abomasal ulcers | Acute onset, sudden collapse, calves two weeks to three months, hand-fed or nursing calves, weakness, recumbency, tachycardia, mild to moderate abdominal distension, mild or no abdominal pain, abdominal splinting occasionally, abnormal peritoneal fluid, feces variable. Laparotomy required; survival about 25%. |
| Torsion of root of mesentery | Sudden onset, found in state of collapse, abdominal pain common, moderate abdominal distension, distended loops of intestine visible and palpable over right flank, blood-stained peritoneal tap, fluid-splashing sounds on palpation and auscultation of right abdomen, scant feces. Emergency surgery. |
| Acute diffuse peritonitis (not due to perforated abomasal ulcer) | Usually in calves under three weeks of age. Toxemia, temperature variable, weak, may be grunting, splinting of abdominal wall, mild abdominal distension, scant feces, fluid-splashing sounds over right flank (due to paralytic ileus), abnormal peritoneal fluid, commonly associated with enteric colibacillosis, polyarthritis and umbilical urachal abscess. Broad spectrum antibiotics. Prognosis is poor. |
| Atresia coli/ani | Calf usually under ten days of age, progressive distension of abdomen, bright and alert for first few days then becomes depressed, no feces only thick mucus from rectum (atresia coli), insertion of tube into rectum may lead to blind end but often blind end is near spiral colon. Surgery indicated but often unrewarding. |
| Intussusception | May have history of diarrhea, now scant blood-stained feces, depressed, will not suck or drink, dehydrated, contour of abdomen may appear normal or slightly distended, fluid-splashing sounds and small ping may be audible, blood-stained peritoneal fluid. Pre-surgical diagnosis often difficult, surgery necessary. Recovery rate is good if diagnose early. |
| Peracute to acute enteritis | Usually in calves under three weeks of age, acute onset of abdominal pain (kicking, stretching), won't suck or drink, may not yet appear dehydrated, temperature variable (if elevated is reliable), mild to moderate abdominal distension, fluid-splashing sounds on auscultation and succussion of abdomen, continuous loud peristaltic sounds on auscultation, diarrheic feces may not be obvious on first examination, digital examination of rectum may stimulate defecation of foul-smelling soft-watery feces, peritoneal tap negative. Treat with fluids and electrolytes for metabolic acidosis and dehydration. Recovery rate is good. |

Dilatation of the abomasum in young calves may be due to pyloric obstruction or the excessive production and accumulation of gas

- pyloric obstruction may follow the eating of indigestible substances, such as baling twine, wood-shavings or cloth rags
- dilatation may occur when calves are fed at irregular intervals on excessive quantities of milk, thereby causing the formation of a rubbery, indigestible curd clot in the abomasum which gradually increases in size.

### Clinical Pointer

Sites caudal to the umbilicus are selected for abdominocentesis to avoid puncturing the abomasum.

Acute volvulus of the abomasum in young calves is characterized by sudden anorexia, vigorous kicking at the abdomen, repeated crouching movements, repeated bellowing, and straining. The heart rate increases to 120–160 bpm. Palpation of the distended abdomen behind the right costal arch is resented and combined auscultation and percussion produce high-pitched tympanic sounds indicative of fluid and gas under pressure.

Abomasal ulceration may occur in young calves at the time when their diet is changed from milk to solid feeds. The incidence appears to be highest in calves stressed by transportation and sale yards. Hairballs occur in the abomasum of suckling beef calves with abomasal ulceration, but the relationship is unclear. Although the majority of cases of ulceration of the abomasum in calves are subclinical and non-hemorrhagic, occasionally there is severe diarrhea with melena, severe depression, shock, and rapid death. On rare occasions, milk-fed calves under 2 weeks of age develop acute ulcers which hemorrhage severely and perforate, setting up acute local peritonitis.

### Rectal examination

A digital rectal examination can provide valuable information about the state of the anus and the nature and amount of feces in the rectum. Atresia ani is characterized by the absence of an anus and gradual distension of the abdomen over a period of days. In atresia coli the anus is present but only mucus is present in the rectum and the abdomen is also distended. Re-examination by rectal examination several hours later will reveal the persistent absence of feces. Medical imaging with a barium enema may reveal the failure of the contrast media to move cranially.

### Feces

Gross examination of the feces can provide valuable information about the location and nature of the lesions of the digestive tract. In the first several days of life the feces of the healthy milk-fed calf will be dark tan-colored and small in quantity. As the calf increases its daily intake of milk and begins to consume other sources of feed the daily amount of feces will increase and the dry matter concentration will increase, making the feces appear more bulky.

The nature of the feces in the rectum of a calf with abdominal pain can provide clues about the possible cause

- small amounts of dark, firm, or pasty feces may indicate the presence of acute intestinal obstruction, such as torsion of the root of the mesentery, intussusception, diffuse peritionitis, or torsion of the abomasum
- foul-smelling pale soft or liquid feces indicate the presence of enteritis or gastrointestinal tympany, associated with dilatation of the abomasum with excessive quantities of fluid, gas and abnormally fermented milk.

The consistency of the feces in acute diarrhea of calves under 30 days of age varies from profuse and liquid to moderate in amount and soft. A profuse liquid diarrhea usually indicates the presence of enteropathy of the small intestines due to enterotoxigenic *Escherichia coli*. Moderate or scant amounts of soft but abnormal mucoid feces commonly indicate enteropathy of the large intestines due to coronavirus infection. The color may be various shades of yellow, green, brown, or red. The yellow, green, and brown coloration does not usually indicate the location or nature of the lesion. The presence of frank blood indicates hemorrhage in the colon or rectum. Occasional streaks of frank blood occur in the feces of diarrheic calves and the source is usually not determined. The presence of dark red blood suggests a lesion of the small intestines. Black tarry feces or melena indicate hemorrhage in the abomasum or upper small intestines, such as the duodenum.

### Clinical Pointer

The presence of large quantities of mucus in the feces suggests a lesion of the large intestines.

Fibrinous casts, which indicate the presence of severe inflammation, appear like 'tan-colored membranes' and may completely cover a bolus of feces or be present in a clump mixed with feces.

## Umbilicus

Diseases of the umbilicus are common in calves in the first few weeks of life. Diseases of the extra-abdominal umbilicus include

- omphalitis resulting in abscess or fistula formation
- omphalitis and hernia, and
- umbilical hernia.

Diseases of the intra-abdominal umbilicus most commonly involve infection of the umbilical remnants, and include

- urachitis
- omphaloarteritis
- omphalophlebitis, and
- omphalourachitis

each of which can result in abscess formation. Such infections may be associated with persistent local infection and toxemia, septicemia, septic arthritis, dysuria, incarceration of the small intestine, and chronic unthriftiness. A patent urachus can also occur but is rare compared to its occurrence in the foal.

Diagnosis of umbilical abnormalities in calves has traditionally been based on history and physical examination. Palpation is the easiest and most commonly used examination technique. Affected calves are usually presented with enlargements of the umbilicus with or without systemic evidence of infection, such as toxemia and fever. Enlargement and inflammation of the extra-abdominal umbilical stalk is easily observed and painful on palpation. The hernial ring of the abdominal wall can be palpated digitally.

Abnormalities of the intra-abdominal umbilicus are not easily assessed by palpation because the abdominal wall of the calf is usually tense and the abnormalities either cannot be felt or circumscribed digitally. The examiner may be able to determine that a palpable mass is present and whether it is situated cranially or caudally, but the extent of the lesion is difficult to evaluate. Often the findings on palpation are inconclusive and the extent of an intra-abdominal umbilical infection can be determined only during surgery or at necropsy. Because of the difficulties with palpation techniques

- abdominal radiography
- fistulography, and
- intravenous urography

have been used as diagnostic techniques. Ultrasonography is now considered as the most useful, non-invasive method of visualizing alterations in the intra-abdominal umbilical structures.

### Involution of umbilical structures

The umbilical remnant structures in the neonatal calf include

- two umbilical arteries
- an umbilical vein, and
- an external umbilical stalk.

The umbilical cord of ruminants is short compared with that of foals, and in the bovine fetus it consists of the allantoic stalk, two arteries, and two veins (Fig. 17.64).

In the bovine fetus the urachus extends from the apex of the urinary bladder to the umbilicus and proceeds to the allantois by way of the umbilical cord. Urine produced by the fetus in utero is voided into the amniotic sac via the urethra, or into the allantoic sac via the urachus. At birth the umbilical cord breaks and the urachus and umbilical arteries immediately retract from the umbilicus into the abdomen, where they normally obliterate. The urachus atrophies and only a scar on the apex of the bladder remains. Failure of the urachus to atrophy has been attributed to congenital abnormalities, abnormal separation of the umbilical cord, and genetic predisposition. The various forms of persistent urachus include

- patent urachus (urachal fistula)
- urachal diverticulum
- urachal cyst, and
- urachal remnant.

In calves diseases of the urachus are usually associated with omphalitis. An ascending infection, acquired during the first few days of life, impairs involution of the urachus and commonly results in abscess formation. Typical signs of urachal infection include dribbling of a purulent discharge from the umbilicus, pollakiuria, and stranguria. Most cases of persistent urachus in calves are infected; non-infected persistent urachus cases are much less common.

In calves with urachal diverticulum and urachal cyst

---

**Clinical Pointer**

Umbilical hernias are characterized by fluctuant painless swellings which are usually easily partially reducible or completely non-reducible.

the edge of the falciform ligament. Immediately after the umbilical cord breaks the stumps of the umbilical arteries close and retract to the level of the urinary bladder and form the round ligaments of the bladder. Shortly after the cord breaks the cranial end of the urachus becomes situated several millimeters closer to the inner umbilical ring than the arteries. The urachus then shrinks and atrophies, leaving a scar on the apex of the bladder.

> ### Clinical Pointer
>
> Urachal cyst should be included in the differential diagnosis of an irreducible umbilical mass in calves. Careful palpation of the umbilicus is indicated to avoid the potential complication of iatrogenic rupture of a urachal cyst.

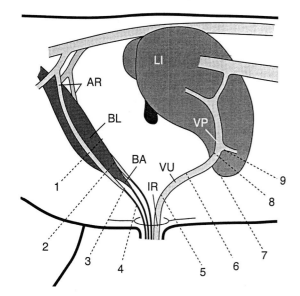

**Fig. 17.64** Umbilical structures of the young calf. The defined positions for ultrasonographic examination of the intra-abdominal umbilical structures. The umbilical arteries (AR) are imaged passing along the side of the urinary bladder (BL) (position 1) and near the bladder apex (BA) (position 2). The urachus (UR) and the umbilical arteries are imaged approximately halfway between the bladder and the inner umbilical ring (IR) (position 3) and directly caudal to the inner umbilical ring (position 4). The umbilical vein (VU) is visualized immediately cranial to the inner umbilical ring (position 5), halfway between the inner umbilical ring and the liver (LI) (position 6), at the caudoventral margin of the liver (position 7), and at the level of the venous sulcus of the liver (position 8). Position 9 shows the junction of the umbilical vein with the left branch of the portal vein (VP). Reproduced with permission from Lischer and Steiner (1993, 1994).

the distal end of the urachus is sealed. The diagnosis is usually made unexpectedly when complications such as cystitis, uroperitoneum, subcutaneous accumulation of urine around the umbilicus, or dysuria develop.

The umbilical arteries and the urachus retract into the abdomen immediately after the umbilical cord breaks. In contrast, the remnants of the umbilical vein remain in the umbilicus and become incorporated into the scarring process. After birth the intra-abdominal part of the umbilical vein often contains a large amount of blood, which gradually coagulates during the first week of life. The lumen of the umbilical vein gradually becomes occluded by the proliferation of connective tissue and by contraction of the vessel wall. This process is normally complete by 3 weeks of age. In some adult animals the atrophied umbilical vein may persist to form the round ligament of the liver along

## Ultrasonography of umbilical structures and abnormalities

Ultrasonography is now used to identify umbilical cord lesions and to detect occult lesions of the internal cord remnants.

The technique can be used to diagnose

- omphalitis with or without abscess formation and without involvement of intra-abdominal structures
- patent urachus
- urachitis with abscess formation with or without bladder involvement
- omphaloarteritis
- omphalophlebitis with or without involvement of the liver
- omphalophlebitis with liver abscess.

The optimum time for surgical correction of internal lesions can also be evaluated.

Normally, after separation of the umbilical cord at birth the urachus retracts into the abdomen and cannot be imaged by ultrasonography caudal to the umbilical ring. During the first 2 days of life the urachus is visible between the two umbilical arteries and cranial to the bladder as a homogeneous hypoechogenic structure without a clearly defined lumen. A persistent urachus can be detected using ultrasonography. A urachal cyst can be traced from the bladder to the umbilicus as a circular structure with an anechoic lumen. A purulent and inflamed urachus has a thickened wall and hyperechoic lumen.

Ultrasonography has been used to identify the internal umbilical structures and the umbilical stalk in clinically normal calves, and to establish a range of

## Advantages of ultrasonography of the umbilical structures

- it is a non-invasive technique that can be used in the standing, non-sedated calf
- there are no known risks
- an experienced clinician can complete the examination in 10 minutes
- calves can be examined in the field
- it can provide a useful description of the extent of internal lesions and of the involvement of other structures, such as the liver and urinary bladder.

normal values for measurement of the umbilical stalk, umbilical arteries, umbilical vein, and urachus. During the first week of life the umbilical vein can be distinctly imaged from the base of the umbilicus to the left branch of the portal vein of the liver. After the third week the vein is only ultrasonographically visible outside the liver. The lumen of the umbilical vein can only be imaged after the first few days of life. The umbilical arteries can best be imaged during the first week of life. The ends of the arteries have no connection to the umbilicus and can be first imaged several centimeters caudal to the base of the umbilicus. Cross-sections of the urachus of the calf with normal umbilical involution are difficult to identify and the identification of a urachal remnant in a calf of any age should be considered abnormal.

## FURTHER READING

Adamson P, Murray MJ. Stomach. In: Traub-Dargatz JL, Brown CM (eds) Equine endoscopy. St. Louis: Mosby, 1990;19–137.

Allen DG. Small animal medicine. Philadelphia: JB Lippincott, 1991; 1062–1064.

Anderson DA, Gaughan EM, St.-Jean G. Normal laparoscopic anatomy of the bovine abdomen. American Journal of Veterinary Research 1993; 54:1170–1176.

Argenzio RA. Functions of the equine large intestine and their inter-relationship in disease. Cornell Veterinarian 1975; 65: 303–330.

Bates B. Physical examination and history taking, 5th edn. Philadelphia: JB Lippincott, 1991.

Becht JL. Physical examination of the horse with colic. In: Robinson NA (ed) Current therapy in equine medicine. Philadelphia: WB Saunders, 1987; 19–22.

Bernard WV, Reed VB, Reimer JM, Humber KA, Orsini JA. Ultrasonographic diagnosis of small intestinal intussusception in three foals. Journal of the American Veterinary Medical Association 1989; 194: 395–397.

Bjorling DE, Prasse KW, Holmes RA. Partial hepatectomy in dogs. Compendium of Continuing Education for the Practicing Veterinarian 1985; 7: 233–239.

Browning GF, Chalmers RM, Snodgrass DR et al. The prevalence of enteric pathogens in diarrhoeic thoroughbred foals in Britain and Ireland. Equine Veterinary Journal 1991; 23: 405–409.

Campbell ML, Ackerman N, Peyton LC. Radiographic gastrointestinal anatomy of the foal. Veterinary Radiology 1984; 5: 194–204.

Center SA. Pathophysiology and laboratory diagnosis of hepatobiliary disorders. In: Ettinger SJ, Feldman EC (eds). Textbook of veterinary internal medicine, 4th edn. Philadelphia: WB Saunders, 1995; 1261–1312.

Cohen ND, Chaffin MK. Assessment and initial management of colic in foals. Compendium of Continuing Education for the Practicing Veterinarian 1995; 17: 93–102.

Cohen ND, Chaffin MK. Causes of diarrhea and enteritis in foals. Compendium of Continuing Education for the Practicing Veterinarian 1995; 17: 568–574.

Darien B. Duodenum. In: Traub-Dargatz JL, Brown CM (eds) Equine endoscopy. St. Louis: Mosby, 1990; 139–144.

Dik JK, Gunsser I. Atlas of diagnostic radiology of the horse, part 3: diseases of the head, neck and throat. Hannover: Schlutereche,1990; 12–71.

Dorland's Illustrated Medical Dictionary, 27th edn. Philadelphia, WB Saunders, 1988.

Edwards DF, Bauer MS, Walker MA, Pardo AD, McCracken MD, Walker TL. Pancreatic masses in seven dogs following acute pancreatitis. American Animal Hospital Association 1990; 26: 189–198.

Embertson RM, Bramlage LR. Clinical uses of the laparoscope in general equine practice. Proceedings of the Annual Convention of the American Association of Equine Practitioners 1992; 38: 165–169.

Farrow CS, Green R, Shively M (eds). Radiology of the cat. St. Louis: Mosby, 1994; 139–217.

Fischer AT. Diagnostic laparoscopy. In: Traub-Dargatz JL, Brown CM (eds) Equine endoscopy. St. Louis: Mosby, 1990; 173–184.

Fischer AT. Standing laparoscopic surgery. Veterinary Clinics of North America (Equine Practice) 1991; 7: 641–647.

Fischer AT, Yarborough TY. Retrograde contrast radiography of the distal portions of the intestinal tract in foals. Journal of the American Veterinary Medical Association 1995; 207: 734–737.

Fischer AT, Kerr LY, O'Brien TR. Radiographic diagnosis of gastrointestinal disorders in the foal. Veterinary Radiology 1987; 28: 42–48.

Galuppo LD, Snyder JR, Pascoe JR. Laparoscopic anatomy of the equine abdomen. American Journal of Veterinary Research 1995; 56: 518–531.

Grindem CB, Fairley NM, Uhlinger CA, Crane SA. Peritoneal fluid values from healthy foals. Equine Veterinary Journal 1990; 22: 359–361.

Hackett RP. Rupture of the urinary bladder in neonatal foals. Compendium of Continuing Education for the Practicing Veterinarian 1984; 6: S488–S494.

Hackett RP. Colonic volvulus and intussusception. In: Robinson NA (ed.) Current therapy in equine medicine. Philadelphia: WB Saunders, 1987; 66–68.

Holstrom SE, Frost P, Gammon RL. Veterinary dental techniques for the small animal practitioner. Philadelphia: WB Saunders, 1992.

Holt PE, Freestone J, Mair TS, Taylor FGR. Renal diseases. In: Higgins AJ, Wright IM (eds) The equine manual. London: WB Saunders, 1995; 576–586.

Hunt E, Tennant BC, Whitlock RH. Interpretation of peritoneal fluid erythrocyte counts in horses with abdominal disease. Proceedings of the Equine Colic Research Symposium 1986; 2: 168–174.

Hunt JM, Gerring EL. Effects of autonomic agonists on equine gastrointestinal electromechanical activity. Proceedings of the Equine Colic Research Symposium 1986; 2: 210–213.

Huskamp B. Displacement of the large colon. In: Robinson NA (ed.) Current therapy in equine medicine. Philadelphia: WB Saunders, 1987; 60–65.

Kelly WR (ed). Veterinary clinical diagnosis, 3rd edn. London: Baillière Tindall, 1984.

King LG, Gelens HCJ. Ascites. Compendium of Continuing Education for the Practicing Veterinarian 1992; 14: 1063–1075.

Kopf N. Rectal examination of the colic patient. In: Robinson NA (ed.) Current therapy in equine medicine. Philadelphia: WB Saunders, 1987; 23–27.

Koterba AM, Brewer BD, Tarplee FA. Clinical and clinico-pathological characteristics of the septicemic neonatal foal: review of 38 cases. Equine Veterinary Journal 1990; 16: 376–383.

Lischer CJ, Steiner A. Ultrasonography of umbilical structures in calves. Part 1: Ultrasonographic description of umbilical involution in clinically healthy calves. Schweizer Archiv Tierheilkunde 1993; 135: 221–230.

Lischer CJ, Steiner A. Ultrasonography of the umbilicus in calves. Part 2: Ultrasonography, diagnosis and treatment of umbilical diseases. Schweizer Archiv Tierheilkunde 1994; 136: 227–241.

McCurnin DM, Poffenbarger EM (eds). Small animal physical diagnosis and clinical procedures. Philadelphia: WB Saunders, 1991; 64–74.

McGrath JP. Exfoliative cytology of equine peritoneal fluid – an adjunct to haematological examination. Proceedings of the International Symposium on Equine Haematology 1976; 2: 408–416.

Malark JA, Peyton LC, Galvin MJ. Effects of blood contamination on equine peritoneal fluid analysis. Journal of the American Veterinary Medical Association 1992; 201: 1545–1548.

Mattson A. Pharyngeal disorders. Veterinary Clinics of North America (Small Animal Practice) 1994; 24 (5): 825–854.

Murray M J. Endoscopic appearance of gastric lesions in foals: 94 cases (1987–1988). Journal of the American Veterinary Medical Association 1989; 195: 1135–1141.

Nappert G, Vrins A, Larybyere M. Gastroduodenal ulceration in foals. Compendium of Continuing Education for the Practicing Veterinarian 1989; 11: 338–345.

Nickel R, Shummer A, Seiferle E. The viscera of the domestic animals. 2nd edn. A. Schummer, R. Nickel and W. O. Sack. Verlag Paul Parey. Springer Verlag. 1979.

Oliver JE, Lorenz MD. Handbook of veterinary neurology, 2nd edn.Philadelphia: WB Saunders, 1993; 27.

Orsini P, Hennet P. Anatomy of the mouth and teeth of the cat. In: Harvey CE (ed) Feline dentistry. Veterinary Clinics of North America (Small Animal Practice) 1992; 22 (6): 1265–1277.

Parry BW. Use of clinical pathology in evaluation of horses with colic. Veterinary Clinics of North America (Equine Practice) 1987; 3: 529–542.

Parry BW, Brownlow MA. Peritoneal fluid. In: Cowell RL, Tyler RD (eds) Cytology and hematology of the horse. Goletta CA: American Veterinary Publications Ltd, 1992; 121–148.

Poffenbarger EM. Gastrointestinal system. In: McCurnin DM, Poffenbarger EM (eds) Small animal physical diagnosis and clinical procedures. Philadelphia: WB Saunders, 1991; 64–74.

Rantanen NW. Diseases of the abdomen. Veterinary Clinics of North America (Equine Practice) 1986; 2: 67–88.

Rebhurs WC, Rumen collapse in cattle. Cornell Veterinarian 1981; 77: 244–250.

Reimer JM. Ultrasonography of umbilical remnant infections in foals. Proceedings of the Annual Convention of the American Association of Equine Practitioners 1993; 39: 247–248.

Reimer JM. Sonographic evaluation of gastrointestinal diseases in foals. Proceedings of the Annual Convention of the American Association of Equine Practitioners 1993; 39: 245–246.

Richardson JD, Lane JG, Waldron KR. Is dentition an accurate indication of the age of a horse? Veterinary Record 1994; 135: 31–34.

Robertson JT. Diseases of the acute abdomen. In: White NA (ed.) The equine acute abdomen. Philadelphia: Lea and Febiger, 1990; 338–418.

Rose RJ, Hodgson DR. Examination of the alimentary tract. In: Rose RJ and Hodgson DR (eds) Manual of equine practice. Philadelphia: WB Saunders, 1993; 192–205.

Ross MW, Hanson RR. Large intestine. In: Auer JA (ed.) Equine surgery. Philadelphia: WB Saunders, 1992; 379–407.

Sack WO. Abdominal topography of a cow with left abomasal displacement. American Journal of Veterinary Research 1968; 29: 1567–1576.

Santschi EH, Slone DE, Frank WM. Use of ultrasound in horses for diagnosis of left dorsal displacement of the large colon and monitoring its non-surgical correction. Veterinary Surgery 1991; 22: 281–284.

Scholes SFE, Vaillant C, Peacock P, Edwards GB, Kelly DF. Diagnosis of grass sickness by ileal biopsy. Veterinary Record 1993; 133: 7–10.

Schummer A, Nickel R, Sack WO. The alimentary canal of the horse. In: Nickel R, Schummer A, Seiferle E (eds) The viscera of the domestic animals, 2nd edn. New York: Springer-Verlag, 1979; 180–203.

Shires GMH. Rectal tears. In: Robinson NE (ed) Current therapy in equine medicine. Philadelphia: WB Saunders, 1987; 75–79.

Sisson S. Equine digestive system. In: Sisson and Grossman's The anatomy of the domestic animals, 5th edn. Vol. 1. Philadelphia: WB Saunders, 1975; 454–497.

Smith DF, Erb HN, Kalaher KM, Rebhun WC. The identification of structures and conditions responsible for right side tympanitic resonance (ping) in adult cattle. Cornell Veterinarian 1982; 72: 180–189.

Smith JE, Erickson HH, DeBowes RM. Changes in circulating equine erythrocytes induced by brief high-speed exercise. Equine Veterinary Journal 1989; 21: 444–446.

Spence J, Aitchison G. Clinical aspects of dental disease in sheep. In Practice 1986; 8(4): 128–135.

Stashak TS. Clinical evaluation of the equine colic patient. Veterinary Clinics of North America (Equine Practice) 1979; 1: 275–287.

Steckel RR. Diagnosis and management of acute abdominal pain (colic). In: Auer JA (ed) Equine surgery. Philadelphia: WB Saunders, 1992; 348–360.

Stober M, Dirksen G. The differential diagnosis of abdominal findings (adspection, rectal examination and exploratory laparotomy) in cattle. Bovine Practitioner 1977; 12: 35–38.

Tietje S, Becker M, Böckenhoff G. Computed tomographic evaluation of head diseases in the horse: 15 cases. Equine Veterinary Journal 1996; 28: 98–105.

Tulleners EP. Complications of abdominocentesis in the horse. Journal of the American Veterinary Medical Association 1983; 182: 232–234.

Vatistas NJ, Snyder JR, Wilson WD, Drake C, Hildebrand S. Surgical treatment for colic in the foal (67 cases): 1980–1992. Equine Veterinary Journal 1996; 28: 139–145.

Walmsley J. Some observations on the value of ageing 5–7 year old horses by examination of their incisor teeth. Equine Veterinary Education 1993; 5: 295–298.

Watson E, Mahaffey MB, Crowell W, Selcer BA, Morris DD, Seginak L. Ultrasonography of the umbilical structures in clinically normal calves. American Journal of Veterinary Research 1994; 55: 773–780.

Wendell Nelson A. Analysis of equine peritoneal fluid. Veterinary Clinics of North America (Equine Practice) 1979; 1: 267–274.

White NA. Surgical exploration of the equine abdomen. In: Moore JN, White NA, Becht JL (eds) Equine acute abdomen. Proceedings of the Veterinary Seminar at the University of Georgia, New Jersey: Veterinary Learning Systems, 1986. Vol 1: pp 52–57.

White NA. Examination and diagnosis of the acute abdomen. In: The equine acute abdomen. Lea and Febiger, PA. 1990; 102–142.

Wilson AD, Ferguson JG. Use of a flexible fiberoptic laparoscope as a diagnostic aid in cattle. Canadian Veterinary Journal 1984; 25: 229–234.

# 18

# Clinical Examination of the Urinary System

*Dogs and Cats – S.I. Rubin*
*Cattle, Sheep, Goats, Horses and Pigs – T.R. Kasari*

The urinary system consists of the kidneys, ureters, bladder, and urethra and is concerned with the production and excretion of urine. The kidneys represent the upper urinary tract; the lower urinary tract consists of the ureters, bladder, and urethra. Most of the clinical manifestations of disease of the urinary tract are due to abnormalities of the lower urinary tract.

## CLINICAL MANIFESTATIONS OF DISEASES OF THE URINARY SYSTEM

**Acute abdominal pain.** Extending or flexing of the back, treading the hindlimbs and kicking at the abdomen may occur in pyelonephritis, and with obstruction of the renal calices or ureters.

**Anuria.** Complete cessation of urine formation by the kidney.

**Azotemia.** A polysystemic toxic syndrome which occurs as a result of abnormal renal function; caused by abnormal quantities of urine constituents in the blood (urea, creatinine and other nitrogenous end-products of protein and amino acid metabolism). Uremia often occurs as the end stage of renal failure. In horses there is depression and chronic diarrhea. In cattle there is somnolence, depression, and recumbency.

**Crystalluria.** The presence of crystals in the urine. The crystals may be present microscopically or grossly. They may occur as gritty substances on preputial hairs, indicating the presence of a large concentration of crystals in the urine, as in animals with urolithiasis.

**Dribbling urine.** A steady, intermittent passage of small volumes of urine, sometimes precipitated by a change in posture or increase in intra-abdominal pressure, reflecting inadequate or lack of sphincter control.

**Dysuria.** Painful or difficult urination, often with grunting and maintaining posture for sometime afterwards. Dysuria is sometimes confused with tenesmus.

**Hematuria.** The presence of blood in urine; it may be grossly visible or microscopic. Urinalysis may be required to differentiate hematuria (red cells present in the urine sediment) from myoglobinuria or hemoglobinuria (red cells not present in urine sediment).

**Inappropriate micturition.** Conscious voiding of urine at inappropriate times or inappropriate locations.

**Nocturia.** Interruption of periods of sleep by the need or urge to urinate.

**Oliguria.** Reduced output of urine.

**Persistent urachus.** Failure of the urachus to obliterate at birth so that urine dribbles from it. Also called pervious or patent urachus.

**Pollakiuria.** Abnormally frequent passage of urine. It may occur with or without an increase in the volume of urine excreted. Commonly associated with disease of the lower urinary tract such as cystitis, the presence of calculi in the bladder, urethritis, and partial obstruction of the urethra.

**Polydipsia.** Consumption of abnormally large volumes of water.

**Polyuria.** Formation and elimination of abnormally large quantities of urine during a specified period of time. Many non-urinary diseases may be associated with polyuria.

**Proteinuria.** The presence of abnormal quantities of protein in the urine. It indicates the presence of glomerutonephritis, amyloidosis or inflammation in the urinary tract or amyloidosis.

**Pyuria.** Pus in the urine. The pus may be visible grossly or only detectable on microscopic examination. It may be in the form of leukocytes in casts and is usually accompanied by bacteria. The pus may originate from the kidneys, ureters, bladder, or urethra, and the reproductive tract. Significant cell numbers suggest inflammatory disease somewhere in the urinary tract. Detection of significant numbers of bacteria in association with pyuria indicates that the inflammatory lesion has been caused or complicated by bacterial infection. The presence of white cells does not aid in localizing the lesion unless there are white cell casts, signifying a renal origin.

**Retention of urine.** Apparent reduction in the frequency of urination occurs temporarily in partial obstruction of the urethra, in spasm of the external sphincter of the bladder, and when there is an inability to adopt a normal posture for urination. Gross distension of the bladder inevitably develops and overrides the obstruction or sphincter spasm, resulting in voiding of small quantities of urine at frequent intervals or urine dribbling from the external urethral orifice. Finding a distended urinary bladder is usually sufficient for recognition of urinary retention. Urethral obstruction often is recognized because difficulty is encountered in passing a urethral catheter. When physical diagnostic methods are inconclusive, radiography or sonography may be necessary to verify or exclude suspected urinary retention.

**Stranguria.** Slow and painful urination associated with disease of the lower urinary tract, including cystitis, vesical calculus, urethral obstruction, and urethritis. The animal strains to pass each drop of urine. Groaning and straining may precede and accompany urination when there is urethral obstruction. In urethritis, groaning and straining occur immediately after urination has ceased, gradually disappearing and not recurring until urination has been repeated.

**Tenesmus.** Excessive straining, usually associated with either defecation or urination. Urinary tenesmus must be differentiated from alimentary tenesmus. A persistent squatting stance following urination in the female dog or male and female cat, bloody urine, dribbling urine or urinary incontinence are signs that suggest that the tenesmus is urinary in origin. Alimentary tenesmus, a hallmark of colorectal disease, indicates urgency to defecate and is characterized by frequent and usually unproductive attempts to defecate. In large animals frequent attempts to urinate, manifested by swishing of the tail, kicking at the abdomen, straining to urinate, sometimes accompanied by groaning, are commonly due to overdistension of the bladder in response to urethral obstruction. Teeth grinding (bruxism) may accompany tenesmus in sheep with obstructive urolithiasis.

**Urinary incontinence.** Lack of voluntary control over the flow of urine owing to inappropriate or incomplete voiding and storage of urine. There are several subsets of incontinence. **Paradoxical incontinence** is induced by bladder or urethral obstruction which allows some urine to leak around the blockage because of the pressure within the bladder. **Overflow incontinence** occurs when the bladder cannot contract but will fill until urine flows passively from the urethra (e.g. lower motor neuron disease).

- **Reflex incontinence** is usually caused by an upper motor neuron lesion and results in the bladder filling and emptying, usually leaving an increased residual volume, but the animal can no longer actively control the process. **Enuresis.** Urinary incontinence that occurs while the animal is asleep and is common in female dogs.

**Urine scalding** (**urinary burn**) of the skin of the perineal region, and sometimes the hindlimbs, occurs due to urine.

# Dogs and Cats

Diseases of the urinary tract are common in both the dog and cat and may affect only a portion of the tract, such as the kidneys or ureters, or may involve the entire urinary system. Clinical findings such as dysuria, pollakiuria and hematuria may localize the abnormality to a segment of the urinary tract such as the bladder, or evidence of systemic illness such as anorexia and vomiting associated with uremia may suggest advanced chronic renal failure.

The objective of the clinical examination is to identify those findings from the history and the physical examination that will aid in localization of the lesion within the urinary tract and assist in making a definitive diagnosis. An accurate diagnosis will facilitate the prognosis and clinical management.

## SIGNALMENT AND HISTORY

The species, sex and age of the animal may suggest diagnostic hypotheses. The history should include information on

- the frequency of urination
- the volume of urine produced
- changes in water intake
- the appearance and odor of the urine.

Polydipsia is usually more easily recognized by the owner than polyuria. It may be helpful for the owner to characterize water consumption in familiar quantitative terms, such as 'cups per day' (250 ml/cup). Some owners may be unable to quantify consumption yet observe that the animal is consuming water in unusual ways, such as drinking out of the toilet bowl, fish tank, or flower pots. In cases where polyuria is verified or suspected, the owner should be asked about possible exposure to a nephrotoxic agent (gentamicin, amphotericin B, non-steroidal anti-inflammatory drugs or ethylene glycol.) Whether or not the animal has been receiving any medication that could cause polyuria and polydipsia (glucocorticoids, diuretics) should be determined. Polydipsia usually occurs if there is significant polyuria.

**Water consumption in dogs and cats**

- normal water consumption in a controlled environment is 6–25 ml/kg/day
- polydipsia is defined as water consumption exceeding 100 ml/kg/day.

Pollakiuria must be differentiated from polyuria. Polyuria may be difficult for the owner to verify or notice and is usually associated with polydipsia. Owners may note a large volume of urine if the dog has 'accidents' in the house. Cat owners may note that the litter pan requires frequent changing because it is soaked with urine.

The clinician attempts to characterize the 'act' of urination. The owner may be able to provide information regarding the diameter of the urine stream and

the ability of the animal to initiate the urination reflex. An animal with a partial obstruction may have difficulty initiating urination and may have an abnormal urine stream. When characterizing abnormalities of urination, the clinician must distinguish between pollakiuria, dysuria, stranguria, and incontinence. Pollakiuria is an important localizing feature of lower urinary tract disease. Dysuria and stranguria are signs localizing to the lower urinary tract. Hematuria may be observed by the owner. In most cases its presence does not have very good localizing value. However, blood at the end of urination or throughout urination may indicate a renal or upper urinary tract problem, whereas blood at the beginning of urination may suggest an abnormality of the urethra or genital tract.

## PHYSICAL EXAMINATION OF THE URINARY TRACT

The urinary tract includes the kidneys, ureters, urinary bladder, and urethra. The kidneys, bladder, and pelvic urethra can be evaluated by physical examination. The prostate gland is part of the sex organs and is commonly examined along with the lower urinary tract. Diagnostic aids such as medical imaging can complement the physical examination to evaluate structures such as the kidneys, ureters, bladder and prostate gland which may not always be accessible by the usual physical examination techniques. Laboratory investigations, including urinalysis, serum biochemistry, hematology, renal function tests such as the endogenous creatinine clearance test, water deprivation tests, cytology, and biopsy of certain tissues, may be necessary to complete the examination.

### Complete physical examination

A complete physical examination should be carried out on small animals with suspected urinary tract disease. This includes a rectal examination and an ocular fundic examination. The state of hydration is evaluated and any evidence of subcutaneous edema or ascites suggestive of the nephrotic syndrome is noted. The oral cavity is examined to evaluate the color of the mucous membranes, ulcers, or tongue-tip necrosis, as

**Urine production in dogs and cats**

- normal urine production is 26–44 ml/kg/day
- polyuria is defined as urine production exceeding 50 ml/kg/day.

> **Clinical Pointer**
>
> Take care to differentiate incontinence from inappropriate micturition. The latter may be
>
> - a symptom of organic disease, such as urinary tract infection or urolithiasis
> - secondary to a polyuric disorder
> - a manifestation of a behavioral problem.

may occur in renal failure. An ocular fundic examination may provide evidence of retinal

- edema
- detachment
- hemorrhage, or
- vascular tortuosity

associated with systemic hypertension secondary to renal disease.

> **Clinical Pointer**
>
> Renal failure and fibrous osteodystrophy in young growing animals can cause enlargement and deformity of the mandible and maxilla (rubber jaw).

### Palpation of abdomen

The abdomen is palpated to evaluate the kidneys for location, size, shape, consistency and pain. The kidneys of the dog are bean-shaped; those of the cat are more spherical. In the dog the kidneys are retroperitoneal and situated on either side of the aorta and caudal vena cava. The right kidney is level with the first three lumbar vertebrae, situated almost entirely under the ribs, and the left kidney is more caudal, at the level of the second, third, and fourth lumbar vertebrae. In the cat the right kidney is situated ventral to the first to the fourth lumbar vertebral transverse processes, whereas the left kidney lies ventral to the second to the fifth lumbar vertebral transverse processes. In most cats both kidneys can be palpated (Fig.18.1), whereas in dogs sometimes only the left kidney can be palpated (Fig. 18.2). The kidneys of the cat are freely movable by palpation of the abdomen and may be mistaken for an abnormal abdominal mass. Enlargement of one or both kidneys due to infectious, neoplastic, or anomalous conditions may facilitate their palpation. Several diseases are associated with renomegaly in the cat, including

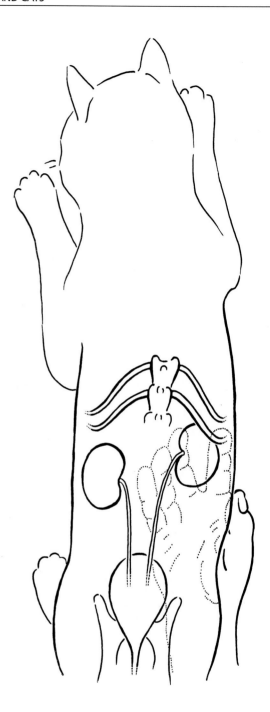

**Fig. 18.1** Both kidneys are readily palpable in most cats and are located in the dorsal portion of the cranial quadrant of the abdomen. This figure illustrates the clinician palpating the right kidney with one hand. During the course of an examination of a cat both kidneys may often be palpated simultaneously, but sometimes each are examined successively.

If the history indicates lower urinary tract disease a digital vaginal examination can be done to assess the vestibule, vagina, and the urethral orifice. In dogs and cats the external urethral orifice can be examined with the aid of a speculum and light source and with chemical restraint. Physical examination of the urethra in male cats is usually limited to inspection of the distal portion of the penile urethra. The urethra of male dogs may be examined by inspection and palpation. The urethral meatus may be examined after exteriorizing the penis from the prepuce. The perineal portion of the urethra in the male dog may be palpated just beneath the skin. Rectal palpation is performed to examine the pelvic urethra in both sexes of dog and cat and the prostate gland in the male dog. As with the bladder, the urethra is palpated and evaluated for position, degree of distension, evidence of pain, thickness of the wall, and the presence of intramural or intraluminal masses. The normal urethra is a smooth, tubular structure on the floor of the pelvis.

## Collection of a urine sample

The collection of a urine sample for analysis is essential for evaluation of the urinary tract. Urine may be collected by natural voiding, urethral catheterization of the bladder, or by cystocentesis. Cystocentesis is the preferred method because it prevents contamination of the sample by the distal urethra and genital tract. However, in animals being examined for evaluation of hematuria, a midstream voided sample is collected first because other collection methods may introduce red blood cells into the sample as a result of trauma.

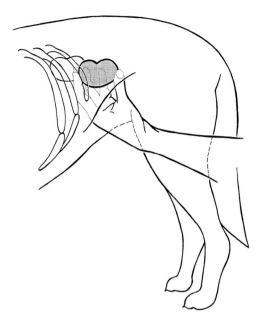

**Fig. 18.2** The left kidney is more caudal and freely movable, and can be palpated in some dogs by deep palpation of the craniodorsal abdomen. The right kidney is not usually palpable in the dog. One or two-handed palpation techniques may be used.

- polycystic kidney disease
- renal lymphosarcoma
- granulomatous nephritis associated with feline infectious peritonitis.

Most chronic diseases, such as chronic interstitial nephritis causing chronic renal failure, are associated with normal or small kidney size.

Normal ureters cannot be evaluated by palpation of the abdomen in the dog and cat. With rare exceptions, abnormal ureters also are not palpable.

The bladder can be palpated in most dogs and cats (Fig. 18.3), unless it is empty or the animal is markedly obese. It is evaluated for position in the abdomen, degree of distension, evidence of pain, thickness of the wall, and the presence of intramural masses such as neoplasms or intraluminal masses such as calculi and blood clots. A full bladder in a clinically dehydrated animal, in the absence of urethral obstruction, suggests the possibility of abnormal renal function or the administration of drugs that impair urinary concentrating ability (diuretics, glucocorticoids).

### Urethra

The urethra of female dogs and cats is difficult to evaluate with routine physical examination techniques.

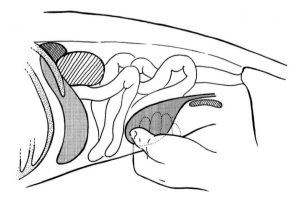

**Fig. 18.3** One-handed technique is best for palpation of the urinary bladder. Very small and very large bladders are usually difficult to feel. A medium-sized bladder is normally palpable in the caudal abdominal quadrant as a smooth, pear-shaped structure.

## Natural voiding

Midstream collection during natural voiding is an acceptable method of collecting a urine sample for routine analysis. The procedure is without risk and can be done by the owner. The disadvantages are that the sample may be contaminated with cells, bacteria, and debris located in the distal urethra, genital tract or on the skin and hair. Nor will the patient always void at the will of the person collecting the sample. Under certain circumstances, such as when verification of the presence of proteinuria or pyuria from a previous sample is desirable, it may be necessary to repeat the analysis of a urine sample collected by either cystocentesis or urethral catheterization. In general, voided samples are less desirable for bacteriological culture than those collected by cystocentesis or urethral catheterization.

## Cystocentesis

Cystocentesis, or puncturing of the bladder with a needle through the abdominal wall to obtain an uncontaminated urine sample, is simple when the bladder is palpable and is generally well tolerated by both dogs and cats.

The procedure is done using a 22 gauge 1" or 1½" needle. Occasionally, 2½" or 3" spinal needles are used for larger dogs. A 10 or 12 ml syringe is used. The procedure can be done in lateral or dorsal recumbency in cats and dogs, or in the standing dog (Figs 18.4, 18.5). Whichever position is used, it is recommended that the needle be inserted through the ventral or ventrolateral wall of the bladder so as to minimize the risk of trauma to the ureters and large abdominal vessels. The needle is directed through the bladder wall at 45° so that an oblique tract will be created, providing an effective seal upon removal. Excessive hair is removed from the cystocentesis site and the skin is wiped with alcohol.

## Lateral cystocentesis

The animal is positioned in lateral recumbency or is standing (Fig. 18.4) and the bladder is palpated to determine its size and location. The bladder is immobilized with the free hand, either from below in lateral recumbency or from the opposite side of the abdomen when the animal is standing, and pressed dorsally and caudally to immobilize it. If the dog is standing it may be useful to have an assistant hold up the flank fold on the side where the needle is to be inserted (Fig. 18.4). The needle is inserted through the skin of the ventro-lateral abdominal wall, abdominal cavity and bladder wall, angling caudomedially, and urine is aspirated into the syringe. If blood or no urine is obtained, aspiration is stopped and the needle withdrawn completely. Attempting to redirect the needle within the abdominal cavity is not recommended. Instead, the needle is replaced with a new sterile one and a second attempt made. If unsuccessful, no further attempts are made for several hours.

## Ventral cystocentesis

The animal is positioned in dorsal recumbency. One or two assistants are often required to restrain and position the patient and the bladder is palpated to determine size

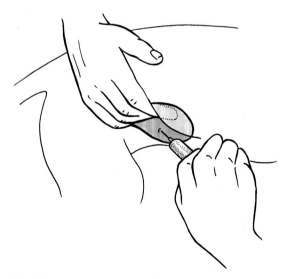

**Fig. 18.4** Lateral cystocentesis: dog is lying in right or left lateral recumbency. The bladder is immobilized dorsally and caudally by pressing it with the clinician's free hand. The procedure is similiar with the dog standing, but the bladder is immobilized by pressing it laterally and caudally. Needle insertion may be facilitated by an assistant holding up the flank fold.

---

### Complications and contraindications of cystocentesis

- complications include hematuria and laceration of the bladder or intestines (the risk of introducing infection is low).
- contraindications include insufficient urine volume to allow digital localization and immobilization of the bladder, and patient resistance to restraint and abdominal palpation.

## Clinical Pointer

For ventral cystocentesis some clinicians advocate dripping alcohol on to the caudal abdomen and inserting the needle at the site of alcohol pooling.

and location. The bladder is stabilized and positioned close to the ventral abdominal wall by compression of the cranial abdomen with the free hand (Fig. 18.5). In female dogs and cats and in male cats the needle is inserted into the abdomen, remaining on the midline.

In the male dog the needle is inserted lateral to the prepuce. Urine is aspirated as described above.

### Urethral catheterization of the bladder

Urethral catheterization of the bladder may be used to obtain a urine sample when cystocentesis is not successful or is contraindicated. Catheterization may also be necessary to relieve a urethral obstruction or to serve as an indwelling bladder catheter. Urethral catheterization is also necessary for radiographic contrast studies of the bladder and urethra. Potential complications of urethral catheterization include trauma, and the introduction of infection.

The entire procedure is done with strict attention to asepsis and a gentle technique. This includes clipping long hairs immediately surrounding the prepuce or vulva and using povidone-iodine or chlorhexidine surgical scrubs to cleanse the surrounding areas, followed by rinsing with sterile saline. Sterile gloves should be used for asepsis and to assist in catheter manipulation. Alternative ways of manipulating the catheter in an aseptic manner without gloves include

- holding the distal end only
- using a sterilized pediatric hemostat
- holding the catheter through its packaging.

Sterile water-based lubricant or lubricant containing a local anesthetic (lidocaine) designed for urological procedures is used on the catheters and specula to minimize trauma and patient discomfort.

### Male dog

The length of catheter necessary to reach the neck of the bladder from the external urethral meatus is estimated and marked with a pen or piece of tape (Fig. 18.6). This prevents the catheter from being advanced too far into the bladder and minimizes the risk of the end becoming knotted or folding back on itself. The patient is restrained in a standing position or in lateral recumbency. The penis is gently extruded from the prepuce by an assistant and cleansed with surgical scrub, followed by a sterile saline rinse (Fig. 18.7). The tip of the catheter is lubricated with sterile water-soluble lubricant or lubricant containing lidocaine, inserted into the urethral orifice and gently advanced towards the bladder. Slight resistance may be encountered as the catheter passes over the ischial arch. It may be necessary to gently aspirate with a syringe if no urine appears when the catheter has been advanced sufficiently to enter the bladder. Unless specifically desired, the first several milliliters of urine are discarded because they may be contaminated with bacteria, debris, and cells from the distal urethra and genital tract. The catheter is withdrawn from the

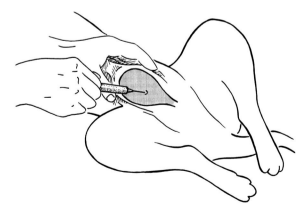

**Fig. 18.5** Ventral cystocentesis. The patient is in dorsal recumbency. The needle is inserted into the abdomen on the midline in female dogs and both male and female cats, and lateral to the midline in male dogs to avoid the penis.

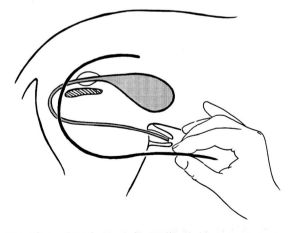

**Fig. 18.6** Estimating the length of the urinary catheter in a male dog.

### Restraint for urethral catheterization in dogs and cats

- most dogs require physical but rarely chemical restraint for this procedure
- most cats require tranquilization or anesthesia – a moribund cat with a urethral obstruction is an exception.

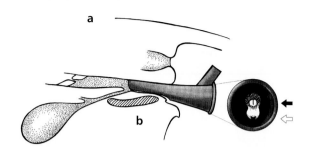

**Fig. 18.8** Female dog. Location of the urethral orifice in ventral wall of vagina. (a) A vaginal speculum (anuscope) is inserted. Looking through the speculum, the external urethral orifice (solid arrow) is approximately 3–5 cm cranial to the ventral commissure of the vulva; the clitoral fossa (open arrow) lies just caudal to the external urethral orifice (b).

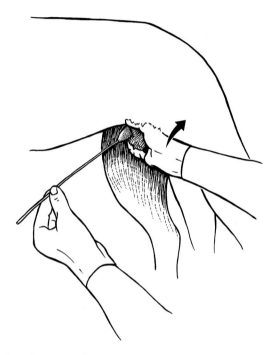

**Fig. 18.7** Extruding the penis from the prepuce in a dog.

urinary tract when the procedure is complete, or is fixed in position for indwelling purposes.

### Female dog – visual technique

The bladder of the female dog is easiest to catheterize when the external urethral orifice can be visualized using some type of light source and a speculum, such as a human nasal speculum, human rectal speculum, otoscope cone, or specula fashioned from plastic syringe cases. Specula with self-contained light sources are the easiest to use. The external urethral orifice is located on a small tubercle in the ventral wall of the vagina (Fig. 18.8). In medium-sized female dogs this is approximately 3–5 cm cranial to the ventral commissure of the vulva. The clitoral fossa is situated caudally to the urethral orifice and must be avoided during catheterization.

The procedure is done with the animal standing or in sternal recumbency, with an assistant restraining the hindquarters

- the vulvar and perineal tissues are prepared and the catheter handled as described above
- the speculum is lubricated and gently inserted into the vagina by initially directing it dorsally and then cranially
- the urethral meatus is visualized and the catheter is introduced through the speculum into the urethral orifice and advanced into the urine bladder
- urine is aspirated with a syringe if none appears when the catheter is advanced into the bladder.

### Female dog – digital technique

This technique may be utilized in female dogs which are large enough to permit digital palpation of the vagina. An assistant is necessary to help restrain the animal in a standing position

- the vaginal and perineal tissues are cleansed with surgical scrub and rinsed with sterile saline
- a lubricated tuberculin syringe (with needle removed) containing 0.3–0.5 ml of topical ophthalmic anesthetic or 0.5% lidocaine is inserted 2–4 cm into the vagina and the anesthetic instilled
- using sterile gloves a lubricated finger is inserted into the vagina and an attempt made to palpate the urethral papilla
- a sterile lubricated urethral catheter is inserted into the vagina, directed dorsal to the clitoral fossa and guided along the midline of the vaginal floor towards the urethral orifice (Fig. 18.9)

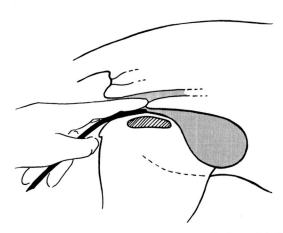

**Fig. 18.9** Urethral catheterization of female dog. Digital technique. The gloved and lubricated finger palpates the urethral papilla on the vaginal floor. The urethral catheter is inserted under the finger and advanced to the urethral papilla, and the catheter is threaded into the urethra and advanced until urine is obtained.

- the catheter is then threaded into the urethra; this can readily be determined when the tip of the catheter vanishes into the floor of the vagina – a common error for inexperienced clinicians is to over-insert the catheter into the vagina, if this occurs, the catheter is withdrawn and the tip redirected towards the urethral orifice
- urine is collected once the catheter has been advanced into the bladder

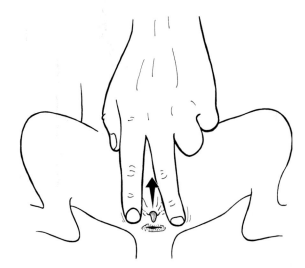

**Fig. 18.10** Extruding the male cat's penis. The prepuce is retracted, exposing the glans of the penis. This is often easiest with the cat in dorsal recumbency with the hindlegs splayed in a 'frog' position.

- a syringe is used to gently aspirate if no urine appears.

### Male cat

The procedure should be attempted without chemical restraint in cats with urethral obstruction who are very ill. Occasionally, a fully conscious cat may be catheterized with tactful manual restraint. For short-term placement, collection of a urine sample or relief of urethral obstruction, an open-ended tomcat catheter (3½ Fr) is satisfactory. For indwelling purposes a soft polypropylene or red rubber infant feeding tube (usually 3½ Fr, occasionally 5 Fr in large cats) may be used. The cat is restrained in lateral or dorsal recumbency

- the penis is extruded by placing a finger on either side of the prepuce and exerting pressure (Fig. 18.10), and cleansed with surgical scrub, followed by a saline rinse
- using surgical gloves, the lubricated catheter is inserted into the urethral orifice
- the catheter is carefully threaded into the urethra, which may be facilitated by extending the penis from the preputial sheath in a caudal direction, with the long axis of the urethra approximately parallel to the vertebral column (Fig. 18.11) – this manipulation will facilitate catheterization by reducing the natural curvature in the distal urethra
- urine is collected once the catheter has been advanced into the bladder
- if no urine appears a syringe is used to gently aspirate
- if an indwelling catheter is needed then a soft feeding tube is recommended.

### Female cat

If chemical restraint is not used, topical anesthetic may be instilled into the vagina with a tuberculin syringe. With the cat in sternal recumbency the procedure may be attempted blindly or visually with the aid of a speculum and light source

- the vaginal and perineal tissues are cleansed with surgical scrub and rinsed with sterile saline
- using sterile gloves the vulvar labia are spread with the fingers and the lubricated catheter inserted into the vagina
- the urethral papilla is located approximately 0.7–1.0 cm cranial to the ventral commissure of the vulva
- the lubricated catheter is advanced cranially while staying on the midline, sliding the catheter along the ventral wall of the vagina until it slips into the urethral orifice – care is taken not to use excessive pressure as it is possible to force the catheter through the vagina/cervix and into the peritoneal cavity

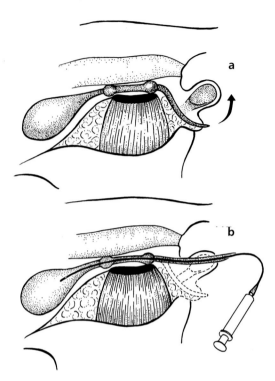

**Fig. 18.11** Positioning the cat's penis so that the urethra is parallel to the vertebral column. (a) The penis in the natural position. (b) The penis extended from the preputial sheath by drawing it in a caudal position, aligning the long axis of the urethra with the long axis of the vertebral column; this minimizes the natural curvature of the caudal portion of the urethra and facilitates catheterization.

- if no urine appears a syringe is used to gently aspirate
- if an indwelling catheter is to be fixed for continuous drainage, a soft feeding tube is recommended.

## MEDICAL IMAGING OF THE URINARY TRACT

### Survey radiography

Survey radiography may be used to evaluate the size, shape, position, and radiographic opacity of the kidneys and the urinary bladder. Radiodense calculi, if present, may be detected in the kidneys, ureters, bladder, and urethra. Survey radiographs are essential as control films prior to contrast radiography. Kidneys, especially the right, may not be distinguishable on survey radiographs even when normal. Preradiography enema and abdominal compression radiography can be useful to enhance visualization of normal structures.

### Contrast radiography

Excretory urography may be employed when the kidneys are not visible on survey abdominal radiographs. Excretory radiography (intravenous urography) also demonstrates renal perfusion, ability of the kidney to concentrate and excrete the contrast agent, filling defects in the renal pelvis, dilation of the renal pelvis and ureter, and ectopic ureters. Positive, negative, and double-contrast cystography can be used to identify the thickness of the bladder wall, luminal filling defects, mucosal irregularities, diverticulae, radiolucent calculi and leakage from and rupture of the bladder. Retrograde positive contrast urethrography and vaginourethrography may identify luminal filling defects, anatomic abnormalities and ruptures.

### Ultrasonography

Ultrasonography is an excellent complement to radiographic examination of the urinary tract and in some cases (e.g. unilateral nephromegaly) may be selected in lieu of contrast radiography. It is useful in demonstrating irregularities of internal architecture, such as a soft tissue mass in the urinary bladder. It can also discriminate solid from fluid-filled lesions within the kidney and define the distribution of lesions (focal, multifocal, diffuse). Renal size can be accurately determined. Ultrasonography may be useful for the detection of calculi, particularly those that are relatively radiolucent (e.g. ammonium acid urate), and can be used to accurately guide the needle during biopsy procedures. Doppler ultrasonography may be used to assess renal blood flow and to distinguish between perfusion deficits and primary renal failure.

---

### Clinical Pointer

Ultrasonography is most beneficial when radiographic definition is reduced

- in the presence of peritoneal effusion
- when contrast radiography provides incomplete information (e.g. non-opacification of one or both kidneys).

---

### Renal biopsy

Renal biopsy is considered when a histological diagnosis is likely to alter patient management. Circumstances would include

- characterization of protein-losing glomerular diseases (e.g. immune-complex glomerulonephritis versus amyloidosis)

- differentiation of acute renal failure from chronic renal failure
- determination of reversibility and prognosis in acute renal failure
- assessing the response to therapy or progression of previously documented renal disease.

This procedure should not be performed without a thorough clinical evaluation of the patient, including assessment of blood clotting ability.

Several methods have been described and include blind percutaneous, keyhole, laparoscopic, open and ultrasound-guided techniques.

> **Contraindications to renal biopsy**
>
> These include a bleeding disorder, a solitary kidney, and renal lesions associated with fluid accumulation (e.g. renal cysts, abscesses, and hydronephrosis).

## Cystoscopy and urethroscopy

Endoscopy can be used to visually verify suspected lesions of the bladder and urethra which may have been identified by radiography and/or ultrasound. Lesions not identified by other methods may be visible during cystoscopy, for example inflammatory conditions of the lower urinary tract. Anatomical defects of the vagina, urethra, and bladder, such as ectopic ureters, may be visible during endoscopic examination. Biopsy samples may be collected accurately with visualization of the lesion(s) and may help to provide a definitive diagnosis.

# Cattle, Sheep, Goats, Horses, and Pigs

Clinical examination of the urinary tract of large animals consists of obtaining a history, performing a distant examination of the external genitalia, visual observation of the act of urination from a distance, examination of the urine, and physical examination of the urinary tract by inspection and palpation.

## Signalment and history

The major clinical and historical findings of disease of the urinary tract include

- painful urination
- abnormal urine in terms of color and consistency
- changes in the volume of urine produced and voided.

Tenesmus or straining is an abnormal behavior consistent with disease of the lower urinary tract, but may also be associated with diseases of the gastrointestinal tract and the nervous system. A history of straining to urinate in young castrated ruminants suggests obstructive urolithiasis. The history may indicate that the animal was straining and dribbling small amounts of urine, or that no urine has been passed for an extended period of time. Although clinical findings of colic, such as restlessness, kicking at the belly, and tail flagging in the horse, are more likely to be indicative of gastrointestinal dysfunction, similar clinical findings in ruminants can reflect pain and discomfort related to the urinary tract as well as the gastrointestinal system. Loss of body condition and weight, inappetence, and anorexia are common in renal disease such as pyelonephritis. Dribbling of urine usually indicates lower urinary tract disease. However, pathological urine dribbling should not be confused with frequent voiding of small quantities as may occur in excitable animals. The voiding of bloody urine commonly indicates lower urinary tract disease. Signs of discomfort such as sudden body or tail movements, vocalization, bruxism, squatting, and treading or kicking with the rear limbs warrant further evaluation of the urinary tract.

## Distant examination

Behavioral aspects of urination vary between the large animal species. Male ruminants may urinate while walking, feeding, or standing still. However, cattle usually assume a posture for urination, characterized by either a firm stance with the legs placed squarely beneath the body, or slightly abducted with subtle extension of the back. The tail may be raised. Urine flows freely in a pulsatile manner from the penile urethra into the preputial cavity and then escapes from the orifice. In steers urine flow is a low-pressure passive event, whereas mature bulls usually void more force-

> **Clinical Pointer**
>
> Rectal prolapse in young castrated ruminants can be caused by straining to urinate; care should be taken not to misdiagnose the cause of the prolapse as gastrointestinal disease.

> ### Clinical Pointer
>
> In the male
>
> - during urination in male large aninmals the skin immediately below the anus and overlying the area of the ischial arch will show rhythmic pulsation
> - pulsation of this skin *without* urine flow from the preputial orifice is abnormal and suggests an obstruction, particularly a urolith, in the penile urethra.

fully and the penis may protrude from the preputial opening. The posture of urination for the ram and buck is characterized by slight caudal placement and flexion of the pelvic limbs.

Female cattle urinate in a stationary position preceded by simultaneous raising of the tail and arching (flexing) of the back. Some cows may actually move their pelvic limbs in a slight caudal direction. Urination is rapid and voluminous. The ewe and doe typically squat to urinate.

The gelding and stallion precede urination by protruding the penis from the prepuce. All male horses demonstrate tail raising, extension of the back and slight flexion movement of the pelvic limbs caudally to present a 'sawhorse' stance. Urine flow is forceful. The mare prepares for urination by arching the back, raising the tail and squatting slightly on the rear limbs. Urination is terminated with dorsal and caudal contractions of the vaginal mucosa to the level of vulvar lips (referred to as 'winking'), presumably to remove residual urine remaining on the floor of the vagina. The mare, stallion, and gelding may groan or grunt during urination. Such vocalization should not be confused with urinary tract pathology, provided urine flows freely and the normal color and consistency are observed.

The boar and barrow flex the back and urinate into the prepuce and preputial diverticulum located in the dorsal wall of the prepuce. The prepuce will visibly distend, simultaneously with preputial rhythmic contractions that force spurts of urine from the preputial orifice. The gilt and sow arch the back shortly before elimination of a straight stream of urine.

The frequency of urination and the amount produced in large animals depends on the quantity of water consumed, together with that produced by metabolic processes and the amount lost by respiration, perspiration, and defecation. Milk production is an important route of water loss in lactating animals, especially dairy cows. Hydration status is influenced by changes in physical activity and by climatic or seasonal events which influence the intake of fluids, nutrients, and electrolytes.

Swine urinate frequently during the day, typically prior to eating, following periods of rest.

Documentation of polyuria and polydipsia is a tedious and time-consuming exercise requiring careful monitoring of total daily fluid intake and urine production. A complete lack of urine production (anuria) may occur in severe acute renal failure, and must be distinguished from the inability to urinate which may occur in obstructive urolithiasis or when there is retention of urine in the bladder. The latter may reflect an inability to adopt the normal posture for urinating, as can occur with abdominal pain. Prolonged recumbency in mature cows and horses may be accompanied by failure to urinate and retention of urine in the bladder. However, in cows the bladder can be emptied with ease by catheterization or by stimulation to urinate with digital pressure on the bladder wall per rectum. Urinary bladder catheterization in recumbent mares is possible but is very difficult in recumbent male horses.

> ### Daily urine volume and frequency
>
> The daily urine volumes and frequencies of the domestic large animal species are
>
> - horses 2–11 liters/day (3–18 ml/kg/day), urinating 4–6 times/day
> - cattle 8–22 liters/day (17–45 ml/kg/day), urinating 9 times/day
> - sheep and goats 0.5–2 liters/day (10–40 ml/kg/day), urinating 9 times/day
> - pigs 2–6 liters/day (5–30 ml/kg/day), urinating 'frequently'.

## PHYSICAL EXAMINATION OF THE URINARY SYSTEM

Both male and female urethrae should be examined with the associated genital organs. The penile urethra is examined indirectly by inspection and palpation of the penis, and by catheterization of the urethra. Physical examination of the male pelvic urethra, bladder, ureters, and kidneys requires rectal palpation, which is possible only in cattle and horses of sufficient body size. The female urethra is examined by palpation and inspection through the vagina. In small ruminants and swine the kidneys may be palpable through the abdominal wall. In normal animals palpation of the external or internal structures of the urinary tract should not elicit sensitivity or discomfort.

## Male urethra

### *Prepuce and penile urethra*

#### General aspects

In large animals the penis and associated urethra can only be inspected along the length of the glans penis to the fornix of the prepuce. However, palpation of the penis is possible along most of its length, with the exception of the segment coursing deeply in the perineal area above the base of the scrotum and below the ischial arch. The normal glans penis and preputial mucosa should have a moist surface and a pink color. The epithelial surface of the glans penis should be smooth, whereas the preputial mucosa has a more wrinkled appearance unless the penis is fully extended. Inflammation of the glans penis (balanoposthitis) is suggested by

- a bright red color
- roughened dry surface
- fine nodular ('pebbly') surface, or
- surface exudation.

#### Bull and steer

The preputial hairs are examined by inspection and palpation for evidence of dryness indicating no recent urination, and the presence of crystals on the hairs indicating crystalluria in urolithiasis. Direct inspection of the prepuce may reveal the dribbling of urine and gross abnormalities such as hematuria. The prepuce is also examined for evidence of inflammation, or maceration of the skin associated with urine scalding.

The penis is palpated for evidence of swelling or painful sites over its entire course, from the prepuce to just above the scrotum and at the ischial arch. Palpation above the scrotum requires some additional dexterity to ensure that all parts of the sigmoid flexure are palpated.

The urethra of the bovine male terminates on the ventrolateral surface of the glans penis. The bull can usually be induced to protrude the penis from the preputial opening by manual massage of its pelvic portion per rectum. Alternatively, the penis can be exteriorized by pushing the sigmoid flexure cranially toward the preputial opening with one hand while simultaneously retracting the prepuce with the other. In contrast, the penis of a steer is virtually impossible to exteriorize.

The patency of the urethra of a mature bull can be determined by inserting a long flexible probe or catheter into the penile urethra after relaxing the penis with an ataractic drug. The presence of a urolith will prevent further passage of the probe at the site of the urolith, and a grating feeling may be appreciated as the probe meets the urolith. Passing a urinary catheter into the bladder of a male bovine often is impossible because of the subischial urethral diverticulum that catches the tip of the catheter.

Obstructive urolithiasis occurs most commonly in young castrated cattle and occasionally in mature bulls. The uroliths or calculi can occur in the renal pelvis, ureter, bladder, and urethra. They commonly lodge in the penile urethra near the attachment of the retractor penis muscles in the distal sigmoid flexure, causing partial or complete obstruction. Animals with partial obstruction have prolonged, painful urination and dribble bloodstained urine. Animals with complete obstruction exhibit frequent tenesmus, with tail switching and shifting of the weight from one hindlimb to the other. Inappetence, depression and rectal prolapse are also common features. Common sequelae of complete obstruction of the urethra include rupture of the urethra and/or bladder. If perforation of the urethra occurs, urine infiltrates the subcutaneous and muscular tissues of the ventral abdominal wall and prepuce, resulting in a prominent swelling of the ventral abdominal wall. Severe cellulitis and extensive necrosis of the skin extending from the scrotum to the prepuce leads to eventual sloughing of the affected skin. Toxemia is common. Extensive involvement of the ventral abdominal wall can result in prolapse of the preputial mucosa in steers and bulls.

---

### Clinical Pointer

Uroliths in cattle commonly lodge in the sigmoid flexure, located immediately dorsal to and deep to the base of the scrotum, palpation dorsal to the scrotum is necessary to detect the painful swelling of the penis.

---

Rupture of the corpus cavernosum during the act of breeding occurs in bulls at the site of attachment of the retractor penis muscles in the distal sigmoid flexure. Like the swelling of a urethral rupture, swelling and subcutaneous edema subsequently develops near the base of the scrotum. However, the resulting penile hematoma tends to occur cranial to the base of the

---

### Rupture of the bladder

When the bladder ruptures, urine accumulates in the peritoneal cavity and the abdomen gradually distends in a bilaterally symmetrical manner, with a prominent fluid wave on tactile percussion of the abdomen.

scrotum, whereas subcutaneous urine accumulation secondary to a ruptured urethra tends to occur slightly caudal to the base of the scrotum, and often becomes more extensively involved over time than the more confined extravasation of blood in the corpus cavernosum. Abscesses and other space-occupying masses can occur in the same area of the perineum and base of scrotum. Ultimately, needle aspiration of the contents may be required to definitively establish a diagnosis.

---

### Clinical Pointer

Care must be taken to differentiate

- abnormal gritty sand-like material from the normal debris adherent to hairs surrounding the preputial orifice of male ruminants
- abnormal material of urinary tract origin from the normal accumulations of dark inspissated mucus and cellular debris (smegma) that surrounds the end of the penile urethra within the urethral sinus of the glans penis (colloquially referred to as a 'bean') of stallions and geldings.

---

### Sheep and goats

The penis of intact and castrated rams and bucks is difficult to exteriorize, but can be accomplished by initially positioning the animal on its hindquarters. The penis then can be exteriorized by pushing the sigmoid flexure (located immediately above and deep to the base of the scrotum) cranially with one hand while simultaneously retracting the prepuce with the other. The urethra of sheep and goats lies in a groove on the ventral surface of the corpus cavernosum and projects 3–4 cm beyond the glans penis, within a tortuous urethral process known as the vermiform appendage. Uroliths commonly lodge in the urethral process or the distal urethra of the glans penis. They are readily identified as a hard nodular mass. The urethra can be examined for calculi by passing a small-bore dog catheter. In castrated males this may be best accomplished after surgical removal of the vermiform appendage under topical anesthesia. Obstruction to the passage of the catheter is often noted by a steady increase in resistance, rather than an abrupt stoppage. Withdrawal of the catheter or gentle flushing with saline may yield calculi. There may be gross swelling of the penis distal to the sigmoid flexure, together with edema of the prepuce and adjacent subcutaneous tissue. In castrated sheep the presence of balanoposthitis is characterized by swelling of the prepuce and painful urination.

### Horses

The penis of the horse can usually be located by inserting a hand into the preputial opening. The penis may subsequently be exteriorized by exerting slow steady retraction with a hand grasping the glans; chemical restraint often is necessary. The urethra terminates as a 2.5 cm free tube (urethral process) within a circular fossa, which opens dorsally into the urethral sinus. This diverticulum is filled with variable amounts of smegma.

### Swine

The penis in the conscious boar and barrow cannot easily be exteriorized, but under sedation it may be exposed with the aid of retractors directed through the preputial opening and blindly attached to the glans. Alternatively, if absolutely necessary, a full-thickness small linear incision can be made through the lateral surface of the prepuce and centered directly over the penis. The penis is then manipulated through this incision. The penis of swine has no glans and is spirally twisted. The urethra appears as a slit on the ventrolateral surface of the penis near its tip.

---

### Clinical Pointer

Mild sedation with phenothiazine ataractics (e.g. acepromazine) will greatly facilitate relaxation of the penis in the bull.

---

## Female urethra

In the female of each animal species the urethra is located on the midline of the floor of the vagina within 10 cm inside the vulvar lips. A suburethral diverticulum is present in the cow, ewe, doe, and sow. The urethral diameter in an adult mare and cow is usually sufficient to allow insertion of a finger. Palpable abnormalities of the female urethra are uncommon.

Debris matted to the vulvar lips and the ventral surface of the tail of any female large animal is unusual and should prompt the examination of the urinary tract and reproductive organs. Maceration of the skin around and below the vulva, with subsequent hair loss, suggests urine scalding.

### Urachus

The urachus normally retracts from the umbilicus within a few hours after birth, allowing the bladder to retract into the pelvic canal. A patent urachus should be suspected in a neonate whenever dribbling of fluid from the umbilicus occurs during urination, or a persistently moist umbilicus is present. External palpation of the abdomen above the umbilicus should reveal a cylindrical structure of variable diameter coursing away in a caudodorsal direction from the ventral midline of the body wall. The neonate may exhibit pain during this palpation and urinalysis may reveal evidence of cystitis.

## Kidneys

Because of the considerable thickness and rigidity of the abdominal wall in mature cattle and horses the kidneys cannot be palpated through the abdominal wall but are palpable by rectal examination. The kidneys of sheep, goats, and pigs are not readily palpable by rectal examination because of the small anus in these animals. They can be evaluated by external abdominal palpation.

### Cattle

In cattle, the kidneys are superficially divided into a variable number (20–25) of lobules. Although fissures separate each kidney lobule, in well nourished cattle the outline of each distinct lobule may not be apparent because of the presence of perirenal fat. Typically, only the caudal half of the normal left kidney (10–12 cm in width and approximately 10 cm thick in the adult) can be palpated on rectal examination ventral to the third, fourth, and fifth lumbar vertebrae. The left kidney may be palpated to the right of the midline if the rumen is full. The normal right kidney cannot be palpated in its more proximal location beneath the last rib and the first two or three lumbar transverse processes. When enlarged, the caudal pole of the right kidney may be palpable in smaller cattle.

> ### Position of the left kidney in cattle
> - in the normal animal, ingesta in the rumen displaces the left kidney to the right of the midline
> - in the anorexic animal, when the size of the rumen is decreased, the left kidney is on or to the left of the midline.

### Sheep and goats

In sheep and goats the kidneys are bean-shaped (7.5 cm long × 5 cm wide × 3 cm thick) without lobulations. In the standing animal (including calves) they can be located using an external palpation technique of placing a hand in the upper margin of each paralumbar fossa immediately behind the last rib,

followed by movement of each hand in a caudomedial direction across the paralumbar fossa. The left kidney should be detected as a freely movable structure dangling a few centimeters below the vertebrae immediately caudal to the last rib. The right kidney may be palpable in the dorsal right paralumbar fossa caudal to the last rib.

### Horse

The left kidney in the horse is bean-shaped (18 cm long × 10–12 cm wide × 5–6 cm thick) with a smooth surface, and is palpable by rectal examination ventral to the last rib and the first two or three lumbar transverse processes. In well conditioned animals extensive perirenal fat accumulation may obscure kidney architecture. The right kidney is somewhat firmly fixed in position ventral to the dorsal part of the last three ribs and the transverse process of the first lumbar vertebra, and is not often palpable by rectal examination. The dorsal surface is related chiefly to the diaphragm, and the ventral surface is contiguous to the liver, pancreas, and cecum. The caudal extremity extends back to the first lumbar transverse process, where it is related to the base of the cecum.

### Swine

The kidneys of swine are smooth textured and bean-shaped (approximately 12.5 cm long × 6–6.5 cm wide) and in animals in good condition are encased in fat. They are located nearly side-by-side ventral to the transverse processes of the first four lumbar vertebrae (middle of each paralumbar fossa). The left kidney may occasionally occupy a position as far caudal as the pelvic inlet. The compact muscling of swine usually precludes adequate external palpation of these structures.

### Abnormal kidneys on rectal palpation

In large animals, enlargement of the kidneys is most likely due to pyelonephritis or hydronephrosis. Amyloidosis can also cause kidney enlargement, particularly in cattle, and is accompanied by marked proteinuria and, if advanced, anasarca due to hypoproteinemia. In cattle, the normal lobulation of the kidneys is usually lost with pyelonephritis and hydronephrosis, but not with amyloidosis. In addition, in pyelonephritis in cattle and horses, rectal palpation commonly reveals thickening of the wall of the bladder and enlargement of the ureters. Affected animals are characteristically febrile, have lost weight, are depressed and weak, and the urine is reddish to brownish and cloudy owing to hematuria, pyuria, proteinuria, and the presence of other cellular debris.

Other possible causes of kidney enlargement include neoplasms, such as lymphosarcoma, adenoma, and carcinoma, and hematomata and abscessation. In swine embryonal nephroma should be considered when a single kidney has a solitary mass affecting the parenchyma. In instances of perirenal edema, such as *Amaranthus retroflexus* (redroot pigweed) toxicity, and postpartum hemolytic–uremic syndrome kidney surface characteristics may be more difficult to delineate, or there may be crepitation of the tissue surrounding the kidneys.

---

### Clinical Pointer

Reduced Kidney size

- occurs in chronic renal disease
- in young animals suggests a developmental anomaly.

---

## Bladder

### Size and shape

In normal cattle and horses, the bladder is a piriform-shaped structure, narrowest at its attachment with the pelvic urethra that lies on the floor of the pelvis. It is usually not readily palpable by rectal palpation because it remains relatively empty. When empty, the bladder has a firm consistency and is small, with a slightly corrugated serosal surface. Although anchored by its neck to the urethra in the caudal pelvis, the bladder should be otherwise freely movable within the pelvic canal. In the cow and mare the bladder may be more difficult to locate because of the overlying reproductive tract. In small ruminants and swine the bladder has the same features as that of cattle and horses. In sheep and goats with obstructive urolithiasis, the distended bladder may be detected in the caudal part of the ventral abdomen using external abdominal palpation.

A readily palpable bladder may reflect simple retention of urine rather than an abnormality of the urinary tract. In simple retention the bladder wall feels thin, and digital compression should induce urination followed by a marked decrease in its size. A diffusely thickened wall is abnormal and consistent with cystitis, particularly if there are gross changes in the urine, including hematuria, pyuria and proteinuria. Persistent enlargement of the bladder occurs because of

- urethral obstruction
- chronic end-stage cystitis, or
- neuromuscular dysfunction.

Inability to completely retract the bladder into the caudal pelvis or to completely encircle its rounded cranial end (apex) is abnormal. When this occurs, adhesions or persistent urachal ligament should be suspected. The persistent ligament maintains tension on the bladder, leading to incomplete filling and emptying.

### Rupture

Rupture of the bladder in large animals can occur at any age, including the neonate at parturition. Complete obstruction of the urethra due to urolithiasis in castrated ruminants is a common cause of bladder rupture. Initially no abnormal clinical signs may be noted, with the exception of a reduction in or absence of urine production. However, accumulated urine in the peritoneal cavity will eventually result in a bilaterally symmetrical distended ventral abdomen ('water belly'). The magnitude of distension is dependent upon the amount of urine accumulated. In a noticeably distended abdomen a corresponding fluid wave can usually be elicited by tactile percussion. Depression, weakness, and dehydration usually accompany the abdominal changes.

In ruminants, simultaneous ruminal atony may alter the abdominal contour so that the left abdomen appears more distended than the right. However, the fluid wave is still present. Rectal palpation of the bladder may be unrewarding in detecting the site of the tear in the bladder wall, depending upon the size of the tear and the relative amount of urine retained. Tears usually occur on both surfaces of the bladder, usually near the apex.

Rupture of the urinary bladder occurs in newborn foals at birth. Most affected foals are

- male
- born without a complicated parturition
- appear normal in the early neonatal period.

Within 24–48 hours there is anorexia, depression, tachycardia, polypnea, and progressive abdominal distension and frequent straining, which can produce small quantities of normal urine. Abdominocentesis reveals large quantities of fluid which is usually uniformly clear and very pale yellow, with a low specific gravity.

In a newborn male foal with a suspected ruptured bladder indirect evidence can be substantiated by urethral catheterization. In neonatal male ruminants and swine this can be attempted but is very difficult. Dyes can be placed in the bladder via such a catheter to determine whether the material enters the peritoneal space through a tear in the bladder. These techniques are cumbersome and unreliable, and analysis of a sample of peritoneal fluid for a high (higher than circulating) concentration of creatinine is most reliable to detect uroperitoneum.

## Paralysis

Paralysis of the bladder is uncommon in large animals. Most cases are associated with neurological disease. There is retention of urine with overflow incontinence, resulting in dribbling. The bladder is enlarged on rectal examination and can be expressed by manual compression. In horses, chronic distension of the bladder leads to the accumulation of a sludge of calcium carbonate crystals (sabbulous urolithiasis). Urine stasis produces ideal conditions for bacterial growth and cystitis is a common sequela.

> ### Overdistension of the bladder
>
> Chronic overdistension of the bladder can cause multiple pinpoint lesions in the bladder wall resulting in leakage of urine into the peritoneal cavity. Structures normally palpable rectally in the abdomen may become less discernible because of accumulated urine in the abdomen.

## Prolapse

Although uncommon, eversion and prolapse of the urinary bladder has occurred in all female large animals, often associated with parturition. In bladder eversion the mucosal surface of the bladder is exposed as a rounded mass protruding through the vulvar lips. It is often edematous, red, and congested. Eversion develops when the urethra dilates sufficiently to allow mucosa to telescope through the urethral lumen. In contrast, with bladder prolapse the serosal surface of the bladder is visualized: it tends to have a pinker color and linear corrugations. A vaginal tear must be present to allow prolapse of the bladder. Both conditions are accompanied by straining.

## Masses and lumps

Benign (papilloma, adenoma) and neoplastic (carcinoma) epithelial tumors and non-epithelial tumors of a benign (leiomyoma, fibroma, rhabdomyoma) and neoplastic (leiomyosarcoma, fibrosarcoma, rhabdomyosarcoma) nature affect the bladder of all domestic large animal species. Tumors do not ordinarily become apparent until adulthood. Palpation alone of solitary or multiple masses affecting the bladder is unsatisfactory to differentiate between tumor types.

> ### Clinical Pointer
>
> Biopsy of a bladder tumor is essential to establish a definitive diagnosis of the tumor type.

Palpable hard round masses of variable sizes that are movable within the lumen of the bladder are most likely uroliths. Bladder uroliths are most common in horses. They cause intermittent mechanical obstruction to the outflow of urine. Ruminants also accumulate siliceous calculi in the bladder and renal pelvis, but their small size generally precludes detection within the bladder by rectal palpation.

## Ureters

The left and right ureters in normal cattle and horses are virtually impossible to palpate because of their small (6–8 mm) diameter and their subperitoneal course along the pelvic musculature to the bladder. However, the terminal end of each ureter may be detected in the dorsal wall of the bladder near the neck. The ureters in small ruminants and swine follow the same general course to the bladder as those of cattle and horses.

Owing to the retroperitoneal location of the right kidney and ureter along the majority of its length, rupture of the right kidney and/or corresponding ureter should be considered as a differential diagnosis when swelling is palpable in the area of the right paralumbar fossa.

> ### Abnormal ureters
>
> If the ureters are palpable there is likely to be an abnormality
>
> - bilateral enlargement is caused by an inflammatory process such as pyelonephritis, ureteritis, or cystitis
> - unilateral enlargement is caused by a ureteral urolith, abscess, or hematoma.

## COLLECTION OF URINE

### Without catheterization of bladder

A urine sample can be obtained during spontaneous or induced urination. Urination occurs frequently in large animals immediately after standing following periods of recumbent rest.

Urination can be induced in most of the large domestic animals.

- In the cow, urination may be induced by gentle rhythmic stroking of the skin immediately below the vulva; it is usually successful if the animal has not just urinated. During the act of stroking the animal should not be unduly restrained or otherwise touched, and the tail need not be held. This allows the cow to posture normally for urination.
- Male cattle may urinate following rhythmic stroking of the hairs of the preputial orifice, or alternatively stroking the hairs with warm water-soaked paper towels for several minutes.
- The horse may urinate after reintroduction into a stall with fresh or urine-soaked bedding following an exercise period.
- The boar or barrow may urinate in response to a stream of warm water directed to the prepuce.
- Urination can be induced in most ewes and rams by manually occluding the nostrils for up to 30–45 seconds until the animal begins to struggle. When the occlusion is relieved the animal usually squats and urinates.

## Urethral catheterization of bladder

In some species urine can be obtained by urethral catheterization. The use of a clean, sterilized catheter in good condition, placement of adequate sterilized aqueous lubricant on the catheter tip prior to insertion, and the practice of an aseptic technique are all required for successful catheter placement. A rigid catheter can be used for females but a pliable catheter should be used for males as they have such a long urethra.

Care should be taken that infection is not introduced into the urinary tract by the catheter, and to avoid trauma to the urethral mucosa. Urine samples, when required for chemical and microscopic examination, should be collected in clean, sterile containers. Passing a catheter is the most effective method of determining the state of patency of the urethra. When it is reasonable to suspect the occurrence of obstruction with possible perforation, or urethritis, the further pain created by catheterization can be controlled by prior administration of a suitable analgesic or narcotic drug.

### Females

#### Mare

Mares can be catheterized with ease. The vulva and skin immediately below it are thoroughly cleansed with soap and water. The lubricated hand is inserted into the vagina and the external urethral orifice is located on the midline on the ventral aspect of the vagina 10–12 cm from the vulva. A rigid metal urinary catheter with a slightly curved end (mare urinary catheter, 8 mm × 30 cm) works well for this procedure. The urethral orifice is identified with one finger and the catheter guided into the urethra and directly into the bladder, when urine should flow from the catheter. A vestibular fold is present just cranial to the urethral opening that can complicate insertion of a urinary catheter.

#### Cow

The bladder of the cow can be catheterized by initially locating the external urethral orifice, a narrow slit on the ventral floor of the vagina about 10–12 cm cranial to the vulva. Ventral to this is the suburethral diverticulum, a small pouch directed cranioventrally and up to 2 cm in diameter.

Several different catheters can be used to catheterize the cow bladder. A plastic insemination rod, a rigid metal mare urethral catheter, and flexible rubber catheters with a pointed, bolded end (such as Immingers bovine urinary catheter 5 mm × 30 cm) are all satisfactory.

One finger is inserted into the suburethral diverticulum and then slowly retracted while applying gentle upward pressure on the roof of the suburethral diverticulum, until the urethral opening is identified in the roof of the entrance of the suburethral diverticulum. Keeping the tip of the finger at the urethral opening, the catheter (held with the other hand) is moved cranially along the palmar surface of the finger into the urethral lumen. If the catheter is in the urethra it will continue to move forward easily into the bladder, at which time urine will usually flow.

Traumatic injury to the suburethral diverticulum is possible if the catheter is incorrectly placed. It has been suggested (with little supporting evidence) that bovine pyelonephritis may be a consequence of bladder catheterization, but these claims are not well founded. Clean, sterilized catheters in good condition should be used.

#### Ewe and sow

The vulva in the ewe, doe, and sow is too small to permit easy visualization of the urethra, although suitable illuminated specula may help, especially in the sow. The presence of a small suburethral diverticulum in the ewe makes it challenging to direct the tip of the catheter into the urethra. A bitch urinary catheter, 3.4 mm × 26.67 cm, can easily be directed along the palmar surface of the finger and into the urethra in small ruminants and sows. Once the catheter has been introduced into the urethra, slight elevation off the floor of the pelvis often facilitates easier passage into the bladder

### Males

#### Stallion and gelding

The urethra of the stallion can easily be catheterized to the level of the bladder using a plastic or rubber catheter (6 mm × 137 cm). In fractious animals, tranquilization often is necessary to ensure that this procedure is completed in an aseptic manner and with minimal risk of injury to the clinician. It is sometimes difficult or impossible to withdraw the penis from the prepuce without prior administration of a tranquilizing drug to relax the retractor penis muscles.

> **Clinical Pointer** ✳
>
> Because of the considerable length of the urethra in male horses, use a catheter which is sufficiently rigid but also sufficiently flexible to be directed around the ischial arch by an assistant. The instrument should be well lubricated before use and the penis cleansed with soap and water.

#### Bull and steer

In order to pass a urethral catheter successfully in the bull or steer it is necessary to relax the retractor penis muscles sufficiently to withdraw the penis from the preputial cavity. This requires the use of a pudendal nerve block; ataractic drugs may be effective in some cases. A polyethylene catheter of the type used for intracardiac catheterization is suitable, provided it is sufficiently long (290 cm), with a small diameter (3.0–5.0 mm), and has a rounded tip. Boars cannot be catheterized because the penis is inaccessible. In rams and bucks the urethral process must be stabilized digitally in order to introduce the tip of a catheter (1.5–2.0 mm) into the urethra. The sub-ischial diverticulum referred to above can prevent catheterizing the bladder successfully in these patients.

## MEDICAL IMAGING

The large abdominal size of adult cattle and horses precludes the routine use of radiography to evaluate the urinary system. Survey films can be obtained from small ruminants, swine, and neonatal calves and foals, to show the size and location of kidneys and bladder. Fluoroscopy or intravenous pyelography can be valuable in these animals to

- evaluate excretory function
- localize obstructions
- delineate the location of masses
- outline the kidneys, ureters, and bladder.

Positive contrast and double-contrast radiography or fluoroscopy can be successfully performed to evaluate the penile urethra of neonates, small ruminants, and swine.

Ultrasonography is useful in assessing the size and location of urinary tract structures and lesions in adult cattle and horses, as well as small ruminants, swine, and neonates of all large animal species.

The normal ultrasonographic anatomy of aspects of the urinary tract has been described for the horse (Pennick et al 1986, Rantanen 1986), (Fig. 18.13) cattle (Braun 1991) and sheep (Braun et al 1992) .

> **Clinical Pointer** ✳
>
> Ultrasonography is particularly useful in examining the left and right (non-palpable) kidneys in cattle and horses.

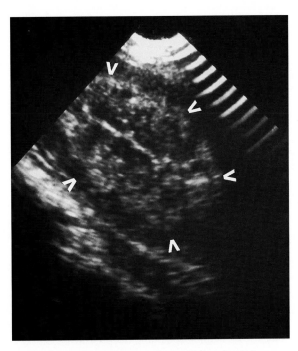

**Fig. 18.13** Ultrasound scan of a normal equine kidney (arrow heads). A hyperechoic cortex is evident. The mixed-signal medulla includes hyperechoic terminal recesses. (Scan courtesy of Dr Bruce McGorum, University of Edinburgh.)

More recently, renograms using nuclear medicine techniques have been helpful in evaluating the glomerular filtration rate of kidneys, as well as detecting pathology in all domestic large animal species. However, because of the equipment constraints and design MRI and CT have been relegated to large animal neonates, small ruminants, and young swine.

## ENDOSCOPY

Endoscopic examination of the bladder (cystoscopy) can be done successfully in all female large animals as well as the stallion and gelding. Passage of the endoscope into the bladder is accomplished using similar techniques as previously described for catheterization of these species.

Endoscopic inspection of the bladder mucosa is helpful in identifying sources of hemorrhage, such as ulcerative lesions or masses (e.g. tumors, intramural abscesses, and hematomas), surface characteristics of the mucosa, the presence of ectopic structures, as well as inspection of ureteral openings. The latter can be viewed with the aid of a flexible endoscope that can be retroflexed 180°, as the paired ureters lie close together on the dorsum of the trigone of the bladder. Urine will be seen to flow in waves through both ureters.

---

### Clinical Pointer ✳

Endoscopy

To ensure an unobstructed endoscopic view of the bladder mucosa and ureteral openings, the bladder must be devoid of urine prior to inflation with air. Problems can occur with bubble formation if the air used for inflation passes through urine.

---

## KIDNEY BIOPSY

As a general rule, because of the relatively small portion of tissue obtained by biopsy instruments renal biopsies should be reserved for diffuse processes affecting the kidneys where histopathological evaluation can help establish a diagnosis. A kidney biopsy may also be helpful in guiding the prognosis.

Commonly used biopsy instruments are

- the Tru-Cut biopsy needle (Travenol Laboratories, Inc., Deerfield, IL), and

- the Franklin-modified Vim Silverman needle (Mueller & Co., Chicago, IL).

The procedure can be done blindly or with the aid of ultrasound. Descriptions of the procedure for horses (Bayley et al 1980, Modransky 1986, Osborne et al 1968), cattle (Osborne et al 1968), sheep (Mitchell & Williams 1975) and swine (Hatfield et al 1975) have been previously reported.

### Appearance and analysis of urine

#### Gross appearance

Urine should have a characteristic yellow color, its intensity varying according to the degree of hydration. Urine is translucent when dilute, as in neonates, and yellow-green when concentrated. In all species but the horse the urine should be watery and relatively transparent. Horse urine is typically viscid and cloudy because of the high mucus and calcium carbonate content.

Urine can be tested for several constituents in the field using commercial reagent strips that test for several different substances. High concentrations of protein occur in the urine of cattle with pyelonephritis and cystitis, and in ischemic muscle necrosis in the downer cow syndrome. Abnormal coloration may be indicative of an alteration in the ability of the kidney to concentrate urine, pyuria, hematuria, hemoglobinuria, or myoglobinuria. Laboratory analysis is needed to differentiate between hemoglobinuria and myoglobinuria.

#### Urinalysis

A midstream urine sample should be used for laboratory analysis. Components of a urinalysis include determination of specific gravity, analysis of biochemical components, and cytological evaluation of urine sediment. Specific gravity determination (using a hand-

---

### The location of hemorrhage in hematuria

The location of the hemorrhage may be determined by observing when the blood first appears during voiding

- blood at the initiation of urination suggests a urethral problem
- blood throughout urination suggests kidney involvement
- blood at the end of urination suggests bladder involvement.

held refractometer) is most helpful in detecting renal dysfunction.

A specific gravity (1.008–1.012) in the general range of plasma osmolality (isosthenuria) is possible to obtain in any animal with normal kidney function. However, a second sample is warranted to assess the functional competence of the kidneys, as continuous isosthenuria is characteristic of primary renal involvement. This finding is particularly suggestive of primary renal tubulointerstitial disease if the patient cannot conserve body water when clinical dehydration (enophthalmia, skin 'tenting') is exhibited along with blood biochemistry changes consistent with tubulointerstitial disease (see below).

A specific gravity reading above plasma osmolality (hypersthenuria) indicates that the kidney has functional renal tubules and the ability to remove solute, whereas hyposthenuria indicates that the renal tubules are not reabsorbing water. In the absence of dehydration and biochemical evidence of compromised renal tubular function, hyposthenuria may be a reflection of recent excessive water consumption or diabetes insipidus. Drugs such as diuretics can also cause transient hyposthenuria.

Hypersthenuria can be a reflection of

- decreased glomerular filtration rate and prerenal dysfunction, as in dehydration and hypovolemia
- obstructive uropathy, or
- fever.

### Clinical Pointer

- Pathological hyposthenuria occurs in severe acute or end-stage renal disease
- Physiological hyposthenuria occurs in neonates and young animals drinking a lot of milk.

The presence of pus, blood, casts, and other solids will also elevate the specific gravity of urine.

Cytological evaluation provides information as to possible causes of discolored urine (red blood cells, leukocytes) or other abnormalities (mineral crystals, bacteria, tumor cells). Commercial urine test strips make the determination of a number of biochemical tests (pH, blood, glucose, ketones, protein, bilirubin, urobilinogen) simple and provide further insight into specific urinary problems (proteinuria due to inflammation, amyloidosis or glomerulonephritis), or suggest clinical problems not necessarily specific to the urinary system (altered systemic acid–base balance, diabetes mellitus, hepatitis).

Casts are cylindrical bodies ('tubular casts') appearing in urine and indicate an inflammatory or pathological process in the renal tubules. The casts may be of

- protein alone (hyaline cast)
- granular material (granular cast)
- tubular epithelial cells (epithelial casts)
- blood (blood cast), or
- leukocytes (leukocyte casts).

Waxy and fatty casts also occur.

## Serum biochemistry

The presence of azotemia (elevated urea nitrogen and creatinine) and abnormal serum electrolyte (sodium, chloride, calcium, phosphorus, potassium, magnesium) concentrations, together with urine sample analysis, should always be determined in the clinical evaluation of patients suspected to have renal disease.

Azotemia of prerenal origin is characterized by physiological oliguria. Urine obtained and analyzed from patients exhibiting prerenal azotemia shows physiologically appropriate characteristics evidenced by

- a noticeably high concentration (specific gravity greatly above plasma osmolality of 1.008–1.012)
- a relative lack of sodium (urine sodium <10 mEq/l or fractional excretion sodium <1% see below)
- a relative abundance of urea (urine urea:serum urea ratio > 20), and
- a relative abundance of creatinine (urine creatinine:serum creatinine ratio > 30).

The ratio of urine osmolality:plasma osmolality is between 1.0 and 3.0. In contrast, when acute renal failure is present, azotemia occurs with physiologically inappropriate characteristics of urine: not highly concentrated (specific gravity 1.008–1.015), relatively urea and creatinine poor (urine urea:serum urea ratio <10; urine creatinine:serum creatinine ratio <5) and relatively sodium rich (urine sodium >25 mEq/l; fractional excretion sodium > 1%). In ruminants with acute renal failure the ratios of urine urea:serum urea may deviate greatly from the above owing to their ability to activate urea recycling through the rumen. Practically, urine specific gravity is usually used with serum urea nitrogen and creatinine concentrations to determine the existence of prerenal versus renal azotemia.

Serum electrolyte alterations reflective of acute renal failure include hyponatremia, hypochloremia, and hypermagnesemia. Hypocalcemia and hyperphosphatemia typically occur in ruminants, whereas horses typically exhibit hypercalcemia and hypophosphatemia. Potassium values can vary greatly, depending on the acid–base status of the animal and, in the case of ruminants, whether potassium is being exchanged for sodium in the saliva.

Although postrenal in location, urolithiasis-induced bladder rupture with uroperitoneum also causes azotemia and electrolyte changes similar to primary renal disease. The similarity in changes develops because the peritoneum, being a semipermeable membrane, allows dialysis of fluid and solute between fluid (urine) in the peritoneal cavity and the interstitial space (blood); each solute moves down its concentration gradient (Fig. 18.12). Consequently, as normal urine is relatively poor in most electrolytes but rich in urea nitrogen and creatinine, and blood is relatively rich in electrolytes but poor in urea nitrogen and creatinine, self-dialysis results in the following serum changes

- hyponatremia
- hypochloremia
- azotemia
- hypocalcemia (hypercalcemia in the horse)
- hyperphosphatemia (hypophosphatemia in the horse), and most likely
- hyperkalemia.

Affected adult animals also exhibit dehydration as a result of extracellular fluid migrating to the more hyperosmolar environment in the peritoneal cavity.

In animals with a ruptured bladder urea nitrogen tends to equilibrate much faster between peritoneal fluid (urine) and blood than does creatinine. When urine is the fluid occupying the peritoneal cavity, a simultaneous analysis of creatinine concentration of this fluid and blood should yield a creatinine concentration at least twice that of blood. In foals and other neonates with a ruptured bladder there is hyponatremia, hypochloremia, and hypherkalemia. The equilibration of a large volume of dilute urine that is low in sodium and chloride and high in potassium across the large surface area of the peritoneum rapidly results in these abnormalities. A state of overhydration occurs so that clinical dehydration usually is not apparent.

In glomerular disease (glomerulonephritis, amyloidosis) hypoproteinemia is accompanied by heavy proteinuria. Azotemia and electrolyte changes may be minimal until late in the disease course. Kidney enlargement often accompanies amyloidosis.

### Urinary enzymology

γ-Glutamyl transpeptidase (GGT) activity has been used in the horse as a sensitive early indicator of tubular damage. A ratio of urine GGT to creatinine should be determined. In normal horses this is 25. A ratio > 25 indicates that active tubular cell damage is occurring.

---

### Chronic renal failure (CRF)

- biochemical changes occur similar to those of acute tubulointerstitial renal failure
- proteinuria occurs if glomerular function is reduced
- the kidneys may be shrunken and body condition poor
- there may be abnormal fluid accumulations (if heavy proteinuria is present) such as subcutaneous edema, ascites, hydrothorax
- polyuria and polydipsia may be evident.

---

**Urine fractional excretion of sodium (FENa)**
Fractional excretion of sodium has proved useful in horses to differentiate prerenal from renal azotemia. Sodium and creatinine concentrations are obtained from urine and serum and then the FENa is determined using the following formula

$$\frac{\text{Urine Na}}{\text{Serum Na}} \times \frac{\text{Serum creatinine}}{\text{Urine creatinine}} = \text{FENa}$$

A fractional excretion less than 1% is supportive of prerenal azotemia and normal tubular function, whereas values > 1% are supportive of renal azotemia and tubular dysfunction.

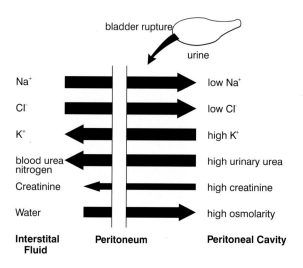

**Fig. 18.12** Movement of fluid and urine components in the pathogenesis of peritoneal self-dialysis following rupture of the urinary bladder (Donecker and Bellamy 1982).

# FURTHER READING

Barsanti JA. Diagnostic procedures in urology. Veterinary Clinics of North America 1984;14: 3–14.

Bayley WM, Paradis MR, Reed SM. Equine renal biopsy: indications, technic, interpretation and complications. Modern Veterinary Practice 1980; 61: 763–768.

Benjamin MM. Urinalysis. In: Benjamin (ed) Outline of veterinary clinical pathology, 3rd edn. Ames IA: Iowa State University Press, 1978;180–212.

Braun U. Ultrasonographic examination of the right kidney in cows. American Journal of Veterinary Research 1991; 52: 1933–1939.

Braun U, Schefer U, Gerber D. Ultrasonography of the urinary tract of female sheep. American Journal of Veterinary Research 1992; 53: 1734–1739.

Chew DJ et al. Vagino-urethro-cystoscopy in female dogs and cats. Proc 12th Ann Vet Med Forum, Am Col Vet Int Med, San Francisco, 1994; 472–473.

Crow SE, Walshaw SO. Manual of clinical procedures in the dog and cat. Philadelphia: JB Lippincott, 1987.

DiBartola SP. Clinical approach and laboratory evaluation of renal disease. In: Ettinger SJ, Feldman ED (eds) Textbook of veterinary internal medicine, 4th edn. Philadelphia: WB Saunders, 1995; 1706–1719.

Donecker JM, Bellamy JEC. Blood chemical abnormalities in cattle with ruptured bladders and ruptured urethras. Canadian Veterinary Journal 1982; 23: 355–377.

Gans JH, Mercer PF. The kidneys. In: Swenson MJ (ed) Dukes' physiology of domestic animals, 10th edn. Ithaca NY: Comstock Publishing, 1984; 507–536.

Getty R. The anatomy of the domestic animals, 5th edn. Vols 1 and 2. Philadelphia: WB Saunders, 1975.

Hafez ESE. The behavior of domestic animals, 3rd edn. London: Baillière Tindall, 1975.

Hatfield PJ, Cameron JS, Cadenhead A. Renal biopsy in the pig. Research in Veterinary Science 1975; 19: 88–89.

Holt PE. Color atlas of small animal urology. London: Times Mirror Publishers, 1994.

Kasari TR. Omphalitis and its sequelae in ruminants. In: Howard JL (ed.) Current veterinary therapy. Food animal practice, 3rd edn. Philadelphia: WB Saunders, 1993; 101–103.

McCurnin DM, Poffenbarger EM. Small animal physical diagnosis and clinical procedures. Philadelphia: WB Saunders, 1991.

Mitchell B, Williams JT. Technique for biopsy of renal cortex in sheep. Veterinary Record 1975; 96: 405.

Modransky PD. Ultrasound-guided renal and hepatic biopsy techniques. Veterinary Clinics of North America (Equine Practice) 1986; 2: 115–126.

Osborne CA, Fahning ML, Schultz RH et al. Percutaneous renal biopsy in the cow and horse. Journal of the American Veterinary Medical Association 1968; 153: 563–570.

Osborne CA, Finco DR. Canine and feline nephrology and urology. Baltimore: Williams & Wilkins, 1995.

Pennick DG, Eisenberg HM, Teuscher EE et al. Equine renal ultrasonography: normal and abnormal. Veterinary Radiology 1986; 27: 81–84.

Rantanen NW. Diseases of the kidneys. Veterinary Clinics of North America (Equine Practice) 1986; 2: 89–103.

# 19
# Clinical Examination of the Nervous System

*R. Bagley*
*I. Mayhew*

## CLINICAL MANIFESTATIONS OF DISEASES OF THE NERVOUS SYSTEM

**Aimless wandering** Persistant walking in random directions for no reason [eg escape or food].

**Anisocoria** Unequal pupil size.

**Anosmia** Lack of sense of smell.

**Areflexia** Lack of reflex action.

**Arthrogryposis** Rigidity or restricted movement of multiple joints.

**Ataxia** Lack of coordination.

**Atonia** (flaccidity) Absent muscle tone; limbs are often limp.

**Babinski reflex** Flexion of digits in response to physical stimulation of the palmer/planter surface of the foot/pastern.

**Blindness** Inability to see; can be due to ophthalmologic or neurological disorders.

**Cataplexy** Abrupt attacks of muscular weakness and hypotonia.

**Circling** Compulsively moving in a circle; can be a sign of either forebrain or vestibular disease.

**Coma** Animal is unresponsive to both environmental and painful stimuli.

**Compulsive behavior** Repetitive, stereotypic behavior; an example would be an animal that compulsively chases its tail.

**Compulsive walking** Persistant walking for no reason [eg escape of food], often stereotypically such as in a circle.

**Corneal ulcer** Loss of corneal integrity; often the result of poor corneal sensation, corneal dryness, or inability to protect the eye through blinking.

**Crossed-extensor reflex** With a patient in lateral recumbency, eliciting a flexion reflex in the upper limb results in extension of the lower limb; seen with disease of the upper motor neuron.

**Dazzle reflex** Abrupt closure of eyelids when a bright light is flashed onto the retina.

**Deafness** Lack of hearing.

**Decerebellate rigidity** Opisthotonos with thoracic limb extension and flexion of the pelvic limbs up under the body caused by contraction of the sublumbar muscles. Mental status is normal.

**Decerebrate rigidity** Opisthotonos and extension of all limbs; usually the animal is stuporous or comatose.

**Dementia/delirium** Mentally disorientated or disassociated from its environment.

**Disuse muscle atrophy** Loss of muscle mass due to lack of appropriate use of a muscle. Associated with UMN or orthopedic disease. Usually less severe and more slowly evolving than neurogenic atrophy.

**Dropped jaw** Inability to close the jaw.

**Dullness, depression** Mild decrease in the animal's mental acuity.

**Dysmetria** Improper measurement of range and force of voluntary movement.

**Dysosmia** Decreased or abnormal sense of smell.

**Dysphagia** Difficulty in eating or swallowing.

**Facial asymmetry** Unequal facial expression; usually due to disease of the facial nerve.

**Facial paralysis** Lack of movement of muscles innervated by the facial nerve.

**Fasciculations** Small, local, involuntary muscle contractions visible under the skin. These represent spontaneous discharge of a number of muscle fibers innervated by a single motor nerve fiber.

**Head pressing** Persistent or repeated pushing with the head against a fixed object; usually a sign of intracranial disease.

**Head tilt** The median plane of the head is rotated from its normal perpendicular relationship with the dorsal plane, the head being tilted to one side. If the animal is viewed from the front, the head appears tilted to one side.

**Head turn** An abnormal posture where the head is directed toward the caudal ('looking backward') rather than the cranial ('looking forward') aspects of the animal. The median plane of the head usually remains perpendicular to the ground.

**Hemifacial spasm** Persistent contraction of the muscles of facial expression on one side; most often associated with chronic disease of the facial nerve.

**Hemiparesis** Partial loss of voluntary movement in the limb(s) on one side of the body.

**Hemiplegia** Total loss of voluntary movement in the limb(s) on one side of the body.

**Horner's Syndrome** Sympathetic denervation of the contents of the bony orbit; ptosis, miosis and enophthalmus [see Ch.20: Visual System].

**Hypalgesia** (hypoesthesia) Decreased sensitivity to stimulation (pain).

**Hyperesthesia** Increased sensitivity to stimulation; painful.

**Hypermetria** Voluntary muscular movement results in overreaching of the intended goal, often resulting in high-stepping.

**Hyperreflexia** Increase in the magnitude of the reflex action.

**Hypertonia** Increase in muscle tone; often results in extension of the limbs.

**Hypoaesthesia** Decreased responsiveness to a noxious stimulus; synonymous with hypalgesia.

**Hypometria** Voluntary movement falls short of the intended goal.

**Hyporeflexia** Decrease in the magnitude of the reflex action.

**Hypotonia** Decrease in muscle tone.

**Incontinence** Inability to store urine or feces normally.

**Knuckling** Flexing or buckling on lower limb joints when supporting weight.

**Kyphosis** An abnormal flexion primarily of the thoracolumbar vertebrae; results in a 'hunchback' appearance.

**Lameness** Reduced ability or desire to bear weight on a limb because of pain or a mechanical restriction of normal joint movement.

**Lordosis** Abnormal extension of the vertebral column, particularly in the thoracolumbar region; this results in a 'dipped-back' appearance.

**Lower motor neuron (LMN) disease.** Degree of paralysis and loss of reflex arc function (areflexia) with muscle hypotonia and muscle wasting.

**Lower motor neuron bladder** Characterized by a large bladder, with poor detrusor and sphincter tone, therefore easy to express manually.

**Megaesophagus** Dilated esophagus due to numerous causes; often seen with cranial nerve, muscle and neuromuscular junction disease.

**Miosis** A smaller than normal pupil; constriction of the pupil.

**Muscle atrophy** Decreased size of the muscle due to decrease of size or loss of muscle fibers.

**Mydriasis** A larger than normal pupil; dilation of the pupil.

**Myoclonus** Shock-like contraction of a portion of a muscle, an entire muscle or a muscle group.

**Myotonia** Persistent muscle contraction following voluntary or external initiation.

**Narcolepsy** Excessive daytime sleep; usually manifested as episodic periods of sleep.

**Nerve root signature** A persistent or episodic non-weightbearing lameness, presumably the result of nerve irritation and pain.

**Neurogenic muscle atrophy** Usually severe atrophy that evolves quickly after an LMN lesion.

**Neurotropic keratitis** Loss of corneal integrity due to loss of innervation from the trigeminal nerve.

**Nystagmus** Oscillatory eye movements having a fast and a slow phase; can occur at rest (spontaneous) or when the head position is changed (positional).

**Ophthalmoplegia** Paralysis of orbital muscle function; globe and iris do not move in total ophthalmoplegia [see Ch.20: Visual System].

**Opisthotonos** Abnormal posture where the head and neck are extended dorsally toward the back; often the thoracic limbs are extended.

**Pain** A sensation of discomfort or distress; clinical signs of pain are inferred in animals based upon behavior and physiological changes.

**Paralysis** Inability to move voluntarily.

**Paraparesis** Partial loss of voluntary movement in the pelvic limbs; weak in the hind limbs.

**Paraplegia** Total loss of voluntary movement in the pelvic limbs.

**Paresis** Weakness resulting from neurologic dysfunction.

**Proprioceptive deficit** Poor correction to normal posture when body parts [limbs] are in an abnormal position [stance]

**Ptosis** Drooping of the upper eyelid.

**Reflex** An act that occurs without conscious control. The patellar or knee-jerk reflex is an example.

**Reflex arc** The necessary components for a reflex to occur. Includes the afferent (sensory) receptor, the afferent (sensory) peripheral nerve, the motor neuron cell body, the efferent (motor) peripheral nerve, the neuromuscular junction, and the muscle.

**Reflex myoclonus** Characterized by episodic, stimulation-evoked extensor rigidity of part of or the whole body.

**Schiff–Sherrington posture** Thoracic limb extension with intact tone and reflexes in the pelvic limbs; results from a severe third thoracic (T3) to third lumbar (L3) spinal cord segment lesion that interrupts the ascending inhibitory impulses to the extensor muscles of the thoracic limbs.

**Scoliosis** An abnormal lateral deviation of the vertebral column.

**Seizure** Intermittent motor events that tend to recur. With a generalized seizure the animal falls to its side, has rhythmic jerking of the head or limbs, followed by paddling or running motions. *Convulsions, fits, ictus* are synonyms.

**Semicoma (stupor)** Animal is unresponsive to environmental stimuli but remains responsive to painful stimuli.

**Shivering** Involuntary trembling or quivering.

**Spasticity** Increased extensor tone of muscles, most often seen in the limbs.

**Star-gazing** Extended-head and neck posture; mild opisthotonus.

**Stiffness** Decreased range of motion and step length when moving.

**Strabismus** Abnormal eye position; can occur at rest (resting) or when the head position is changed (positional).

**Tetanus** Severe, persistent extensor rigidity of the limbs, neck, trunk and tail.

**Tetraparesis** Partial loss of voluntary movement in the thoracic and pelvic limbs; weak in all 4 limbs

**Tetraplegia** Total loss of voluntary movement in the thoracic and pelvic limbs; animal is clinically recumbent.

**Toe dragging** Dragging of toes when moving; usually indicates flexor weakness or paresis.

**Tongue paresis/paralysis** Inability to use the tongue normally; often associated with disease of the hypoglossal nerve.

**Torticollis** A contracted state of the cervical muscles producing twisting of the neck and head.

**Tremor** Involuntary to and fro movement of the body or a part of the body.

**Upper motor neuron (UMN) disease** Degrees of paralysis with intact reflex arc function, normal to increased muscle tone and only disuse muscle atrophy.

**Upper motor neuron bladder** Characterized by a large bladder, with good detrusor and sphincter tone, therefore difficult to express manually.

**Vestibular syndrome** Signs referable to lack of vestibular function including staggering, leaning, falling, head tilt, nystagmus and strabismus.

**Weakness** Non-specific term meaning inability to perform muscle activity normally; can result from disease of a variety of body systems.

**Wide-based stance** Standing with the limbs placed more laterally than usual.

**Yawning** Laborious inhalation with exaggerated opening of the jaws; can be a sign of cerebral disease in large animals.

# INTRODUCTION

The clinical evaluation of animals suspected of having nervous system disease requires a fundamental knowledge of neuroanatomy and neurophysiology. More important is an understanding of how discrete elements within the nervous system are integrated, interrelate and interact for the animal to perform various normal functions. Logical evaluation of normal nervous system function will allow one to:

- determine if the nervous system is abnormal,
- determine the neuroanatomical sites of involvement
- formulate a realistic differential diagnosis, therapeutic plan, and prognosis.

The purpose of this chapter is to familiarize the clinician with the clinical examination of the nervous system in domestic animals.

# FUNCTIONAL COMPONENTS OF THE NERVOUS SYSTEM

The major components of the nervous system include

- the brain
- nerves arising from the brain (cranial nerves)
- the spinal cord
- peripheral spinal nerves.

These components are connected to and interact with each other in order to control most bodily functions.

## Functions controlled by the brain

- consciousness (mental status, awareness)
- behavior
- voluntary and reflex movements of the head, body, and limbs
- vital functions such as sleeping, eating, drinking, and breathing
- conscious recognition of senses (seeing, hearing, taste, touch, and pain).

### Brain

The brain is housed within the skull. Using the level of the tentorium cerebelli as a dividing point, the brain can be separated into the structures rostral to the tentorium cerebelli (i.e the supratentorial structures, also called the forebrain) and structures caudal to the tentorium (i.e. the infratentorial structures) (Fig. 19.1). This anatomical division is also convenient for dividing the brain into areas that have similar functions (functional areas).

#### Supratentorial structures

Supratentorial structures provide for many **conscious** functions, such as vision and voluntary movement.

Portions of the cerebral hemispheres (e.g. the parietal cortex) sense where the limbs and head are in space. Recognition of the orientation of the body in relation to gravity is referred to as proprioception. The diencephalon (hypothalamus and thalamus) controls many autonomic and basic life-support functions (e.g. eating, drinking, body temperature regulation).

## Supratentorial structures

- cerebral hemispheres
- basal nuclei
- diencephalon.

## Infratentorial structures

- mid brain
- pons
- medulla oblongata
- cerebellum.

### Brain stem/cranial nerves

The brain stem contains the groups of neurons (nuclei) that make up many of the cranial nerves (III–XII), as well as the reticular activating system (which via the cerebral cortex keeps the body in an alert and awake state). Recognition of the need for and the drive to maintain breathing is controlled by areas within the

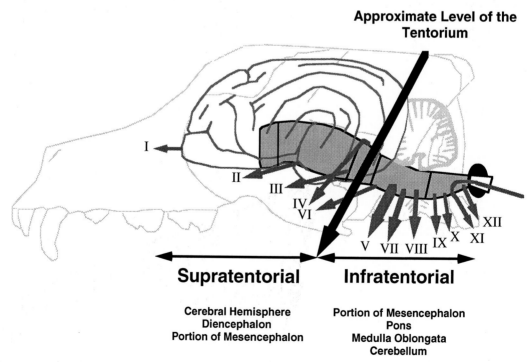

**Approximate Level of the Tentorium**

I
II
III
IV
VI
V VII VIII IX X XI XII

**Supratentorial**

Cerebral Hemisphere
Diencephalon
Portion of Mesencephalon

**Infratentorial**

Portion of Mesencephalon
Pons
Medulla Oblongata
Cerebellum

**Fig. 19.1** Schematic representation of the division between the supratentorial and infratentorial spaces occurring approximately at the level of the tentorium cerebelli.

caudal brain stem. Many ascending and descending neural pathways important for movement also course through, or originate within, the brain stem.

The cerebellum, which is immediately dorsal to pons and medulla oblongata, smoothes and coordinates movements and is important for **unconscious** control of proprioceptive functions.

## Spinal cord

The spinal cord houses pathways that connect the brain to the peripheral nerves. It contains variable numbers of spinal cord segments, depending upon the species. These are anatomically divided as follows

- cervical (C): 8 segments
- thoracic (T): 13–18 segments
- lumbar (L): 5–7 segments
- sacral (S): 3–6 segments
- caudal (Ca): 5+ segments.

Clinical signs of spinal cord dysfunction often manifest as abnormalities of limb strength and movement (Table 19.1).

**Table 19.1.  General clinical syndromes resulting from lesions of the five functional areas of the spinal cord**

| Spinal segments | Clinical signs |
|---|---|
| C1 – C5 | – Tetraparesis/plegia, +/–neck pain<br>Normal to exaggerated spinal reflexes |
| C6 – T2 | – Tetraparesis/plegia, +/–neck pain<br>Decreased to absent thoracic limb spinal reflexes<br>Normal to exaggerated spinal reflexes – pelvic limbs |
| T3 – L3 | – Paraparesis/plegia, +/–back pain<br>Normal thoracic limb spinal reflexes<br>Normal to exaggerated pelvic limbs spinal reflexes |
| L4 – S3 | – Paraparesis/plegia, +/–lower back pain<br>Normal thoracic limbs spinal reflexes<br>Decreased to absent spinal reflexes – pelvic limbs |
| Caudal | – Paresis/plegia of tail<br>Decreased tail tone<br>Decreased tail sensation |

## Peripheral nerves

The peripheral nerves arise from within the spinal cord (motor nerves) or nerve root ganglia (sensory nerves) and bring information from (sensory), or carry information to (motor) parts of the body such as the muscles of the limbs (Table 19.2). Motor nerves provide stimulation to the muscles through a special connection known as the **neuromuscular junction**. The motor component of these nerves forms the final pathway whereby information from the brain is conveyed to the body in order to perform a function, such as muscle movement. Components of the clinical neurological examination are used to test the complex normal interactions of these structures to determine whether the nervous system is working properly.

# THE NEUROLOGICAL EXAMINATION

Because the differential diagnosis, diagnostic plan, treatment plan, and prognosis are heavily dependent upon lesion localization, the neurological examination is the foundation of accurate clinical management of animals with neurological disease. Often diseases affect discrete portions of the nervous system, and clinical signs reflect this focal abnormality. Some diseases, however, affect multiple areas. Clinical signs will usually reflect the diffuse nature of such lesions.

After localization of the problem and consideration of the signalment and historical disease course, a realistic differential diagnosis list can be formulated. Diagnostic tests are next chosen to ascertain the ultimate diagnosis. An accurate diagnosis provides information important for the formulation of a treatment plan and realistic prognosis for the owner.

A complete neurological examination is the most important diagnostic step to successfully evaluate an animal suspected of having neurological disease. To ensure completeness of examination and to have a record for future comparison, all aspects of the examination should be recorded. An evaluation form listing the neurological tests performed and their outcome is often helpful (Fig. 19.2a, b). For large animals a

---

### Goals of the neurological examination

The goals of the neurological examination are

- to establish that disease involves the nervous system and
- to determine the location of the lesion(s) within the nervous system.

**Table 19.2.** Origin and motor innervation of the major spinal nerves to the limbs of dogs (Adapted from deLahunta, A. Veterinary neuroanatomy and clinical neurology, 2nd edn. Philadelphia: WB Saunders, 1983)

| Nerve | Spinal cord segments | Muscle innervated | Function of muscles |
|---|---|---|---|
| **Thoracic limb** | | | |
| Suprascapular | C(5)*, 6,7 | Supraspinatus | Shoulder extension |
| | | Infraspinatus | Shoulder flexion or extension |
| Subscapular | C6,7 | Subscapularis | Shoulder extension |
| Musculocutaneous | C6,7,8 | Biceps brachi | Elbow flexion |
| | | Brachialis | |
| | | Coracobrachialis | Shoulder extension and bduction |
| Axillary | C(6), 7,8 | Deltoides | Shoulder flexion and abduction |
| | | Teres major/minor | |
| | | (Subscapularis) | |
| Radial | C7,8,T1, (2) | Triceps | |
| | | Extensor carpi radialis | |
| | | Ulnaris lateralis | Elbow, carpal, and digital extension |
| | | Common digital extensor | |
| | | Lateral digital extensor | |
| Median | C8, T1 (2) | Flexor carpi radialis | Carpal and digital flexion |
| | | Superficial digital flexor | |
| | | (Deep digital flexor) | |
| Ulnar | C8, T1 (2) | Flexor carpi ulnaris | Carpal and digital flexion |
| | | Deep digital flexor | |
| **Pelvic limb** | | | |
| Femoral | L4,5,6 | Iliopsoas | Stifle Extension |
| | | Quadriceps | Coxofemoral flexion |
| | | Sartorius | |
| Obturator | L(4), 5,6 | External obturator | |
| | | Pectineus | Coxofemoral adduction |
| | | Gracilis | |
| | | Adductor | |
| Cranial gluteal | L6,7,S1 | Middle gluteal | |
| | | Deep gluteal | Coxofemoral adduction |
| | | Tensor fascia lata | |
| Caudal gluteal | L7, S(1,2) | Superficial gluteal | Coxofemoral extension |
| | | (Middle gluteal) | |
| Sciatic | L6,7, S1,(2) | Biceps femoris | Stifle flexion |
| | | Semimembranosus | Coxofemoral extension |
| | | Semitendinosus | |
| Common peroneal | L6,7 | Peroneus longus | Hock flexion |
| | | Lateral digital extensor | |
| | | Deep digital extensor | Digital extension |
| | | Cranial tibial | |
| Tibial | L1, S1 | Gastrocnemius | Hock extension |
| | | Popliteus | |
| | | Superficial digital flexor | Digital flexion |
| | | Deep digital flexor | |
| Pudendal (caudal rectal) | S1,2,3 | External anal sphincter | Anal and external urethral sphincter |

* Numbers in brackets denote a normal anatomic variation

systematic approach beginning at the head and ending at the tail is recommended. It is imperative to examine each functional area of the nervous system systematically. Incomplete examination and inaccurate observations are more common causes of incorrect diagnoses than false conclusions based on correct and sufficient facts.

## Signalment

The signalment is important as many diseases are breed, age, or sex associated, for example

- globoid cell leukodystrophy occurs in Cairn terrier dogs and polled Dorset sheep
- congenital cerebellar hypoplasia due to panleukopenia virus infection in cats causes clinical signs which usually begin early in life; with brain neoplasms, clinical signs usually begin later in life
- Golden retriever muscular dystrophy occurs in only males.

Breed-associated diseases of dogs and cats have been previously summarized (Kornegay 1986; Oliver et al 1987; Wheeler 1989; Mayhew 1989; Smith 1996; Oliver and Lorenz 1993; Radostits et al 1994; Braund 1994).

## History

In addition to a general history, questions should address the clinical problem (regarded by the owner or handler as the chief complaint), the duration and clinical course (progressive, unchanged, or improving; persistent or episodic). Video-tapes of the animal when it is abnormal, especially with episodic abnormalities such as seizures, sleep disorders, or lameness, can be an invaluable tool to allow the veterinarian to observe abnormal posture and activity.

Historical questioning needs to be adapted for each individual animal after clarification of the presenting problem. Depending upon the presenting complaint specific questions can be formulated for each case.

With episodic clinical signs the relationship of the signs to eating should be noted. Thus signs occuring very soon after eating are more often seen with hepatic encephalopathy, whereas signs seen long after eating may be associated with hypoglycemia.

## Distant subjective assessment

A subjective observation and evaluation can be made by viewing the animal from a distance as the history is obtained.

During examination normal animals are usually somewhat apprehensive of the veterinarian or the hospital environment. Consequently they usually

> ### Some relevant clinical history questions
>
> - Has the animal been exposed to toxic substances?
> - Have any related or in-contact animals been affected by similar problems?
> - Was the onset sudden or insidious?
> - Is the condition static, improving, or worsening?
> - Are the symptoms continuous or episodic?
> - Is there any coexisting disease?
> - What is the animal's diet, any recent changes?
> - Is there a history of recent travel (e.g. exposure to endemic infectious agents)?
> - What is the vaccination status (e.g. canine distemper, rabies)?
> - Are any recent drug therapies significant (e.g. metronidazole toxicity to the vestibular system in dogs and cats)?

remain alert and aware of what is happening and will look at or orient themselves toward someone entering the examination area. Prior observations by the owner or handler are often necessary to clarify the personality of an individual animal and discover how the animal has acted in similar situations in the past. Comments such as 'this animal is much less responsive than usual', or 'this animal is always calm when seen by a veterinarian' are often helpful.

Abnormal posturing and movement are usually observed at this stage. Animals may wander, head press, or become somnolent (Fig. 19.3). Animals with severe brain-stem, spinal cord, or peripheral nerve disease often will not be able to stand and walk.

## Level of consciousness (mental status) and behavior

For an animal to be alert and oriented to its environment two basic components of the nervous system must be functioning normally

> ### Clinical Pointer
>
> At first the animal should be observed unrestrained and, if possible, in its normal environment. This 'distant observation' may reveal important information that may be missed if a close physical examination is undertaken too quickly.
>
> Dogs and cats can be allowed to move freely around the consulting room at this stage. If spinal injury is suspected unrestricted movement is contraindicated.

# Neurological Examination

## *Washington State University College of Veterinary Medicine*

**Date:**

**Time:**

**History:**

**Subjective:**

**Mental Status:** (Circle)

Alert          Depressed      Demented

Disorientated  Stuporous      Comatose

**Posture:** (circle)   Normal

Head Tilt (L/R)   Head Turn (L/R)          Falling

Tremor        Tetany

Decerebrate   Decerebellate

Schiff Sherrington

Other:

**Gait:**                    Normal

Ataxia         Trunkal   All    Pelvic

Paretic        Tetra  Para  Hemi  Mono

Plegic         Tetra  Para  Hemi  Mono

Lame           LT    RT    LP    RP

Shortstrided/stiff    T     P     All

Unable to stand       T     P     All

**Postural Reactions:**

0=absent, 1=reduced, 2=normal, 3=exaggerated

| | | L | R |
|---|---|---|---|
| Conscious | Thoracic | _____ | _____ |
| Proprioception | Pelvic | _____ | _____ |
| Hopping | Thoracic | _____ | _____ |
| | Pelvic | _____ | _____ |
| Wheelbarrowing | Thoracic | _____ | _____ |
| | Pelvic | _____ | _____ |
| Hemistand/walk | Thoracic | _____ | _____ |
| | Pelvic | _____ | _____ |
| Placing | Thoracic | _____ | _____ |
| | Pelvic | _____ | _____ |
| Extensor Postural | Thoracic | _____ | _____ |
| | Pelvic | _____ | _____ |

**Clinician**_____

**Cranial Nerves**                    L        R

Smell (CN I)                       ____    ____

Menace  Response (CN II + VII)     ____    ____

Pupils Size (at Rest) Right    Left

Pupil response to Light

Light in Left eye

Light in Right eye

Fundus

Strabismus, resting (III, IV, VI)       ____    ____

Strabismus, positional                  ____    ____
(III, IV, VI, VIII)

Nystagmus (VIII) -(Circle )

Spontaneous-                              None

| | L | R |
|---|---|---|
| | Horizontal | Horizontal |
| | Rotary | Rotary |
| | Vertical | Vertical |
| Positional | Y or N | |
| Changing | Y or N | L        R |

Oculovestibular                         ____    ____
(VIII, III, IV, VI)

Facial sensation (V)                    ____    ____

Mastication (V)                         ____    ____

Ocular Sensation (V)                    ____    ____

Facial Symmetry (VII)                   ____    ____

Palpebral (V + VII)                     ____    ____

Swallowing (IX, X)                      ____    ____

Trapezius Muscle (XI)                   ____    ____

Tongue (XII)                            ____    ____

Fig. 19.2a

## Spinal Reflexes:

0=absent, 1=reduced, 2=normal, 3=exaggerated, 4=clonus

|  | L | R |
|---|---|---|
| **Thoracic Limb** | | |
| Biceps (C6 - C8) | _____ | _____ |
| Triceps (C7- T2) | _____ | _____ |
| Extensor Carpi radialis (C7 -T2) | _____ | _____ |
| Flexion (C6 -T2) | _____ | _____ |
| **Pelvic Limb** | | |
| Patella (L4 -L6) | _____ | _____ |
| Cranial Tibial (L6 - S1) | _____ | _____ |
| Gastrocnemius (L6 - S1) | _____ | _____ |
| Flexion (L6 - S1) | _____ | _____ |
| Perineal (S1 - 3) | _____ | _____ |

## Atrophy:

## Urination

| | | |
|---|---|---|
| Voluntary | Yes | No |
| Bladder distended? | Yes | No |
| Ease of expression? | Yes | No |

## Sensation:

| | | |
|---|---|---|
| Hyperesthesia | Cervical | None |
| | Thoracic | |
| | Thoracolumbar | Other |
| | Lumbar | |
| | Lumbosacral | |
| | Caudal | |

Cutaneous trunci
    Normal

<u>T2 T3 T4 T5 T6 T7 T8 T9 T10 T11 T12 T13 L1 L2 L3 L4</u>

| Deep pain | T | P | Tail |
|---|---|---|---|
| | + - | + - | + - |

## Comments:

## Neuroanatomic diagnosis:
### (Circle)

| | | L | R |
|---|---|---|---|
| Forebrain | | L | R |
| Brain stem | | L | R |
| Cerebellum | | L | R |
| Vestibular | Central  Peripheral | L | R |
| Spinal cord Segments | | L | R |

        C1-5
        C6-T2
        T3-L3
        L4 - S1
        S1 -3
        Caudal
Generalized neuromuscular
Peripheral Nerve (Name)

_____

## Differential Diagnosis:

## Diagnostic Testing:

Signature: _____

**Fig. 19.2a** (cont'd)

**b**      **LARGE ANIMAL NEUROLOGICAL EXAMINATION**

Case No. ...............................................................

Owner's Name: ...................................................

Tel. No: .............................. Fax No: ...........................

Animal's Name .....................................................

Species ............................................... Age .........................

Breed ................................................ Sex ........................

VFS Clinician ......................................................

Ref. Vet. ..................................Tel. No. .......................

Fax No. ................................. **AFFIX LABEL HERE**

**Large Animal Hospital**

Department of Veterinary Clinical Studies
Royal (Dick) School of Veterinary Studies
Veterinary Field Station
Easter Bush
Roslin, Midlothian EH25 9RG

Telephone   0131 650 6253
Accounts     0131 650 6238
After hours 0131 650 2257
Fax          0131 650 8824

*THE UNIVERSITY OF EDINBURGH*

**HISTORY:**

**PHYSICAL EXAMINATION:**

**NEUROLOGICAL EXAMINATION**

**HEAD**

| Behaviour: | | Head Posture: |
| Mental Status: | | Head Coordination: |

Cranial Nerves:

| Eyes | LEFT | RIGHT | | | LEFT | RIGHT |
|---|---|---|---|---|---|---|
| *Ophthalmic Examination:* | | | **Vestibular-ear** | | | |
| *Vision ; II:* | | | *Eye drop, normal/abnormal:* | | | |
| *Menace ; II-VII, Cerebellum:* | | | *Nystagmus; normal, vestibular:* | | | |
| *Puplis, PLR; II-III:* | | | *abnormal:* | | | |
| *Horners; Symp:* | | | *Blindfold:* | | | |
| *Strabismus; III, IV, VI, VIII:* | | | **Tongue** | | | |
| **Face** | | | *Tone, mass; XII, cerebrum:* | | | |
| *Sensation; Vs, cerebrum:* | | | **Pharynx,** Larynx | | | |
| *Muscle mass, jaw tone; Vm:* | | | *Voice; IX, X:* | | | |
| *Ear, eye, nose, lip reflex; V-VII:* | | | *Swallow; IX, X, cerebrum:* | | | |
| *Expression; VII, cerebrum* | | | *Endoscopy:* | | | |
| *Sweating Symp:* | | | *Slap test:* | | | |

| GAIT | LEFT | | RIGHT | |
|---|---|---|---|---|
| | FORE | HIND | FORE | HIND |
| **Paresis:** | | | | |
| **Ataxia:** | | | | |
| **Hypometria:** | | | | |
| **Hypermetria:** | | | | |
| **Posture:** | | | | |
| **Total deficit:** | | | | |
| **NECK & FORELIMBS:** (localising signs) | | | | |
| **TRUNK & HINDLIMBS:** (localising signs) | | | | |
| **TAIL & ANUS & RECTAL:** | | | | |

**ASSESSMENT**

| SITE OF LESION(S): | **General sites** (circle): cerebrum, brainstem, peripheral cranial nerves, cerebellum, spinal cord, peripheral nerves, muscles, skeleton |
| | **Specific site:** |
| **CAUSE OF LESION(S):** | |

**PLAN**

| DIAGNOSTIC: | |
| THERAPEUTIC: | |
| PROGNOSITC: | |

SIG. .............................................................    DATE: ......... / ......... / .........    CHARGE .....................................    IGM/rh/NEUROA.DOC

**Fig. 19.2** (a, pages 500–501) Form for recording the neurological examination of small animals. (b, above) Form for recording the neurological examination of large animals.

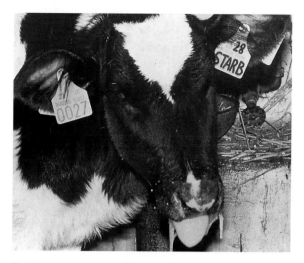

**Fig. 19.3** Abnormal behavior with an extended head posture and slight left head turn, along with dorsal rotation of the eyeballs ("star-gazing") in a depressed adult cow. These signs are consistent with the thalamic–hypothalamic syndrome associated with basilar empyema (pituitary abscess).

**Table 19.3. Categories of consciousness (mental status) in animals from least severely affected to most severely affected**

| | |
|---|---|
| Alert | – Normal |
| Depressed | – Quiet, unwilling to perform normally but responsive to environmental stimuli |
| Delerium, dementia | – Responsive to environmental stimuli, but responses are not clearly directed to the stimuli |
| Semicomatose stuporous | – Remains unresponsive to environmental stimulation but responsive to painful sensation |
| Comatose | – Non-responsive to either environmental or painful stimulation |

- the **cerebral cortex** is the ultimate source of awareness
- the **ascending reticular activating system** (ARAS) within the brain stem receives input from the environment via all parts of the body and sends stimuli to the cerebral cortex to maintain a wakeful state.

Abnormalities of consciousness reflect either a primary (e.g. encephalitis) or secondary (e.g. hepatic encephalopathy) supratentorial or brain-stem abnormality.

Various categories of consciousness can be identified (Table 19.3). Consciousness is interpreted as normal when certain stimuli evoke a similar response in the animal being examined as would be expected in normal animals. As individual animals may react differently to the same environmental stimuli, comments from the owner or handler regarding the animal's usual responsiveness are often helpful.

**Coma** is the most severe state of impaired consciousness. Animals are recumbent and have no response to any external stimuli, including stimuli that are painful.

Animals with **semicoma** or **stupor** are similarly not responsive to external stimuli, but their responsiveness to painful stimuli remains. Reactions to these stimuli may, however, not clearly be directed toward the stimuli. **Depression**, **delirium**, and **dementia** are terms taken from human medicine to describe abnormal

demeanors associated with psychological abnormalities. They suggest a state of altered consciousness or personality change that is not as severe as stupor and coma, and are used figuratively rather than literally when describing animal activity. As it is impossible to determine what an animal is thinking, these terms may be inappropriate for use in veterinary medicine. On the other hand, unusual activity can be seen with focal or diffuse cerebral disease.

**Narcolepsy** refers to excessive daytime sleepiness that is usually episodic and results in abnormal consciousness.

**Cataplexy** is periodic muscular hypotonia. An abnormal sleep/wake cycle is suspected to be present in both cataplexy and narcolepsy.

Sleep appears to be controlled by areas within the reticular formation of the brain stem. Acute onset of

## Some signs of focal or diffuse cerebral disease

- continuous yawning in horses (hepatoencephalopathy)
- frantic and compulsive locomotion in horses (moldy corn poisoning – leukoencephalomalacia)
- jaw clamping and personality changes in dogs (hypocalcemia)
- constant bellowing in cattle (lead poisoning; rabies)
- backwards running in pigs (salt intoxication – eosinophilic encephalopathy).

sleep, sometimes occurring with specific stimuli (such as eating), is characteristic of narcolepsy. Disordered neurotransmitter metabolism or abnormalities of the reticular activating system are thought to be responsible for this disorder, but a true cause is not known.

Breeds predisposed to narcolepsy include

- Doberman Pinscher
- Labrador retriever
- miniature Poodle
- Dachshund
- Beagle
- Saint Bernard
- Shetland ponies.

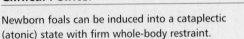

### Clinical Pointer ✳

Newborn foals can be induced into a cataleptic (atonic) state with firm whole-body restraint.

Clinical signs usually begin at a young age, but dogs as old as 7 years have been diagnosed with this disorder. An adult-onset progressive sleep disorder occurs in horses of many breeds.

## Posture and body position at rest

Posture is evaluated at rest and as the animal adopts or is placed in various positions throughout the examination. Posture of

- the head
- the limbs
- the trunk.

is assessed

### Abnormal posture of the head

With a **head tilt** the median plane of the head is rotated from its normal perpendicular relationship with the dorsal plane as though the head is tilted to one side (Fig. 19.4). If the animal is viewed from the front, one side of the head is directed more ventrally than the other. When severe, the head tilt may be associated with rolling or falling toward the side of the tilt.

A head tilt is most often associated with disease of the vestibular system. The tilt is usually directed toward the side of the lesion, especially when the lesion occurs in the peripheral vestibular apparatus. Occasionally, with central lesions involving the caudal cerebellar peduncle or flocculonodular lobe, the head tilt is directed away from the side of the lesion: the so-called **paradoxical vestibular syndrome**.

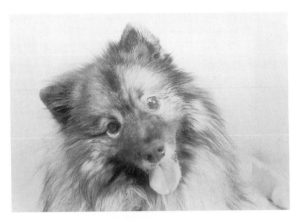

**Fig. 19.4** Dog with a right head tilt.

The **adversive syndrome** consists of a **head turn** and circling. A head turn is an abnormal posture where the head is directed toward the caudal ('looking backward') rather than the cranial ('looking forward') aspects of the animal (Fig. 19.5). The median plane of the head remains perpendicular to the ground. This occurs most often with supratentorial lesions. The head turn and circling are usually directed toward the side of a unilateral supratentorial lesion. A similar abnormality, termed hemi-inattention or hemineglect, may be seen when an animal will only eat from one side of the food container.

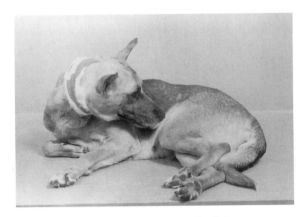

**Fig. 19.5** Left head turn in a dog with a left supratentorial lesion.

### Clinical Pointer ✳

Head tilts, turns, and circling are often directed *towards* the side of a unilateral lesion.

With some vestibular disorders a head tilt and a head and neck turn can occur together. In such instances assessment for a head tilt should be made only when the neck is held straight on the median plane.

## Abnormal posture of the limbs

Standing with the limbs placed more laterally than usual is a **wide-based stance** and may be associated with a variety of lesions of the nervous system, especially those involving the vestibular system, cerebellum, and spinal cord (Fig. 19.6). This posture may be an attempt by the animal to support itself against gravity, preventing it falling to one side or the other.

**Spasticity** can be seen at rest or while moving, and is usually associated with disease of the central nervous system motor pathways. In a recumbent animal spasticity and/or opisthotonos can be seen in numerous situations. These include decerebrate rigidity, decerebellate rigidity, and Schiff–Sherrington posture.

**Decerebrate rigidity** is characterized by opisthotonos (extreme dorsal extension of the head and neck towards the back) and extension of all limbs. Usually the animal is stuporous or comatose. This is caused by the loss of descending input from supratentorial structures to the medullary centers normally responsible for flexion of the limbs, and is seen with severe brain-stem lesions.

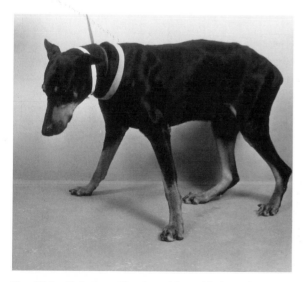

**Fig. 19.6** Doberman Pinscher with a wide-base thoracic limb stance. Also the head is held lower to the ground and the neck is straight in relation to the back. This dog had a C6–C7 extradural spinal compressive lesion.

**Decerebellate rigidity** is characterized by opisthotonus with thoracic limb extension and flexion of the pelvic limbs up under the body owing to contraction of the sublumbar muscles. Mental status is normal. This posture is associated with cerebellar disease. If the lesion involves the ventral aspects of the cerebellum, extensor rigidity of all limbs is seen. This posture can occur episodically, when it may be referred to as 'cerebellar seizures'.

**Schiff–Sherrington posture (phenomenon)** is characterized by thoracic limb extension with normal tone and reflexes in the pelvic limbs. This results from a severe third thoracic (T3) to third lumbar (L3) spinal cord segment lesion that interrupts the ascending inhibitory impulses from the lumbar region to the extensor muscles of the thoracic limbs. Except for extension, the thoracic limbs are neurologically normal. This feature, along with the results of the pelvic limb examination, should help differentiate this posture from extensor rigidity occurring as a result of an abnormality of the central pathways cranial to the sixth cervical (C6) spinal cord segment. The Schiff–Sherrington posture occurs only rarely, in large animals.

Severe extensor rigidity of the limbs, neck, trunk, and tail is characteristic of **tetanus** (Fig. 19.7). Classically a 'sawhorse' stance is seen. Facial muscle contraction may result in a 'tense' facial expression termed risus sardonicus. Although tetanus usually affects the entire body, localized tetanus involving only one limb is occasionally noted.

In some instances of chronic disease of the motor neuron cell body or peripheral nerve that results in muscle atrophy and fibrosis, one or both pelvic limbs may be held in chronic extension. This posture is often seen with toxoplasmosis or neosporosis infection in young dogs. Likewise, in utero crowding and, more frequently, lower motor neuron insults such as viral infection and toxins, can result in congenital limb and vertebral contractures (arthrogryposis) in most species. This is especially true in cattle (crooked calf disease) and horses (contracted foal disease).

Muscle weakness can also result in flaccid limbs: the animal tends to 'buckle' in the limbs and lie down, and when passively manipulated the limbs have reduced to absent tone (i.e. like a 'wet noodle'). These signs are more often associated with motor neuron cell body, peripheral nerve, neuromuscular junction, or muscle diseases.

A persistent or episodic non-weightbearing lameness, presumably the result of nerve irritation and pain, is termed **nerve root signature**. This most often involves a thoracic limb and is commonly associated with cervical disk disease (Fig. 19.8). A similar abnormality can involve the pelvic limb. In general animals

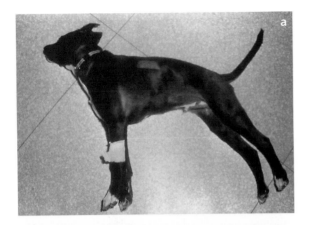

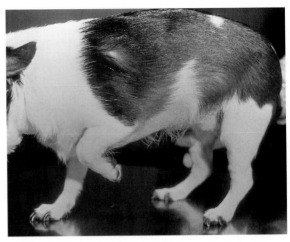

Fig. 19.8 Nerve root signature of the thoracic limb in a dog due to hydro/syringomyelia.

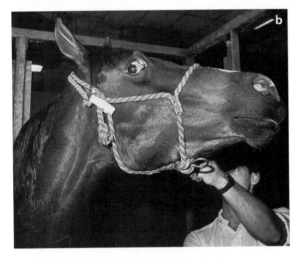

**Fig. 19.7** (a) Dog with persistent generalized extensor rigidity characteristic of generalized tetanus. (Courtesy of Michael Moore, Washington State University, College of Veterinary Medicine). (b) This adult horse with tetanus demonstrates the characteristic abnormal facial expression, with stiff ear posture, flared nares, tight lips and muzzle, and particularly medial angulation of the dorsal palpebral margin and protrusion of the membrana nictitans associated with retraction of the eyeball.

that carry limbs have orthopedic disease, whereas those that drag limbs have neurological disease. Nerve root signature is an exception to this generalization. Involvement of the sympathetic innervation of a limb (reflex sympathetic dystrophy) may cause profound disuse of one limb in horses.

Dancing Doberman syndrome is a special situation of limb carriage characterized by alternating pelvic limb flexion when the animal is standing. A peripheral neuropathy or myopathy of the pelvic limb nerves is suspected. This is similar to shivering and spastic syndrome in adult horses and cattle, respectively, where

one or both hindlimbs is intermittently held in various abnormally flexed or extended positions, with or without muscle trembling.

---

**Clinical Pointer**

Limb carried → orthopedic problem
Limb dragged → neurological problem
But nerve root signature is an exception!

---

### Abnormal posture of the trunk

**Scoliosis**, an abnormal lateral deviation of the vertebral column, often occurs secondary to intramedullary spinal cord lesions such as syringo- or hydromyelia. **Kyphosis**, an abnormal flexion primarily of the thoracolumbar vertebral column, results in a 'hunchback' appearance. This posture can be noted with back, or more commonly, cervical pain. Animals with cervical pain will also often keep their neck muscles rigid and their head lowered to the ground. Doberman Pinschers with cervical vertebral malformation/malarticulation and large animals with C1–2 subluxation and osteomyelitis will often keep the neck straight in relation to the back, presumably as a result of pain, or possibly to relieve some of the associated spinal cord compression (see Fig. 19.6). Animals that have dysfunction or pain in either the cranial or caudal halves of the body may attempt to shift their weight backward or forward, respectively.

**Lordosis** is abnormal extension of the vertebral column, particularly in the thoracolumbar region. This results in a 'dipped back' appearance of the vertebral column when the animal is viewed from the side. This posture is uncommon but may be a characteristic of old horses.

## Involuntary movements

These are abnormal movements that start, stop, recur, or persist without the animal's voluntary control. They may occur at rest or during activity. Involuntary movements include tremor, myoclonus, and seizure.

**Tremor** is an involuntary, rhythmic oscillatory movement of all or part of the body. It results from the alternate or synchronous contraction of reciprocally innervated antagonistic muscles. True tremor ceases with sleep. Tremor can be localized to one body area or be generalized to involve the whole body. Localized tremor usually involves the head or pelvic limbs. A tremor that is more obvious when an animal tries to perform a task (e.g. such as eating) is referred to as intention tremor and is most commonly associated with cerebellar dysfunction.

**Fasciculations** are small local involuntary muscle contractions visible under the skin. These represent spontaneous discharge of a number of muscle fibers innervated by a single motor nerve fiber. Accordingly, fasciculation may occur with lesions affecting

- motor neuron cell bodies
- peripheral nerves
- neuromuscular junctions
- muscle tissue.

**Myoclonus** is a shock-like contraction of one muscle or a group of muscles. Clinically it is seen as explosive movement of part of the body, particularly limb flexion. Myoclonia most often affects a thoracic limb, but a pelvic limb, or even the facial muscles, may be involved. In dogs it is usually a sequela to distemper infection, which establishes a pacemaker-like depolarization of local motor neurons (Breazile et al 1966). Once established, myoclonus usually persists in a regular pattern, occurring every few seconds, and will often persist even when the animal is under light anesthesia. In some cases after long periods (years) myoclonus may resolve.

**Reflex myoclonus** is characterized by episodic stimulation-evoked extensor rigidity of muscle groups or the entire body and is most commonly seen in Labrador retrievers and polled Hereford calves. Other breeds, such as Dalmatian dogs and Peruvian Paso foals, are occasionally affected. As this is a congenital disorder young (weeks to months of age) animals are affected. Several of these syndromes are caused by a deficit in inhibitory glycine receptors.

**Seizures** are an important and common sign of intracranial neurological disease. A seizure is a transitory paroxysmal disturbance of brain function that is sudden in onset, ceases spontaneously, and has a tendency to recur. Clinically, the most common type of seizure seen is a generalized abnormality wherein the animal falls to its side, has rhythmic jerking of the head or limbs, followed by paddling or running motions. This is referred to as a generalized tonic–clonic seizure and is usually accompanied by autonomic disturbances such as urination, salivation, and defecation.

Focal seizures result in movements that remain localized to one body region. This may be characterized by twitching of a single limb or of one side of the face. Focal seizures can be distinguished from myoclonus, for example, as the former are usually more episodic, infrequent, and less rhythmic.

---

### Clinical Pointer

Tremor → disappears in unconscious states
Intention tremor → cerebellar disease
Myoclonia → persists in light anesthesia
Focal seizure → episodic, non-rhythmic pattern

---

Bizarre behavior may be a manifestation of a seizure disorder, possibly initiated in components of the limbic system (temporal lobe epilepsy). 'Fly biting' is one example and may be more common in breeds such as the Cavalier King Charles spaniel. At one extreme even some gastrointestinal abnormalities such as vomiting have been suggested to be the result of seizure activity. Other behavior disorders, such as flank sucking or tail biting, may result from a seizure focus, but definitive proof is lacking.

## Gait

The term gait refers to the method of moving the limbs and body in order to get from one place to another and is commonly defined as a regularly repeating series of limb movements during walking or running. The nervous system controls the actions of the muscles, bones, joints, and associated connective tissue important for this function. Normal walking is produced by central nervous system control of stepping reflexes. Each limb alternates between extension and flexion. The vestibulospinal and reticulospinal tracts are facilitatory to the extensor muscles, important for maintenance of body posture against gravity (the stance or propulsive phase). The corticospinal and the rubrospinal tracts are facilitatory to the flexor muscles, important for the protraction (swing or flight) phase of limb movement.

Locomotion is thought to be controlled at the level of the brain stem, but a discrete anatomic gait center (nucleus) has not been identified. Supratentorial (forebrain) structures are important for voluntary control, mainly of intricate movements. The cerebellum, although not necessary for the initiation of movement, is important for coordination. Cerebellar influences coordinate and smooth body movements by controlling the rate, range and force of limb motion. The cerebellum is most likely responsible for inhibition of the flexor component of gait.

### Abnormalities of gait

Abnormalities of gait include
- ataxia
- dysmetria
- spasticity
- stiffness
- myotonia
- paresis
- lameness.

**Ataxia** is a lack of coordination and can involve the head, body, or limbs. Animals with ataxia are incoordinated in their motion, usually with jerky, irregular limb movements when walking or running. This gives the appearance that the animal does not know where the limbs are being placed. They often will sway from side to side and sometimes fall. Ataxia can result from a variety of anatomic lesions within the nervous system, most commonly the cerebellum, vestibular system, and spinal cord sensory pathways. Ataxia without weakness or loss of conscious proprioception usually implies cerebellar or cerebellar pathway disease.

**Dysmetria** indicates improper measurement of range and force in muscular acts. Dysmetria can include the characteristics of **hypometria** and **hypermetria**. With hypermetria voluntary muscular movement results in overreaching of the intended goal, often resulting in high-stepping (Fig. 19.9). With hypometria voluntary movement falls short of the intended goal, resulting in stiff, tin-soldier-like movements, particularly in the thoracic limbs. Both of these abnormalities are most commonly seen with lesions involving the cerebellum or spinocerebellar pathways. In hypermetria the loss of cerebellar input, which normally dampens the flexion phase of gait, results in the exaggerated movement.

**Spasticity** is a state of increased muscle tone and commonly occurs with lesions of the white matter tracts of the brain stem and spinal cord. This is observed in the gait as stiffness or floating (failure to adequately flex the limbs during gait). Hypometria and spasticity are clinically difficult to distinguish. Palpation of the muscles with the limbs placed in a relaxed position will reveal the hypertonia of spasticity.

**Stiffness** associated with decreased step length is commonly seen with diseases of the peripheral neuro-

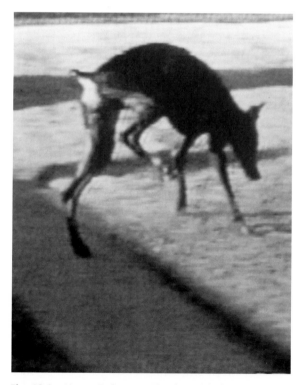

**Fig. 19.9** Young Doberman Pinscher with dysmetria (hypermetria) of the right pelvic limb due to cerebellar disease.

muscular apparatus (motor neuron cell body, nerve roots, peripheral nerve, neuromuscular junction, and muscle). A similar appearance may occur in animals with limb pain, primarily as a consequence of orthopedic disease such as polyarthritis and laminitis.

Animals with neuromuscular disease may also have a stiff, stilted, choppy gait due primarily to muscle weakness. These abnormalities may be episodic in, for example, canine myasthenia gravis and hyperkalemic periodic paralysis of horses, and occur as the level of exercise is increased.

**Myotonia** refers to persistent muscle contraction following voluntary or external initiation. Animals with myotonia often have a stiff gait. The muscles may dimple when percussed (struck with a reflex hammer). Myotonia occurs as a congenital problem in various breeds of dogs, such as the Chow-Chow. The excessive muscle contraction is thought to be due to an abnormal muscle cell membrane supporting persistent depolarization.

Various syndromes, including **Scotty Cramp** in dogs, **spastic paresis** in calves (Fig. 19.10), **spastic syndrome** in cattle, and **stringhalt** in horses, are characterized by continual or paroxysmal muscular hypertonicity. In many instances signs may be precipitated by excitement or exercise. Some of these diseases are inherited as a recessive trait, but an underlying mechanism is not always known.

**Paresis,** or neurological weakness, indicates decreased motor effort without complete paralysis. Paresis is noted in an animal while it is moving, when it drags a limb, or scuffs the dorsum of the paw or hoof when walking or running. Sometimes, however, paresis is only evident when other aspects such as postural reactions are tested (see postural reaction tests). Varying degrees of paresis exist; some animals retain the ability to walk, whereas others are unable to support their weight. With paresis,

however, some voluntary motion remains. Observation of abnormal toenail and hoof wear may be a clue to underlying flexor paresis (Fig. 19.11). Extensor weakness in large animals can be detected readily by pushing down on the lumbar region or by pulling the tail to each side in turn, all while the patient is walking forward.

**Lameness** is an abnormal gait wherein there is reduced ability or desire to bear weight on a limb because of pain or a mechanical restriction of normal joint movement. It is usually associated with pain in the limb from musculoskeletal disease, but may result from nerve root disease (see nerve root signature). If limbs are painful or weak the weight may be shifted to normal limbs.

### Clinical evaluation of abnormalities of gait

Clinical evaluation of gait involves observation of the animal's movements during walking, and, when indicated, at faster paces. This is best accomplished by having a handler walk the animal over a flat, non-slippery area.

Central nervous system lesions result in irregular and uncoordinated gaits and a tendency for the animal to sway from side to side. Some may fall to one side. The feet may contact the ground with increased force.

---

### Assessing gait

- assess whether the gait is normal or abnormal
- if the gait is abnormal, then assess whether the stride length is normal, increased, or decreased
- note the presence of any lameness.

---

Doberman pinschers with cervical vertebral malformation/malarticulation, for example, may overflex the hock joints during weightbearing, presumably as a result of extensor weakness.

Animals with disease of the motor neuron cell body, peripheral nerves, neuromuscular junction, and muscle, take short, choppy steps. Some have a kyphotic posture. They may tire easily and appear unwilling to perform tasks. Animals with orthopedic disease may have a similar gait abnormality. The presence of normal conscious proprioception should suggest underlying orthopedic disease. Poor limb perfusion, such as from a partial bilateral iliac arterial thrombus or from a right-to-left patent ductus arteriosus (PDA), may also result in a short, choppy pelvic limb gait. The clinical signs in these situations may worsen with exercise, as in myasthenia gravis. Differential cyanosis (the cranial parts of body being

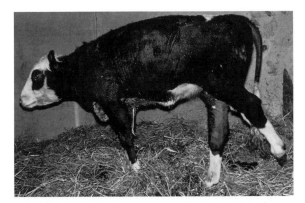

**Fig. 19.10** Yearling beef calf with prominent upright limb posture and spastic caudal thrusting of the left pelvic limb consistent with spastic paresis.

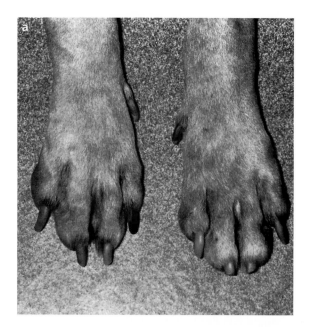

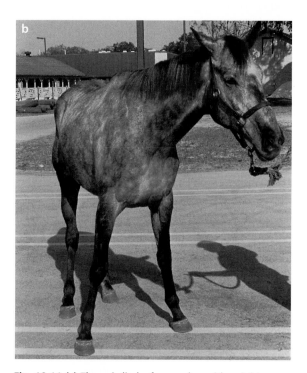

**Fig. 19.11** (a) Thoracic limbs from a dog with a right forebrain lesion. Note the excessive wear of the nails of the left foot compared to the right. This dog had an associated left hemiparesis. (b) Conscious proprioceptive deficits in this horse are demonstrated by the adoption of abnormal foot placement after maneuvering in a circle. In addition, there is evidence of flexor weakness, with wearing of the front of the hooves due to dragging of the toes.

normally perfused and the caudal aspects being cyanotic) may be seen with the reverse-shunting PDA. Animals with vertebral pain may also have a short stride and be reluctant to move.

Depending upon where the lesion affects the nervous system the gait may be altered to differing degrees. Supratentorial disease will often not affect the gait. Wide circling toward the side of a unilateral forebrain lesion is common. Spasticity may be noticed, the limbs (primarily a thoracic limb on the side opposite a unilateral lesion) appearing stiff, with a floating and overreaching action.

Lesions of the brain stem and cervical spinal cord will often have dramatic effects on gait, frequently impairing the ability to even stand and generate a gait. If the lesion occurs unilaterally, ipsilateral paresis of a thoracic and pelvic limb (hemiparesis) is noted. If pathways are affected bilaterally, all four limbs (tetraparesis) may be affected. Spinal reflexes are normal to exaggerated, reflecting the central nervous system origin of the lesion.

With cervical spinal lesions the pelvic limbs may appear more obviously affected than the thoracic limbs. Various explanations exist for this finding.

1. There are quantitatively more afferent and efferent pathways influencing thoracic compared to pelvic limb function.
2. The pelvic limbs are further from the center of gravity.
3. Tracts coursing to the pelvic limbs are located more superficially in the spinal cord than those coursing to the thoracic limbs, rendering them more susceptible to damage from extradural compressive lesions.

The last explanation is based upon the somatotopic orientation of spinal cord tracts, wherein tracts influencing specific body areas lie in specific anatomically discrete areas of the brain and spinal cord.

Somatotopic organization may also be the explanation as to why some animals with cervical spinal cord lesions present with paresis that is worse in the thoracic limbs than in the pelvic limbs. This presentation, termed **central cord syndrome** or **cruciate paralysis** in humans, implies that the more centrally (medially) located tracts influencing thoracic limb function are preferentially

---

**Clinical Pointer**

Normal or increased step length → CNS lesion
Shortened step length → orthopedic or neuromuscular lesion

involved with the disease process, compared to the more peripherally placed tracts traveling to and from the pelvic limbs. Both intramedullary spinal lesions, such as syringomyelia or hydromyelia, and extradural compressive lesions can result in this abnormality.

Lesions of peripheral nerves can also affect limb movement (see Table 19.2). Lesions of the femoral nerve result in an inability to extend the stifle and support weight. An affected animal may have difficulty bringing the limbs forward and may 'bunny-hop', or be short-strided in the affected limb. 'Bunny-hopping' is the simultaneous advancement of the pelvic limbs and has classically been associated with spinal cord disease, such as spinal dysraphism or myelodysplasia. However, animals with orthopedic disease (such as bilateral hip dysplasia or stifle osteochondrosis) may have the same gait abnormality. With abnormalities of the femoral nerve the animal is unable to extend the stifle and bear weight thus adopting a crouched posture.

Lesions of the obturator nerve often do not affect gait in dogs and cats. If an animal is placed on a slippery surface, however, the affected pelvic limb(s) may slide laterally with weightbearing.

Lesions of the sciatic nerve result in a characteristic gait wherein the distal foot is almost 'thrown' forward by the movements of the more proximal muscles of the limb. When the animal is weightbearing the hock joint may overflex, resulting in the 'dropped hock' appearance. A similar appearance can be seen with avulsion of the gastrocnemius tendon. With lesions of the cranial gluteal nerve the stifle may become abducted during the stance phase of gait.

If the radial nerve is affected the animal cannot extend the carpus normally. If the lesion occurs proximally in the radial nerve, the elbow may be held more ventrally than normal. If the musculocutaneous nerve is intact the limb may be carried off the ground with the elbow flexed.

With individual lesions of the medial, ulnar, musculo-cutaneous, and suprascapular nerves gait is usually

> ### Presenting patterns of peripheral nerve lesions
>
> Femoral nerve → 'bunny-hopping' gait; stifle extension not possible; crouched posture
> Obturator nerve → abduction of pelvic limbs (especially on slippery surfaces)
> Sciatic nerve → 'thrown foot' gait; 'dropped hocks'
> Radial nerve → carpal extension not possible; ventral elbow position with proximal lesions
> Median, ulnar, musculocutaneous and suprascapular nerves → not individually essential for normal gait.

unaffected. With medial and ulnar lesions the carpal joint may be overextended. With musculocutaneous nerve paralysis elbow flexion is poor and this joint may be held overextended.

## Postural reactions

Postural reactions are tests of an animal's ability to recognize that a limb is in an abnormal position and to replace it in the correct position. To perform these reactions the bulk of the nervous system needs to be functioning normally, i.e. proprioceptive and motor pathways to the body part being tested should be intact.

### Conscious proprioception testing

Proprioception is the ability of the animal to know where the limbs and other body parts are with respect to the trunk and to gravity. Conscious proprioception testing ('knuckling') is used to determine whether the animal is conscious of where a limb is placed (Figs 19.12, 19.13).

Another way to test conscious proprioception in small animals is by using a paper slide test. A piece of paper is placed under the weightbearing foot and

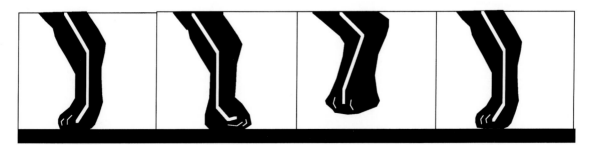

**Fig. 19.12** Normal conscious proprioceptive response of a dog. (Left to right) The paw is placed in an abnormal position and the animal rapidly replaces it in the normal position.

## Conscious proprioception test

- animal in standing position
- turn one paw so that dorsum contacts the ground surface
- assess time taken to return paw to normal position
- repeat for other limbs
- the paw position is corrected immediately in normal animals, any delay implies neurologic disease.

## Hopping test

- animal in standing position
- weight displaced on to one limb and the animal is then pushed laterally over this limb (see text for method in small and large animals)
- should hop when center of gravity moves laterally over the weightbearing limb as the animal accommodates to the new body position
- repeat test for contralateral limb.

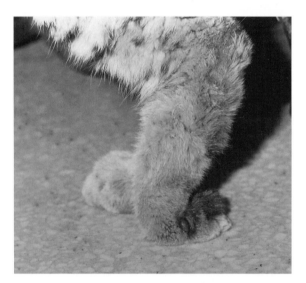

**Fig. 19.13**  Deficit of conscious proprioception. When the paw is turned on its dorsum the animal fails to replace the paw quickly to the normal position.

## Clinical Pointer

Animals with neuromuscular weakness such as myasthenia gravis will not be able to hop normally when most of their weight is placed on one limb, but will hop normally when the examiner supports most of the animal's weight. This is because the animal with neuromuscular junction disease is conscious of when it needs to move and may attempt to move, but does not have the muscular strength to complete the task.

slowly pulled laterally by the examiner. As the limb is slid progressively laterally the animal will pick it up and replace it in its original position. This helps in evaluating conscious proprioception, but may better test proximal rather than distal limb proprioception.

As these tests are difficult to perform and do not work well in large animals, conscious proprioception deficits usually become evident by forcing the animal to place the limbs in awkward positions while turning, walking or backing, and determining that the limb is left in the abnormal stance for an excessive period of time (Fig.19.11b).

### Hopping

Hopping tests proprioception, strength, and voluntary movement. Hopping is tested on a single limb at a time. The animal's weight is placed exclusively on one limb and the body forced in one direction (Fig. 19.14a, b).

For small animals the examiner usually stands lateral to the animal and picks up all limbs but the one to be tested. The most reliable direction to have the animal hop for ease of interpretation is laterally (towards the limb being tested), as even normal animals will move awkwardly when forced in other directions. In adult large animals and large dogs it is acceptable (and practical) to hold up one forelimb and push the animal laterally on the weightbearing limb (Fig. 19.14c). A delay in hopping is abnormal. As both central and peripheral motor as well as sensory (proprioceptive) pathways are necessary for hopping to be performed normally, a hopping deficit suggests a neurological abnormality. Some animals with cerebellar or vestibular pathway lesions may have exaggerated limb movement when hopping (Fig. 19.15).

### Wheelbarrowing, hemiwalking, extensor postural thrust

If an animal has obvious abnormalities on conscious proprioceptive testing and hopping, it is not necessary to perform these additional tests as no further information will be obtained. The tests can, however, be performed if conscious proprioception and hopping yield equivocal results, or in large dogs where single-limb hopping is physically difficult for the examiner to perform. They are not practical in adult horses and cattle.

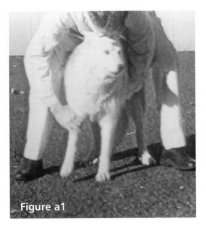

Figure a1

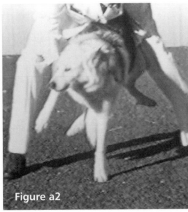

Figure a2

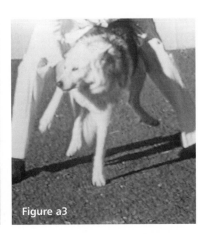

Figure a3

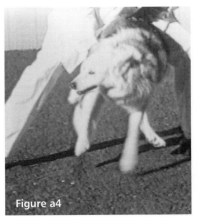

Figure a4

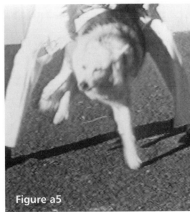

Figure a5

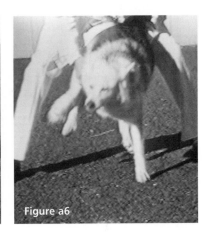

Figure a6

**Fig. 19.14a** Normal hopping response in a dog.

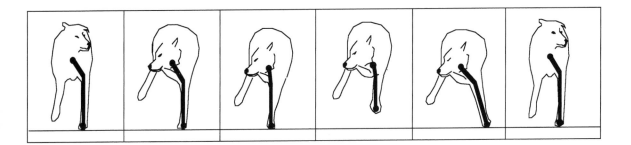

**Fig 19.14b** Schematic representation of the same response showing the shifting of weight distribution and the center of gravity (black lines).

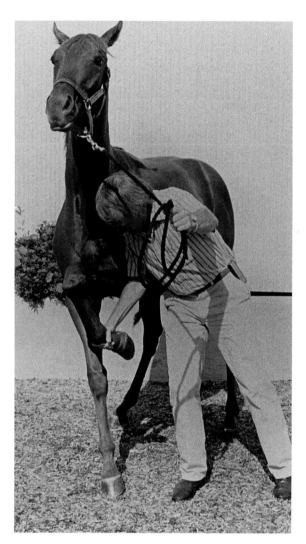

**Fig 19.14c** Hopping on one thoracic limb at a time in an adult horse can be accomplished by lifting one limb and pushing against the shoulder to make the horse move away from the handler. Subtle degrees of weakness may be evident that are not seen at normal gait.

### Placing reactions

Testing of placing reactions is most practical for smaller animals that can easily be held off the ground. Non-visual, tactile placing reactions are assessed first. Non-visual placing yields information similar to hopping and conscious proprioception tests concerning the integrity of the nervous system. Visual placing may help in defining a visual deficit. Normal tactile placing with a deficit in visual placing indicates a lesion in the visual pathways.

### Wheelbarrowing test

- animal in standing position
- raise the front or rear of the animal so that the weight is placed on either both pelvic or both thoracic limbs
- force the animal to move the body forward (when testing the thoracic limbs) or backward (when testing the pelvic limbs)
- the animal should make normal walking movements in the limbs touching the ground.

Wheelbarrowing of the thoracic limbs, especially if the head is concurrently held extended by the examiner, may be very helpful in testing for subtle thoracic limb paresis not revealed by other tests.

### Hemiwalking test

- animal in standing position
- hold up a thoracic and pelvic limb on one side and force the animal laterally in the opposite direction
- when the animal is moved laterally, the limbs contacting the ground should move laterally to accommodate this new body position
- a modified type of hemiwalking can be performed in large animals by pulling the tail to one side while the animal is moving forward
- lack of resistance to tail pulling indicates weakness; awkward, ataxic limb movements may be seen when the tail is released abruptly (weakness and proprioceptive deficits may also become evident when pulling the head collar and tail simultaneously).

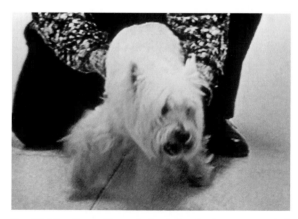

**Fig. 19.15** Dog with cerebellar lesion having exaggerated limb movement when hopped to the right.

## *Abnormal postural reactions*

Many neural pathways are necessary for normal conscious proprioception. Information is sent from the limb to the cortex for conscious recognition of where that limb is in space. Functionally, these pathways cross to the opposite side in the region of the caudal mesencephalon and rostral pons (Fig. 19.16). A unilateral lesion rostral to this region (i.e. in the supratentorial area) will therefore result in conscious proprioception deficits on the contralateral side of the body. A unilateral lesion caudal to this region (i.e. the caudal brain stem, spinal cord, or peripheral nerve) will result in evaluation of gait and ipsilateral deficits.

If postural reaction testing reveals abnormalities of limb function these abnormalities are described as follows

- **paraparesis** is gait and/or postural abnormalities in the pelvic limbs bilaterally
- **monoparesis** is gait and/or postural abnormalities in only one limb
- **tetraparesis** is gait and/or postural abnormalities of all four limbs
- **hemiparesis** is gait and/or postural abnormalities of a thoracic and pelvic limb on the same side.

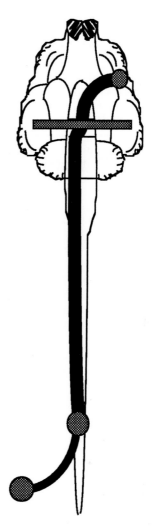

**Fig. 19.16** The functional cross-over for conscious proprioception at the caudal mesencephalon, rostral pons junction (level of dotted bar).

There is currently no descriptive term for bilateral postural reaction abnormalities of the thoracic limbs only.

## Cranial nerve examination

The cranial nerves are evaluated systematically, some being assessed individually and some in functional groups.

### *Olfactory cranial nerve – (CN) I: smell*

Smell can be assessed by placing a substance that is aromatic (e.g. baby food) but non-irritating around the nasal opening so the vapors can be exposed to the nasal mucosa. This should evoke a behavioral response (turning away, contraction of the facial muscles, sniffing) that indicates the animal recognizes the substance. Irritating substances will excite the sensory (free nerve) endings of the trigeminal nerve (CN V).

The olfactory behavioral response may be used to test for the presence or absence of olfaction and can be combined with electroencephalographic monitoring to provide a more objective measure of smell. Odors used include eugenol, a pure olfactory nerve stimulant, and benzaldehyde, which stimulates both olfactory and trigmenial receptors.

Anosmia (loss of smell) is most often recognized secondary to bilateral nasal passage disease. Unilateral lesions in the forebrain will not cause anosmia as smell is recognized bilaterally in the brain. Occasionally bilateral rostral forebrain disease involving the olfactory areas can affect smell. Viral infections such as distemper and parainfluenza may also cause anosmia. Clinically, dysosmia (abnormal smell) is difficult to determine unless further objective testing with various compounds is performed.

## Optic – CN II: vision

Cranial nerve II function can be assessed in many ways, the simplest being evaluation of the **menace response**.

---

### Menace response test

- make a menacing gesture (move the hand quickly toward the eye)
- look for the normal blinking response (closure of the palpebral fissure)
- guard against touching the vibrissae of the face around the eye or creating air currents that will contact the eye, as this will excite sensory receptors of the trigeminal nerve (CN V) and cause reflex blinking (resulting in misinterpretation of the menace response)
- perform the menace response independently in each eye while the opposite eye is covered to prevent visual information being projected to the opposite eye (in large animals, where the visual fields are sufficiently isolated from one another, it is usually not necessary to cover the non-tested eye).

---

An understanding of functional neuroanatomy is important for accurate localization of lesions affecting the visual pathways. The menace response tests CN II

---

### Clinical Pointer

Some species, such as rabbits, do not have a menace response.

---

(as part of the afferent pathway) and CN VII (the efferent pathway responsible for blinking). Input from the cerebellum is also necessary for the normal menace response (Fig. 19.17).

When a hand is brought toward the eye the image is first projected through the globe to the retina. Electrochemical receptors in the retina are excited and the impulses generated are projected into the optic nerve. The image is next projected from the retina through the optic nerve to the optic chiasm. In dogs 75% of the optic nerve fibers cross at the chiasm to

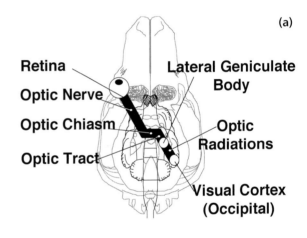

(a)

Retina
Optic Nerve
Optic Chiasm
Optic Tract
Lateral Geniculate Body
Optic Radiations
Visual Cortex (Occipital)

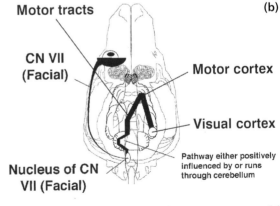

(b)

Motor tracts
CN VII (Facial)
Nucleus of CN VII (Facial)
Motor cortex
Visual cortex
Pathway either positively influenced by or runs through cerebellum

Fig. 19.17 Pathway necessary for the menace response. (a) Indicates affected pathways of occipital (visual) cortex. (b) indicates efferent pathways to facial nucleus via motor paths.

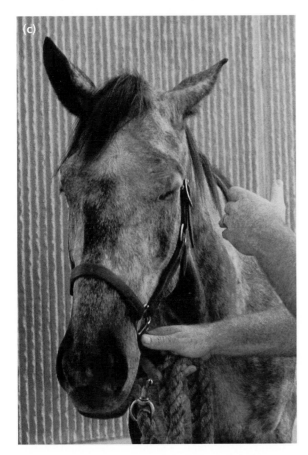

**Fig. 19.17** (c) A typical menace response with closure of the eyelids in response to a mild visual threat using the hand. A right-sided optic tract or occipital lobe lesion in this horse could result in the menace response being absent in the left eye but normal pupillary light reflexes being maintained.

enter the contralateral optic tract (65% in cats; 90% or more in cows, horses, pigs, sheep, and goats). From a practical point of view in large animals the menace response tests fibers that cross to the opposite visual cortex.

After passing through the chiasm the impulse is projected through the optic tract, lateral geniculate nucleus (in the thalamus), and optic radiations to the visual cortex in the occipital lobe. The object is now recognized by the brain to be present in the visual field.

The afferent pathway for the menace response, then, courses from the eye to the occipital cortex. The efferent portion of this response is mediated through CN VII (facial nerve), resulting in closure of the eyelid.

How the information for eyelid closure projects anatomically from the visual cortex, via motor

pathways, to the contralateral nucleus of CN VII is not completely understood. It is known that this pathway either synapses in, or is positively influenced by, the cerebellum, as animals with cerebellar disease will lack a menace response. Some such animals will withdraw the head from a threatening gesture (without eyelid closure) and may still blink in response to a bright light shone in the eyes (dazzle reflex) (Oliver, Hoerlein & Mayhew 1987). With unilateral cerebellar disease animals will have an ipsilateral menace deficit with normal vision and normal CN VII function.

Other tests of vision are more subjective. Rolling an object in the visual fields of an animal is not a good test of vision as other senses such as hearing may be elicited simultaneously. Even though humans may not be able to hear such objects moving, dogs, because of their relatively superior sense of hearing, may well do so and subsequently orient to the stimulus. Dropping cotton balls in the visual fields may be a better substitute, but some animals will not respond to these objects consistently. Making the animal walk through an unfamiliar obstacle course may be the best test of vision. If only a single eye is blind, blindfolding of the normal eye may be necessary.

### Oculomotor – CN III: pupils

**Assessment of the pupils at rest**

Examination of the pupils can be helpful in assessing abnormalities of the visual pathway, CN III (oculomotor nerve) and the sympathetic system. When stimulated, CN III constricts the pupil and the sympathetic system

---

**Mydriasis**

- dilated, poorly, or non-responsive pupil
- indicates parasympathetic denervation (CN III) or loss of muscle tone of the iris
- parasympatholytic drugs (e.g. atropine) applied to the eye will dilate the pupil, effect may last for several days
- primary disease of the iris such as iris atrophy is common in older animals, especially dogs – a dyscoric pupil and an irregular pupillary margin may be clues of underlying iris disease
- intraocular diseases such as synechia and glaucoma can result in a dilated pupil – this is rare in domestic animals
- dysautonomia occurs in dogs, cats, and horses (grass sickness); in addition to other clinical signs such as vomiting and constipation, dilated poorly to unresponsive pupils may be seen.

### Miosis

Miosis is indicated by smaller than normal pupil size and may be caused by

- iridic vascular congestion and edema associated with anterior uveitis
- painful conditions of the cornea, a bilateral phenomenon mediated through CN V (**oculosensory pupillary reflex**)
- instillation of parasympathomimetic drugs into the eye.

dilates the pupil. Initially the pupils are assessed for size and symmetry. It is important to consider the amount of light in the examination area when making these assessments. A pupil that is smaller than normal is **miotic**; a pupil larger than normal is **mydriatic**.

Fear and apprehension will result in dilated pupils. Unequal pupil size is referred to as anisocoria. Diseases of the eye (see Chapter 20) should be ruled out prior to neurological assessment.

Species differences regarding pupil appearance should be recognized

- dogs have round pupils
- cats have vertically directed elliptical shaped pupils
- horses, cattle, sheep, and goats have horizontally directed elliptical or ovoid pupils.

### Anisocoria

Anisocoria is resting inequality in pupil size. To determine which pupil is abnormal place the animal in both bright light (daylight) and darkness and note changes in pupil size.

- with a lesion of the sympathetic system the affected pupil will not dilate fully in the dark
- with a CN III lesion the abnormal pupil will not constrict in the light.

An abnormality of sympathetic innervation to an eye can result in a miotic pupil alone, or in signs of complete sympathetic denervation of the orbit that is (**Horner's syndrome**) (Fig. 19.18). Clinical signs of Horner's syndrome include

- miotic pupil
- prolapsed third eyelid
- ptosis
- enophthalmos
- peripheral vasodilation.

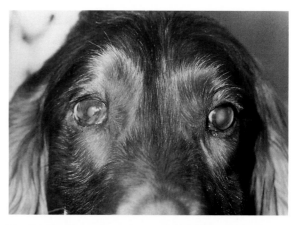

**Fig. 19.18**   Horner's syndrome of the right eye of a dog. Miosis and prolapse of the nictitating membrane are noted.

All species except the horse show decreased sweating in sympathetically denervated skin, whereas in the horse characteristically there is hyperhidrosis (Table 19.4).

A lesion anywhere along the sympathetic pathway (Fig. 19.19) can result in these clinical signs. Various causes for Horner's syndrome in dogs and cats have been described (Kern et al 1989; Morgan and Sanotti 1989).

**Pupillary light reflex (PLR)**
When a bright light is shone into one eye, both pupils should constrict. This is known as the pupillary light

**Table 19.4.   Clinical signs of Horner's syndrome in various species (all ipsilateral to lesion)**

**Dogs and cats**
Miosis
Ptosis
Enopthalmos
Protrusion of third eyelid
Vasodilation on side of the head

**Horse**
Ptosis is most consistent
Miosis is less obvious (greater constriction in affected eye)
Sweating of the face and cranial neck
Protrusion of third eyelid sometimes present

**Cattle, sheep and goats**
Ptosis most consistent
Miosis less obvious (greater constriction in affected eye)
Distension of vessels of ear
Decreased sweating on muzzle (cattle)

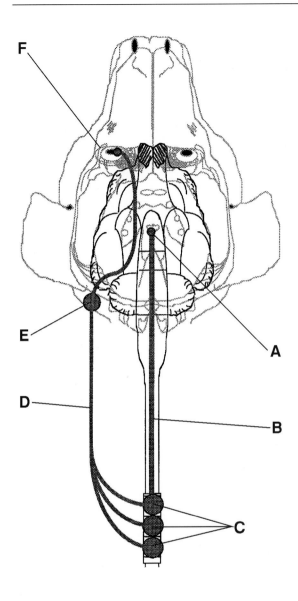

**Fig. 19.19** Pathway for sympathetic innervation to the eye. Upper motor neurons (A) from the hypothalamus descend the spinal cord in the lateral lectomertospinal spinal pathway (B) to synapse on cell bodies of preganglionic neurons in the T1–3 intermediate gray matter (C). Preganglionic neurons course cranially in the cervical sympathetic trunk (part of the vagosympathetic trunk) (D) to synapse in the cranial cervical ganglion (medial to the origin of the digastric muscle and ventromedially to the tympanic bulla) (E). Postganglionic fibers form a nerve plexus around the carotid artery, course through the middle ear, enter the skull and course along the ventral aspect of the skull. They then exit the skull through the orbital fissure and project to the ciliary body and iris dilator muscle of the eye (F).

reflex and is used to assess portions of the afferent visual pathway to approximately the level of the lateral geniculate nucleus in the thalamus. Cranial nerve III (oculomotor) is responsible for the efferent portion of this reflex, constriction of the pupil. A direct pupillary constrictor response occurs in the stimulated eye. Constriction of the opposite pupil is known as the consensual response.

When performing the PLR examination, especially if a poor-quality light source is used, the stimulated pupil may be seen to dilate slightly during continued stimulation. This is referred to as **pupillary escape** or accommodation. Rhythmic contraction and subsequent dilation of the pupil is called **hippus**. Although the clinical significance of this finding is debatable, some clinicians feel it is indicative of CNS disease.

> ### Clinical Pointer
>
> The direct PLR is more powerful than the direct (consensual) PLR. Thus, when moving a bright light quickly from one fundus to the other, in the eye that temporaneously receives the light stimulus the pupil constricts, even though it is partially constricted from a consensual response. This is the *swinging light test* and is useful when examining large animals.

When a bright light is initially flashed into the eye a blink response may occur. This is referred to as the **dazzle reflex** and probably does not involve the forebrain but is restricted to the brain-stem. With forebrain disease this reflex may be more prominent, suggesting release (lack of inhibition) of the reflex from higher control.

Fundic examination is important to determine retinal integrity and to look for clues to systemic abnormalities that may secondarily affect the central nervous system. Fundic examination will also allow visualization of a portion of the optic nerve to assess for abnormalities such as papilledema, and vascular engorgement seen with meningitis in ungulates.

**Pupillary changes with central nervous system disease**

With bilateral, usually severe, cerebrocortical disease the pupils will often be smaller than normal, i.e. miotic.

Many focal and diffuse cerebral lesions result in unilateral or bilateral cerebral swelling. If unilateral transtentorial occipital herniation occurs the ipsilateral pupil will dilate and become non-responsive to light, either directly or indirectly, because of pressure exerted on CN III. As the midbrain is compressed fixed midrange pupils will occur. Bilateral involvement results in bilateral involvement of the pupils.

## Ocular movement – CN III, IV, and VI

Cranial nerves III, IV, and VI function together to produce normal ocular movement. They are often evaluated concurrently.

### Oculomotor – CN III: eye movement, pupillary constriction

The motor function of CN III can be assessed by observing the position of the eye at rest. If the motor function is abnormal the eye may be deviated from a normal position. This is termed **strabismus**. Lesions of this portion of CN III produce a lateral and ventral strabismus and also ptosis due to paralysis of the levator palpebrae muscle (Figs 19.20, 19.21). Both of these signs are rarely, if ever, seen alone in large animals.

In some instances dysfunction of the oculomotor nerve will not result in a strabismus, but the eye will be unable to move normally (Fig. 19.21). When a normal animal's head is moved laterally the eyes will attempt to maintain direction towards the area where the animal was initially looking (straight ahead). This will result in a slow drifting of the eyes in the direction opposite the movement. As the head continues to be moved laterally the extraocular muscles, influenced by the vestibular system, will produce a quick movement of the eyes in the direction of head movement. This slow/quick eye movement will be continued in succession as the head is continually moved laterally and is referred to as induced vestibular or physiological nystagmus, or the oculovestibular response.

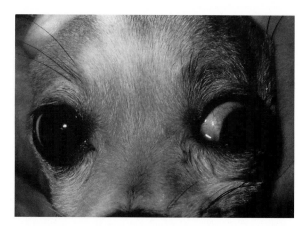

**Fig. 19.20** Dog with a resting ventral lateral strabismus of the left eye indicative of an ipsilateral oculomotor nerve lesion.

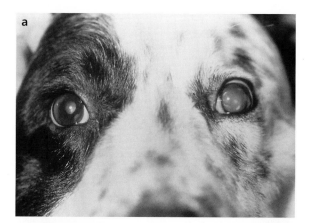

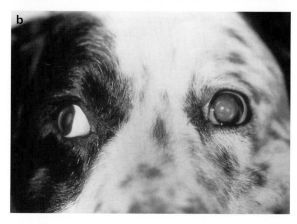

**Fig. 19.21** Dog shown (a) at rest and (b) when attempting to move the eyes to the right in the direction of an auditory stimulus. At rest the left pupil is dilated and non-responsive, however, vision is normal. When attempting to move the eyes the left eye cannot move medially indicative of an oculomotor nerve lesion.

### Clinical Pointer ✳

In addition to oculovestibular testing, motor function of the extraocular muscles can be determined by holding the animal's head fixed in a normal position while simultaneously creating a stimulus (auditory or visual) for the animal to look in various directions

- the animal's head is held still and a loud noise created slightly outside the limits of the animal's lateral visual field
- most often this kind of stimulus will result in the animal looking in the direction of the stimulus, an animal with CN III motor dysfunction may not be able to move the affected eye in a medial direction (Fig. 19.21).

### Trochlear – CN IV: ocular movement

Lesions of the trochlear nerve or nucleus cause a contralateral dorsomedial strabismus. In species with a round pupil no strabismus is seen. Fundic examination of the retina with a direct ophthalmoscope, however, reveals the superior retinal vessels to be deviated laterally. If indirect visualization is used the superior retinal vessels will be seen to be directed medially.

As cats have a vertical pupil the dorsal aspect of the vertical pupil is deviated laterally with such a lesion. Isolated lesions of this nerve are extremely rare in all animals. Bilateral dorsomedial strabismus occurs in several diffuse encephalopathies in ruminants, such as polioencephalomalacia, but it is unclear whether this is due to a true bilateral trochlear lesion or not (Fig. 19.22).

### Abducent – CN VI: ocular movement

Disease of CN VI results in a ventromedial strabismus. The eyeball cannot be abducted fully and may not be able to be retracted within the orbit. Isolated lesions of CN VI are uncommon in all species.

### Clinical abnormalities – CN III, IV, and VI combined

Paralysis of all the muscles responsible for eye movement is known as **complete ophthalmoplegia**. Cranial nerves III, IV, VI, the sympathetic innervation and CN V (ophthalmic branch) lie ventral in the skull within the cavernous venous sinus, which encircles the pituitary fossa. These nerves all exit the skull through the orbital fissure. Lesions on the floor of the skull in this area, such as basilar empyema (pituitary abscess) in ruminants and horses, may damage this combination of nerves and result in the '**cavernous sinus syndrome**'

Strabismus seen only when the head is forced into an abnormal orientation is termed **positional strabismus** and is most easily evoked by extending the head and neck and elevating the nose. As the head is moved vestibular receptors in the inner ear are stimulated and via the medial longitudinal fasciculus in the brain stem, the cranial nerves to extraocular muscles are either excited or inhibited to keep the eyes focused in the direction of head movement (Fig. 19.23). In small animals, as the head is extended the eyes will tend to remain normally positioned in the orbit and subsequently appear to be looking dorsally at the ceiling. In large animals the eyeballs are lower in the bony orbit, giving a normal 'eye drop' when the nose is elevated. If one or both eyes deviate from these normal positions this is termed a positional strabismus. Most commonly the abnormal eye will deviate more ventrally, and this is most easily appreciated by observing the more prominent dorsal sclera of the affected eye (Fig. 19.24). As there often is no eye deviation at rest this finding

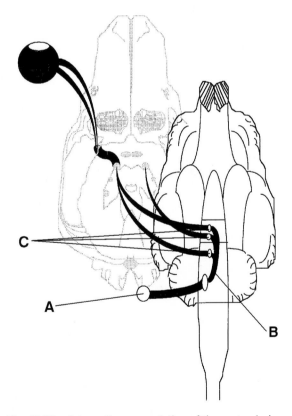

**Fig. 19.23** Schematic representation of the anatomical association between the vestibular receptors and the cranial nerves that provide for extraocular muscle function. A. Vestibular receptors in the ear. B. Medial longitudinal fasciculus. C. Cranial nerve nuclei (III,IV and VI) innervating the extraocular muscles of the eye.

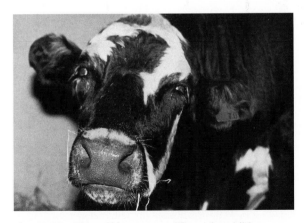

**Fig. 19.22** This calf has acute coliform choroiditis, ependymitis, and meningitis. As with many diffuse cerebral diseases there is evidence of a dorsomedial rotation of the globe mimicking trochlear (CN IV) nerve paralysis.

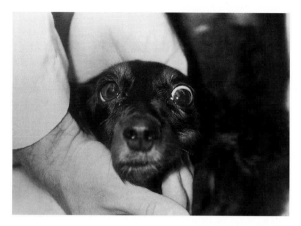

**Fig. 19.24** Positional strabismus in the left eye of a dog with a vestibular system abnormality. The head is extended dorsally and is being observed from above. The left eye is rotated ventrally and laterally.

implies that the vestibular input to CNs III, IV, and VI is abnormal. This clinical abnormality is almost always associated with an ipsilateral, central (such as listeriosis), or peripheral (such as otitis interna) vestibular lesion.

---

**Clinical Pointer** ✳

Siamese cats can have strabismus (usually esotropia or cross-eyed appearance) caused by congenitally abnormal visual projection pathways (Fig. 19.25). An inherited divergent strabismus also occurs in Holstein cattle.

---

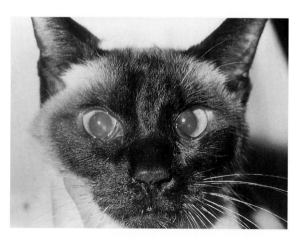

**Fig. 19.25** Esotropic ('cross-eyed') appearance of a Siamese cat. This cat also had fine pendulous oscillating eye movements at rest.

### Trigeminal – CN V: facial sensation, motor to muscles of mastication

The trigeminal nerve supplies sensory innervation to the head and motor innervation to the muscles of mastication. There are three major branches of this nerve

- ophthalmic
- maxillary
- mandibular.

The ophthalmic branch of CN V is sensory to the eye and surrounding skin. It can be assessed by testing for a palpebral reflex (afferent, CN V; efferent, CN VII) (Fig. 19.26) and by testing for corneal sensation (Fig. 19.27). When the medial canthus of the eye is touched the animal should quickly close the palpebral fissure (**palpebral reflex**). If the cornea itself is touched the animal usually retracts the eye in the orbit (**corneal reflex**) as well as blinking (**palpebral reflex**). Normal CN V innervation of the cornea is also needed to maintain the corneal epithelium. If sensory CN V innervation to the cornea is lost a neurotropic keratitis can develop and tear secretion may decrease owing to the loss of afferent stimulation for lacrimation. Tear secretion will usually be decreased but not absent, as CN VII is intact. The ipsilateral nasal mucosa may become dry for similar reasons.

The **maxillary branch** supplies sensory innervation to the maxillary area. This function is assessed by touching the external nasal mucosa, preferably with the animal's eyes covered. Two events occur with the stimulus. A direct CN V to ipsilateral CN VII (facial)

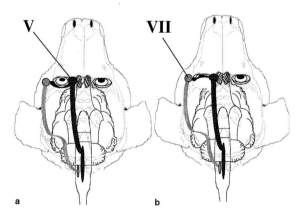

**Fig. 19.26** Pathways needed for a normal palpebral reflex. (a) The afferent impulse is projected centrally in CN V (ophthalmic branch) to synapse on the ipsilateral facial nerve nucleus. (b) The efferent response (closing of the palpebral fissure) is carried in CN VII.

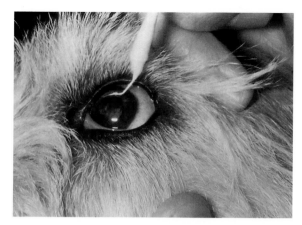

**Fig. 19.27** Corneal sensation being tested with the fine fibers of a cotton swab.

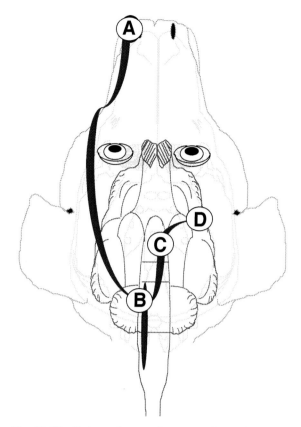

**Fig. 19.28** Pathway for conscious recognition of facial sensation. (A) Stimulus is recognized and projected through CN V (maxillary branch) to the ipsilateral CN V sensory nucleus (B). This is projected to the contralateral thalamus via the trigmenial lemniscus (C). From the thalamus information is projected to the ipsilateral (contralateral to the stimulus) parietal cortex (D) for conscious recognition.

reflex arc is evoked, resulting in ipsilateral movement (usually twitching) of the muscles of facial expression (blinking, wrinkling of the facial muscles). This component is a subcortical (subconscious) reflex. The second event is a consciously mediated movement of the head away from the stimulus. This requires conscious recognition of the stimulus via pathways projecting to the contralateral thalamus and parietal cortex (Fig. 19.28). An animal with a CN V maxillary branch lesion will have neither the facial reflex nor a conscious response to the stimulus. An animal with a forebrain disease should have the reflex component (i.e. blinking or licking when the stimulus is applied), but will not consciously move the head away from the stimulus applied to the side of face contralateral to the forebrain lesion (Fig. 19.29).

The **mandibular branch** of CN V is assessed by stimulating the skin overlying the mandibular area and also by assessing for muscle tone, function, and atrophy of the temporal and masseter muscles. Pinching of the skin with a hemostat should result in the animal pulling its head away from the stimulus. This can be inconsistent, especially in stoic animals. The temporalis and masseter muscles are palpated to assess muscle atrophy. Opening the mouth and assessing for jaw closure will aid in determining tone in these muscles. An animal with bilateral mandibular nerve disease will have a **dropped jaw** and be unable to close its mouth (Fig. 19.30).

Unilateral dysfunction of all three branches of CN V is almost always associated with a peripheral CN V lesion (outside the brain stem) because the nuclear areas of V are so extensive within the brain stem that a lesion causing destruction of all of them would be incompatible with life.

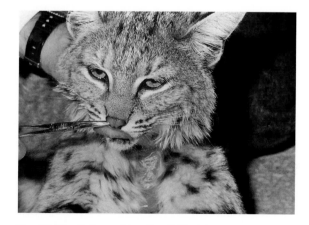

**Fig. 19.29** Bobcat with reflex (licking) but no conscious recognition of an irritating stimulus applied to the nostril. This is indicative of a contralateral forebrain lesion.

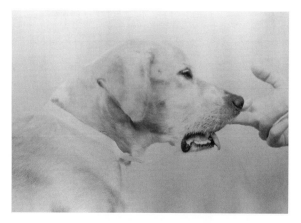

Fig. 19.30 Dog with bilateral mandibular nerve disease with a dropped jaw and inability to close the mouth.

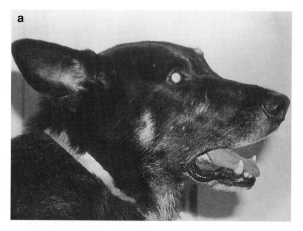

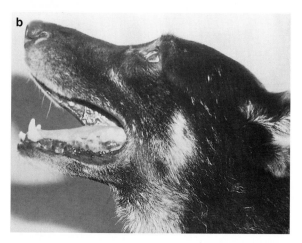

## Facial – CN VII: motor to muscles of facial expression, taste, salivation, and skin sensation inside ear

The facial nerve has branches coursing to the lacrimal gland (major petrosal nerve), the salivary glands and tongue (chorda tympani branch), and the muscles of facial expression (buccal and auriculopalpebral branches). Clinical signs of a lesion of the facial nerve usually include paresis or paralysis of facial muscles, resulting in facial asymmetry (Fig. 19.31). Damage to the buccal branches alone causes the lips to droop and the nose to be pulled **towards** the normal side. This is most readily seen in horses, where the normally functioning facial muscles are relatively strong. Damage to the auriculopalpebral branch causes paresis of the ear and eyelid.

Facial nerve motor function is most easily assessed by testing the palpebral reflex: the medial aspect of the palpebral fissure is lightly touched and the animal blinks rapidly and completely. Touch is sensed through CN V, ophthalmic branch, and the muscle contraction is elicited through CN VII. If the lateral periorbital region is touched afferent stimuli are projected in the maxillary branch of CN V. Animals with an abnormality of CN VII function will not be able to close the palpebral fissure when this reflex is initiated. The menace response will also be decreased or absent, but the animal will have normal vision. When testing the menace response it may be noticed that the eye can be retracted in the bony orbit, indicating that the afferent components of this response are intact.

Fig. 19.31 Dog with left-sided facial muscle paresis (a) due to a CN VII abnormality. The normal side is present for comparison (b).

A lesion of the facial nerve can be localized using knowledge of where this nerve branches after exiting the brain stem

- with lesions distal to the stylomastoid foramen innervation to the facial muscles will be abnormal; however, taste, lacrimation, and innervation of the stapedius muscle will be normal

### Clinical Pointer ✳

In large animals ptosis is a prominent feature of facial nerve paralysis and is probably due to loss of tone in the musculature dorsal to the eyelids. The palpebral fissure is widened in small animals with facial paresis/paralysis.

- with lesions in the petrosal bone, innervation to the facial muscles will be abnormal and the function of the other areas may or may not be affected
- intracranial extramedullary lesions will result in all CN VII functions being abnormal
- brain-stem nuclear lesions usually result in abnormal function of the facial muscles and stapedius muscle, with variable effects on taste and lacrimation
- discrete brain-stem lesions, such as from ruminant listeriosis and equine protozoal myeloencephalitis, can result in paresis of selected facial muscles, such as those of the muzzle but not those to the eyelids or ear.

With facial nerve irritation a facial muscle spasm resulting in continual contraction of the muscles of facial expression can be seen (Roberts & Vainisi 1967)(Fig. 19.32). Similar clinical features are noted with chronic facial nerve paralysis that has resulted in fibrosis and resultant contracture of the ipsilateral facial muscles.

Supratentorial lesions may also result in facial paresis. At least in the horse, poor facial muscle movement associated with a taut facial expression can result from thalamic and cerebral lesions. This abnormality is usually seen on the side of the face ipsilateral to the lesion.

### Parasympathetic function of CN VII
This portion of the facial nerve is primarily responsible for lacrimal gland secretion. Keratoconjunctivitis sicca (KCS) or dry eye may be seen with involvement of this nerve. Lesions distal to the facial canal in the temporal bone, however, will not affect these fibers. Salivation can be crudely assessed by examining for a moist buccal mucosa.

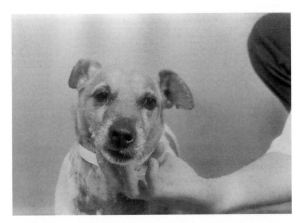

**Fig. 19.32** Dog with contraction of the right muscles of facial expression indicative of hemifacial spasm. Notice the smaller palpebral fissure and contracted ear on this side.

### Taste
Taste is difficult to test clinically, being a subjective sensation similar to smell. An atropine-soaked cotton-tipped applicator swab touched to the tongue may evoke a conscious response (jerking the head away from the stimulus) and salivation, suggesting the presence of some normally functioning taste fibers.

## Vestibulocochlear – CN VIII: equilibrium, balance, and hearing

### Clinical evaluation of balance
Clinical signs of vestibular disease include

- ataxia/staggering
- head tilt
- nystagmus
- eye deviations.

Some of these signs are present at rest and do not have to be elicited. Vomiting is uncommon but is occasionally recognized in small animals with vestibular dysfunction. Anorexia in association with vestibular disease in animals may reflect occult nausea.

The vestibular system can be abnormal as a result of disease of CN VIII (peripheral) or its nuclear regions (central). Every attempt should be made to determine initially whether the vestibular abnormality is due to a central or a peripheral lesion (Table 19.5), as differential diagnoses and prognosis are quite different for each.

Any head tilt is usually directed towards the side of the lesion, except those associated with some central

**Table 19.5. Characteristics of central and peripheral vestibular diseases**

| Abnormality noted | Central disease | Peripheral disease |
|---|---|---|
| Nystagmus (spontaneous) | Horizontal Rotatory Vertical | Horizontal Rotatory |
| (positional) | Changing | Constant |
| Head tilt | Present | Present |
| Cranial nerve deficits | Any other than VII | VII |
| Horner's syndrome | +/− | +/− |
| Paresis and postural reaction deficits of limbs | Present | Absent |

## Clinical Pointer

*Slow phase* of nystagmus usually moves eye towards the side of the lesion
*Fast phase* of nystagmus returns eye to its original position.

lesions (paradoxical vestibular syndrome). In association, the neck and head may be rotated towards the affected side. The presence or direction of a head tilt alone does not help to localize the lesion within the vestibular system.

Nystagmus is a spontaneous eye movement that has both a fast and a slow phase. When the vestibular system is abnormal the eyes have a tendency to be drawn to one side, usually toward the side of the lesion (slow phase). There is an overriding brain-stem compensatory mechanism which then rapidly moves the eyes back to their initial location (fast phase). The direction of the nystagmus is named in relation to the fast phase of movement and in the direction of movement – horizontal, vertical, or rotatory.

With unilateral central vestibular lesions hemiparesis may be seen ipsilateral to the lesion. Hemiparesis is determined by assessing gait and postural reactions. Extensor tone in the limbs on the affected side may be decreased. Recumbent animals often prefer to lie on the affected side, and if placed on the normal side will tend to roll toward the affected side. Occasionally hemiparesis is found on the side of the body opposite to the direction of the head tilt (paradoxical vestibular syndrome); the lesion is on the side of the body ipsilateral to the hemiparesis.

With vestibular lesions the oculovestibular response may be abnormal. In animals with bilateral vestibular abnormalities no oculovestibular response is elicited upon head movement. The head may swing from side to side in wide excursions during spontaneous movement.

## Nystagmus

The character of nystagmus may help to localize the lesion

- horizontal or rotatory nystagmus → peripheral or central vestibular disease
- vertical nystagmus → central vestibular disease
- with a peripheral lesion the direction of the fast phase of nystagmus is always directed away from the side of the lesion.

**Clinical assessment of hearing**
Hearing can be evaluated subjectively by creating a loud noise (without creating other vibration currents) and assessing for ear (Pryer's reflex), eye, and other body movements suggesting that the animal heard the sound. Bilateral deafness will result in no clinical response to sound. Unilateral deafness may be more difficult, if not impossible, to determine using this type of testing. The most objective test of hearing currently available is brain-stem auditory evoked potential (BAEP or BAER) testing (see Ancillary testing).

Occasionally a sound can actually be heard emanating from an animal's ear (otoacoustic emission). The cause of this interesting phenomenon is not known.

## Glossopharyngeal – CN IX: pharyngeal sensation and movement (with CN X), salivation, taste

Lesions of CN IX cause swallowing difficulty and pharyngeal muscle abnormalities. To evaluate this function a gag or swallow reflex is stimulated by placing a finger, hand, or tube in the caudal aspect of the animal's pharynx. The animal should gag, pushing the stimulating object out of the area with the caudal aspect of the tongue. It should not be done in aggressive animals or those where a zoonotic disease such as rabies is suspected.

A less consistent way of inducing a swallow reflex is by massaging the laryngeal/pharyngeal/hyoid area externally after gently pulling on, then releasing, the tongue. Dysfunction is suggested when the animal does not attempt to gag or swallow with stimulation of the pharynx. In affected animals the examiner may be able to palpate the epiglottis without a response.

**Glossopharyngeal neuralgia** is paroxysmal pain in the throat or tonsillar region commonly provoked by swallowing, vocalizing, chewing or yawning. This may also be associated with bradycardia and syncope, presumably due to triggering of cardiovascular regulatory fibers by afferent pain impulses.

## Clinical Pointer

Many diffuse and focal forebrain lesions in large animals result in apparent dysphagia, with food being held in, and dropping from, the mouth and/or nares. This is regarded as an upper motor neuron or supranuclear dysfunction. With pharyngeal stimulus, such as passage of a stomach tube, affected animals are able to swallow reflexly.

## *Vagus – CN X: laryngeal sensation, laryngeal movement, salivation, and other autonomic functions*

Lesions involving these functions of CN X (along with the accessory branch of CN XI and the recurrent laryngeal nerve), result in paralysis of intrinsic laryngeal muscles.

Unilateral lesions result in no clinical signs at rest but interfere with inspiration during forced exercise, particularly in horses. Bilateral lesions result in paralysis of the larynx, with inspiratory stridor, dyspnea and cyanosis, and sometimes abnormal esophageal function.

The thoracolaryngeal (slap) reflex is an interesting and repeatable CN X reflex in horses. By slapping the dorsal thorax, reflex movement of the contralateral intrinsic laryngeal musculature can be palpated dorsolaterally on the larynx and seen endoscopically as an adduction of the contralateral arytenoid cartilage (Fig. 19.33). Cervical spinal cord, caudal brain stem, vagal nerve, recurrent laryngeal nerve, and laryngeal lesions can all interfere with this reflex. The most common cause of exercise-associated inspiratory noise and thoracolaryngeal areflexia is severe idiopathic left recurrent laryngeal paralysis in tall horses.

Laryngeal function in small animals can be assessed under light anesthesia using a laryngoscope to depress the caudal tongue out of the way. The movement of the arytenoid folds should be assessed during respiration. Normally, these folds abduct during inspiration: failure to do so is evidence of laryngeal paralysis.

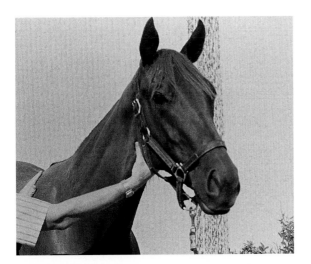

**Fig. 19.33** The thoracolaryngeal reflex can be tested manually or with the aid of a fiberoptic endoscope. Laryngeal movement can be palpated or seen endoscopically contralateral to a sharp slap applied to the dorsal thoracic region, particularly just caudal to the withers as shown.

## *Spinal Accessory – CN XI: motor innervation to trapezius muscle*

Lesions in this nerve result in atrophy of the trapezius muscle. Decreased resistance to lateral passive movement of the head and neck contralateral to the side of the lesion may be noted. In chronic cases the neck may be deviated toward the affected side. Such signs are difficult to detect in large animals.

## *Hypoglossal – CN XII: motor to the tongue*

Clinical signs of CN XII disease include problems with deglutition, prehension, mastication, and vocalization. The tongue will be weak or paralyzed. With unilateral lesions in dogs the tongue will be pushed toward the side of the lesion by the intact muscles on the normal side. With a chronic unilateral hypoglossal lesion the tongue will protrude toward the side of the lesion (ipsilateral) and there may be atrophy (ipsilateral) (Fig. 19.34). Atrophy may occur on the affected side. Occasionally, lesions of forebrain controlling centers will result in very poor use of the tongue.

### Spinal reflexes

To help in interpreting results of spinal reflex testing, an understanding of the concepts of **upper motor neuron** (UMN) and **lower motor neuron** (LMN) are important (Fig. 19.35). An UMN is a neuron or group of neurons that does not exit the central nervous system and influences, either positively or negatively, the LMN. The UMN usually exerts an inhibitory or damping influence on spinal reflexes. Clinical signs of

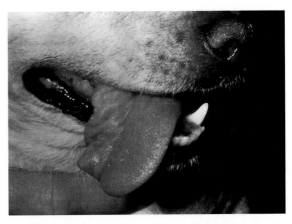

**Fig. 19.34** Dog with signs of a chronic unilateral CN XII abnormality. The tongue is deviated toward the side of the lesion and this side of the tongue is atrophied.

> ### Clinical Pointer
>
> UMN lesion → hyperreflexia; hypertonia then *chronic* muscle atrophy (from disuse)
>
> LMN lesion → hyporeflexia; hypotonia and *acute* muscle atrophy (neurogenic).

UMN lesions thus include exaggerated (hyperreflexia) or normal reflexes, and exaggerated (hypertonia) or normal muscle tone. If muscle atrophy occurs secondary to a lesion of the UMN it is due to the improper use of the affected muscles resulting from poor nervous system control (disuse atrophy). Because this atrophy is the result of poor muscle use it evolves slowly, often over weeks to months, and is milder than that seen with LMN disease. Tone of the limbs can be determined by the degree of resistance to passive movement of a limb, being normal to increased in animals with UMN lesions.

The LMN is analogous to the motor portion of the reflex arc and includes the motor neuron cell bodies of the brain stem and spinal cord, the peripheral motor

nerves, and the effector organs (muscles). Clinical signs of LMN disease include hyporeflexia to areflexia, and hypotonia to atonia, the latter being referred to as flaccidity. Because the connection between the peripheral nerve and the muscle is required to maintain muscle mass, atrophy that occurs after a complete peripheral nerve injury is severe (neurogenic atrophy) and evolves over a short period of time. This may be present within 5 days of a severe peripheral nerve injury in small animals. Neurogenic atrophy may take longer to evolve in large animals presumably because of their larger size (longer nerves).

As the entire nervous system is necessary for the performance of postural reactions, lesions involving either or both the UMN and LMN can result in postural testing deficits and in weakness. Evaluation of spinal reflexes is ultimately important in determining whether lesions resulting in paresis or paralysis affect the UMN or the LMN portions of the nervous system.

## Reflex function

Reflex functions are involuntary activities that do not require conscious thought. A sensory receptor is stimulated, with information traveling in an afferent (sensory) nerve. This nerve will synapse (connect), either directly or indirectly through interneurons, on an efferent (motor) nerve, which travels to the organ to be stimulated. With most spinally mediated reflexes the organ to be stimulated is a muscle. This direct pathway involving afferent and efferent nerves is commonly referred to as a reflex arc. Stimulation of the afferent nerve results in a stereotypic motor response.

### Thoracic limb reflexes

Spinal reflexes of the thoracic limb include the extensor carpi radialis, biceps, triceps, and withdrawal or flexion reflexes (Moore 1993) (see Table 19.2). The extensor carpi radialis and the triceps reflexes assess the radial nerve with cell bodies in the spinal cord

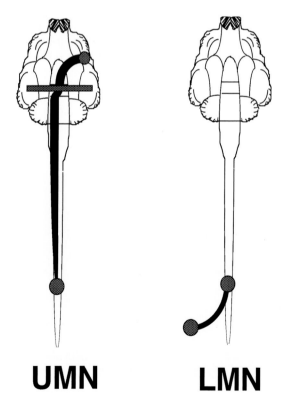

**Fig. 19.35** Schematic representation of an UMN and a LMN.

> ### Patellar reflex: a simple spinal reflex
>
> - stretching of the middle patellar tendon (by tapping with a reflex hammer or similar instrument) provides a sensory stimulus which results in excitation of the femoral nerve
> - this results in contraction of the quadriceps muscle
> - the quadriceps contraction extends the stifle and produces the 'kick' or 'knee jerk'.

segments C7–T1. The biceps reflex assesses the musculocutaneous nerve (C6–C8). These reflexes are elicited by percussing the muscle belly or tendon of insertion of the individual muscles and observing for the appropriate muscular response. When the extensor carpi radialis is percussed the carpus should extend slightly owing to contraction of this muscle. When the triceps is percussed, slight elbow extension is observed. When the biceps muscle is stimulated, slight elbow flexion may be seen. With the latter reflex, movement may be slight and not visualized. The examiner may, however, feel the muscle contract by placing a finger over it during percussion.

The withdrawal reflex is elicited by pinching the skin of the foot or pastern region with a hemostat and looking for flexion of the carpal and elbow joints in order to move the distal limb away from the stimulus. This reflex assesses all major nerves of the thoracic limb, including the radial, ulnar, median, musculocutaneous, and axillary nerves. A decreased or poor response is seen when the animal cannot adequately flex all limb joints and thus pull the limb away from the stimulus (Fig. 19.36).

### Pelvic limb reflexes

Reflexes assessed in the pelvic limb include the patellar, cranial tibial, gastrocnemius, and withdrawal or flexion reflexes (see Table 19.2). The patellar reflex assesses the femoral nerve, which arises from the L4–L6 spinal cord segments.

The cranial tibial and gastrocnemius reflexes assess the sciatic nerve (spinal segments L6–S1), specifically the peroneal and tibial branches respectively.

The withdrawal reflex of the pelvic limb also assesses the integrity of the sciatic nerve (spinal segments L6–S1). As in the thoracic limb, the reflex is elicited by pinching the skin of the foot and looking for flexion of the hip, hock, and stifle joints to move the foot away from the stimulus. Decreased ability to flex the hock is usually the most notable abnormality when sciatic disease is present (Fig. 19.37). Sometimes with sciatic disease the patellar reflex may concurrently appear hyperreflexic. This is not due to an additional UMN lesion, but results from loss of sciatic nerve innervation to muscles which function as antagonists to this reflex (pseudohyperreflexia). Spinal reflexes are usually graded in the following manner.

---

### Thoracic limb reflexes

- extensor carpi radialis reflex → slight carpus extension
- triceps reflex → slight elbow extension
- biceps reflex → slight elbow flexion (since the movement is slight it may not be visualized but the muscle contraction may be felt by placing a finger over the muscle during percussion).

---

### Pelvic limb reflexes

- patellar reflex → stifle extension
- cranial tibial reflex → slight hock flexion
- gastrocnemius reflex → hock extension.

---

### Anal reflexes

To assess function of this reflex the perianal area is

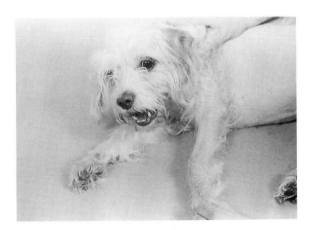

**Fig. 19.36** Dog with poor withdrawal reflex of the left thoracic limb. The animal consciously recognizes the stimulus (vocalizes) but is unable to withdraw the limb.

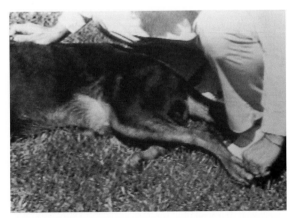

**Fig. 19.37** Dog having decreased hock flexion during the performance of the withdrawal reflex. This is indicative of sciatic nerve disease.

stimulated briskly and a brisk contraction of the anal orifice is observed (anal reflex). This reflex is mediated through the pudendal nerve to the anal sphincter. The pudendal nerve arises from the S1–S3 spinal cord segments. Anal contraction can also be elicited by squeezing the penis of a male dog or the clitoris of a bitch. In some instances rectal examination or palpation to assess the tone of the anal sphincter may be useful. With anal stimulation the tail will often be flexed concurrently, although a light stimulus can result in reflex tail elevation (tail reflex).

## Spinal reflex evaluation

When evaluating spinal reflex function the presence or absence as well as the magnitude of response is important. Spinal reflexes are usually graded in the following manner.

| | | |
|---|---|---|
| 0 | = | absent |
| 1 | = | depressed |
| 2 | = | normal |
| 3 | = | exaggerated |
| 4 | = | exaggerated with alternate muscular contraction and relaxation in rapid succession (clonus) |

Grading of a reflex is somewhat subjective based on the examiner's experience and therefore will vary slightly between examiners. It is most important to determine whether the reflexes are at least present or not. In instances of paresis this should allow differentiation between disease of the descending central motor pathways (UMN) or of the reflex arc (LMN).

For a reflex to be clinically useful it needs to be both easily assessed and consistently present in normal animals. Of all of these spinal reflexes the patellar, flexion (both thoracic and pelvic), and anal are the most helpful, as the others are found only inconsistently. All are very prominent in newborn animals, especially foals, calves, lambs, and kids (Fig. 19.38).

In most dogs with neurological disease postural reactions will be abnormal concurrently with reflex changes. An animal that has changes in reflex function, especially increased reflexes without concurrent postural reaction abnormalities, probably is normal.

## Other reflex functions

The cutaneous trunci reflex tests superficial pain receptors, the spinal cord and the lateral thoracic nerves. It is tested by pinching or prodding the skin over the lateral thoracolumbar trunk. The efferent response is contraction of the cutaneous trunci muscles bilaterally.

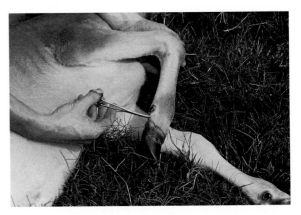

**Fig. 19.38** Normal flexor reflex in a young calf. A crossed-extensor reflex with reciprocal extension of the lower limb is also present. This is normal for neonates and disappears in several days to weeks.

The receptor in the specific dermatomal distribution is excited by the stimulus, which sends an impulse through the dorsal sensory afferent nerve to the spinal cord, where this pathway becomes bilateral. The impulse travels cranially in the spinal cord to reach the cell bodies of the lateral thoracic nerves in the ventral gray matter of the C8–T1 spinal cord segments. The lateral thoracic nerves exit the spinal cord and course to the cutaneous trunci muscles.

The cutaneous trunci reflex is most helpful when evaluating T2–L3 lesions and those involving the brachial plexus.

Although there is some debate as to the exact dermatomal distribution in the flank area, it appears clinically in dogs that the T12 to L1–L2 dermatomes are distributed from the last rib to the cranial border of the wing of the ilium. Therefore, a dog with a normal cutaneous trunci reflex and UMN paresis of the pelvic limbs has a lesion in the L1–L3 spinal cord segments.

With a unilateral brachial plexus injury contraction of the cutaneous trunci muscle may occur only on the side opposite the lesion, regardless of which side of the

---

### Clinical Pointer

With lesions in the T2–L3 area, the cutaneous trunci reflex will be lost caudal to the spinal segment involved. Since the nerves innervating the skin in the thoracolumbar area originate cranial to the area of skin innervated, the lesion is approximately 1–3 vertebral segments cranial to where the cutaneous trunci reflex is lost.

body is stimulated. Because of this the spinal pathways for this reflex are assumed to be intact.

Local cervical reflexes, similar to the cutaneous trunci reflex, can be useful to help localize cervical lesions in large animals. Tapping the lateral neck results in cutaneous coli muscle contraction and often a contraction of other (e.g. sternocephalicus and brachiocephalicus) neck muscles. This local cervical reflex is most prominent in horses and foals and may involve segmental cervical spinal cord sensory and motor systems, nerves of the brachial plexus and the spinal accessory (CN XI) nerve. Also, in horses contraction of the labial, eyelid, and ear muscles occurs in response to tapping the lateral skin of the neck. The complete pathways for this reflex are not fully understood but may be due to anastomotic connections between the facial nerve and the C2–C6 dorsal spinal nerve branches.

Tone can be assessed by passively flexing and extending the limbs. Increased to normal tone (spasticity) is noted with UMN lesions, making it difficult to move the limb passively. With LMN lesions tone is decreased or absent (flaccidity). In this instance the limb may feel like a 'wet noodle' when passively moved.

When the withdrawal reflex is tested some animals with UMN lesions may extend the opposite limb. This is termed the **crossed extensor reflex**. To assess this accurately, the animal is placed in lateral recumbency and the up limb is tested for the withdrawal reflex and the down limb is observed for abnormal extension. When an animal is standing the crossed extensor reflex is normally active, so that as one limb is flexed towards the body the opposite limb extends to maintain body position against gravity. When the animal is lying on its side, however, UMN influences will prevent this from occurring, except in neonates where this reflex is normal (Fig. 19.38). Damage to descending UMN pathways that normally dampen this reflex allows contralateral extension to occur. The crossed extensor reflex is more often seen when the inciting lesion has been present for a long time. This abnormal reflex can occur in either the pelvic or thoracic limbs. If in the pelvic limbs the causative lesion is cranial to the L3 spinal segments if in the thoracic limb then the lesion is cranial to C6 spinal segment.

The **Babinski reflex** is another abnormal reflex, commonly observed in human beings and sometimes in dogs with UMN disease. When the ventral foot or paw stroked, such as with the handle end of a reflex hammer, the toes normally curl (flex) toward the sole of the foot. With UMN lesions, when the sole of the foot is stroked the toes may extend and flare outwards. This is referred to as a positive Babinski reflex. It may be seen in dogs with UMN lesions but is inconsistent.

## Muscle evaluation

Skeletal muscles are evaluated for atrophy by visual inspection and palpation and compared for size, consistency and tone on both sides simultaneously. This is most easily accomplished in the standing animal.

Disuse atrophy may occur with UMN lesions and is generally slow to progress and less severe than LMN atrophy. It is, however, difficult to distinguish disuse from neurogenic atrophy based on physical characteristics alone. Localized atrophy within a single muscle group suggests a neurogenic cause; however, in some instances, such as infraspinatus contracture, a primary myopathic cause is present. With sciatic disease there is usually atrophy of the cranial tibial muscles. Significant paravertebral muscle atrophy is often associated with diskospondylitis. In horses selective muscle atrophy is commonly a hallmark of myeloencephalitis caused by *Sarcocytis neurona* (equine protozoal myeloencephalitis).

At the same time as the muscles are palpated for atrophy the rest of the body can be examined for palpable abnormalities. A fontanelle may indicate associated hydrocephalus. Tumors of bone and vertebral incongruities may be noted. Focally painful areas may indicate nerve compression or vertebral osteomyelitis (see under Hyperesthesia below).

## Clinical assessment of urination

Urination is an important function of the nervous system that is commonly misunderstood. Urination can be thought of as a local spinal reflex under UMN control, similar to other spinal reflexes.

Conscious urination involves the cerebral cortex. Unconscious urination involves the brain stem and the parasympathetic and sympathetic systems within the spinal cord and peripheral nerves. Simply put, the sympathetic system prevents and the parasympathetic system allows urination.

The pelvic nerve cell bodies, which supply parasympathetic lower motor neuron innervation to the detrusor and bladder neck (internal urethral sphincter), are located in the intermediate gray matter of the S1–S3 spinal cord segments. The pudendal nerve provides somatic innervation to the striated muscle of the external urethral sphincter. These cell bodies are located in the same area as for the pelvic nerve. The hypogastric nerve provides sympathetic innervation to the bladder. These cell bodies are located in the L1–L4 spinal cord segments.

Sensory receptors are located in the wall of the bladder and are responsive to stretching and/or pressure. Information from these receptors travels in the afferent pelvic nerve entering the sacral spinal cord. The afferent cell bodies of the pelvic nerve are in the spinal ganglia of the S1–S3 segments. Axons of the pelvic nerve either terminate on interneurons in the gray matter of the sacral spinal cord, or ascend in projection pathways to the brain.

The pelvic nerve axons terminate on interneurons, which then terminate on the cell bodies of the preganglionic pelvic nerve of the parasympathetic system, which results in contraction of the detrusor muscle (smooth muscle of the bladder). Additional interneurons synapse on pudendal efferent nerves innervating the striated muscle of the urethra to inhibit its activity.

Voluntary urination is initiated in the cerebral cortex, with descending impulses going to the pudendal nerve to either excite or inhibit the external urethral sphincter. The cerebellum is normally inhibitory to urination.

### Neurogenic abnormalities of urination

With ascending sensory pathway involvement the bladder may not be recognized as being full. With descending motor pathway (UMN) involvement bladder emptying is interrupted. These will both result in a large bladder. Because the local peripheral nerves (S1–S3 spinal cord segments) to the bladder are not impaired the bladder has good tone (i.e. it feels turgid), and because of hyperreflexia of the bladder outflow region the UMN bladder is difficult to express. This is the same concept as hyperreflexia of the patellar reflex seen with UMN lesions. After about 2 weeks reflex bladder expression may begin to occur.

Additionally with such lesions, poor coordination between the phases of urination may occur (i.e. poor synchrony between detrusor contraction and urethral sphincter relaxation). Affected animals may begin to urinate normally, but then stop abruptly before the bladder is completely empty. This abnormal urinary pattern is referred to as reflex dyssynergia.

With LMN lesions affecting the sacral spinal segments or associated peripheral nerves the bladder is again large because the ascending and descending information cannot project through the damaged peripheral nerves. Bladder tone is decreased and the bladder feels flaccid (jelly-like). Also, the bladder is easily expressed because the local tonic reflex to maintain tone in the outflow tract is not present.

In horses a paralyzed bladder with urinary overflow usually indicates a LMN (sacral segment or nerve) lesion and is seen most often with polyneuritis, sacral fractures, and equine herpes virus 1 vasculitis-associated myelopathy.

### Clinical Pointer

UMN bladder → large and tense, difficult to express; reflex dysynergia possible
LMN bladder → large and flaccid, easy to express.

### Defecation

With lesions affecting the sacral spinal segments or associated caudal rectal nerves contraction of the colon may be ineffective, leading to constipation, obstipation, megacolon or incontinence. With UMN lesions reflex defecation persists and is usually adequate for evacuating stool from the colon.

### Evaluation of pain and sensation

Because pain is a subjective sensory experience, and because animals cannot verbally communicate their feelings, recognition of pain in animals is more difficult than in humans. The presence of both physiological and behavioral responses associated with pain in human beings can be taken to indicate that pain is present in animals.

### Superficial pain sensation

Two types of pain sensations are evaluated in animals. Superficial pain sensation is conscious recognition by the animal that the skin is being pinched or pricked. Such evaluation is often subjective, however, as many animals respond inconsistently to superficial pain stimulation. Deep pain sensation is used to describe conscious recognition of stimulation of pain receptors

### Behavioral and physiological indications of pain in animals

- abnormal activity (increased or decreased)
- abnormal sleep patterns
- changes in posture, orientation of body toward source of pain
- aggression
- 'guarding' an area by muscle tension
- disuse of an area
- vocalization
- increased temperature
- tachycardia
- tachypnea
- increased blood pressure.

deeper within the body, such as those associated with the periosteum of bone (see below). Although still subjective, the results of testing for deep pain sensation are more quantifiable than those for superficial pain sensation.

A two-step pinch technique is used to assess cutaneous sensation in all species

- first lightly tent a small area of skin between the jaws of a hemostat (step 1)
- pause till the animal settles
- squeeze briskly to elicit reactions indicating conscious recognition of this stimulus, i.e. vocalization or a quick orienting of the head toward the stimulated area.

The entire area of skin innervated by a single nerve is termed a **dermatome**. An area of skin innervated by only one nerve is termed the **autonomous zone** for that nerve. It is important when trying to determine the number of peripheral nerves involved in a disease to stimulate only the autonomous zones of the peripheral nerves. Autonomous areas have been determined for dogs and horses and are based upon fixed anatomical points. Individual variations in innervation patterns and skin movement overlying these points can lead to false assessments.

With increasing severity of nervous system injury superficial pain perception is lost before deep pain sensation. However, superficial pain sensation may be hard to elicit in stoic animals and can be impossible to evaluate reliably and consistently in adult horses and cattle. In some instances, such as brachial plexus injury, assessment of areas where superficial sensation is absent may be helpful in evaluating which peripheral nerves are affected. It may also be important for localization of disease to a single nerve, for example when a nerve sheath tumor is present.

## Hyperesthesia

Hyperesthesia is defined as increased sensitivity to stimulation. This term is commonly used to describe areas of the body that appear unusually painful when palpated or manipulated. Hyperesthesia can be very helpful in localizing lesions and formulating differential diagnoses, especially with spinal cord disease (Fig. 19.39). Finding a focal area of hyperesthesia is often helpful to localize a lesion to within a few spinal cord segments. Widespread vertebral pain, however, is more indicative of diffuse disease, such as meningitis.

Hyperesthesia associated with minimal pressure stimulation of the paws is characteristic of polyradiculoneuritis (Coonhound paralysis). Conversely, animals with primary disease of the sensory nerves may have

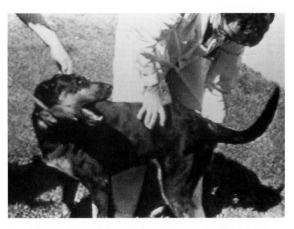

**Fig. 19.39** Dog with caudal lumbar hyperesthesia upon palpation. The lesion was associated with a compressive spinal lesion in this area.

decreased or absent skin sensation. Such animals may self-mutilate, presumably because of this lack of sensation.

## Deep pain sensation

The presence or absence of deep pain sensation (pain elicited by pressure on periosteum) is important for prognosis, as with a severe spinal cord lesion this sensation is the last function to be lost. Fibers that carry deep pain perception are small myelinated or unmyelinated axons that are less susceptible to the effects of pressure, and these tracts cross and recross widely in the spinal cord. Therefore, a near complete functional or anatomical transection of the cord is necessary to account for complete loss of deep pain sensation.

Deep pain is assessed by placing increasing pressure with a hemostat or similar instrument on the toe or pastern region of the affected foot and looking for either vocalizing, attempts to bite the examiner, or immediate orientation of the body toward the area of stimulation. If one of these does not occur, deep pain is absent. The examiner must be somewhat brutal with this testing if there is any doubt about the presence or absence of deep pain sensation. The prognosis is so very different if even a little pain sensation is present (some hope) compared to absolute analgesia (grave outlook).

If an animal only withdraws its limb from such a stimulus it must not be concluded that deep pain perception is present. Such withdrawal is a purely reflex action and will be present even in an animal that has its spinal cord transected cranial to the level being tested. For the examiner to know that the animal has deep pain sensation, a conscious behavioral response (vocalizing, trying to bite, or immediate orientation of the body towards the area of stimulation) must be clearly observed.

## NEUROANATOMICAL DIAGNOSIS

By the time the neurological examination is complete the examiner should be able to localize the lesion within the nervous system.

## Clinical signs of disease in specific functional areas

### Supratentorial/forebrain

The structures located rostral to the level of the tentorium cerebelli include

- cerebral hemispheres
- basal nuclei
- diencephalon (thalamus and hypothalamus)
- part of the mesencephalon.

The terms forebrain or prosencephalon are used by some authors to indicate these similarly functioning structures. These are the higher cortical and subcortical centers controlling conscious and unconscious responses.

When a disease process involves the supratentorial structures, the following clinical signs are possible

- blindness and menace deficits with normal PLR and CN VII function contralateral to a unilateral lesion
- postural reaction deficits (contralateral to a unilateral lesion)
- consciousness abnormalities
- abnormal behavior (head pressing, wandering, bellowing)
- seizures
- circling (usually toward the side of the lesion)
- head turn (usually toward the side of the lesion).

A tendency to circle may be seen in animals with disease involving either the supratentorial (forebrain) or vestibular areas. Usually, but not always, animals circle toward the side of a unilateral forebrain or vestibular lesion. Animals with vestibular disease tend to circle in tighter, smaller circles compared to the wider circling seen with supratentorial lesions.

Severely altered consciousness usually indicates significant central nervous system dysfunction and requires emergency evaluation. Metabolic derangements from numerous causes (for example hypoglycemia) may alter consciousness, and so a complete systemic as well as neurological evaluation is imperative.

Severe bilateral cerebral hemispheric disease is necessary to markedly alter consciousness. In comparison, a smaller lesion in the rostral brain stem can result in a substantial decrease in consciousness. In a comatose animal there are various indicators of brain-stem function that need to be assessed including

- other cranial nerves
- respiratory pattern
- pupil size and reactivity
- ocular movements.

Structural intracranial causes of coma usually result in focal neurological signs. A history of neurological abnormalities prior to the onset of coma may be helpful in making this distinction. Abrupt onset of coma, especially after brain trauma, usually indicates brain-stem involvement. Animals with brain-stem involvement resulting in coma have a poorer overall prognosis.

**Seizures** often result from a supratentorial (forebrain) abnormality and must be differentiated from other episodic disturbances, including cataplexy/narcolepsy, syncope, weakness, vestibular disturbances, intermittent cerebellar dysfunction, tetany and tremor.

Focal seizures are of value in localizing the seizure focus to a particular side of the brain, as they often occur in the side opposite to a lesion. Focal seizures are more often associated with localized structural brain disease.

Clinical evaluation initially depends upon two important features

- age at onset of the first seizure
- the presence of interictal neurological deficits.

Idiopathic seizures (idiopathic epilepsy) begin between 1 and 4 years of age. A dog that begins having seizures at 9 years of age, therefore, most likely does not have idiopathic epilepsy. Idiopathic epilepsy occurs in certain breeds of dogs, such as

- Beagle
- Belgian tervuren
- German shepherd
- Kieshound
- Collie
- Saint Bernard
- Golden retriever
- Irish setter
- American Cocker spaniel
- wire-haired Fox terrier
- Alaskan malamute
- Siberian husky
- miniature Poodle.

In horses no equivalent of adult-onset inherited epilepsy has been documented, but in a few breeds of cattle it has. Young Arabian foals can have adolescent benign epilepsy. Many of these foals, however, will recover completely following anticonvulsant therapy for a few weeks to months.

Idiopathic seizures are not associated with interictal (between seizures) neurological deficits. Obvious deficits found upon neurological examination in animals with seizures suggest a structural cause. Some animals, however, may have reversible neurological deficits, especially blindness, during the postictal period. These deficits usually resolve within 48 hours, but at times may last for days after the seizure. Knowledge of when the seizure(s) occurred in relation to the examination, its duration, and severity is important for this determination to be made.

## Infratentorial/brain stem

Embryologically the brain stem extends from the diencephalon to the myelencephalon. Lesions of the diencephalon and part of the rostral mesencephalon result in clinical signs that are difficult to distinguish from lesions of the cerebral cortex. These structures are therefore placed functionally with the supratentorial or forebrain areas. For this discussion the brain stem includes part of the mesencephalon (midbrain), the metencephalon (pons) and the myelencephalon (medulla oblongata).

The brain stem is particularly important for wakefulness, normal cardiopulmonary function, generation of gait and normal cranial nerve function. Clinical signs of brain-stem disease include

- cranial nerve deficits (CNs III–XII)
- paresis (ipsilateral to unilateral lesion)
- sensorium abnormalities
- cardiac and respiratory abnormalities
- sleep abnormalities (narcolepsy/cataplexy)
- gait abnormalities (ataxia and paresis ipsilateral to a unilateral lesion)
- recumbency is often present.

## Infratentorial/cerebellum

The cerebellum can also be divided functionally along its sagittal axis as follows.

1. MEDIAL ZONE includes the vermis and fastigial nucleus – important for regulation of tone for posture, locomotion, and equilibrium.
2. INTERMEDIATE ZONE includes the paravermal cortex and interposital nucleus – important for adjusting tone and posture for more skilled movement.
3. LATERAL ZONE includes the lateral hemispheres and the lateral (dentate) nucleus – important for regulation of skilled movement.

---

**Causes of seizures**

- structural brain abnormality
- metabolic abnormalities: (a) endogenous, e.g. hepatic encephalopathy, (b) exogenous, e.g. toxin exposure
- no apparent cause (idiopathic epilepsy).

Because of its unique function clinical signs of cerebellar disease are often characteristic and include

- ataxia and dysmetria
- intention tremor
- menace deficits with normal vision and normal CN VII function
- decerebellate rigidity
- vestibular signs
- pupillary abnormalities
- increased frequency of urination.

Unilateral lesions of the cerebellum result in ipsilateral clinical signs. **Ataxia** and **dysmetria** are commonly, but not exclusively, seen with disease of the cerebellum. The animal's strength is normal with cerebellar disease alone, but movements may be somewhat delayed or compensations may be exaggerated (see Figs 19.9 and 19.15). If the head is elevated and released it may descend further ventrally than normal (rebound phenomenon).

An **intention tremor** is one that begins or worsens as the animal intends to perform a task in a goal-oriented manner. It may involve the whole body but is most obvious in the head, which usually moves up and down at a frequency of 2–4 oscillations/second. This type of tremor is exaggerated by tasks such as visual fixation or smelling.

Involvement of the flocculonodular lobe or fastigial area may result in a **vestibular disturbance** characterized by lack of balance, nystagmus, and a broad-based gait. The nystagmus may only be seen when the head is flexed to one side, with the fast phase directed toward the side of the tilt. A pendulous eye movement (eyes oscillate from side to side) may also be seen with cerebellar disease.

A **menace deficit** with normal vision and normal CN VII function can be seen ipsilateral to a unilateral cerebellar lesion, as cerebellar influence is needed for performance of this response (Fig. 19.17).

Occasionally animals with cerebellar disease may adopt abnormal postures but maintain normal mentation. The rostral cerebellar lobe is inhibitory to stretch in the antigravity muscles, and lesions here may result in opisthotonos with the thoracic limbs extended (**decerebellate posture**). The pelvic limbs are usually flexed forward under the body by hypertonia of the hypaxial muscles that flex the coxofemoral joints. If the lesion also involves the ventral lobules the pelvic limbs may be in rigid extension. Reflexes are usually exaggerated.

With unilateral lesions of the fastigial or interposital nuclei a pupillary dilation which is slowly responsive to light may be seen. Occasionally, the third eyelid may protrude and the palpebral fissure may be enlarged. Such pupillary dilation occurs in the eye ipsilateral to

an interposital nuclear lesion and contralateral to a fastigial nuclear lesion.

The cerebellum normally has an inhibitory influence on urination. Rarely a cerebellar lesion will result in frequent urination due to loss of this inhibitory input.

A cerebellar lesion of the caudal cerebellar peduncle or flocculonodular lobules may cause clinical signs of vestibular disease. The head tilt in this instance is to the side **away** from the lesion, prompting a diagnosis of **paradoxical vestibular syndrome**. Postural reaction deficits ipsilateral to the lesion will help to localize the lesion to the correct side.

### Infratentorial/vestibular system

Clinical signs of vestibular system disease and the differentiation between central and peripheral disease are described under CN VIII (see Table 19.5).

### Spinal cord disease

With spinal cord disease it is important first to determine which limbs are affected and if the reflexes reflect UMN or LMN disease. After obtaining this information the examiner should be able to localize the lesion into one of five spinal cord regions (see Table 19.1).

Abnormalities of the C1–C5 spinal segments result in tetraparesis. Progression to tetraplegia (total lack of voluntary movement in all limbs) is uncommonly seen as concurrent involvement of pathways important for respiratory function are compromised and death becomes imminent. If the lesion occurs unilaterally within the spinal cord hemiparesis is found ipsilateral to the lesion. Cervical hyperesthesia is common with extradural compressive lesions and inflammatory vertebral (diskospondylitis and osteomyelitis) and spinal cord (meningitis or myelitis) diseases. Horner's syndrome may be present as a result of involvement of the descending sympathetic fibers in the lateral tectotegmental spinal tract (Fig. 19.19). In horses such involvement also results in vasodilatation and sweating on the entire ipsilateral side of the body. Reflexes in the affected limbs, being normal to exaggerated, will reflect UMN disease.

With C6–T2 spinal segment (cervical intumescence) involvement tetraparesis may also result. Reflexes in the pelvic limbs will remain UMN in character, whereas those in the thoracic limbs may have characteristics of LMN involvement. In large animals, because of the smaller proportion of LMN (gray matter) to UMN (white matter) involvement with similar focal compressive lesions, signs of LMN disease such as marked weakness, hyporeflexia and muscle atrophy are much less evident than in small animals. If the lesion is unilateral a hemiparesis is seen, with similar reflex changes. Horner's syndrome may be present as the preganglionic cell bodies and nerves are associated with the caudal cervical intumescence (Fig. 19.19). In horses hyperhidrosis may or may not be present. If the lesion involves the C8–T1 segments or nerves the cutaneous trunci reflex may be abnormal. If the lesion is unilateral the ipsilateral cutaneous trunci muscle will not contract with stimulation on either side of the body. The unaffected side should still contract with stimulation on either side confirming the integrity of the T3–L3 spinal segments.

Lesions of the T3–L3 spinal segments will result in paraparesis or paraplegia. Reflexes in the pelvic limbs will be UMN in character. The cutaneous trunci reflex may be absent caudal to the cranial extent of the lesion. With severe lesions a Schiff–Sherrington posture may be seen. This is rare in large animals. With extradural compressive and inflammatory diseases there is often focal hyperesthesia in the area of the lesion. With unilateral lesions a UMN monoparesis of the pelvic limb may be found.

Disease of the L4–S3 spinal segments (lumbar intumescence) may also result in paraparesis or paraplegia. Pelvic limb reflexes will be LMN in character. Depending upon which area of the intumescence is involved, specific reflexes may be abnormal (Table 19.2). With a lesion of the L4–L6 segments (femoral nerve outflow) the patellar reflex will be reduced or absent. Quadriceps muscle atrophy may be evident. Sensation on the medial aspect of the pelvic limb may be reduced or absent owing to involvement of the saphenous nerve, which is a sensory branch of the femoral nerve.

With lesions of the L6–S2 spinal segments (sciatic nerve) the withdrawal reflex is reduced or absent. The patellar reflex may appear exaggerated owing to loss of antagonist muscles to this reflex as a result of sciatic involvement. Atrophy of the muscles innervated by the sciatic nerve will result, and is often most obvious in the cranial tibial muscle.

If the S1–S3 spinal segments are abnormal, bladder, anus, and terminal colon dysfunction is seen. The bladder will have characteristics reflecting a LMN lesion. Lesions of the caudal spinal segments result in reduced or absent tail movement, tone, and sensation.

### Neuromuscular junction (NMJ), peripheral nerve and muscle disease

Lower motor neuron signs, particularly weakness, are seen in the affected parts of the body. Horses with marked weakness often stand with all feet close together and will constantly shift the weight from limb to limb. In animals still standing the gait is usually short-strided and choppy. Limbs may appear floppy and flaccid, and may tremble and buckle with weight-bearing. Heavy animals, especially horses, show marked muscle tremor which may become quite violent before the animal becomes recumbent. With some diseases weakness is exacerbated with exercise (e.g. myasthenia gravis) or when more weight is placed on a limb. Muscle weakness may be seen in visceral structures such as the esophagus.

If LMN disease is suspected it is useful to evaluate conscious proprioception when the animal is fully weightbearing and again when its weight is supported by the examiner. Some diseases affect only the motor portion of the peripheral nerves: neuromuscular diseases are one such example. Animals with disease of the neuromuscular junction or muscle may have postural reaction deficits during weightbearing that are not evident when the weight is supported. With many peripheral nerve and spinal cord lesions both motor weakness and sensory ataxia occur concurrently. Postural reaction abnormalities will therefore be seen regardless of weightbearing status.

With many LMN diseases spinal reflexes are reduced or absent. Tone in the limbs is poor and there is very little resistance to passive manipulation by the examiner.

---

### Clinical Pointer

In some neuromuscular diseases, such as myopathies and myasthenia gravis, spinal reflexes are normal.

---

Other signs of nervous system weakness, such as megaesophagus, dysphagia, facial muscle weakness, dysphonia, and respiratory abnormalities, may be seen. Many of the cranial nerves are motor nerves and can be affected by polyneuropathies and junctional disease.

Individual peripheral nerves (Table 19.2) may be selectively involved with various pathological processes. Evaluation of the distribution of sensory loss may be helpful in this localization.

## DIFFERENTIAL DIAGNOSIS

After the neuroanatomical diagnosis has been determined a differential diagnosis should be formulated. Diseases considered should have signs consistent with the neuroanatomical diagnosis. For example, seizures in a dog would not be caused by intervertebral disk disease, as seizures are caused by diseases of the fore-brain. Description of specific diseases are beyond the scope of this chapter but are described in the numerous veterinary textbooks.

## ANCILLARY TESTING

### Intracranial disease

If a lesion is suspected to involve the brain (forebrain, brain stem, or cerebellum) in small animals an advanced imaging study such as **computed tomography** (**CT**) or **magnetic resonance imaging** (**MRI**) is used to assess the structural integrity of these areas. These studies are non-invasive but do require anesthesia. **Survey radiographs** of the skull are useful in instances of skull fracture or middle ear (bulla) disease; however, they do not allow for assessment of nervous system parenchyma.

**Cerebrospinal fluid** (**CSF**) analysis is helpful primarily to determine the presence of inflammatory diseases. Collection techniques for spinal fluid have been reviewed (deLahunta 1983). While CSF analysis is often helpful in determining the presence of nervous system disease, used alone it does not often make for a specific etiologic diagnosis.

**Electroencephalography** (**EEG**) records electrical activity associated with the forebrain structures. This may be useful during evaluation of seizures, narcolepsy, and encephalopathies, but often yields little information concerning the specific disease process compared to advanced imaging techniques. Recording the **brain-stem auditory evoked potential** (**BAEP**) may be helpful in determining the presence of intact hearing pathways and may also provide some information about the integrity of central (brain stem) projection pathways associated with hearing.

When an extramedullary cranial nerve abnormality is suspected, **electromyography** (**EMG**) of the facial or head muscles may be used to assess the extent of the abnormality and localize the process to specific cranial nerves. MRI gives the best visualization of individual cranial nerves.

In some instances topical pharmacological testing is used to localize pupillary abnormalities resulting from autonomic disease due to either pre- or postganglionic lesions. Such testing, however, is often inconclusive.

### Spinal cord disease

**Survey radiology** and **myelography** are often used to evaluate spinal cord lesions. Survey radiographs are often diagnostic in instances of bone infection (diskospondylitis), trauma (fracture, luxation, subluxation) and neoplasia. Diseases that affect the spinal cord often require myelography.

---

### Myelography

- a contrast agent is injected into the subarachnoid space after a spinal tap has been performed
- the contrast agent outlines the spinal cord, which is normally not seen on survey radiographs
- myelography is used to delineate compressive or expansile lesions of the spinal cord.

---

Cerebrospinal fluid should be assessed to exclude inflammatory diseases, particularly meningitis and myelitis. Ideally, CSF should be collected caudal to the suspected lesion. Advanced imaging studies may yield additional information as CT provides better delineation of bony structures, whereas MRI yields superior images of the soft tissue. **Evoked potentials** (**spinal evoked potentials, somatosensory evoked potentials**) provide supportive information as to lesion location and possible severity.

### Peripheral nerve, neuromuscular junction, or muscle disease

Disease involving the peripheral nerves, neuromuscular junctions, or muscles is initially evaluated with **electromyographic studies** (**EMG, nerve conduction velocity**). Specific disease etiologies, however, may not be able to be determined as end-stage nerve and muscle disease from a variety of diseases may appear similar.

---

### CSF tap/spinal tap

- a spinal needle is inserted into the subarachnoid space either in the cerebellomedullary cistern or in the lumber area
- in general, collection of spinal fluid caudal to the level of the lesion is most accurate for diagnosis
- fluid is analyzed for cellularity, protein content, and cell morphology
- protein electrophoresis on CSF can give additional information concerning the integrity of the blood–brain barrier and local production of immunoglobulins
- detecting the presence of *Sarcocystis neurona* antibodies and selected protein sequences in CSF is very useful in the diagnosis of equine protozoal myeloencephalitis.

---

## Assessment of nerves and muscles

- special electrical testing such as repetitive stimulation and single-fiber EMG, may be necessary when neuromuscular disease is suspected
- late potentials (F waves, H waves) are used to assess the integrity of the more proximal peripheral nerve and nerve roots
- serum p-2 (myelin protein) antibody titers have been useful to detect circulating antibodies against this component of myelin in horses suspected of having immune-associated polyneuritis
- antiacetylcholine receptor antibodies may be found in serum of animals with acquired myasthenia gravis
- serum creatine kinase may be elevated by diseases causing muscle membrane damage
- muscle and nerve biopsy will give objective morphological data as to the disease process.

# REFERENCES AND FURTHER READING

Bagley RS. Tremor syndromes in dogs: diagnosis and treatment. Journal of Small Animal Practice 1992; 33: 485–490.

Bagley RS, Pluhar GE, Alexander JE. Lateral intervertebral disk extrusion causing lameness in a dog. Journal of the American Veterinary Medical Association 1994; 205: 181–183.

Bailey CS, Kitchell RL. Cutaneous sensory testing in the dog. Journal of Veterinary Internal Medicine 1987; 1: 128–135.

Bonneau NH, Olivieri M, Breton L. Avulsion of the gastrocnemius tendon in the dog causing flexion of the hock and digits. Journal of the American Animal Hospital Association 1983; 19: 717–722.

Braund KG. Nerve and muscle biopsy techniques. Progress in Veterinary Neurology 1991; 2: 35–56.

Braund KG. Clinical syndromes in veterinary neurology, 2nd edn. St. Louis: Mosby, 1994.

Breazile JE, Blaugh BS, Nail N. Experimental study of canine distemper myoclonus. American Journal of Veterinary Research 1966; 27: 1375–1379.

Breitschwerdt EB, Breazile JE, Broadhurst JJ. Clinical and electroencephalographic findings associated with ten cases of suspected limbic epilepsy in the dog. Journal of the American Animal Hospital Association 1979; 15: 37–50.

Child G, Higgins RJ, Cuddon PA. Acquired scoliosis associated with hydromyelia and syringomyelia in two dogs. Journal of the American Veterinary Medical Association 1986; 189: 909–912.

Chrisman CL. Dancing Doberman disease: Clinical finding and prognosis. Progress in Veterinary Neurology 1990;1:83–90.

Chrisman CL. Problems in small animal neurology. Philadelphia: Lea & Febiger, 1991.

Collins BK, O'Brien D. Autonomic dysfunction of the eye. Seminars in Veterinary Medicine and Surgery 1990; 5: 24–36.

Colter SB. Stupor and coma. Progress in Veterinary Neurology 1990; 1: 137–145.

Cummings JF, deLahunta A, Winn SS. Acral mutilation and nociceptive loss in English Pointer dogs. A canine sensory neuropathy. Acta Neuropathologica (Berlin) 1981; 53: 119–127.

DeJong RN. Introduction. In: The neurologic examination, 3rd edn. New York: Harper & Row, 1967; 6.

deLahunta A. Comparative cerebellar disease in domestic animals. The Compendium of Continuing Education for the Practicing Veterinarian 1980; 2: 8–19.

deLahunta A. Veterinary neuroanatomy and clinical neurology, 2nd ed. Philadelphia: WB Saunders, 1983.

Easton TA. On the normal use of reflexes. American Scientist 1972; 60: 591–599.

Farrow BRH. Generalized tremor syndrome. In: Kirk RW (ed) Current veterinary therapy IX. Philadelphia: WB Saunders, 1986; 800–801.

Fischer A, Obermaier G. Brainstem auditory-evoked potentials and neuropathologic correlates in 26 dogs with brain tumor. Journal of Veterinary Internal Medicine 1994; 8: 363–368.

Fox JG, Averill DF, Hallett M, Schunk K. Familial reflex myoclonus in labrador retrievers. American Journal of Veterinary Research 1984; 45: 2367–2370.

Griffiths IR. Neurological examination of the limbs and the body. In: Wheeler SJ (ed) Manual of small animal neurology. West Sussex: British Small Animal Veterinary Association, 1989; 35.

Guilford WG, Shaw DP, O'Brien DP, Maxwell VD. Fecal incontinence, urinary incontinence, and priapism associated with multifocal distemper encephalomyelitis in a dog. Journal of the American Veterinary Medical Association 1990; 197: 90–92.

Gundlach AL, Dodd PR, Grabara CSG et al. Deficit of spinal cord glycine/strychnine receptors in inherited myoclonus of Poll Hereford calves. Science 1988; 241: 1807–1810.

Gundlach AL, Kortz G, Burazin TCD et al. Deficit of inhibitory glycine receptors in spinal cord from Peruvian Pasos: evidence for an equine form of inherited myoclonus. Brain Research 1993; 628: 263–270.

Hansen B. Recognition of acute pain and distress in the dog. Proceedings of the Eighth Annual Veterinary Medicine Forum, Washington DC, May 1990; 773–776.

Hendricks JC, Morrison AR. Normal and abnormal sleep in mammals. Journal of the American Veterinary Medical Association 1981; 178: 121–126.

Holliday TA. Clinical signs of acute and chronic experimental lesions of the cerebellum. Veterinary Science Communications 1979/1980; 3:259–277.

Holliday TA. Unilateral neglect (hemi-inattention) syndrome in dogs. Proceedings of the Ninth Annual Veterinary Medicine Forum. New Orleans, May 1991; 819–821.

Holliday TA. Electrodiagnostic evaluation, somatosensory evoked potentials and electromyography. Veterinary Clinics of North America (Small Animal Practice) 1992; 22: 833–857.

Hopkins AL, Howard JF, Wheeler SJ, Kornegay JN. Stimulated single fibre electromyography in normal dogs. Journal of Small Animal Practice 1993; 34: 271–276.

Johnson BW. Congenitally abnormal visual pathways of Siamese cats. The Compendium of Continuing Education for the Practicing Veterinarian 1991; 13: 374–377.

Joseph RJ. Vestibular eye movement revisited. Proceedings of the Tenth Annual Veterinary Medicine Forum. San Diego, May 1992; 762–764.

Kern TJ, Aromando MC, Erb HN. Horner's syndrome in dogs and cats: 100 cases (1975–1985). Journal of the American Veterinary Medical Association 1989; 195: 369–373.

King AS. Physiological and clinical anatomy of the domestic mammals. Oxford: Oxford University Press, 1987.

Knecht CD, Redding RW, Wilson S. Characteristics of F and H waves of ulnar and tibial nerves in cats: reference values. American Journal of Veterinary Research 1985; 46: 977–979.

Kornegay JN. Management of animals with neurologic disease. In: Kornegay JN (ed) Neurologic disorders – contemporary issues in small animal practice. New York: Churchill Livingstone, 1986; 3.

Kornegay JN, Oliver JE, Gorgacz EJ. Clinicopathologic features of brain herniation in animals. Journal of the American Veterinary Medical Association 1983; 182: 1111–1116.

Latshaw WK. A model for the neural control of locomotion. Journal of the American Animal Hospital Association 1974; 10: 598–607.

Lewis GT, Blanchard GL, Trapp AL, DeCamp CE. Ophthalmoplegia caused by thyroid adenocarcinoma invasion of the cavernous sinuses in the dog. Journal of the American Animal Hospital Association 1984; 20: 805–812.

McCormick DA, Thompson RF. Cerebellum: essential involvement in the classically conditioned eyelid response. Science 1984; 223: 296–299.

Malik R, Church DB, Maddison JE, Farrow BR. Three cases of local tetanus. Journal of Small Animal Practice 1989a; 30, 469–473.

Malik R, Ho S, Church DB. The normal response to repetitive motor nerve stimulation in dogs. Journal of Small Animal Practice 1989b; 30: 20–26.

March PA, Knowles K, Thalhammer JG. Reflex myoclonus in two labrador retriever littermates: a clinical, electrophysiological, and pathological study. Progress in Veterinary Neurology 1993; 4: 19–24.

Mayhew IG. Large animal neurology. Philadelphia: Lea & Febiger, 1989.

Moore MP. Approach to the patient with spinal disease. Veterinary Clinics of North America (Small Animal Practice) 1992; 22: 751–780.

Moreau PM. Neurological examination of the cranial nerves. In: Wheeler SJ (ed) Manual of small animal neurology. West Sussex: British Small Animal Veterinary Association, 1989; 13.

Morgan RV, Zanotti SW. Horner's syndrome in dogs and cats: 49 cases (1980–1986). Journal of the American Veterinary Medical Association 1989; 194: 1096–1099.

Myers LJ. Dysosmia of the dog in clinical veterinary medicine. Progress in Veterinary Neurology 1990; 1: 171–179.

Neer T M. Horner's syndrome: anatomy, diagnosis and causes. The Compendium of Continuing Education for the Practicing Veterinarian 1984; 6: 740–746.

Neer T M, Carter JD. Anisocoria in dogs and cats: ocular and neurologic causes. The Compendium of Continuing Education for the Practicing Veterinarian 1987; 9: 817–823.

O'Brien D. Brain damage and behavior. Proceedings of the Eleventh Annual Veterinary Medicine Forum. Washington DC, May 1993; 542–545.

Oliver JE, Lorenz MD. Handbook of veterinary neurology. Philadelphia: WB Saunders, 1993.

Oliver JE, Hoerlein BF, Mayhew IG. Veterinary neurology. Philadelphia: WB Saunders, 1987.

Palmer AC. Clinical and pathological aspects of cervical disc protrusion and primary tumors of the cervical spinal cord in the dog. Journal of Small Animal Practice 1970; 11: 63–67.

Palmer AC, Malinowski W, Barnet KC. Clinical signs including papilloedema associated with brain tumors in twenty-one dogs. Journal of Small Animal Practice 1974; 15: 359–386.

Parker AJ. Behavioral changes of organic neurologic origin. Progress in Veterinary Neurology 1990; 1: 123–131.

Perdrizet JA, Dinsmore P. Pituitary abscess syndrome. The Compendium of Continuing Education for the Practicing Veterinarian 1986; 8: s311–s318.

Prata RG, Stoll SG. Ventral decompression and fusion for the treatment of cervical disk disease in the dog. Journal of the American Animal Hospital Association 1973; 9: 462–472.

Radostits OM, Gay CC, Blood DC, Hinchcliff K. Veterinary medicine, 9th edn. WB Saunders, 2000.

Reilly L, Habecker P, Beech J et al. Pituitary abscess and basilar empyema in 4 horses. Equine Veterinary Journal 1994; 26: 424–426.

Roberts SR, Vainisi SJ. Hemifacial spasm in dogs. Journal of the American Veterinary Medical Association 1967; 150: 381–385.

Scagliotti RH. Neuro-ophthalmology. Progress in Veterinary Neurology 1990; 1: 157–170.

Sharp NJH, Nash AS, Griffiths IR. Feline dysautonomia (the Key–Gaskell syndrome): a clinical and pathological study of forty cases. Journal of Small Animal Practice 1984; 25: 599–615.

Shelton GD, Willard MD, Cardinette GH, Lindstrom J. Acquired myasthenia gravis, selective involvement of esophageal, pharyngeal, and facial muscles. Journal of Veterinary Internal Medicine 1990; 4: 281–284.

Shores A, Vaughn DM, Holland M, Smith B, Simpson ST, Burns J. Glossopharyngeal neuralgia syndrome in a dog. Journal of the American Animal Hospital Association 1991; 27: 101–104.

Sims MH. Hearing loss in small animals: occurrence and diagnosis. In: Kirk RW (ed) Current veterinary therapy X. Philadelphia: WB Saunders, 1989; 805–811.

Sims MH, Selcer RR: Occurrence and evaluation of a reflex-evoked muscle potential (H reflex) in the normal dog. American Journal of Veterinary Research 1981; 42: 975–983.

Sims MH, Brace JJ, Arthur DA, Harvey RC. Otoacoustic emission in a dog. Journal of the American Veterinary Medical Association 1991; 198: 1017–1018.

Smith BP (ed) Large animal internal medicine, 2nd edn. St. Louis: CV Mosby, 1996.

Spaulding KS, Sharp NJH. Ultrasonographic imaging of the lateral cerebral ventricles in the dog. Veterinary Radiology 1990; 31: 59–64.

Steiss JE. Linear regression to determine the relationship between F-wave latency and limb length in control dogs. American Journal of Veterinary Research 1984; 45: 2649–2650.

Steiss JE, Cox NR, Hathcock JT. Brain stem auditory-evoked response abnormalities in 14 dogs with confirmed central nervous system lesions. Journal of Veterinary Internal Medicine 1994; 8: 293–298.

Thompson CE, Kornegay JN, Stevens JB. Analysis of cerebrospinal fluid from the cerebellomedullary and lumbar cistern of dogs with focal neurologic disease:145 cases (1985–1987). Journal of the American Veterinary Medical Association 1990; 196: 1841–1844.

Thompson HS, Franceschetti AT, Thompson PM. Hippus, semantic and historic considerations of the word. American Journal of Ophthalmology 1971; 71: 1116–1120.

Wheeler SJ. Breed related neurological disorders. In: Wheeler SJ (ed) Manual of small animal neurology. West Sussex: British Small Animal Veterinary Association, 1989; 287.

Wise LA, Lappin MR. A syndrome resembling feline dysautonomia (Key–Gaskell syndrome) in a dog. Journal of the American Veterinary Medical Association 1991; 12: 2103–2106.

# 20

# Clinical Examination of the Visual System

*B. Grahn*

## CLINICAL MANIFESTATIONS OF OCULAR DISEASE

**Anisocoria** Pupils of unequal size which may vary in bright (photopic) and dim (scotopic) light conditions or remain static. Anisocoria is a manifestation of ocular, autonomic nerve, cranial nerve or central nervous system diseases.

**Ankyloblepharon** Fusion of the eyelids. This is a congenital anomaly where the eyelid fissure fails to develop. It is physiological for the first 7–14 days in kittens and puppies.

**Aphakic crescent** Crescent moon appearance that occurs when the lens is subluxated. The crescent appears between the lens border, where the zonulae have ruptured, and the pupillary margin of the iris.

**Aqueous flare** A faint smoke-like beam in the aqueous humor that can be visualized when a very focal bright light is directed through the anterior chamber of an eye with uveitis. This is possible because the blood–aqueous barrier has been disrupted. Protein and cells that have leaked into the aqueous humor stop some of the light and create the beam.

**Blepharitis** Inflammation of the eyelids. The lids appear swollen and hyperemic, and ocular discharge is usually present on the skin.

**Blepharospasm** Spasmodic eyelid closure which is due to contraction of the orbicularis oculi muscle. This develops secondary to ocular irritation and is an important indicator of ocular pain.

**Blindness** An inability to see, manifested by a lack of a menace reflex and bumping into objects in a maze. Blindness may be due to peripheral (ocular, optic nerve) or central (central nervous system) diseases.

**Buphthalmos** Enlargement of the eye due to stretching of the fibrous tunic. Buphthalmos is synonymous with concurrent or previous glaucoma.

**Cataract** An opacity in the lens. Cataracts develop when the lenticular fibers are disrupted secondary to osmotic changes and overhydration or protein denaturation. They may be categorized as incipient (small), immature (a tapetal reflex can be visualized), mature (tapetal reflex is not visible), hypermature (a wrinkled lens due to resorption of liquid lens material) and intumescent (swollen).

**Chemosis** Conjunctival edema. It appears as a swollen, pale conjunctiva and is a common manifestation of infectious, inflammatory or neoplastic conditions of the conjunctiva and eyelids.

**Choroidal mass** A proliferation of pigmented or non-pigmented tissue in the choroid which may be discrete or generalized. It usually displaces the retina over the mass into the vitreous. These masses may occur with primary or metastatic neoplasms or inflammation. Retinal detachments, edema, cellular infiltrates and hemorrhage are often associated with choroidal masses.

**Ciliary mass** A proliferation of tissue in the ciliary body which may be discrete or generalized. A ciliary mass may develop with primary or metastatic neoplasia, cyst, or inflammation.

**Coloboma** A congenital hole or fissure that may be present in any ocular tissue and represents a failure of tissue development. Typical colobomata occur along the embryonic fissure (6 o'clock position), and those present in other locations are designated atypical.

**Conjunctival hemorrhage** A collection of blood in the conjunctiva, which can vary from petechiae to ecchymosis. Conjunctival hemorrhage occurs secondary to systemic diseases, including viral or bacterial infections, coagulation disorders, neoplasia or trauma; or to local ocular inflammatory, infectious or neoplastic disorders.

**Conjunctival hyperemia** Engorgement of the conjunctival blood vessels (red eye), a non-specific clinical manifestation of inflammation of the eye and orbit.

**Conjunctival mass** A proliferation of tissue in the conjunctiva. The mass may be a neoplasm, teratoma or inflammatory growth.

**Corneal facet** An epithelium-lined corneal depression that develops after a deep corneal stromal ulcer has healed. The cornea around and beneath the facet is usually scarred and stromal vascularization is commonly present. Fluorescein staining is negative, which allows differentiation from a corneal ulcer.

**Corneal mass** A proliferation of tissue in the cornea. These masses may be neoplasms that extend into the cornea from the limbus, teratomas, cysts or inflammatory growths.

**Corneal opacity** A loss of translucency of the cornea. Opacities develop secondary to infiltrates such as edema, tears, minerals, lipids, blood vessels, cells or pigment. They may be discrete and vary in size (nebula or macula), or be diffuse.

**Dyscoria** An abnormally shaped pupil. Dyscoria may be congenital, secondary to iridal anomalies including iris coloboma or persistent pupillary membranes, or develop with acquired conditions including uveitis and anterior or posterior synechiae or iris atrophy.

**Ectropion** Eversion of the eyelid margin. Ectropion may be congenital when eyelid margins are excessive. It may develop with cicatrization of scar tissue after eyelid trauma.

**Enophthalmos** Recession of the eye into the orbit. This may develop secondary to a loss of sympathetic innervation to the eye (Horner's syndrome), loss of orbital fat, orbital scar tissue, dehydration, anterior orbital neoplasia, or contraction of the retractor bulbi muscle in response to painful or threatening conditions.

**Entropion** Inversion or turning inward of the margin of the eyelid. It may be congenital, or develop secondary to a combination of orbicularis muscle contracture and abnormal eyelid fissure, or as a result of cicatrization of scar tissue after eyelid and conjunctival trauma.

**Epiphora** An overflow of tears on to the eyelids and facial skin. It is the result of either increased tear flow (lacrimation) or decreased tear drainage. Lacrimation in animals usually occurs in response to inflammatory anterior segment disorders. Decreased tear drainage occurs secondary to obstruction, stenosis or aplasia of the ventral puncta, ventral canaliculus or nasolacrimal duct.

**Episclera or scleral mass** A proliferation of tissue in the episclera or sclera. This may occur with a metastatic or locally invasive neoplasm, cyst or inflammation.

**Exophthalmos** Protrusion of an eye out of the orbit. It develops secondary to orbital inflammation (cellulitis, abscess, adenitis, myositis, osteomyelitis), neoplasia, cyst, salivary mucocele, vascular anomaly or emphysema. Exophthalmos is an important differential diagnosis for buphthalmos. The eye is of normal size in the former but enlarged in the latter.

**Eyelid mass** A discrete or generalized swelling of the eyelid. It may be a clinical manifestation of neoplasia, cysts or inflammatory disease.

**Hemeralopia** Day blindness, which is manifested by impaired vision in bright light. It occurs when the cone photoreceptor function is impaired and is an inherited disorder in the Alaskan Malamute and Miniature Poodle dog.

**Horner's Syndrome** Sympathetic denervation of the orbit seen as ptosis, miosis, enophthalmos, and protrusion of the third eyelid. It can be accompanied by excessive facial sweating in the horse.

**Hyphema** Blood in the anterior chamber, which occurs secondary to a breakdown of the blood aqueous barrier (uveitis). Common etiologies include ocular trauma, inflammation, intraocular neoplasia, coagulopathies and retinal detachment.

**Hypopyon** A collection of purulent material which usually settles in the ventral anterior chamber. It may develop with severe uveitis, ulcerative keratitis or panophthalmitis.

**Iridal atrophy** A loss of iris tissue that occurs with age. It may occur around the pupillary margin and result in dyscoria (irregular pupil) or diffusely over the stroma, leaving the iris with a lace-like appearance if it is retroilluminated in the tapetal reflex.

**Iridal depigmentation** A lightening of the iris color, which may be focal or diffuse. Iridal depigmentation develops secondary to cell infiltration into the iris and disruption of the iris melanocytes. Iridal depigmentation may be multifocal when it develops over follicles of lymphocytes and plasma cells in chronic uveitis, or generalized when associated with diffuse neoplastic cell infiltration (lymphoma) or immune-mediated melanocyte destruction (Vogt–Koyanagi–Harada-like syndrome of dogs).

**Iridal hemorrhage** Leakage of blood into the iris, which is indicative of a breakdown of the blood–iris barrier. This is a manifestation of uveitis. Common etiologies include coagulopathies, neoplasia, infectious diseases, inflammatory and traumatic conditions.

**Iridal hyperpigmentation** A darkening of the iris which may be focal or diffuse. Focal hyperpigmentation is a clinical manifestation of some neoplasms (melanoma) or benign conditions (freckles and nevi). Diffuse hyperpigmentation develops with chronic uveitis in most domestic animals, and diffuse iris melanoma in the cat.

**Iridal mass** A proliferation of tissue in the iris, which may be discrete or generalized. An iridal mass may occur with a primary ocular or metastatic neoplasm, cyst or inflammation.

**Iridodenesis** Trembling of the iris. It develops when the iris loses support secondary to lens subluxation or luxation.

**Keratoconus** A conical projection of the cornea due to stromal degeneration.

**Keratotic precipitates** Clumps of leukocytes and fibrin that are adherent to the corneal endothelium. They appear as pale yellow opacities on the ventral corneal endothelium and develop secondary to uveitis.

**Lenticonus** An anterior or posterior conical projection of the lens. This is a congenital lenticular maldevelopment. Occasionally trauma and cataracts will alter the lens and resemble lenticonus.

**Leukocoria** A white pupil. This is usually a manifestation of a cataract. Occasionally inflammatory infiltrates in the anterior chamber may resemble leukocoria.

**Microphthalmia** A congenitally small eye. The microphthalmic eye may be visual or blind and may be an incidental finding or part of multiple ocular anomalies. It is an important differential diagnosis for phthisis bulbi.

**Miosis** Constriction of the pupil. This develops secondary to uveitis or a loss of sympathetic innervation to the iris (Horner's syndrome). Miosis can be induced with topical or systemic drugs, such as parasympathomimetics or opiates.

**Mydriasis** Dilatation of the pupil. Mydriasis may occur with glaucoma, loss of parasympathetic innervation to the iris, stimulation of the sympathetic innervation to the iris, or hypoplasia or atrophy of the iris constrictor muscle. It may also be induced with topical or systemic drugs, including parasympatholytics and adrenergics.

**Nyctalopia** Blindness that is present in dim light (scotopic). This occurs when the rod photoreceptors are impaired. It is an early clinical sign of vitamin A deficiency in cattle and photoreceptor degeneration in horses, dogs and cats.

**Ocular discharge** The collection of a serous, hemorrhagic, mucoid or purulent material on the eyelids, conjunctiva and cornea. It is a common non-specific manifestation of eyelid, conjunctival, corneal, scleral, uveal or orbital disease.

**Ophthalmoplegia** Paralysis of all the extraocular or intraocular muscles. **O. externa** is paralysis of all the extraocular skeletal muscles and **O. interna** is paralysis of the intraocular smooth muscles. Ophthalmoplegia is manifested as an immobile eye or iris and may occur with extraocular and intraocular muscle or nerve dysfunction.

**Optic disk swelling** Protrusion of the optic disk into the vitreous, usually accompanied by generalized disk pallor and a decrease in the size of the optic disk pit. A swollen optic disk develops secondary to optic nerve edema and infiltration with inflammatory or neoplastic cells.

**Papillitis** Optic disk inflammation, which is manifested as swelling, pale color, loss of the optic pit and hemorrhage. Papillitis is consistent with the diagnosis of **optic neuritis**.

**Persistent pupillary membranes (PPM)** Congenital vascular remnants of the tunica vasculosa lentis. They appear as small, pigmented vascular strands which attach to the iris, lens or cornea. They are important differential diagnoses for synechiae.

**Photophobia** Avoidance of brightly lit (photopic) conditions. Blepharospasm, retraction of the globe and prolapse of the third eyelid are present and represent discomfort associated with eye orbital or adnexal disease.

**Phthisis bulbi** A shrunken disorganized and atrophic globe. This develops secondary to chronic uveitis. It is an important differential diagnosis for microphthalmia (congenitally small eye).

**Ptosis** A droopy eyelid. Ptosis occurs with dysfunction of the eyelid levator muscles or their motor nerves, or a lack of sympathetic innervation to the orbit (Horner's syndrome).

**Red eye** Engorgement and hyperemia of the conjunctival and episcleral blood vessels. This vascular congestion is a non-specific sign of keratitis, uveitis, glaucoma, conjunctivitis, episcleritis or orbital disease.

**Retinal atrophy** A loss of retinal tissue which is manifested by diminished retinal blood vessels, tapetal hyperreflectivity and focal non-tapetal pigment changes. Retinal atrophy is synonymous with the term retinal degeneration. It may be generalized or it may be focal.

**Retinal cysts** Pale gray cysts are commonly seen in the peripheral retina at the pars plana. They represent a localized collection of fluid within the peripheral retina near the junction of the ciliary epithelium. They are incidental findings with minimal clinical significance.

**Retinal detachment** A separation of the retina from the retinal pigment epithelium. The detachment may be focal or complete and is categorized as rhegmatogenous (associated with a retinal tear) or non-rhegmatogenous. Focal detachments appear as dull, often gray, subtle projections of the retina into the vitreous. Complete detachments resemble a flower with the gray strands of retina suspended like petals from the optic disk. Retinal detachments may be congenital or develop later in life secondary to ocular or systemic disease.

**Retinal opacities** A loss of retinal translucency develops when the retina is infiltrated with cells or fluids (edema).

**Staphyloma** A bulging corneal or scleral defect lined with uveal tissue.

**Strabismus** Malalignment of the eyes. This may be unilateral or bilateral and is a manifestation of congenital or acquired disorders of the visual pathway or the extraocular muscles or their nerve supply. **Esotropia** is medial, **exotropia** is lateral, **hypertropia** is dorsal and **hypotropia** is ventral deviation of the eye.

**Synchysis scintillans** Tinsel-like appearance of cholesterol crystals in liquefied vitreous. This develops secondary to hyalitis and previous vitreous hemorrhage.

**Synechiae** Adhesions of the iris which appear as irregularly shaped, pigmented strands to the cornea (**anterior synechiae**) or the lens (**posterior synechiae**). They develop secondary to previous or concurrent uveitis. They are differential diagnoses for persistent pupillary membranes (PPM).

**Tapetal hyperreflectivity** An increased reflection of light from the tapetum. It may be focal or generalized and is consistent with retinal degeneration.

**Tapetal hyporeflectivity** A decreased reflection of light from the tapetum. It may be focal or diffuse and is a manifestation of cellular or fluid infiltrate into or beneath the retina.

**Third eyelid prolapse** A protrusion of the nictitating membrane. This may occur in response to retraction of the globe, atrophy of orbital structures, displacement of the globe or to a loss of sympathetic orbital tone (Horner's syndrome).

**Vitreous opacities** A loss of translucency of the vitreous. This may be focal or complete and prevent visualization of the fundus. These opacities occur secondary to cellular infiltrates (hemorrhage, leucocytes, scar tissue, blood vessels, neoplastic cells), protein exudation, mineral and lipid deposits (asteroid hyalosis), or congenital defects (persistent hyperplastic primary vitreous and persistent hyaloid artery).

**Vitreous syneresis** Liquefaction of the vitreous which appears as white focal opacities. They will settle in clear vitreous fluid and there is a loss of the normal faint white vitreous veils. This develops secondary to inflammation (uveitis and hyalitis) and degeneration of the vitreous.

## CLINICAL EXAMINATION OF THE EYES OF DOMESTIC ANIMALS

Veterinarians play an integral role in the delivery of ophthalmic care as primary and referral clinicians. The purpose of this chapter is to describe the clinical examination of the eye, orbit, and adnexa (ancillary tissues, including lacrimal and salivary glands, fat, extraocular skeletal and smooth muscles, blood vessels, and nerves) of the horse, cow, sheep, goat, pig, dog, and cat (Fig. 20.1). Some comparative aspects of the ophthalmic examination of each species and ocular conditions that should be referred to an ophthalmologist are also described. The ophthalmic examination is an extension of the physical examination. The clinician collects a history and signalment, and completes a physical examination before initiating the ocular examination.

### Facilities and diagnostic equipment

To complete an ophthalmic examination, an examination room and a variety of instruments, diagnostic materials and drugs are required. A quiet room with controlled lighting, allowing for complete darkness, is essential. Brightly illuminated (photopic) conditions result in numerous reflections that preclude a thorough intraocular examination. Controlled illumination

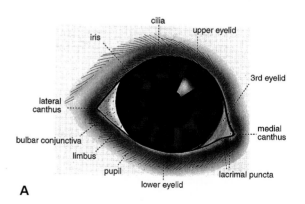

**A**

**Fig. 20.1** (a) The external gross anatomy of the eye of a dog.

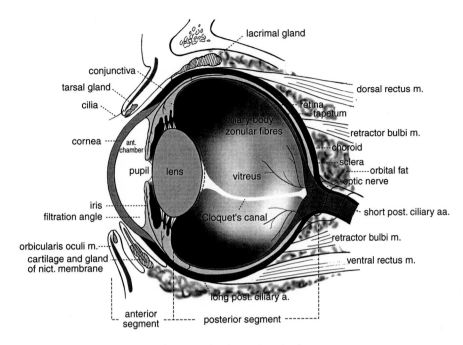

**Fig 20.1 (b)** Gross anatomy of the cross-section of an eye of a domestic animal.

allows evaluation of pupil symmetry and maze tests in photopic and dimly lit (scotopic) conditions. Under field conditions, such as on a farm, a darkened stall or covering the animal's head with a blanket will suffice. The required items for ophthalmic examination are listed in Table 20.1 and shown in Figs 20.2–20.7.

A handheld biomicroscope (Fig. 20.8) and indirect ophthalmoscope (Fig. 20.9) are optional instruments which are being more commonly used in veterinary clinics. These instruments require practice and patience to master, but they enhance the veterinarian's ability to complete a thorough ocular examination in all species. Sterile culture swabs and glass slides are needed for culture of samples and cytology. Preprinted

records assist in the completion of a thorough eye examination (Fig. 20.10).

## History

The owner of an animal with ocular disease may have noticed some of the clinical manifestations of disease described at the beginning of this chapter. Ocular discharge, red eye, painful eye, color changes, alterations in size or shape of the globe or pupil, and blindness are common presenting complaints. The owner's observations may allow the clinician to establish a provisional problem list and collect a thorough and specific ocular history. It is important to determine

- the duration of clinical signs
- the rate of development of the condition
- whether there is unilateral or bilateral involvement.

Additional useful historical information includes

- whether the condition is slowly or rapidly improving or deteriorating
- whether discharge or color changes have occurred over time
- if the animal has other injuries or systemic diseases
- was the animal being medicated, and
- is there a familial history of ocular disease.

| Table 20.1. Equipment and materials required to complete an ocular examination |
|---|
| Transilluminator |
| Direct ophthalmoscope |
| Converging lens |
| Indentation tonometer (small animals) |
| Applanation tonometer (large animals) |
| Schirmer Tear Tests |
| Fluorescein stain |
| Topical ocular anesthetics, injectable local anesthetics and sedatives (large animal) |
| Topical mydriatic and eyewash solutions |

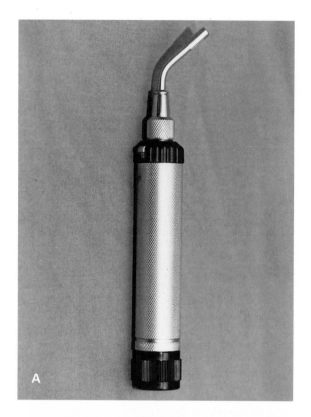

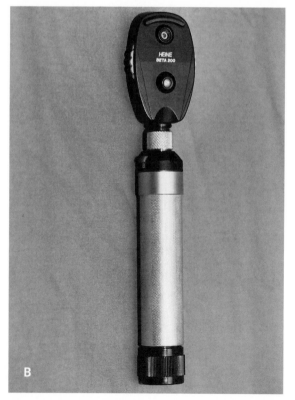

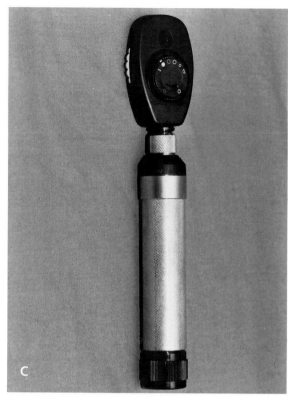

**Fig. 20.2** **(A)** Transilluminator attached to the Heine rechargeable direct ophthalmoscope handpiece. This light source is excellent for anterior and posterior segment evaluation. **(B)** Examiner's side of the *Heine Beta 200* direct ophthalmoscope. **(C)** Patient's side of the *Heine Beta 200* direct ophthalmoscope.

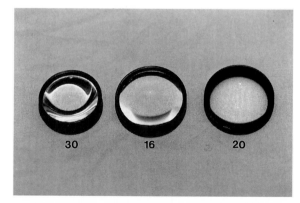

**Fig. 20.3** Heine converging lenses, used for indirect ophthalmoscopy. The 20 is used for routine examinations, the 16 provides increased fundic magnification and the 30 is selected when the pupil size is restricted.

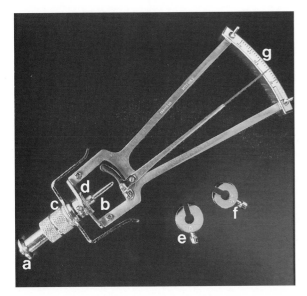

**Fig. 20.4** Schiotz tonometer, an indentation tonometer. Note **(a)** the corneal reception plate and **(b)** indentation pin, **(c)** examiner's handles attached to the sliding collaret, **(d)** the 5.5 g weight plate, **(e)** the 7.5 and **(f)** 10 g weights, and **(g)** the Schiotz scale.

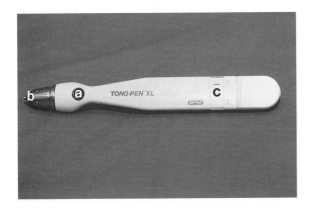

**Fig. 20.5** Tonopen II, an applanation tonometer. Note the power button **(a)** and applanation tip **(b)**, which must be covered by an examination condom prior to use. **(c)** The intraocular pressure display window.

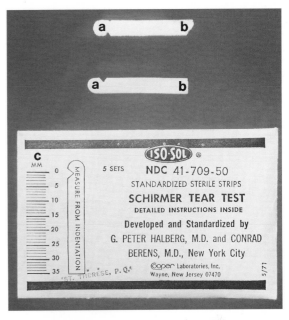

**Fig. 20.6** Schirmer tear test strips. Note the notched end **(a)** that will be folded and inserted into the lower conjunctival fornix, the slashed and square ends of the strips **(b)** and the measuring guide for determining millimeters of wetting **(c)**.

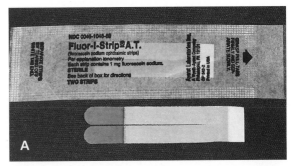

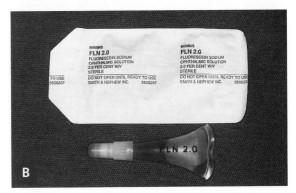

**Fig. 20.7** **(A)** Fluorescein-impregnated strips. **(B)** Liquid fluorescein.

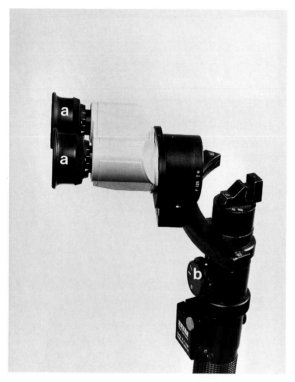

**Fig. 20.8** A handheld Zeiss biomicroscope. Note the moveable eye pieces **(a)** and light control dial **(b)**.

| WCVM Ophthalmology Examination | | |
|---|---|---|
| MAZE TESTING: | PHOTOPIC | SCOTOPIC |
| | OD | OS |
| MENACE | | |
| PALPEBRAL | | |
| PLR     DIR | | |
| CONS | | |
| OCCULO-CEPHALIC | | |
| STT | | |
| IOP | | |
| GONIOSCOPY | | |
| FL. STAIN. | | |
| NASOLACRIMAL | | |

OD (RIGHT)    OS (LEFT)

GLOBE/ORBIT

LIDS

CONJUNCTIVA/
NICITATING MEMBRANE

CORNEA

ANTERIOR CHAMBER

IRIS

PUPIL

LENS

T    N    P    A    A    P    N    T

FUNDUS

**Fig. 20.10** An ophthalmic examination record.

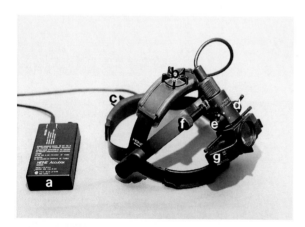

**Fig. 20.9** A *Heine Omega 200* indirect ophthalmoscope. Note the rechargeable power pack **(a)**, circumferential headband adjuster **(b)**, the vertical headband adjuster **(c)**, the light aperture size lever **(d)**, the light filter control lever **(e)**, the control knob for angulation of the eyepieces **(f)**, and the teaching mirror viewing ports **(g)**.

## Signalment

The breed, age, and sex of an animal provide useful clues for the diagnosis and prognosis of many eye diseases.

### Breed

Many breeds of domestic animals are predisposed to or are known to inherit specific diseases of the eye. Examples include optic nerve coloboma of Charolais cattle congenital night blindness of Appaloosa horses, glucocerebroside storage disease in Yorkshire pigs, Chédiak-Higashi syndrome of Persian cats, and primary lens luxations of Terrier dogs.

For a complete review of inherited ocular conditions of the dog the reader is referred to Rubin (1989).

### Age

The age of the animal is often relevant to the diagnosis of the ocular condition. Examples of this are the development of nyctalopia and visual impairment in puppies and kittens with photoreceptor dysplasia, leukocoria in Morgan foals or Jersey calves with congenital cataracts and the progressive development of visual impairment late in life with photoreceptor degeneration in the Miniature Poodle dog. Kittens and puppies have their eyelids fused together (ankyloblepharon) for the first 7–14 days of life, which prevents examination of the eye. Vision is limited in neonate as visual pathways and the eye continue to develop during the first months of life. The retina and choroid of the cat and dog are not fully developed until approximately 3 months of age. The menace reflex is a learned reflex and it is usually not present until the animal is a few weeks old.

## Sex

X-linked progressive retinal atrophy has been reported in the male Siberian Husky and is an example of a gender-related eye disease.

## Ophthalmic examination

To prevent one part of the examination interfering with another it should be carried out in the following order

- distant examination and preliminary diagnostic tests
- neuro-ophthalmic examination
- ocular diagnostic tests
- intraocular examination.

## Distant ocular examination and preliminary diagnostic tests

The examination begins by observing the animal from a distance. It is important to note the reaction to new surroundings. If blindness or impaired vision appear likely from the history or physical examination, the animal is observed during navigation of an obstacle course (maze testing) in photopic (light) and scotopic (dark) conditions. An obstacle course is completed by placing a number of boxes, hay bales or similar objects randomly across the animal's pen or examining room and walking the animal through the maze (Fig. 20.11).

---

### Neonatal vision

In the neonate vision is limited as visual pathways and the eye continue to develop during the first months of life

- the retina and choroid of the cat and dog are not fully developed until approximately 3 months of age
- the menace reflex is a learned reflex and is usually not present until the animal is a few days to weeks old.

---

Stumbling into and over objects in a new environment is a clue to impaired vision. The eyes are next observed simultaneously, at a distance of approximately 2 m, through a direct ophthalmoscope or with the aid of a transilluminator in both photopic and scotopic conditions. The light reflection from the fundi will retroilluminate the pupillary margins. Subtle dyscoria, strabismus, or anisocoria, which may change in photopic and scotopic conditions, are readily visible in the tapetal reflex (Fig. 20.12).

Animals will require restraint to complete the remainder of the examination. Standing restraint stocks are appropriate for horses, and cattle are suitably restrained in stanchion devices or with a halter. Sheep can be held and goats are manually restrained with a halter. Pigs are consistently difficult to examine. If small they may be handheld by an assistant; large pigs are held by a wire hog holder or rope. Dogs and cats are held by an assistant on an examining room table. Ocular discharge, swellings, and changes in color and symmetry are noted and the details recorded on the medical record. If an ocular discharge is present a sample may be submitted for virus isolation, bacterial and fungal cultures, and cytological examination. A sterile culture swab is placed on the ocular discharge or lesion while the eyelids are held open (Fig. 20.13). This prevents lid contact and potential contamination of the

---

### Some inherited ocular conditions

- optic nerve coloboma of Charolais cattle
- congenital night blindness of Appaloosa horses
- glucocerebroside storage disease in Yorkshire pigs
- Chédiak–Higashi syndrome of Persian cats
- primary lens luxation of terrier dogs.

---

### Pupillary assessment in the absence of a tapetum

- albinos or animals with a subalbinotic pigmentation often lack a tapetum, but the red reflex from the choroidal vessels is usually adequate to illuminate the pupil and allow this distant pupillary assessment
- pigs lacks a tapetum, but their pigmented fundi preclude the use of this form of pupillary assessment.

swab. Samples for cytology are collected in a similar fashion using a spatula or premoistened sterile swab which is then rolled across a glass slide.

The examination continues with a direct visual inspection of the orbital and eyelid region. The symmetry and position of eyelids and globes are noted. The orbital rims and eyelids are palpated, and the eyes are gently retropulsed into the orbits by digital pressure through the eyelids (Fig. 20.14). This retropulsion alone allows indirect assessment of orbital contents. Orbital masses will restrict retropulsion of the globe and usually cause exophthalmos and prolapse of the third eyelid. The eyelids from the lateral to the medial canthus are examined next. They are gently everted bilaterally to allow examination of the palpebral conjunctiva, tarsal glands, bulbar conjunctiva and episclera. Abnormal hairs or masses are noted if they are detected. The palpebral surface of the third eyelid is examined. To examine the bulbar surface of the third eyelid the leading edge is gently reflected (Fig. 20.15b) with a scleral indentation probe (Fig. 20.15a). Several small follicles are normally visible on the bulbar surface of the third eyelid. The distant and superficial examination of the eyes, orbits and adnexa and preliminary laboratory tests are now complete.

*Neuro-ophthalmic examination*

This examination evaluates the

- menace
- direct and consensual pupillary light
- palpebral, and
- vestibular

ocular reflexes, which are recorded as present or

absent. They evaluate all or part of the

- optic
- oculomotor
- trochlear
- trigeminal
- abducens
- facial, and
- vestibular

nerves and the sympathetic and parasympathetic ocular innervation. The neuro-ophthalmic examination is completed prior to administering sedatives or tranquilizers, topical anesthetics, mydriatic drugs, and regional nerve blocks, as these may prevent or interfere with interpretation of the reflexes. The corneal reflex (touching the cornea to elicit a blink) is not required because of the inherent danger of producing corneal ulceration and the lack of additional useful neurological information.

**Menace reflex and the dropped cotton ball test**

The menace reflex is elicited by making a direct and sudden hand motion across the visual field of the ipsilateral eye while the contralateral eye is covered (Fig. 20.16). The normal response is a blink. Care must be taken to avoid creating air waves which will activate the palpebral reflex. The optic nerve is the afferent and the facial nerve is the efferent pathway of this reflex. A functional orbicularis oculi muscle is also required. This is a learned reflex that may be absent in neonates. A blind animal will respond to facial hair contact by blinking.

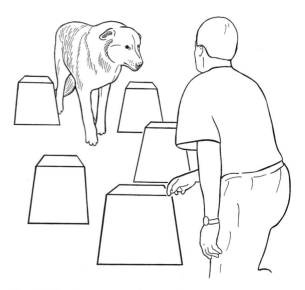

**Fig. 20.11** A maze test where a dog traverses an obstacle course of boxes to get to the owner while the veterinarian observes.

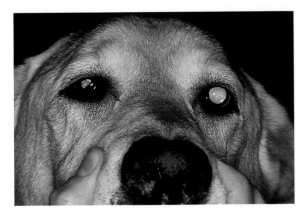

**Fig. 20.12** Tapetal reflex illumination of the pupils of a dog with Horner's syndrome. Note how obvious the anisocoria with left miosis, ptosis, and third eyelid prolapse is with tapetal retroillumination.

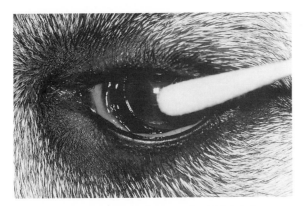

**Fig. 20.13** A moistened culture swab which is being placed on the cornea of a dog, without eyelid contact.

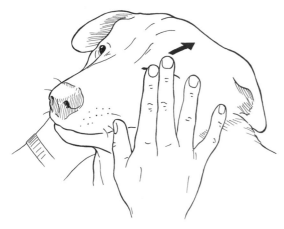

**Fig. 20.14** Retropulsion of the globe into the orbit by moving the eye with the index and middle fingers through closed eyelids. The movement of each eye is compared to subjectively evaluate orbital contents.

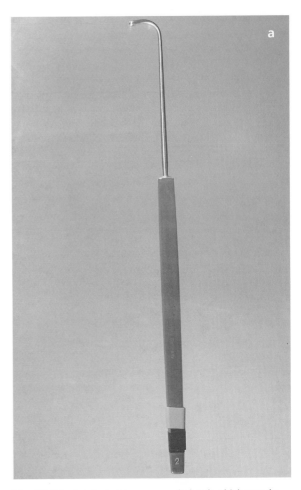

**Fig. 20.15** **(a)** A strabismus muscle hook which may be used to gently reflect the eyelids, explore the conjunctival fornix and indent the sclera as an aid to examination of the peripheral retina. **(b)** The hook is being used to gently reflect the third eyelid of a horse to allow examination of its bulbar surface.

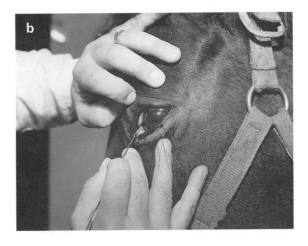

False negative menace reflexes may occur in the docile and complaisant but visual animal. These animals are evaluated by dropping a cotton ball from above the ipsilateral eye while the contralateral eye is covered (Fig. 20.17). The visual eye will usually track the falling object as it flutters through the visual field. When unilateral blindness is suspected on the basis of an absent menace reflex and visual tracking, the scotopic and photopic maze test is repeated with a patch covering or temporary tarsorraphy performed on each eye in turn. All the above only provide crude assessments of vision but they represent the only methods available to the veterinarian.

> ### Clinical Pointer ✳
>
> Place a clear plexiglass plate between the examiner's hand and the animal's visual pathway to prevent false positive menace reflexes in blind animals by stopping air currents and direct facial hair contact.

### Direct and consensual pupillary light reflexes

The direct pupillary light reflex (dPLR) is elicited by shining a bright light through the pupil and observing a prompt pupillary constriction in that eye (Fig. 20.18). This reflex requires

- photoreceptor activation
- the ipsilateral optic nerve as an afferent pathway
- the parasympathetic pathway in the ipsilateral oculomotor nerve as an efferent pathway, and
- a functional ipsilateral iris constrictor muscle.

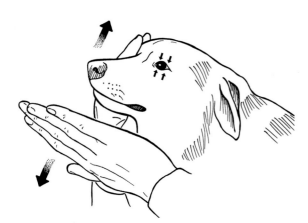

**Fig. 20.16** The menace reflex is elicited by directing a threatening hand motion across the visual pathway of one eye while the other is covered. It is very important to avoid contact between facial hair and the hand or air currents during this process as either will elicit the palpebral reflex.

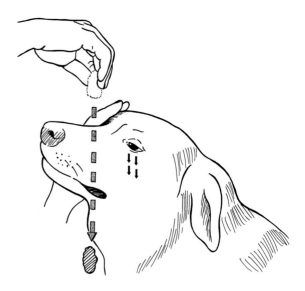

**Fig. 20.17** The dropped cotton ball test is performed by dropping an object through the animal's visual field and observing that eye follow the object while the other is covered.

> ### Clinical Pointer ✳
>
> The lateral position of the globes and darkly pigmented irides of the horse, cow, sheep, and goat make evaluation of the cPLR difficult for one clinician to detect. An assistant is therefore required to simultaneously evaluate the cPLR in these species.

The consensual pupillary light reflex (cPLR) is elicited by observing the contralateral pupil while a focal bright light is directed through the ipsilateral pupil (Fig. 20.18). The cPLR requires

- photoreceptor activation
- an ipsilateral optic nerve as an afferent pathway
- a contralateral parasympathetic pathway in the oculomotor nerve as an efferent pathway
- a functional contralateral iris constrictor muscle.

The cPLR occurs because of decussation of some of the optic nerve fibers at the optic chiasm and pretectal region. A dPLR and cPLR are frequently present in blind animals. This occurs when blindness is the result of a central (brain) lesion. It also occurs when the blindness is the result of retinal or optic nerve disease, where a few functional photoreceptors and optic nerve axons remain. The dPLR and cPLR require only a limited number of photoreceptors and optic nerve axons compared to the large number required for vision.

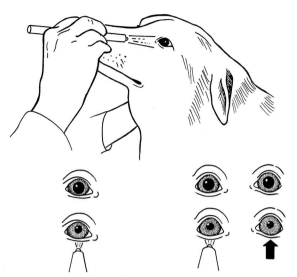

**Fig. 20.18**  The direct pupillary light reflex is a contraction of the ipsilateral pupil when a bright light is shone through it (left). The consensual pupillary light reflex is contraction of the contralateral pupil to that light (right).

### Palpebral reflex

The palpebral reflex is elicited by touching the medial and then the lateral canthus of both eyes (Fig. 20.19). The normal response to eyelid contact is a blink. Failure to blink indicates a lesion in the nerve pathway or the target muscle of this reflex. The afferent nerves for this reflex include the ophthalmic branch of the trigeminal nerve from the medial canthus and the maxillary branch of the trigeminal nerve from the lateral canthus. The efferent nerve is the auriculopalpebral branch of the facial nerve. A functional orbicularis oculi muscle is also required to complete the reflex.

### Vestibular ocular reflex

This reflex is elicited by moving the animal's head from side to side, then up and down while observing the lateral and vertical movements of the eye (Fig. 20.20). It requires functional oculomotor and abducens nerves, a vestibular system and most of the extraocular muscles. The oculomotor nerve supplies the ventral, medial, and dorsal rectus muscles, and the abducens nerve supplies the lateral rectus muscle. Dysfunction of these nerves, their respective extraocular muscles, or the vestibular system will alter the lateral or vertical eye motions of this reflex.

## Ocular diagnostic tests

Once the distant ocular and neuro-ophthalmic examinations are completed the animal is restrained to permit completion of the ocular diagnostic tests. Cattle and horses require sedation and an auriculopalpebral nerve block. Intravenous tranquilizers such as xylazine

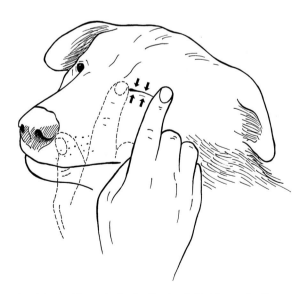

**Fig. 20.19**  The palpebral reflex is elicited by contacting the medial and lateral canthus with the index finger: the normal response is eyelid closure.

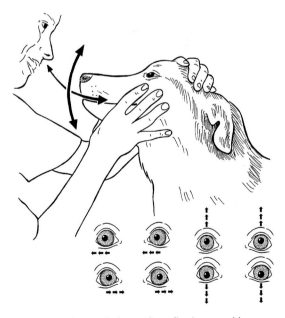

**Fig. 20.20**  The vestibular ocular reflex is created by moving the animal's head from side to side while observing the eyes, which will move together in saccades with the fast motion in the direction of the head movement.

or acepromazine are appropriate to limit continual head motion. A subcutaneous injection of lidocaine over the auriculopalpebral nerve will eliminate the forceful closure of the eyelids and allow an accurate assessment of the ocular diagnostic tests and intraocular examination. Depending on their size and demeanor, the sheep, goat, and pig, and the fractious dog and cat, may require sedation. Ketamine or oxymorphone are excellent choices in the dog and cat because they affect eye and lid position only minimally.

### Clinical Pointer ✱

Avoid using ketamine as a sedative when glaucoma is suspected because it may increase the intraocular pressure.

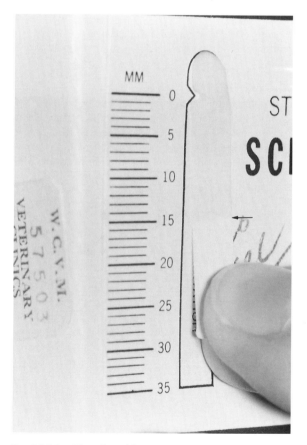

**Fig. 20.21**   A Schirmer tear strip placed in the ventral medial conjunctival fornix of a dog; it will be left there for 1 minute to stimulate and absorb the reflex tears.

### Schirmer tear test

This test evaluates reflex tear production in millimeters of wetting on a paper strip. The strips can be manufactured from No. 40 Whatman filter paper, or are available commercially (Fig. 20.6).

1. One strip is slashed obliquely at one end and the other is square to allow identification of the right and left eye when they are simultaneously removed from the eyes.
2. One end of each strip is notched (Fig. 20.6) and the strips are folded at this notch, without direct finger contact to avoid grease or oil contamination of the absorptive end.
3. The folded ends are placed in the ventral conjunctival fornix of both eyes and are left for 1 minute (Fig. 20.21).
4. The strips are then removed and immediately placed on a measuring gauge to determine the millimeters of wetting per minute (Fig. 20.22).

Cattle, sheep, goats, and horses usually produce copious quantities of tears, often exceeding 20–30 mm of wetting in 30 seconds. Schirmer tear test values less than 5 mm in the cat and 10 mm in other domestic animals are indicative of diminished production of the aqueous portion of tears and support the diagnosis of keratoconjunctivitis sicca.

### Schirmer tear test values

Values less than 5 mm in the cat and 10 mm in other domestic animals are indicative of diminished production of the aqueous portion of tears and suggest keratoconjunctivitis sicca.

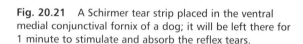

**Fig. 20.22**   After the Schirmer tear strip has been in the ventral conjunctival fornix for 1 minute (**Fig. 20.21**) it is removed and immediately placed on a measuring gauge and the millimeters of wetting are determined. In this example these are approximately 15 mm (arrow), which is within the normal reference range of 10–25 mm.

The phenol red thread tear test has been suggested as an alternative, perhaps superior, assay of tear production in cats; however, its use in veterinary medicine to date is limited by a lack of commercial availability. A Schirmer tear test II has been reported. This measures basal tear secretion after the conjunctiva and cornea have been topically anesthetized, but it has limited clinical application.

**Fluorescein stain**

Fluorescein staining is applied topically, as an impregnated paper strip on the cornea and conjunctiva (Fig. 20.23) to

- detect ulcers
- assess the integrity of corneal perforations (Seidal test), and
- determine the quality of the tear film (tear breakup time).

Fluorescein is hydrophilic and readily stains the tear film. It also stains the corneal stroma and conjunctival substantia propria when the lipophilic epithelial barriers are broken (ulcers). Fluorescein dye is commercially available as an impregnated strip and as a liquid in minim containers (Fig. 20.7a,b). When using the strips follow a standard procedure.

1. Physiological eye wash is allowed to run over the fluorescein-impregnated end to form a drop.
2. One drop of liquid fluorescein from this strip or the minim container is placed on to the upper bulbar conjunctiva of each eye (Fig. 20.23).
3. The corneal and conjunctival surfaces are promptly and thoroughly rinsed with a physiological eyewash solution. Thorough rinsing is required to remove the stain from corneal and conjunctival mucus or corneal facets, to prevent false positive interpretation.
4. The surfaces of the cornea and conjunctiva are examined in scotopic conditions with cobalt blue filtered or ultraviolet light (Woods lamp). These forms of light induce fluorescence of the stain and enhance detection of corneal and conjunctival ulcers (Fig. 20.24).

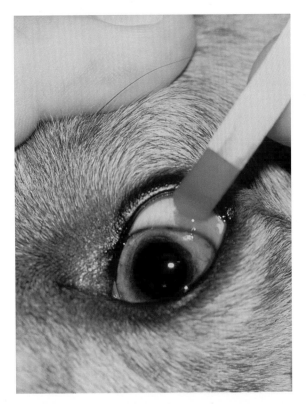

**Fig. 20.23** A drop of liquid fluorescein is placed on the bulbar conjunctiva.

---

**Clinical Pointer**

Specimens for immune fluorescent antibody testing should be collected prior to using fluorescein because false positive assays have been reported after its use.

**Tonometry**

Tonometry is the estimation of intraocular pressure and is an essential diagnostic test in all ocular examina-tions. The cornea is anesthetized by 1–2 drops of topical corneal anesthetic and the tonometer is positioned over the central cornea while the eyelids are restrained. For accurate estimation of intraocular pressure

- consistent head restraint
- careful tonometer positioning
- corneal anesthesia, and, in horses and cattle
- sedation and auricular palpebral nerve blocks

are required. Head position, impaired venous return from the head due to excessive neck restraint, and digital pressure on the eyelids, globe, and orbit during tonometry may elevate the intraocular pressure.

Indentation tonometers (Shiotz) (Fig. 20.4) are useful for estimating the intraocular pressure in

---

**Clinical Pointer**

Indentation tonometry is contraindicated in perforated and potentially perforated eyes.

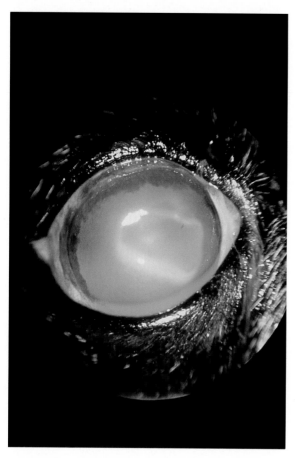

**Fig. 20.24** A corneal ulcer that has been stained with fluorescein, rinsed with eyewash and illuminated with cobalt filtered light.

smaller animals (dog, cat), who tolerate muzzle elevation and repeated vertical placements of a Shiotz tonometer on to the cornea (Fig. 20.25). For accurate estimation of intraocular pressures, an average of three readings is calculated on each eye with the 5.5 g weight on the Schiotz tonometer. The average Shiotz readings are converted to mmHg with a conversion table that has been developed for the dog and cat (Table 20.2). If the averaged readings estimate the intraocular pressure between 25 and 35 mmHg then the procedure is repeated with a 7.5 g weight and, if necessary, a 10 g weight to ensure consistent estimations in either the normal or the glaucomatous range.

In order for the Schiotz tonometer to function well it must be dismantled, cleaned with alcohol and a pipe cleaner, and dried after each use.

Applanation tonometers (Fig. 20.5) estimate the intraocular pressure by flattening a predetermined corneal surface area. The force of this flattening is automatically converted by the tonometer into intraocular pressure in mmHg. They are required for measuring intraocular pressure in horses and cattle, and are also appropriate for the sheep, goat, pig, dog, and cat. The tonometer is positioned perpendicular to the curved cornea surface and the condom-covered tip gently touches the epithelium (Fig. 20.26) repeatedly until an automatically averaged reading with less than 5% error is attained. The condom is left on the instrument after each usage and is replaced with a sterile one prior to the next examination. This protects the delicate tip during storage. Unfortunately these tonometers are expensive and currently unavailable to most veterinarians.

### Intraocular examination

#### Examination of the anterior segment (cornea, anterior and posterior chamber, iris, and lens) by direct and retroillumination

The examining room is completely darkened for this procedure. A focal light is directed at the cornea and the entire cornea examined for clarity and curvature. The iris and the anterior chamber are examined similarly, by directing the light both acutely and obtusely into the eye. Pupillary dilatation is required for a complete examination of the lens, posterior chamber and posterior segment with a direct ophthalmoscope, transilluminator or indirect ophthalmoscope and converging lens. Mydriasis is achieved by topical corneal administration of a mydriatic. Tropicamide (0.5% solution) is the preferred agent in domestic animals because of its fast onset of action, short duration, and lack of cycloplegia (ciliary muscle paresis). One drop is placed on each cornea and this is repeated in 10 minutes. Within 20 minutes the pupils should be dilated and will remain so for approximately 4 hours.

---

### Intraocular pressures

- normal pressure range in the dog, cat, cattle, sheep, and goat is 15–30 mmHg
- normal pressure range in the horse is 15–35 mmHg
- there is usually less than 8 mmHg difference between normal eyes
- elevated intraocular pressure confirms the diagnosis of glaucoma
- decreased intraocular pressure in an intact globe is usually consistent with the diagnosis of uveitis.

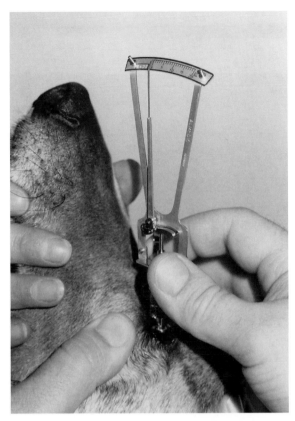

**Fig. 20.25** Placement of the Schiotz tonometer on a dog's cornea. Note the vertical instrument and the Shiotz reading (0). The tonometer reading will be measured three times, averaged, and then converted to mmHg by a conversion table (Table 20.2). In this case the average of the three Schiotz readings was 1; using the conversion table this is an intraocular pressure of 42 mmHg, which is consistent with the diagnosis of glaucoma.

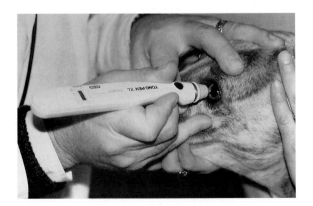

**Fig. 20.26** The applanation tonometer is positioned on to the central cornea of a dog and the tip will be repeatedly gently touched to the cornea until an average reading is established.

When a focal light is directed through the dilated pupil in scotopic conditions three light reflections can be seen. These are the Purkinje–Sanson images (Fig. 20.27) and represent reflection of light from the

- cornea
- anterior lens capsule, and
- posterior lens capsule.

The position of these three reflections allows the examiner to determine the approximate position of lesions in the clear ocular media. For example, a lesion in the anterior lens capsule may obliterate the second or third Purkinje–Sanson image, whereas a lesion in the cornea may obliterate all three reflections.

The biomicroscope (slit lamp) is a combination of a mobile light source and a microscope that utilizes the Purkinje–Sanson images and permits a thorough examination of the anterior segment. The biomicroscope allows magnified examination of the cornea, iris, anterior and posterior chambers, lens, and anterior vitreous. This instrument is available as table-mounted or handheld models. The handheld version (Fig. 20.8) is preferred for examination of the anterior segment in the horse, cattle, sheep, goat, pig, dog, and cat, but it is a difficult instrument to master and is not readily available. The clinician is encouraged to read the following introductory references on biomicroscopy (Martin 1969a,b,c) before using the instrument. However, a careful examination of the anterior segment with a focal light source, directly and with retroillumination, will suffice and allow visualization of most of the intraocular lesions that are detectable with a biomicroscope.

**Examination of the eye with the direct ophthalmoscope**

A direct ophthalmoscope (Fig. 20.2B,C) may be used for examining the entire eye using the following procedure.

1. The direct ophthalmoscopic examination occurs in close proximity to the eye.
2. The power source to the ophthalmoscope is activated by depressing the red button on the neck of the instrument and rotating it clockwise.
3. The diopter wheel on the examiner's side of the instrument is rotated until a 0 diopter lens is noted in the lens aperture (Fig. 20.28A).
4. The large light spot and no filters (Fig. 20.28B) are selected and the eyebrow piece is placed on the examiner's eyebrow.
5. To achieve retinal focus with the 0 diopter lens in position, the instrument is held approximately 2–3 cm from the surface of the animal's eye.

**Table 20.2.    Shiotz conversion table for the dog and cat**

| Schiotz Scale Reading | Values in cats | | | Values in dogs | | |
|---|---|---|---|---|---|---|
| | IOP (mm Hg) 5.5 g wt. | IOP (mm Hg) 7.5 g wt. | IOP (mm Hg) 10.0 g wt. | IOP (mm Hg) 5.5 g wt. | IOP (mm Hg) 7.5 g wt. | IOP (mm Hg) 10.0 g wt. |
| 0.5 | 44 | 73 | – | 46 | 61 | 75 |
| 1.0 | 42 | 71 | – | 44 | 59 | 73 |
| 1.5 | 40 | 68 | – | 43 | 56 | 70 |
| 2.0 | 37 | 65 | 80 | 40 | 53 | 66 |
| 2.5 | 33 | 61 | 76 | 33 | 47 | 61 |
| 3.0 | 30 | 56 | 71 | 26 | 40 | 55 |
| 3.5 | 27 | 48 | 66 | 23 | 35 | 49 |
| 4.0 | 25 | 42 | 61 | 21 | 32 | 44 |
| 4.5 | 24 | 37 | 56 | 20 | 29 | 41 |
| 5.0 | 22 | 34 | 51 | 19 | 27 | 38 |
| 5.5 | 21 | 31 | 47 | 18 | 26 | 36 |
| 6.0 | 20 | 29 | 44 | 17 | 24 | 33 |
| 6.5 | 18 | 27 | 40 | 16 | 23 | 31 |
| 7.0 | – | 25 | 37 | 15 | 22 | 30 |
| 7.5 | 17 | 24 | 35 | – | 20 | 28 |
| 8.0 | 16 | 22 | 33 | 14 | 19 | 27 |
| 8.5 | 15 | 21 | 31 | 13 | – | 25 |
| 9.0 | 14 | 20 | 29 | – | 18 | 24 |
| 9.5 | 13 | 19 | 27 | 12 | 17 | 23 |
| 10.0 | – | 18 | 25 | – | 16 | 22 |
| 10.5 | – | 17 | 23 | 11 | 15 | 21 |
| 11.0 | 12 | 16 | 22 | – | – | 20 |
| 11.5 | 11 | 15 | 20 | 10 | 14 | 19 |
| 12.0 | – | 14 | 19 | – | 13 | 18 |
| 12.5 | 10 | 13 | 18 | – | – | 17 |
| 13.0 | – | 12 | 17 | – | 12 | 16 |
| 13.5 | 9 | – | 15 | 8 | 11 | 15 |
| 14.0 | – | 11 | 14 | – | – | – |
| 14.5 | 8 | 10 | 13 | – | 10 | 14 |
| 15.0 | – | – | 12 | 7 | – | 13 |
| 15.5 | – | 9 | 11 | – | 9 | 12 |
| 16.0 | 7 | 8 | 10 | – | – | – |
| 16.5 | – | – | 9 | 6 | 8 | 11 |
| 17.0 | 6 | 7 | 8 | – | – | 10 |
| 17.5 | – | 6 | 7 | – | 7 | – |
| 18.0 | – | – | 6 | 5 | – | 9 |
| 18.5 | 5 | 5 | 5 | – | 6 | – |
| 19.0 | – | – | – | – | – | 8 |
| 20.0 | – | – | – | – | 5 | – |

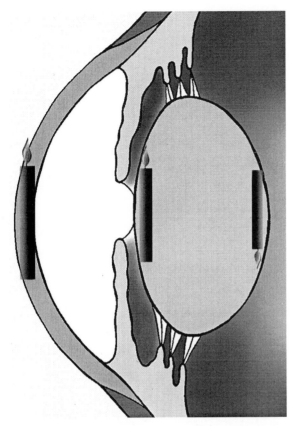

**Fig. 20.27** The Purkinje–Sanson images as depicted by a candle reflection in the cornea, anterior lens capsule and posterior lens capsule. These are reflections of light which are present when a light is directed into the eye. They are very important in localizing the position of an opacity in the eye.

### Retroillumination

- this occurs when a light is directed through the pupil and the reflection off the tapetum illuminates the anterior segment
- retroillumination after pupillary dilatation is essential for the detection and localization of small opacities in the anterior segment of the eye
- opacities or masses detected in the cornea, anterior or posterior chamber, and lens, or changes in the iris color or pupil shape are noted
- if possible, photographs of anterior segment lesions are obtained as they are useful for long-term evaluation.

6. The patients' right eye may be examined with the examiner's right eye, and the left eye with the examiner's left eye (Fig. 20.29A,B).
7. Initially, the optic disk is located by examination of the central and medial fundus.
8. Once the disk is identified, its color and contour are noted, and retinal vessels are observed as they cross over the disk.
9. The posterior ocular segment is examined in quadrants. In species that have a holangiotic (completely vascularized) retina, such as cattle, sheep, goats, pigs, dogs, and cats, the retinal vessels divide the fundus into quadrants. The horse has a paurangiotic retina, which means that the retinal vessels are limited to the periphery of the optic disk. The fundic quadrants are therefore established arbitrarily.
10. Each quadrant is examined, starting at the optic disk and progressing outwards to the ora ciliaris retina.

The structures to be examined in the fundus include

- the retina (which is normally translucent)
- retinal blood vessels, and
- the tapetum and non-tapetal region.

### Clinical Pointer

Direct ophthalmoscopy has the inherent disadvantage of providing high magnification – approximately 15 times – and makes complete examination of the entire ocular structure tedious and difficult.

When the fundus is subalbinotic or the animal is an albino, the lack of pigment allows examination of the choroidal vessels and portions of the sclera. Retinal or optic disk lesions are recorded in detail or, if possible, photographed with a fundic camera.

Domestic animals have variable tapetal patterns and colors, optic disk shapes, and retinal blood vessel patterns. Typical fundic patterns of the horse, cattle, sheep, goat, pig, dog and cat are shown in Figures 20.30–20.38.

After the fundic examination is complete the diopter wheel may be moved clockwise with the index finger. This moves a series of positive diopter lenses through the viewing field and allows the examiner to focus on closer objects (vitreous, lens), provided the distance between the direct ophthalmoscope and the animal is constant. As each structure is identified it is examined in a quadrant fashion, starting in the center and

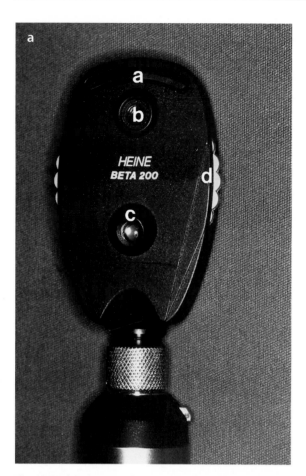

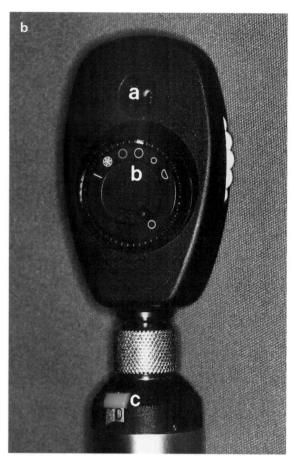

**Fig. 20.28 (a)** Close-up photograph of the direct ophthalmoscope from the examiners' side. Note the eyebrow rest (a), viewing aperture (b), the diopter indicator window (c) and the diopter wheel (d). **(b)** Close-up photograph of the direct ophthalmoscope from the patients' side. Note the light aperture (a), light filter and aperture control wheel (b) and the power control switch (c).

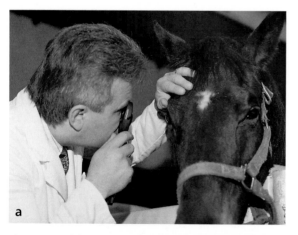

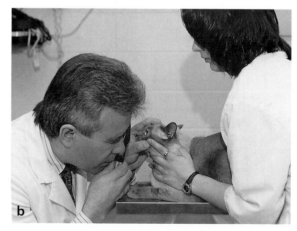

**Fig. 20.29** **(a)** A direct ophthalmoscope being used to examine a horse's eye. Note the close proximity of the examiner to the horse. The examiner uses his right eye to examine the horses' right eye. **(b)** A direct ophthalmoscope being used to examine a cats' left eye. Note that the examiner's left eye is used to examine the cats' left eye.

moving laterally. Lesions are drawn or photographed and described in the medical record.

### Indirect ophthalmoscopic examination of the posterior segment (vitreous and fundus)

Indirect ophthalmoscopy is performed by shining a focal light from a transilluminator (Fig. 20.2a) or from a binocular head set (Fig. 20.9) through a converging lens (Fig. 20.3) and the animal's pupil at arm's length in scotopic conditions (Figs 20.39, 20.40 on page 568). The converging lens is held approximately 6–8 cm from the animal's eye. The fundic image seen is an **inverted** mirror image that is only minimally magnified (2–4 times). The headset with a self-contained light source provides binocular evaluation with superior depth perception of the fundus through the converging lens, and allows the examiner to use one hand to restrain the animal's head.

---

### Clinical Pointer ✳

Indirect ophthalmoscopy requires practice to master but is the method of choice for fundic examination in all domestic species. The low magnification allows a quick and complete examination of the vitreous and fundus.

---

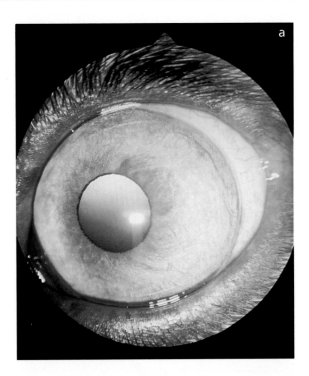

The indirect examination proceeds as described for direct ophthalmoscopy by identification of the optic disk. The disk, fundus, and vitreous are then examined in quadrants. The appearance of the fundus varies widely between and within species and individual animals. Photographs of normal fundi are provided for each domestic animal described in this chapter (Figs 20.30–20.38). The vitreous is usually examined last by moving the converging lens away from the cornea to focus anterior to the retina.

## Ancillary diagnostic testing

Several ancillary diagnostic tests may be required after the initial examination is completed. These include

- nasolacrimal duct flushing
- special stains, and
- imaging techniques.

---

### Normal vitreous

The normal vitreous is identified as faint white veils of collagen fibers suspended in clear fluid. It is the most difficult portion of the posterior segment to visualize.

---

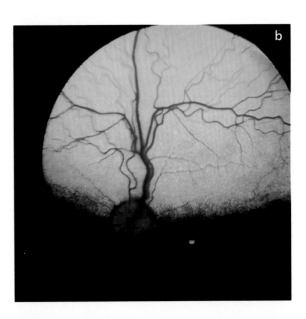

**Fig. 20.30** **(a)** The anterior segment of a normal pigmented dog eye. Note the three color bands in the iris, the round pupil and the yellow tapetal reflex. **(b)** Fundus photograph of the dog in **(a)**. Note the blue-green tapetum, the dark non-tapetal region, and the numerous retinal veins and arteries extending over the retina from the optic disk.

563

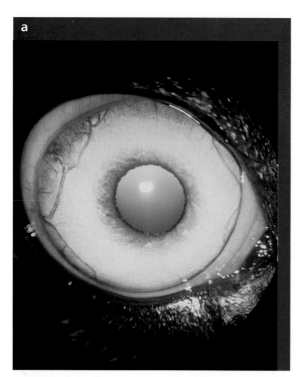

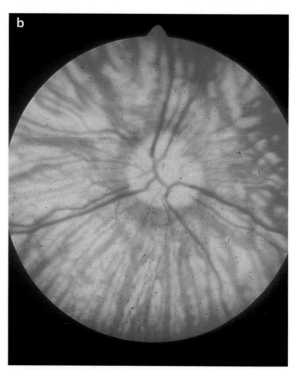

**Fig. 20.31** (a) Anterior segment of a normal dog with a poorly pigmented (subalbinotic) eye. Note the blue iris with three distinct color bands, and the pink fundic reflex visible in the pupil. (b) Fundus photograph of the normal dog in (a). Note the lack of tapetum and the extension of red retinal veins and arteries from the optic disk across the retina, which overlies the orange-red choroidal blood vessels. The faint yellow streaks between the choroidal vessels are sclera that lie underneath the choroid. The sclera and choroid are clearly seen in this dog because of a lack of pigment and tapetum.

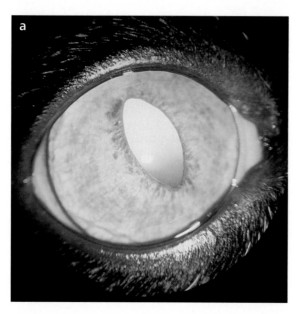

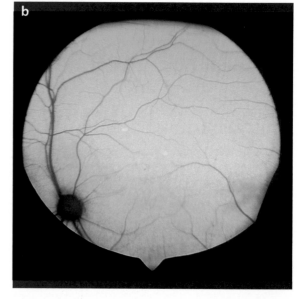

**Fig. 20.32** (a) Anterior segment of a normal domestic short-haired cat. Note the pale yellow iris, the oval pupil and the yellow tapetal reflex. (b) Fundus photograph of the cat in (a). Note the large yellow tapetum, the small round optic disk and the retinal veins and arteries that extend from the optic disk across the retina.

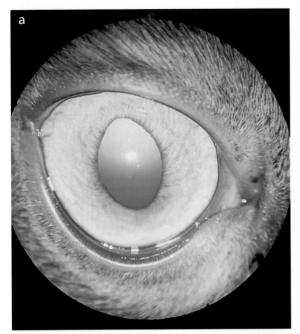
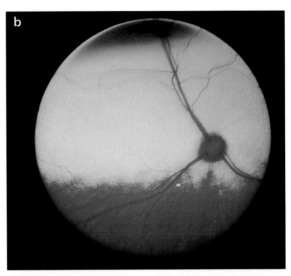

**Fig. 20.33** (a) Anterior segment of a normal cat with a subalbinotic eye. Note the blue iris, oval pupil and the reddish tapetal reflex. (b) Fundus photograph of the cat in (a). Note the bright yellow tapetum, the pale round optic disk, the red retinal blood vessels extending from the disk across the retina, and the lack of pigment in the non-tapetal area, which exposes the orange-red choroidal vessels and small strips of sclera.

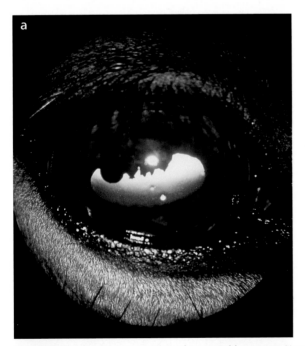
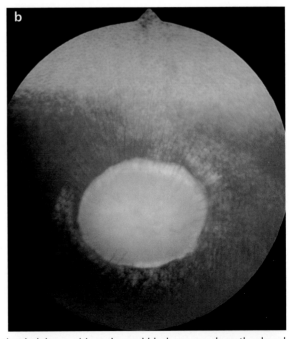

**Fig. 20.34** (a) Anterior segment of a normal horse eye. Note the dark brown iris and round black masses along the dorsal edge of the pupil (corpora nigra), and the yellow tapetal reflex. (b) Fundus photograph of the horse in (a). Note the oval salmon-pink optic disk with small retinal blood vessels that extend only a few millimeters across the retina (paurangiotic). A few orange choroidal blood vessels are also visible around the optic disk. The tapetum is partially seen as a blue crescent above the optic disk and the non-tapetal region is dark brown.

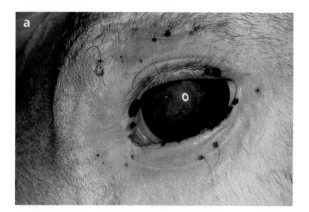

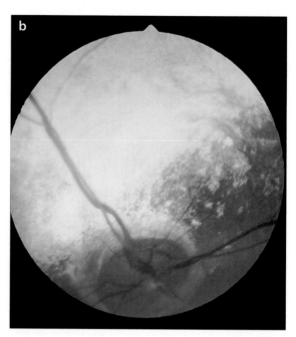

**Fig. 20.35** **(a)** Anterior segment of a normal cow's eye. Note the dark brown iris, oval pupil, and corpora nigra along its dorsal border. **(b)** Fundus photograph of the cow's eye in **(a)**. Note the large gray (poorly myelinated) optic disk, the large retinal veins which twist around one another as they extend over the retina, the small straight retinal arteries visible over the blue tapetum, and the brown non-tapetal region. The white strip centered on the disk is a remnant of the primary vitreous.

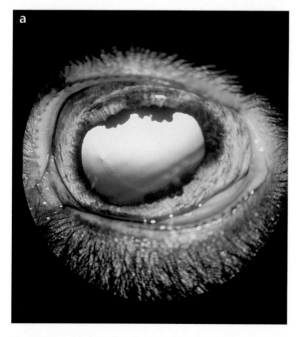

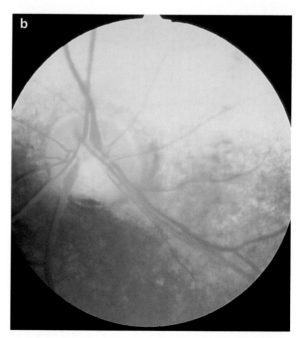

**Fig. 20.36** **(a)** Anterior segment of a normal sheep's eye. Note the dark brown iris, the corpora nigra and the oval pupil. **(b)** Fundus photograph of the sheep's eye in **(a)**. Note the oval bean-shaped optic disk, red retinal blood vessels, blue tapetum, and the dark brown non-tapetal region.

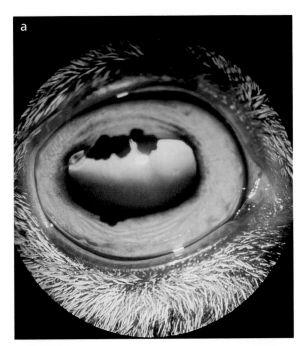

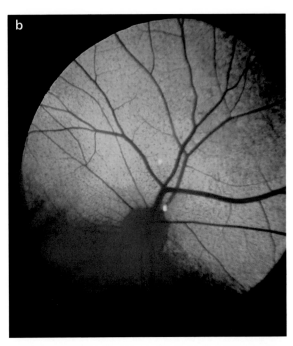

**Fig. 20.37**  (a) Anterior segment of a goat's eye. Note the yellow iris, oval pupil with corpora nigra along its dorsal and ventral margin, and the tapetal reflex. (b) Fundus photograph of the goat's eye in (a). Note the round dark optic disk, red retinal blood vessels, blue tapetum, and dark brown non-tapetal region.

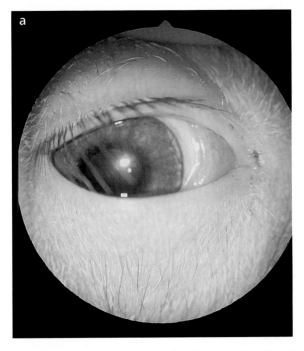

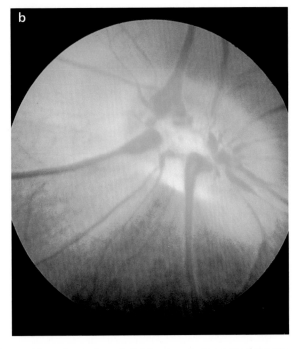

**Fig. 20.38 (a)** Anterior segment of a pig's eye. Note the pale brown iris and round pupil. **(b)** Fundus photograph of the pig in **(a)**. Note the white streaks of myelin and red retinal blood vessels emanating from the oval optic disk. There is no tapetum (normal for the pig), and brown pigment covers the choroidal vessels.

### Nasolacrimal cannulation and flushing

The nasolacrimal drainage system is normally present for each eye and includes a superior and inferior puncta and canaliculi, and a nasolacrimal duct (Fig. 20.41). Tears flow across the cornea with the assistance

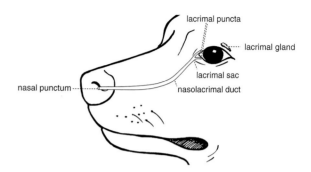

**Fig. 20.41** The nasolacrimal drainage system of the dog. Note the dorsal and ventral puncta and canaliculi which join to form the nasolacrimal duct, which drains into the ventral nostril.

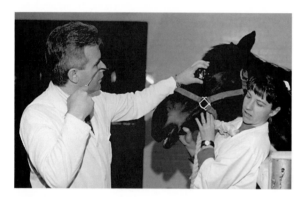

**Fig. 20.39** Indirect ophthalmoscopy where the examiner is using a transilluminator to direct light through a 20 diopter converging lens to examine a horse's fundus. Note the arm's length position away from the horse.

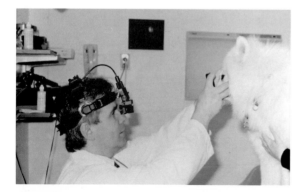

**Fig. 20.40** Indirect ophthalmoscopy using a binocular indirect headset. Note that the examiner is positioned at arms' length from the dog while directing a beam of light through the examination lens and pupil.

of the eyelids. Gravity and a slight negative pressure in the nasolacrimal canaliculi (induced by contraction of the orbicularis oculi muscle) result in tear flow through the puncta and canaliculi, and out of the nasolacrimal duct into the nostril.

Chronic epiphora and ocular discharge are clinical signs that warrant nasolacrimal flushing, which may be completed in a normo- or retrograde fashion to evaluate the patency of the drainage system. Conjunctival, canaliculus, and nasolacrimal duct anesthesia are attained by placement of topical anesthetic solution.

Normograde flushing is performed in small animals with a curved lacrimal cannula or a 20–24 gauge intravenous catheter without the stylet (Fig. 20.42). A syringe containing sterile eyewash is attached to the catheter or lacrimal cannula, which is inserted into the inferior or superior lacrimal puncta and the eyewash is injected (Fig. 20.43). Gentle pressure should evoke a stream of eyewash out of the contralateral puncta, if it is present and not obstructed. The injection is continued after the contralateral puncta has been gently occluded. With occlusion of the other puncta, continued injection should evoke a prompt swallowing reflex or a stream of fluid from the ipsilateral nasal opening, depending on the head position.

An inability to flush the nasolacrimal duct normogradely is an indication for a retrograde flush. This is

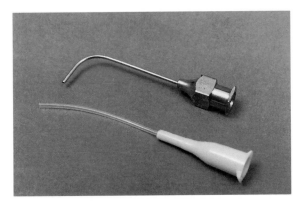

**Fig. 20.42** A metal nasolacrimal cannula and an intravenous catheter without the stylet.

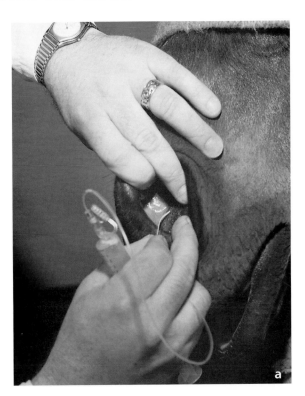

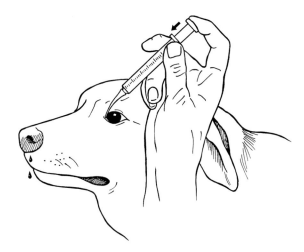

**Fig. 20.43** A normograde nasolacrimal flush in a dog. The upper puncta and canaliculi have been cannulated with a 24 gauge intravenous catheter and eyewash solution is being injected and seen exiting the nostril.

completed after identification and cannulation of the nasolacrimal duct orifice in the ventral lateral nostril (Fig. 20.44 a,b,c). A 6 Fr silastic feeding catheter is appropriate for the horse and smaller soft feeding tubes or catheters will suffice in other species. Eyewash is flushed up the nasolacrimal duct and occluding debris is usually dislodged. Discharge material that is flushed or backwashed from the nasolacrimal system may be retrieved for laboratory examination.

**Fig. 20.44** **(a)** Cannulation of the left nasolacrimal duct orifice in a horse with a #5 silicone feeding tube. **(b)** The feeding tube is stabilized in the nasolacrimal duct by digital pressure and the eyewash solution is slowly injected retrogradely.

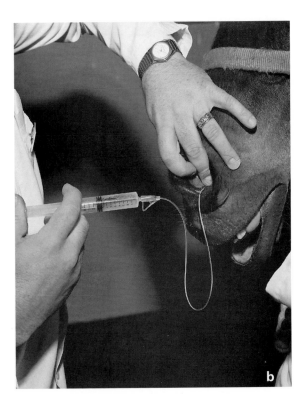

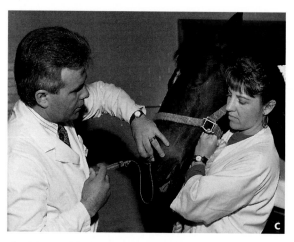

Fig. 20.44 (c) The horse is just starting to blink as tears and eyewash solution begin to well up in the medial canthus. This confirms a patent left nasolacrimal duct in this horse.

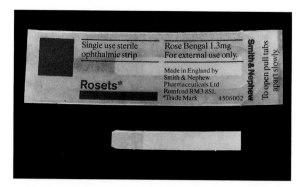

Figure 20.45 Rose Bengal-impregnated strip.

## Special stains

### Rose Bengal

This stain is available commercially as an impregnated paper strip (Fig. 20.45). Rose Bengal is a supravital dye used to stain necrotic or degenerating epithelial cells. It is applied to the surface of the eye as a solution and promptly rinsed away with liberal volumes of eyewash. The stained cornea is then examined with unfiltered light. Interpretation can be difficult because excess stain has been reported to penetrate normal corneal epithelium even after minimal topical exposure, thereby creating false positive staining. It has been used to confirm multifocal punctate erosions in herpes virus keratitis.

### Clinical Pointer ✳

Rose Bengal stain has antiviral and antibacterial properties, and all cultures should be collected before it is used.

### Tear break-up time (BUT)

This is similar to the fluorescein staining procedure, except that the concentrated dye is allowed to pool on the horizontally positioned cornea while the animal's eyelids are restrained to prevent the blink reflex. With the aid of a biomicroscope or direct ophthalmoscope and a cobalt blue filter in scotopic conditions, the thick green stain on the cornea is observed while the examination is timed. When tear evaporation and break-up

of the green tear surface is detected, the time is noted. Tear break-up times less than 10 seconds in the dog have been reported to be associated with qualitative tear film abnormalities (lipid or mucin deficiencies).

### Clinical Pointer ✳

The tear break-up time test has not been reported in the horse or food animals, but it is recommended in animals with a diffuse keratitis of unknown etiology and normal Schirmer tear tests.

### Seidel's test

This test is used to confirm leakage of aqueous humor from corneal perforations. Several drops of concentrated fluorescein are placed onto the cornea and the stained tear film around the suspect perforation is observed under cobalt blue filtered light as described for the tear BUT. Small black rivulets of aqueous humor will be noted streaming into the fluorescein stain around a leaking corneal perforation. If these rivulets are not detected around the perforation, **gentle** pressure may be applied to the eye through the eyelids while the perforated area is observed.

### Leaking corneal perforations

Leaking corneal perforations require prompt surgical closure.

## Imaging and additional examination techniques

Additional diagnostic and ophthalmologic procedures allows the veterinary ophthalmologist to complete in-depth examinations.

### Gonioscopy

Gonioscopy is examination of the filtration angle. It is recommended when glaucoma is present or impending, and when inflammatory or neoplastic masses are present at the limbus, base of the iris or ciliary body. Only a small portion of the lateral and medial filtration angle is directly visible in cattle, horses and sheep. Gonioscopy lenses are required for complete examination of the filtration angle in all domestic species except the cat, where the entire angle is visible by direct examination. An introductory reference on gonioscopy is recommended reading (Martin 1969d).

### Ultrasonography

Complete opacification of the cornea precludes direct examination of the contents of the eye. A mature cortical cataract or mass in the anterior chamber or vitreous may preclude visualization of the posterior segment. Ultrasound, CT, and MRI allow detailed examination of the eye and orbit despite such opacities. Intraocular or orbital masses observed with these types of imaging may require

- fine needle aspiration and cytological examination, or
- orbital exploration, biopsy, and histological examination

to establish a diagnosis. These are difficult procedures with inherent risks and referral to an ophthalmologist is recommended.

### Electroretinography

The electrical activity generated by varied portions of the retina after light stimulation of the photoreceptors can be examined by electroretinography and oscillatory potentials. These techniques are invaluable aids for the ophthalmic surgeon prior to cataract removal, as they allow assessment of the electrophysiology of the retina through an opaque lens.

### Other procedures

Fluorescein angiography is used primarily as a research tool in animals to study the blood–ocular barrier. The outflow of aqueous humor from the eye has been measured by tonography. The thickness of the cornea may be accurately measured by pachymetry. This equipment is sophisticated, expensive, and not required for primary ophthalmic care.

## Referrals to Certified Veterinary Ophthalmologists

Veterinary clinicians who require further information on these specialized ophthalmic examination procedures are encouraged to consult the introductory references provided. Referral to a veterinary ophthalmologist should be considered when the diagnosis cannot be established, when glaucoma, ocular perforation, blindness, ocular or orbital masses are present, and when intraocular surgery is required.

## FURTHER READING

Acland GM, Blanton SH, Hersfield B, Aguirre GD. XLPRA: a canine retinal degeneration inherited as an X-linked trait. American Journal of Medical Genetics 1994; 52: 27–33.

Aguirre G, Alligood J, O'Brien P, Buyukmihci N. Pathogenesis of rod–cone degeneration in Miniature poodles. Investigative Ophthalmology and Visual Science 1982; 23: 610–630.

Barnett KC, Ogden AL. Ocular coloboma in Charolais cattle. Veterinary Record 1972; 91: 592.

Beech J, Aguirre G, Gross S. Congenital nuclear cataracts in the Morgan horse. Journal of the American Veterinary Medical Association 1984; 184: 1363–1365.

Brown M, Brightman A, Davidson H, Moore-Dickson T, Butine M. The phenol red thread tear test in cats. Proceedings of the American College of Veterinary Ophthalmology 1994; 25: 33–34.

Brightman A. Rose Bengal: an ocular pharmacology update. Proceedings of the American College of Veterinary Ophthalmology 1993; 24: 16–17.

Buyukmihci N, Aguirre G, Marshall J. Retinal degeneration in the dog III. Development of the retina in rod–cone dysplasia. Experimental Eye Research 1980; 30: 575–591.

Calia CM, Kirschner SE, Baer KE, Stefanacci JD. The use of computed tomography scan for the evaluation of orbital disease in cats and dogs. Prog Veterinary Comp Ophthalmol 1994; 4: 24–30.

Collier LL, King EJ, Prieur DJ. Tapetal degeneration in cats with Chediak–Higashi syndrome. Current Eye Research 1985; 4: 767–773.

Craig EL. Fluorescein and other dyes. In: Mauger TF, Craig EL (eds) Havener's ocular pharmacology, 6th edn. London: Mosby, 1994; 451–467.

Curtis R, Barnett KC. Primary lens luxations in the dog. Journal of Small Animal Practice 1980; 21: 657–668.

Curtis R, Barnett KC, Leon A. An early onset retinal dystrophy with dominant inheritance in the Abyssinian cat. Investi Ophthalmol Vis Sci 1987; 28: 131–139.

da Silva Curiel JMA, Nasisse MP, Hook R, Wilson HH, Collins BK, Mandell CP. Topical fluorescein dye: effects on immunofluorescent antibody tests for feline herpesvirus keratoconjunctivitis. Prog Veterinary Comp Ophthalmol 1991; 1: 99–104.

Dziezyc J, Hager DA. Ocular ultrasonography in veterinary medicine. Seminars in Veterinary Medicine and Surgery 1988; 3: 1–9.

Gelatt KN. Ophthalmic examination and diagnostic procedures. In: Gelatt KN (ed) Veterinary ophthalmology, 2nd edn. London: Lea & Febiger, 1991; 196–197.

Gelatt KN, Gwin RM, Peiffer RL, Gum GG. Tonography in the normal and glaucomatous beagle. American Journal of Veterinary Research 1977; 38: 515–520.

Gelatt KN, Henderson JD, Steffen GR. Fluorescein angiography of the normal and diseased ocular fundi of the laboratory dog. Journal of the American Veterinary Medical Association 1976; 169: 980–984.

Gilger BC, Whitley RD, McLaughlin SA, Wright JC, Drane JW. Canine corneal thickness measured by ultrasonic pachymetry. American Journal of Veterinary Research 1991; 52: 1570–1572.

Grahn BH, Stewart WA, Towner RA, Noseworthy MD. Magnetic resonance imaging of the canine and feline eye, orbit, and optic nerves and its clinical application. Canadian Veterinary Journal 1993; 34: 418–424.

Martin CL. Slit lamp examination of the normal canine anterior segment. Part I. Introduction and techniques. Journal of Small Animal Practice 1969a; 10: 143–149.

Martin CL. Slit lamp examination of the normal canine anterior ocular segment. Part II. Description. Journal of Small Animal Practice 1969b; 10: 151–162.

Martin CL. Slit lamp examination of the normal canine anterior segment. Part III. Discussion and summary. Journal of Small Animal Practice 1969c; 10: 163–169.

Martin CL. Gonioscopy and anatomical correlation of the drainage angles of the dog. Journal of Small Animal Practice 1969d; 10: 171–184.

Marts BS, Bryan GM, Prieur DJ. Schirmer teat test measurements and lysozyme concentration of equine tears. Journal of Equine Medicine and Surgery 1977; 1: 427–430.

Moore CP, Wilsman NJ, Nordheim EV, Majors LJ, Collier LL. Density and distribution of canine conjunctival goblet cells. Investigative Ophthalmology and Visual Science 1987; 28: 1925–1932.

Roat ME, Romanowski E, Araullo-Cruz T, Gordon J. The antiviral effect of rose bengal and fluorescein. Archives of Ophthalmology 1987; 105: 1415–1417.

Rubin LF. Inherited eye diseases in purebred dogs. London: Williams and Wilkins, 1989.

Rubin LF. Clinical electroretinography in dogs. Journal of the American Veterinary Medical Association 1967; 151: 1456–1469.

Sims MH, Brooks DE. Changes in oscillatory potentials in the canine electroretinogram during dark adaptation. American Journal of Veterinary Research 1990; 51: 1580–1586.

Slatter D. Fundamentals of veterinary ophthalmology, 2nd edn. London: WB Saunders, 1990; 585–592.

Water L, Barnett KC. Tear function in cats. Proceedings of the American College of Veterinary Ophthalmology 1993; 24:15.

Whiteley RD, Moore CP. Ocular diagnostic and therapeutic techniques in food animals. Veterinary Clinics of North America (Large Animal Practice) 1984; 6: 569.

Witzel DA, Riis RC, Rebhun WC, Hillman RB. Night blindness in the Appaloosa. Journal of Equine Medicine and Surgery 1977; 1:383–386.

# 21
# Clinical Examination of the Musculoskeletal System

*Small Animals – G.L. Flo*
*Horse and Foal – S.J. Dyson*
*Cattle – M.L. Doherty*

## CLINICAL MANIFESTATIONS OF DISEASES OF THE MUSCULOSKELETAL SYSTEM

**Abnormal posture** Any deviation from a posture in which the body is naturally straight, the head held up so that both eyes look straight ahead and weight is borne equally on all four limbs. Abnormal postures are adopted intermittently by animals in pain; in neurological disease the abnormality is usually continuous.

**Ataxia** Irregular deviations from normal movement patterns of body parts (usually limbs). Most often due to neurological disease.

**Bench knee** The metacarpus is set relatively lateral to the central limb axis of the antebrachium and carpus. Also known as an offset knee.

**Bone fracture** Break in the continuity of a bone.

- **Closed** fracture is one which does not result in an open wound.
- **Complete** fracture is a total disruption of bone, usually accompanied by marked displacement of the fractured ends. Swelling, crepitus, pain and instability are usually present.
- **Greenstick** fracture is one in which one side of the bone is broken, the other side bent. Usually occurs in young animals and although there may be pain and lameness swelling may be minimal.
- **Open or compound** fracture is one in which a skin wound communicates with the site of the break; osteomyelitis is a common complication.

- **Stable** fracture is one where interlocking fragments resist shortening and bending forces with little motion at the fracture site upon palpation.
- **Unstable** fractures (e.g. comminuted, oblique) are very mobile upon palpation.

**Bucked shins** Swelling on the dorsal aspect of the third metacarpal bones, associated with remodelling of the dorsal cortex of the bone due to periostitis or an incomplete dorsal cortical fracture.

**Buttress foot** An abnormally pointed foot with swelling at the dorsal aspect of the coronary band, usually associated with extensive new bone formation on the dorsal aspect of the distal interphalangeal joint.

**Calk** The heel end of the shoe is folded back on itself through 90°.

**Circumduction** Circular movement of a limb during the swinging or non-weightbearing phase of the stride or step.

**Cold back** Excessive thoracolumbar extension (lordosis) when a horse is saddled or mounted.

**Comes out of the shoulder** The position of the neck relative to the horse's trunk. A 'well set-on neck' is positioned high relative to the thorax.

**Crepitation or crepitus** Crackling or grating sound heard or sensation felt when the ends of fractured bones are rubbed together, or when soft tissues are moved over prominences such as orthopedic pins or suture knots. Joint crepitation from cartilage erosion and periarticular osteophyte production also occurs with advanced degenerative joint disease. Similar joint 'noises' may also be normal in some lax joints such as the carpus or distal hock joints.

**Curby hocks** Convex swelling or enlargement on the plantar aspect of the calcaneus. Curby hocks describes an unusually curved appearance in this area.

**Downer cow** Any cow which has been clinically recumbent with parturient paresis and remains recumbent for up to 24 hours, even following two treatments, and there is no clinical evidence of systemic disease or physical injury of the musculoskeletal system to account for the persistent recumbency. The term is also used generally to refer to cattle which are persistently recumbent for any cause.

**Dropped elbow** The elbow and carpus are held flexed, owing to loss of extensor function of at least the triceps musculature.

**Entheseophyte** New bone deposited at the site of a joint capsule or ligament insertion.

**Exostosis** A benign bony outgrowth, characteristically capped by cartilage, which projects from the surface of a bone. Exostoses are frequently due to trauma to ligaments or tendons at their points of attachment to bone.

**Fasciculation** A jerky, flickering, involuntary contraction of skeletal muscle fibers which is visible and palpable under the skin and associated with a spontaneous discharge of a number of muscle fibers innervated by a single motor nerve fiber.

**Flaccidity** A loss of tone of skeletal muscle associated with reduced reflex arcs and decreased muscle tone. Flaccid paralysis of the limb musculature is commonly due to diseases of lower motor neurons.

**Grass rings** Prominent parallel horizontal rings on the hoof wall which develop in association with changes in nutrition and growth of the hoof wall.

**Head bob or nod** Elevation of the head when a painful forelimb is placed on the ground. The head returns to its normal position when the affected limb is non-weightbearing.

**Hyperextension** Extension of a limb or part of limb beyond its normal limit.

**Hyperflexion** Flexion of a limb or part of a limb beyond its normal limit.

**Hypermobility** Abnormal mobility of a joint or a limb associated with a fracture, luxation or defects in the joint support system of ligaments and tendons.

**Hypertonia** Increase in muscle tone.

**Hypotonia** Decrease in muscle tone.

**Joint buckling** Sudden 'giving way' or collapse of a joint upon weightbearing, usually occurring with instability or pain. Luxating patella with resultant buckling of the stifle joint is an example of instability.

**Joint contracture** Abnormal angulation of a joint associated with resistance to passive flexion or extension of a joint, usually produced by fibrosis of muscle or other soft tissue surrounding muscles or joints.

**Joint hypermobility or laxity** Excessive movement of a joint. There may be excessive flexion or extension or lateral movement.

**Joint instability** Abnormal joint movement resulting in sliding, subluxation, luxation or angulation of two joint surfaces.

**Knock-down hip** Ventral and/or axial displacement or both of all or part of a tuber coxa due to a fracture and resulting in an abnormally flattened or lowered tuber coxae or both.

**Kyphosis** Flexion of the vertebral column, usually the thoracolumbar part. A roached, arched or dorsally convex back.

**Lameness** Lameness, or limping, is an alteration in an animal's normal stance or gait most commonly, though not exclusively, associated with musculoskeletal pain. It is often manifested as a halting or irregular gait. Lameness may be due to disease of the muscles, bones, joints, soft tissues or nervous system.

**Limb deformity** Limb disfigurement or malalignment. It may result from trauma, asynchronous bone growth, and conformational or genetic defects.

**Limb trembling** Involuntary shaking or shivering of a limb, usually due to weakness or pain.

**Lordosis** Extension of the vertebral column, usually the thoracolumbar part. A dipped or abnormally dorsally concave back.

**Luxation or dislocation** Displacement of the bones from a joint resulting in a deviation from the normal angle of the joint.

**Muscle atrophy** Decrease in muscle mass. This may be due to lack of use caused by chronic pain immobilization (disuse atrophy), or loss of innervation to the muscle (neurogenic atrophy) or muscle disease (myogenic atrophy). Generalized muscle atrophy occurs in emaciation.

**Musculoskeletal pain** An expression of discomfort, distress or agony resulting from the stimulation of specialized nerve endings in the musculoskeletal system, including bones, joints, muscles, tendons and ligaments. The animal may be reluctant to stand, reluctant to walk, or manifest discomfort such as anxious facial expression, limb withdrawal or aggression if an affected part of the musculoskeletal system is palpated or passively moved. There may be limping or non-weight-bearing, distressed vocalizations and behavioral changes.

**Non-weightbearing** Lack of or reluctance to bearing weight on a limb.

**Offset knee** The metacarpus is set on relatively lateral to the central limb axis of the antebrachium and carpus. Also known as a bench knee.

**On the bit** The International Equestrian Federation (FEI) definition is: 'a horse is said to be "on the bit" when the hocks are correctly placed, the neck is more or less raised and arched according to the stage of training and the extension or collection of the pace, and it accepts the bit with a light and soft contact and submissiveness throughout. The head should remain in a steady position, as a rule slightly in front of the vertical, with a supple poll as the highest point of the neck and no resistance should be offered to the rider'.

**On the forehand** The horse's weight is excessively loaded on the forelimbs owing to inadequate engagement of the hindlimbs. The hindlimbs are not moving sufficiently underneath the body and not carrying adequate weight.

**Overtrack** A horse overtracks if each hindfoot is placed beyond (in front of) the imprint of the ipsilateral front foot.

**Plaiting** As each hindlimb is advanced it deviates axially, so that viewed from behind the hindlimbs appear to cross over each other.

**Plantigrade stance** Abnormal posture in which the heel (fibular tarsal bone) touches the ground surface upon weightbearing. Humans and bears normally have a plantigrade stance. In dogs this is a deformity resulting from hock trauma, such as Achilles tendon rupture.

**Radius curvus** Bowing of the radius secondary to disturbance of the distal ulnar growth plate, resulting in valgus deformity of the carpus.

**Recumbency** The state of lying down and being unable or unwilling to stand, even with encouragement.

- **Sternal recumbency** The animal is lying on its ventral thorax and abdomen with the forelimbs flexed, one each side of the sternum, and will not or cannot stand when encouraged to do so. The hindlimbs are slightly flexed; the upper hindlimb is held next to the lateral abdomen, the distal part of the lower hindlimb is visible under the abdomen. The head may be held normally or folded back onto the flank in the 'sleeping position.'

- **Lateral recumbency** The animal is lying on one side or the other with the fore and hindlimbs stretched out laterally; the animal will not stand when encouraged but it may be possible to roll it into sternal recumbency. The head and neck are commonly extended.

**Scoliosis** Lateral deviation of the vertebral column.

**Spasticity** A state of increased muscle tone, exaggerated reflex arcs and/or spasms of skeletal muscles resulting in jerky, awkward movements. Spasticity of the limb musculature is most commonly due to lesions of upper motor neurons.

**Splint** Bony enlargement along the second and fourth metacarpal/tarsal bones.

**Stiffness** Restriction of joint motion and reduction in flexibility of limb motion.

**Swelling** Increase in size or volume of a body part or area not due to cell proliferation.

**Torticollis** Deviation of the vertebral column on more than one plane.

**Track up** A horse tracks up if each hindfoot is placed in the path of the imprint of the ipsilateral front foot.

**Valgus** Bent outward. Deformity in which the part distal to the named joint is angulated laterally away from the midline of the body (abaxially). Genu (knee) valgum is 'knock-kneed'; the limb distal to the knee is deviated away from the midline of the body.

**Varus** Bent medially (axially). Deformity in which the part distal to the named joint is angulated toward the midline of the body. Genu varum is 'bowlegged'; the limb distal to the knee is deviated toward the midline of the body.

**Weakness** Weakness or paresis is a loss of muscle strength which may be due to a muscular, neuromuscular or neurological abnormality. It is characterized by a sluggish gait, lowering of the head, dragging of feet leading to worn hooves and claws, and a tendency towards recumbency. There is reluctance or difficulty in rising, and a disinclination to move and then only slowly.

**Weightbearing lameness** Lameness in which the animal will bear some weight on the affected limb.

# Small Animals

## MUSCULOSKELETAL SYSTEM FUNCTION AND DYSFUNCTION

The musculoskeletal system provides the body with a means of support and locomotion. The skeleton furnishes protection, support, and levers for muscular action. The muscular system provides power for moving the skeleton. Tendons are fibrous connective tissues that unite muscles to bone, whereas ligaments are bands of collagen uniting bone to bone. Synovial joints, or articulations, facilitate skeletal movement. The nervous system controls and integrates the functions of the musculoskeletal system.

Diseases of the muscle usually result in

- varying degrees of weakness
- a painful and stiff gait
- pain on palpation
- joint contracture with difficulty in passive flexion and extension of the joints
- disuse muscle atrophy.

Diseases of bone may result in varying degrees of lameness, pain on palpation of the affected bone, and localized or diffuse enlargement of the bone. Fractures are characterized by varying degrees of pain with or without obvious swellings and deformity of the affected part. Fractures of the long bones of limbs usually result in a sudden onset of lameness. Fractures of the mandible or ribs result in painful mastication or breathing. Fractures of the vertebrae may cause spinal cord compression, resulting in paresis or paralysis.

Diseases of the joints may result in enlargement of the affected joint, decreased range of motion, pain on palpation, a stiff and painful gait, and malalignment when there is luxation. Rupture of cruciate ligaments may result in palpable stifle joint instability.

---

**Clinical Pointer** ✳

Musculoskeletal disease may be localized or generalized

- polymyositis causes generalized muscle pain and stiffness
- myositis of the masticatory muscles is characterized by pain, muscle atrophy, and fibrosis resulting in an inability to open the mouth.

---

Clinical examination of the musculoskeletal system includes history taking, physical examination, and the use of ancillary diagnostic tests. The first objective is to determine whether the lesion is due to disease of the bone, joint, muscle, or other soft tissues.

## HISTORY TAKING

The general aspects of history taking are described in an earlier chapter. However, when disease of the musculoskeletal system of small animals is suspected there are some special aspects of history taking.

### Signalment

Musculoskeletal diseases of small animals may be specifically associated with age, gender, species and breed, and the signalment may suggest diagnostic possibilities, such as bone tumors in giant-breed dogs.

#### Species

Cats develop fewer developmental orthopedic conditions than dogs. Occasionally luxating patella and hip dysplasia occur in cats.

#### Age

Certain diseases or conditions are peculiar to specific age groups. For example, 'swimmer puppy' or 'kitten syndrome' is a self-limiting (i.e. gets better by itself) condition particularly affecting the pelvic limbs in which there is a delay in the animal's ability to stand or walk by 21 days of age. The limbs project laterally from the body and forward motion is accomplished by lateral paddling motions. Permanent dorsoventral flattening of the thorax can occur. In dogs, osteochondrosis (OCD) is a developmental bone and cartilage problem typically manifesting clinical signs by the time the animal is 6–8 months of age. The condition begins in the growing dog and often results in permanent joint disease.

Congenital diseases usually are clinically evident in early life (Fig. 21.1). Older animals are predisposed to degenerative joint disease following trauma or congenital conditions, such as hip dysplasia or OCD. Bone and soft tissue tumors occur more frequently in older animals.

#### Breed

Hip dysplasia is most often seen in large to giant breeds of dogs, whereas patellar luxation occurs most frequently in toy breeds such as the Poodle.

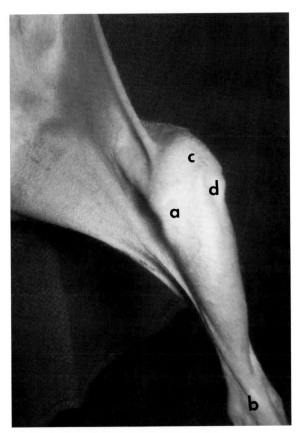

**Fig. 21.1** Cranial–caudal view of the left stifle of a 10-month-old Yorkshire Terrier with medial patellar ectopia. Note the malalignment of the tibial tubercle (a), hock (b), femoral trochlea (c) and fibular head (d).

Normal conformations of the various breeds of dog are very different. Breed standards for conformation are established by the dog and cat show clubs.

Chondrodystrophied breeds (Basset Hound, Dachshund) have shortened bones and often bowed legs, whereas sporting dogs have long straight bones and joints that do not deviate from midline when viewed from a cranial or caudal perspective. Valgus of the carpus may be normal for the Basset Hound, but in straight-legged breeds may result from physeal

---

### Legg–Calvé–Perthes disease

This disease (avascular necrosis of the femoral head and neck) affects young toy breeds of dog. It does not occur in large breeds nor does it begin in mature dogs.

---

### Clinical Pointer

A thorough knowledge of normal breed conformation is essential for detecting disease conditions.

---

trauma, elbow disease, or congenitally poor conformation (Fig. 21.2). Conformational variations present two different clinical problems

- those that predispose to malfunction or are a result of bone or joint disease
- those that are of concern to owners wishing to breed or show the animals.

Severe genu valgum ('knock-knee') in large breeds may result in lateral patellar luxation and marked disability, whereas in less severe cases the mild deformity may cause the dog to be eliminated from show competition.

## CHIEF COMPLAINT

The chief complaint is what the owner perceives to be the animal's major problem, which may be inapparent when the animal is examined. Musculoskeletal pain may cause behavioral changes, including inappetence, irritability, unusual licking of an area, restlessness, withdrawal from family activities, or poor athletic performance.

### Present illness

Specific questions include

- date or age of onset
- rapidity of onset
- recurrency of episodes
- possibility of trauma
- identification of the limb or limbs involved
- factors that worsen or improve the problem (weather, exercise, upon arising, response to medications such as analgesics, anti-inflammatory drugs or antibiotics, rest or weight changes)
- similar problems in other household animals or littermates.

### Disease history

Inquiries should be made about any previous surgery, orthopedic disease, other diseases, allergies or drug reactions, and any problems with sedatives or anesthetics.

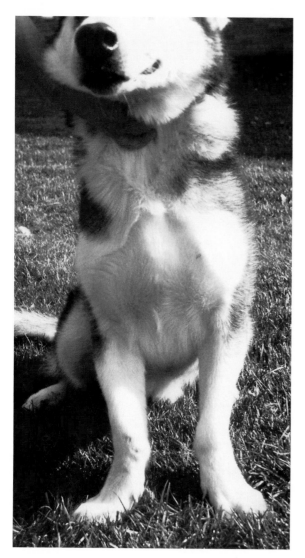

**Fig. 21.2** Valgus deformity of both carpi (carpal joints), resulting in external rotation of the forepaw in a dwarf Malamute puppy.

## Family, travel, diet and environmental history

Helpful information in patients with musculoskeletal complaints includes the presence of factors such as other household pets and children in the family that can contribute to the cause or alter therapeutic measures. Other pertinent information includes whether the animal has been to geographical locations where bone or joint disease is common. For example, Lyme disease is more prevalent in the northeastern USA.

> **Clinical Pointer** ✳
>
> It is important to ask the owner if the animal is used for showing or performance trials.

### Nutrition

The nature and amount of the diet should be determined.

1. Florid rickets associated with hypovitaminosis D or inadequate dietary mineral intake is rare, but is commonly blamed as resulting in unthrifty puppies or kittens.
2. Nutritional secondary hyperparathyroidism is a result of nutritional imbalances during the growth stages of puppies and kittens fed an all-meat diet and is characterized clinically by multiple fractures from trivial trauma to the softened bones.
3. Feeding excess vitamin A (liver diet) to cats causes painful bony proliferations around cervical vertebrae and major joints.

Fortunately, education of pet owners has reduced the occurrence of these diseases.

> **Overnutrition**
>
> Overnutritiion and feeding of unnecessary dietary vitamin and mineral supplements is currently of greater clinical importance in dogs and cats than deficient diets. Accelerated skeletal growth and body weight lead to bone disease, especially in large breeds.

Hip dysplasia and osteochondrosis are thought to be strongly influenced by diet. Obesity appears to accelerate joint wear and tear and is believed to predispose dogs to rupture of the cranial cruciate ligament.

## PHYSICAL EXAMINATION

The musculoskeletal system is examined by visual inspection, palpation, tests for range of movement, and the use of ancillary diagnostic aids.

### Distant examination of the standing animal

The animal is first examined by visual inspection from a distance. Demeanor, disposition, and body condition and conformation are observed and evaluated. The distant examination includes a particular distant examination of body regions: head and neck, thorax, abdomen, vertebral column, and limbs. There are specific criteria to note.

- **Head and neck carriage** – a dog with cervical disk disease may hold its head and neck in a lowered position and be reluctant to move the head ('guarded position').
- **Bowing or abnormal angulation of limbs and joints** – this occurs with growth plate (physeal) injury and untreated long bone fractures. Achilles tendon rupture results in a plantigrade stance.
- **Slope of the back and tail carriage** – a dog with lumbar disk disease or prostatic pain may arch the lumbosacral area (kyphosis) or tuck the tail under the hindquarters.
- **Swellings or asymmetry of one limb or part of a limb** compared to the contralateral limb. Swellings caused by tumors or trauma are often best discovered from a distance by noting asymmetry of paired parts. Muscle atrophy and subluxation from unilateral hip dysplasia are best observed from facing the hindquarters.
- **Ability to bear weight** – painful conditions usually cause the animal to bear less weight on the affected side. The toe spread is less than in the unaffected contralateral limb.

## Examination of gait

Encouraging the dog to walk or trot, preferably while controlled on a leash, will usually help to identify the affected limb. The animal is walked toward and away from the examiner and the gait is observed from the rear, front, and side. A faster gait, turning tight circles, stair walking, and observation of the recumbent animal rising may all be helpful to detect occult lameness.

Cats are usually uncooperative because they are not leash-trained and their gait can best be observed by allowing them to walk around the examination room.

Abnormalities of gait include

- dropping and raising of the head (head bob)
- limping
- dragging of the toes
- exaggerated toeing in or out
- limb circumduction
- joint buckling
- joint noises
- limb trembling
- limb carrying and lifting
- uneven weightbearing on a limb.

> ### Clinical Pointer ✳
>
> Avoid muzzling or sedating an uncooperative, aggressive, or fearful patient if possible as this may alter the gait or pain response to physical movements.

A head bob during the gait is common in dogs with forelimb lameness. The head becomes elevated when the affected limb strikes the ground and returns to its normal position when the non-lame limb lands on the ground. Toeing in or out of one foot may indicate pain or some loss of range of motion. Dogs with elbow pain often toe out (valgum of the carpus). However, if toeing out is bilateral it could represent a conformational deformity (Fig. 21.2) rather than a painful condition. Sudden joint buckling may occur with patellar luxation.

> ### Limb circumduction
>
> This is a circular outward swinging of the limb and can be caused by contracture of the infraspinatus tendon in the forelimb. This injury occurs in hunting breeds.

Meniscal injury with cruciate ligament rupture can occasionally produce an audible click or snap, similar to human knuckle cracking. Limb trembling may be a sign of pain or of weakness after exercise. Lifting of the limb or incomplete weightbearing is usually a sign of pain and is the most reliable indicator for identifying the affected limb. Dragging of the toenails may be seen and heard and indicates

- generalized weakness
- neurologic disease, or
- unilateral limb dysfunction.

## Close examination of the standing animal

The close physical examination should be systematic and proceed from inspection to palpation and then to tests of range of movement of joints and limbs. Evaluation of the standing animal allows comparison with contralateral regions and structures.

Clinical manifestations of musculoskeletal dysfunction detectable in the standing animal include enlargements of bone, muscle, joints and other soft tissues, muscle atrophy, and malalignment of joints.

Enlargements of bones, joints, muscles, and other associated soft tissue may be discrete or diffuse. Discrete swellings or 'lumps' are obvious deviations from the surrounding tissues and are usually composed of abnormal tissue. Diffuse swelling of a limb may be due to inadequate lymphatic drainage in the proximal part of the limb, such as is seen in animals in prolonged recumbency or those with proximal fractures. Diffuse swelling may also be subtle and the underlying structures may not be as clearly identifiable as in the contralateral normal limb.

Muscle atrophy usually results from chronic disuse or denervation. Its presence, however subtle, helps identify the affected limb when lameness is obscure. Atrophy is detected directly when the circumference of the muscle can be grasped (for example, the triceps brachii), or indirectly when the muscle cannot be grasped (for example infraspinatus). When atrophied muscles lie adjacent to bones, bony prominences become more apparent. Atrophy of specific muscles from chronic pain or lameness does *not* usually help localize the source of that pain. Severe and selective muscle atrophy often indicates neurological dysfunction.

Malalignment of joints may be the result of congenital defects or be due to trauma. When specific bones or parts of bones surrounding joints are malpositioned, the areas distal to those joints are affected. For example, when the patella luxates medially, the tibial tubercle and the paw are malaligned (Fig. 21.1).

### Thoracic limb

The anatomical landmarks for examination of the thoracic limb in the standing animal are depicted in Fig. 21.3.

The examination proceeds from the proximal to the distal regions of the limb as follows.

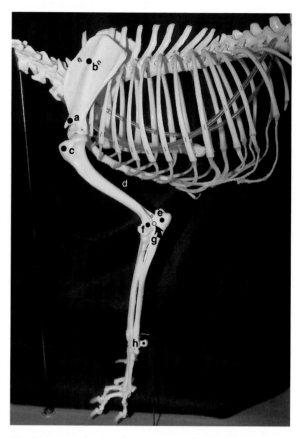

**Fig. 21.3**  The landmarks to note on the forelimb of a standing animal include: acromion (a) and spine (b) of the scapula, greater tubercle of the humerus (c), triceps brachii region of the midhumerus (d), olecranon (e), lateral epicondyle of the humerus (f), the region between e and f (g), and the accessory carpal bone (h).

1. The hands are placed over the animal's neck with the thumbs on the dorsal midline and the fingers extending over each side to detect muscle atrophy and spasms.
2. The hands then move methodically over all portions of the forelimb, palpating muscles, bony prominences, and joints as they are encountered.
3. Palpation progresses over each humerus, elbow, radius and ulna, carpus, and paw.
4. Comparisons between both limbs are noted as the examiner feels and looks for swelling, atrophy, or other changes.

Atrophy from chronic forelimb lameness is often palpable in the region of the suprascapular muscles. To discern this, the thumb and index finger straddle the acromion of the scapula (Fig. 21.4) and the spinous process is traced dorsally. As the suprascapular muscles

### Enlargements of the musculoskeletal system

- enlargement of bone is usually associated with neoplasia or trauma
- enlargement of joints usually results from trauma, inflammation and, rarely, neoplasia
- enlargements of muscles and soft tissue are usually caused by trauma, inflammation, or neoplasia.

decrease in bulk, the bony acromial process, and often the spinous process, become more prominent. If the acromion of the affected limb appears less distinct than that on the normal side, swelling (inflammation, neoplasia) of the infraspinatus muscle or lateral displacement of the humeral head from traumatic luxation is suspected. The greater tubercle of the humerus is palpated and any enlargement or swelling indicative of tumor of the proximal humerus is noted.

The elbow region is palpated for any abnormality, particularly swelling or atrophy of the triceps brachii. Next, the distance between the lateral and medial epicondyles of the humerus is noted. An increased distance may indicate a fracture, dislocation, or arthritis. Thumb pressure is then applied between the lateral epicondyle and olecranon (Fig. 21.5). A bulge under the normally thin anconeal muscle suggests joint effusion or fibrosis. A bony ridge between the lateral epicondyle and the olecranon indicates the presence of osteophytes from elbow osteoarthritis.

The radiocarpal joint lies cranially to the readily palpable accessory carpal bone. Joint swelling is detected by moving the thumb vertically over the cranial aspect of the joint. Bony enlargement or swelling of the distal radius occurs with bone tumor.

The metacarpal and paw regions are palpated for swelling and the toes observed for redness or malalignment compared to the adjacent toes and those of the opposite paw. With less weightbearing the paw appears smaller, and may actually be smaller as a result of tissue atrophy.

Conscious proprioception of the forelimb is tested (see Chapter 19).

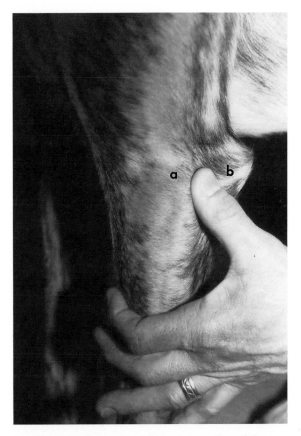

**Fig. 21.5** The best area to determine swelling of the elbow joint is on the lateral aspect of the forelimb between the lateral epicondyle of the humerus (a) and the olecranon (b). The thumb palpates for any 'bulge' or mass which is not present in normal animals.

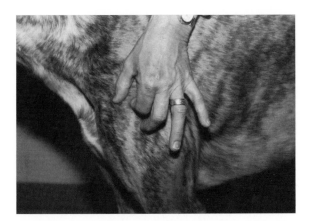

**Fig. 21.4** The thumb and index finger straddle the acromial process to assess muscle atrophy.

### Thorax and abdomen

The common abnormalities occurring in the thoracolumbar regions are swellings and painful areas, and paresis or paralysis of the pelvic limbs. The anatomical landmarks of importance include

- the ribs
- dorsal vertebral spinous processes, and
- the xiphoid cartilage of the sternum.

The examiner's hands are moved simultaneously over the dorsal, lateral, and ventral areas, palpating the entire trunk thoroughly. Any swelling detected in the thoracic region is palpated for firmness, attachments and origin. Any swelling of ribs is palpated to determine whether there is a firm connection to the underlying ribs. In the abdominal wall it is often possible to 'reduce' a swelling, which indicates an abdominal hernia. The thoracolumbar dorsal spinous processes are palpated to

<table>
<tr><td>

**Clinical Pointer** ✳

Compare tissues with surrounding structures as well as with the normal side to detect enlargements or masses.

</td><td>

**Clinical Pointer** ✳

A fracture of the ilium may cause swelling of the gluteal muscles between the wing of the ilium and the trochanter major.

</td></tr>
</table>

detect pain, malalignment, or any anatomical deviation. Pain can be elicited in intervertebral disk disease, injury, inflammation, and neoplasia.

### Pelvis and pelvic limb

The anatomical landmarks for examination of the pelvis and pelvic limbs are depicted in Fig. 21.6.

Beginning on the dorsum, the cranial, lateral, and caudal aspects of the pelvis are palpated, followed by palpation of the pelvic limbs. Digital pressure is applied on the dorsal spinous processes over the sacral region to elicit discomfort. Pain in this area may indicate lumbosacral disease.

Enlargements of muscle and bone may be palpable in the pelvic region. Swelling of the gluteal muscles between the wing of the ilium and the trochanter major is detected by moving the fingers between these two points. Swelling surrounding the proximal femur can be the result of a fracture or tumor. Crepitation may be elicited by applying digital pressure over fractured bones or puncture wounds of the skin. The trochanter major region is either enlarged or is less distinct than on the normal side when the surrounding soft tissue swells. A more prominent but normally positioned trochanter major could indicate muscle atrophy. An elevated or abnormally positioned trochanter is often due to coxofemoral luxation or avascular necrosis of the femoral head and neck (Legg–Calvé–Perthes disease). To detect these abnormalities imaginary points are placed on the wing of the ilium, greater trochanter, and tuber ischii to form a triangle (Fig. 21.7). When the coxofemoral joint is luxated craniodorsally the trochanter major rides proximally, which causes the triangle to become more acute (Fig. 21.7). This is the most common traumatic coxofemoral luxation seen in small animals.

To evaluate limb length discrepancy in small animals

- place the thumbs between the trochanters major and tuber ischii on each side
- with both tuber ischii positioned parallel to the table or floor, elevate the hindquarters and completely extend the hindlimbs (Fig. 21.8).

Normally, both paws are on the same level with one another. With a craniodorsal coxofemoral luxation or Legg–Calvé–Perthes disease the abnormal side will appear shortened. The paw will be more proximal than the paw on the normal side.

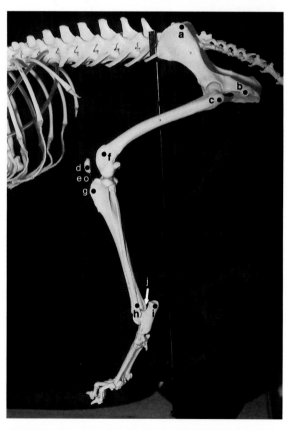

**Fig. 21.6** Important landmarks for the pelvic limb of the standing animal include: wing of the ilium (a), tuber ischii (b), trochanter major (c), patella (d), straight patellar ligament region (e), width of the femoral condyles (f), tibial tubercle (g), distal tibia (h), fibular tarsal bone (i), and the space between h and i (j).

---

**Acetabular fracture**

A trochanter major that is less distinct on one side than the other could be due to an acetabular fracture which has allowed the head of the femur to push inward and narrow the pelvic canal.

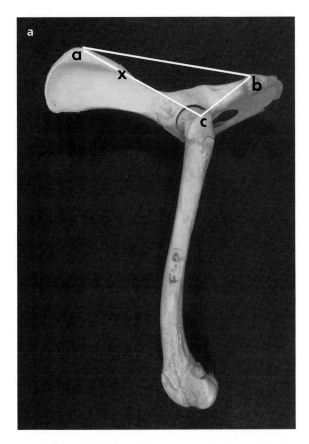
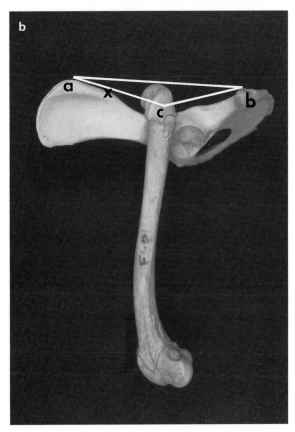

**Fig. 21.7** **(a)** Imaginary points are placed on the wing of the ilium (a), tuber ischii (b) and trochanter major (c) to form a triangle (x). **(b)** With craniodorsal coxofemoral luxation the triangle becomes more acute (x), especially when compared to the opposite side.

The femorotibial (stifle) area is examined next. Swelling, malalignment, and malpositioning of the bony prominences indicate abnormalities. The tibial tubercles, which are obvious in dogs but less so in cats, are palpated and compared. The patella is located 1–4 cm proximal to the tubercle, depending on the animal's size. When the tubercle deviates medially or laterally from the straight axis of the limb (Figs 21.1 and 21.9) it could indicate patellar luxation or torsion of the femoral and tibial condyles, as seen with genu valgum. The patella normally lies in the middle of the femoral condyles in the midlongitudinal axis of the limb. The examiner traces each patellar ligament proximally to locate the patella. The thickness and distinctness of the patellar ligament is assessed. Normally, the cranial two-thirds of the circumference of the taut patellar ligament in the normal standing animal is palpable (Fig. 21.10). Joint swelling origi-

nates caudally to the patellar ligament, and as swelling increases cranially it engulfs the caudal aspect of the ligament, making it less distinct upon palpation when two-thirds of the diameter of the ligament cannot be palpated. In addition, joint swelling from fibrosis and bony remodeling widens the medial to lateral, femoral, and tibial condylar distances (Fig. 21.11A,B).

The tibiotarsal (hock) joint and the Achilles tendon are then examined. Any increased width of the distal tibia is noted. Hock joint swelling is detected using the thumb and index finger to palpate between the distal caudal tibia and the fibular tarsal bone (Fig. 21.12).

Examination of the metatarsus and the digits is similar to that described for the forelimb.

Examination for conscious proprioception of the rear toes is then carried out (see Chapter 19).

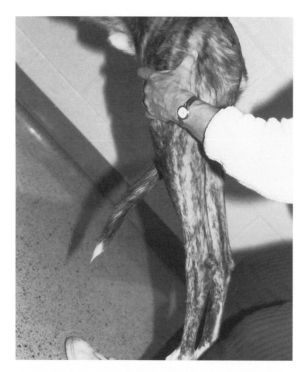

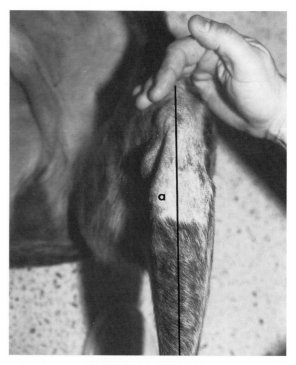

**Fig. 21.8** To ascertain limb length discrepancy the rear limbs are grasped with the thumbs positioned between the trochanters major and the tuber ischii. The femurs are pulled backward keeping the stifles straight while both tuber ischii are positioned parallel with the table or floor.

**Fig. 21.9** The tibial tubercle (a) is deviated medially from the midline of the long axis of the limb. The vertical line approximates the midline axis of the rear limb.

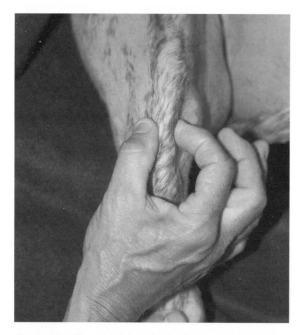

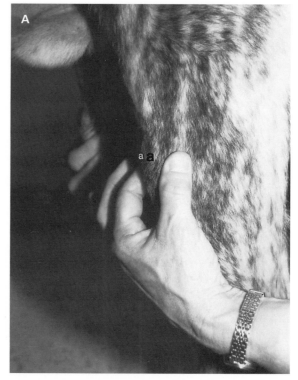

**Fig. 21.10** The cranial two-thirds of the patellar ligament are palpable with the thumb and index finger.

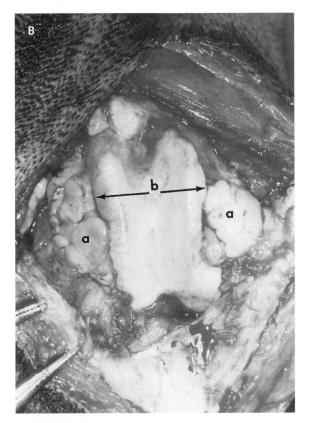

**Fig. 21.11** Palpation for normal femoral condylar width is performed 1–3 cm caudal to the patella. **(A)** Lateral view (a, patella). **(B)** In arthritic stifle joints osteophytes (a) proliferate along the edges of the femoral condyles, increasing the width between the normal condylar ridges (b). An arthrotomy has been performed and the patella has been luxated.

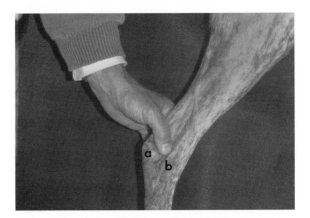

**Fig. 21.12** Tibiotarsal (hock) joint swelling is detected by palpating between fibular tarsal bone (a) and the caudal edge of distal tibia and the fibula using the thumb and index finger.

## Clinical Pointer

- skin and bone are the only structures palpable in the normal hock joint
- the presence of a firm, non-bony mass indicates joint swelling
- swelling of the normally pencil-like and symmetrical Achilles tendon suggests either inflammation, or partial or total rupture of this tendon.

# EXAMINATION OF THE ANIMAL PLACED IN RECUMBENCY

A thorough examination of the limbs, including the bones, joints, and muscles, and tests for range of movements of the joints, is possible with the animal placed in lateral recumbency. This position

- encourages the animal to relax
- allows patient restraint, and
- permits examination of the normal side without forcing weightbearing on the painful limb.

Eliciting a painful response on palpation of the limb aids in location of the lesion but is unnecessary when the abnormal area is obvious. The presence or absence of a painful response is *not* conclusive evidence of abnormality: stoic or excited animals may not react to painful stimuli. A painful response from a particular movement may be due to referred pain or generalized agitation of a non-painful patient. When a painful reaction occurs the movement producing it is gently repeated with all other areas held as steady as possible to minimize a referred reaction. Swellings can usually be more thoroughly examined in the recumbent than in the standing animal. Joint malalignment, although detectable in the standing animal, is also evaluated more precisely when the limbs are manipulated through several ranges of motion.

If pain interferes with necessary diagnostic manipulations, sedation may be necessary. Sedation can mask the presence of intra-articular or musculoskeletal pain, therefore it is probably best to use sedation after the examiner is satisfied that no abnormality will be missed because of its use.

## Clinical Pointer

Examine the normal limb first and then move to the affected limb, examining the suspected area last to ensure thoroughness and patient cooperation.

Muscles, bones, joints, ligaments, and tendons may be directly palpated for size, consistency, symmetry, the presence of painful responses, and continuity. Continuity of muscles and tendons is tested by direct palpation during passive motion. Continuity of superficial ligaments is tested by applying a tension force across a joint while digitally palpating the ligament, noting its tautness (or lack of it) or abnormal joint motion.

---

### Indirect palpation

- bones are indirectly palpated for stability and crepitus by grasping bone ends and applying bending or rotary movements
- joints are indirectly palpated for stability and crepitus and for evidence of painful responses by applying valgus, varus, abduction, adduction, cranial, caudal, medial, and lateral forces by grasping the bone ends above and below the joint being tested.

---

## Bones

The long bones of the limbs are examined for their shape and outline. Swellings of bones may be localized or diffuse. Fractures occurring in healthy bones commonly involve the long bones and are usually due to trauma. On examination for suspected fractures it is essential to establish whether the fracture is open (compound) or closed. In open fractures the bone communicates with the surface of the skin, either because the primary injury has broken the overlying skin or because deformation at the fracture site has caused the bone ends to penetrate the skin. Deformity is an obvious feature in many fractures.

---

### Clinical Pointer

Certain fractures, such as those of the femoral head and pelvic girdle, may show little deformity or clinical examination.

---

Most fractures of long bones are characterized by local pain and swelling, unless the overlying muscle mass is large. Bony crepitus is a typical feature of fractures. Localization of the source of the crepitus may require repeated careful passive flexion, extension, and rotation of the limb to identify the point of maximum intensity.

### Clinical Pointer

Take care in examining a suspected fracture as the fractured bone may also injure adjacent soft tissues, including the nerve and blood supply to the limb.

---

Joint instability and suspected fractures are always palpated gently as overmanipulation or rough handling can cause significant pain and worsen the problem. For example, a simple fracture mishandled during examination could become an open fracture. Discovery of instability in a painful swollen midhumeral region of a cat helps differentiate fracture from abscess or soft tissue tumor. To palpate for bone instability the examiner grasps the proximal humerus with one hand and the distal humerus with the other, and then applies a varus or valgus bending maneuver as well as rotation. After the instability and/or pain has been localized to a particular area, radiographs will provide valuable and less traumatic fracture evaluation than further manipulation.

## Joints

Examination of the joints should proceed from inspection to palpation and then to tests of range of movement. The joint may be enlarged or malaligned. Palpation may reveal pain or increased warmth.

Swelling is an important finding. All swollen joints should be palpated and ballotted. This will allow detection of

- the presence of fluid
- differentiation between simple effusion, synovial thickening, and capsule or bony enlargement, and
- determination as to whether the swelling is confined to the joint or is periarticular.

Joint effusions usually have a characteristically smooth outline and fluctuation is often demonstrable. Digital compression of one side of a distended joint capsule will result in a corresponding distension of the opposite side. Pain or swelling at only one joint margin may actually be arising in adjacent ligaments or tendons.

When examining joints for range of movement it is usually sufficient to estimate the degree of limitation based on comparison with the normal side. There is a wide variation in the range of normal joint movement. Excessive laxity or hypermobility is demonstrated by passive flexion and extension of the joint. Both active and passive movement should be assessed. Active movement, however, may give a poor estimation of true range of movement because of muscle spasm due to pain. If on attempted active movement pain is severe and other findings suggest fracture, neither active nor passive movement should be attempted. In testing the range of passive movement gentleness must be exercised, particularly in the case of painful joints.

Limitation of joint movement may be due to

- pain
- muscle spasm
- contracture of soft tissues
- inflammation
- increased thickness of the capsules or periarticular structures
- effusion into the joint space
- bony growths
- bony ankylosis
- mechanical factors such as a displaced or ruptured meniscus, or to
- painful conditions unrelated to the joint.

Decreased ranges of joint motion and soft tissue contracture occur in joints, muscles, and tendons and are a result of injury and fibrosis. Previous long bone fracture, chronic arthritis, chronic joint dislocation, ischemia, and neurological dysfunction can all cause temporary or permanent changes in joint motion or result in soft tissue contracture. For example, after intramedullary pin repair of a femoral fracture and placement of the limb in external coaptation, it is common for the stifle to develop a temporary, reduced range of motion.

Crepitus associated with a joint abnormality is either felt or heard as the affected limb is passively flexed or extended. Crepitus is transmitted by bone and resounds throughout an affected limb. Localization of the source requires careful and repeated palpation of the entire length of the limb in an attempt to determine the site of maximum intensity. When crepitus is elicited while examining the stifle joint, the examiner must be certain that its origin is in the stifle joint and not in the hip joint. The grinding noise elicited by manipulation of a dysplastic hip joint is abnormal, but not all such noises are crepitus or abnormal. For instance, normal 'clicks' often misinterpreted as crepitus occur with manipulations of the shoulder and hock joints.

---

### Soft tissue contracture

Contracture of the infraspinatus muscle is an example of the contracture of a specific muscle occurring after injury to the scapulohumeral (shoulder) area in hunting dogs.

---

## Muscle

Muscles are examined by inspection, palpation of the muscle mass, and by range of movement of the limb. Muscle bulk is best estimated clinically by inspection and palpation.

---

### Abnormalities in muscle bulk

- wasted or atrophic muscles → smaller, softer, and more flabby than normal when actively contracted
- wasted and fibrotic muscles → hard and inelastic, shorter and contracted, and difficult to stretch passively.

---

Muscle tone is the state of tension or contraction of muscles and is present in normal healthy animals. The degree of tone is estimated by handling the limbs and moving them passively at their various joints. The maintenance of muscle tone depends on spinal reflex arcs, and if this reflex arc is injured tone is diminished or lost. Hypotonia occurs in lower motor neuron disease. Hypertonia or spasticity occurs in upper motor neuron disease. These abnormalities are discussed in Chapter 19.

## Thoracic limb

Depending on the size of the animal, the thoracic limb can be examined with the animal on a table or on the floor. A methodical examination begins at the distal aspect of the limb and proceeds proximally, including the forepaw, forearm, elbow joint, arm, shoulder joint, and scapula. Those areas known to be painful are examined last. Any instability, swelling and abnormal noises are noted.

---

### Clinical Pointer

Flexion and extension of the major joints may help to relax the animal.

---

### Forepaw

The forepaw includes the carpus, metacarpus, and the phalanges. The toenails are examined for fracture, discoloration, pain, malalignment, and unusual wear. Abnormal nail wear can occur when the nails strike the ground abnormally owing to neurological dysfunction or malposition of the foot. The dorsal aspects of the digits are inspected for abnormalities of the skin and are palpated for swelling. The volar (bottom) surface of the toe pads and interdigital webbing are examined for discoloration, swelling, abrasion, or laceration. The digits are flexed and extended to evaluate range of motion, the presence of crepitus and any painful responses. Laceration of digital flexor tendons can produce malaligned toes. Tendons are palpated for normal tautness and continuity. Fractures of the proximal sesamoid bones can cause swelling caudal to the distal metacarpal bones. The metacarpal bones may sustain trauma. Proliferative bony and edematous soft tissue changes (hypertrophic osteopathy) can accompany intrathoracic neoplasia or occur for unknown reasons.

The carpus is flexed and extended while observing for pain, crepitus, and instability. The cranial or dorsal aspect of the carpal joint is found by first identifying the base of the readily palpable accessory carpal bone, which lies at the same level as the dorsal aspect of the joint. As the joint is flexed the thumb can identify the joint space created when the radius and radial carpal bone normally move apart. Swelling of the joint capsule lying over this region can be identified. This can occur from trauma or from inflammatory joint conditions such as rheumatoid arthritis. The collateral ligaments of the carpus lie medial and lateral to the joint. To test their integrity a valgus (outward bowing) or varus (inward bowing) stress is applied across the sides of the joint while the thumb or index finger is placed over and parallel to the ligaments. Normal ligaments become taut with this maneuver but with their rupture the joint opens abnormally.

> ### Clinical Pointer ✳
>
> Some normal carpal (and tarsal) joints produce clicks during manipulation and this should not be interpreted as crepitus.

### Antebrachium (forearm) and cubital (elbow joint) area

Applying pressure over the forearm muscles may elicit a painful response when musculoskeletal disease is present. The examiner flexes and extends the elbow with one hand grasping the forearm while the other palpates between the lateral epicondyle and olecranon for crepitus. Hyperextension of the elbow may elicit a painful response when an ununited anconeal process is present. Elbow flexion is facilitated in tense animals by first flexing the carpus. The bone between the lateral aspect of the lateral humeral epicondyle and olecranon normally slopes backward with no prominences, but osteophytes from elbow arthritis can form on the caudal lateral epicondylar ridge, creating an extra bony structure which is palpable between the lateral epicondyle and the olecranon. This is detected by moving the thumb between the two structures. While internally and externally rotating the forearm, digital pressure applied at the medial joint line may produce pain accompanying such conditions as fragmented coronoid process or osteochondritis dissecans.

### Brachium (arm) and scapulohumeral (shoulder) joint

The cranial and caudal arm muscles are gently squeezed to detect any painful response. Flexion and extension of the shoulder joint elicits a painful response in diseases such as osteochondritis dissecans of the humeral head. These movements are accomplished by grasping the forearm with one hand and placing the other hand cranially across the shoulder joint (Fig. 21.13). Crepitus may indicate luxation or fracture of the joint.

Bicipital tendinitis and/or rupture causes pain when the abnormal biceps brachii becomes taut. Stimulating this discomfort requires the elbow to be held in extension while the entire limb is pulled in a caudal direction along the thoracic wall. Simultaneous digital pressure applied on the proximal part of the medial intertubercular groove of the proximal humerus may also produce pain (Fig. 21.14).

Contracture of the infraspinatus muscle, a condition seen in hunting dogs, causes loss of shoulder extension and produces an abnormal circumduction of the forelimb when the animal walks. The forelimb can

> ### Evaluation of the scapulohumeral joint for luxation
>
> - using one hand grasp the animal's distal humerus
> - place the other hand over the scapular region
> - apply a medial and lateral force across the shoulder, causing a sliding motion of the humeral head
> - crepitus can be felt when luxation (or fracture) is present
> - sedation or anesthesia may be necessary to successfully detect abnormal shoulder instability
> - if there is an acromial fracture a cranial–caudal digital force on the acromial process may elicit a painful response.

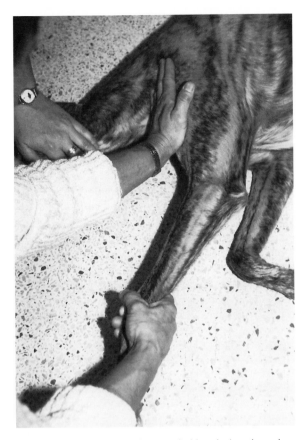

**Fig. 21.13** The shoulder is extended by placing the palm of one hand across the cranial aspect of the shoulder joint while the other hand pulls the limb forward.

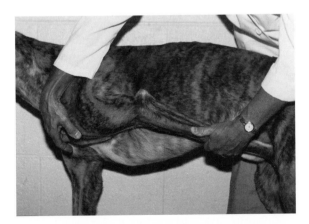

**Fig. 21.14** To elicit pain from an abnormal bicipital tendon the elbow is extended and the entire foreleg pulled caudally, parallel to the thorax. Digital pressure is applied to the proximal tendon region.

extend because the scapula moves on the thoracic wall, but to discern whether the shoulder joint itself is able to move normally, the thumb and index finger of one hand grasp the acromion while the other hand holds the elbow region so that the shoulder joint can be flexed and extended. Minimal or no shoulder extension occurs with contracture of the infraspinatus tendon.

Fractures, neoplasia, and inflammation of the scapular region cause swelling of the surrounding soft tissues. Manipulating the scapular spine is helpful in producing a painful response with scapular fracture.

Because bone pain from panosteitis and tumor is often intense, long bone palpation is performed last. Bony structures to be palpated are the

- distal radius
- distal and proximal ulna
- distal and proximal humerus
- spine of the scapula.

Bone examination begins distally and proceeds proximally up the limb with gentle pinching or compression. Comparing painful responses from examining the affected bones with the normal limb is helpful in determining whether the painful response is significant. The examiner's fingers push gently through muscle planes to find the underlying bone, to which pressure is applied. In this way digital pressure to muscles is avoided, which helps differentiate muscle from bone pain. However, it is difficult to attribute a painful response only from bone when it is surrounded by thick muscle, as is found in the midhumeral regions.

## Abdominal wall

A more precise evaluation of abdominal wall swellings is possible in a recumbent than in a standing animal. Digital and manual palpation of enlargements of the abdomen may elicit pain, and the enlargements can be evaluated for any attachment to surrounding structures.

> ### Clinical Pointer
>
> Roll the animal on its back to allow a more thorough visual and tactile inspection of the ventral thoracic and abdominal walls, especially when neoplasia or hernia may be present.

## Pelvis and pelvic limb

The pelvic limb is systematically examined by proceeding from distal to proximal regions and including the hindpaw, tibial region, stifle joint, femoral region, coxofemoral joint, and pelvis. Again, known areas of pain are examined last.

### Hindpaw

The hindpaw includes the tarsus, metatarsus, and phalanges. Examination of the metatarsal bones and phalanges is identical to that for the forepaw. The tarsus has three joint levels

- the tarsocrural (hock or tibiotarsal)
- the intertarsal, and
- the tarsometatarsal joints.

Traumatic, congenital, and inflammatory conditions affecting these regions cause swelling, instability, malalignment, pain, and crepitus. To examine for these abnormalities, varus and valgus stresses, and flexion and extension movements are applied at each joint level while attempting to immobilize other levels. Thumbs and fingers placed craniocaudally and medio-laterally across each joint line allow palpation of any instability as the bones slide across one another, and of any abnormal positioning of bones. With arthritic changes the tarsocrural (hock) joint has decreased range of motion, especially compared to the normal contralateral joint. Tarsocrural joint swelling, first detected with the animal standing, and the Achilles tendon can now be more precisely examined when the joint is manipulated.

The Achilles tendon is best examined during hock and phalangeal movement. Partial rupture, laceration and rheumatoid arthritis are causes of Achilles tendon dysfunction. Toe flexor tendons are examined for continuity by extending the toes while palpating caudally over the tendons.

### Tibial region and stifle joint

The tibial area is gently compressed for the detection of pain. Any swelling initially detected in the standing patient is now more precisely evaluated.

Specific manipulations of the stifle joint are used to elicit pain, produce crepitus or any abnormal noises, identify instability, and evaluate swellings more thoroughly. Abnormalities encountered in the stifle joint include

- patellar luxation
- cruciate ligament rupture
- meniscal injury
- avulsion and luxation of the long digital extensor tendon
- fracture
- osteochondritis dissecans of the femoral condyles
- infective and, less commonly, neoplastic conditions.

Patellar luxation is a common clinical problem and may be lateral, medial, or both. It may be ectopic (luxated, Fig. 21.1) or recurrent (luxating). The position of the tibial tubercle is more thoroughly evaluated during the manipulations. An ectopic patella is located by tracing the patellar ligament proximally from its insertion on the tibial tubercle. Joint flexion and extension also assist in locating the ectopic patella. Ectopic patellas may be movable or immovable. Evaluation of patellar mobility and location of the tibial tubercle assist the surgeon in planning corrective procedures.

To displace the patella medially one hand is used to extend the stifle while the foot is internally (medially) rotated and the thumb of the opposite hand pushes the patella medially (Fig. 21.15A). Medial–lateral movement of the patella within the trochlea or trochlear groove is not abnormal, but luxation out of the trochlea is. If no luxation occurs the joint is slightly flexed and the patella again pushed medially. If the patella luxates out of the trochlea the stifle sponta-neously flexes. Any luxations produced should be reduced by reversing the above described maneuvers. Conversely, to luxate the patella laterally the stifle is slightly flexed while the paw is externally rotated. Lateral digital pressure against the patella pushes it out of position (Fig. 21.15B).

---

### Drawer movement

- this is the abnormal cranial and caudal sliding of the tibia in relation to the femur
- rotary motion of the tibia on the femur can be normal and should not be mistaken for drawer movement
- large-breed puppies may have normal 'puppy drawer' until 6–12 months of age
- mature animals have essentially no drawer movement.

---

### Clinical Pointer

A common cause of tarsocrural (hock) joint swelling in large dogs is osteochondritis dissecans.

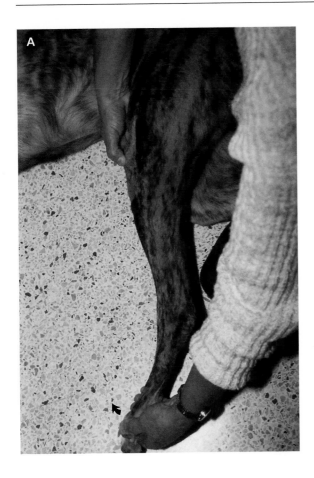

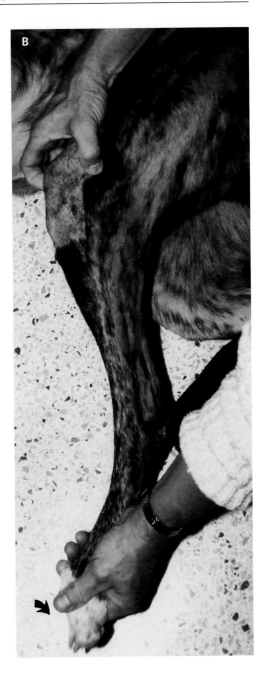

**Fig. 21.15** **(A)** The patella can be luxated medially by extending the stifle, internally rotating the paw (arrow), and pushing the patella medially with the thumb. **(B)** Lateral luxation is accomplished by flexing the stifle slightly, rotating the paw externally (arrow) and pushing the patella laterally using the index finger.

Ligament damage in the stifle results from trauma and most commonly occurs spontaneously, with no external injury. Gentle manipulation of a normal stifle is not painful. Dogs and cats with unstable stifle joints may resent palpation and require sedation to determine the extent of the injury.

The cranial cruciate ligament is the most common ligament to rupture or partially rupture. With acute rupture the tibia may slide cranially 3–8 mm, but with a tense animal, chronic rupture or partial tear of the ligament the amount of drawer movement is lessened. With significant stifle joint injury, such as vehicular trauma, the caudal cruciate and collateral ligaments may also rupture, thereby increasing the amount of joint instability.

Direct drawer movement is produced with the patient in lateral recumbency and the examiner standing behind the animal to produce the proper forces to detect instability. The limb is flexed and extended several times to relax the patient. The fingers are always placed around bony, *not* muscular, structures, because muscle manipulation will result in a false drawer movement. The index finger of one hand is placed on the cranial proximal patellar region and the thumb is placed *caudally* on the lateral fabella. The index finger of the other hand is placed on the cranial aspect of the tibial crest and the thumb placed *caudally* on the fibular head (Fig. 21.16). The examiner's wrists are kept straight during the maneuver. Once the hands are positioned the stifle is held in slight flexion while the tibia is pushed forward and pulled backward several times, gently but quickly, in order to perceive the movement. The maneuver is then repeated with the stifle held in extension, and repeated again in 90° flexion. Large or giant breeds of dog usually require this maneuver to be performed while they are lying on the floor. Stabilizing the distal limb while drawer

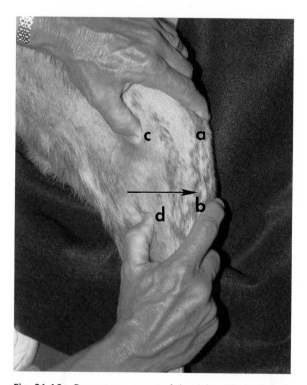

**Fig. 21.16** Drawer movement of the right stifle is elicited by placing the index finger of the left hand proximal to the patella (a) and the thumb caudal to the lateral fabella (c). The index finger of the right hand is placed on the tibial tubercle and crest (b), and the thumb is placed caudal to the head of the fibula (d). The femur is held steady while the tibia is quickly pushed cranially (arrow) and then pulled caudally. This is attempted in extension, slight flexion and moderate flexion.

### Clinical Pointer

When creating drawer movement in a patient, proper finger positioning is essential to produce the correct force. If the thumb is placed laterally rather than caudally the skin moves, causing misinterpretation of drawer movement.

movement is performed is helpful and can be accomplished by an assistant holding the distal metatarsal region, or by the examiner placing their own ankle under the dog's hock. The force used to produce direct drawer movement may be painful in affected animals. Indirect cranial drawer movement is accomplished by the tibial compression test, which has the advantage of being non-painful. The gastrocnemius muscle originates on the distal femur, crosses the stifle joint, and inserts on the calcaneus. When stretched the gastrocnemius compresses the femur and tibia together. With an intact cruciate ligament no abnormal movement occurs, but when the cranial cruciate ligament is ruptured the tibia slides forward.

The tibial compression test is performed with the stifle held in slight flexion

- the palm of one hand is placed over the cranial stifle, including the tibial tubercle
- the other hand extends the foot as far as possible (Fig. 21.17)
- with cranial cruciate rupture the tibia slides forward and the movement is detected by the hand located over the stifle and tibial tubercle.

This maneuver is performed quickly several times. Determining whether the tibia slides forward is more subjective than with direct drawer assessment.

Meniscal injury often occurs with cruciate ligament damage. To assess for meniscal injury the stifle is flexed and extended, this is repeated with the tibial tubercle both internally and externally rotated. A palpable click, clunk, snap, or grating sound is very suggestive of meniscal injury.

Other stifle conditions, such as

- long digital extensor avulsion
- joint fracture

### Clinical Pointer

The tibial compression test can be used when direct drawer maneuvers cause sufficient pain to cause the patient to become uncooperative.

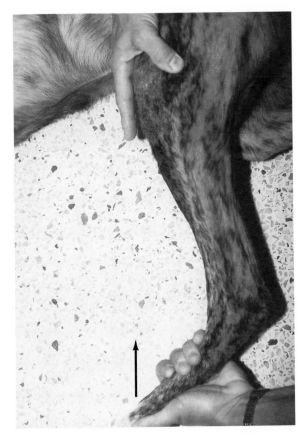

**Fig. 21.17** The cranial tibial thrust is an indirect mechanism to detect drawer motion. It is accomplished by steadying the left stifle joint with the right hand while the hock and metatarsus are flexed with the left hand (arrow). When the right hand is placed across the stifle joint it detects the tibial tubercle moving forward relative to the femur.

- osteochondritis dissecans
- inflammatory joint disease, and
- joint neoplasia

usually produce joint capsule swelling. In addition, avulsion of the long digital extensor tendon causes a lump of firm or bony material lateral and distal to the level of the patella. Radiography is an important diagnostic tool to differentiate these clinical problems.

## Femur and coxofemoral (hip) joint

The coxofemoral joint is composed of the femoral head and neck and the acetabulum. The trochanter major, wing of the ilium, and tuber ischii are helpful landmarks. The femur is palpated from distal to proximal regions, noting swelling, atrophy, or pain. The hip joint is moved through a normal range of motion to detect any pain, crepitus, decreased range of motion, or instability. The hip joint is a common site for

- fracture
- traumatic dislocation, and
- congenital disorders such as Legg–Calvé–Perthes disease and hip dysplasia

which can all result in osteoarthritis (degenerative joint disease). The evaluation of luxated coxofemoral joints has been discussed in the examination of the standing animal.

Crepitus from hip fracture, arthritis, subluxation, or dislocation may be palpable during hip flexion and extension. Less prominent crepitus from hip dysplasia may be heard by the examiner placing an ear over the trochanter major while the hip joint is moved through a range of motion. The use of a stethoscope can be used to hear crepitus, but harsh hair noises often obliterate crepitant sounds.

Assessment of hip instability is often not possible in the painful, awake animal. Although malpositioning of bones can be appreciated in a dog with traumatic luxation of the coxofemoral joint, assessment of instability and manipulation to produce instability is usually too painful in the conscious animal. In young dogs with hip dysplasia, however, some instability may be detected; occasionally sedation is needed for a thorough examination. There are two ways to produce the instability.

1. The 'sign of Ortolani' is a noise or palpable 'thud' produced when the subluxated femoral head is suddenly replaced in the acetabulum. To perform this maneuver the stifle is slightly adducted with one hand while an upward or proximal force is slowly applied. The other palm stabilizes the pelvis with the first two fingers resting on the trochanter major. Stifle abduction while downward pressure is applied to the trochanter major causes reduction and a resultant palpable and sometimes audible 'thud' (Fig. 21.18 A,B). The sign may also be produced bilaterally simultaneously. With the dog in dorsal recumbency the stifles are adducted and pushed proximally. Abduction causes reduction of the femoral heads and production of the noise.

### Clinical Pointer

Applying proximal pressure at the stifle region compresses the abnormal cartilages of the femoral head and acetabulum, and accentuates the crepitant sound from hip dysplasia. Take care to distinguish the fine grating noises produced by cartilaginous degeneration of the coxofemoral joint from haircoat noises.

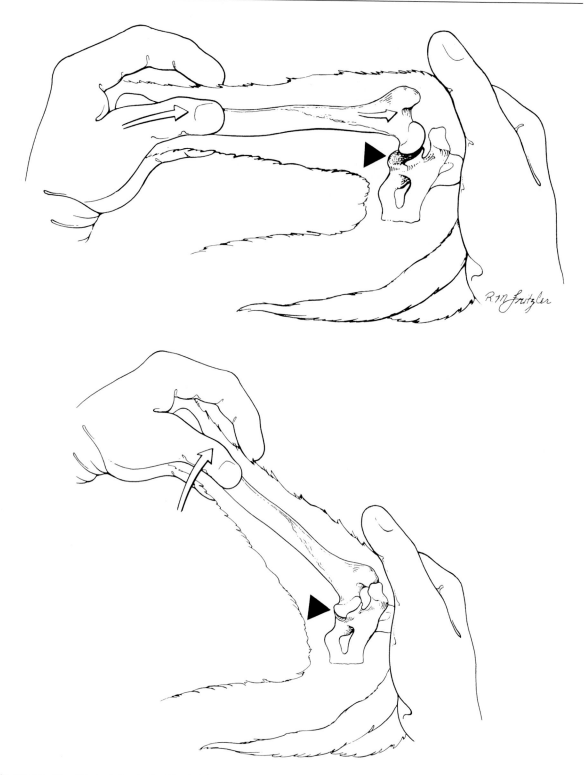

**Fig. 21.18** The Ortolani sign is the 'thud' felt and sometimes heard as a lax hip which has been subluxated returns to the acetabulum. **(A)** The distal femur is forced proximally (white open arrows) to subluxate the coxofemoral joint (solid arrowhead). **(B)** The stifle is abducted (white arrow) and reduces (solid arrow head) the subluxated hip joint.

2. A second method to detect coxofemoral laxity in the laterally recumbent animal is to position the femur parallel to the table by grasping the thigh. The femoral head is alternately lifted and relaxed. The other hand stabilizes the pelvis while the first two fingers press down on the trochanter major when thigh pressure is relaxed. Pressure is released when the femoral head is lifted. The procedure is repeated several times. A 'thud' as well as an estimation of the distance of subluxation can be detected in unstable hips. The force on the thigh muscles needed to produce the subluxation is often painful in both normal and abnormal hip joints.

To ensure patient cooperation throughout the examination, suspected painful conditions (panosteitis, fracture) and painful maneuvers are evaluated last.

To isolate bone pain, bone is pressed in areas least covered by muscle (medial tibia, distal, and proximal femur).

---

### Clinical Pointer

Palpate the muscles and long bones from distal to proximal.

---

The pelvic bones, including the wings of the ilium, ischium, and pubis, are palpated for instability, pain, and crepitus. Digital rectal examination often helps to delineate fractures, especially of the pubis. Occasionally rectal examination reveals

- coxofemoral crepitus
- fracture fragments impinging on the pelvic canal, or
- swelling within the abdominal wall or retroperitoneal area.

The tail is palpated for swelling, crepitus, deformity, and pain. Congenital coccygeal hemivertebrae cause corkscrew tails in Bulldog or Pug-type breeds. One hemivertebra is often responsible for a 'kink' in the tail.

## ANCILLARY DIAGNOSTIC TESTS

Trauma and congenital disorders are the most common causes of musculoskeletal abnormalities in dogs and cats. Often the physical examination provides enough information to arrive at a presumptive diagnosis. Depending on the seriousness and chronicity of the musculoskeletal signs, additional diagnostic tests or procedures may be needed to arrive at a definitive diagnosis. These include medical imaging, arthrocentesis and laboratory examination of synovial fluid, biopsy of muscle, bone and synovial membrane tissues, exploratory surgery, arthroscopy, and clinical pathology.

### Medical imaging

#### Radiography

This remains the most common diagnostic tool to evaluate disorders of the musculoskeletal system. It is especially useful in detecting and evaluating fractures and tumors of bones, joint diseases, and abnormal physical examination findings.

#### Computed tomography (CT)

CT is a specialized medical imaging modality in which a three-dimensional image of a body structure is computer constructed from a series of plane cross-sectional images made along an axis. It is most frequently used in diagnosing vertebral, and skull abnormalities, but it is also very useful to demonstrate fragmented or fissured coronoid processes in dogs' elbows (Fig. 21.19).

---

### Pros and cons of CT

- CT eliminates the complication of bony superimposition in radiographic imaging and allows detailed visualization
- CT equipment is expensive, requires anesthesia in animals, and is not readily available to most veterinarians.

---

#### Magnetic resonance imaging (MRI)

MRI is a non-invasive diagnostic technique that delineates soft tissue structures much better than does CT. MRI is based on the nuclear magnetic resonance of atoms within the body induced to move and emit radiowaves by the application of magnetic fields. Cost limits its use in veterinary medicine.

#### Nuclear imaging (NI)

Nuclear imaging uses radioactive materials in the diagnosis of disease. Depending on the organ to be investigated, a specific radioactive substance is administered intravenously to a sedated patient. Radioactive

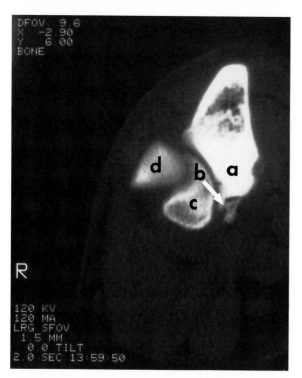

**Fig. 21.19** Cross-sectional CT image of a dog's elbow at the level of the coronoid process surface. Note the separate fragment that is usually not appreciated on conventional radiographic views. (a) Coronoid process. (b) Separate fragment. (c) Radial head. (d) Lateral humeral condyle.

decay emits gamma radiation which is then detected by a scintillation crystal. These counts are transmitted to a dedicated computer for image production. Radioactive materials will selectively accumulate in an area of active vascularity (e.g. inflammation) and open growth plates, where they can be detected by the gamma camera. The specific radiopharmaceutical used in veterinary medicine is technetium-99m ($^{99m}$Tc). It is taken up by soft tissues within 4–8 minutes and then by bone in 2–8 hours, which necessitates scanning during these times.

Nuclear imaging helps detect bone tumors as well as bony and soft tissue inflammation. At present it has limited application in small animals because of cost and lack of availability.

---

### Clinical Pointer ✳

For safety reasons an animal undergoing nuclear imaging must be housed for at least 12 hours in special holding facilities for radiation decay to occur.

---

### Arthrocentesis

Arthrocentesis is the puncture of a joint cavity, usually to aspirate joint fluid for laboratory evaluation of

- total and differential white blood cell count
- protein concentration
- viscosity
- the presence of microorganisms.

A 20–22 gauge needle and a 5 ml syringe are used. Specific techniques for individual joints are described elsewhere.

Evaluation of joint fluid can distinguish between inflammatory (infection or immune-mediated) and non-inflammatory (traumatic or congenital) joint disease. The technique is also used for the instillation of therapeutic or diagnostic agents into the joint. Radio-opaque substances are injected into a joint for contrast radiography. Arthrography is most often done in the scapulohumeral joint to diagnose bicipital tendinitis or the presence of cartilaginous flaps or loose osteochondral bodies (joint mice) in osteochondritis dissecans.

### Biopsy

Biopsy of muscle, bone, and synovial membrane involves the removal of a small piece of these various tissues for histopathological examination. Biopsy may reveal inflammatory or degenerative diseases of muscle, tumor, infection, or foreign body. Special histochemical techniques may be used to characterize particular pathological changes.

### Clinical pathology

Hormonal and enzyme assay and serology are used to evaluate the patient for systemic illness associated with musculoskeletal disease, such as systemic lupus erythematosus, rheumatoid arthritis, septicemia, endocrine disorders (hypothyroidism, hyperadrenocorticism) and Lyme disease. Cytological examination of lymph nodes and masses involving a limb or joint is often helpful.

### Exploratory surgery

When the diagnosis is uncertain it may be necessary to explore a suspected anatomical area surgically in order to determine the nature and extent of the abnormality. This provides an opportunity to obtain biopsy specimens, make a diagnosis, and possibly correct any abnormalities detected. For example, in a dog with a swollen stifle joint without drawer movement an exploratory arthrotomy may reveal

- a partial tear of the cranial cruciate ligament

- synovial tumor
- synovial chondrometaplasia, or
- inflammatory joint disease.

### *Arthroscopy*

Arthroscopy is the examination of a joint with an arthroscope, which is a narrow-gauge rigid endoscope used only for joints. Joint cavities are dilated with fluid prior to insertion of the arthroscope. Besides gross inspection of the joint, surgical maneuvers may be performed using highly specialized instruments. Although useful in humans and horses, patient size and the unavailability of arthroscopic surgical equipment limit its practical application in small animals.

# Horse and Foal

## INTRODUCTION

There are many reasons why a veterinarian may be asked to assess some aspect of the musculoskeletal system of a horse. Evaluation of conformation may be required to assess the correctness of a yearling destined for the sales; to determine the significance or otherwise of a suspected abnormality of conformation (e.g. carpal valgus) with respect to both the horse's future soundness and its future athletic capabilities; and to assess whether the abnormality is potentially correctable. Lameness or poor performance requires a comprehensive evaluation of the musculoskeletal system, bearing in mind that more than one problem can occur concurrently. At a prepurchase evaluation the purchaser requires assessment of conformation and swellings, the presence or absence of lameness, and the likelihood of future lameness. The development of a swelling calls for an assessment of its likely functional significance and determination as to whether or not treatment might alleviate the swelling.

Clinical signs, possibly indicative of a disorder of the musculoskeletal system, include

- a gait abnormality

### Gait abnormalities

Not all gait abnormalities are due to lameness – stumbling or a toe drag may be associated with, but not synonymous with, lameness. Depression, weakness, lack of fitness, and tiredness can all cause gait abnormalities.

- a reluctance or inability to move
- an unusual posture at rest
- a tendency to lie down more than usual
- the development of a localized or diffuse swelling, and
- a localized area of heat or patchy sweating.

Lameness is characterized by abnormal load bearing on one or more of the limbs and is generally associated with either pain involving the musculoskeletal system or mechanical dysfunction, or both. In addition there may be abnormal limb flight or foot placement, and irregularity of rhythm and movement of the head and neck or pelvis. Lameness due to pain or mechanical dysfunction must be differentiated from abnormal weightbearing due to neurological dysfunction. Lameness, stiffness, reluctance to move, an abnormal posture, and lying down for prolonged periods are not unique to musculoskeletal disorders. Thoracic pain, pain in the groin region due to a scirrhous cord or mastitis, and other systemic diseases must also be considered.

If the examination is performed because of lameness or poor performance it is helpful to obtain an accurate history. This should include the signalment of the horse. A small pony, kept at pasture, which is reluctant to move is likely to have laminitis. A foal with sudden-

### Some relevant facts to determine during the examination

- the duration of clinical signs
- whether the horse is in work and if the lameness alters with work
- whether the lameness was sudden or insidious in onset
- how the lameness has altered since its onset
- whether the owner has noted any abnormal swellings or posture of the animal
- whether there have been difficulties in picking up one or more limbs
- whether or not the horse has experienced difficulty in getting up from lying down.

onset severe lameness probably has a subsolar abscess or a septic joint, although the owner may think that the dam trod on the foot. A yearling with distension of the femoropatellar joint capsule may have osteochondrosis.

Any history of trauma should be recorded. It is helpful to know when the horse was last shod, whether any treatment has been given and, if so, the response and whether other clinical abnormalities have been observed. For example, a horse presenting with poor performance following recent nasal discharge and/or depressed appetite may have muscle soreness following equine influenza virus infection.

A systematic approach to examination should be adopted whenever possible. If the whole horse is routinely examined, including all four limbs, the examiner is constantly familiar with normal variations and has an excellent opportunity to review anatomy. Careful comparison of pairs of limbs facilitates the identification of subtle problems and permits recognition of subclinical problems that may be clinically important.

It can be particularly valuable to examine the horse undisturbed in its home environment, either in the stable or in a paddock, assessing it in a relaxed state to give the best opportunity to detect abnormalities of posture. While in the stable a comprehensive visual assessment and palpation of the entire body can be done. Each limb should be assessed in both weight-bearing and non-weightbearing positions. Although a general assessment of both conformation and muscle symmetry can be carried out in a stable, these are best assessed with the horse standing outside on a firm level surface. Evaluation of gait should ideally be performed

- in hand on a hard surface
- on the lunge on both soft and hard surfaces, and
- while the animal is being ridden.

Flexion tests are an integral part of all lameness and prepurchase evaluations.

### Clinical Pointer

A regular routine order of examination is helpful to ensure that nothing is missed.

During the examination the clinician should repeatedly be questioning what is a normal variant, what is abnormal but of unlikely clinical importance, and what is clinically abnormal. Swellings may develop unassociated with lameness, but the absence of detectable heat, pain, or swelling associated with a

### Clinical Pointer

The foot cannot be evaluated adequately with a shoe on – detailed foot examination necessitates removal of the shoe.

structure does not preclude that structure from being the primary source of pain and therefore a cause of lameness. A bony exostosis involving the second or fourth metacarpal bones (i.e. a 'splint') may develop without lameness. Distension of the femoropatellar joint capsule, due to underlying osteochondrosis, may be present without detectable lameness, although lameness may develop subsequently. In contrast, lameness may be alleviated by intra-articular analgesia of a metacarpophalangeal joint, despite the absence of joint capsule distension, pain on passive manipulation of the joint, joint stiffness, or accentuation of lameness by flexion. Differentiation should be made whenever possible between primary musculoskeletal problems and neurological abnormalities.

The order in which an examination is carried out and the depth of examination will be dictated by the history and severity of clinical signs, remembering that common diseases should be considered first.

### Clinical Pointer

Sudden-onset severe forelimb lameness associated with a bounding digital pulse is probably caused by a subsolar abscess, only a cursory examination of the other limbs is indicated.

If the history or clinical signs are suggestive of a fracture then exercise should be minimal, as there is a risk of making the fracture worse. However, many investigations merit an appraisal of the entire musculoskeletal system. Reliance must not be placed entirely on the owner's assessment of which is the lame limb and, similarly, some aspects of the given history may be misleading.

## CONFORMATION

Conformation should be assessed with the horse standing squarely on a firm level surface. The animal should be assessed from the side, front, and rear. A general impression of the proportion of size of the head, neck, back, and limbs should be formed. An unusually large head may predispose the horse to working 'on the forehand', i.e. to load the forelimbs excessively. The thickness of the throat region may influence how easily the horse can flex its head relative to the neck, and thus the ease of working 'on the bit'. This refers to the correct angulation between the horse's head and neck, and acceptance of the bit. The shape of the neck and the position of the neck relative to the trunk will also influence the head and neck carriage. The shape of the wither and the curvature of the back will influence where the saddle, and therefore the rider, will sit. The shape of the horse's 'barrel' (the circumference of the thorax) determines where the rider's leg will naturally be positioned and thus influences how easy it is for the rider to be balanced with the horse. Each limb of an adult horse should be relatively straight in the sagittal and transverse planes, so the central axis of each limb should also be straight. The foot should be symmetrically positioned about the central limb axis.

> ### Normal development of conformation
>
> Patterns of normal development must be appreciated when evaluating a foal's conformation and deciding whether or not intervention by corrective foot trimming, the application of a glue-on shoe, or surgery may be required.

## The foal

A young foal has a very narrow chest and relatively base-wide stance (Fig. 21.20). It has a tendency towards carpal valgus (axial deviation of the carpi, or knock knees) and having the carpi rotated outwards. As the foal matures the chest broadens, the carpi rotate inwards to face straight forwards, and the foal looks progressively less knock-kneed.

## The yearling

Most yearlings grow rapidly, but the speed of growth may appear to differ in different parts of the body. Frequently the hindquarters of a yearling or 2-year-old are significantly higher than the forequarters. In other aspects, the conformation of a yearling is much closer to that of an adult than a foal. Thus it is easier to predict the ultimate conformation of an individual as an adult. There are many inter-horse variations both within and between breeds, and there is no uniformly correct conformation. Good conformation essentially reflects symmetry and balance.

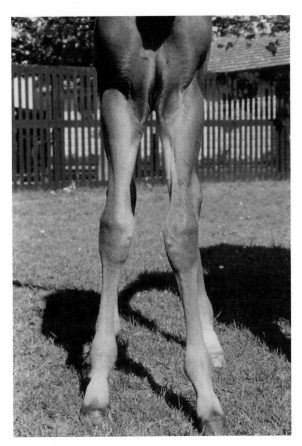

**Fig. 21.20** Narrow chest conformation and base-wide stance typical of a neonatal foal.

> ### Clinical Pointer
>
> - defects in conformation can be masked in an overweight individual
> - unacceptable aspects of conformation may appear in a horse in poor condition.

Thus a horse may have kyphosis due to prominence of the summits of the dorsal spinous processes and the tubera sacrale, but this may be inapparent when the horse is in good bodily condition.

## The adult

Conformation should be considered in the light of the breed. For example, the rather lordotic (dipped back) conformation and prominent tubera sacrale typical of many Arabian horses might be considered a fault in a Thoroughbred. If a horse is being purchased as a potential show animal or for breeding purposes it is important that the purchaser is informed of any abnormalities of conformation. However, conformation is far more important with respect to the horse's athletic ability and potential soundness. A metacarpus being set on relatively lateral to the central limb axis of the antebrachium (offset or bench knee) will predispose to the development of splints. A straight conformation of the hock, hyperextension of the hind fetlock or both, may predispose to suspensory apparatus disease. However, it must be recognized that there are relatively few studies investigating the long-term relationship between either conformation and performance ability or conformation and lameness. Two common conformational foot abnormalities are illustrated in Figs 21.21 and 21.22.

> ### Conformation and ability
>
> The relatively straight conformation and angle of the pelvis of a Thoroughbred can adversely affect the horse's natural ability to engage the hindlimbs for dressage compared to a Danish Warmblood.

## VISUAL APPRAISAL OF THE TRUNK AND LIMBS

The horse is examined visually to determine the presence of abnormal swellings. It is important to view systematically from all angles to identify slight abnormalities of limb contour. The left–right symmetry of the forelimb and hindlimb musculature should also be assessed. To evaluate forelimb musculature the horse should stand on a firm level surface precisely squarely in front, while loading both hindlimbs. Visual and tactile inspections of the left and right muscles are carried out simultaneously so that subtle differences are detected. Although mild atrophy of the shoulder musculature may be seen in association with any chronic forelimb lameness, marked wastage usually reflects an upper forelimb lameness related to the shoulder or elbow, or neurogenic atrophy. To assess hindlimb musculature the hind feet should be exactly level, bearing weight evenly, with the trunk straight. Any pattern of muscle wastage should be carefully assessed. With chronic hindlimb lameness there is usually a generalized loss of bulk to the gluteal muscle group. The involvement of other muscle groups may suggest a central (e.g. equine protozoal myelitis) or peripheral neurological disease. An abnormal contour of the semimembranosus or semitendinosus muscles or both can be associated with fibrotic or ossifying myopathy.

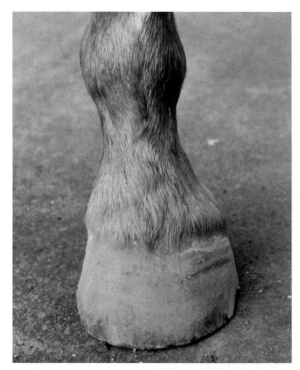

**Fig. 21.21** The central axis of the foot and pastern is lateral to the central limb axis of the proximal limb. Lateral is to the right.

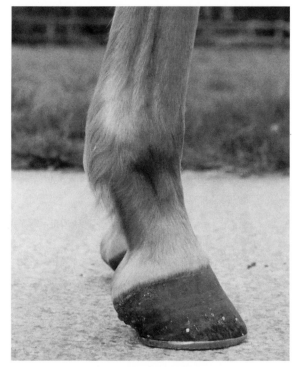

**Fig. 21.22** Upright pastern foot axis.

Assessment of the hindquarters should also include evaluation of the levelness and symmetry of the tubera coxae and tubera sacrale. The horse must be standing squarely behind. It may be helpful to have two assistants place fingers extended horizontally on to the dorsal tuberosity of each tuber coxae or to apply light-colored tape to obtain a true impression (Fig. 21.23). In most normal horses the tubera coxae are relatively level, although slight asymmetry of the tubera sacrale is a common incidental finding, unassociated with any detectable gait abnormality. Marked asymmetry of the tubera sacrale with levelness of the tubera coxae usually reflects a fracture, current or previous, of the ilial wing or the ilial shaft, or both, which may or may not involve the sacroiliac joint by itself. If both the tubera sacrale and the tubera coxae are asymmetrical this probably reflects injury to the sacroiliac joint(s), whereas if the tubera sacrale are level and the tubera coxae are not (knock-down hip) this usually indicates a fracture of the tuber coxae.

Hoof growth is reflected by horizontal rings on the hoof wall. These tend to be more prominent at times of rapid growth due to improved nutrition. This can result in so-called grass rings, i.e. prominent parallel horizontal rings on the hoof wall. Hoof growth also alters as a result of laminitis: there tends to be more rapid growth at the heel, so the hoof rings diverge at the heel and the foot orientation alters owing to an excessively high heel. Foot shape can also change because of disease within the foot: a space-occupying lesion such as a keratoma may alter the contour of the hoof wall. The foot may assume a buttress shape (pointed dorsally) in association with degenerative joint disease of the distal interphalangeal joint or new bone on the extensor process of the distal phalanx, referred to as pyramidal disease. Changes in hindfoot shape are much less commonly appreciated in association with lameness, except as a result of a space-occupying lesion.

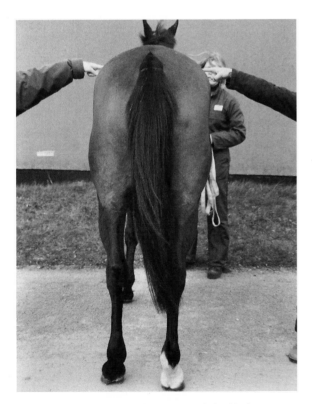

**Fig. 21.23** Assessment of symmetry of the hindquarter musculature, and the levelness of the tubera coxae. The horse must be standing squarely, evenly loading the hindlimbs, on a flat level surface.

**Asymmetry of the shape and size of the front feet**

- this is generally an acquired abnormality
- it may develop as a result of chronic lameness – there is a tendency for the foot of the lame or lamer limb to become more narrow and upright, the frog clefts become deeper, and the contralateral foot becomes flatter and slightly broader
- a narrow, upright, so-called boxy foot can develop extremely rapidly, and remain a permanent feature, as a result of a distal interphalangeal joint flexural deformity.

## POSTURE

A normal horse usually stands bearing weight evenly between both forelimbs, with the limbs relatively vertical. When grazing the forelimbs are straddled alternately, still bearing weight on each. However, horses commonly shift weight alternately between each hindlimb, resting each in turn. The rested limb is usually positioned in front of the weight-bearing limb, with slight weight applied only on the toe.

If one forelimb is placed in front of the other the horse is said to **point**. The pointed limb is generally less loaded than the contralateral limb and slight elevation of the heel can sometimes be seen. This usually signifies palmar foot pain, which may also result in the horse standing with the forelimbs vertical with bedding stacked under the heel, resulting in slight flexion of the distal limb joints. Horses with adhesions of the accessory ligament of the deep digital flexor tendon (the inferior check ligament) to adjacent structures may stand with the fetlock slightly flexed. In contrast, a horse with forelimb laminitis may stand with the forelimbs slightly outstretched and the weight rocked back on the heels (Fig. 21.24). If all four limbs are involved they may be positioned unusually far underneath the body. A horse which has received trauma to the shoulder region may stand with its weight slightly inclined towards the contralateral limb, giving a false impression of asymmetry of the pectoral musculature. If the shoulder intermittently bulges outwards, reflecting loss of stability, this is usually due to trauma to the brachial plexus. Massive swelling in the shoulder region and an abnormally straight forelimb may indicate subluxation or luxation of the scapulohumeral joint.

---

### Dropped elbow posture

A horse standing with the elbow and carpus of one forelimb semiflexed (the dropped elbow posture) is typical of

- a fractured olecranon
- radial nerve paralysis
- brachial plexus injury or, less frequently,
- triceps myopathy.

---

Trauma to the base of the neck often results in an abnormally low head and neck posture.

A horse with severe stifle pain will often semiflex the limb, bearing weight only on the toe. However, this must not be confused with foot pain, with which the horse may stand similarly. Young horses with bilateral stifle pain associated with osteochondrosis may stand with an unusually straight hindlimb conformation and a rather kyphotic (roached) back. A foal with excessively flexed (curby) hocks that appear never to straighten may have incomplete ossification of the small tarsal bones.

The posture of a horse with exertional myopathy depends which muscles are most severely affected

- if only one hindlimb is affected it is usually rested
- if both are involved the horse may shift weight from one to the other with the back slightly arched.

---

### Clinical Pointer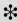

Femoral nerve paralysis results in an inability to extend the stifle, hock, and fetlock, so that the horse appears to crouch with the pelvis flexed on the vertebral column, especially if affected bilaterally. Nettle stings can produce a similar posture for 1–2 hours!

---

If the horse stands with a hindlimb extended caudally this is almost pathognomonic for upward fixation of the patella (Fig. 21.25). An unusually straight posture of a hindlimb, with apparent shortening, may be the result of luxation of the coxofemoral joint.

## PALPATION OF THE NECK, LIMBS AND BACK

Palpation of the neck, back, and limbs should be done in a systematic and methodical manner so that no abnormality is missed. The aims are to identify areas of heat, swelling, muscle tension, crepitus or pain, and to determine the significance of these findings.

---

### Clinical Pointer

Horses commonly shift weight alternately between each hindlimb, resting each in turn. To rest a single hindlimb persistently is rather unusual.

---

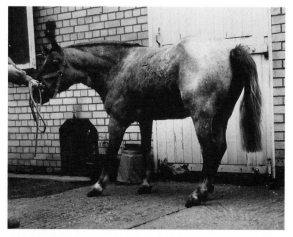

**Fig. 21.24** Posture associated with bilateral forelimb laminitis.

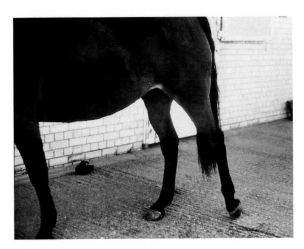

**Fig. 21.25** Stance almost pathognomonic of upward fixation of the patella. The patella may become lodged in this position. Pushing the horse backwards may help to release it.

## Neck

The neck is palpated with each hand running simultaneously down the sides to detect areas of swelling or muscle loss. Many normal horses have slightly asymmetrical development of the neck musculature. Firm pressure is applied at the level of each vertebra on both sides. Most normal horses will not react, therefore evidence of pain is usually clinically significant. The musculature is palpated carefully to identify tension or pain. Many normal horses will resent firm pressure applied to the caudal aspect of the brachiocephalicus muscles. Neck flexibility can be assessed by grasping the nose and twisting the neck first to one side and then the other. Some horses naturally resist this and it is easier to assess flexibility by holding a bowl of feed under the horse's nose and moving it round to the shoulder. A normal horse can usually turn its neck easily so that feed can be reached from the shoulder. The ease with which a horse can lower its head to the ground is best assessed by observing it eating from the ground. If the horse stands with the limbs straddled abnormally (i.e. wide apart from side to side, or from back to front) in order to reach the ground, this usually indicates caudal neck pain. The head and neck should also be manually elevated: if this induces pain the horse may rear up or reverse rapidly.

---

**Clinical Pointer**

Palpate each forelimb and hindlimb in both weightbearing and non-weightbearing positions.

---

Areas of swelling or pain are sometimes most easily detected when the limb is non-weightbearing. For example, slight rounding of the margins of the superficial digital flexor tendon, indicative of current or previous injury, is best appreciated in the non-weightbearing position, as is pain on pressure applied to the margins of the superficial digital flexor tendon. Joint flexibility and pain on passive motion (flexion, rotation or both) can only be assessed with the limb non-weightbearing. Abnormal joint laxity due to collateral ligament injury can usually only be appreciated if the joint is stressed when non-weightbearing.

## Forelimbs

### Shoulder and elbow

Starting proximally, the shoulder musculature is palpated, comparing left and right sides and assessing the prominence of the scapular spine. The cranial aspect of the distal scapula is palpated: abnormal thickening in this area may be due to a fracture of the supraglenoid tubercle. Firm pressure is applied over the cranial proximal humerus in the region of the intertubercular (bicipital) bursa. The presence of pain usually reflects bursitis or bicipital tendonitis, but the absence of detectable pain does not preclude these diagnoses. Pain may also be induced by forced retraction of the limb. By moving the limb slowly backwards and forwards with the investigator's ear close to the shoulder, crepitus due to an intra-articular fracture may be heard. The triceps musculature is assessed and the olecranon firmly grasped. Pain may reflect a fracture of the olecranon. Distension of either the shoulder or elbow joint capsules is extremely difficult to assess except in foals.

---

**Clinical Pointer**

When examining the elbow joint be aware of the close proximity of the joint capsule to the skin surface laterally, and the consequent danger of penetrating wounds in this area resulting in synovial sepsis.

---

### Forearm and carpus

The muscles of the antebrachium are palpated. Atrophy generally reflects either chronic severe lameness or a neurological problem. The dorsal aspect of the carpus is carefully assessed. Soft tissue swellings here are common and must be carefully differentiated. Longitudinal swellings usually reflect distension of one of the extensor tendon sheaths with or without enlargement or disruption of an extensor tendon. Rupture of the extensor carpi radialis is not uncommon in foals. Tendon sheaths in this location are usually not palpable unless distended. Slight fullness of the antebrachiocarpal or middle carpal joint capsules results in more horizontally organized swellings, usually best detected by palpation, ballotting fluid from one side of the joint to the other. Distension of these joint capsules is sometimes also detectable on the palmarolateral aspect of the carpus. The precise location of the swelling should be determined by palpation with the limb semiflexed (Fig. 21.26). An unusually doughy feel to the capsule usually reflects synovial proliferation. There may also be a crackling sensation of soft tissue crepitus. Small outpouchings are sometimes palpable in association with chronic joint disease. More diffuse swellings generally represent subcutaneous edema, hemorrhage, fibrosis or a false bursa. Distension of the carpal sheath is usually most easily detectable on the medial aspect of the limb, both proximal to the carpus and distal, extending to the junction of the proximal and middle thirds of the metacarpus.

With the limb non-weightbearing the carpus can be flexed. In the normal horse the back of the fetlock comes into contact with the back of the elbow region (Fig. 21.26). Flexion may be restricted because of pain, mechanical constraints, or both, e.g. periarticular or joint capsule fibrosis or both. By placing the distal limb between the examiner's legs (Fig. 21.27), both hands can be used to carefully palpate

- the antebrachiocarpal and middle carpal joint capsules
- the distal dorsal radius and the proximal and distal borders of the proximal row of carpal bones
- the proximal border of the distal row of carpal bones.

Joint capsule distension in this location is generally clinically significant, as is restricted flexibility or pain on flexion or palpation. Pain on palpation of the borders of the carpal bones may reflect a fracture or, less commonly, degenerative joint disease. Palpable distension of the carpal sheath is also usually clinically significant, and may be due to effusion, synovitis, and/or tendonitis.

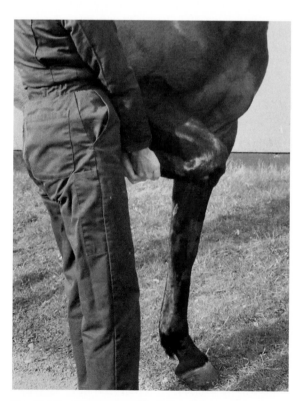

**Fig. 21.26** Assessment of flexibility of the carpus. Note the elbow is flexed concurrently.

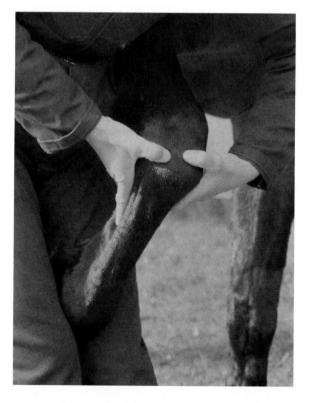

**Fig. 21.27** Palpation of the carpal joints.

## Metacarpal region

With the horse bearing full weight on the limb, the thumb and first finger of each hand are moved along the dorsal and palmar borders of the suspensory ligament and each branch, medially and laterally, to assess size. Enlargement reflects previous or current injury. Diffuse swelling in the proximal third of the metacarpus dorsal to the superficial digital flexor tendon usually reflects enlargement of the accessory ligament of the deep digital flexor tendon due to current or previous injury.

The palmar contour of the metacarpus is normally straight. Swelling confined to the palmar aspect usually reflects peritendinous edema or tendon injury, and must not be ignored even if it disperses with local therapy. Localized heat may reflect tendonitis even in the absence of detectable enlargement of the superficial digital flexor tendon. Careful comparison is made with the contralateral limb. Localized heat may be masked if the limbs have been bandaged or are very hairy. Subtle differences in surface temperature are best appreciated if the limbs are clipped. With the limb non-weightbearing pressure should be applied over the proximal aspect of the suspensory ligament, medially and laterally, rolling away the deep digital flexor tendon and its accessory ligament. Pain may reflect proximal suspensory desmitis or an avulsion fracture at the origin of the suspensory ligament. The margins of the suspensory ligament are palpated gently at first to assess their demarcation (Fig. 21.28). Rounding of the margins usually reflects previous or current injury. Abnormal stiffness of the ligament indicates previous injury. Firm pressure applied to the margins may elicit pain, but be aware that most horses will react if excessive pressure is applied.

The amount of soreness should also be related to recent work. Very hard work may result in transient soreness of the suspensory ligaments without detectable structural abnormalities. Firm pressure should also be applied over each suspensory ligament branch and at their insertions on the proximal sesamoid bones. Each of the accessory ligaments of the deep digital flexor tendon, the deep digital flexor tendon, and the superficial digital flexor tendon should be palpated similarly, bearing in mind that the

> **Clinical Pointer**
>
> Always compare a horse's reaction to palpation of one limb with that of the contralateral limb as there is considerable variability between horses in their reaction.

absence of pain on palpation does not preclude a significant tendon injury. Enlargement of a tendon or ligament, rounding of its margins or pain on pressure may reflect previous or current injury.

The dorsal aspect of the metacarpus should be palpated firmly, particularly in racehorses: localized soreness, especially in the middle third, may reflect periosteal disease (sore or bucked shins). The contour of the second and fourth metacarpal bones is carefully assessed for the presence of enlargements, pain on palpation, or both due to periostitis or a fracture. Pain is most easily assessed with the limb lifted. The ease with which the suspensory ligament can be separated from the second and fourth metacarpal bones can also be assessed. Impingement of an exostosis may result in suspensory ligament soreness and/or adhesions.

Enlargement of the digital flexor tendon sheath (tendinous windgall) is a common incidental finding, but if it develops suddenly in association with lameness, or is asymmetrical, it is likely to be of clinical importance. As with any synovial structure, differentiation should be made between effusion and synovial thickening. The 'tightness' of the palmar annular ligament should be carefully assessed. Notching of the palmar

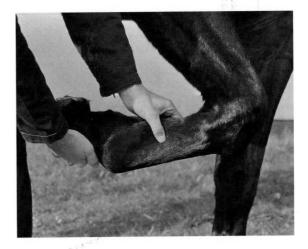

**Fig. 21.28** Palpation of the suspensory ligament to assess size, flexibility, demarcation of its margins, and the presence or absence of pain.

> **Clinical Pointer**
>
> Enlargement of the medial palmar vein is a common finding in association with any source of distal limb pain.

contour of the limb at the level of the palmar annular ligament is usually indicative of significant constriction of the digital flexor tendon sheath.

### Fetlock region

Distension of the metacarpophalangeal joint capsule may be appreciated both dorsally and in the palmar pouch – the recess between the third metacarpal bone and the suspensory ligament. Joint capsule distension may reflect underlying significant joint disease, but not invariably so. Some horses, especially those with upright pastern conformation, seem prone to joint capsule distension. Apparent pain on flexion of the fetlock joint is not necessarily specific for the joint: horses with primary suspensory ligament disease frequently react positively to fetlock flexion. Restricted flexibility is a common incidental finding, especially in older horses, and is usually bilaterally symmetrical. A marked difference in flexibility between right and left limbs, or unusual stiffness in a young horse, is probably clinically important. With the limb non-weightbearing, firm pressure should be applied over the dorso-proximal aspect of the proximal phalanx. Pain on pressure may be the only clinical indication of an incomplete sagittal fracture of the dorsoproximal aspect of the proximal phalanx.

The digital pulse amplitudes are most easily assessed at the level of either the fetlock or the pastern by holding the thumb and fingers over the vessels. Pressing too hard will obliterate the pulse. A careful comparison should be made both between limbs and between medial and lateral sides.

> ### Changes in the digital pulse
>
> - if the horse is without shoes the pulse amplitudes tend to be stronger than in the same horse when shod
> - bounding pulse amplitudes, similar medially and laterally, are characteristic of laminitis
> - an increase in pulse intensity on one side is often seen in association with a subsolar abscess or nail bind (pressure on the sensitive laminae by a nail placed too close)
> - chronic palmar foot pain can result in enlarged vessels.

### Pastern

The contours of the pastern should be carefully assessed. Firm swellings are not necessarily

synonymous with bony swellings and often cannot be evaluated further without radiography or ultrasonography. Distension of the proximal interphalangeal joint capsule is rarely appreciated, but filling on the dorsal midline immediately proximal to the coronary band usually indicates distension of the distal interphalangeal joint capsule. Distension of the distal outpouching of the digital flexor tendon sheath on the palmar aspect of the pastern is often an incidental finding of no importance. Firm soft tissue swellings on the palmar aspect of the pastern can be difficult to distinguish by palpation alone. A midline swelling most likely reflects subcutaneous fibrosis or enlargement of the deep digital flexor tendon, whereas swelling restricted to either the medial or the lateral aspect is more likely to indicate subcutaneous fibrosis or damage to either a distal sesamoidean ligament or a branch of the superficial digital flexor tendon.

The flexibility and symmetry of the cartilages of the foot are assessed. If there is any possibility that the horse may previously have had a palmar digital neurectomy, the pastern region should be inspected carefully for the presence of surgical scars. This may be facilitated by fine clipping of the hair. In addition, firm pressure should be applied to the heel region using, for example, the tips of artery forceps, to establish whether or not there is normal sensation. The coronary band should be carefully assessed. A focal area of heat, pain, or softness may indicate the site of impending drainage of a subsolar abscess. Depression of the entire coronary band is seen in association with distal movement (sinking) of the distal phalanx due to laminitis.

> ### Clinical Pointer
>
> Mineralization of the foot cartilages tends to be much more extensive in heavier horses.

### Foot

Detailed examination of the foot is best done after removal of the shoe, but in most cases it is preferable to delay this until the horse has been examined moving as it may be foot sore without shoes and the hoof wall may crack. Percussion and pressure applied to the foot with hoof testers can be very usefully carried out at this stage. Percussion is applied to the wall of the foot, a localized reaction possibly reflecting

- nail bind
- inflamed laminae, or
- a submural abscess.

The most accurate way of assessing the response to pressure applied with hoof testers is to place the foot between the examiner's legs, as if for shoeing. The hoof testers are applied using both hands, starting at one side of the foot and moving carefully around it applying pressure across the wall and sole (Fig. 21.29). Pressure is applied gently at first because pain in association with a subsolar abscess may be profound. However, the absence of pain on firm pressure does not preclude the presence of an abscess. Pain may be detected by a variable response: from a subtle slight withdrawal of the limb to a vigorous snatching or the horse rearing upwards. The handler may notice the horse lay its ears back or threaten to bite. Pain on pressure with hoof testers may reflect

- subsolar bruising or hemorrhage
- a subsolar abscess
- thrush
- fracture of the distal phalanx, or
- laminitis.

It is important to map out both the area and the degree of pain to determine the most likely cause. The size of hoof testers used, the examiner's strength and the

temperament of the horse all will influence the response. Using 'short-armed' hoof testers a positive response is usually significant, whereas with 'long-armed' hoof testers some normal horses will show a withdrawal response.

The site and degree of a swelling may not accurately reflect the primary site and cause of lameness. Diffuse filling of the limb from the carpus distally is commonly seen associated with a subsolar hoof abscess. Other common causes include cellulitis, suspensory ligament desmitis, or a fracture of the second or fourth metacarpal bones. Fractures of both these bones may occur concurrent to suspensory desmitis. The degree of swelling may interfere with accurate palpation and it may be preferable to use ancillary diagnostic aids such as radiography and ultrasonography to determine the cause. Alternatively, symptomatic treatment could be used to reduce the swelling and then the limb reappraised.

If a limb is extremely hairy, this prohibits accurate palpation and valuable information may be missed unless the limb is finely clipped. After clipping it may be possible to identify, for example, distension of the digital flexor tendon sheath and associated constriction by the palmar annular ligament, which might otherwise have been missed.

## Hindquarters

The hindlimb is approached similarly to the forelimb, starting by palpating the musculature of the hindquarters searching for an area of pain and abnormal swelling, or texture. An area of abnormal firmness in the semimembranosus or semitendinosus muscles may be due to fibrotic or ossifying myopathy.

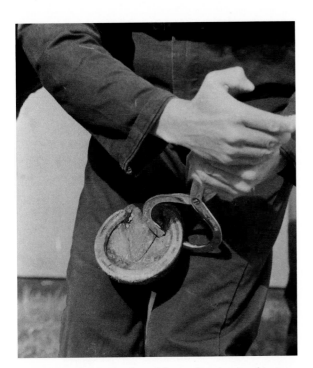

**Fig. 21.29** Determination of foot pain using hoof testers. The examiner should bend his knees in towards the horse to avoid excessive outward rotation of the carpus, which may itself induce discomfort.

### Clinical Pointer

If a pelvic fracture is suspected it may be helpful to auscultate over each hindquarter using a stethoscope to detect crepitus.

Firm pressure is applied over the tubera sacrale. The normal horse resists this, but if there is pain the horse usually sinks abnormally and may grunt. This may reflect sacroiliac pain or damage to the ilium. Soreness of the tuber ischium, or abnormal swelling, especially if combined with soreness of the semimembranosus and semitendinosus muscles, may reflect an ischial fracture. With chronic ischial fracture there may be muscle wastage around the tail head on the affected side.

## Stifle and crus

The stifle region is most easily assessed by locating the tibial crest and then moving proximally and identifying the middle, medial, and lateral patellar ligaments, the tendon of the long digital extensor muscle, and the lateral and medial collateral ligaments of the femorotibial joint. The middle patellar ligament is larger than the medial and lateral patellar ligaments. The collateral ligaments of the femorotibial joint are relatively flat. Distension of either the femorotibial or femoropatellar joint capsules is usually readily appreciated, but should be distinguished from periarticular soft tissue swelling. All are generally of clinical importance; however, owing to the potential communication between the joint compartments the site(s) of joint capsule distension may not be specific. The position of the patella should be noted. Lateral displacement occurs occasionally in foals and young horses and is associated with severe lameness. The patella should be firmly palpated and pushed upwards. If there is a tendency towards delayed release of the patella from this upward position, slightly abnormal movement may be appreciated. In addition, by grasping the tail and rocking the horse from side to side the patella may be seen to move rather jerkily. The region of the medial patellar ligament should be carefully palpated to detect a surgical scar. Thickening of the ligament or periligamentous thickening is indicative of a previous medial patellar desmotomy. Firm pressure applied to the patella and trochleas of the femur may elicit pain following localized severe bruising or a fracture.

> ## Cruciate ligament injury
>
> It is impossible to palpate the menisci and the cruciate ligaments and essentially impossible to elicit a 'drawer' response in horses with cruciate ligament injury.

A horse with stifle pain may resist full flexion of the stifle, or alternatively may lift the limb exaggeratedly during flexion. Because of the reciprocal apparatus of the hindlimb, the hock, stifle, and hip joints are flexed simultaneously, and in a normal horse the dorsal aspect of the fetlock can be raised close to the stifle (Fig. 21.30).

Cracking or clicking noises, presumed to be ligamentous in origin, are sometimes heard, especially in the stifle region, but generally these are not clinically important.

> ## Clinical Pointer
>
> A horse may be unwilling to allow a limb to be held in flexion because it either
>
> - has pain in the flexed limb, or
> - resents standing on the contralateral limb.

The tibia has minimal soft tissue covering medially and firm percussion may elicit pain in a young Thoroughbred with a stress or fatigue fracture, although in many cases the response will be negative. Pain on palpation of the tibial crest may indicate a fracture, especially in the presence of localized soft tissue swelling. The saphenous vein is readily seen on the medial aspect of the crus (the gaskin or second thigh).

## Hock

In the distal one-third of the crus, the gastrocnemius tendon wraps around the lateral border of the superficial digital flexor tendon and comes to lie cranially.

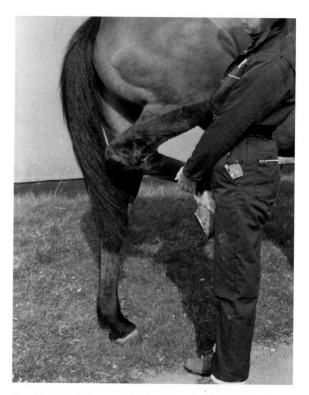

**Fig. 21.30**  Assessment of flexibility of the proximal joints of the hindlimb. Also the position for a proximal hindlimb flexion test (also called hock flexion test).

Distension of the gastrocnemius bursa between the gastrocnemius tendon and the superficial digital flexor tendon, or the calcaneal bursa under the insertion of gastrocnemius muscle, or a slightly bulging (capped) hock appearance, may reflect gastrocnemius tendonitis. However, all these swellings may be seen as incidental findings. Soft tissue swellings in this area can be difficult to identify precisely by visual appraisal and palpation. Distension of the tarsal sheath (true thoroughpin) usually produces swelling both medially and laterally. This often develops transiently in young horses unassociated with lameness. It should be possible to ballotte fluid from the dorsomedial outpouching of the tarsocrural joint capsule to the caudolateral outpouching (Fig. 21.31).

Although mild distension of the tarsocrural joint may occur without other clinical signs, it may be seen in association with lameness or poor performance due to osteochondrosis, collateral ligament desmitis or degenerative joint disease of the talocalcaneal–centroquatral (proximal intertarsal) joint.

Pressure should be applied to the medial and lateral malleoli of the tibia. It is sometimes possible to detect both crepitus and pain associated with an avulsion fracture of the attachments of the deep or superficial, medial or lateral collateral ligaments. Firm

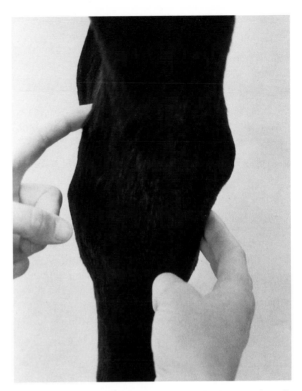

**Fig. 21.31** Distension of the tarsocrural joint capsule. It is possible to ballotte fluid from the dorsomedial to the caudolateral outpouching.

enlargement on the medial aspect of the hock at the level of the central and third tarsal bones may reflect new bone formation, but is more likely to be an overlying soft tissue reaction and may or may not reflect degenerative joint disease of the distal hock joints. Significance of this is best assessed using local analgesic techniques, radiography, and occasionally ultrasonography. In the presence of diffuse soft tissue swelling over the tuber calcaneus the position of the superficial digital flexor tendon should be carefully checked: displacement occurs laterally more often than medially. Enlargement on the plantar aspect of the calcaneus or the proximal metatarsus should be carefully assessed to differentiate abnormal prominence of the base (head) of the fourth metatarsal bone, with or without slight displacement of the superficial digital flexor tendon, from other soft tissue enlargements, such as superficial or deep digital flexor tendonitis, plantar ligament desmitis, and subcutaneous fibrosis. Differentiation of the latter conditions is usually only possible using ultrasonography.

Examination of the remainder of the distal hindlimb is similar to the forelimb, although distension, enlargement or both of the digital flexor tendon sheath (windgall) is seen more commonly as an incidental finding in hindlimbs rather than forelimbs.

## Back

Back pain may develop as a primary problem causing poor performance and gait abnormalities or may be secondary to lameness, especially of the hindlimb. Conformational abnormalities such as

- kyphosis (arched back), and
- lordosis (dipped back)

may be present without associated clinical signs. The ease with which the summits of the dorsal spinous processes in the thoracolumbar region can be palpated depends on the conformation of the horse and the development of the longissimus dorsi muscles, which should be aligned straightly. Poorly developed muscles may lead to prominence of the summits of the dorsal spinous processes in the caudal thoracic and cranial lumbar regions and apparent kyphosis.

> ### Clinical Pointer
>
> If scoliosis (twisted back) is suspected it is helpful to mark the summits of the dorsal spinous processes with tape and view the horse from above.

The longissimus dorsi muscles are generally reasonably soft in the normal horse standing at rest. Abnormal firmness is usually due to muscle spasm, either primary or secondary, although it may reflect apprehension. Firm stroking may elicit muscle fasciculations in regions of soreness. The flexibility of the thoracolumbar region can be assessed by stimulating flexion (arching) by firm stroking of the gluteal musculature from cranially to caudally. Extension (dipping) is stimulated by firm pressure applied over the dorsal midline in the thoracolumbar region. Flexibility to the left and right is evoked by dorsoventral firm stroking on each side of the thoracolumbar region and the hindquarters. This is best done using artery forceps. Most normal horses will repeatedly flex and extend the thoracolumbar region without becoming agitated, with the longissimus dorsi muscles remaining relaxed. Possible indicators of pain are

- abnormal tension in the longissimus dorsi muscles
- kicking
- laying the ears back
- biting

- holding the back stiffly, and
- flexing the hindlimbs rather than extending the back.

However, the reactions must be interpreted in the light of the horse's temperament. The horse should be as relaxed as possible during this examination; normal Thoroughbreds may react excessively as a reflection of their temperament, rather than back pain.

Rib soreness or pain associated with the sternum occasionally causes gait or behavioral abnormalities, such as abnormal dipping of the back when the horse is saddled or mounted (cold back behavior). A complete examination should include firm palpation of these structures. The inguinal region should also be assessed as castration reactions and mastitis may cause hindlimb stiffness or overt lameness.

## Rectal examination

A rectal examination should be done systematically, feeling the 'floor' of the pelvis, the pelvic brim, and the shafts of the ilia to assess contour, the presence of swellings such as a hematoma, or the presence of pain. If a fracture of the pelvis is suspected the horse should be rocked from side to side, or walked a few steps, to see whether crepitus can be appreciated. In a normal horse the pelvic contours are symmetrical. Asymmetry may reflect

- a hematoma
- fibrosis
- callus formation, or
- a displaced fracture.

Abnormal swelling, pain, and crepitus usually reflect a fracture, although the absence of these signs does not preclude a fracture. The ilial wings cannot reliably be assessed per rectum and an abnormality of the coxofemoral joint will only be detected if there is a displaced articular fracture. Firm pressure should be applied to the psoas muscles. Pain usually reflects

> ### Indications for rectal examination
>
> These include
>
> - cases with a sudden onset of severe hindlimb lameness associated with a fracture of the pubic bone, ischium, and the caudal ilium, or severe muscle damage
> - cases of intermittent hindlimb lameness which develops during exercise and improves rapidly with rest, associated with aortoiliac thrombosis.

primary or secondary injury. The size, firmness, shape and pulsations of the aorta and iliac arteries should be assessed. In the normal horse these vessels have obvious pulsations and can be compressed. In association with thrombosis the vessels may have an abnormal contour, or be unusually firm. The inguinal ring areas should be carefully evaluated, especially in colts.

---

### Clinical Pointer

During rectal examination;

- identify the ventral bony protrusion of the lumbosacral articulation about 2–4 cm caudal to the terminal aorta
- just behind this on the plateau of the sacrum is the predilection site for a fractured sacrum (S2)
- palpate here for evidence of a fracture or callus formation.

---

## ASSESSMENT OF GAIT

Accurate assessment of gait can be very difficult if a horse is overly fresh or exuberant. Provided a fracture is not suspected based on the history and preliminary clinical examination, it may be helpful to lunge the horse first to encourage it to settle. The handler should be encouraged to wear a helmet and gloves for protection. In some circumstances mild sedation with an $\alpha_2$ agonist drug can be very helpful. When the horse is being led in hand it is important that the handler allows as much freedom as possible while maintaining control. Many owners may be unable to restrain their horses adequately in a head collar, and a bridle may be preferable. However, the reins should be held sufficiently loose so that there is minimal interference with head and neck movement. The horse must trot freely, preferably with the handler running at the shoulder. If the horse is unwilling, encouragement with a lunge whip is helpful. Assessment of gait is difficult unless the horse is moving freely at a steady speed. This may of course be difficult to achieve in a foal, which is generally best assessed moving freely and following its dam. It is important both to observe and listen to the horse moving.

### Walking

The horse should first be assessed moving at the walk. The relatively slow sequence of footfalls gives time to assess carefully limb flight and foot placement. The

---

### Clinical Pointer

Rhythm irregularities in the gait, or asymmetrical loading forces, are most easily appreciated by sound and best assessed with the horse moving on a concrete or tarmac surface, which must be sufficiently rough so that the horse moves confidently, without fear of slipping.

---

horse should be viewed from the front, from the side, and from behind. For the inexperienced observer it is probably best to focus on different parts of the horse independently, assessing first

- the forelimbs, then
- the head and neck movement, and finally
- the hindlimbs.

There is considerable variation in limb flight and foot placement between horses and between left and right limbs of horses, not necessarily related to lameness. Many horses when viewed from the front will have an axial or abaxial deviation in limb or foot flight of one or both forelimbs. Some normal horses move with their hindlimbs very far apart, whereas others move closely behind. Familiarity with the normal and its variations is important.

At both the walk and trot assess

- the flight of each limb
- the height of the arc of foot flight
- foot placement
- the degree of fetlock extension
- the placement of each hind foot relative to the imprint of each front foot.

---

### At the walk

- a forelimb may be swung outwards a little to avoid carpal flexion in association with carpal pain
- a horse with palmar foot pain may tend to land toe first
- a horse with diffuse foot pain may land with the foot flatter, or even heel first
- fetlock extension may be reduced in association with fetlock pain
- lameness may induce a shortened length of the cranial phase of the stride so that the horse fails to track up
- abrupt slapping of one hindlimb to the ground is typical of ossifying or fibrotic myopathy, this is most easily detected at the walk.

A normal horse will place each hind foot in the imprint of the ipsilateral front foot (track up), or place each hind foot beyond or in front of the imprint of the ipsilateral front foot (over track).

The horse is observed carefully as it turns to change direction. A horse with foot pain will often appear most lame when turning. Horses with more proximal limb pain usually turn much more normally. Gait abnormalities may be due to either musculoskeletal problems or to neurological dysfunction, when signs of ataxia, dysmetria, and weakness may be present. Assessing the horse turning in small circles to the left and to the right, and stepping backwards, can be helpful in determining such abnormalities.

1. A horse with proximal forelimb pain (shoulder or elbow) may be unwilling to abduct or adduct the lame limb when turned in small circles.
2. A horse with neck pain will hold the neck stiffly.
3. A horse with meniscal pain, or pain associated with the collateral or cruciate ligaments of the femorotibial joint, may resent turning on the affected hindlimb.
4. Neurological abnormalities such as circumduction may be seen.
5. Some gait abnormalities, for example shivering, may only be apparent when the horse steps backwards.

## Trotting

At the trot the horse normally moves in a regular two-time rhythm. At a normal trot the limbs are moved in diagonal pairs, so that the horse alternately bears weight on the left hind and right forelimbs, then the right hind and left forelimbs. If the horse paces it also moves in a two-time rhythm, bearing weight alternately on the left hind and left forelimbs, and then the right hind and right forelimbs. If the horse trots too quickly subtle irregularities of rhythm reflecting lameness may be missed. Time should be spent watching and listening to the horse trotting several times at different speeds. This is best assessed moving on a firm, level, non-slip surface so that the horse trots confidently, in order that the rhythm of footfall and any toe drag can be clearly heard. A horse without shoes may be foot-sore and move very cautiously, making evaluation of any concurrent lameness difficult. It may be best to reassess the horse when it has been trimmed and shod. Appreciation of stride length and lift to the stride is very important. Some normal horses move with great elevation, bouncing from diagonal to diagonal, with a long stride. Others move in a more restricted fashion. Without prior knowledge of the horse detection of a slight shortening in stride or decreased lift, often signi-

fying a bilateral forelimb lameness, can be difficult. Similarly, appreciation of subtle bilateral hindlimb lameness, characterized by slightly reduced hindlimb impulsion, may be difficult. Lameness associated with a palmar cortical fatigue fracture of the third metacarpal bone characteristically deteriorates the further the horse trots each time before turning around, especially on a hard surface. Some lamenesses are very inconsistent in degree both within and between examinations, and it is very important to appreciate this before proceeding with local analgesic diagnostic techniques.

## Forelimb lameness

A normal horse keeps the head and neck relatively steady at the trot, although a horse with a naturally short stride may appear to have slight movement of the head and neck from side to side in rhythm with the trot.

*Forelimb lameness is characterized by a drop or nod of the head when the sound (or less lame) limb is bearing weight, and lifting of the head during weightbearing on the lame (or lamer) limb. Lifting of the head when the lame limb is weightbearing may be particularly exaggerated with shoulder pain or severe distal limb pain.*

Bilateral forelimb lameness of similar degree may be characterized by a short striding gait, with minimal suspension between diagonal limb placements. The head and neck may remain still.

## Hindlimb lameness

A normal horse has symmetrical movement of each hindquarter. Asymmetrical musculature between the left and right hindquarters may give a false impression of asymmetrical movement. Focusing on the tubera coxae rather than the hindquarters per se is the most accurate way of assessing movement.

> ### Common causes of bilateral forelimb lameness
>
> These include
>
> - navicular syndrome
> - proximal suspensory desmitis, and
> - middle or antebrachiocarpal joint pain (in Thoroughbred or Quarterhorse racehorses).
>
> The trainer may complain of the horse having "lost its action" rather than appreciating an overt lameness by observing the horse to move with symmetrically shorter strides than normal.

*Hindlimb lameness is usually characterized by increased movement of the hindquarter of the lame or most lame limb, due to increased lifting, increased sinking, or both.*

There is frequently a stiff limb flight, typical of many hindlimb lamenesses regardless of the site of pain, owing to the reciprocal apparatus of the hindlimb. The height of arc of foot flight is often reduced, frequently resulting in toe drag. However, toe drag is not necessarily synonymous with lameness: some lazy or unfit horses may toe drag. Limited hindlimb impulsion, stiffness or a failure to move straight on two tracks may all indicate bilateral hindlimb lameness. If hindlimb lameness is moderate to severe then there may be an associated head nod, so that superficially the horse may appear to be lame on the ipsilateral forelimb. The head nods as the lame hindlimb and contralateral forelimb bear weight. The horse effectively rocks forward on to the sound (or less lame) contralateral forelimb to reduce loadbearing on the lame hindlimb.

Hindlimb lamenesses vary considerably in their appearance on the lunge and there are few general rules to assist the clinician. Many horses with hindlimb lameness will be unwilling to properly engage the hindlimbs, and show a tendency to hop or break into canter rather than trot freely forwards with good hindlimb impulsion. Another reason to work the horse on the lunge is to see whether or not the lameness improves with exercise; this is important to appreciate if local analgesic techniques are to be employed. Mild neurological gait abnormalities may also become more apparent as the horse tires. A normal horse swings the back freely so that the tail also swings from side to side. In association with back pain the horse may hold its back and tail stiffly, or hold the tail to one side. The longissimus dorsi muscles may appear to tense abnormally. Hindlimb impulsion may be limited, at both the trot and the canter, which may result in a 'bunny-hopping' gait behind at canter. This is not, however, pathognomonic of back pain: a horse with bilateral hind fetlock pain may have a bunny-hopping type gait.

### Clinical Pointer

Occasionally a horse with hindlimb lameness will move on three tracks with the pelvis held to one side of midline, or move so closely as to plait the feet on protraction (each hindlimb appears to cross over each other if viewed from behind).

### Clinical Pointer

- most foot lamenesses appear worst on a hard surface
- lameness associated with a soft tissue injury, such as proximal suspensory desmitis, is often worst on a soft surface.

## Lunging

Lameness is frequently accentuated, and in some cases may only be detectable, with the horse exercising on a circle. The horse is best assessed moving freely on the lunge rather than being led in circles, and ideally should be examined on both soft and hard surfaces, as this may alter the degree of lameness. The horse should not be lunged on a tarmac or concrete surface if it is excessively exuberant, as it may inadvertently slip and fall. It should be lunged on the soft first until it has settled.

## Ridden exercise

Lameness may only be evident as reduced performance, for example unwillingness to work on the bit. The horse may carry its head higher than normal, or extend its nose, or both, rather than flex normally at the poll. Some lamenesses, especially hindlimb, may only be apparent when the horse is ridden. However, a rider may complicate the issue, especially if inexperienced. Movement of the rider's hands may induce movement of the head and neck. A heavy rider, out of balance with the horse, may induce apparent hindlimb lameness. If the horse is unduly restricted by the reins, not ridden forwards sufficiently, or both, it may appear to have a very restricted gait either in front, behind or both, with or without an irregular rhythm. Thus some lamenesses are actually induced by inappropriate riding, and it can be helpful to see the horse ridden both by the regular rider, the trainer or both, and an independent, skillful rider. Tact and diplomacy may be required!

Hindlimb lamenesses usually are accentuated when, while trotting, the rider sits on the diagonal of the lame

### Lameness on a circle

- forelimb lamenesses are most commonly, but not always, accentuated with the most lame limb on the inside of a circle
- lameness associated with proximal suspensory desmitis, shoulder pain, or pain restricted to the medial aspect of the foot or pastern is often worse with the lamer limb on the outside of a circle.

limb, compared to the opposite diagonal. Thus if the horse is lame on the left hindlimb, lameness is worst when the rider sits on the right fore/left hind diagonal.

---

### Clinical Pointer

As some lamenesses, in particular hindlimb lamenesses, are only apparent when the horse is ridden, ridden exercise should be an integral part of a prepurchase assessment.

---

### Grading lameness

It is helpful to develop a grading system when assessing lameness, and to record the degree of lameness so that comparisons can be made with subsequent examinations, and before and after flexion tests or nerve blocks. It is probably most accurate to grade lameness independently in each circumstance; the horse is assessed on each rein

---

### A simple grading system for lameness

0 = no lameness detectable
1 = mild lameness
2 = moderate lameness
3 = severe lameness
4 = non-weightbearing lameness.

---

- at the walk in hand
- at the trot in hand
- on the lunge on a soft surface
- on the lunge on a hard surface, and
- when ridden.

When possible, each limb should be graded independently, but this may be difficult with bilateral forelimb or hindlimb lameness, especially if each limb is affected similarly. The usefulness of any system relies principally on its repeatability rather than the precise number of grades used.

However, it may be necessary at times to subdivide the grades to be more precise and to indicate variability in degree within an examination. The use of more precise guidelines, such as extent of head nod, can be misleading as the characteristics of lameness vary considerably depending on the source of pain, whether one or more limbs is affected, and the circumstances under which the horse is examined.

Owners tend to expect that the source of pain and therefore lameness can be accurately determined by analysis of gait. However, although certain characteristics of gait can be highly suggestive of the general source of pain, they are often not specific. Even with high-speed cinematography the precise focus of pain cannot usually be determined.

---

### Clinical Pointer

Lameness due to many different sites of pain can appear similar, especially in the hindlimb.

---

Thus visual gait analysis is unquestionably useful for general localization of pain in some cases, and may guide the clinician towards what to do next, but not invariably so.

### Flexion tests

A flexion test involves holding one or more joints in a flexed position for approximately 45–60 seconds. The degree of lameness at the trot is then immediately assessed. Flexion may cause pain from

- stretching of tissues around the joint
- compression, or
- alteration of blood flow.

Accentuation of lameness after flexion is suggestive of a problem involving the flexed joints.

Flexion tests may be helpful in identifying the lame limb or the source of pain, but can be confusing. Some normal horses will take several lame steps after flexion of the distal joints (metacarpophalangeal and interphalangeal) of each forelimb. A similar response in each forelimb can usually be regarded as normal, but a difference between each limb or prolonged lameness probably reflects an underlying problem. Most normal horses do not show lameness after carpal or hock flexion, or flexion of the hind fetlocks, but the degree of response will obviously depend on the duration of flexion and the force applied.

The front fetlock should be flexed by facing the rear and holding the foot by the toe (Fig. 21.32); in this way

---

### Clinical Pointer

Lameness can be induced in any horse by excessive flexion! It is helpful always to use a consistent technique.

---

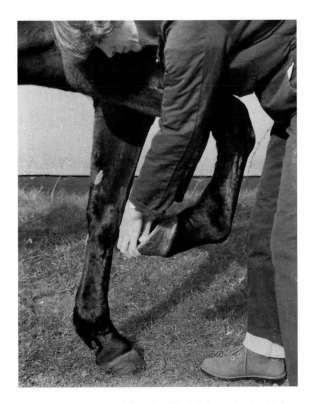

**Fig. 21.32** Flexion of the distal limb joints of a forelimb, the fetlock flexion test.

phalangeal joints. An alternative, more specific technique is to hold the fetlock in flexion by grasping the proximal pastern. Carpal flexion (see Fig. 21.26) is also non-specific, as the elbow is flexed concurrently. Forelimb protraction occasionally accentuates lameness associated with the shoulder joint, whereas retraction may increase lameness associated with pain involving the tendon of the biceps brachii and/or the intertubercular bursa.

Hindlimb flexion tests are also non-specific, particularly because of the reciprocal apparatus. Flexion of the hock (see Fig. 21.30) by holding the distal metatarsus flexes the stifle and hip joints concurrently. Holding the limb in the 'shoeing' position by grasping the foot and keeping it as close to the ground as possible, stresses principally the fetlock and interphalangeal joints (Fig. 21.33). If the limb is held in a similar but slightly higher position by supporting the distal crus, the stifle is stressed (Fig. 21.34). However, it is quite common for a lame horse to respond to more than one type of flexion test in the lame limb, especially the hindlimbs. Protraction, retraction, and abduction of the hindlimb are rather non-specific tests and in the author's experience have not proved very useful.

if the horse moves it is easy to stay with it safely. Moderate force is applied for approximately 45–60 seconds and the horse is then trotted. It is better that it walk for a couple of steps first, rather than bound off at a trot (or canter!). A positive response is assessed as the production or accentuation of lameness for five or more strides. The sound or less lame limb is routinely flexed first to avoid a sustained positive response to flexion of the lamer limb, thus masking the response to flexion of the contralateral limb. A positive response does not necessarily reflect the primary source of pain. A positive response to fetlock flexion may be alleviated by intra-articular analgesia, although the baseline lameness may remain unaltered. Fetlock flexion using the technique described above also stresses the inter-

### Clinical Pointer ✳

Occasionally a paradoxical increase in lameness is seen in the lame limb after any manipulative test of the sound or less lame limb, owing to increased load-bearing on the lame limb.

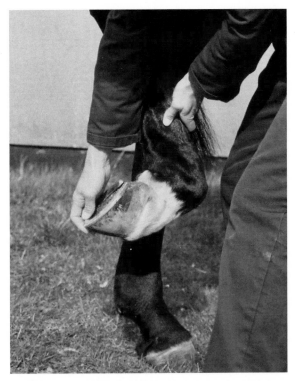

**Fig. 21.33** Flexion of the hindlimb distal limb joints. Note the stifle is also partially flexed.

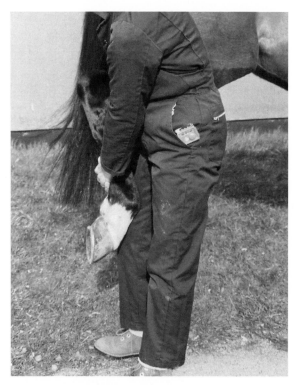

**Fig. 21.34** Stifle flexion test.

## Other provocative tests

### The wedge test

Lameness associated with any source or cause of pain in the palmar aspect of the foot may be accentuated by elevating the toe of the lame limb on a plank of wood while picking up the contralateral limb. This wedge test is performed for approximately 1 minute.

Squeezing a painful structure, such as the body of the suspensory ligament, or applying pressure over a painful structure, such as a fractured second metacarpal bone (splint) may accentuate lameness. Similarly, squeezing the wall and sole of the foot with hoof testers may accentuate lameness associated with a painful focus in that region.

## DETAILED EXAMINATION OF THE FOOT

Foot balance can be critical to soundness, even though there are many sound horses with mild to severe

imbalance. Ideally each foot should be set on symmetrically about the central limb axis. The coronary band is equidistant from the solar surface on the medial and lateral sides of the foot. Viewed from the side, an imaginary perpendicular line from the center of the radius of curvature of the distal interphalangeal joint to the ground should approximately bisect the solar surface of the foot (Fig. 21.35). If the toe is abnormally long there is considerably more foot in front of this imaginary line than behind, predisposing to overload of the back of the foot, i.e. dorsopalmar imbalance. The pastern foot axis is ideally straight, although there is considerable variation between horses in the precise angle. A broken forward or backward pastern foot axis may be the result of inappropriate trimming and shoeing. Mediolateral imbalance is best assessed with the following procedure

- view the horse from the front and assess the pastern and shape of the foot relative to the central limb axis
- pick up the limb and hold it by the proximal metacarpus underneath the thorax, allowing it to hang down naturally in the sagittal plane of the horse's body (Fig. 21.36)
- observe the ground-bearing surface, it should be perpendicular to a line bisecting the metacarpus.

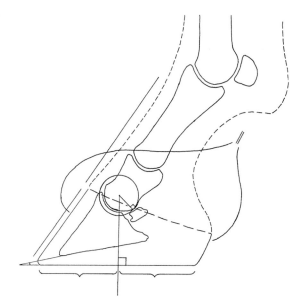

**Fig. 21.35** Diagrammatic representation of assessment of dorsopalmar foot balance. A perpendicular line from the center of the radius of curvature of the distal interphalangeal joint to the ground should approximately bisect the solar surface of the foot.

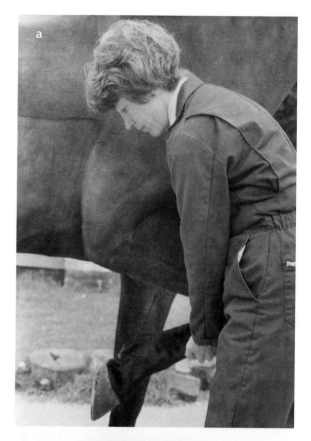

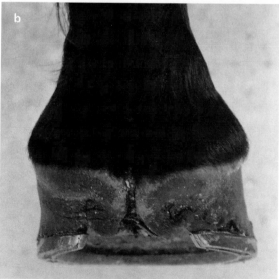

**Fig. 21.36** **(a)** Assessment of foot balance. The limb must be allowed to hang freely in the sagittal plane, held in the proximal metacarpal region. **(b)** The relative heights of the bulbs of the heel, the medial/lateral symmetry and the position of the foot relative to the central limb axis should be evaluated.

Hooves that have been trimmed so that one bulb of the heel is effectively lower than the other, are predisposed to overload. In turn, this or the natural foot placement of the horse may result in the coronary band being displaced proximally at one bulb. Frequently the wall on this side becomes steeper and the contralateral wall flares. In severe cases there may be a deep groove and physical instability between the two bulbs (sheared heels), so that each bulb can be grasped and moved independently (Fig. 21.37). This is usually associated with lameness.

The shoe itself must also be assessed, both for the appropriateness of its design and fit, and for abnormal wear. If the branches of the shoes are too short, or are set slightly inside the outer edge of the wall at the heel, this predisposes to the development of corns and other causes of palmar foot pain. The presence of a heel calk may predispose to localized bruising, especially if unilateral. Abnormal wear of the toe of a front shoe may reflect palmar foot pain. Hindlimb lameness often results in abnormal wear both of the toe of the shoe and the foot.

The foot can only be evaluated in its entirety after removal of the shoe. This is most easily achieved using

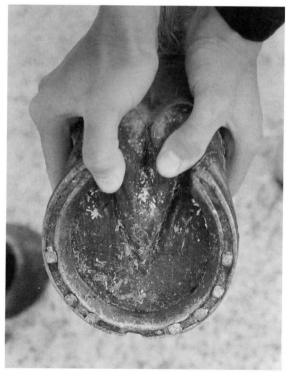

**Fig. 21.37** Assessment of stability of the bulbs of the heel. The thumbs of the investigator's hands press in opposite directions.

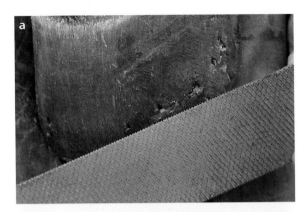

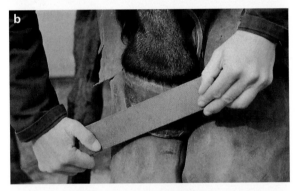

> ## Clinical Pointer ✳
>
> Abnormal wear of the lateral branch of the shoe indicates distal joint hock pain. An affected horse tends to swing its limb underneath the body and then stab it outwards as the foot is placed to the ground.

a rasp and pincers; nail pullers can also be useful. The foot is picked up and pulled forwards and balanced on the investigator's thighs. The rasp edge is run under the bottom edge of the clenches (Fig. 21.38a), and then the rasp is run firmly over the clenches (Fig. 21.38b). The limb is then pulled backwards and placed between or on the investigator's legs, depending on whether it is a forelimb or a hindlimb. Using pincers the medial and lateral branches of the shoe are each levered forwards from the back to loosen the nails (Fig. 21.38c). The nails can then each be removed individually with the pincers or, if they are very tight, using nail pullers. After levering the shoe upwards it may be helpful to then tap it down, to assist nail removal. This technique allows the shoe to be removed with both minimal force and pain while maintaining hoof wall integrity.

After shoe removal it is easier to assess conformation of the solar surface of the foot: its degree of concavity (undue flatness may predispose to bruising), the quality of the horn and the thickness of the wall (a very thin wall may predispose to nail bind). Deviation of the white line may be due to a space-occupying lesion such as a keratoma. Areas of redness indicative of previous or current subsolar hemorrhage or bruising are usually only apparent following paring of the sole with a sharp hoof knife. However, the absence of redness does not preclude the presence of deep-seated bruising. Necrotic material over the frog should be removed. This is usually associated with a malodorous black discharge (thrush) and, if sensitive tissues are affected, may cause lameness. These sensitive tissues must be exposed to allow adequate cleaning and resolution of infection. Instability between the hoof wall and the underlying foot can only be appreciated following shoe removal and the use of hoof testers. Cavitatory defects at the white line that occur commonly at the toe (seedy

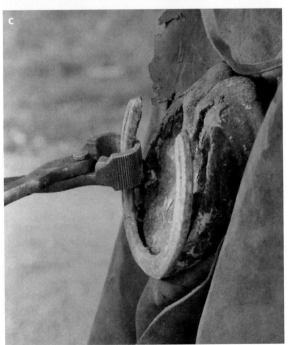

> ## Clinical Pointer ✳
>
> - pain during removal of a nail may indicate nail bind
> - a horse with nail bind will often be lamer immediately after removal of the shoe.

**Fig. 21.38** Removal of the shoe by **(a)** rasping underneath the clenches; **(b)** rasping over the clenches; **(c)** levering the shoe from the back forwards to loosen the nails, which can be removed individually.

toe) are often incidental abnormalities unassociated with lameness. If the defect extends a considerable distance proximally, resulting in hoof wall instability, the gait may be compromised.

Defects in the hoof wall may or may not cause lameness. Vertical hoof wall cracks extending from the solar surface proximally, especially at the quarter or closer to the heel bulb, may cause pain and therefore lameness or poor performance. Short vertical hoof wall cracks are a common feature of unshod horses, especially if inadequately trimmed. These are generally not associated with lameness but may be portals for entry of infection. Horizontal hoof wall cracks are less likely to be associated with lameness but generally reflect previous trauma to the coronary band or hoof wall. Previous trauma to the coronary band may result in permanent deformity of the hoof wall contour, e.g. bulging, but this is rarely associated with lameness.

## ASSESSMENT OF FINDINGS: WHAT TO DO NEXT

If the history is of a sudden-onset moderate to severe lameness associated with increased amplitude of the digital pulses and obvious pain when turning, this is highly suggestive of foot pain, even if the response to pressure and percussion with hoof testers is equivocal or negative. Such conditions as

- nail bind
- subsolar abscess
- subsolar hemorrhage, or
- fracture of the distal phalanx should be suspected.

Removal of the shoe is indicated to facilitate further exploration of the foot. This may result in resolution of the lameness. If no abnormality can be found then it is advisable to soak or poultice the foot for several days and then reassess it, especially if the horn is very hard.

---

### Subsolar abscesses

- if a subsolar abscess is suspected explore the foot carefully
- identify the area of suspected pain using hoof testers and then pare away the sole
- follow any black area until it terminates or until a pus-filled cavity is found
- desensitize the foot with perineural analgesia if necessary
- areas of abnormally soft sole, discoloration, or both, indicate pockets of subsolar hemorrhage.

---

If lameness persists, radiographic examination is indicated.

### Radiography

If a fracture is suspected based on the history and clinical signs, then the area should be radiographed.

In some areas, such as the ilium, a suspected fracture is best confirmed by ultrasonography. In the case of a suspected stress or fatigue fracture of the humerus, radius, or tibia, nuclear scintigraphic evaluation is indicated.

Radiography may also be helpful prior to performing local analgesia. If one or more of the distal hock joints is suspected as the primary source of pain, based on the way the horse moves and the response to flexion tests, radiography may give useful information to determine which is the most appropriate nerve block to perform to confirm the source.

### Ultrasonography

Ultrasonographic examination may give more detailed and accurate information about an area of diffuse swelling, distension of a tendon sheath, an enlarged or painful tendon or ligament, or an area of localized heat. Comparison with the contralateral limb is invaluable.

### Local analgesia or nerve blocks

In many cases there will be no clues as to the source of pain, in which case selective local analgesic techniques are required.

Perineural analgesia may potentially relieve pain both distal and proximal to the site of injection. A palmar nerve block at the level of the base of the proximal sesamoid bones may relieve pain from the fetlock joint. Nerve blocks may only improve lameness rather than alleviate it fully, either with a single source of pain or when there is a concurrent, more proximal, painful focus. In association with severe pain, improvements in lameness may be barely detectable. Thus nerve blocks must be interpreted carefully in the light of both the history and the results of clinical evaluation. In other situations a focus of joint pain may be suspected. It is reasonable to perform intra-articular

---

### Clinical Pointer

If a fracture is suspected do not use local analgesia – more normal loading of the limb may result in catastrophic deterioration of any fracture.

---

### Nerve blocks

- use nerve blocks when the source of pain is unknown
- start distally and work in a proximal direction.

analgesia as the first technique, to rule in or out the particular joint as the primary source of pain and hence the lameness.

Having established the region of pain, the area should be examined radiographically and, when indicated, ultrasonographically. If the findings are negative or inconclusive, arthroscopic evaluation of a joint or nuclear scintigraphic evaluation of an area may be indicated. Nuclear scintigraphy can also be useful in selected cases in which the lameness cannot be altered by local analgesic techniques.

### Serum muscle enzymes

If a horse has a history and clinical signs indicative of exertional rhabdomyolysis (tying up) then a blood sample should be collected for analysis of creatine kinase (CK) and aspartoaminotransferase (AST) activities to confirm the diagnosis

- CK peaks at approximately 6 hours after an episode of myopathy and declines relatively rapidly
- AST peaks at about 24 hours and falls slowly.

The degree of elevation of CK and AST does not necessarily accurately reflect the severity of clinical signs. A doubling of CK concentration may be significant. It should be borne in mind that some rise in CK and AST can be seen after strenuous exercise in unfit horses, and in young Thoroughbreds in training.

### Clinical Pointer

If the history is suggestive of repetitive tying-up episodes

- measure CK and AST levels at rest
- perform an exercise test stressing the horse to the maximum of its fitness, then
- reassess CK and AST levels at 1 and 6–12 hours after exercise.

### Arthrocentesis and synovial fluid analysis

Sudden-onset distension of a synovial structure (joint capsule or tendon sheath), with or without localized edema, and moderate to severe lameness is highly suggestive of infection and a synovial fluid sample should be collected into EDTA, and into culture medium for bacterial culture. Its color and consistency can be assessed grossly. Although red discoloration may reflect trauma or contamination during sampling, brown discoloration is usually indicative of sepsis. Rapid clotting is also typical of sepsis. A smear should be obtained to assess the predominant cell type and a Gram stain performed. In a normal joint mononuclear cells predominate, whereas in association with infection polymorphonuclear leukocytes are the major cell type. With infection the total white blood cell count is usually higher than 10 000 cells/µl (10 x 10⁹/l). The synovial fluid total protein concentration, red and white blood cell count, and differential white blood cell count should be estimated. It is important to determine the relative proportions of red and white blood cells in order to assess whether an elevated white cell count is genuine or reflects blood contamination.

### Hemarthrosis

- hemarthrosis can cause sudden-onset severe lameness
- diagnosis is confirmed by arthrocentesis
- removal of blood from the joint can also result in rapid relief of lameness.

If sepsis is suspected therapy should be initiated immediately.

## SPECIAL CONSIDERATIONS FOR FOALS

In foals up to 6 months of age suffering a sudden onset of lameness the possibility of an infected joint must always be excluded first. A postulated history of the mare having trodden on the foal is almost invariably a red herring. Joint infection is nearly always associated with joint capsule distension, with or without periarticular soft tissue swelling. Thus all joints should be carefully assessed by visual inspection and palpation, as infection may be multifocal. The whole animal should be considered, as umbilical infection for example may have been the primary bacterial source for joint infection. A young foal unfamiliar with being regularly handled is very much more difficult to assess.

Small-armed hoof testers rather than a large instrument are much more appropriate for assessing foot pain in foals.

# EXAMINATION OF A RECUMBENT HORSE

A horse which is recumbent following a fall, or which has become recumbent following the sudden or gradual development of a gait abnormality, may have a musculoskeletal problem. It is important to obtain an accurate history, establishing what happened before the horse became recumbent, noting also the ground conditions and the environmental temperature and humidity.

1. If the animal fell on its neck it may have fractured a cervical vertebra and damaged the spinal cord
2. If it became recumbent during exercise, then establish how much exercise had been done and if the animal was moving normally before the fall
3. If the horse fell at the end of an endurance race in hot, humid conditions it may have exertional rhabdomyolysis, possibly complicated by heatstroke or exhaustion.

It is also important to establish whether or not the horse has had any gait abnormalities on previous occasions. A horse which has 'tied up' previously or had evidence of hyperkalemic periodic paralysis, or signs suggestive of aortoiliacofemoral thrombosis, is likely to have a recurrent problem.

A systematic clinical examination is performed to try to determine why the horse is recumbent, bearing in mind that in an exercising horse there are a number of potential causes including

- respiratory distress (the horse is 'winded')
- a fracture or fractures
- major muscle trauma or avulsion
- exertional rhabdomyolysis syndrome
- atypical myoglobinuria
- cardiovascular insufficiency
- severe internal hemorrhage
- neurological trauma to the brain or spinal cord
- the horse is physically stuck
- hyperthermia and exhaustion
- hyperkalemic periodic paralysis
- aortoiliacofemoral thrombosis.
- protozoal myeloencephalitis

If the horse was found recumbent with no preceding exercise other differentials should include neurological diseases, such as equine herpesvirus-1 myelopathy. Therefore the clinical examination should include comprehensive neurological and cardiovascular examinations using the following procedure

1. establish that the airway is patent and the horse is breathing adequately
2. assess the head, including pupillary light and blink reflexes
3. determine the color of the mucous membranes
4. measure the pulse and respiratory rates
5. evaluate the demeanor of the horse, being aware that it may have sustained a life-threatening fracture yet be calm, with little evidence of pain
6. note any spontaneous attempts to move the limbs or to lift the head and neck
7. palpate the muscles, hard muscles are suggestive of exertional rhabdomyolysis, but severely damaged muscles may still feel normal
8. palpate and auscultate the limbs to determine the presence of swelling or crepitus
9. palpate the pelvic region per rectum to assess the integrity of the pelvis, the presence of swelling due to hemorrhage, and the shape of the aorta, its texture and pulse.

Trauma as the result of a fall may result in a fracture or major muscle trauma. If the horse has sustained a proximal limb fracture and the injured limb is underneath, it may be unable to rise. If the horse is rolled on to its other side, or into sternal recumbency, it may get up spontaneously and then it may be possible to reach a diagnosis. Most limb fractures that result in an inability to rise are associated with obvious crepitus, instability of the limb or both, if the limb is on the up side.

> ### Pelvic fractures
>
> - these can be difficult to diagnose, especially if the ilium is involved
> - they are not palpable per rectum and may be associated with severance of a major vessel and severe, fatal internal hemorrhage (rupture of a major muscle group may also result in severe internal hemorrhage)
> - repeated evaluation of the pulse rate and quality, the color of the mucous membranes, and capillary refill time is therefore important.

If there is no obvious diagnosis the entire examination should be repeated, several times if necessary. Serum samples for serial determinations of creatine kinase concentrations can be saved.

# PRINCIPLES OF LOCAL ANALGESIA

Perineural local analgesia, ring blocks, intrasynovial analgesia, and intrathecal analgesia are integral parts of many lameness investigations, either to identify or to confirm the site or sites of pain. Before performing any form of local anesthesia it is important to establish the consistency of lameness. If lameness is only slight and tends to improve spontaneously with exercise, interpretation of a nerve block is difficult. Very severe lameness, although consistent, may be improved only marginally by local analgesia.

The order in which local analgesic techniques should be performed is determined by the presenting clinical signs and the skill of the investigator. An experienced clinician may be reasonably confident that pain arises from the middle carpal joint, and therefore proceed directly to intra-articular analgesia, whereas it may well behove an inexperienced practitioner to start with desensitization of the foot region and proceed stepwise proximally.

## Specificity of local analgesic blocks

Local analgesic techniques are not necessarily either specific or reliable and false negative and false positive results can occur. For example, a palmar digital nerve block immediately proximal to the cartilages of the foot may relieve pain from the proximal interphalangeal joint, despite apparently achieving cutaneous desensitization of the heel region only. This is presumably due to proximal diffusion of local anesthetic solution. Improvement in lameness associated with the foot may be obtained paradoxically despite the persistence of cutaneous sensation in the heel region. However, lameness associated with the navicular bone and related structures is sometimes unaffected by apparent desensitization of the palmar aspect of the foot following palmar digital nerve blocks (Table 21.1), whereas significant improvement is seen after perineural analgesia of the palmar nerves at the level of the proximal sesamoid bones. Failure of adequate desensitization of an area following perineural analgesia may be due to

- intravascular
- intralymphatic, or
- intrasynovial injection.

False negative results may also be due to

- a mechanical component to lameness, or
- to a more proximal source of innervation of the painful structure(s).

False positive results may also be seen. For example, perineural analgesia of the palmar metacarpal nerves performed immediately distal to the carpus may substantially improve lameness, although the primary source is the middle carpal joint. This may be due either to inadvertent deposition of local anesthetic solution into the palmar distal outpouchings of the middle carpal joint capsule, or to proximal diffusion. False negative results may also be seen after intra-articular analgesia due to subchondral bone pain, or after intrathecal analgesia due to adhesion formation, intratendinous pain, or both.

## Speed of response to analgesic blocks

Perineural analgesia depends on the local anesthetic solution diffusing into the nerve, and with larger nerves this takes longer. Therefore, the response to tibial and fibular nerve blocks or median and ulnar nerve blocks is generally slower than for more distal limb nerve blocks. The delayed response may also be due in part to less precise deposition of the local anesthetic solution because of the deeper location of the nerves.

1. The effect of distal limb nerve blocks (distal to the carpus or tarsus) should be assessed 5–10 minutes, and up to 30 minutes, after injection
2. Proximal limb nerve blocks should be assessed at 20-minute intervals up to 1 hour.

The response to intra-articular analgesia is also variable. Although improvement may be seen very rapidly within 10 minutes of injection, in large joints such as the femoropatellar the response may be delayed to up to 30 minutes. If extrasynovial structures such as the cruciate ligaments are damaged the response may be further delayed.

There is some controversy as to whether a horse should be walked or stood still after performing a nerve block and before assessing the response. For a perineural block to be as specific as possible it seems logical to stand the horse still to minimize diffusion of the anesthetic solution away from the site of injection. However, spread of the solution throughout a joint or tendon sheath may be facilitated by walking.

## Degree of improvement in lameness

Although there may be only one source of pain, perineural or intrasynovial analgesia may result in improvement in lameness rather than its alleviation.

The decision to proceed with further nerve blocks should be based on clinical signs, the degree of improvement in lameness, and clinical experience.

**Table 21.1.** Site of commonly used nerve blocks and alternative nomenclature

| Site | Name of nerve block | Alternative name(s) |
|---|---|---|
| Digital nerves immediately proximal to the cartilages of the foot | Distal digital | Palmar digital |
| Digital nerves at the level of the base of the proximal sesamoid bones | Proximal digital | Palmar abaxial sesamoid |
| Palmar (plantar) nerves at junction of proximal and distal halves of metacarpus (metatarsus) | Palmar (mid-metacarpus) | } 4-point block |
| Palmar (plantar) metacarpal (metatarsal) nerves distal to 'button' of second or fourth metacarpal (metatarsal) bones | Palmar metacarpal | |
| Palmar nerves immediately distal to carpus | Palmar (subcarpal) | |
| Palmar metacarpal nerves immediately distal to carpus | Palmar metacarpal (subcarpal) | |
| Deep branch of ulnar nerve at level of accessory carpal bone | Ulnar | Lateral palmar |
| Ulnar nerve proximal to accessory carpal bone, between flexor carpi ulnaris and ulnaris lateralis | Ulnar | |
| Dorsal metatarsal nerves at level of 'button' of second or fourth metatarsal bones | Dorsal metatarsal | 6-point block (when combined with plantar mid-metatarsus and plantar metatarsal) |
| Plantar nerves immediately distal to tarsus | Plantar (subtarsal) | |
| Plantar metatarsal nerves immediately distal to tarsus | Plantar metatarsal (subtarsal) | |
| Tibial nerve cranial to common calcaneal tendon | Tibial | |
| Deep and superficial fibular nerves | Fibular | Peroneal |

## Clinical Pointer

Remember that there may be more than one source of pain, for example palmar foot pain and pain associated with the metacarpophalangeal joint or the proximal aspect of the suspensory ligament frequently occur together.

## Safety

Performing analgesic blocks is potentially hazardous to the horse, the handler, and the veterinarian. To minimize risks to all concerned it is important that a suitable environment in which to perform the injections is selected. The horse must be adequately restrained. The limb should be prepared appropriately and a non- or low-irritant local anesthetic solution used to minimize the risks and severity of any postinjection reaction.

## Choice of local anesthetic solution

Mepivacaine is the least irritant of the short-acting local anesthetic solutions currently available and is the drug of choice in most situations. The incidence of

## Communication with the owner

- give a clear explanation of the procedure and its expected outcome to the owner, handler, or both, so that they know what is going on and understand why it is necessary
- this is particularly important when dealing with difficult horses, when the owner must be made aware why firm restraint is essential
- this is also important when it is necessary to perform multiple blocks as lack of tolerance can become an important feature in this situation
- inform the owner of the limitations of local anesthetic techniques as well as their value, to avoid misunderstandings
- inform the owner of the potential cost of the investigation.

## Bupivacaine

Bupivacaine is the drug of choice when an anesthetic solution with a longer action than mepivacaine is required, for example

- when investigating a horse with concurrent lameness in two or more limbs
- if the horse is exceedingly fractious.

local inflammatory reactions at the site(s) of injection is relatively low and the degree of any reaction comparatively small. However, if repeated attempts at needle insertion are made, or excessively large volumes of anesthetic solution used, soft tissue reactions are likely to develop, especially if local hemorrhage has been induced. If a low-grade bacterial infection is induced swellings are likely to persist. Prilocaine is also acceptable, although there tends to be a higher incidence of postinjection reactions. The frequency of adverse reactions after injection of lignocaine is comparatively high. Although the aim of any local anesthetic technique is to localize as closely as possible the source(s) of pain, and epinephrine will theoretically tend to restrict diffusion by causing local vasoconstriction, it can make the anesthetic solution persist for longer and thereby increase the risk of an adverse reaction. Therefore, the use of mepivacaine without epinephrine is strongly recommended. It is a relatively rapidly acting drug whose maximum effect tends to persist for 1–3 hours.

To enhance specificity of the block, needle placement should be as precise as possible. This requires the cooperation of the horse, adequate restraint, and accurate knowledge of anatomy. Practice on cadaver limbs at unfamiliar sites of injection is invaluable. The volume of local anesthetic solution should be as small as possible and is determined by both the precision of needle placement relative to the site of the nerve and the size of the nerve. Perineural analgesia of the nerves distal to the carpus and tarsus is usually effective within 10 minutes of injection, although loss of reaction to firm pressure may precede complete pain relief. Effective blockade of the larger

nerves proximal to the carpus and tarsus usually takes longer, from 20 minutes up to 1 hour occasionally.

### Testing a block

Before assessing whether lameness is improved the potential efficacy of the block should be assessed. Following blockade of the palmar nerves at the level of the proximal sesamoid bones, the foot and part of the pastern should be assessed. If the horse previously reacted to hoof testers this reaction should now be diminished or absent. There should be no reaction to firm pressure applied around the coronary band, although reaction to light touch may persist transiently. The reaction is best tested by approaching the horse from the opposite side to that which has been blocked. The eye on that side is covered so that the horse does not anticipate the approach. Firm pressure is applied around the coronary band using blunt-ended instruments, such as artery forceps for a forelimb or the hook of a window pole when assessing a hindlimb. Some hyperreactive horses will anticipate and it may be necessary to test each limb repeatedly and compare reactions, and to assess the reaction to pressure with the limb non-weightbearing. An apprehensive horse may snatch up the nerve-blocked limb, and so it is wise for the examiner to avoid positioning the head in a vulnerable position underneath the patient. Sensation at the level of the fetlock should persist.

Blockade of the palmar metacarpal or plantar metatarsal nerves should reduce the reaction to firm palpation of the margins of the suspensory ligament and its branches distal to the site of injection. Perineural analgesia of both the palmar or plantar metacarpal or metatarsal nerves in the metacarpus or metatarsus should reduce any reaction to passive manipulation of the fetlock, and reduced joint stiffness may be detected. If a bilateral nerve block has been performed (i.e. both medial and lateral palmar nerves blocked), but sensation is reduced only unilaterally, it is always worth assessing the effect on lameness. A unilateral block may have a significant effect. If it apparently does, it should be checked that the block is not now effective bilaterally.

## Reassessment of lameness

Although there may be apparent complete superficial desensitization, relief of pain sometimes takes a little longer, the horse may therefore still be lame when first trotted, but may improve progressively thereafter. Thus the horse must be re-evaluated trotting up and down several times. The investigator must, however, be cognisant of the possibility of local anesthetic solution diffusing further from the original site of injection with time.

### Clinical Pointer

- always reassess the horse under the circumstances in which it appeared most lame
- reassess on both the left and right reins – lameness may appear in another limb
- following relief of pain from a forelimb, assess for hindlimb lameness, a previously subtle lameness may become much more apparent.

The reaction to the nerve block should be assessed in the light of clinical signs. If, for example, the gait was highly suggestive of foot pain, but lameness persisted despite apparent desensitization of the foot, there may be

- an additional deeper nerve supply – nerves may enter the deep digital flexor tendon proximally
- a mechanical component to the lameness
- laminar or other sources of severe pain that can be difficult to alleviate fully
- more than one source of pain, including proximal to the site of injection
- pain persisting despite eliminating reaction to deep pressure
- a previous neurectomy.

In this situation it is worth reassessing the lameness after an additional 10 minutes, and considering repeating the block either then or on a subsequent occasion. Responses to specific nerve blocks may vary from day to day.

### Clinical Pointer

Nerve blocks are best not performed in the face of a local inflammatory reaction or infection, as this can alter the pH and thus the efficacy of the local anesthetic solution.

If some reaction to deep pressure persists then the deposition of local anesthetic solution was probably imprecise, or local fibrosis limited or prohibited its diffusion into the nerve. The nerve block should therefore be repeated.

If lameness is improved but not fully alleviated the decision whether to proceed to more proximal nerve blocks is a difficult one, based on

- the degree of improvement
- the degree of residual lameness
- clinical signs, and
- patient tolerance.

It is quite common for moderate to severe lameness due to a single cause to be significantly improved but not fully alleviated. However, persistence of moderate lameness despite significant improvement usually indicates a second concurrent problem.

## Intrasynovial injection

### Limitations to intrasynovial injection of local anesthetic

- the speed of response is extremely variable, ranging from 10 to 45 minutes
- the response may be limited if there is severe articular cartilage pathology and associated subchondral bone pain
- if the articular cartilage is completely intact and the pain is principally subchondral in origin a false negative response may be obtained
- the response may be delayed if the primary site of damage is extrasynovial, such as damage to the cruciate ligaments of the stifle.

Occasionally, lameness associated with apparent intra-articular pain is unaffected by local anesthetic solution but is significantly improved by intra-articular corticosteroids. Multiple adhesions within a tendon sheath may result in only partial improvement in lameness.

Ideally, synovial fluid should always be withdrawn prior to injection of a synovial structure to ensure that the needle is correctly positioned. However, it may be difficult to retrieve synovial fluid from the

- proximal interphalangeal joint
- coxofemoral joint
- compartments of the stifle
- centrodistal joint

unless there is an increased volume present. In these joints easy retrieval of large volumes of synovial fluid is generally indicative of underlying pathology, even if the response to local analgesia is minimal.

## Restraint

Horses are generally most easily handled in an enclosed environment and so nerve blocks are best performed indoors. A stable with bedding is not ideal, neither is a concrete surface, especially when dealing with an awkward horse. Occasionally a horse may slip or try to throw itself to the ground. The ideal situation is a large stable with a non-slip rubber-type floor. Many horses tolerate the needle insertion well, but if it starts to fidget or becomes fractious then restraint using a neck twitch, nose twitch or both, or a chain shank placed over the gum, is recommended. Some horses will not tolerate a twitch. Picking up the contralateral forelimb when blocking a forelimb, or the ipsilateral forelimb when blocking a hindlimb, may be helpful. However, a horse can still kick standing on two limbs and especially when a forelimb is being blocked with the contralateral limb picked up, the horse may be inclined to jump towards the investigator. When blocking hindlimbs it may be helpful to confine the horse in stocks to prevent it from sidling.

> ### Clinical Pointer
>
> It is hazardous to perform a nerve block in a stable with bedding (e.g. straw, shavings, or paper) because of the risk of dropping and never finding a needle. If this occurs and the needle cannot be found the entire bedding should be removed. Needles left in the bedding may result in catastrophic penetrating injuries of the solar surfaces of the feet.

Sometimes it is necessary to sacrifice potential specificity for safety; it may be necessary to inject local anesthetic as the needle is advanced, before the desired site is reached. Occasionally nerve blocks cannot be performed safely in an unsedated horse. Sedation with $\alpha_2$ agonists such as xylazine or detomidine may allay the horse's anxiety but its tendency to kick or strike may become less predictable. Combined with butorphanol, the results are more predictable; however, the horse generally cannot be safely trotted until at least 20 minutes after injection. The doses of xylazine, detomidine, and butorphanol used generally have no significant effect on the pain causing lameness, although limb flight may be slightly altered. If very heavy sedation is required there will be a longer delay before lameness can be reassessed. Bupivacaine should

be used to ensure that the block is likely to still be effective, but the possibility of the local anesthetic diffusing to a distant site must be borne in mind. In some circumstances it may be useful to use short-acting corticosteroids by an intra-articular route, and reassess the lameness 2–3 days after injection.

> ### Clinical Pointer
>
> Many horses will behave much better if handled by someone other than the owner, and in the absence of the owner. In this situation the owner must be handled delicately!

## Injection technique

The needle should always be inserted detached from the syringe. If it is in a blood vessel, blood usually appears spontaneously in the needle hub; the needle should be withdrawn or redirected slightly, or both, before attaching the syringe. Further aspiration is only indicated to check whether or not the needle is within a synovial cavity, e.g. the palmar distal outpouchings of the middle carpal joint capsule. The needle should be as small as possible to minimize pain, but ultimately there must be a compromise between

- safety
- speed of injection, and
- the risks of breaking very fine-gauge needles.

> ### Needles and syringes used for nerve block
>
> - the syringe should be as small as is compatible with the volume of local anesthetic being used
> - it is helpful to withdraw the solution from the bottle or vial using a 14 or 16 G needle, and to use a smaller gauge needle for injection
> - if the larger needle is left in the bottle the syringe can easily be topped up if problems arise during injection
> - it is always helpful to draw up a slightly larger volume of solution than that predictably required in case some is misplaced or squirts out from the needle–syringe junction
> - syringes with acentric nozzles are easier to position closely adjacent to the limb.

Whether the needle is inserted with the limb weight-bearing or lifted depends on the site of injection and the temperament of the horse. Ideally both needle and syringe should be supported during injection, to try and maintain the position of the needle, and so the clinician is already prepared to detach the syringe if the horse starts to move, to reduce the risk of premature withdrawal.

---

### Clinical Pointer

Following nerve blocks in the metacarpal and metatarsal regions bandage the limb for the following 12 hours or so to minimize the risks of postinjection swelling. At other sites this is unnecessary.

---

Prior to performing perineural blocks the area should be thoroughly cleansed with antiseptic. If the horse is very hairy accurate palpation may be difficult and therefore clipping will be beneficial. If there is danger of penetrating a synovial cavity the area should be fully clipped and surgically scrubbed. When performing intra-articular or intrathecal blocks a small area around the site of needle insertion should be clipped and then scrubbed surgically. Before any nerve block gross dirt, shavings, or dust should be removed from the body surface, to avoid this falling on to the injection site.

If hemorrhage is induced after needle withdrawal, firm pressure should be applied to the area until the bleeding stops. With a difficult horse it may be best to tape a wad of cotton wool over the area.

With the precautions outlined above the risk of adverse reactions developing is very small. However, if an area is not adequately cleansed prior to perineural analgesia there is a small risk of introducing infection, resulting in persistent filling of the limb with or without heat. This generally responds satisfactorily to broad-spectrum systemic antimicrobial therapy for approximately 5 days. If there is acute exacerbation of lameness within 24–48 hours after intrasynovial injection, sepsis must always be considered and treated accordingly. If a horse has not recently been vaccinated against tetanus, tetanus prophylaxis should be administered.

Multiple nerve blocks can generally be done safely in a single limb within a day. However, the efficacy of perineural blocks performed proximal to the carpus and tarsus is best assessed without distal limb nerve blocks in place.

## Order of injections

Although in principle, analgesic blocks should be done sequentially from distal to proximal, in some instances it is acceptable to alter this order based on the results of the clinical evaluation. The clinician should decide which is the most appropriate question to ask, and then select the most appropriate local analgesic technique to answer the question as specifically as possible.

1. If there is distension of the metacarpophalangeal joint capsule, pain on manipulation of the joint and accentuation of lameness after flexion, and no indication of foot pain, it is appropriate to ask whether the fetlock is the primary source of pain and therefore do intra-articular analgesia first.
2. If a horse with hindlimb lameness has no clinical evidence of an abnormality in the fetlock or distal limb it is often appropriate to start with perineural analgesia of the plantar nerves (at the middle to distal third of the metatarsus), plantar metatarsal nerves distal to the buttons of the second and fourth metatarsal bones, and the dorsal metatarsal nerves (six-point block) to eliminate the fetlock and distal limb as sources of pain.
3. If the horse is very difficult to handle the dorsal metatarsal nerve block can be excluded.

If the horse is lame in more than one limb the most lame one is evaluated first, followed by the less lame limb(s). Although many lamenesses occur bilaterally, bilateral lameness does not always have identical causes in each limb. If the lameness is extremely subtle and the owner reports that it has previously been more obvious, it may be helpful to work the horse to accentuate it. This will facilitate interpretation of the nerve blocks. The owner may be concerned that working the horse may result in irreversible deterioration in the underlying condition. They should be reassured that this is comparatively unlikely and that by working the horse it is more likely that an accurate diagnosis will be reached.

It is beyond the scope of this book to describe the technique for each individual nerve block. However, it is important to recognize that nerve blocks are time-

---

### The duration of nerve blocks

- this depends on the site of injection and the volume of local anesthetic used
- after perineural analgesia it takes 3–5 hours before baseline lameness returns, although cutaneous sensation may be restored more quickly
- this must be considered if either more proximal or more selective nerve blocks or intra-articular analgesia is to be done later the same day.

consuming and should not be done in a hurry: adequate time must be allowed for the block to be effective. Once lameness has successfully been alleviated in one limb it may become apparent in another, necessitating further nerve blocks. The owner should be made aware of this and the potential cost of the investigation. Occasionally, analgesic blocks (regional and intrasynovial) can be done throughout a limb with no improvement in lameness. Nuclear scintigraphic examination may then be indicated.

## IMAGING TECHNIQUES

### Radiography

Radiography is a potentially very useful ancillary aid to diagnosis but it is vital that an adequate number of high-quality views of the area under investigation are obtained. Poor-quality radiographs, or a failure to obtain specific views, may provide misleading information. It is difficult to be categorical about which views are required, but generally a minimum of four projections

- dorsopalmar
- lateromedial
- dorsolateral–palmaromedial oblique, and
- dorsomedial–palmarolateral oblique

are necessary for comprehensive evaluation of most joint views. It is important to maintain a flexible approach to radiographic examination based not only on the clinical signs but also on the signalment of the horse. For example, in Thoroughbred racehorses lesions of the third carpal bone detectable only in dorsoproximal–dorsodistal oblique (skyline) views are frequently encountered, whereas in a mature showjumper this projection is rarely useful. Multiple similar oblique views obtained with slight differences in angle may be required to detect a sagittal fracture of the dorsoproximal aspect of the proximal phalanx. Soft exposures are needed to identify periosteal new bone formation, and even then it may only be visible if the radiograph is viewed over high-intensity illumination.

The limitations of radiography must also be recognized.

> ### Clinical Pointer
>
> Radiography is more valuable when done at a clinic rather than out in the field, so that additional views at different angles or at different exposures can be obtained in an effort to identify a lesion.

1. There must be a 40% change in bone density before it can be recognized radiographically.
2. A non-displaced fissure fracture may be inapparent until lysis along the fracture line – a natural part of the healing process – has occurred within the first 10 days after injury.
3. Periosteal new bone is usually detectable only 10 days or more after the original insult to the periosteum. Thus in the acute phase of injury radiographs may appear normal despite the presence of significant bony lesions.
4. Joint pain, or pain associated with, for example, the navicular bone, can be present without associated radiological abnormalities.
5. Some radiological abnormalities can be seen without associated clinical signs, although their interpretation is not always straightforward. For example, small well rounded bony opacities on the dorsoproximal aspect of the proximal phalanx can be present coincidentally, but also may be a cause of lameness.
6. Entheseous new bone formation (new bone at the site of a joint capsule or ligament insertion) on the palmar aspect of the proximal phalanx at the site of insertion of the middle distal sesamoidean ligaments is frequently seen as an incidental radiological abnormality unassociated with lameness, but occasionally is seen in conjunction with active desmitis.
7. Modelling of the dorsoproximal aspect of the proximal phalanx may be associated with lameness in a young Thoroughbred flat racehorse, but be present without clinical signs in a mature Thoroughbred used for showjumping. Flattening of the lateral trochlea of the femur, a sign synonymous with osteochondrosis, can be present without associated clinical signs.

It is important that the owner is made aware of the limitations of radiographic interpretation with respect to both lameness investigations and prepurchase evaluations.

Obtaining good radiographs requires attention to detail. The area to be examined should be prepared by removing mud and other debris, including manure, and, in the case of the foot, removal of the shoe and thorough paring of the foot. The frog clefts and central sulcus should be packed with a radiodense substance with a similar density to hoof horn, such as children's plastic dough. This prevents the frog clefts causing radiolucent artefacts superimposed over the navicular bone and distal phalanx. The limb should be positioned appropriately, and this may be facilitated by the use of sedation. Radiographs should be examined systematically to determine whether there are any abnormalities of the soft tissues, the shape or contour of any bone, the opacity of each bone, and the width and opacity of joint spaces.

Any abnormality should be described in radiological terms and then the pathological process or processes which might cause that change should be determined. This may then be related to a specific condition and to the clinical signs. The radiological technique of spotting lesions can be dangerous and often leads to misdiagnosis. It is frequently useful to compare postulated lesions with comparable sites in the contralateral limb.

## Ultrasonography

Diagnostic ultrasonography can be used to assess

- tendons and ligaments
- bone surfaces
- synovial structures
- blood vessels
- other soft tissue swelling.

High-quality images are essential for accurate diagnosis.

## Clinical Pointer

Hair traps air which is a poor conductor of ultrasound waves → poor-quality pictures, therefore clip or shave the area to be examined first.

After thorough washing of the area a liberal amount of coupling gel should be applied and given an adequate time to soak in. For routine examinations of the metacarpus, metatarsus and pastern, a 7.5 MHz transducer is required to ensure high image resolution. A stand-off head as a separate or an integral part of the transducer is usually required for optimal image quality of the most superficial structures. It is a good principle to examine the entire length of all the tendons and ligaments, even if clinical signs are indicative of a specific injury or a lesion is found in one structure, as more than one structure may be damaged concurrently. Lesions may occur bilaterally despite unilateral clinical signs, therefore examination of both forelimbs or both hindlimbs is helpful and can also provide a 'normal' comparison.

Artefacts are frequently encountered as a result of either

- poor scanning technique
- hyperechoic foci causing shadowing, or
- an inability to evaluate all structures in focus simultaneously.

The ultrasound beam must be perpendicular to the structure for optimal image quality. Each structure should be examined carefully to assess its shape, size, clarity of contour, and echogenicity. If the gain controls are too high subtle lesions may be missed. Enlargement of a structure compared to the contralateral limb and subtle alterations in 'fiber pattern' are sometimes the only abnormalities detectable ultrasonographically.

Settings on the ultrasound machine giving the best images for tendons and ligaments are not identical to those for assessing muscle or deeper bony structures, and so familiarity with the machine controls is clearly important.

## Arthroscopy/tenoscopy

The absence of significant radiological abnormalities associated with a joint does not preclude that joint as a source of pain.

Arthroscopy does not allow comprehensive evaluation of all aspects of all joints, but does permit visual evaluation of

- a proportion of the articular surfaces
- the synovial membrane
- intra-articular ligaments (e.g. the medial palmar intercarpal ligament)
- extra-articular ligaments (e.g. the cranial crucial ligament)
- the meniscal cartilages of the femorotibial joint
- the meniscal ligaments.

In addition, fractures not detectable radiographically may be identified. Thus using arthroscopy a specific diagnosis for the cause of pain and therefore the lameness may be identified. Tendon sheaths may also be examined, providing information complementary to that obtained by ultrasonography.

## Nuclear scintigraphy

Nuclear scintigraphy is an ancillary aid to diagnosis rather than a primary diagnostic technique, except in an immature athletic horse in which a stress or fatigue fracture is suspected, or a dangerous horse in which nerve blocks cannot safely be performed.

Although hand-held scintillation counters have proved useful in evaluation of the musculoskeletal system of immature athletes, a gamma camera with high-quality image resolution and collimation is much more versatile and accurate, provided that an adequate number of counts are made. This may require general anesthesia.

Recently performed nerve blocks may confound the results, so ideally 10–14 days should elapse after multiple nerve blocks have been performed, prior to scintigraphic examination. Very low-grade chronic lamenesses are less likely to yield positive results than more acute injuries. Even so, the results may be confusing and several 'hot spots' may be identified at different locations in a particular horse, yet their significance may be extremely difficult to assess.

## Magnetic resonance imaging

Magnetic resonance imaging (MRI) is an imaging technique for the future. Although anatomical studies of cadaver limbs have been performed, the technique is not currently widely available for clinical use. However, it has tremendous potential for the evaluation of tendons, ligaments, and joints, especially for structures within the hoof capsule.

## Thermography

Thermography is another non-invasive technique that can provide additional information in conjunction with other diagnostic techniques. Areas of abnormal heat or cold may be detected and this may facilitate localization of the source of pain. However, images of anatomical structures per se are not obtained.

# OTHER NON-INVASIVE TECHNIQUES

A number of other non-invasive diagnostic techniques alleged to measure alterations in local magnetic currents have been marketed, but their accuracy and usefulness remain to be validated.

## Faradism

Faradism is a method of stimulating muscles to contract and relax. The strength of contraction is proportional to the strength of the stimulus, although this can be influenced by the presence of muscle pain. A sore muscle can usually be detected because it responds to a lesser degree of stimulation, and the muscle contraction and relaxation is less smooth than in a normal muscle. Thus soreness in superficial muscles can be detected.

## Electromyography

Electromyography can be useful in a limited number of cases in which there is an unusual pattern of muscle atrophy associated with lameness. Thus it can be useful in confirming a diagnosis of damage to the brachial plexus. It is also useful for the diagnosis of neuromuscular disorders such as myotonia. The most accurate recordings are usually obtained with the horse under general anesthesia, although some muscle groups, such as those of the hindquarters, can be adequately assessed with the horse standing.

## Force plates, high-speed treadmills

In recent years force plates and high-speed treadmills, in conjunction with high-speed cinematography, have been used for gait evaluation. These more sophisticated techniques can be useful in detecting subtle asymmetries of gait, but are not a substitute for other methods of investigation and do not themselves lead to a specific diagnosis of the source or sources of pain.

## CONCLUSIONS

Comprehensive evaluation of the musculoskeletal system requires a systematic approach. Enough time should be available for a thorough examination. There is no substitute for accurate clinical evaluation, and the results of nerve blocks, radiography and ultrasonography should always be interpreted in the light of clinical examination. Results should be documented carefully. Interpretation of results requires familiarity with the normal and its variations and a thorough knowledge of anatomy. Repeated examinations will sometimes yield results when the first assessment was negative. Correlation of palpation findings with imaging techniques such as ultrasonography should improve palpation skills. The investigator will find that time spent in dissection of cadaver limbs is always invaluable.

# Cattle

The musculoskeletal system supports the body and allows normal locomotion and posture. Lameness is the most important clinical manifestation of disease of this system and surveys of dairy herds have shown that between 25% and 30% of cows are affected by lameness each year. The causes of economic losses due to lameness include

- reduced milk yield
- increased calving-to-conception interval
- increased rate of involuntary culling.

There are also welfare implications for painful conditions of such high morbidity. Lameness also affects the breeding soundness of beef bulls, which can influence the reproductive performance of the herd.

Lameness may be due to abnormalities of bones, muscles, joints, tendons and feet. The first step in the clinical examination is to decide if the animal is lame. The location of the lesion is then determined and the type of lesion considered before a prognosis is made or appropriate treatment recommended. The emphasis in this section will be on those aspects of the clinical examination that are relevant to identification of the origin of a lameness problem. Diseases of the nervous system also cause gait abnormalities and these are discussed in Chapter 19.

## HISTORY TAKING

Accurate history taking is an essential component of the clinical examination of a lame animal and may provide clues as to the precise cause of the lameness.

### Signalment

The age, sex, breed and purpose for which the animal is being kept may provide clues about the cause of some types of lameness

- congenital defects such as arthrogryposis are apparent at birth
- osteochondrosis and physitis are diseases of young, rapidly growing cattle
- spastic paresis is most common in calves between 2 and 9 months of age
- dorsal patellar luxation is generally a disease of mature cattle
- interdigital fibromata have been associated with the Hereford breed
- hip dysplasia is predominantly associated with the Charolais breed.

### Environment

Lameness in the high-producing dairy cow is related to certain housing conditions, particularly floor surfaces, and to the feeds and feeding program. Continuously wet pasture conditions are associated with a high incidence of lameness of dairy cows in certain countries with high rainfall.

Satisfactory claw health is partially mediated through the increased lying time in cattle given access to comfortable cubicles or stalls, although excessive stall moisture may also contribute to lameness problems. Penetration of the white line is more likely in cows driven roughly over cattle tracks from pasture or concrete surfaces that contain loose sharp aggregate. Cows kept in straw-bedded areas spend more time recumbent, have fewer problems with ulceration of the sole and white line lesions, but are more susceptible to infectious digital disease, such as interdigital necrobacillosis.

Certain farms and even certain pastures are associated with an increased incidence of clostridial disease, and in particular, tetanus and blackleg. Examination of ryegrass seed heads in outbreaks of lameness associated with ergotism may reveal the presence of black sclerotia. Outbreaks of interdigital necrobacillosis during the summer months are associated with cattle standing in wet, muddy pastures. Fractures of the pedal bone are also more common in dry summers when cattle are grazing on hard ground.

## Nutrition

Diets with a high ratio of concentrate to silage in early lactation may be associated with a high incidence of solar ulceration in dairy cows. Physitis of the metacarpal and metatarsal bones is a cause of lameness in copper-deficient nursing beef calves, and enzootic muscular dystrophy may occur in nursing beef calves and in yearling cattle associated with diets deficient in vitamin E and selenium.

## Owner's complaint

Dairy farmers may identify several lame cows for examination. Specific details of the type of lameness are uncommon, and farmers will identify cows that are stiff or slow coming into the parlor for milking. A detectable reduction in the milk yield of individual cows is not a common finding until the lameness is severe. Details of any management changes, such as

- turnout on to pasture
- traumatic incidents, or
- recent estrus activity

should be ascertained. Histories for individual lame pedigree heifers or bulls, particularly those intended for show purposes, are usually more detailed.

## Onset and course of lameness

The date of onset and duration of the lameness should be determined.

| Sudden onset lameness | Slow onset lameness |
|---|---|
| Traumatic events | Solar ulcers |
| – fractures | White line lesions |
| Infectious digital conditions | Septic conditions |
| – interdigital necrobacillosis | – septic arthritides |
| – digital dermatitis | |
| – foot-and-mouth disease | |
| Acute laminitis | |

Minor traumatic sprains to joints, ligaments, and tendons show a gradual improvement over a period of several days.

## Numbers of animals affected

The numbers of affected animals may suggest a herd problem. Digital dermatitis and foot-and-mouth disease are acute-onset diseases with high morbidity rates. Ulceration of the sole and white line lesions are diseases of insidious onset with high morbidity rates. Lameness associated with fractures, interdigital fibromata and bovine viral diarrhea–mucosal disease are usually sporadic conditions with low morbidity rates. With the exception of the clostridial diseases such as blackleg, bovine lameness is rarely associated with a high mortality rate.

# CLINICAL EXAMINATION OF THE STANDING ANIMAL

## General clinical examination

A routine general clinical examination is necessary for any lame animal. All body systems should be examined for evidence of abnormalities. Lameness may be secondary to disease of body systems other than the musculoskeletal system. Polysynovitis and tenosynovitis may occur secondary to endocarditis, causing a shifting lameness because of multiple joint and tendon sheath involvement. The enlarged and painful mammary gland in summer mastitis interferes with normal locomotion, resulting in abduction of the hindlimb. Generalized stiffness and reluctance to move associated with grunting is present in acute localized peritonitis and may be present in the acute stages of photosensitization, particularly if the unpigmented skin around the coronary band is involved.

Diseases of the musculoskeletal system may result in secondary abnormalities of other body systems. Loud stertorous breathing in a calf in the first few months of life may indicate tracheal stenosis caused by fracture of the cranial ribs. Auscultation and palpation will differentiate the case from laryngeal dyspnea and may reveal evidence of a bone callus at or near the thoracic inlet. Tachypnea associated with exercise intolerance may be due to myopathy associated with selenium–vitamin E deficiency, or reflect severe pain associated with septic arthritis or acute laminitis.

The umbilicus of lame calves with arthritis should be examined for evidence of swelling, pain, and purulent discharge, as it may have been the portal of entry of infection.

## Distant examination of the standing animal

The animal is first examined from a distance, ideally while it is standing on a clean, level surface in natural daylight. Unless restrained in a stanchion or tied, cattle will not remain motionless for long periods and so patience is required when performing this examination. In the normal standing posture the head is held up so that both eyes look straight ahead and the weight appears to be borne equally on all four limbs. The animal is examined visually in an orderly fashion from head to tail on each side of its body and from in front and behind to assess:

1. symmetry of the body around the median plane comparing each limb with the contralateral limb for signs of asymmetry in the relative sizes and shapes of joints, bones, tendons, and muscle masses.
2. each limb from the foot proximally to the withers or pelvis, recording the presence of any swellings or discharges.
3. the overall shape and the length of the claws scrutinizing the heels and the coronary band for evidence of swelling or exudation. Dorsal rotation of the toe with sinking at the heel suggests that rupture of the deep flexor tendon has occurred as a sequel to deep digital sepsis.

Conformation refers to the proportional shape or contour of the animal. The normal tibiotarsal–metatarsal angle is between 129° and 134°. A straight hock, with an angle in excess of 160°, has been associated with an increased incidence of arthritis of the stifle joint (gonitis). The conformational changes associated with lactation, in which the hindlimbs are displaced laterally because of the bulk of the udder, may contribute to the pathogenesis of lesions involving the lateral claws of the hind feet. Judgment of conformation is very subjective and practical and accurate methods of assessment have not been developed.

If the animal is recumbent when first approached, take note of its lying position. Cattle in sternal recumbency normally lie with the slightly flexed hindlimbs stretched out on the same side of the body. Lame cows usually adopt a sternal lying position, in which the painful hindlimb is uppermost and the normal limb is folded under the ventral abdomen. This reduces contact pressure between the painful limb and the ground. In severe cases animals will rest the lame hind foot on the lower rail of the cubicle or stall.

Recumbent animals should be coaxed to stand and the act of standing should be observed closely for difficulties

- cattle normally bear weight first on the hindlimbs; using their sternum as a fulcrum they then lurch forward, moving the head up and down in order to shift weight on to the knees of the forelimbs
- an animal that begins to rise by bearing weight on its forelimbs suggests an abnormality of the hindlimbs
- cattle with painful foot conditions are reluctant to rise when encouraged to do so, and will stand for only a few minutes before returning to a more comfortable lying position.

---

### Clinical Pointer

A majority of beef bulls in AI studs which were rejected on the basis of conformational defects were found to be affected with laminitis.

---

### *Abnormal postures in the standing animal*

Any specific abnormal postures of the standing animal are noted and may provide clues to the location of a painful lesion. Cattle adopt abnormal postures to relieve pain or because of structural abnormalities of the musculoskeletal or nervous systems. Painful lesions of the feet are usually localized to one of the two claws, and animals adopt postures that reduce the weight borne on the painful claw, or even part of a painful claw.

---

### Painful lesions of the claws

- painful lesions involving the medial claw result in **adduction** of the limb across the midline, allowing the lateral claw to bear more weight
- painful lesions of the lateral claw result in **abduction** of the limb away from the midline to allow the medial claw to bear more weight.

Cattle with bilateral or unilateral fractures of the medial pedal bone in the front limbs adduct the limb to relieve weightbearing on the medial claw. This crossed-leg forelimb posture may also be associated with other painful conditions affecting the medial claw in the front feet, and has been observed in cattle with acute laminitis (Fig. 21.39).

Fracture of the lateral pedal bone of the front limb results in abduction of the limb; the affected limb is also held cranially to allow the contralateral limb to bear more weight. Similarly, cattle with painful ulceration of the lateral claw of the hindlimb tend to stand with the lame hind foot abducted and stretched forward.

When an animal is standing with the toe of one limb only lightly and intermittently touching the ground, it usually indicates lameness associated with severe pain (Fig. 21.40). Conditions that lead to this posture include

- penetration of the sole by a foreign body, leading to the collection of pus between the wall and the third phalanx
- septic pedal arthritis
- severe cases of digital dermatitis.

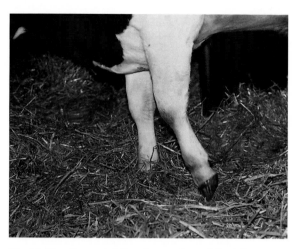

**Fig. 21.40** Non-weightbearing posture of the left forelimb due to foreign body penetration of the sole.

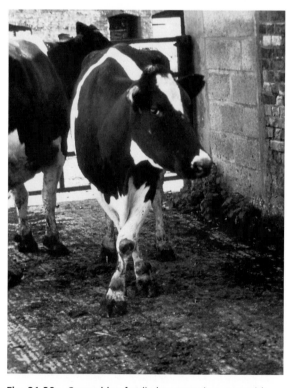

**Fig. 21.39** Crossed-leg forelimb posture in a cow with painful lesions of the medial claws. (Courtesy of Mr R. Blowey, Wood Veterinary Group, Gloucester, UK.

Cattle also stand with the toes of the hind feet on the edge of a cubicle or stall to reduce the weight borne by painful heels. Paddling behavior, in which weight is continuously shifted from one foot to another, is associated with pain in more than one foot and is most noticeable in the hindlimbs. It is characteristic of acute laminitis and bilateral hindlimb claw lesions.

Knuckling is overflexion of the fetlock joint so that weight is borne on the dorsal surface of the flexed fetlock joint (Fig. 21.41). It may be caused by neurological or structural abnormalities. An association between hindlimb knuckling and the presence of laminitis in young pedigree beef bulls has been reported. Knuckling is also evident in newborn calves with arthrogryposis. However, flaccidity of the limb is not a feature of this condition, which is characterized by stiffness and difficulty in or inability to manually extend the limb.

Marked overextension of the hindlimb is characteristic of spastic paresis (Fig. 21.42). Caudal hyperextension of one or both hindlimbs is also a feature of the spastic syndrome. The episodic character of the spastic syndrome contrasts with the constant progressive signs of spastic paresis. In addition, spastic paresis occurs mainly in calves from 3 to 6 months of age, whereas the onset of the spastic syndrome is

**Clinical Pointer**

Dragging of both hind feet with knuckling of the fetlocks is a feature of ankylosing spondylosis in old bulls, particularly those held in AI studs.

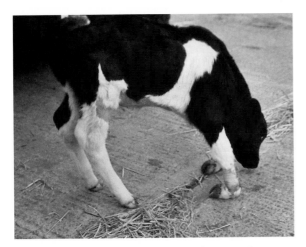

**Fig. 21.41**    Knuckling in a calf with arthrogryposis.

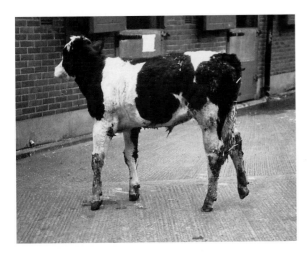

**Fig. 21.42**    Overextension of the right hindlimb in spastic paresis.

usually between 3 and 7 years. However, animals with arthritis of the stifle joint (gonitis) or those with dorsal luxation of the patella may adopt this posture. Arching of the back (kyphosis) may be associated with a physical deformity of the vertebrae, but may also reflect acute abdominal pain. Abnormal persistent elevation of the tail head is seen in both spastic paresis and tetanus. The generalized nature of the stiffness and the presence of ruminal tympany and prolapse of the third eyelid in tetanus are important differentiating features of these diseases.

Marked overflexion of the hindlimb with a dropped hock is characteristic of rupture of the gastrocnemius muscle or the Achilles tendon.

## Examination of gait

The objective of examination of the gait is to determine in which limb or limbs the animal is lame. This is followed by location of the lesion causing the lameness.

Evaluation of the gait of lame cattle is much more elementary than the advanced diagnostic testing used commonly to evaluate the lame horse. Halter-trained horses are usually led to walk and trot for gait analysis, and nerve blocks are used extensively to localize lesions. Only halter-trained cattle can be led to walk for evaluation of their gait and nerve blocks are not used routinely. However, examination is essential and the gait of dairy cows can be examined as they are gathered from pasture, or as they enter a chute for further examination. Every reasonable effort should be made to encourage the animal to walk in order to manifest the lameness for detailed examination.

Ideally the lame animal is examined while it is walking on a clean, level, hard surface. Unless they have been trained for the purpose of showing adult cattle can rarely be halter led. A lame calf or bull can usually be encouraged to walk in an enclosure so that the characteristics of the lameness can be evaluated. If the animal cannot be led, it should be placed in an enclosed area and encouraged by vocal and physical stimulation to walk. The gait is examined

- with the animal walking away from the examiner
- while walking towards the examiner, and
- from both sides.

In the case of fractious animals this examination must be done from a safe vantage point.

The stride of walking cattle consists of swinging and supporting phases. After the foot is lifted the limb enters the swinging phase; the foot is then placed on the ground, entering the supporting phase of the stride (period of contact with the ground). In normal cattle the gait should be relatively even, with no marked abduction or adduction of the limb.

A severely lame cow will prefer recumbency. If forced to walk, it will do so to relieve weightbearing on the affected limb.

With painful lesions of the lateral claw the limb is abducted and more weight is placed on the medial claw

> **Clinical Pointer**
>
> Abnormalities of gait, like those of posture, commonly reflect a natural attempt by an animal to relieve pain.

during the supporting phase of the stride. The supporting phase will also be shorter than normal. With painful conditions of the medial claw the limb is adducted at the walk and more weight is borne on the lateral claw; the supporting phase is also reduced. This shortened supporting phase is identifiable as a 'tenderness' of gait, in which the feet are placed carefully on the ground and lifted again as quickly as possible. Tenderness of gait is associated with painful conditions of the feet, such as bilateral ulceration of the sole, white line lesions or interdigital ulceration caused by BVD-MD virus. The most common claw lesions resulting in lameness are solar ulcer and white line disease. It is not possible to differentiate these conditions by examining the gait, however the degree of lameness associated with sole ulceration is generally more severe. Animals with painful upper limb conditions, particularly arthritis of the stifle and hip joint, reduce the range of motion of the painful joint by decreasing the length of the swinging period of the gait.

Examination of lame cattle from a distance usually allows the identification of an abnormality of gait associated with a specific limb or limbs. Stiffness, on the other hand, is a generalized problem. When viewing a stiff animal from a distance it may not be possible to localize it to a particular limb. Stiffness is common to many forms of lameness, such as

- polyarthritis
- myopathy and
- tetanus.

It is characterized by

- a reluctance to move voluntarily
- a reduction in the range of motion of a joint
- a shortened stride length
- reduced flexibility of the limbs or vertebrae.

Stiffness of gait may also be associated with abdominal, thoracic, or even cutaneous pain. An initial visual examination will rarely identify the musculoskeletal system as the source of the stiffness.

Like stiffness, weakness of gait is also a generalized phenomenon which cannot be localized to a particular limb. Weakness is a general loss of motor function due to a muscular, neuromuscular or neurological abnormality. Any factor that depresses normal muscle metabolism may result in generalized muscle weakness. Weakness is seen in toxemic, emaciated or severely anemic animals, as well as in acidotic or dehydrated, hyperkalemic patients. The gait is characterized by flexion of the neck, and dragging of the feet leading to worn hooves. Weak cattle have difficulty negotiating obstacles and tire quickly, frequently becoming recumbent.

> ### Some abnormalities of gait associated with certain diseases
>
> - femoral nerve paralysis → flexion of joints genuflexion, or a marked ventral sinking of a flexed hindlimb at a walk (Fig. 21. 43)
> - dorsal luxation of the patella → caudal extension of one hindlimb, followed by sudden cranial jerking of the limb associated with a distinct clicking sound
> - dislocation of the coxofemoral joint → outward rotation of the stifle on the affected side at a walk, the greater trochanter of the femur appears higher and much more prominent on the normal side
> - hip dysplasia → swaying, or an excessive lateral movement of both hindquarters

The severity of lameness in dairy cows can be graded using a scoring system. Wells and others (1993) scored clinical lameness from 0 to 4. Cattle with score 0 had no gait abnormality and exhibited no reluctance to walk. Severe gait abnormality (score 3) was characterized by marked gait asymmetry. Animals with a score of 4 were recumbent.

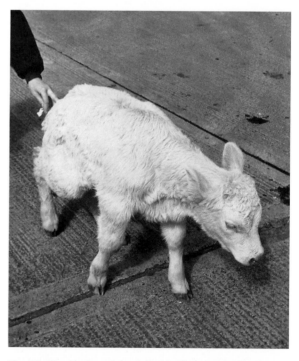

**Fig. 21.43** Flexion of the right hindlimb in a calf with femoral nerve paralysis. (Courtesy of Ms A. Healy, Faculty of Veterinary Medicine, University College Dublin, Ireland.)

## Close physical examination

### Techniques of physical examination

The basic techniques used in the close physical examination of the musculoskeletal system are

- palpation
- manipulation
- passive flexion and extension
- auscultation, and
- percussion.

#### Palpation

Palpation is the gentle handling of muscles, tendons, ligaments, joints and bones to determine consistency and to detect evidence of heat, pain or swelling. Palpation to detect consistency and pain generally involves the application of pressure between the thumb and index finger (Fig. 21.44). Increased temperature and swelling of the tissues is detected using the palm of the hand (Fig. 21.45). Terms used to describe the consistency of tissue following palpation include

- doughy, when the structure pits on pressure as in edema
- firm, when the structure has the consistency of normal liver

- hard, when the consistency is bone-like
- fluctuating, when the structure is soft, elastic and undulates on pressure but does not retain the imprint of the fingers
- emphysematous, when the structure is puffy and swollen and moves and crackles under pressure because of the presence of gas in the tissue.

The perception of pain requires the involvement of ascending pathways traveling to the thalamus and the sensory cerebral cortex. The withdrawal of a limb in response to stimulation of a local reflex arc may occur with or without a cerebral response, such as vocalization or moving the whole body away from the stimulus. The animal's head should be observed while

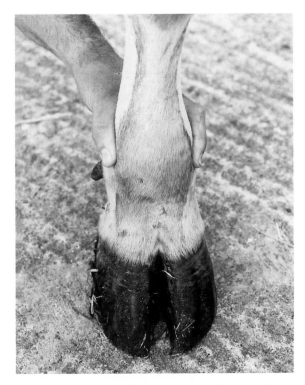

**Fig. 21.44** Palpation of the fetlock joint of the forelimb.

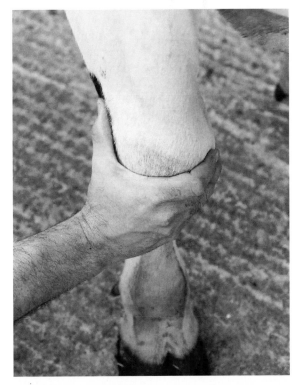

**Fig. 21.45** Examination of the fetlock joint of the forelimb for evidence of heat or swelling.

performing palpation to detect any change in facial expression. Some animals are excitable and will react to only the slightest touch; others exhibit stoicism and tolerate higher pain thresholds. The size of the structure being palpated, its anatomical location and the size of the animal also influence the sensitivity of the pain test. Accurate assessment of pain in a hip joint using palpation is virtually impossible in mature animals, and assessment of musculoskeletal pain in a large mature bull can be difficult, depending on the location of the lesion, because of

- the large size of these animals
- their difficult temperament, and
- the need to be aware of personal safety.

These limitations must be considered when examining large bulls. An enlarged joint in the absence of detectable pain may be the only clue available to facilitate further investigations using arthrocentesis or radiography.

### Manipulation

Manipulation involves the use of both hands and is the gentle application of force in lateral, medial, dorsal and palmar (plantar) directions at joint surfaces and over bones to detect abnormal mobility, pain or crepitus (Fig. 21.46).

### Passive flexion and extension

This is the manual flexion and extension of joints to detect abnormal or reduced mobility, pain or crepitus. It is a simple and easy procedure in young calves which can be handled easily. However, unlike horses, adult cattle do not facilitate manual lifting of the limb and so this technique is physically difficult unless the animal is clinically recumbent or a casting table is available. Where possible, the limb is stabilized proximal to the joint being examined with one hand and the joint is flexed and extended with the other (Fig. 21.47). Passive flexion and extension can be attempted with the use of leg-lifting devices, but meaningful interpretation of the findings is difficult. If the fore- or hindlimb of an adult animal can be lifted easily, it frequently indicates evidence of a severe musculoskeletal problem (e.g. tendon rupture).

### Auscultation and percussion

Auscultation and percussion are useful for the diagnosis of fractures and for the detection of crepitus in arthritic joints, particularly the stifle and hip joints. The area over the joint is auscultated with or without a stethoscope when the joint is being passively flexed and extended (Fig. 21.48). Confident assessment of crepitus

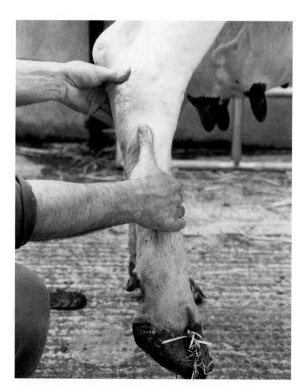

**Fig. 21.46** Manipulation of the hock joint.

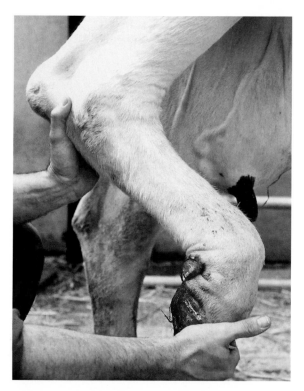

**Fig. 21.47** Passive flexion of the fetlock joint in the hindlimb.

during the auscultation of moving joints requires experience, as 'clicks' and 'pops' are frequently detected during manipulation of normal joints.

Percussion sound is not transmitted along the shaft of a fractured long bone, and percussion and auscultation above and below a suspected fracture site is a useful aid to diagnosis. In the case of a suspected fractured femur the bell of the stethoscope is placed over the greater trochanter and a metallic object is used to tap a pleximeter plate held next to the metatarsal bone. In the presence of a femoral fracture sound transmission is significantly reduced or absent compared to transmission along the normal limb.

### Examination of joints

Joint size is assessed both visually and by palpation, and by comparing the joint being examined with the equivalent joint on the contralateral limb.

When presented with an enlarged joint in association with lameness, it is most important first to decide exactly which structures are involved in the swelling (Fig. 21.49). The swelling may be due to distension of the joint capsule and periosteal reaction, or inflammation of periarticular structures such as bursae, tendon sheaths and subcutaneous tissue. Inflammation of the growth plates proximal or distal to the joint may also appear as an enlarged joint.

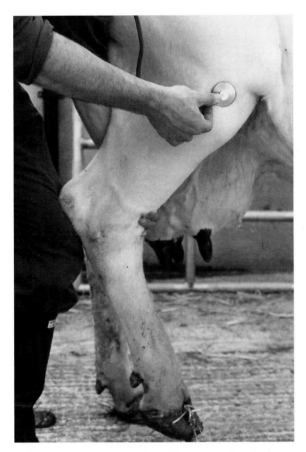

**Fig. 21.48** Auscultation while flexing the stifle joint in a cow with gonitis.

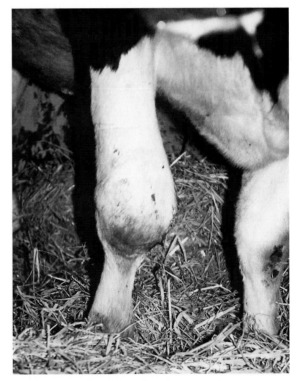

**Fig. 21.49** Swelling over the area of the right carpal joint in a cow.

Deciding exactly which structures are involved requires a thorough knowledge or review of the anatomy of the joint, but it should be possible following careful visual examination, palpation and manipulation. Inflammation and enlargement of the growth plate is detectable as a hard painful circumferential swelling several centimeters proximal to the joint. Enlargement of the growth plates of the metacarpus and metatarsus is the most commonly encountered. The degree of pain associated with these growth plate enlargements is variable. Pain is severe in septic physitis associated with *Salmonella dublin*, whereas that in copper-deficiency physitis is less marked.

Once a decision has been reached that enlargement of the joint is due to distension of the joint capsule and arthritis, it is important to decide whether the arthritis is septic or non-septic, as this will greatly influence any treatment and prognosis. Reaching a tentative diagnosis of septic arthritis in joints distal to the hip and shoulder joints should be possible without the need for radiological investigation.

## Examination of bones

Physical examination of bones requires careful palpation to detect exostoses, discontinuities, hypermobility, crepitus, and pain. Fractures are characterized by excess mobility, loss of function, and crepitus. Crepitus is detected by manipulation or passive flexion and extension, and results from the rubbing together of the fractured ends of bone. Crepitus is a reliable clinical finding in the detection of fractures but it may be difficult to detect in mature, heavily muscled cattle. Furthermore, the fractured ends of the bone are often distracted, or muscle intervenes so that crepitus cannot be produced. Detection of pain may be useful in diagnosing incomplete fractures, such as short oblique fractures of the lower midshaft of long bones in calves. Enlargement of the metaphyseal aspects of long bones in calves may be associated with osteomyelitis and is characterized by lameness and marked pain on palpation of the affected site.

## Examination of muscles

Normal muscle has a smooth surface and a soft, rubbery consistency that undulates on pressure but which does not retain the imprint of the fingers. Swelling of muscle may be due to hypertrophy, myositis or myopathy. When there is localized swelling associated with muscle masses, careful palpation is necessary to distinguish hematomata (rarely a cause of lameness) and localized cellulitis from swelling associated with the muscle tissue itself, such as in clostridial or non-specific bacterial myositis. A circumscribed hardening in a muscle may be an abscess, a granuloma or, rarely, a tumor.

Passive flexion and extension of the limb allows assessment of muscle tone (flaccidity and spasticity).

---

### Septic arthritis

Septic arthritis is characterized by severe lameness. In cases of hindlimb lameness there is often marked atrophy of the semimembranosus and semitendinosus muscles. Palpation of the joint capsule reveals pain and marked distension, the pain is marked when the joint is manipulated.

The severity of pain associated with septic arthritis is an important diagnostic finding and may be severe enough to be accompanied by excess salivation and tachypnea.

The presence of a purulent sinus discharge supports the diagnosis. Collection and examination of synovia is easily performed, typically in septic arthritis the synovia is grossly turbid and there may be pus within the joint.

---

### Non-septic arthritis

The degree of pain and swelling associated with non-septic arthritis is less marked. Degenerative joint disease is insidious in onset and exacerbated by moderate exercise and manipulation of the affected limb. With the exception of a slight blood-tinged appearance, the examination of synovial fluid in cases of degenerative arthritis usually reveals no remarkable gross abnormalities.

---

### Clostridial myositis

- is characterized by emphysematous crackling associated with swelling and crepitant edema over a muscle mass
- lameness and severe mental depression are usually present
- the swelling is warm and painful to the touch in the early stages but soon becomes cool and painless.

Note that subcutaneous emphysema over the withers due to alveolar rupture may be present in atypical interstitial pneumonia and verminous pneumonia.

Prominent flaccidity is most commonly associated with neurological disease.

---

### Clinical Pointer

Botulism is characterized by a progressive flaccid paralysis commencing at the hindlimbs and extending cranially to involve the forelimbs, leading to recumbency and death.

---

Increased muscle tone (spasticity) may be so marked that the limb cannot be flexed without considerable effort. Spasticity of the limbs can be associated with lesions of the spinal cord. Generalized spasticity of skeletal muscles is seen in tetanus, and in hypomagnesemic tetany.

### Procedure for the physical examination

Physical examination of the musculoskeletal system requires a precise knowledge of topographic anatomy and involves a detailed examination of muscle masses, bones, joints, ligaments, and tendons. The examination usually begins at the head and continues in an orderly fashion toward the tail on each side of the animal's body.

### Skull and neck

The head is viewed from the frontal aspect and laterally for symmetry. The bony skeleton of the skull is then palpated. The frontal sinuses are percussed and the temporomandibular joint is examined for mobility and pain by opening and closing the jaw, and by palpation over the area of articulation. Note the alignment of the maxillae and mandible when closing the jaw and assess the integrity of the mandibular symphysis by manipulation. Bony swellings of the mandible and maxilla are most commonly associated with actinomycosis or, rarely, with tumors. The muscles of the neck and the ligamentum nuchae are palpated for evidence of swelling or crepitation. Injection-site abscesses are not uncommon in the depth of the neck musculature.

The atlanto-occipital joint is flexed and extended and the neck manipulated both from side to side and dorsally and ventrally to detect crepitus or pain. In calves with cervical osteomyelitis manipulation and deep palpation over the spinous processes of the affected vertebrae may elicit vocalization. Torticollis, an abnormal twisting of the neck, may also indicate the presence of painful lesions of the cervical vertebrae.

### Forelimbs

Examination of any limb should commence at its distal portion. Palpation and manipulation of the coronary band proceeds proximally to the withers, with examination of the joints, bones, muscle masses, and tendons for evidence of heat, pain, or swelling. Where possible, the joints are passively flexed and extended to detect abnormal or reduced mobility, pain, or crepitus.

#### Joints

Joint capsule distension is relatively easily detected in the fetlock (palmar aspect), carpus (dorsal aspect), and elbow (lateral aspect), but more difficult to determine in the shoulder joint. In cattle septic arthritis is the most common cause of joint enlargement, and in the forelimb the fetlock and carpal joints are the most common sites for septic arthritis proximal to the coronary band. The detection of distension of some joint capsules, such as the coxofemoral, shoulder, and elbow joints, is difficult because they are covered by tendons, ligaments, and muscle.

Lameness is frequently associated with lesions of the elbow or shoulder joints. However, detection of crepitus in either of these may indicate the presence of degenerative joint disease. Physical examination of the shoulder joint is difficult in adult cattle. Where possible, the joint should be examined by flexion, extension, and rotation. Direct pressure should also be applied over the joint with the palm of the hand and the fingers. The shoulder joint may click following this type of direct pressure and this should not be a diagnostic basis for luxation. Shoulder joint luxation is extemely rare and is characterized by severe lameness, joint swelling, and limb shortening.

#### Bones

Using the thumb and index finger, firm pressure is applied along the cortex of the entire shafts of the long bones to detect swelling, crepitus, or pain. Multiple

---

### Arthrogryposis

Calves with arthrogryposis frequently develop a swelling dorsal to the carpal joints, this swelling

- results from excess weightbearing
- is painless to touch (unless damage to the skin allows the entry of infection)
- is due to serous enlargement of the bursa (hygroma) between the skin and the extensor tendons, and
- the joint space and joint capsule are not distended.

---

easily palpable exostoses of the shafts of long bones are characteristic of chronic fluorosis. In neonatal calves the proximal phalanx should be carefully examined for fractures, that occur as a sequela to excessive obstetric traction. Complete fractures of the metacarpus are relatively easily diagnosed and are characterized by pain, swelling, crepitus, malalignment, and abnormal mobility.

Complete fractures of the humerus in cattle are also relatively easily diagnosed. Evidence of radial nerve damage may be a useful aid to diagnosis of incomplete fractures of the humeral shaft.

*Muscles*

Flaccidity of the forelimb muscles is associated with neurological diseases such as radial nerve injury and osteomyelitis of the cervical vertebrae. Fasciculation of the flexor and extensor muscles of the forelimbs is present in many diseases, including hypomagnesemic tetany.

*Skin*

The presence of any skin wounds or discharges is noted. Decubital ulcers of the skin over bony prominences occur commonly in recumbent animals. A purulent sinus discharge and soft tissue swelling over bone may indicate a sequestrum. If the bone is visible the presence of dull, gray necrotic bone suggests the presence of a sequestrum. Cool extremities are associated with terminal dry gangrene (ergotism, *Salmonella dublin* thrombosis) and frozen feet. Subtle changes in the texture of unpigmented skin associated with the early stages of photosensitization may also be detected on palpation. Palpable engorgement of the superficial veins between fetlock and carpus is a feature of acute laminitis.

**Thorax and abdomen**

The ribs are palpated for evidence of excess mobility, exostosis, callus, or pain. Cattle with enzootic nutritional myopathy dystrophy involving the intercostal muscles and the diaphragm may be affected with tachypnea and dyspnea. The dorsal and transverse processes of the thoracic and lumbar vertebrae are palpated to detect excess mobility and crepitus associated with fractures,

---

> ### Clinical Pointer
>
> Unilateral enlargement of the prescapular lymph node is a useful indicator of infectious arthritis of the joints of the forelimbs. In the hindlimbs the joints drain to the popliteal lymph nodes which are not readily palpable in adult cattle.

which may occur in young calves. Diagnostic manipulation of the thoracolumbar vertebrae in adult cattle is not possible. Localized soft tissue swellings are rarely associated with vertebral disease, the clinical signs of which usually relate to pressure on the spinal cord.

The dorsolumbar and abdominal muscles are palpated for changes in size, consistency, and the presence of pain.

**Hindlimbs and pelvis**

Both hindlimbs are examined in a similar manner to the forelimbs.

*Joints*

Proximal to the coronary band, septic arthritis is most common in the fetlock and hock joints. Septic gonitis (stifle joint) is an occasional cause of lameness in calves and sepsis of the hip joint is rare. Joint capsule distension is relatively easily detected in the fetlock joint (plantar aspect). Enlargement of the joint capsule of the hock joint is most easily palpated on the dorsomedial aspect and may be present as a relatively painless serous arthritis in cases of spastic paresis.

Tarsal hygromata are relatively common painless swellings of acquired subcutaneous bursa over the lateral aspect of the hock. They occur in herds where the cubicles or stalls are too small, and where cubicles are not covered with comfortable bedding or rubber mats. Extension to the joint capsule following injury to the skin may result in suppurative tarsitis, characterized by severe lameness.

---

> ### Enzootic nutritional myopathy
>
> Useful diagnostic findings of enzootic nutritional myopathy of calves include
>
> - enlarged, hard, or board-like bilateral dorsolumbar muscle masses
> - involvement of the shoulder and gluteal muscles
> - the presence of muscle fasciculation
> - stiffness
> - a tendency towards recumbency.

---

> ### Clinical Pointer
>
> Considerable care should be taken not to confuse growth plate fractures of the metacarpus with arthritis of the fetlock joint. The growth plate is immediately proximal to the joint and radiographs may be necessary to confirm the diagnosis.

Distension of the capsule of the stifle joint is most readily detected as a bulging between the middle and medial patellar ligaments. In a normal animal there should be no such distension, and a gap should be detected between the middle and medial and the middle and lateral patellar ligaments. Extensive diverticula of the joint capsule extend proximally between the quadriceps femoris muscle and the femur, and distally in the extensor groove of the tibia. Distension of the joint capsule may result in swelling of these diverticula, which may initially appear unrelated to the stifle joint. In advanced cases of septic or degenerative gonitis palpation reveals severe pain and gross enlargement compared to the contralateral stifle joint.

Rupture of the cranial cruciate ligament is an occasional cause of lameness in older cattle, and in particular bulls. It is characterized by

- relatively sudden onset, moderate to severe lameness
- excessive movement of the joint
- clicking on the supporting phase of the stride
- marked joint capsule distension
- the detection of pain and crepitus on manipulation.

Although a positive drawer test (distinct sliding movement between tibia and femur) in the standing bovine has been described in the literature, testing of this phenomenon in mature bulls weighing 1000 kg or more which are non-weightbearing is unrealistic. The diagnosis is more reliably based on the clinical findings described above, the presence of excessive amounts of blood-tinged joint fluid aspirate, and radiological examination.

The patella should be tested for position and laxity. Normally the patella should not be easily moved by manipulation; a freely movable patella associated with laxity of the patellar ligaments is an important diagnostic feature of femoral nerve paralysis in calves in the first few weeks of life. In dorsal luxation of the patella, palpation of the stifle joint reveals the dorsal position of the patella and the prominence of its ligaments.

Physical examination of the coxofemoral joint is difficult. The area over the greater trochanter should always be carefully palpated. With the animal standing, one hand should be placed over the greater trochanter and (physical size allowing) the animal pushed so that it is bearing more weight on the contralateral limb. The animal should then be allowed to take weight again on the limb being palpated. In hip dysplasia crepitus characterized by a clicking sensation, associated with the movement of the greater trochanter dorsally, may be felt or heard as weight is borne on the limb. This test can be performed in young bulls up to

12 months of age. In advanced cases of coxofemoral arthritis associated with hip dysplasia obvious crepitus may be auscultated over the hip joint when the animal is walked. Detection of dislocation of the hip joint is discussed in the section on the recumbent animal.

*Bones*

The first phalanx and metatarsus are examined as described for the forelimb. Fractures of the femur, and particularly of the femoral head, are relatively difficult to diagnose. This is particularly so in mature cattle and/or where there is marked muscle swelling and hematoma formation at the fracture site. The limb shortening associated with muscle contraction may be a useful aid to the diagnosis of femoral fractures in younger animals. Radiographic examination is often necessary to confirm femoral fractures. However, it is useful to perform an auscultation–percussion technique to facilitate diagnosis.

The pelvis is examined for symmetry. Where appropriate, a rectal examination is an essential part of the physical examination and pelvic abnormalities such as exostosis, pain, and crepitus may be detected in arthritis of the coxofemoral joint and in fractures of the pubic symphysis. Fractures of the tubera coxae (knocked-down hip) are common and are easily detected as a visual abnormality. They rarely cause problems unless a sequestrum is produced. In dairy cows the tubera coxae are common sites for hematomata resulting from trauma in the milking parlor or in the stalls. Other pelvic fractures are rare and usually associated with direct trauma, or following mounting by another cow. Fractures of the shaft of the ilium result in severe lameness, with limb dragging and abnormal pelvic contour. Fractures of the body of the ischium and pubis invariably involve the obturator foramen. They are associated with pelvic instability and marked pain, and may be confirmed by rectal examination.

*Muscles*

The gluteal muscles are palpated for signs of swelling and hardness consistent with myopathy.

Varying degrees of atrophy of the semimembranous and semitendinous muscles are present in septic arthritides of the hindlimb. Marked atrophy of the quadriceps femoris muscle is a characteristic feature of femoral nerve paralysis in neonatal calves. It develops within a few days, and examination of the limb reveals the prominence of a femur lacking significant muscle cover. Aplasia of the quadriceps muscle has been reported in neonatal beef calves and its presence at birth should help distinguish it from acquired (obstetrical) femoral nerve paralysis. The chronic pain associated with hip arthritis in cattle with fluorosis leads to atrophy of the hindlimb musculature and a compensatory hypertrophy of the muscles of the shoulder as weight is shifted cranially from the hindlimbs to the forelimbs. The muscle masses of the hindlimb are also common sites for the presence of crepitation in cases of blackleg.

---

### Clinical Pointer

The gluteal muscles should not be used routinely for intramuscular injections. However, injection site abscesses are not uncommon findings in this area.

---

**Tendons**

Examination of the deep and superficial flexor tendons for evidence of septic tenosynovitis is important in the assessment of cattle with septic pedal arthritis. This condition is most common in the hindlimb. Septic tenosynovitis proximal to the proposed level of amputation (usually the distal end of the first phalanx) indicates a poor candidate for surgery. Septic tenosynovitis is characterized by severe pain and palpation is greatly resented. Cellulitis (inflammation of subcutaneous tissue planes) is marked by moderate pain; the swelling involves the subcutaneous tissue around the whole limb and is not confined to the area of the flexor tendon sheaths. Subcutaneous non-inflammatory edema pits on pressure and is not associated with any significant degree of pain.

Rupture of the gastrocnemius tendon may occur in periparturient cows, particularly those struggling to rise following treatment for hypocalcemia. It is characterized by severe lameness, a 'dropped' hock and, in many cases, an inability to rise. Palpation of the tendon is not particularly painful but reveals evidence of marked swelling and edema.

**Feet**

Approximately 90% of lameness in dairy cattle is due to lesions in the feet, and of these almost 90% involve the claws of the hindlimbs. When investigating lameness in an individual animal, examination of the musculoskeletal system must always be accompanied by detailed examination of all feet. A thorough knowledge of the regional anatomy and normal conformation of the bovine foot is therefore essential.

*Regional anatomy of the feet*

Each foot has two claws, each of which contains the terminal phalanges of the main digits and two accessory claws for the vestigial digits (dew claws).

Externally, each claw consists of four components

- the periople
- the horn of the wall
- the horn of the sole, and
- the bulb.

The horn of the claw is a modification of the superficial layer of the epidermis. The periople is the hairless band of soft horn that separates the claw wall from the skin at the coronary band (the line of transition between skin and claw). It is responsible for the smooth waxy coating over healthy hooves.

The white line represents the junction between the horn of the wall and the horn of the sole. It consists of immature, non-pigmented horn which is incompletely keratinized and considerably weaker than the horn of either the wall or the sole. The white line is therefore vulnerable to penetration by dirt and grit, which may allow the introduction of infection into the sensitive laminae of the foot, resulting in inflammation and lameness. The axial groove (a groove at the junction of the axial horn of the sole and the wall) is of functional importance in that penetration of horn in that region rapidly leads to sepsis of the anatomically contiguous navicular bursa and deep flexor tendon sheath. The anatomical structures of the foot are illustrated in Figures 21.50–21.52.

*Restraint*

Adequate restraint is essential to facilitate proper examination of the feet, which requires that the limb and foot be lifted off the ground. To minimize personal injury, each limb is lifted using ropes or pulleys, with the animal suitably restrained in a chute. Simple lifting of the limb with ropes has been widely replaced by the use of quick-release claw-lifting devices, such as that illustrated in Figure 21.53. The hindlimb is lifted by placing the rope immediately proximal to the hock and operating the ratchet until the limb is in the desired position. Lifting and examination of the forefeet is more difficult, as access is often restricted by the horizontal bars of the chute. The front limb may be lifted using a claw-lifting device if the rope is placed immediately distal to the carpal joint. This procedure is greatly facilitated by the presence of a side gate at the front of the chute which can be opened to allow access to the front feet. Casting tables are also becoming popular for the examination and trimming of feet in cattle. Limb-lifting devices will suffice for the average-sized dairy cow or yearling bull. Unless the animal is extremely fractious there is no need for sedation. If this is necessary, light sedation with xylazine may be performed to ensure that the animal remains standing. In cases where foot lesions are particularly painful and

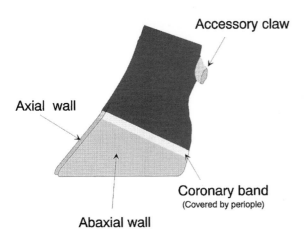

**Fig. 21.50**   Lateral view of the bovine foot.

Labels: Accessory claw, Axial wall, Coronary band (Covered by periople), Abaxial wall

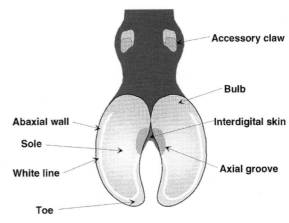

**Fig. 21.51**   Palmar/plantar view of the bovine foot.

Labels: Accessory claw, Bulb, Abaxial wall, Interdigital skin, Sole, White line, Axial groove, Axial groove, Toe

extensive and deep paring of the foot is necessary, regional intravenous analgesia can be quickly done and is recommended (Fig. 21.54).

Examination of the feet of mature bulls requires special restraint. If available, the use of a casting table

designed for foot trimming is ideal for large cattle, including bulls. Limb-lifting devices such as that illustrated are only suitable for young bulls up to the age of 12 months. If a casting table is not available, proper examination of the feet of mature bulls may require

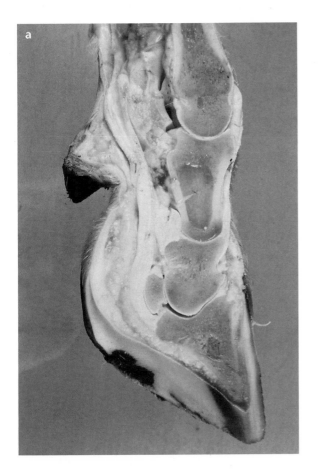

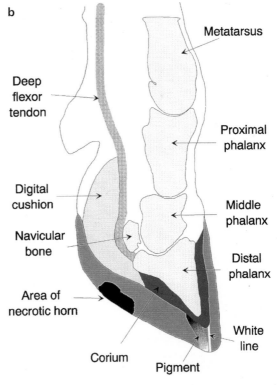

Labels: Metatarsus, Deep flexor tendon, Proximal phalanx, Digital cushion, Middle phalanx, Navicular bone, Area of necrotic horn, Distal phalanx, Corium, Pigment, White line

**Fig. 21.52**   (a) Longitudinal section of the digit. (b) Longitudinal section of the digit illustrating the important anatomical features.

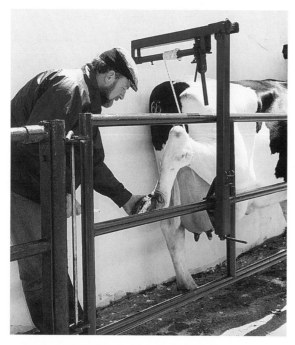

**Fig. 21.53** Lifting the limb for examination of the foot using a hoist. (Ballindee Engineering Ltd, Co. Cork, Ireland.)

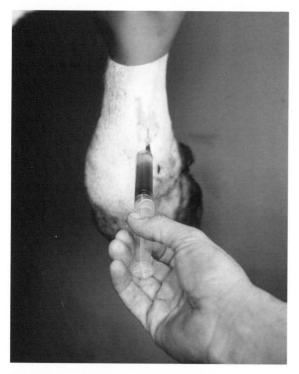

**Fig. 21.54** Intravenous regional anesthesia. A tourniquet has been placed below the hock and 20 ml of lidocaine is introduced into the lateral metatarsal vein.

casting using xylazine or a combination of xylazine and casting ropes.

> ### The use of xylazine for casting mature bulls
>
> - the animal must be properly fasted and the dose accurately calculated and adhered to
> - the procedure is best performed in a spacious well-bedded area or, weather permitting, in a paddock
> - the animals must be kept calm in the 15–20 minutes following the intramuscular administration of xylazine or the efficacy of the drug will be impaired resulting in an unsatisfactory examination.

*Diagnostic procedure for physical examination of the foot*
It is essential that there is good light and that sharp and effective claw knives and claw clippers are available (Fig. 21.55).

1. The limb is lifted and the claws cleaned.
2. The soles of the claw are examined noting the relative length, breadth, and depth of each claw.
3. Examination continues to the wall of each claw from the side and from in front, noting the relative lengths of the claws and the presence of any cracks in the horn.
4. Each claw is flexed and extended at the level of the first interphalangeal joint to test for evidence of pain.

Various systems have been used for recording the lesions of bovine digital disease. The predilection sites of some of the more common foot lesions in cattle are illustrated in Figure 21.56. A form for lesion recording which is based on the anatomical regions shown in Figures 21.50 and 21.51 is illustrated in Figure 21.57. The site and nature of foot lesions can be recorded using the lesion codes and a simple drawing style. Details of history, clinical signs, treatment, and control could be recorded on the reverse side of a form of this type, as described by Mills et al (1986).

> ### Clinical Pointer
>
> The pus associated with foot abscesses is generally small in quantity, watery in consistency, and black or pale yellow in color. Unless the claws are kept clean during paring, detection of this type of pus would be extremely difficult.

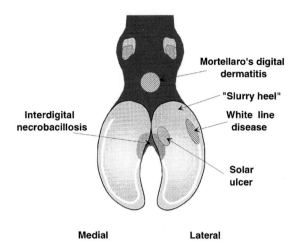

Fig. 21.56 The predilection sites for the common causes of foot lameness.

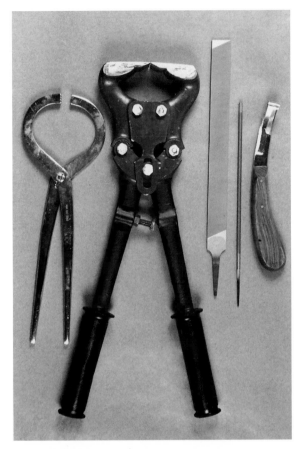

**Fig. 21.55** Equipment for diagnostic foot paring; (left to right) hoof testers, hoof clippers, flat and round files and double-edged knife.

The following areas are examined in the order described and any lesions associated with each area are recorded.

*Area of skin between bulb and accessory claws* This area is frequently covered by a crust of fecal material which should be carefully cleaned away, as this is a predilection site for the raw circumscribed lesions of Mortellaro's digital dermatitis (Fig. 21.56). The lesions of digital dermatitis are usually painful and palpation over them will evince a marked withdrawal response. The junction between the skin and horn at the base of the accessory claw is an occasional site for ulceration caused by BVD-MD virus or infection with *Fusobacterium necrophorum*.

*Interdigital skin* This skin generally has a pock-marked appearance, is relatively smooth, and palpation of the interdigital space should not elicit a withdrawal

response. Pain on palpation of the interdigital space is present in

- interdigital necrobacillosis
- ulceration due to BVD-MD virus, and
- foot-and-mouth disease.

Severe swelling and fissuring of the skin of the interdigital digital area is characteristic of interdigital necrobacillosis. The erosions and ulcers associated with mucosal disease are usually linear or elliptical in shape. They fail to heal, are discrete and very painful when palpated. The interdigital area is examined for the presence of interdigital fibromata, granulation tissue, and foreign bodies.

*Coronary band* Inspection and palpation of the coronary band along its length is essential. Swelling may indicate localized inflammation or the presence of deep infection within the claw. In normal cattle there should be no evidence of pain, swelling, exudation, or separation along the length of the coronary band. Hard, severely painful swelling of the dorsal coronary band, particularly in association with the fistulation of creamy pus, is characteristic of septic arthritis of the distal interphalangeal joint (Fig. 21.58). Soft, fluctuating swelling of the coronary band

> ### Clinical Pointer
>
> The interdigital area should be examined with a light source to avoid overlooking any lesions.

Date:     Client:                    Case No.:
Age:     Sex:     Breed:
Lactation status:

LF

LATERAL                    MEDIAL

RF

LATERAL                    MEDIAL

LH

LATERAL                    MEDIAL

RH

MEDIAL                    LATERAL

**Lesion code:**

| | | | |
|---|---|---|---|
| A - solar ulcer | G - interdigital necrobacillosis | N - horizontal sand crack | T - other: |
| B - white line lesion | H - interdigital fibroma | O - vertical sand crack | |
| C - white line abscess | J - heel erosion | P - hoof wall deformity | |
| D - punctured sole | K - skin ulceration | Q - horn overgrowth | |
| E - foreign body | L - skin hyperplasia | R - pus fistulation | |
| F - solar hemorrhage | M - digital dermatitis | S - deep sepsis | |

**Fig. 21.57** Form for recording foot lesions.

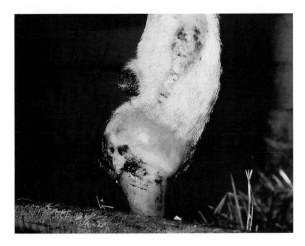

**Fig. 21.58**  Hard, painful coronary band swelling in septic pedal arthritis of the hind limb.

associated with a moderate degree of pain is a feature of acute laminitis. Localized separation of horn of the wall from the sensitive lamina at the abaxial coronary band with the exudation of black watery pus may be a sequel to an abaxial white line abscess. Separation of the horn of the wall along the complete length of the coronary band, which may be accompanied by thimbling, occurs in severe laminitis and in chronic selenium toxicity.

*Abaxial wall* Inspection of the abaxial horn of the wall is made for evidence of horizontal and vertical sand cracks. Areas of diffuse hemorrhage in the wall of unpigmented horn might suggest the presence of laminitis. The marked distortion to the horn of the wall caused by the rings or horizontal grooves of chronic laminitis gives the claw a buckled appearance when viewed from the side.

*Bulbs of the foot* (heels) In cattle with unpigmented heel horn, erythematous reaction may be visible, in association with heat, pain, and swelling in cases of septic navicular bursitis, solar abscess or severe heel erosion ('slurry heel') associated with *Dichelobacter (Bacteroides) nodosus* infection. Horn cover on the bulb is relatively thin (Fig. 21.52a), so is lightly scraped and should not be pared radically. Instead, lightly scrape this area with the hoof knife to remove areas of necrotic horn and to explore any fissures or tracks. A probe can be used during paring to explore the extent of any cavity and the sensitivity of any area of fissured horn. If there is extensive erosion with underrunning of horn from the heels toward the toe, this flap of horn must be removed. Paring away this underrun sole usually reveals a cavity of black necrotic material sandwiched

between the superficial flap of solar horn and a lower, softer layer of juvenile solar horn, and may expose the presence of an axial ulcer of the solar horn.

*Sole* When initially examined the lateral claw of the dairy cow, because of its greater loadbearing, is usually longer, broader, and deeper than that of the medial claw. A superficial layer of horn must initially be pared away with the hoof knife from both claws before the sole can be properly clinically assessed. The white line – normally a grayish-white color then can be examined along its entire length for any black necrotic lesions of white line disease or for the presence of hemorrhage reflecting either traumatic or metabolic laminitis. The predilection site for white line lesions causing lameness is that portion of the abaxial white line at the sole–heel junction (Fig. 21.56). All black necrotic areas are pared away, no matter how insignificant they appear, on both the white line and the solar horn, until either healthy horn, sensitive lamina or pus is detected. The type of pus found when paring the sole is of clinical significance

- thin, watery, brownish (occasionally golden yellow) pus is associated with white line abscessation and foreign body penetration of the sole
- thick creamy pus suggests lameness of long duration, with involvement of deep structures of the foot such as the distal interphalangeal joint or the navicular bursa.

## Clinical Pointer

It is *always* essential to pare away horn from the point of the toe with claw clippers, as pus within the sole frequently gathers towards the toe in cases of abscessation. To gauge how much horn to pare at that site it is useful to know that the length from the coronary band to the toe is approximately 7 cm (one hand's breadth) in the adult dairy cow.

Adequate drainage of a solar abscess produces a certain amount of bleeding, which is necessary and advantageous for the healing process. However, the sole must not be over-pared and the amount of bleeding created should be kept to a minimum. The blunt end of the hoof knife or firm thumb pressure is useful in determining the extent to which the horn has been pared.

1. At the commencement of paring, pressure usually reveals a hard, unyielding sole.
2. Once thinning of the horn has occurred pressure over the area will reveal a 'give', or a feeling of yielding over the sole.

3. If this area of thinner horn is not associated with a marked pain response on palpation, the operator should stop paring at this point for fear of causing unnecessary bleeding.
4. Also if pinpoint areas of hemorrhage become visible through the horn, paring should cease.
5. If, however, pressure over the area of thinner horn is associated with significant pain, very gentle scraping using the seeking end of the knife should be continued, as an area of abscessation may be present below the horn.

A marked withdrawal in response to pressure on the sole is an important criterion in the diagnosis of a solar abscess. The sole is tested for evidence of pain by applying pressure with claw testers, the blunt curved end of a claw knife, or even firm thumb pressure. One jaw of the claw testers is placed on the sole and the other on the abaxial wall of the claw and moderate pressure is applied. The sole should be tested in this way from the toe towards the heel:

- extreme pain towards the toe may indicate a solar abscess
- fractures of the pedal bone and navicular bursitis tend to be most painful towards the caudal third of the sole.

The claws should be manipulated, flexed, and extended. In septic arthritis of the distal interphalangeal joint and in fractures of the distal phalanx, flexion and extension will elicit a pain response.

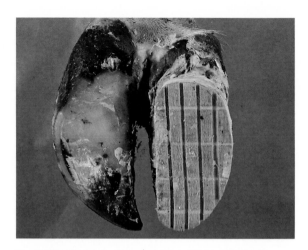

**Fig. 21.59** Placing a shoe on a sound claw can aid the diagnosis of pedal fractures. (Technovit, Kulzer Ltd, Germany.)

> ### Clinical Pointer ✳
>
> Solar ulcers are rarely visible when the foot is first lifted – they are usually discovered only after a superficial layer of solar horn has been pared away, particularly if there has been underrunning of the horn from the heel toward the toe.

If pus has not been detected within the sole following these procedures but severe pain is still obvious on pressure testing of the claw, fracture of the pedal bone should be suspected. Placing a shoe on the opposite, normal claw should relieve much of the pain associated with pedal bone fracture, and can be an aid to diagnosis of this condition (Fig. 21.59).

The axial sole of the lateral claw is the predilection site for ulcers (Fig. 21.56).

Areas of solar hemorrhage (reddish colored areas which are only easily visible in unpigmented horn) may be diffuse or focal. Focal areas of solar hemorrhage are commonly found on the sole of the foot and are usually attributable to bruising by stones or associated with a shift in weightbearing away from a painful area of claw. Diffuse solar hemorrhage, particularly if it involves claws on all feet, is more likely to be have resulted from nutritional or toxemic laminitis. Areas of black pigmented horn (Fig. 21.52) on a white sole should not be confused with solar hemorrhage. Paring of pigmented horn does not result in any marked change in the appearance of the pigment within the horn. Paring over areas of solar hemorrhage leads to a change in appearance of the area being pared; the area of hemorrhage within the horn changes hue and frequently disappears, leaving healthy horn beneath. Paring over an area of hemorrhage may lead to the discovery of a larger area of friable hemorrhagic horn indicative of a developing solar ulcer.

The aim of diagnostic foot paring is to detect any abnormalities of the claws. If the examination fails to reveal any specific lesion the claws must be pared to restore them to approximately normal shape and size. Studies of gait in cattle have shown that weight is normally borne on the heels and the abaxial surfaces of the sole. The normal weightbearing areas are illustrated (Fig. 21.60). A concave axial area of solar horn exists in the normal animal and paring the sole to recreate this anatomy and restore the normal weightbearing areas should be attempted. The depth of horn on the solar surface of the lateral claw is lowered so that it is approximately level with the solar horn of the medial claw. Use of the claw clippers is made to restore the length from the coronary band to the toe to approximately 7 cm. Details of these routine paring techniques are described by Toussaint Raven (1985) and Blowey (1993).

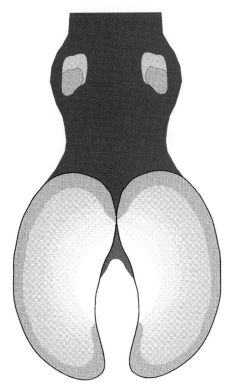

**Fig. 21.60** The weightbearing surfaces of the foot, indicated by shading.

## EXAMINATION OF THE CLINICALLY RECUMBENT ANIMAL

Cattle that are unable or unwilling to stand are clinically recumbent and are commonly known as 'downer cattle'. The most common form of downer cow syndrome is in mature lactating dairy cattle which develop parturient paresis within a few days after parturition and do not stand following adequate calcium therapy. However, recumbency can occur in all classes and ages of cattle due to a variety of diseases and circumstances, and often without any history to explain the recumbency.

One of the first objectives in the examination of recumbent cattle is to determine whether the recumbency is due to muscle weakness because of disease of the body as a whole, such as metabolic disease or toxemia from many different causes, or to primary diseases of the musculoskeletal or nervous system. However, because of the large size of adult cattle it is often very difficult to carry out a thorough clinical examination. Therefore, detection of the cause of recumbency can be challenging. It is also necessary to predict the likelihood that the animal will be able to

stand following specific or general therapy, or if the prognosis is unfavorable regardless of therapy. Because of increasing societal concerns about the humane aspects of handling and care of recumbent animals, the veterinarian has an obligation to make every reasonable effort to determine the cause of the recumbency and to make appropriate recommendations. More and more countries are drafting legislation for the disposition of recumbent animals, which will include strict guidelines for the handling and transportation of such animals from the farm.

Normal cattle in sternal or lateral recumbency will usually stand when encouraged to do so. Clinically recumbent animals or 'downer cattle' will not stand because of either an inability or a lack of desire to stand, or both. Primary diseases of the musculoskeletal system that may cause recumbency include diseases of muscle, bones, joints, and feet. An inability to stand because of muscle weakness may be due to primary nutritional myopathy. Secondary causes of muscle weakness include toxemia, dehydration, shock, and ischemic necrosis resulting from prolonged recumbency. Metabolic disease such as parturient paresis is a common cause of recumbency in mature lactating dairy cattle, usually within 48 hours after parturition. Arthropathies and polysynovitis can also result in recumbency. Cattle with severe acute laminitis may be able to stand if coaxed, but prefer to remain recumbent because of painful feet. Fractures of long bones such as the femur or humerus commonly result in recumbency, especially in large adult cattle; calves with fractures of the long bones may be able to stand and walk.

Clinical examination of the recumbent animal follows the same principles and orderly routine as that described for the standing animal. However, it is phys-

---

### Downer cows

The downer cow is one that has been recumbent for more than 24 hours. This often is because of a combination of muscle and nerve damage following parturition. These primary factors are then complicated by the effects of pressure on the main muscle masses (crush-compartmentalization), leading to edema and necrosis.

- nerve damage includes damage to the sciatic over the ventral sacral ridge and caudal to the proximal femur
- muscle damage, particularly tearing of the adductor muscles as these cows attempt to rise, also plays a role.

ically more demanding and may require the assistance of several people to roll the animal from one side to the other to allow examination of the entire animal. The following description places emphasis on those aspects of the examination relevant to determining the cause of the recumbency. Some aspects of neurological examination will be mentioned, but the details are given in Chapter 19.

## History

Taking an appropriate and adequate history is vital when examining a recumbent animal. The age, reproductive status, nutritional history, and any current disease may provide clues as to the possible cause of the recumbency. The downer cow syndrome is most common in adult female cattle from 2 days before to 10 days after parturition as a complication of prolonged recumbency associated with parturient paresis. The length of time the animal has been recumbent and whether recumbency was associated with dystocia, traumatic incidents, or any other specific illness such as hypocalcemia are important initial considerations. Previous treatment for hypocalcemia and the bodily condition of the animal prior to calving are relevant to the diagnosis of the downer cow syndrome and severe ketosis caused by the fatty liver syndrome. The cause of recumbency may be difficult to determine in animals which are found recumbent without any history of preceding illness or abnormality to account for the recumbency. In other situations the history is highly suggestive:

- a recent history of unaccustomed exercise in well-nourished beef calves found suddenly recumbent suggests acute enzootic nutritional myopathy
- a sudden onset of recumbency in pregnant beef cattle just prior to parturition and during inclement weather in the spring may suggest hypocalcemia
- a lactating dairy cow with peracute coliform mastitis may become recumbent within 24 hours of the onset of the mastitis.

## Distant examination

The position and posture of the recumbent animal are carefully noted. Cattle in sternal recumbency normally lie on their ventral thorax and abdomen with the forelimbs flexed on each side of the sternum. The position of the hindlimbs is noted (in sternal recumbency the upper hindlimb is that which is opposite to the side the animal is lying on). Normally the upper hindlimb is slightly flexed and held next to the abdomen. The

distal part of the lower hindlimb is also positioned and visible under the abdomen. The head and neck may be held normally or folded back on the flank in the 'sleeping posture'. Cattle in lateral recumbency normally lie with the neck outstretched and the forelimbs and hindlimbs fully extended, and are still able to move them.

If one or both hindlimbs is extended cranially, reaching up to the elbow joint, dislocation of the hip joints with or without rupture of the teres ligament should be suspected. Dislocation of the coxofemoral joint occurs most commonly in a craniodorsal direction, and there is usually marked shortening of the affected limb. In a frog-legged position, common in the downer cow syndrome following parturient paresis, both hindlimbs are partially flexed and extended caudally. These animals are frequently able to creep around a box stall or enclosure. There are usually varying degrees of adductor muscle and obturator nerve injury due to complications of parturient hypocalcemia and/or dystocia. With vertebral lesions caudal to the second thoracic vertebrae, which are uncommon, affected cattle commonly assume a dog-sitting posture. They have normal use of the forelimbs but may display either flaccid or spastic paralysis of the hindlimbs.

The bodily condition of the recumbent animal may provide some diagnostic clues. Severe muscle weakness associated with chronic protein–energy malnutrition may lead to recumbency in beef cows in late pregnancy. These cows are emaciated, do not exhibit ketosis, and remain alert.

The first step is to decide whether the animal is clinically recumbent. Normal cattle will usually stand promptly when touched or prodded. How readily this occurs reflects factors such as the age, sex, breed, and temperament of the animal

- free-range beef cattle will usually stand and move away before one is close enough to encourage them to do so
- dairy cows are more likely to remain recumbent when first approached
- bulls should always be approached with caution, however, they are generally more reluctant than cows to stand when encouraged
- neonatal calves frequently remain in sternal or lateral recumbency when approached.

Cattle which remain in lateral or sternal recumbency when approached should be encouraged to stand by vocal stimulation, by gentle physical stimulation (prodding or slapping the back and hindquarters), or by a combination of both. Nudging the animal over the thorax with the knee is also effective. Battery-operated cattle prods can be effective as a point stimulus but must be used humanely and judiciously. If the animal does not get up following reasonable coaxing efforts, it may be considered clinically recumbent (Fig. 21.61).

Some recumbent cattle may attempt to stand but are unsuccessful. Close observation of such attempts may provide an indication of the nature of the recumbency. In trying to stand they may move themselves forward with the hindlimbs projected caudally in a frog-legged position. Lactating recumbent cows that scramble about on the ground when stimulated are known as 'creeper cows'. As they continue to creep, their hindlimb movements will displace any bedding and eventually they may be in contact with the floor surface of a box stall. The continued struggling to stand or to creep frequently continues and exacerbates the recumbency. Decubital ulcers commonly develop over bony prominences of the hindlimbs. Some animals are able to lift their hindquarters marginally off the ground and, with a little assistance by lifting on the tail, are able to stand if the ground surface provides a good footing.

Recumbent animals which are able to stand for a few moments can be examined further in the standing position for their ability to bear weight on any or all four limbs, and those parts of the limbs that were not accessible during recumbency can be examined in detail.

### General appearance (mental state)

The demeanor of the recumbent animal can be classed as

- alert and reactive
- dull and depressed, or
- hyperesthetic.

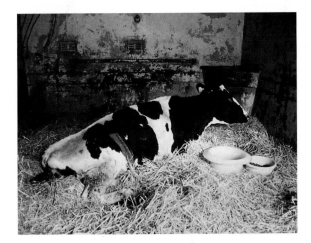

**Fig. 21.61** The clinically recumbent cow.

Alert recumbent cattle are more likely to be affected with primary musculoskeletal disease or disease of the central nervous system below the level of the foramen magnum. The depressed recumbent animal is unresponsive to physical or auditory stimuli, is usually inappetent, and may adopt a permanent sleeping posture with its head folded caudally into its flank. Variable degrees of clinical depression and recumbency are associated with

- dehydration
- toxemia
- metabolic disease
- severe acid–base imbalance
- shock, or
- nervous system disease.

Hyperesthesia is common in recumbent cattle with hypomagnesemic tetany and lead poisoning.

> ### Assisting recumbent animals to stand requires:
>
> - sufficient space in front of the animal so that it can pivot itself on its sternum and lurch forward with its head and neck – part of the standing act of cattle
> - good footing on the ground surface – solid dirt floors, deep sand, rough wooden floors, pasture, or deep wet and soggy bedding in a box stall provide the best footing
> - hip lifters, cattle slings, or other humane lifting devices to be used judiciously, only with animals that are almost able to stand on their own. If, when lifted, the animal bears no weight itself it should be let back down onto a well-bedded ground surface until there is evidence that it will bear weight on its own.

### Close physical examination

#### General clinical examination

Animals in lateral recumbency should be placed and propped up in sternal recumbency for the clinical examination and for their comfort. A routine clinical examination of all body systems is recommended to exclude the common diseases that may result in clinical recumbency. This includes

- rectal temperature
- state of hydration and of the mucous membranes
- auscultation of the heart and lungs

- examination of the abdomen, particularly the state of the rumen and ruminal contractions
- rectal examination
- examination of the reproductive tract and mammary gland.

The major objective is to determine whether the animal has a primary or secondary illness severe enough to cause recumbency. Any disease resulting in severe toxemia, septicemia, cardiovascular insufficiency, severe dehydration or severe acid–base imbalance can cause muscle weakness and recumbency.

## Mammary gland

Examination of the mammary gland is essential and can only be properly performed by rolling the cow from one side to the other. Each teat and quarter must be examined carefully by palpation, and the milk from each gland examined using a strip cup. Toxemic mastitis is a common cause of recumbency in dairy cows immediately after calving. Changes in the mammary gland secretion may be subtle in cattle with peracute coliform mastitis, which is a common cause of recumbency, and the use of a strip-cup and a familiarity with the appearance of normal colostrum and the early changes in gross appearance of the milk are important.

---

### Urinalysis in recumbent cattle

Urine is always collected from recumbent cattle and examined for the presence of ketones, protein, and globin.

- ketonemia associated with severe fatty liver disease may lead to recumbency in cows immediately before and after calving
- proteinuria and (myo/hemo) globinuria may indicate the degree of muscle injury and associated renal disease due to myoglobin tubular nephrosis.

---

## Reproductive tract

The reproductive tract must be examined both vaginally and rectally. A manual examination of the vagina and uterus may reveal evidence of large blood clots and evidence of uterine laceration. Hemorrhagic shock associated with intra-abdominal bleeding from a ruptured middle uterine artery must not overlooked. There are usually no outward signs of blood loss. Severe toxemic metritis is marked by a putrid reddish-brown vaginal discharge and the presence of an enlarged uterus on rectal palpation. Hydrops allantois may be a cause of recumbency in late pregnancy and is characterized by excessive amounts of fluid in the uterus.

## Rectal examination

It may be awkward to do a rectal examination in a recumbent animal because of its position, and the information obtained usually is not as useful or reliable as in the standing animal. However, evidence of diffuse peritonitis, acute intestinal obstruction, and other severe abnormalities may be present. The bony skeleton, including the sacrum, sacroiliac junction, the body of the iliac bone, the medial part of the acetabulum, obturator foramen, and the pelvic symphysis, is palpated methodically for evidence of bony displacement, pain, or crepitus. In caudoventral luxation of the coxofemoral joint the femoral head may occasionally be palpated in the obturator foramen.

## Musculoskeletal system

All parts of the musculoskeletal system must be examined. This requires recumbent animals to be gently rolled from one side to the other to allow examination of both sides and all four limbs while in lateral recumbency.

## Head and neck

The examination should begin at the animal's head and proceed in a systematic manner towards the hindquarters. The carriage of the head and neck is noted for any evidence of deviation or rotation. The head and neck are passively moved from side to side and dorsoventrally in an attempt to detect pain in animals with cervical vertebral lesions.

## Forelimbs

Each forelimb is palpated, manipulated, and passively flexed and extended, and visually inspected from the coronary band proximally to the shoulder for evidence of pain, swelling, or fractures. The long bones, including their epiphyses, are palpated over their entire length. Each joint is palpated for evidence of pain or swelling. Acute polysynovitis may be present and not clinically obvious on cursory examination. The joint capsules must be palpated carefully and repeatedly, and any painful response noted. The muscles are palpated for evidence of swelling or increased firmness, and the tone of the forelimbs is evaluated as normal, flaccid, or hypertonic.

## Hindlimbs

Most of the abnormalities causing recumbency occur in the hindlimbs. The position of each hindlimb relative to the trunk is noted first. The limbs may be extended cranially, laterally, or caudally. Each hindlimb is palpated, manipulated, and passively flexed and extended, and visually inspected from the coronary band proximally to the hip joint for evidence of pain, swelling, or fractures. For passive abduction the extended limb is held at the level of the foot and gently abducted as far as possible. For circumduction the extended limb is held at the foot and moved in a circular direction cranially, laterally, and caudally, circumscribing a circle as large as is gently possible. This circular movement will assist in the detection of fractures of the shaft of the femur and femoral head, and dislocation of the coxofemoral joint. This commonly requires an assistant, who moves the limb while the examiner feels and listens for abnormalities at the level of the hip joint. The ability to manually abduct a hindlimb beyond normal range is an indication of a major abnormality.

With dislocation of the coxofemoral joint some cows are recumbent and unable to rise, whereas others stand and are capable of moving around. Recumbent cows are usually in sternal recumbency and the affected limb is excessively abducted. In standing cows the affected limb is usually extended, often difficult to flex, and often rotated about its long axis. The diagnostic criteria are

- sudden onset of lameness with the affected limb extended and possibly rotated
- displacement of the greater trochanter of the femur from its normal position relative to the ischiatic tuber and coxal tuber of the pelvis
- ability to manually abduct the limb beyond its normal range
- crepitus in the hip on abduction and rotation of the limb
- ability to palpate the femoral head per rectum or per vaginum against the cranial border of the ilium or pubis in cases of cranioventral dislocation, or in the obturator foramen in cases of caudoventral dislocation.

Fracture of the femur is characterized by marked swelling of soft tissues at the fracture site, pain on palpation, and crepitus on movement of the limb. However, some femoral fractures are not easily detectable because the thickness and spasm of the surrounding muscle masses may inhibit crepitus. In some cases detection may be facilitated using the auscultation–percussion techniques described above. The flexor withdrawal reflex of each hindlimb is tested by squeezing the coronary band with hemostats, needle holders or pliers.

The muscles of the hindlimb are palpated for evidence of increased firmness or hardness, indicating acute myopathy. In some calves with acute nutritional myopathy, the hamstring muscles may be firmer than normal or even board-like, but these physical findings are very unusual. In some cases it is not possible to palpate muscle changes which may be severe enough to result in recumbency. For example, it is not possible to palpate the ischemic necrosis and hemorrhage of the medial thigh muscles in mature downer cattle as a complication of parturient paresis. Rupture of the gastrocnemius muscle, in contrast, usually results in a marked swelling of the affected muscle, which is visible and palpable as a firm diffuse swollen structure. The degree of ischemic necrosis of muscle can be determined only by measurement of serum levels of creatine phosphokinase.

Acute myopathy due to infectious causes such as clostridiosis, or trauma due to fractures of long bones such as the femur, is characterized by enlargement and increased firmness and hardness of muscle masses. In blackleg the affected part will be

- swollen
- crepitant because of the presence of gas, and
- cool to touch in the late stages.

The intramuscular injection of irritating substances into the hamstring muscles of young calves may result in severe myositis, characterized by hindlimb lameness and recumbency and marked swelling of the affected muscles. Intramuscular hematomas in dicoumarol poisoning are characterized by lameness and enlargement of the affected muscle masses, which are easily visible and palpable.

**Feet**

Cattle may be recumbent because of severely painful conditions of the feet and it is essential that all four feet are examined carefully by visual inspection and digital palpation, with special emphasis on the coronary band, for evidence of pain. The claws should be examined with hoof testers and trimmed if necessary, as described earlier.

## Neurological examination

A neurological examination must be performed on every clinically recumbent animal to exclude the possibility that lesions of the nervous system may be the cause of the recumbency. The extent of the examination is limited by the size of the animal. Recumbent young calves can usually be handled easily and assisted to stand to test placing reflexes and muscle strength, along with other neurological tests. In contrast, recumbent adult cattle are difficult to handle and roll from side to side, and the neurological examination is limited to testing the

- cranial nerves
- flexor withdrawal reflexes, and
- other spinal reflexes.

# ANCILLARY DIAGNOSTIC AIDS

Ancillary tests have a role in confirming the diagnosis. However, in the context of commercial dairy or beef cattle, economic limitations restrict the use of many of these tests, and the skills of physical examination are more important in the day-to-day examination of the bovine musculoskeletal system. Tests should only be used to confirm diagnoses. They will be necessary when dealing with valuable pedigree cattle or in the investigation of herd problems with a nutritional basis, such as outbreaks of vitamin E–selenium myopathy or copper deficiency physitis.

## Serum biochemistry

The serum levels of both creatinine phosphokinase (CK) and glutathione peroxidase (GSH-PX) are useful aids for the diagnosis of vitamin E–selenium deficiency myopathies. Creatinine phosphokinase is highly specific for cardiac and skeletal muscle and serum levels are elevated following the myodegeneration caused by vitamin E–selenium deficiency myopathy. In cattle CK has a half-life of between 2 and 4 hours; plasma levels fall quickly, but remain a useful guide to the previous occurrence of muscle damage for a period of 3 days. There is a direct relationship between GSH-PX activity of blood and the selenium levels of the blood and tissues of cattle.

The sequential levels of plasma CK, aspartate aminotransferase (AST) and urea levels have a significance to assessing prognosis in the downer cow. Increasing levels of CK, AST, and urea over the 3 days following initial examination usually indicates a poor prognosis. Serum copper levels are frequently below the normal range in physeal lameness due to copper deficiency in beef calves on deficient diets.

## Collection and examination of synovial fluid (arthrocentesis), Synoviocentesis

The collection and laboratory examination of synovial fluid is indicated when arthropathy is suspected. This relatively easy procedure is one of the most useful ancillary aids to diagnosis. Arthrocentesis requires an initial review of the normal anatomy of the joint and its capsule, and the various sites for synovial fluid collection are illustrated by Greenhough et al (1981). In septic arthritis, distension of the joint capsule is frequently present, facilitating a successful procedure. Arthrocentesis should be performed aseptically. A small area of skin over the distended joint capsule is surgically prepared. With the exception of the shoulder

and hip joints, collection of synovial fluid may be performed with a minimum of restraint in most cattle. However, in fractious animals, and for collection of fluid from the shoulder or hip joints, xylazine sedation or even general anesthesia may be required.

There is no need to infiltrate the area with local anesthetic. A sterile hypodermic needle is gently inserted through the skin into the joint space. The length and gauge of needle differ with the individual joint location, being approximately

- 5–6 cm long for all sites distal to the carpus and tarsus, and
- up to 16 cm long for the shoulder and hip joints.

A needle of at least 18 gauge with a short bevel and equipped with a stylet is preferred. However, when the synovial fluid is of a thick, tenacious consistency, a 14 or 16 gauge needle may be required. Using a sterile syringe 5 to 10 ml of synovial fluid are aspirated then transferred to a tube containing EDTA and into a sterile container for the appropriate bacteriological or mycoplasmal culture. A decrease in synovial glucose levels is associated with the glycolytic activity of neutrophils, and glucose levels may be estimated in samples collected into fluoride oxalate tubes. Occasionally blood is observed in the sample and it is important to differentiate this from hemorrhage that occurred prior to or during aspiration

- with acute traumatic arthritis the sample is diffusely hemorrhagic
- samples that are streaked with whole blood usually indicate hemorrhage at the time of collection.

Synovial fluid is examined cytologically, for protein concentration, and cultured for bacteria and mycoplasma. It may be difficult to culture bacterial pathogens from the synovial fluid of joints in which there is clinical evidence of acute infectious arthritis. Biopsy of the synovial membrane from such joints may reveal the presence of pathogens. However, infection may be assumed to be present within the joint if the synovial-fluid

---

### Appearance of synovial fluid

- normal synovial fluid is transparent, odorless, pale yellow, and slightly viscid but does not clot
- in disease conditions synovial fluid may be slightly turbid to purulent in consistency
- in septic arthritis gross discoloration and turbidity give a reasonably accurate indication of the numbers of leukocytes present.

has a greatly increased leukocyte count and the clinical examination otherwise supports a diagnosis of septic arthritis.

Aspiration of tendon sheath and bursal synovial fluid may be attempted and the fluid examined similarly to joint synovial fluid. This may be useful in assessing sepsis of the sheaths of the superficial and deep flexor tendons proximal to the proposed level of amputation in candidates for digital amputation. Aspiration of synovia from the distended sheath of the flexor tendons may be attempted immediately proximal to the annular (palmar/plantar) ligament of the fetlock joint.

## Medical imaging

### Radiography

Radiography is used in the diagnosis of

- fractures
- physitis
- osteomyelitis, and
- septic and degenerative arthritis

and provides valuable information on prognosis in these cases. It also has a role in the successful reduction and treatment of fractures and dislocations, and is particularly useful in the investigation of joints or bones which are inaccessible to either physical examination or the collection of synovial fluid. The precise type of fracture can only be determined by radiography; physeal separation of the femoral head in neonatal calves is a diagnosis that would be impossible without radiography. The various views and positioning used in bovine radiography are illustrated by Bargai et al (1988).

Cervical vertebral osteomyelitis is a cause of recumbency in calves which requires confirmatory radiological diagnosis using lateral views of the neck (Fig. 21.62). In suspected septic arthritis of the distal interphalangeal joint, lateromedial views of the foot may be difficult to interpret because of superimposition of the digits, the dorsopalmar (plantar) views are of most use. Definitive diagnosis of fracture of the pedal bone requires the use of an interdigital film (Fig. 21.63).

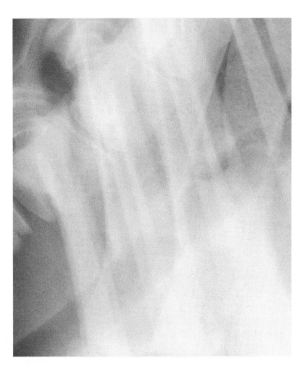

**Fig. 21.62** Cervical osteomyelitis. Most of the sixth cervical vertebral body has been lysed, with its remnants extruded ventrally. There is also lysis of the cranial epiphysis of the seventh cervical vertebra. (Courtesy of Ms H. McAllister, Faculty of Veterinary Medicine, University College Dublin, Ireland.)

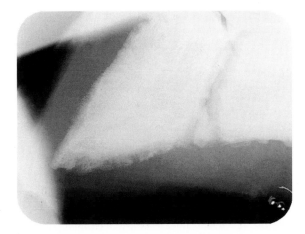

**Fig. 21.63** Lateral claw pedal bone fracture. A radiolucent linear opacity runs parallel to the dorsal aspect of the distal phalanx from the distal interphalangeal joint to its solar surface. (Courtesy of Ms C. Skelly, Faculty of Veterinary Medicine, University College Dublin, Ireland.)

## Clinical Pointer

The large muscle masses of adult cattle restrict the application of diagnostic bovine radiography. Adequate examination of the shoulder and hip joints in adult cattle requires the use of high-output X-ray machines following general anesthesia.

## Arthroscopy

Arthroscopy involves examination of the surfaces of joint cavities following the insertion of a fiberoptic scope into the joint space (or atherosynovial structure). A constant flow of sterile Ringer's solution through the sleeve of the joint distends the joint and carries blood and debris away from the joint. Arthroscopy has had limited application in the investigation of bovine lameness and is undertaken to acquire more information about a particular area of articular surface. It has been particularly applied to the stifle joint, and facilitates the appreciation of cranial and caudal cruciate ligament rupture and the presence of degenerative joint disease. Osteochondrosis is a cause of lameness in growing cattle, and stifle or shoulder joint arthroscopy may have a role in identifying cartilage degeneration in cases of osteochondrosis where radiographically detectable erosion of subchondral bone has not occurred.

## Ultrasonography

Ultrasonography is used primarily to produce images of joints, ligaments, and tendons, but can also be used to examine the soft tissues of the limbs for the presence of non-palpable foreign bodies, abscesses, or cysts. Septic tenosynovitis of the superficial and deep flexor tendons proximal to the fetlock joint in cases of septic pedal arthritis and navicular bursitis would usually indicate that the animal was a poor candidate for surgical amputation at the level of the first phalanx. Ultrasonography can be used to examine the flexor tendons and their sheaths proximal to the coronary band to determine whether or not sepsis has extended proximally. In this way limb swelling associated with peritendinous edema could be differentiated from that involving sepsis of the tendon sheaths themselves.

## Scintigraphy

Scintigraphic imaging may also have a diagnostic role in clinical lameness in which radiographs have failed to demonstrate pathology.

## Muscle biopsy

The use of skeletal muscle biopsy techniques for the diagnosis of myodegeneration in cattle has been reviewed by Bradley (1978).

In acute myodegenerative diseases, such as vitamin E–selenium deficiency myopathy, the biopsy should be taken as early as possible after the onset of clinical signs

> **Clinical Pointer**
>
> Sites for muscle biopsy must not have been previously used for intramuscular injection.

and a heparinized blood sample for estimation of plasma CPK and GSH-PX levels taken simultaneously. However, in neurogenic muscle atrophy little of diagnostic value is seen until 10 days or more from the onset of clinical signs, and some delay in sampling would be beneficial. Bradley (1978) recommends biopsy of the proximal part of the biceps femoris muscle and the flexor muscles of the forelimbs as the most useful in the diagnosis of vitamin E–selenium deficiency myopathy.

Muscle biopsies can be collected using needle biopsy or simple surgical techniques, and an aseptic surgical procedure.

In cases of vitamin E–selenium deficiency myopathy, areas of coagulative necrosis are evident. Neurogenic, disuse, and cachetic atrophy have unique histological appearances.

## ACKNOWLEDGEMENT

Mr. Eamonn Fitzpatrick, Department of Veterinary Anatomy, for his help in producing the illustrations and Mr. Paul Stanley, Department of Large Animal Clinical Studies, for his photgraphic assistance.

## FURTHER READING

Adams R. The musculoskeletal system. In: McKinnon A, Voss J (eds) Equine reproduction. Philadelphia: Lea and Febiger, 1993; 1060–1075.

American Kennel Club. The complete dog book, 18th edn. New York: Howell Book House, 1992.

Andrews AH. The "downer cow". In Practice 1986; 18: 187.

Arkins S. Lameness in dairy cows. Irish Veterinary Journal 1981; 35: 163–170.

Back, W. Development of equine locomotion from foal to adult. The Netherlands: Harry Otter Addix, Wijk bij Dvurstede, 1994.

Bardet JF. Lameness. In: Ettinger SJ, Feldman EC (eds) Textbook of veterinary internal medicine, 4th edn. Philadelphia: WB Saunders, 1995; 136–143.

Bargai U, Pharr JW, Morgan JP. Bovine radiology. Ames, Iowa: Iowa State University Press, 1989.

Bentley H, Dyson S. Practical ultrasound physics – how to make optimal use of your machine. Equine Veterinary Education 1991; 3: 227–231.

Blowey R. Cattle lameness and hoofcare; an illustrated guide. Ipswich: Farming Press, 1993.

Booth JM. Lameness and mastitis losses. Veterinary Record 1989; 125: 161.

Bradley R. Skeletal muscle biopsy techniques in animals for histochemical and ultrastructural examination and especially for the diagnosis of myogeneration in cattle. British Veterinary Journal 1978; 134: 434–444.

Bramlage L, Embertson R. Observations on the evaluation and selection of foal limb deformities for surgical treatment. Proceedings of the American Association of Equine Practice 1990; 36: 273–279.

Brinker WO, Piermattei DL, Flo GL. Diagnosis and treatment of orthopedic conditions of the hindlimb. In: Piermattei DL, Flo GL (eds) Handbook of small animal orthopedics and fracture treatment, 3rd edn. Philadelphia: WB Saunders, 1997.

Butler J, Colles C, Dyson S, Kold S, Poulos P. Clinical radiology of the horse. Oxford: Blackwell Scientific, 1993.

O'Callaghan M, Seeherman H. Scintigraphic screening of lameness and the benefits of combining imaging methods. Proceedings of the American Association of Equine Practice 1991; 37: 301–314.

Chalman JA, Butler HC. Coxofemoral joint laxity and the Ortolani sign. Journal of the American Animal Hospital Association 1985;21: 671–676.

Clarkson MJ, Downham DY, Faull WB et al. Incidence and prevalence of lameness in dairy cattle. Veterinary Record 1996; 138: 563–567.

Colbern G. Diagnostic nerve block procedures. The Compendium on Continuing Education for the Practicing Veterinarian 1984; 6: S611–S622.

Cox VS. Pathogenesis of the downer cow syndrome. Veterinary Record 1982; 111: 76–79.

Doherty ML. Laminitis in beef bulls. Veterinary Record 1987; 121: 134.

Doherty ML, Bassett HF, Markey B, Healy AM, Sammin D. Severe foot lameness in cattle associated with invasive spirochaetes. Irish Veterinary Journal 1998; 51: 195–198.

Dyson S. Nerve blocks and lameness diagnosis in the horse. In Practice 1984; 6: 102–107.

Dyson S (ed) Tendon and ligament injuries: Part I. Veterinary Clinics of North America (Equine Practice) 1994; 10(2).

Dyson S (ed) Tendon and ligament injuries: Part II. Veterinary Clinics of North America (Equine Practice) 1995; 11(2).

Emery L, Miller J, Van Hoosen N. Horseshoeing theory and hoof care. Philadelphia: Lea & Febiger, 1977.

Greenough PR, Gracek ZJ. A preliminary report on a laminitis like condition occurring in bulls under feeding trials. 5th International Symposium On Disorders Of The Ruminant Digit, Dublin, Ireland, 1986.

Greenough PR (ed), Weaver AD (assoc ed) Lameness in cattle 3rd edn. Philadelphia: WB Saunders,1997

Healey AM, Doherty ML, Monaghan ML, McCallister Cervico-thoracic vertebral osteomyelitis in 14 cases. Veterinary Journal 1997; 154: 227–232.

Henderson RA, Milton JL. The tibial compression mechanism: a diagnostic aid in stifle injuries. Journal of the American Animal Hospital Association 1978;14: 474–479.

Holmström M, Magnusson L-E, Philipsson J. Variation in conformation of Swedish Warmblood horses and conformational characteristics of elite sport horses. Equine Veterinary Journal 1990; 22: 186–193.

Hurtig MB. Recent developments in the use of athroscopy in cattle Symposium on bovine lameness and orthopedics. Veterinary Clinics of North America 1985;1: 175–197.

Jeffcott L. Diagnosis of back problems in the horse. The Compendium on Continuing Education for the Practicing Veterinarian 1981; 3: S134–S143.

Johnson KA, Watson ADJ, Page RL. Skeletal diseases. In: Ettinger SJ, Feldman EC (eds) Textbook of veterinary internal medicine, 4th edn. Philadelphia: WB Saunders, 1995; 2077–2103.

Leach D. Non-invasive technology for assessment of equine locomotion. The Compendium on Continuing Education for the Practicing Veterinarian 1987; 9: 1124–1135.

Leonard FC, O'Connell J, O'Farrell K. Effect of different housing conditions on behaviour and foot lesions in Friesian heifers. Veterinary Record 1994; 134: 490–494.

Logue DN, Offer JE, Kempson SA. Lameness in dairy cattle. Irish Veterinary Journal 1993;46: 47.

McIlwraith CW. Diagnostic and surgical arthroscopy in the horse, 2nd edn. Philadelphia: Lea & Febiger, 1990.

Mills LL, Leach DH, Smart ME, Greenough PR. A system for the recording of clinical data as an aid in the diagnosis of bovine digital disease. Canadian Veterinary Journal 1986; 27: 293–300.

Oetzel GR, Berger LL. The Compendium on Continuing Education for the Practicing Veterinarian 1986; 8 (1): S16–S22.

Peterse DJ, Korver S, Oldenbroek JK, Talmon FP. Relationship between levels of concentrate feeding and incidence of sole ulcers in dairy cattle. Veterinary Record 1984; 115: 629–630.

Prescott JRR, Collins JA, Jackson PGG. Scintigraphic imaging of a degenerative arthropathy in the shoulder of a nine-month-old Hereford bull. Veterinary Record 1998; 143: 81–82.

Rantanen A, McKinnon A (ed) Diagnostic ultrasonography of the horse. Baltimore: Williams & Wilkins, 1998.

Richardson DC. Developmental orthopedics: nutritional influences in the dog. In: Ettinger SJ, Feldman EC (eds) Textbook of veterinary internal medicine, 4th edn. Philadelphia: WB Saunders, 1995; 252–257.

Riser WH, Brodey RS, Shirer JF. Osteodystrophy in mature cats: a nutritional disease. Journal of the American Veterinary Radiology Society 1968; IX: 37–45.

Stashak T (ed) Adam's Lameness in horses, 4th edn. Philadelphia: Lea & Febiger, 1987.

Scott GB. Studies of the gait of Friesian heifer cattle. Veterinary Record 1988; 123: 245–248.

Toussaunt Raven E. Cattle footcare and claw trimming. Ipswich: Farming Press, 1985.

Vermunt JJ, Greenough PR. Lesions associated with subclinical laminitis of the claws of dairy calves in two management systems. British Veterinary Journal 1995; 151: 391–399.

Wallace MS, Davidson AP. Abnormalities in pregnancy, parturition, and the periparturient period. In: Ettinger SJ, Feldman EC (eds) Textbook of veterinary internal medicine, 4th edn. Philadelphia: WB Saunders, 1995;1614–1623.

Wells GAH, Hawkins SAC, O'Toole DT et al. Spastic syndrome in a Holstein bull: a histologic study. Veterinary Pathology 1987; 24: 345–353.

Wells SJ, Trent AM, Marsh WE, Robinson RA. Prevalence and severity of lameness in lactating dairy cows in a sample of Minnesota and Wisconsin herds. Journal of the American Veterinary Medical Association 1993; 202: 78–82.

Wells SJ, Trent AM, Marsh WE, Williamson NB, Robinson RA. Some risk factors associated with clinical lameness in dairy herds in Minnesota and Wisconsin. Veterinary Record 1995; 136: 537.

Wyn-Jones G. Equine lameness. Oxford: Blackwell Scientific, 1988.

# 22
# Clinical Examination of the Reproductive System

*Dogs and Cats – K. Post*
*The Mare – M.M. LeBlanc*
*The Stallion – M.M. LeBlanc*
*Ruminants – J.G.W. Wenzel*
*Swine – J.G.W. Wenzel*

## CLINICAL MANIFESTATIONS OF DISEASES OF THE REPRODUCTIVE TRACT

**Abortion** Premature expulsion from the uterus of the products of conception before the fetus is viable.

**Agalactia** Absence or failure of the secretion of milk (lack of milk production in the mammae or failure of milk letdown).

**Balanitis** Inflammation of the glans penis.

**Balanoposthitis** Inflammation of both the glans penis and prepuce.

**Cervical adhesions** Spider web-like strands of tissue criss-crossing within the cervical canal or extending over the external os.

**Cervical laceration** Loss of tissue due to a tear in the external cervical os.

**Cryptorchidism** Failure of one or both testes to migrate to the normal position within the scrotum. Position of testes can be abdominal or inguinal.

**Dyspareunia** Painful or difficult coitus.

**Dystocia** Difficult, prolonged parturition or the inability to expel the fetus from the uterus through the birth canal.

**Eclampsia (puerperal tetany)** A metabolic disease in lactating bitches characterized by a reduction in the concentration of ionized calcium in the extracellular fluids. It may be seen at parturition. The typical signs are the induction of tonic or tonoclonic contractions of skeletal muscle.

**Enlarged scrotum** Increase in size of the scrotum due to fluid.

**Failure to conceive (repeat breeder syndrome)** Inability to become pregnant.

**Fertility** The ability to reproduce in a normal and regular manner.

**Fluid accumulation (uterine)** Hypoechogenic or non-echogenic area within the uterine lumen as visualized by ultrasonography during diestrus or early pregnancy which is associated with infertility.

**Freemartin** is a sterile female born co-twin with a male.

**Hemospermia** Blood in semen.

**Hypogalactia** Deficiency of milk secretion.

**Hypogonadism** Abnormally decreased functional activity of the testes, with retardation of growth and sexual development.

**Hypospadia** The urethra opens on the ventral aspect of the penis, caudal to the normal urethral orifice.

**Impotence** Inability of the male to achieve or maintain an erection of sufficient rigidity to perform intercourse successfully.

**Infertility** Temporary inability to conceive and produce viable offspring.

**Interestrous interval** The period between the start of two subsequent estrous cycles.

**Intraestrous interval** The period between the end of estrus and the start of the next proestrus.

**Irregular estrus** Estrus occurring at abnormal intervals or abnormal behavior signs.

**Libido** The sexual desire or sexual drive, vigor and enthusiasm.

**Lochia** The normal vaginal discharge seen during the first 3 weeks after parturition, initially consisting of a large amount of blood and later becoming more serous.

**Lymphatic lacunae** Pooling of lymph within uterine lymphatics, resulting in fluid accumulation within the interstitial spaces and within the uterine lumen.

**Monorchidism** The condition of having only one testis in the scrotum, often referred to as unilateral cryptorchidism.

**Mummification of fetus** The shrivelling of the soft tissues around the skeleton of a dead fetus.

**Nymphomania** Prolonged signs of estrus or estrus occuring at abnormally short intervals.

**Paraphimosis** Inability to retract the penis into the sheath.

**Penile paralysis** Most commonly traumatic in origin, paralysis results from swelling, edema and increased weight on the penile structures.

**Periglandular fibrosis** Fibrosis surrounding the endometrial glands which prevents the glands from secreting uterine milk, resulting in early embryonic death.

**Persistent frenulum** A fold of the prepuce which fails to separate during maturation from its attachment to the glans penis.

**Phantom tie** During copulation in the dog the bulbis glandis becomes engorged before entering the vestibule and therefore unable to enter it; also known as an outside tie.

**Phimosis** Inability to extend the penis from the sheath.

**Pneumovagina** Aspiration of air into the vestibulum and vagina, resulting in inflammation of the vagina and uterus and possibly infertility.

**Posthitis** Inflammation of the prepuce.

**Postpartum hemorrhage** Bleeding from the uterine artery into the abdomen, the uterine wall or broad ligament after parturition.

**Preputial discharge** Secretion from the prepuce other than smegma, which is bloody to purulent in nature.

**Priapism** Persistent abnormal erection of the penis, accompanied by pain and tenderness.

**Primary uterine inertia** Failure of the uterine muscles to respond to hormonal stimuli, lack of the development of receptors on muscle, or an actual lack or failure of release or imbalance of hormones, with the end result that parturition is not initiated.

**Prolapse** Eversion of a tubular organ to the outside, with the connotation that it cannot be retracted voluntarily (uterine and vaginal prolapses).

**Prolonged diestrus** Failure to exhibit estrous behavior every 16–18 days during the cyclic season.

**Puberty** Age at which the reproductive organs become functional and reproduction could occur.

**Pyometra** Long-standing accumulation of pus within the uterine lumen, associated with cervical or uterine adhesions and an inability of the uterus to empty itself (closed pyometra). Hyperechoic material will be visualized within the uterus on ultrasonography of animals may drip pus from the vulval lips for a period of time (open pyometra).

**Reduced fertility** Ability to reproduce, but at a rate below what is considered regular and normal for that breed.

**Retained placenta** Retention of fetal membranes for more than the expected period for that species.

**Rugae** Palpable thick ridges that are present on the involuting uterus for the first 15–20 days postpartum.

**Scrotal hernia** Entrapment of intestine or omentum within the scrotum, usually within the vaginal tunic.

**Secondary uterine inertia** A prolonged dystocia, or in some animals, after 1 or 2 normal deliveries muscle contractions cease, even though more fetuses are present in the uterus.

**Silent heat** Lack of observed signs of estrus. Absence of sanguineous vaginal discharge, or signs of receptivity to mating.

**Smegma** A thick cheesy secretion consisting principally of desquamated epithelial cells, and found chiefly about the prepuce and penis of male dogs and horses.

**Split heat** An apparently normal proestrus without ovulation followed within 1–8 weeks by a normal ovulatory heat cycle.

**Squamous papillomas** Multiple small (1–2 mm) gray cauliflower-like cutaneous growths that may be found on the prepuce and penis.

**Stallion-like behavior** Mare exhibits mounting behavior, vocalization, herding of a group of mares, flehmen response and aggressiveness toward other horses.

**Sterility** Permanent inability to conceive and produce viable offspring.

**Stillbirth** Delivery of a dead fetus.

**Subfertility** Less than normal reproductive capacity.

**Superfecundation** Presence of fetuses sired by different males within the maternal uterus at one time.

**Superfetation** The fertilization and subsequent presence of fetuses of different ages within the uterus. Occurs when a pregnant female comes into estrus and is bred when a fetus is already present in the uterus.

**Tenesmus** Straining as if to urinate or defecate.

**Testicular torsion** Rotation of the spermatic cord resulting in either a non-pathogenic ($< 180°$ torsion) to a severely painful condition ($> 360°$) that will adversely affect fertility.

**Tie** During copulation in dogs the bulbus glandis of the penis becomes engorged and the vestibule constriction muscle clasps behind the bulbar part of the gland, making withdrawal of the penis impossible (inside tie).

**Unobserved estrus** Lack of observed estrus due to absence of the endocrinologic cycle, absence of behavioral signs, or untimely observation on the part of humans.

**Urospermia** Contamination of ejaculated semen with urine.

**Uterine rupture** A laceration in the uterus due to complications with parturition or movement of the fetus within the uterus during the birth process.

**Uterine torsion** A twist of the uterine body and horns during late pregnancy of greater than 180°. One broad ligament will be crossed over the uterus, will be tense and will elicit pain on palpation.

**Vaginal discharge** Appearance of an abnormal substance dripping from the vulval lips.

**Vaginal hyperemia** A red, glistening appearance to the vaginal walls.

**Vaginal varicosities** Enlarged, protruding blood vessels within the vaginal or vestibular walls that may rupture and bleed, usually most prominent in heavily pregnant mares.

**Vestibulovaginal reflux** The presence of urine or urine crystals within the vaginal vault, usually observed on vaginal speculum examination during estrus or within the first weeks postpartum.

# Dogs and Cats

The reproductive system of the dog and the cat consists of the external and internal genitalia. In the female the mammary glands are often examined as part of the external genitalia.

The clinical examination of the reproductive tract is an extension of the general physical examination and the clinician must have a good understanding of the normal reproductive anatomy and physiology of the species. A prebreeding examination is best performed approximately 1 month before expected onset of proestrus.

## ANATOMY OF THE FEMALE GENITALIA
(FIGS 22.1, 22.2)

The ovaries are elongated, flattened and situated about 1–2 cm caudal to the corresponding kidney. In the bitch they are about 2 cm long and 1–5 cm thick, varying with the size of the breed, and in the queen they are about 8–9 mm long. The ovaries are suspended by the mesovaria at about the level of the third or fourth lumbar vertebra. In the bitch the ovary is completely enveloped by the ovarian bursa, whereas in the queen it is only partly enclosed.

The uterine tubes (oviducts) in the bitch are 6–10 cm long and begin with the fimbriae ventral to the entrance of the ovarian bursa. In the queen the uterine tubes are 4–5 cm in length.

The uterine horns in both the bitch and queen are long, uniform in diameter, and lie entirely within the abdomen. The uterine horns of the bitch are 10–15 cm in length with a diameter of 5–10 mm, depending upon the breed. In the queen, length and diameter are 8–10 cm and 3–4 mm, respectively.

The uterine body is short in both the bitch and queen (2–3 cm). The cervix of the bitch is about 1–1.5 cm long and projects ventrally into the cranial vagina. In the queen the cervix represents a hard oval knot.

| Female genitalia | Male genitalia |
|---|---|
| • ovaries | • scrotum |
| • uterine tubes (oviducts) | • two testes |
| • uterus | • epididymides |
| • cervix | • deferent ducts |
| • vagina | • spermatic cord |
| • vestibule | • prostate gland |
| • vulva | • penis |
| | • urethra |

The vagina of the bitch is relatively long and its mucous membranes form longitudinal folds (rugae), allowing for a great expansion in diameter. Smaller transverse folds connecting the longitudinal folds permit craniocaudal stretching of the vagina. The fornix vaginae is a small recess between the floor of the cranial vagina and the semicylindrical intravaginal part of the cervix. Caudally, the vagina ends just cranial to the urethral opening, at which point the vestibule begins (vaginovestibular junction). The vestibule is the space connecting the vagina with the external genital opening. It is variable in size, depending on the size of the animal and whether or not she is pregnant. In the bitch the clitoris is relatively large and lies on the ventral floor of the vestibule.

The vulva or external genitalia consists of the vestibule, clitoris and labia. The labia are round, often pigmented and covered with hair, and form the external boundary of the vulva.

### Mammary glands

The applied anatomy of the mammary glands in dogs and cats is found in Chapter 23. The examination of the mammary glands consists of inspection and palpation and, when considered necessary, microscopic examination of milk samples. Both the superficial and deeper parts of each mammary gland are palpated and compared for size and symmetry.

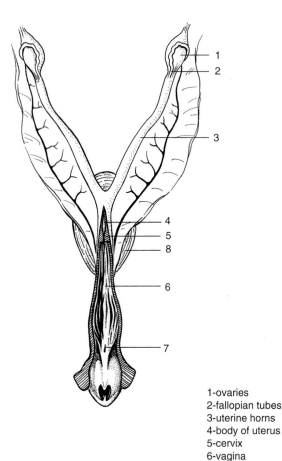

1-ovaries
2-fallopian tubes
3-uterine horns
4-body of uterus
5-cervix
6-vagina
7-vestibule
8-bladder

**Fig. 22.1** Anatomy of the genital organs of the bitch. The body of the uterus, vagina and vestibule have been opened dorsally. Dorsal aspect.

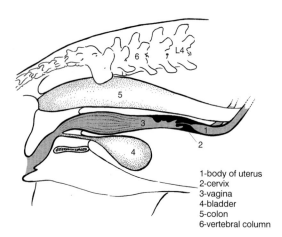

1-body of uterus
2-cervix
3-vagina
4-bladder
5-colon
6-vertebral column

**Fig. 22.2** Anatomy of the genital and urinary organs of the bitch. Right lateral aspect.

Skin lesions over mammary glands have the potential to spread to the secretory tissues.

## ANATOMY OF THE MALE GENITALIA

The scrotum of the dog is situated between the thighs and is visible from behind. In the cat it is just ventral to the anus. In the dog the almost spherical testes are relatively small and are positioned obliquely, so that the cranial pole points cranioventrally. Two testes should be palpable within the scrotum by 8 weeks of age in both dogs and cats. The epididymis is attached to the dorsolateral surface of the testis and is continuous at its tail with the ductus deferens. The ductus deferens is incorporated in the slender spermatic cord which enters the superficial inguinal ring, passes through the inguinal canal and enters the abdominal cavity through the vaginal ring.

---

### The prostate gland

- the prostate gland of the dog is spherical, smooth and divided into right and left lobes which completely surround the urethra
- in the cat the prostate gland has an uneven surface and covers the urethra dorsally and laterally only.

---

The penis of the dog is almost cylindrical and extends cranially. The osseous part is formed by the os penis, which develops after birth. In large breeds it may be as long as 10–12 cm. On the ventral surface of the os is a groove containing the urethra.

The glans penis surrounds the slender distal part of the os penis, whereas the bulbus glandis surrounds the thick proximal portion. The bulbus glandis is capable of considerable distension during penile erection and contributes to the so-called 'tie' during coitus, which may last up to 20–30 minutes. The prepuce of the dog is fairly well separated from the abdominal wall but remains attached to it by a median skin fold. The distal part of the prepuce is free and forms a complete cylindrical fold with a tapered preputial orifice.

The cat's penis has a peculiar orientation, with its urethral orifice facing caudodorsally while the dorsum of the penis faces cranioventrally. The os penis is only 0.1 cm in length and points distally. The free part of the penis is conical and studded with small cornified papillae or spines. These develop between 2 and 6 months of age and regress following castration.

# PHYSIOLOGY OF THE REPRODUCTIVE TRACT

The normal estrous cycle of the dog and cat is divided into

- proestrus
- estrus
- diestrus, and
- anestrus.

## Dog

### Proestrus

Proestrus lasts an average of 7–10 days, with a range of 4–25 days. At the beginning of proestrus the vulva rapidly increases in size due to edema formation. Occasionally a brownish mucoid-like vaginal discharge will be observed just prior to the vulvar enlargement. This changes to a hemorrhagic discharge which persists throughout proestrus. Toward the end of proestrus the color changes from red to pink. The erythrocytes in the discharge originate from the uterus, probably as a result of diapedesis and subepithelial capillary rupture within the endometrium. The quantity of discharge varies between animals (from large amounts to almost nothing). During proestrus the bitch is sexually attractive to the male but will not stand to be mounted. Although males are attracted to the female in early proestrus (probably owing to pheromones in the vaginal discharge), she is not receptive. As proestrus progresses, receptivity increases. Some may even allow mounting, and toward the end of proestrus intromission and ejaculation occasionally occur.

### Estrus

Estrus is marked by an abrupt appearance of sexual receptivity. The typical signs are

- presentation of the hindquarters to the male
- reflex deviation of the tail
- elevation of the perineum, and
- a display of the vulva.

The vulvar edema reaches its maximum and becomes more flaccid in consistency. The vaginal discharge becomes straw colored, although in some bitches it remains hemorrhagic throughout estrus and, in some cases, into diestrus. Estrus lasts an average of 3–7 days, with a range of 2–15 days. Ovulation takes place during the first few days.

---

### Ovulation

The young bitch may ovulate as early as the first day, whereas older animals tend to ovulate later, between days 2 and 5 of estrus (average day 3). This is probably because older bitches become sexually receptive sooner than young ones and is not due to any hormonal differences.

---

Ovulation of all Graafian follicles usually takes approximately 24–48 hours to complete and fertilization cannot take place until the first polar body has been formed.

### Diestrus

Diestrus is the phase of the cycle that occurs after the cessation of standing heat, when the reproductive tract is under the influence of increasing and decreasing levels of progesterone from the developing and regressing corpus luteum. The onset of diestrus is difficult to define in the bitch, as she may still be sexually receptive during the first few days of this phase. Exfoliative vaginal cytology is used to indicate the onset of diestrus. The size of the vulva decreases but it usually returns to its normal size and consistency during mid- or late diestrus. The vaginal discharge becomes mucoid in nature and may even appear to be mucopurulent. The quantity diminishes at approximately the same rate as the size of the vulva.

### Anestrus

The onset of anestrus in the non-pregnant bitch is difficult to describe, but endocrinologically it starts when progesterone has reached basal concentration again. Clinically there is no difference between an ovariohysterectomized and an anestrous bitch. The vulvar lips are soft and small and can be covered for a large part by the dorsal skin fold. There is no discharge. This period is often referred to as the quiescent phase, although neither the ovary nor the pituitary gland is quiescent during anestrus. Anestrus lasts from 4 to 5 months, with a range of 2–9 months.

## Cat

### Proestrus

The onset of proestrus is indicated when the queen shows continuous rubbing of the head and neck on various objects. There is no vaginal discharge and vulvar edema is not pronounced. During proestrus, a period lasting 1–2 days, the female will not permit the male to breed her.

## Estrus

The onset of estrus is characterized by receptivity toward the male. Behavioral changes include

- crouching with the forelimbs pressed to the ground, with the hindquarters elevated, and lateral deviation of tail
- presentation of the vulva for mating
- restlessness, and
- vocalization.

---

### Clinical Pointer

Many owners confuse the signs of normal mating behavior in cats with signs of pain.

---

Once breeding occurs the queen will ovulate and stop estrous behavior. The duration of estrus is 3–20 days if coitus does not occur.

---

### Postestrus

Postestrus is the period that follows one estrus and precedes the next in queens that have not been induced to ovulate.

---

## Diestrus

Diestrus is the period after induced ovulation. It lasts approximately 40 days in the non-pregnant animal and approximately 60 days in the pregnant animal. Cycling resumes 7–10 days following the end of diestrus in both pregnant and non-pregnant queens. Lactation and suckling will delay the onset of cyclicity until 2–3 weeks post weaning. It is possible that during the postpartum estrus the queen will not ovulate, even after multiple breedings.

## Anestrus

Anestrus is the absence of cyclicity normally seen during October, November, and December. Changes in photoperiod will affect cyclic activity during this time.

## CLINICAL EXAMINATION

The objectives of clinical examination of the reproductive tract are

- to assess anatomical defects
- to determine the stage of the estrous cycle
- to recognize the existence of reproductive system disease.

A systematic clinical examination of all other body systems precedes the detailed examination of the reproductive tract.

### Signalment

In the bitch sexual maturity or puberty is reached in the smaller breeds between 6 and 10 months of age, and in larger breeds as late as 18–24 months. Some animals may not show the first cycle (silent heat). In the latter case there is little vulvar discharge and swelling and the onset of the cycle may go unnoticed by the owner. In long-haired dogs vaginal discharge may be more difficult to observe. The bitch that licks her vulvar region excessively may make it more difficult for the owner to determine the onset of the first estrous cycle. If bitches are housed together there is the possibility of synchrony in the onset of estrus, or the first estrous cycle may be encountered earlier. Free-roaming bitches may show a first estrous cycle that is earlier in onset than in bitches of the same breed that are kennelled or kept indoors.

---

### The estrous cycle in dogs

- normally dogs cycle throughout the year
- sexual activity may be slightly increased from February to May
- there may be a slightly more quiescent period between June and September
- the average interestrous interval is 7 months, but there are breed differences, the German Shepherd may cycle every 4–5 months, whereas the Basenji cycles once a year
- dogs will cycle throughout life.

---

Breeding is recommended between 2 and 6 years of age. After 6 years of age detrimental variables occur, such as

- increased birth defects
- parturition problems
- decreased conception rate and smaller litter size
- increased puppy mortality
- increased interestrous interval
- increased pathological conditions of the uterus.

The older male dog may develop prostate problems, testicular degeneration, and other abnormal conditions with decreased sperm numbers. Senile changes may start occurring at 5–6 years of age in some cases.

In smaller breeds there are usually fewer but relatively heavier puppies delivered per litter than in larger breeds. The narrow pelvis, large head, and wide shoulders found in brachycephalic breeds have an effect on the progress of parturition and often cause dystocia.

In cats the first estrous cycle is normally noted at 5–9 months of age, with a range from 4 to 21 months. Most cats reach puberty at a body weight of 2.3–2.5 kg, but a delay can be expected if pubertal age is attained during the period of the year when most cats are anestrus.

---

### Clinical Pointer

It has been reported that long-haired cats tend to have delayed puberty compared to short-haired cats.

---

The queen is considered to be seasonally polyestrous. Under natural conditions sexual activity commences with increasing day length. A seasonal effect is not noted when cats are maintained under conditions of constant day length.

## History taking for evaluation of reproductive performance

Evaluation for infertility in the bitch should not begin until 2 years of age, when puberty has been reached in all breeds. Elements of the history that are of particular importance are

- dates of proestrus
- onset of proestrus during previous cycles
- dates of copulations
- fertility status of the males used
- timing of ovulation
- dates of delivery
- litter size of any previous pregnancies
- presence of previous reproductive disease, such as pyometra.

It is important to know whether the bitch has been treated to postpone or suppress heat, or if she has been treated with progestins for skin conditions. Signs of underlying disease such as hypothyroidism (lethargy, weight gain, bilateral alopecia) or hyperadrenocorticism (polydipsia, polyuria) are recorded. It is important to distinguish between the normal and abnormal discharge from the vulva. Normal physiological discharges occur during the estrous cycle, at the time of parturition and during the postpartum period.

---

### Inhibition of spermatogenesis

Spermatogenesis is interrupted by environmental overheating and medications such as

sex steroids
anabolic steroids
glucocorticoids
ketoconazole
cimetidine, and
anticancer medication.

---

The normal postparturient discharge (2–3 weeks) is greenish in color for 1–3 days, then changes to a reddish, rusty color, and finally to colorless and mucoid. In the male it is important to obtain information regarding the use of the dog (sports or competition).

Many dogs with poor libido have been given exogenous testosterone, which in turn can result in azoospermia in previously fertile males. Past breeding history includes

- *Brucella canis* titer
- results of past semen analysis
- past libido
- number of breedings per bitch
- type of breeding (artificial insemination or natural)
- method of timing breedings
- pregnancy diagnosis
- number of puppies sired.

History taking in the cat is similar to that in the dog.

---

### Fertility

- fertility is best indicated if the male has recently sired, or the bitch has whelped, a litter of normal puppies
- acquired infertility is considered if the animal has sired or produced a normal litter, but a number of cycles have passed without offspring
- congenital infertility or infertility since puberty must be considered if no litters have been obtained using proper breeding management.

## Clinical examination of the female external genitalia

A general physical examination is done prior to examination of the reproductive tract. The size of the external genitalia can increase as a result of

- pregnancy
- pyometra, or
- reproductive hormones.

> ## Clinical Pointer ✳
>
> - the normal uterus cannot be palpated in the queen
> - if the uterus can be palpated, note its diameter and turgidity
> - the cervix can be palpated during proestrus and estrus as a firm, walnut-shaped organ in the caudal abdomen.

Palpation should be gentle, otherwise the animal will show sensitivity which may be interpreted as tenderness. With one hand steadying the queen or small bitch in a standing position, the other hand may palpate from below.

Pregnancy is first detectable at 3 weeks in the queen and at 4 weeks in the bitch after breeding. Information on pregnancy diagnosis is described later. Endometrial hyperplasia, neoplastic changes and fluid distension are pathological changes of the uterus that may be detected on palpation. A uterus tensely distended with pus is at risk of rupture. This occasionally occurs during examination.

The external genitalia are examined by direct inspection for the presence of any skin eruption, change in pigmentation, and vaginal discharge. The position and size of the vulva and infolding of the mucocutaneous junction is noted. If there is a vulvar discharge, a cranial vaginal aerobic bacterial culture specimen is collected. This should be done before any manipulation in the vulva or vagina, as it is important to prevent the secondary introduction of organisms. The mucous membranes of the caudal vulva are exposed to view by parting the labia with the hands or the thumb and index finger of one hand. The deeper parts of the vulva along the vagina are examined by introducing a suitable vaginoscope, such as a pediatric proctoscope or fiberoptic endoscope; the latter, may enable one to inspect the external os of the cervix. The vulvar and vaginal mucosa is examined for evidence of

- hyperemia
- papular nodules
- pustules
- vesicles
- erosions
- ulcers
- hemorrhage
- urine pooling
- other discharges, and
- sites of trauma.

> ## Palpation of the vestibule and vagina
>
> In bitches it is important to digitally palpate the vestibule and vagina. A sterile glove and lubricant are used to facilitate insertion of the index finger in a dorsocranial direction. This is not possible in queens It is important to determine the presence of any strictures and masses which may be missed during endoscopy.

## Vaginal swab cultures

The aerobic bacterial culture must be interpreted cautiously as almost all normal bitches will yield a bacterial flora. This is composed of microorganisms that usually exist in symbiosis and which therefore protect the host from infections. In about 15–20% of cases a pure culture is obtained; in ±5% the result is negative. The aerobic bacteria isolated from the vagina depend upon the breed of dog and the stage of the reproductive cycle.

Although anaerobic bacteria can also be isolated from the vagina of normal bitches, the numbers appear to be fewer than aerobic bacteria unless reproductive disease is present (i.e. anaerobic overgrowth due to conformation, foreign bodies, or rectovaginal fistula). Although the canine and feline vagina contains normal flora, the uterus does not.

Before obtaining a sample for culture the vulva must be cleansed. The swab specimen must be obtained through a vaginal speculum, such as a sterile otoscope cone (Fig. 22.3). The capsule of the commercial swab, containing transport medium, is broken and the swab is then inserted into the cranial portion of the vagina. A guard swab, such as a Teigland, can be used without a speculum, but these swabs are very long and difficult to manipulate (Fig. 22.4). It is important to obtain a bacterial culture when the cervix is open, as in proestrus, estrus, postpartum, or in open-cervix pyometra. At this time a moistened Q-tip can be inserted and a specimen for vaginal cytology obtained as well.

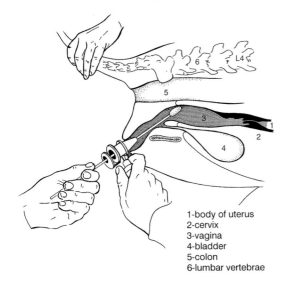

1-body of uterus
2-cervix
3-vagina
4-bladder
5-colon
6-lumbar vertebrae

**Fig. 22.3** Placement of an intravaginal otoscope cone and a Q-tip to obtain a vaginal cytology sample from the dorsal vaginal wall of the bitch.

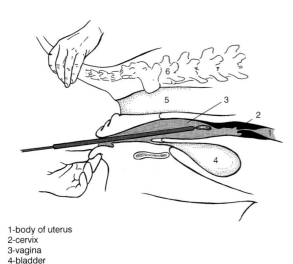

1-body of uterus
2-cervix
3-vagina
4-bladder
5-colon
6-lumbar vertebrae

**Fig. 22.4** Placement of an intravaginal guarded swab to obtain a culture of the cranial vagina and external cervical os of the bitch.

## Vaginal smear cytology

The cytological changes in a vaginal smear can be used to

- monitor or detect abnormalities in the stages of the estrous cycle
- determine the time to breed

- detect mismating
- determine the nature of vaginal discharge, and
- sometimes determine the existence of other reproductive disorders.

Vaginal cytology is not a valuable diagnostic aid for uterine disease. Smear collection is performed with a saline-moistened cotton swab and a speculum or otoscopic cone. The labia of the vulva are separated with one hand and the otoscope cone inserted with the other in a craniodorsal direction. The otoscope cone is held in place, the moistened cotton swab is introduced through the cone and cells are collected by touching the vaginal mucosa. The swab is withdrawn through the otoscope cone, which is then withdrawn. After withdrawal the swab is rolled on to a prelabeled microscope slide and, if a trichrome stain is used, fixed immediately. If stains such as Wright's and Wright–Giemsa are used the smear can be air-dried.

Coverslipping will prolong the storage time of the slides. Interpretation of the smear includes detecting the presence or absence of

- erythrocytes
- leukocytes
- intracellular and extracellular bacteria
- mucus
- debris, and
- epithelial cells.

The epithelial cells consist of the immature basal cell which gives rise to all of the epithelial cells observed in a vaginal smear. Basal cells are rarely observed in a vaginal smear; normally, the parabasal cells are the smallest epithelial cells observed. Other epithelial cells with increasing maturity are the intermediate, nucleated superficial and non-nucleated superficial cells or squames. Other cell types found in vaginal smears are metestrum cells, which are parabasal cells that contain a neutrophil in the cytoplasm and are seen

### Foam cells

Foam cells are parabasal cells that contain vacuoles in the cytoplasm.

during diestrus, but also at any time whenever neutrophils are present.

## Proestrus and estrus

During early proestrus the cells become more differentiated and types encountered include superficial, intermediate, and parabasal epithelial cells. Erythrocytes are also present, and neutrophils may be seen during the first few days. By midproestrus the neutrophils are absent, as are the parabasal and intermediate cells. In late proestrus virtually only superficial cells are present in the smear, although red blood cells may still be seen. Late proestrus and early estrus are difficult to distinguish with vaginal smears. In both there is a disappearance of debris, with only pyknotic and anuclear superficial cells being present. Midestrus is characterized by the presence of superficial cells, most of which are anuclear, and the background of the smear is clean and clear. Erythrocytes may or may not be present during estrus.

## Diestrus

There are numerous cells of the intermediate and parabasal variety. A few superficial cells may be seen during metestrus. A characteristic phenomenon is the high number of neutrophils at the beginning of this phase. If parabasal or intermediate cells are infiltrated by white blood cells they are referred to as metestrus cells. Foam cells – parabasal cells that contain cytoplasmic vacuoles – may also be seen during this phase of the cycle.

## Anestrus

Very few cells are usually encountered during this phase. Those present are usually of the intermediate and parabasal type. Neutrophils may be present.

Vaginal cytology in the cat is similar to that described in the bitch, except that erythrocytes are not usually seen in proestrus, and metestrum cells and foam cells are not seen in cats. Leukocytes may or may not be seen during metestrus.

> ### Clinical Pointer
>
> Ovulation may occur as a result of vaginal stimulation in the cat, therefore the technique of obtaining a vaginal smear may induce ovulation.

## Vaginal endoscopy

Vaginal endoscopy of the caudal reproductive tract is a method of examining the mucosa of the vagina and vestibule and vulva of the bitch. In cats this procedure is difficult because of the small size of the vagina. A human pediatric proctoscope is the ideal instrument for visual examination of the vagina, but all small-diameter rigid or flexible fiberoptoscopes are appropriate. Minimal restraint, or reassurance by the owner or assistant, is adequate to allow examination of most bitches. The assistant supports the abdomen to keep the dog standing.

> ### Clinical Pointer
>
> If a bitch suffering from vaginitis objects to vaginal endoscopy, general anesthesia is indicated.

A full bladder or impacted rectum may occasionally displace the reproductive tract, or provoke discomfort during vaginoscopy. The scope is inserted in an aseptic manner to minimize the danger of carrying bacteria and debris from the vulva to the cranial vagina. To take account of the slope of the vestibule and the change of direction of the reproductive tract at the vestibulovaginal junction in the individual bitch, the scope is first directed dorsocranially within the vestibule. It can be readily advanced with gentle pressure through the vestibulovaginal junction. The cessation of resistance, normally present in all bitches at the vestibulovaginal junction, indicates that the scope has entered the vaginal lumen. If excessive resistance is encountered the vestibule should be re-examined for the presence of a pathological or congenital abnormality, such as an imperforate hymen. When the vaginal folds fill the lumen, as in early proestrus, the endoscope may have to be partially withdrawn and readvanced to guide it through the lumen. When guided correctly, little resistance is encountered until the scope arrives at the narrower paracervix. In some bitches, particularly those with a long vagina that falls steeply over the pubic brim into the abdomen, slight distension of the vagina with air aids visualization of the mucosa.

Several stages of the estrous cycle are detectable from the endoscopic appearance of the posturerine tract. During anestrus the tract has a relatively simple, featureless appearance. During proestrus the mucous membranes become edematous and folds increase in size as a result of rising estrogen. During estrus there is maximal paleness and angulated appearance to the mucous membrane folds. This peak angulated period is the time to recommend as optimum for natural and artificial insemination, and likely conception. During early diestrus a patchy hyperemia, low, simple plicate folds, and rosettes of folds are recognizable. As cornified layers are shed at the end of estrus and the start of diestrus, small ulcerated areas may be seen.

## Rectal examination

A digital rectal palpation is recommended in both dog and cat. In the female the wall of the pelvis is examined to evaluate for symmetry, old fractures, irregularities, narrowing of the pelvic canal, and to determine whether tumors are present, especially in the dorsal wall of the vagina. Rectal examination may be helpful if vaginal palpation is impossible as a result of narrowing or extensive tumor growth. It is difficult in the cat because of its size.

## Pregnancy diagnosis

Bitches and queens show a relatively large variation in gestation length. This variation is seen not only within a breed, but also an individual may show different gestation lengths during subsequent pregnancies. In the bitch this variation can be minimized with the use of vaginal cytology. The gestation length from the onset of diestrus is 56–58 days, and from the luteinizing hormone (LH) peak is 64–66 days.

Pregnancy in the bitch is diagnosed by abdominal palpation at about 28–32 days from the LH peak. The

blastocysts are about 2–4 cm in diameter at this stage and can be palpated as distinct, round, and very smooth enlargements in the uterus. In the cat abdominal palpation can be done 21–25 days after the LH peak. Abdominal palpation may be difficult or even impossible in timid, nervous, or obese animals, or those with a small number of fetuses. Palpation is inaccurate for assessing fetal number and viability.

Radiography after day 45 in both dog and cat is a much more accurate method of counting the number of fetuses than ultrasonography. Fetal death can be assessed with radiographs 12–48 hours after the fetuses died. Signs of fetal death are

- overlap of fetal skull bones
- collapse of fetal vertebrae
- hyperextension of limbs, and
- intrafetal gas.

It is normal for a physiological anemia to develop during pregnancy, caused primarily by increased plasma volume. In the dog the hematocrit level may decrease to less than 0.35 l/l at parturition (normal 0.37–0.55 l/l). This physiological decline is dependent upon the number of fetuses, with the greatest decrease occurring in large litters. Pregnancy in the bitch may induce an insensitivity to insulin and a carbohydrate intolerance, resulting in transient hyperglycemia and glucosuria. Immune function and coagulation factors may be altered.

## Physical examination of the male genitalia

A complete physical examination is done of all body systems. The male must be carefully examined for any abnormalities that will interfere with its libido or ability to mount or achieve intromission.

---

### Reluctance to mount

Dogs with any type of intervertebral disk or joint disease may be reluctant to mount. If these conditions are not heritable such dogs can be used in artificial insemination programs.

---

Obesity, scrotal skin diseases, and endocrine disorders are other problems that may adversely influence fertility.

With the animal restrained on its back the penis and prepuce are inspected visually and palpated for abnormalities, such as

- persistent frenulum
- hypospadias, or
- restricted preputial orifice.

The prepuce is retracted and the non-erect penis protruded. This is essential for the detection of ulcers, scars, nodules, or signs of inflammation. A small amount of discharge (smegma) may accumulate normally under the prepuce. The shaft of the penis can be milked to allow some discharge out of the urethral meatus for examination. The penis is palpated between the thumb and first two fingers and any tenderness, induration, or other abnormality recorded. The os penis is palpated for signs of fractures and congenital abnormalities. The scrotum and scrotal skin is inspected for dermatitis, swelling, lumps, or venous engorgement. Using the thumb and first two fingers, the testes are palpated for size, symmetry, shape, consistency, and tenderness. Pressure on the testes normally produces a deep visceral pain. Although testicular size will vary widely between breeds, size can be measured with calipers and recorded for comparative purposes at later examinations.

The epididymides are palpated next. The head of the epididymis is located on the craniolateral aspect of the testicle and the body runs caudally along the dorsolateral aspect. At the caudal pole of the testicle the tail of the epididymis proceeds medially toward the spermatic cord, which can be palpated until it enters the external inguinal ring.

---

### Disorders of the testes

- softening of the testes indicates testicular degeneration, hypoplasia, or atrophy
- increased hardness indicates testicular fibrosis, neoplasia, inflammation, or the presence of a prosthesis.

---

### Transillumination of the scrotum

This can be used to examine any swelling in the scrotum other than the testicle. The room is darkened and the beam of a strong penlight is shone from behind the scrotum through the mass

- swellings containing serous fluids transilluminate with a red glow
- swellings containing blood or tissue, such as normal testes, a tumor, and most hernias, do not transilluminate.

---

The prostate, the major accessory sex gland, is responsible for the volume of the canine ejaculate. The prostate of the dog is bilobed and, in the adult, is located at the pelvic inlet on the symphysis. The precise location varies according to breed, size of the prostate, age, and distension of the urinary bladder. The two lobes are separated by a dorsal medium septum and completely surround the urethra. The prostate gland is examined by digital rectal examination with concurrent abdominal palpation to determine size, the presence of pain, location, consistency and texture. Prostatic hypertrophy, a common finding in older intact male dogs, results in a greatly enlarged gland which extends into the abdominal cavity. In some cases palpation may be facilitated by having the animal's front limbs elevated and, using the free hand under the abdomen to elevate the prostate toward the pelvic inlet and palpate the gland per rectum.

---

### Clinical Pointer

In Scottish Terriers the prostate is four times larger than in other breeds of the same size.

---

### Semen collection

Semen collection and evaluation is an important procedure in the evaluation of the male dog. A sexual rest of 5–7 days is indicated before collection. If a male dog has not been evaluated for at least 1 month it is recommended to collect semen once or twice, disregard these collections and then collect a sample for evaluation. Collection can be accomplished by different means. In almost all cases a teaser bitch in any stage of her cycle, preferably proestrus or estrus, will provide the necessary stimulation. If a teaser bitch is not available, a commercially available pheromone or previously frozen and thawed vaginal swab from a disease-free estral bitch can be applied to the perineal area of a bitch. A room is reserved where collection can take place. A non-slip rubber mat to provide adequate safe footing for the dogs is needed. Three people are required

- the handler holds the teaser bitch in a standing position
- a second person holds the male dog
- a third person collects the semen.

When the male and female dogs are brought into the collection room they are allowed to play together for a few minutes. The male's attention is directed toward the female so that he will not urinate before mounting. Licking and smelling the bitch's vulvar area creates a partial erection and protrusion of the penis. The semen collector, if right-handed, kneels at the male dog's left side; the handlers of the male and female dogs are also on the left side. The collector holds the artificial vagina (AV) in the left hand and the right hand is used to move the prepuce up and down the shaft of the penis while directing it into the AV. Once a semierection has been obtained and the bulbus glandis starts to engorge, the prepuce is pushed behind the bulbus glandis with a sliding action of the collector's hand. When this is accomplished, the penis is gripped with moderate pressure between forefinger and thumb just caudal to the gland. This act mimics the copulatory lock. Using the other three fingers a pulsating pressure is applied directly on the bulbus. Most male dogs ejaculate the presperm (clear) semen during the thrusting movements. The dog will cease thrusting, almost abruptly, and will attempt to dismount and lift one leg over the arm of the collector thus directing the penis backwards between the rear legs. At this time the second, sperm-rich (milky white) fraction is obtained. The first and second fractions are often collected together. After emitting the sperm-rich second fraction the dog will begin to emit the third fraction, originating from the prostate gland. The third fraction is clear and is collected to obtain an adequate sample for appropriate microscopic analysis. After the sample has been collected the AV is carefully removed and a water-soluble lubricant applied to the penis to prevent drying of the mucosa.

The male dog is carefully watched in the collection room until the erection has completely subsided and the entire penis is back within the preputial sheath.

On occasion it is possible that a total erection will occur before the prepuce is pushed over the bulbus glandis. In this case it is necessary to separate the animals until the erection subsides. The process is then reinitiated, attempting to slide the prepuce back at an earlier stage in the collection procedure. It is important not to do this too quickly, as some dogs

## Clinical Pointer

In long-haired breeds it is important to make sure that the prepuce does not invert and cause injury or paraphimosis.

resent this and seem to enjoy the initial stimulation of the penis and gland through the preputial sheath.

The AV used is a conical latex or plastic sheath that contacts with the engorged penis and closely simulates the natural process of mating. The sheath is adjusted to the size of the penis by folding the top. It is important to have the tip of the penis as far down in the sheath as possible, as the latex will make the spermatozoa immotile upon contact. A collection tube is attached to the sheath.

## Clinical Pointer

Do not collect the first few drops of ejaculate if the dog urinates just prior to collection, in this case delay placing the collection apparatus until after the start of ejaculation.

### Criteria for semen evaluation

- **Color** The semen sample should be cloudy to milky white. Yellow discoloration indicates urine contamination or a purulent exudate. Red or brown indicates blood from the reproductive tract.
- **Volume** The first two fractions average 0.5–6 ml, depending upon the breed.
- **pH** The third fraction normally has a pH between 6.5 and 7.0.
- **Motility** This should be assessed as total, progressive, and speed (slow, medium, fast).
- **Concentration** depends upon the amount of third fraction that is collected.
- **Total sperm number** should exceed 200 million in the ejaculate.
- **Morphology** under an oil immersion lens allows sperm cells to be divided into normal sperm are those with head abnormalities, those with midpiece abnormalities, and tail abnormalities.
- **Cytology** A drop of raw semen is placed on a glass slide, processed as for a blood smear and allowed to air dry. The slide is then stained and the presence of RBCs, WBCs, epithelial cells, other cells, and bacteria noted. If a large number of WBCs or bacteria are noted, bacterial culture is indicated.

Other tests that may be indicated are urine analysis, brucellosis testing, seminal alkaline phosphatase, hormonal assays, epididymal aspirate, testicular biopsy, and chromosomal karyotyping. These tests are useful when there is oligospermia or azoospermia, or if differentiating between primary and secondary hypogonadism is important.

# The Mare

The use of radioimmunoassays, molecular biology, and ultrasonography in equine reproduction has resulted in an explosion of new scientific information. New technologies, such as the shipment of cooled semen and insemination with frozen/thawed semen, are now commonly used in veterinary practice. These scientific advancements require that the veterinarian excel in the skills needed for clinical examination of the reproductive tract. Such skills include taking an accurate history, performing thorough rectal, vaginal, and ultrasound examinations and, if needed, procuring uterine cytology samples for culture and biopsy.

## HISTORY

Evaluating a complete history of the reproductive performance of the mare prior to examination is essential for

- making a diagnosis
- giving a prognosis, and
- selecting appropriate treatments.

Because improper management is often the principal cause of infertility, a complete history is needed if no physical causes of infertility are found in the examination. Reviewing the history frequently reveals the cause of the problem. The ideal breeding history includes a sequential, year-by-year account of the mare's entire working and breeding career. Unfortunately this is rarely obtained because mares frequently change owners and many owners keep incomplete records.

The length of the performance career, race or show training, and the ages when it began and finished should be noted. Drugs, stress, or injuries incurred during performance may adversely affect cyclic patterns, behavior, and body condition. Behavioral attitudes developed in training may also compromise reproductive performance in the young mare for several months after arrival at the breeding farm. Mares that are to be bred may be housed at facilities that lack a stallion, making estrus detection difficult.

Reproductive data should include

- when the mare was first bred
- the number of years bred
- number of foals carried to term
- difficulties incurred at foaling
- whether the foal was born alive.

---

### The influence of age on the fertility of mares

- young mares, 2–3 years of age, may experience abnormal estrous cycles and have aberrant estrous behavior.
- older, pluriparous mares, more than 15 years of age, may have undergone anatomical changes leading to pneumovagina, refluxing of urine in the cranial vagina, or accumulating fluid within the uterine lumen after breeding.

---

The time of year that the mare was bred and whether she was subjected to artificial lighting needs to be noted. Abortions, placentitis, retained placenta, and early embryonic death need to be recorded. A detailed reproductive history for the preceding 3 years, including teasing and breeding data, is invaluable because it may reveal cyclic patterns. Short cycles suggesting uterine infection, and prolonged diestrual patterns suggesting endocrine dysfunction should be noted. Communication with the management personnel and other veterinarians who have previously attended the mare is helpful as they can supply information on estrous behavior, such as the ease with which estrus was detected, restraint needed to produce signs of estrus, and other behavioral characteristics.

Treatment history, ultrasonographic findings, cytology and culture results, drugs infused into the uterus, and the schedule of drugs administered should be evaluated. Such data will be invaluable when compared with results of a subsequent examination of the reproductive tract. Any response to treatments contributes to the prognosis. Evidence of, or recorded data relating to, previous surgery of the reproductive tract may influence conception or maintenance of pregnancy.

Knowledge of the fertility of the stallion to which the mare has been bred previously and the method by which she was bred is needed. Obtaining information on the number of estrous cycles per conception, the motility of shipped, cooled semen or post-thaw motility of frozen/thawed semen will help identify whether the stallion is contributing to the problem. If cooled or frozen semen is used, insemination must be properly timed if conception is to occur. First-cycle pregnancy rates are highest in mares bred with frozen/thawed semen when the mares are examined every 6 hours to determine ovulation. Such intensive management may be logistically impossible. In addition, some mares may experience an acute prolonged endometritis after being bred with frozen semen, resulting in early embryonic death.

## EXTERNAL EXAMINATION

Prior to examination of the reproductive tract, the general physical condition of the mare should be appraised and any systemic problems that may interfere with fertility noted. In addition to a general appraisal, the perineal and pelvic conformation needs to be thoroughly examined as the anatomical alignment of the perineum is important for reproductive soundness (Fig. 22.5).

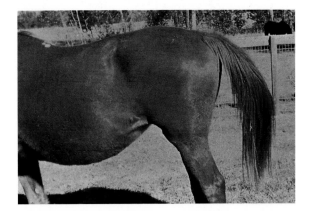

Fig. 22.5  Conformation of mare that exhibits a delay in uterine clearance. Note the flat croup and high tail setting.

> ### Clinical Pointer ✳
>
> Extremes in body condition, from debilitation to obesity, may affect fertility.

Examination of the external genitalia should include the entire perineal area as well as the tail and buttocks, to detect signs of vulval discharge. The vulva is best evaluated during estrus, when relaxation and elongation of the lips are greatest. The integrity of the vulval lips, the angulation of the vulva, and the location of the dorsal commissure of the vulva in relation to the pelvis needs to be evaluated. The vulvar lips should meet evenly and appear full and firm. They function as a seal

> ### Pelvic conformation and fertility
>
> Pelvic conformation is viewed laterally and caudally. Conformational characteristics that correlate with high fertility include
>
> - a long sloping hip
> - tubera sacrale located well dorsal to the tail setting
> - a vulva that is no more than 10° off vertical.
>
> Mares that experience bouts of infertility frequently have conformational defects that lead to pneumovagina, urovagina, and the accumulation of intrauterine fluid (Fig. 22.5), for example
>
> - a flat-topped croup
> - a tail setting that is level with the tubera sacrale
> - a sunken anus.

against external contamination of the uterus (Fig. 22.6), and should lie vertically, with a cranial to caudal slope of no more than 10° from vertical. The dorsal commissure of the vulva should be no more than 4 cm dorsal to the pelvic floor. If it is more than 4 cm the vulva is predisposed to cranioventral rotation, leading to pneumovagina and contamination.

The lips of the vulva should be parted to determine the integrity of the vestibulovaginal sphincter. The sphincter is intact when the labia can be spread slightly without air entering the cranial vagina (Fig. 22.7). By parting the labia, the color and moisture of the vestibular walls can be assessed.

> ### Changes in the vestibular walls
>
> - estrus → a glistening pink to red mucosa
> - anestrus → a pale, dry mucosa
> - inflammation → a dark-red or muddy color
> - progesterone dominance → a white, tacky mucosa.

In older, pluriparous mares the perineal body may be defective. The defect most likely occurs from repeated foalings and poor reproductive conformation, and results in a sunken anus and lack of tissue between the rectum and vagina.

> ### Clinical Pointer ✳
>
> Integrity of the perineal body is assessed by placing one finger (usually the second) into the rectum and the thumb into the vestibule. There should be at least 3 cm of muscular tissue between the two fingers.

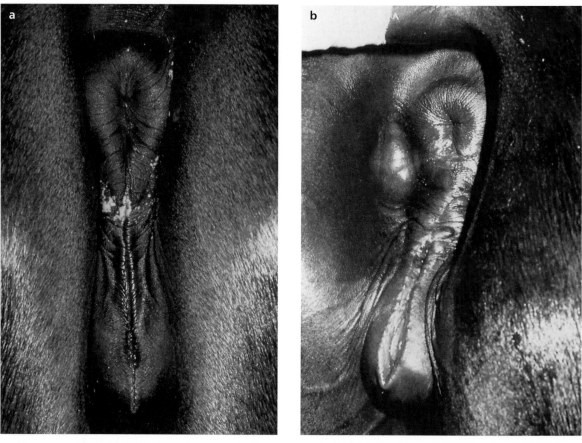

**Fig. 22.6** (a) Normal vulvar conformation. (b) Abnormal vulvar conformation. Note the slant of the upper half of the vulvar lips.

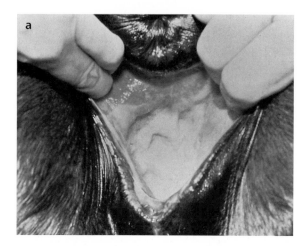

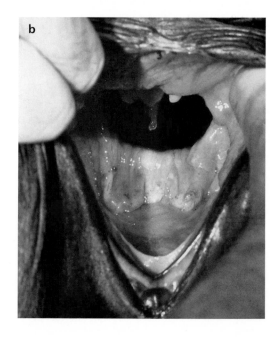

**Fig. 22.7** (a) Normal vestibular vaginal sphincter. (b) Abnormal vestibular vaginal sphincter.

# EXAMINATION OF THE REPRODUCTIVE TRACT BY RECTAL PALPATION

## Restraint

The safety of both veterinarian and mare must be considered prior to rectal palpation. Mares are routinely examined in well designed stocks or backed out of a stall door. Examination in a set of stocks offers the advantage of requiring less restraint, so that the animal is more relaxed for the procedure. However, stocks should be viewed critically for design faults that predispose to injury. Overhead braces are dangerous if the animal rears. A rear door protects the operator but is hazardous if the mare suddenly squats during examination. The preferred technique for examination in box stalls is to restrain the mare with a twitch or lip chain and back her through the stall door so that her hindquarters are in the aisle. The operator can then stand far enough to one side to be protected by the door frame.

It may be necessary to examine a mare in an open field. In this case, the handler and examiner should work on the same side of the mare. The examiner, using the left-hand, should

- stand at the mare's right hip initially
- grasp the base of the tail with the right hand, and
- slowly and deliberately introduce the palpation hand into the mare's rectum.

Once the examination is under way the examiner can move safely to a point close behind the right hindquarter. Muscular movements preparatory to kicking can be anticipated when close contact with the mare is maintained. Chemical restraint may be needed. The $\alpha_2$ agonist drugs should be used in combination with other tranquilizers or opioids when working near the rear of a horse to avoid hypersensitivity over the hindquarters that can occur as an adverse side effect when they are used alone. Combinations of xylazine and acepromazine or xylazine with butorphenol both produce good chemical restraint.

## Technique

Rectal palpation must be performed gently and carefully. Undue pressure against the rectal wall will traumatize the rectal mucosa and may induce a tear. Prior to palpation of any abdominal organ, the examiner should remove all feces from the rectum as far cranially as possible – usually 45–60 cm – with a well lubricated arm. The rectal wall should feel snug and pliable around the hand as the fingers are opened and closed. If there is air in the rectum the rectal wall will feel like a tense drum.

Some mares may forcibly strain during examination, and should be palpated with caution. Adding 50–100 ml of 2% lidocaine to the lubricant and infusing 100–200 ml of the mixture into the rectum improves relaxation.

---

### Clinical Pointer

To avoid causing a rectal tear during palpation

- ensure adequate restraint
- use gentle pressure
- use ample lubrication
- make sure that sleeves are free from irritating seams
- remove air from the rectum.

---

The genitalia should be examined systematically, using the same routine for each examination. A suggested technique is to first identify the uterus and follow it laterally to locate the ovaries.

1. The examiner cups the hand by bending the wrist and fingers and gently pulls the relaxed rectal wall caudally and slightly ventrally.
2. As the hand nears the pelvis the non gravid uterus will be felt as a soft, pliable, and relatively flat tissue lying transversely in the caudal abdomen.
3. The uterus is generally 4–7 cm wide and 2–5 cm thick (Fig. 22.8).
4. In older pluriparous mares the uterus will be found ventral to the pelvis.
5. In young nulliparous animals it may be located slightly dorsal to the pelvis.
6. In the postpartum mare, the uterus will be large, 9–14 cm in diameter, and will be located more ventrally and cranially than the non-pregnant uterus.

Once identified, the uterus should be held in the examiner's hand by curling the fingers over the cranial portion and resting the tips of the fingers on its ventral, caudal aspect. The palm should lie over the cranial, dorsal edge.

To palpate the uterine horns and ovaries the hand is moved laterally up the uterine horn. To grasp an ovary, the examiner must reach in a craniolateral and usually dorsal direction. There is a space of 5–10 cm between the most lateral aspect of the uterine horn that is palpable and the ovary, so if the ovary cannot be grasped the uterine horn must be reidentified and the process repeated. The ovary is a round to kidney-shaped firm mass attached to the uterine horn by the utero-ovarian ligament. It is suspended by the broad ligament of the uterus along its dorsum, with the attachment continuing both medially and laterally. The caudal aspect of the ovary is free of ligamentous attachments. If the ovary is small it can be held in the hand and completely evaluated. If large it can be stabilized against the iliac shaft and evaluated in portions. The ovary is then rotated on its mesovarian attachment, in either a cranial to caudal or a lateral to medial direction, to palpate that part of the ovary lying next to the iliac shaft. The uterus is reidentified and the other ovary examined in a similar fashion.

After examining both ovaries, the uterine body and the cervix are palpated. To locate the cervix the hand is retracted slowly from the rectum while gentle pressure is placed on the rectal floor with the fingertips. The cervix will feel like a firm, cylindrical structure, caudal to the uterine body. Unlike in the cow, it is not possible to pick up the cervix.

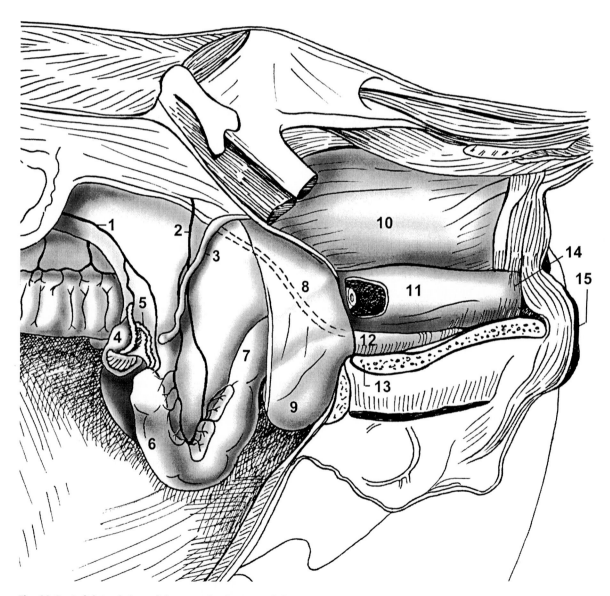

**Fig. 22.8** Left lateral view of the reproductive tract of the mare. 1, ovarian artery; 2, uterine artery; 3, round ligament of uterus; 4, left ovary; 5, left uterine oviduct; 6, left uterine horn; 7, uterine body; 8, cervix; 9, bladder; 10 rectum; 11, vagina; 12, urethra; 13, pelvic brim; 14, vaginal vestibule; 15, clitoris.

## Ovarian palpation

The entire surface of the ovary must be palpated to identify landmarks and important structures. This is accomplished by holding the ovary in the palm of the hand. The thumb, index finger, and middle finger may then explore the pole of the ovary lying in the hand and its greater curvature or center. The opposite pole is best evaluated by turning the entire ovary 180° on its mesovarial attachment and repeating the above process. The cranial and caudal poles are identified by locating the free edge of the mesovarium, which attaches to the cranial half of the ovary. The ovulation fossa, a sharp indentation in the ovarian stroma, is medial and slightly ventral when the ovary is in cranio-caudal alignment.

Two functional structures of the ovary can be identified by rectal palpation

- the follicle, and
- the corpus hemorrhagicum.

Follicles are fluid-filled symmetrical structures which, as they mature, project above the ovarian surface. Their size may vary from 10 to 60 mm or larger, depending on the stage of the estrous cycle. As ovulation approaches a 'shoulder' forms around the base of the growing follicle and increases its angle. The turgidity of the follicle generally changes with maturity, progressing from firm and thick-walled to fluctuant and thin-walled. On the first or second day of estrus the dominant follicle will range from 30 to 40 mm in diameter and increase in size by 3–5 mm daily until it ovulates, at which time it will be 38–60 mm in diameter.

The size of ovarian structures, turgidity data, and uterine tone need to be recorded for all examinations. In addition, teasing records, which describe the mare's clinical behavior when presented to a stallion, should be used to correlate palpation findings with clinical behavior and to time ovulation. Follicle size can be estimated in finger widths, millimeters, or inches. Knowledge of the width of one's fingertips or the distance from the fingertips to the various phalangeal joints is necessary before assigning numbers to structures. Some subjective method of assigning values for turgidity is also helpful.

Determination of the time of ovulation is important because the ovum is viable for only a few hours (probably 8) after ovulation. Collapse of the follicle is generally assumed to be the time of ovulation. Typically this collapse is felt as a crater or pit at the location of the follicle. When palpating this crater the mare responds to the local pain involved by tensing the flank muscles on that side or raising the limb.

> ### Predicting the time of ovulation
>
> The time of ovulation is predicted using a combination of
>
> - follicular size
> - projection from the surface
> - turgidity.
>
> None of these observations is absolute. Small ovaries, as found in young mares, are prone to ovulate smaller follicles than large ovaries of pluriparous mares. Occasionally a follicle that is still firm and tense ovulates with no prior change in turgidity. All the criteria for maturity must be correlated, using sequential examinations to track changes.

The borders of the crater are sharp and the cavity feels empty for about 8 hours. As the hemorrhage of ovulation organizes into a clot to form the corpus hemorrhagicum, the mushy consistency of the cavity becomes progressively firmer until 24 hours after ovulation. After 24 hours the crater may redistend with clot and serum, suggesting the presence of another follicle on palpation. The consistency of the corpus hemorrhagicum in this stage has been likened to that of a ripe plum, and the size is smaller than the original follicle. These changes are best evaluated by repeated rectal examinations or by ultrasonography.

> ### Clinical Pointer
>
> If the mare has ovulated within the last 24–48 hours some confusion between follicle and corpus hemorrhagicum may occur. The presence of other estral signs and the tone of the uterus are used to distinguish between the two.

The mature corpus luteum (5 days postovulation) is seldom detectable by rectal palpation, as retraction deep into the ovarian stroma occurs rather quickly. The corpus luteum can be identified by ultrasonography or by the presence of elevated serum progesterone levels.

The ovaries will change their size and shape during the year, as will the number of palpable follicles present. To determine if an ovary is abnormal, the time of year, the age, and clinical appearance of the mare and uterine findings must be taken into consideration. The most common ovarian abnormality is a granulosa cell tumor. Classically mares will have one extremely large ovary (> 100 mm in diameter) and one extremely small one (< 30 mm in diameter). Clinically the mare may show signs of estrus, may be in anestrus or be nymphomaniac. Variations in ovarian findings on rectal palpation are summarized in Table 22.1.

## Uterine palpation – non-pregnant uterus

The non-pregnant uterus is palpated to determine its size, tone, consistency, and general conformation, followed by a detailed examination for abnormalities. The initial impression is best gained by cupping the fingers over the cranial brim of the uterus, with the palm on the dorsal aspect, and by moving the hand laterally and medially from the tip of one uterine horn to the other. Uterine size is estimated by encircling the organ with the index finger and thumb, and estimating the diameter of each horn and the body.

Evaluation of uterine tone helps determine the stage of the estrous cycle (Tables 22.1, 22.2). The effect of progesterone on the uterus increases tissue density, causing a tubular, compact feeling on palpation. In proestrus and estrus the tubularity of diestrus progresses to relaxation. Circulating estrogens produce uterine edema, spreading the tissues of the endometrium and myometrium. The palpator detects this edema as a soft thickening of the uterus. There is also the impression that the thickened wall could be easily compressed between the fingers.

In anestrus the uterus becomes flaccid, thin-walled, and often quite indistinct. Endometrial atrophy is the prominent anatomic feature of this stage. The novice veterinarian may experience difficulty in tracing the entire uterus in anestrus owing to thinning of the wall.

After foaling the uterus will be large, thick walled, and muscular for 7–14 days. The previously pregnant horn will range in size from 70 to 140 mm in diameter, depending on how soon after parturition the mare is examined. The non-gravid horn will be 40–80 mm in diameter. The normal postpartum uterus will have palpable ridges over its serosa (rugae).

---

### Metritis

Mares with metritis have a thin-walled flaccid uterus without palpable rugae. Fluid may be palpable and can be moved from one horn to the other. As the metritis subsides uterine tone will become muscular, the wall will thicken and rugae will be present.

---

Specific changes in the conformation and consistency of the uterus should be noted. Enlargements and thinning of the ventral aspect in the area of the junction of the horn and body may indicate myometrial fibrosis or endometrial atrophy. Palpation of a

---

**Table 22.1.** Palpable changes of the ovaries and uterus and behavior of the non-pregnant, non-cycling mare according to the seasons of the year*

| Ovaries | Season | Tubular tract | Behavior | Other findings | Probable cause |
|---|---|---|---|---|---|
| Normal size, active, may have follicles | Summer | Excellent tone | Rejects stallion | None | Spontaneous prolonged corpus luteum |
| Normal size, active | Spring | Poor tone | Passive or irregular estrus | Pale, dry cervical and vaginal mucosa | Transition from anestrus to ovulatory stage |
| Small, inactive | Winter | Flaccid | Passive or irregular estrus | Pale, dry cervical and vaginal mucosa | Winter anestrus |
| Very small, inactive | Any | Infantile | Passive | Small body size | Gonadal dysgenesis |
| One ovary enlarged, other ovary smaller than normal | Any | Variable (flaccid) | Masculine (aggressive) or constant estrus | No ovulation fossa on large ovary | Secreting ovarian tumor |

* From Colahan, PT et al. Equine medicine and surgery, 4th edn. Goleta, CA: American Veterinary Publications, 1991, with permission.

**Table 22.2.** Endocrine, physical and behavioral changes during the estrous cycle of the mare[*]

| Stage of cycle | Endocrine changes | | | Physical changes | | |
|---|---|---|---|---|---|---|
| | Pituitary | Ovary | Ovary | Tubular tract | Behavioral changes |
| Early estrus | FSH rise | Estrogen rise | Follicle develops | Uterine edema, cervical relaxation | Beginning receptivity |
| Late estrus | LH surge | Estrogen peak | Follicle matures | Maximum uterine edema and cervical relaxation | Strong receptivity |
| Ovulation | LH near peak | Estrogen fall begins, progesterone rise begins | Follicle collapses, fresh 'crater' palpable | Uterine contraction, cervix still relaxed | Variable, usually still receptive |
| Early diestrus | LH fading | Progesterone climbing | CH palpable | Firm uterine tone | Rejects stallion |
| Mid-cycle | FSH rise | Progesterone peak | May detect follicular activity, CL may be palpable | Maximum uterine tone, cervix firm | Rejects stallion |
| Late diestrus | | Luteolysis: rapid demise of CL causes progesterone fall | No palpable changes | Early softening of uterus | Rejects stallion |

[*] From Colahan, PT et al. Equine medicine and surgery, 4th edn. Goleta, CA: American Publications, 1991, with permission.
FSH = follicle stimulating hormone
LH = luteinizing hormone
CH = corpus hemorrhagicum
CL = corpus luteum

thickened and edematous uterine wall during diestrus may be correlated with lymphatic stasis or lacunae. If abnormalities are palpated then further diagnostic procedures, particularly endometrial biopsy and ultrasonography, are indicated.

## Uterine palpation – pregnant uterus

As early as 17 or 18 days post ovulation there are characteristic changes in uterine and cervical tone in pregnant mares that can be used to differentiate the pregnant mare from the mare in diestrus. The cervix elongates, is firm and tubular. The uterine wall has considerable tone and has the texture of a high-pressure water hose. These changes are more pronounced than those produced by progesterone in mid-diestrus, and are most probably due to the combination of progesterone and estrogen.

To confirm pregnancy, the actual conceptus in its chorionic vesicle must be identified. At 17–18 days the vesicle may feel like a distinct, fluid-filled spherical structure on the ventral aspect of the uterus, usually at the base of one of the two horns. Because the vesicle is about 2.5 cm in diameter, considerable proficiency is required to define it. At this time the uterine horns may appear to be 'curled' owing to the prolonged progesterone influence. A curled horn is commonly mistaken for the chorionic vesicle.

The conceptus grows slowly, with the vesicle reaching 3 cm in diameter at 25 days and 4.0–4.5 cm at 30 days. Different-sized fruit are commonly used to compare the size and thus the gestational age of the vesicle

- at 28 days it is the size of a small lime
- at 35 days a lemon
- at 42 days an orange
- at 49 days a grapefruit
- at 56 days a cantaloupe

By 90 days the pregnant horn is the size of a small football and has dropped in the abdomen. To locate the vesicle between 18 and 50 days of gestation the ventral aspect of the uterus must be palpated, as little dorsal distension occurs during this period. The fingers must be flexed over the cranial margin of the uterus and must reach well under the uterine body and horns. Both margins of the vesicle are quite distinct, making an abrupt junction with the non-gravid portion of the uterus. A common error at this stage is not extending the fingers caudally enough under the edge of the uterus, thus missing the vesicle.

After 45 days of gestation uterine tone begins to diminish, especially in the area of the vesicle. Interpretation of rectal findings of mares bred on foal heat (first postpartum estrus) may be confusing, as the formerly pregnant horn will not be completely involuted. If the mare loses the conceptus the uterus becomes soft, doughy and flaccid, and the cervix shortens, widens and loses its tone.

---

### Clinical Pointer

Care must be taken so as not to confuse the bladder with a chorionic vesicle of 45–80 days of age.

---

After 50 days' gestation it may be difficult to completely evaluate both uterine horns, as the uterus extends cranially over the pelvic brim and is too large and heavy to retract. From the time the uterus attains this position until the fetus can be palpated consistently (120–150 days), positive pregnancy diagnosis by rectal palpation becomes somewhat more difficult. The first step in examining such mares by rectal palpation is to grasp one ovary and the broad ligament and by moving the cupped hand medially, attempting to 'slip' the uterus caudally into the pelvic cavity

- a non-gravid uterus can be elevated, allowing palpation in its entirety
- a gravid uterus fails to respond to this maneuver and gentle caudal traction.

Frequently only the non-gravid horn can be palpated: the gravid horn will slip out of reach. If the uterus is not

retractable the hand is placed flat on the dorsal surface of the uterus and its fluid content confirmed by ballottement. If the uterine wall feels thin and pliable and if the fluid is not viscous, a positive diagnosis of pregnancy can be made. The bladder wall is much thinner than that of the pregnant uterus. A more definitive diagnosis can always be made by ultrasonography.

## Cervical palpation

The cervix is palpated by pressing it firmly against the pelvis with the fingertips. The effects of estrogen and progesterone on the cervix are similar to those on the uterus. Estrogens produce cervical softening, shortening, and edema. Late in estrus, prior to ovulation, the cervix is so soft that it readily flattens against the pelvis. The diestrual cervix is long, tubular, and readily palpable. In anestrus the cervix becomes soft and indistinct.

## Vaginoscopic examination

The entire vagina and external cervical os can be inspected visually through a vaginal speculum using a bright light source, allowing dilatation of the vagina with air. The degree of cervical relaxation and the character of uterine, cervical, and vaginal secretions can be evaluated. Anatomical abnormalities of the area and those caused by trauma also are easily detected.

Preparation of the mare for vaginal examination requires restraint in a suitable location, preferably out of direct sunlight. The tail should be wrapped and the perineal area carefully washed with a non-irritating soap to remove external contaminants. After ample rinsing, the labia should be blotted dry and clean moist cotton used to wipe the inner edges. In many examination procedures the speculum examination is followed by obtaining endometrial samples for culture, cytology, and histopathology. Aseptic preparation of the vulva is more important in these procedures to prevent uterine contamination.

A sterile instrument such as a plastic, cardboard, or glass tubular speculum is usually used for vaginal examination. These types of specula are inexpensive and disposable, or are easily sterilized. Alternatively, the trivalve metal Caslick's speculum may also be used. This provides excellent visibility of the cervix and anterior vagina and is used for evaluation of cervical tears, rectovaginal fistulas, and assessment of the integrity of urethral extensions. It is, however, cumbersome to sterilize and relatively expensive. A bright beam of focused light is needed to assess the vaginal walls and cervix. Light sources include penlights, halogen illuminators attached to either long- or short-handled transilluminators, and flashlights.

If used in conjunction with teasing and rectal palpation vaginoscopic examination helps determine the stage of the estrous cycle. In estrus the cervix progressively softens and drops toward the floor of the distended vagina. At the time of maximal relaxation the cervix appears completely flattened on the vaginal floor, especially in pluriparous mares. In maiden and younger mares the cervix usually relaxes to a lesser degree. Estrogen secretion by the developing follicle also produces edema, mucus secretion and hyperemia of both the cervical and vaginal mucosa. Early in estrus it is common for the external cervical os to have edematous folds of mucosa that resolve as ovulation approaches. The degree of mucus secretion correlates with follicular development, and is seen as increased shininess of the cervical and vaginal mucosal surfaces. Judging the degree of hyperemia is important in evaluating the cervix and vagina for inflammatory and physiological changes.

### Clinical Pointer

During estrus, artifactual reddening is quickly produced when air contacts the cervical and vaginal tissues, so an evaluation for color will be made shortly after the vagina is dilated.

In diestrus the cervical and vaginal surfaces become pale and dry. The color of the membranes is typically gray, with a yellowish cast. The external cervical os projects into the cranial vagina from high on the wall and is tightly contracted, lending itself to the terms high, dry and tight, and rosebud. The appearance of the cervix correlates well with its elongated shape and firm consistency on rectal examination.

In pregnancy the cervix may be intensely white and tightly closed. On vaginal speculum examination it is located high on the vaginal wall, midway between the vaginal floor and vaginal ceiling. It is white and tightly closed, and appears like a rosebud. Vaginal secretions are thick and sticky. In late pregnancy the mucosa of the vaginal wall is covered by a thick, sticky, exudate which prevents the usual ballooning effect caused by introducing a speculum. It is sometimes difficult to visualize the cervical os late in pregnancy because it is pulled cranioventrally. Inactive ovaries are commonly found in winter anestrus and in conditions of gonadal dysgenesis. Cervical and vaginal color in anestrus is blanched, almost white. The cervix becomes atonic and flaccid, and often gapes open to reveal the uterine lumen.

### Clinical Pointer

In anestrus, blood vessels are scarce on the vaginal wall and little hyperemia occurs after exposure to air.

## Exudates and physical abnormalities

The source of exudates seen at the lips of the vulva can usually be determined by vaginoscopy. Inflammatory changes, such as mucosal hyperemia and suppurative exudates, are often discovered by visual examination. These changes are seen most frequently on the second or third day of estrus, after the perineum has relaxed under the influence of estrogens and prior to the flushing action of the increased uterine secretions. On speculum examination a grayish, watery to white, purulent exudate may be present on the vaginal floor. Exudate may be seen passing out of the cervical os from the uterus and the vaginal mucosa may be hyperemic. If pneumovagina is present the mucus and exudate will often have a 'foamy' appearance because air has mixed with the mucus.

Vaginal varicosities in the region of the perforated hymen are not uncommon. These may rupture late in pregnancy, causing blood to drip from the vulvar lips. If observed at breeding, the bleeding must be differentiated from vaginal rupture. Varicose veins are detected by speculum examination of the hymen. They usually are 1–2 cm in diameter and the color of venous blood inside a bluish translucent vein wall.

### Urovagina

Urovagina is the pooling of urine in the cranial fornix of the vagina. The fluid may be confirmed to be urine by assessment of its color, smell, osmolality, and urea content. On speculum examination the urine often covers at least a portion of, if not the entire cervix. Inflammatory cells are often mixed with the urine and its salt sediment. In severe cases the urine flows into the uterus when the cervix is relaxed, causing cervicitis and endometritis,

- it is seen in older, multiparous mares that have developed problems associated with pneumovagina, such as a pelvic canal that slopes cranioventrally
- sometimes it is only observed on the day before ovulation, when estrogen levels and perineal relaxation are maximal
- it may be seen during the first postpartum estrus, when the vaginal structures are stretched, relaxed, and pulled forward by the weight of the involuting uterus.

Vaginoscopy can be used to identify:

1. Rectovaginal fistulas – indicated by the presence of a green watery exudate with fecal matter on the vaginal floor. The location of the fistula can be determined by examining the dorsum of the vagina and vestibulum as the speculum is extracted from the vagina. It will appear as a small to large opening containing feces.

2. Persistent hymen – may be present in maiden mares. On vaginal speculum examination it will appear as a thin, bluish-white sheet of tissue covering the cranial aspect of the vestibulovaginal junction. If the hymen is complete the speculum cannot be advanced into the vagina. In fillies that have reached puberty and are having estrous cycles the hymen may bulge out through the lips of the vulva. This is a result of the accumulation in the cranial vagina of uterine fluids produced during estrus.

3. Necrotic vaginitis – may occur as a sequela to dystocia and can be life-threatening. On vaginal speculum examination the vaginal walls will be black and necrotic or gray and granulomatous. There will be a foul odor when the speculum is passed into the vagina.

### Manual examination of the vagina

Evaluation of the mare's genital tract is incomplete without manually exploring the vaginal and cervical lumen. Aseptic technique is essential in these procedures, in preparation of both the mare and the hand and arm of the examiner. A sterile, shoulder-length, latex glove is ideal, but a practical alternative is a clean plastic sleeve with a sterile surgeon's glove applied over it. Lubrication should be with a sterile, water-soluble product. When the gloved hand is introduced into the mare's vagina the labia should be parted with the fingers of the other hand to reduce contamination. The vestibulovaginal junction should be tight, making it difficult for the examiner to pass the hand. If the hand slips easily into the cranial vagina the mare may be predisposed to developing pneumovagina. In maiden mares the vestibulovaginal junction should be palpated to ensure the absence of tissue bands formed by hymen remnants. Such bands could later contribute to a recto-vaginal perforation at parturition.

The cervix should always be palpated directly if a complete reproductive examination is performed. By carefully dilating the external os and then palpating the entire cervical canal, it is possible to locate lacerations and adhesions not evident on vaginoscopy. The cervical os may be torn or the cervical body may be ruptured such that it is permanently overstretched.

> **Clinical Pointer**
>
> Because of the importance of the cervical seal during pregnancy, if a lesion is noted the cervix should be re-examined during diestrus to determine whether it closes completely.

## EXAMINATION OF THE POSTPARTUM MARE AND PLACENTA

The placenta should be passed within 5 hours of foaling. If it is still present 8 hours after foaling the mare needs immediate medical care because she may develop metritis, laminitis, and septicemia. The entire chorioallantois or only a small portion, usually a piece in the tip of one of the two horns, may be retained. If the entire chorioallantois is retained the examiner needs to determine the extent of placental retention and the firmness of its attachment. This can be accomplished by manually exploring the space between the endometrium and the placenta with one hand while twisting the placenta slowly with the other. If the placenta loosens it is lifted out of the uterus. If it remains firmly attached the mare is placed on appropriate antibiotics and non-steroidal anti-inflammatory drugs. The placenta should never be forcefully pulled. The degree of retention should be reassessed daily. If a small piece of placenta is retained it is rarely located by manual examination of the uterine lumen because it is most frequently in the tip of a uterine horn and cannot be reached.

Mares that develop metritis will be dull, depressed, and quiet. The heart and respiratory rates will be increased and intestinal sounds diminished. With increasing severity the mare may exhibit colic, be febrile, and develop laminitis and ileus. The diagnosis of acute metritis is made on a general physical and reproductive examination and clinical pathology parameters

- the uterus will be large, fluid filled, and flaccid
- there will be a fetid, slimy, dark-red, vaginal discharge
- Gram-negative, Gram-positive, and anaerobic bacteria may be isolated
- the circulating total white blood count will frequently drop below $5000/\mu l$ ($5 \times 10^9/l$)
- the fibrinogen will be greater than 5 g/dl (0.5 g/l)
- toxic and immature neutrophils will be present.

The placenta should always be examined for completeness and pathological changes. Both the fetal and maternal sides of the chorioallantois need to be examined. The fetal side will have a bluish-white tinge to it, whereas the maternal side will have a red, velvety, appearance. The placenta should be laid out in an F-shape on a flat surface. There should be no tears in the tips of the horns and both horns must be present. In the case of twin placentas only one horn may be present.

## Clinical Pointer

If a piece of placenta is missing the uterus should be examined and the mare remain under close medical supervision for 3–5 days.

Most pathology is observed on the maternal side of the chorioallantois, frequently in the area of the cervical star. In ascending placentitis or premature placental separation the area surrounding the cervical star may be brown and granular in appearance. A discharge may or may not be present on the placental surface. In a hematogenous placentitis the placental body or horn is most frequently affected. The affected area will be white, brown or black, edematous, and thickened. If placentitis is suspected a uterine culture should be taken. In the case of twins, a large white avillous area where the two placentas abutted will be present. Sections of abnormal and normal-appearing placenta should be collected and placed in formalin for histological interpretation if pathology is suspected. The areas affected and the samples taken should be recorded.

## Clinical Pointer

A Polaroid camera is useful as the photograph can be marked to indicate where the samples of placenta were procured.

## ANCILLARY DIAGNOSTIC AIDS

Diagnostic procedures that are routinely performed to augment the general reproductive tract examination include

- endometrial cytology
- culture of secretions and discharges
- endometrial biopsy
- ultrasonography.

## Endometrial cytology

The presence of neutrophils in a cytological specimen obtained from the uterine lumen indicates an active inflammatory process. Cytological examination of the uterus can be helpful in establishing a diagnosis in chronic or low-grade endometritis, especially if the physical examination does not reveal signs of inflammation, such as hyperemia or exudate.

Various methods for collecting samples of endometrium are available, including swabbing, aspiration, or curettage. To be diagnostically useful and practical under field conditions, the examination must be rapid, simple, and produce consistent results. The following technique is recommended.

1. Samples of endometrium and luminal contents are obtained with the same instrument used to obtain samples for microbiological cultures, a disposable guarded culture instrument with a plastic cap (Kalayjian Industries, Long Beach, CA). The swab in this instrument is guarded by the cap and outer tube as it is passed through the cervix.
2. Once in the uterus the swab is exposed by pushing it against the cap, which snaps open. The cap remains attached to the tube by a plastic stalk.
3. After the swab is saturated for the microbiological sample it is retracted back into the tube.
4. While the swab is still in the uterine lumen the entire tube is rotated briskly several times, causing the cap to collect a sample of endometrium and uterine fluid.
5. As soon as the instrument is withdrawn the cap is cut off and a slide prepared from the fluid and cellular material it contains. This is done by placing the open end of the cap on a slide and tapping it briskly with the index finger to transfer the sample to the slide. The sample is spread gently and allowed to air dry.
6. A simple three-step staining process (Diff-Quik, Harleco) has proved practical and effective for field use. Staining takes a few minutes and slides may be examined wet or allowed to dry for later evaluation. Permanent mounting of a cover slip is recommended for long-term storage of slides.

A specimen that has been properly collected and prepared will have sheets of epithelial cells found throughout the slide. If no epithelial cells are seen there is no assurance that the uterine lining was scraped sufficiently. This problem tends to occur in older, pluriparous mares whose uterus is located ventral to the pelvis. If many neutrophils are seen inflammation is present. Interpretation of the vast majority of samples processed in this manner is straightforward as positive or negative. Occasional samples show few neutrophils. In these cases a ratio of neutrophils to epithelial cells should be calculated. If this is higher than 1 neutrophil to 10 epithelial cells, inflammation may be judged to be significant.

## Culture of secretions and discharges

The secretions and discharges of the reproductive tract can be collected using a variety of techniques. The traditional wire loop method is available, as well as various types of guarded swabs. Samples are collected either through a speculum or by manual insertion to the desired location. Care must be taken to avoid contamination of the uterus with introduced bacteria. Extracorporeal, vulvar, and vaginal contamination are all potential sources of bacteria which can confound interpretation of the results. To eliminate these sources a clean site for examining the mare is selected, the vulvar and perineal areas are prepared aseptically, and only the instrument to sample the uterus is used.

The optimum time to recover uterine pathogens is the first or second day of standing estrus, even if the cervix is not fully relaxed. At that time secretions from the endometrium are increasing, making a moist swab easier to obtain, and the full flushing action of estrus has not yet developed. During diestrus the endometrium is often dry, making bacterial recovery more difficult. Also one may inoculate the uterus with bacteria carried on the hand from the vestibulum. The technique of culturing the uterus in the winter is questionable because the probability of isolating bacteria associated with chronic endometritis is low.

Immediately after collection uterine swabs should be placed directly in the final medium for culture. This will ensure the best culture yield. The number of bacteria declines as the swab dries, and any method that delays drying, such as

- refrigeration
- adding sterile saline to the swab
- placement in a culture transport medium

extends their viability.

It is fairly simple to culture and identify the organisms that cause endometritis. Therapeutic decisions can be made in most cases by grossly inspecting colonies and making Gram stains. Streaking the swab on blood agar plates and one selective Gram-negative medium is adequate, though more sophisticated multiple diagnostic plates are available commercially. Plates are incubated at 37°C (98.6°F), preferably in a candle jar to provide microaerophilic

conditions, and inspected daily. An indication of the number of colonies must be included in the laboratory report. Pure cultures are more significant than mixed ones.

The following organisms, in significant numbers, must be considered pathogenic

- β-hemolytic streptococci
- Hemolytic *E. coli*
- coagulase positive *Staphylococcus* spp.
- *Pseudomonas* spp.
- *Klebsiella* spp.
- *Monilia (Candida)* spp.

Other organisms, when isolated repeatedly, are occasionally suspect in the presence of inflammation. However, α-hemolytic streptococci, coagulase negative staphylococci, and various enteric organisms other than those listed above should generally be viewed as contaminants.

Culture results must be correlated with cytological findings. When cytological findings are persistently positive and cultures are negative, the cause of the inflammation remains to be determined. Other causes of inflammation include

- reflux of urine into the uterus
- pneumovagina, and
- hypersensitivity to antibiotics or chemicals infused into the uterus.

When cultures are positive and cytological findings are repeatedly negative, contamination of the sample is the usual conclusion.

---

### Clinical Pointer

When many mares are examined for uterine pathogens at one farm over a prolonged period it is advantageous to streak culture plates directly on location.

---

## Endometrial biopsy

Histological evaluation of the endometrium is helpful in assessing the degree of inflammation, noting the presence or absence of fibrosis and lymphatic lacunae and evaluating glandular density. Established standards for interpretation make this procedure an integral part of the reproductive examination.

Candidates for endometrial biopsy include

- barren mares with a clinically evident abnormality of the reproductive tract that fail to conceive after repeated breedings to a stallion of known high fertility

- mares with a history of early embryonic death
- mares with a history of acyclicity during the physiological breeding season
- non-pregnant mares presented for fertility evaluation as a part of a prepurchase examination
- mares requiring genital surgery that may not be capable of supporting a pregnancy to term, in these cases the biopsy should be done prior to surgical intervention.

The instrument of choice for obtaining an endometrial biopsy is a 70-cm alligator punch with a basket measuring 20 × 4 × 3 mm, made specifically for uterine biopsy (Pilling, Fort Washington, PA). Endometrial architecture changes with the stage of the cycle and the season of the year. For this reason, the person evaluating the biopsy should be informed of the stage of cycle and physical findings at the time the sample was taken.

After proper preparation of the mare, as described above (see Vaginoscopic examination), the instrument is introduced into the uterus with a gloved hand. The tip is guarded carefully as it passes through the cervix to prevent cervical trauma. When the basket is located well inside the uterine lumen, the hand is withdrawn from the vagina and inserted into the rectum. The instrument is then directed to the uterine area chosen for biopsy. When previously detected focal lesions are present, multiple biopsies are indicated and should include the area(s) in question as well as a portion of endometrium that feels normal. In the absence of palpable focal lesions the base of either horn should be sampled.

The safest method for taking a biopsy is to turn the instrument on its side and press a portion of endometrium between the side walls of the punch with the index finger of the hand in the rectum. If the uterus is pushed into the front of the 20-mm basket there is a chance of cutting through the entire uterus. After removal from the tract the specimen is removed from the basket very gently with a small-gauge hypodermic needle. Rough handling disrupts the luminal epithelium of the sample. The tissue should immediately be placed in fixative. Cellular detail and tissue integrity are best preserved using Bouin's fixative for 12–24 hours, followed by replacement of the Bouin's solution with 80% ethanol; 10% formalin is also used but tends to create more tissue distortion on sectioning. The fixed tissue is trimmed for embedding in paraffin, so that sections are cut perpendicular to the endometrial surface. Paraffin-embedded sections are best stained with hematoxylin and eosin for routine examination. For proper interpretation, specimens need to have at least 1–2 cm of endometrium.

> ## Clinical Pointer ✳
>
> Endometrial biopsies may be obtained at any stage of the estrous cycle because the equine cervix is easily dilated.

The major pathological changes found in endometrial biopsies are

- inflammation
- fibrosis, and
- lymphatic stasis.

To be of diagnostic and prognostic value these changes must be characterized and quantified.

**Endometrial inflammation** This is characterized by increased numbers of inflammatory cells, either in foci or diffused in various areas of the lamina propria. The cellular infiltrate is classified by the predominant cell type

- in acute endometritis the predominant cell type is the polymorphonuclear neutrophil
- in subacute endometritis there is a mixture of neutrophils and lymphocytes
- in chronic endometritis there are lymphocytes, plasma cells, and macrophages.

**Endometrial fibrosis** This occurs most commonly around the glands and appears in response to inflammation or glandular damage, or from other undefined causes. Periglandular fibrosis may interfere with gland function to the extent that glandular support of the early conceptus is altered and causes early embryonic death between 35 and 70 days.

**Lymphatic stasis** This appears as large, fluid-filled spaces lined with endothelial cells. When widespread and accompanied by a jelly-like consistency of the uterus on rectal palpation, this lesion is correlated with reduced fertility. Because large areas of edema may be artificially produced during the biopsy procedure care must be taken to identify the spaces as lymphatics.

When these basic pathological changes are observed they should be evaluated for severity and distribution. This allows mares to be categorized into three diagnostic and prognostic groups.

**Category I** includes mares with an endometrium compatible with conception and capable of supporting a foal to term. Any pathological changes are slight and widely scattered. No endometrial atrophy or hypoplasia is seen on biopsies taken during the physiological breeding season. Mares in category I have a ≥ 70% probability of producing a live foal.

**Category II** includes mares with endometrial changes that reduce the chance of conception and pregnancy maintenance but which are reversible or only moderately severe. Endometrial changes may include combinations of any of the following

- slight to moderate, diffuse cellular infiltrations of superficial layers
- scattered but frequent inflammatory or fibrotic foci throughout the entire lamina propria
- scattered but frequent periglandular fibrosis of individual gland branches of any degree of severity
- ≤ 3 nests of gland branches per low-power field in five fields (fields 5 mm in diameter)
- mild to moderate lymphatic stasis.

Pregnancy rates for mares in this category range from 30% to 70%, depending on the severity of the lesions. Frequently, this category is divided into IIa, that due to inflammation, and IIb, that due to fibrosis. As there is no treatment for fibrosis, mares in category IIb have a lower likelihood of carrying a foal to term.

**Category III** includes mares with endometrial changes that reduce the chances of conception and pregnancy maintenance, and which are essentially irreversible. The endometrium may contain any of the following changes

- widespread periglandular fibrosis of any degree of severity, with ≥ 5 nests in an average low-power field
- widespread, diffuse, severe cellular infiltration of superficial layers
- widespread lymphatic stasis accompanied by palpable changes in the uterus
- endometrial atrophy or hypoplasia with gonadal dysgenesis
- pyometra accompanied by rectally palpable endometrial atrophy or widespread, diffuse, severe inflammatory-cell infiltration.

Mares in category III have less than a 10% chance of becoming pregnant.

**Clinical Pointer**

Care should be taken in declaring a mare sterile on the basis of single or even multiple biopsies.

## Ultrasonography

Ultrasonography has now become an integral part of the examination of the reproductive tract. It can be used to diagnose uterine disease, such as intrauterine fluid, air, and cysts, and to identify ovarian irregularities, such as anovulatory follicles, neoplasia, and hematomas. Also, examination of the ovaries by ultrasonography may aid in determining the stage of the estrous cycle, the status of preovulatory follicles, and development of the corpus luteum. Excellent in-depth reviews of reproductive tract ultrasonography are available.

The procedure and precautions are similar to those for rectal palpation. Feces must be thoroughly removed from the rectum before introducing the transducer, which should be well lubricated, and care should be taken to avoid fecal material attaching to the transducer. Good contact must exist (and be maintained) between the transducer and rectal wall. Air in the rectum or a gas or fluid-filled interposed loop of intestine will result in a distorted image.

A linear array 5 MHz transducer is most frequently used in routine equine reproductive work. Its use enables the operator to detect a conceptus on day 10 (day 0 being the day of ovulation), follicles as small as 3 mm in diameter, and the presence of a corpus luteum (CL) through most of diestrus. A linear array 2.5 or 3 MHz transducer is used to evaluate fetal viability using a transabdominal approach in later pregnancy.

### *Normal anatomy*

The uterus is visualized as a cross-sectional image. With the probe held in a sagittal plane the cranial aspect of the uterus is seen on the right of the ultrasound screen and the caudal aspect on the left. The uterus undergoes dynamic changes due to hormonal influences that can be visualized by ultrasonography. During estrus the uterine horns are well rounded, and both horns and body have an interdigitated pattern of alternating echogenic and non-echogenic areas, similar to the spokes on a wheel or slices of an orange (Fig. 22.9). The areas of decreased echogenicity are the outer edematous portions of endometrial folds. The edema

**A systematic scanning technique**

A systematic scanning technique needs to be developed to eliminate the possibility of missing structures or an embryonic vesicle. One method is to move the probe from

- uterine body to left uterine horn
- left uterine horn to left ovary
- re-examine the left uterine horn and uterine body
- evaluate the right uterine horn and right ovary
- return to the uterine body, and then
- scan the cervix.

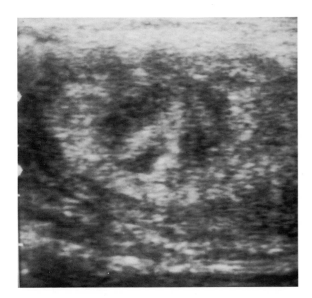

**Fig. 22.9** Ultrasound image of the uterine body on day 3 of estrus. Cranial aspect of the uterus is oriented to the left of the image. Note the interdigitated pattern of alternating echogenic and non-echogenic areas, similar to spokes on a wheel or slices of orange. Scale on left is in cm (from Kobluk, Ames and Goer, 1995, with permission).

is caused by the influence of estrogen. Endometrial folds generally parallel estrogen production and are visible at the end of diestrus, becoming quite prominent as estrus progresses and decreasing or disappearing 12 hours before ovulation. A small amount of fluid may be present normally within the uterine lumen during estrus. Endometrial folds are sometimes seen in early pregnancy, 16–28 days gestation, especially if large follicles are present on the ovaries.

During diestrus the echo texture is more homogeneous and the uterus is well circumscribed. The uterine lumen is often identified by a hyperechogenic white line in the area of apposing endometrial surfaces. During anestrus the uterus is flat and irregular and may contour closely to surrounding abdominal organs. The uterus during pregnancy appears similar to that during diestrus, except that endometrial folds may again appear after day 16 and a vesicle will be present.

Follicles are non-echogenic and appear as black, roughly circumscribed-shaped images. Follicles may appear irregular in shape owing to impending ovulation, or compression by adjacent follicles or luteal structures. Within 24 hours of ovulation a preovulatory follicle softens and becomes teardrop-shaped as it progresses toward the ovulation fossa. After the follicle ruptures a corpus hemorrhagicum forms. It has one of two appearances on ultrasound, either

- it is a uniformly echogenic circumscribed image (Fig. 22.10), or
- it contains a centrally non-echogenic center (Fig. 22.11).

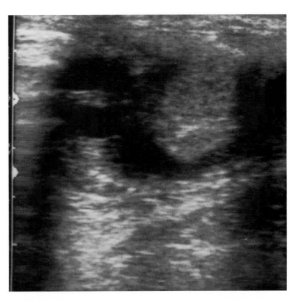

**Fig. 22.10** Ultrasound image of a 48-hour-old corpus hemorrhagicum. The corpus hemorrhagicum is located centrally within the ovary and is surrounded by non-echogenic fluid (from Kobluk, Ames and Goer, 1995, with permission).

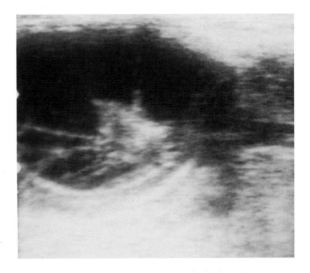

**Fig. 22.11** Corpus hemorrhagicum on day 1 post ovulation that has a non-echogenic central cavity and an echogenic portion with echogenic strands radiating into the fluid-filled central cavity (from Kobluk, Ames and Goer, 1995, with permission).

Echogenic lines attributable to clotting and fibrinization in the central non-echogenic center may be present. The corpus luteum is highly echogenic on the day of ovulation, echogenicity decreases and then plateaus during the first 6 days, and then increases over days 12–16.

## Pregnancy

The first ultrasound examination for pregnancy determination is usually performed between 14 and 20 days after ovulation, even though pregnancy status can be determined as early as day 10. The early equine conceptus, or vesicle, is highly mobile within the uterine lumen and moves between the uterine horns and uterine body from the time it enters the uterus on day 5.5 until days 16–17. Because the vesicle is moving it may be found anywhere within the uterine lumen, from the tip of a horn to the cranial aspect of the cervix. After day 17 the vesicle fixes at the caudal portion of one of the uterine horns near the bifurcation. Fixation of the early conceptus on days 16–17 is apparently caused by increased uterine tone and thickening of the uterine wall, as well as rapid growth of the conceptus.

Initially the vesicle is spherical and rapidly increasing in size. Between days 17 and 26 it becomes irregular in shape and its rate of growth plateaus (Fig. 22.12). Increasing uterine tone on days 16–17, combined with rapid enlargement of the vesicle, may explain this change in shape. After day 26 the vesicle resumes growth but at a slightly slower rate. The embryo is first detected within the vesicle by ultrasound at days 20–25. The heartbeat is commonly detected at about day 22 and is an important indicator of embryo wellbeing.

Location of the embryo within the vesicle varies with gestational age, generally moving from the ventral (day 22) to the dorsal (day 40) aspect of the vesicle. This positional change is caused by expansion of the allantois, with concurrent contraction of the yolk sac. After day 40 the yolk sac degenerates and the umbilical cord elongates from the dorsal pole, permitting the fetus to gravitate to the ventral floor, where it is seen in dorsal recumbency from day 50 onward. Apposition of yolk sac and allantois results in a visible line that is normally oriented horizontally (Fig. 22.13). At times, orientation of the yolk sac and allantois is abnormal and the line is oriented vertically. This does not adversely affect embryo development, but it may be confused with twin vesicles.

## Pathological changes visualized by ultrasonography

Uterine cysts, accumulations of intrauterine fluid, and air can be identified by ultrasonography. Uterine cysts vary in size from 5 to 50 mm and indicate an ongoing

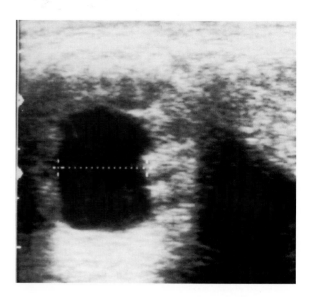

**Fig. 22.12** Ultrasound image of an 18-day embryonic vesicle. Note the irregular shape. Its width is 18 mm (dotted line) (from Kobluk, Ames and Goer, 1995, with permission).

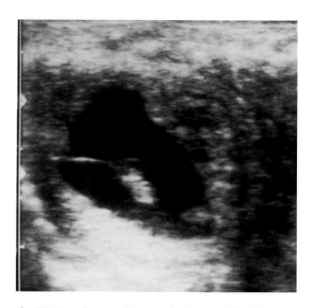

**Fig. 22.13** Ultrasound image of a 28-day-old embryo. The developing allantois is dorsal and the regressing yolk sac is ventral (from Kobluk, Ames and Goer, 1995, with permission).

degenerative process within the endometrium. There may be many small cysts that appear to be embedded within the endometrium, or just a single, large cyst containing many partitions.

Fluid present within the uterus during diestrus and the early postovulatory period has been associated with early embryonic death, endometritis, and decreased conception rates. A small amount of fluid in the uterine lumen during estrus does not appear to adversely affect fertility. Air within the uterus appears as multiple hyperechogenic reflections. If present during estrus or directly after ovulation, the mare should be closely examined for pneumovagina.

Anovulatory follicles, luteinized unruptured follicles, persistent corpus luteum, tumors and hematomas can be identified by ultrasonography. Anovulatory follicles result when preovulatory follicles grow to an unusual size (70–100 mm), fail to ovulate, fill with blood, and gradually recede. These follicles are distinctly echogenic, with criss-crossing fibrin-like strands without significant luteal tissue around the periphery. The granulosa theca cell tumor (GCT) (Fig. 22.14) and the teratoma are the two most common ovarian tumors

ovarian enlargement, the presence or absence of the ovulation fossa, the size of the contralateral ovary, and the concentration of inhibin in plasma.

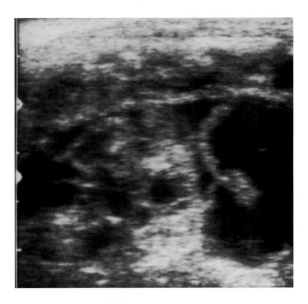

**Fig. 22.14** Granulosa cell theca tumor. Note the motheaten or cystic appearance (reprinted from Kobluk, Ames and Goer, 1995, with permission).

---

### Intraluminal cysts versus an embryo

It is helpful to record the presence of intraluminal cysts visualized by ultrasonography because they may be confused with an embryo. Characteristics of the embryo that can be used to differentiate the two include

- early mobility (days 10–16)
- the presence of specular reflection on the upper and lower surfaces of the vesicle
- spherical appearance without partitions
- growth rate.

---

and characteristically have a "honeycomb" appearance, with multiple small non-echogenic areas separated by echogenic trabeculae. However, the GCT can be highly variable in appearance, some containing one to two cysts (60–88 mm in diameter; Fig. 22.14), others being homogeneously dense throughout. Measurement of plasma inhibin concentrations can be used to diagnose GCT definitively. An ovarian hematoma can be confused with a GCT because they appear similar on ultrasound, and some GCTs have hematomas within their stroma. Frequently, hematomas appear uniformly echogenic. Some may appear as lucid areas separated by trabeculae (Fig. 22.15), similar to those of a multicystic GCT (Fig. 22.14). Diagnosis of GCT and hematomas must be made on the basis of clinical signs, the rapidity of

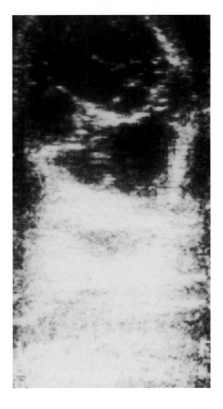

**Fig. 22.15** Ultrasound image of a hematoma (from Kobluk, Ames and Goer, 1995, with permission).

# The Stallion

## INTRODUCTION

The reproductive tract of the stallion is examined primarily to evaluate fertility potential and to diagnose gross abnormalities of the external genitalia. It is critical that the examination is thorough and results are properly recorded, as findings are frequently used for sale purposes, for obtaining fertility insurance, or for making recommendations on breeding management.

Rectal examinations are not routinely performed because of the inherent risks to both the examiner and the stallion. This chapter describes physical examination procedures, discusses semen collection and evaluation and presents the Breeding Soundness Examination guidelines established by the Society for Theriogenology for categorizing a stallion's breeding potential.

A complete history detailing the medical problems, injuries, and vaccinations and drug therapy the stallion has received over the past 6 months needs to be recorded. It should also include the dates of the performance career, and the present use of the stallion. Previous breeding performance, including

- first-cycle conception rates
- pregnancy rate for the year
- libido
- mating behavior, and
- any abnormalities encountered during breeding

need to be recorded. Results of previous fertility examinations and past breeding management should be evaluated and compared to the present findings, especially if the stallion has decreased fertility.

A general physical examination should be performed at the initial evaluation. Mismanagement, inadequate nutrition, or a medical disorder may lead secondarily to a deterioration in semen quality.

---

### Examination of the stallion for breeding purposes

The examination should include

- evaluation of the external genitalia
- evaluation of libido
- assessment of ability to mate
- collection of semen to determine sperm numbers, progressive motility, and morphology.

---

### Identification of the stallion

The animal must be positively identified by noting

- name
- age
- breed
- registration number
- lip tattoo
- hide brands
- color markings
- hair whorls.

A photograph is a particularly helpful permanent record, especially when sale of the horse is involved.

---

Particular attention should be directed to auscultation of the heart and evaluation of the eyes and gait. Observation of the stallion moving freely in a small paddock allows one to identify any musculoskeletal problems, such as chronic degenerative joint disease, laminitis, or back disorders. Potentially heritable traits such as cryptorchidism, brachygnathia, or wobbler syndrome need to be recorded. Supporting clinical laboratory data should be collected if there is debate about any of the physical examination findings.

## EXAMINATION OF EXTERNAL GENITALIA

The scrotum, testicles, epididymis, penis, and prepuce are examined routinely by manual palpation. Ultrasonography or endoscopy can be used to complement the examination.

### Scrotum and its contents

The external genitalia can be examined by placing the animal in a set of stocks with the side bars located above the ventral abdomen. This allows the examiner to grasp the scrotum below the bar while either standing or bending down next to the horse's flank. If stocks are not available the horse may be backed into a padded corner. A twitch on the nose or chain over the upper

---

### Clinical Pointer

It is often easier to examine the scrotum and spermatic cords after semen collection, when a stallion is usually more manageable.

gum (lip chain) is useful in diverting the horse's attention during examination. The examiner needs to move slowly and stay close to the stallion while palpating the scrotum and its contents. A preferred technique is to approach the horse from the left just caudal to its shoulder, grasp the mane at the withers with the left hand and, keeping close contact with the body, slide the right hand medially along the ventral abdominal wall until the scrotum is grasped. Many stallions will squeal, flinch, and suck the scrotum up close to their body. A few will kick out. However, if the examiner remains in contact with the horse's body and moves the hand slowly most stallions will tolerate the examination. Once the animal has relaxed both hands can be used to palpate the scrotal contents.

The scrotum in the stallion is pendulous, smooth, thin, elastic, and hairless (Fig. 22.16). During manual palpation, or in extremely cold temperatures, it may be drawn toward the body by voluntary contractions of the cremaster muscles. Both testes and attached epididymides should be freely movable within their respective scrotal pouches. There should be no free fluid within the scrotum (hydrocele), nor should there be any extraneous tissue within the sac (scrotal hernia). The scrotum should be free of scars and granulomatous lesions.

The testes should be palpated carefully to determine their general shape, size, orientation, and texture. Normal testes are oval and turgid, similar in size and with a smooth surface. Testicular parenchyma should bulge slightly between the fingers when compressed. The testes lie horizontally, with the head of the epididymis closely apposed in a cranial position (Fig. 22.17). The body of the epididymis is loosely apposed on the dorsolateral surface of the testis, with the tail located on the caudal pole of the testis. The epididymis

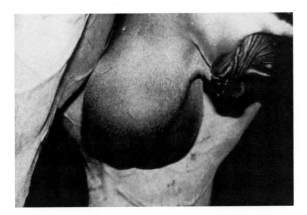

**Fig. 22.16** Scrotum of a stallion containing two testes and their attached epididymides.

---

### Clinical Pointer

It is not uncommon for some stallions to have one of the testes rotated 180° without the animal showing any pain or its having a negative effect on fertility.

---

should have a soft, spongy texture. There should be no firm nodules, heat, or pain on palpation. The prominent tail of the epididymis and the remnant of the gubernaculum (caudal ligament of the epididymis) serve as landmarks for orientation of the testis. The caudal ligament palpates as a small (1–2 cm) fibrous nodule adjacent to the epididymal tail that is attached to the caudal pole of the testis.

A small portion of the spermatic cord can be palpated through the neck of the scrotum, although its specific contents are not always definable. The two cords should be of equal size and uniform in diameter (2–3 cm). Acute pain in this area is usually associated with inguinal herniation or torsion of the spermatic cord.

## Penis and prepuce

The penis and prepuce are best examined by stimulating penile tumescence through exposing the stallion to an estrous mare. The penis can be examined while the horse urinates, or it may be allowed to protrude under the influence of a tranquilizer. Because phenothiazine-derivative tranquilizers have been incriminated in some cases of paralytic paraphimosis, they should not be used indiscriminately. The penis can be grasped proximal to the glans and then rinsed with warm water and cotton to remove smegma and debris prior to inspection. Good illumination at floor level is essential, as is good restraint because the stallion may be unaccustomed to such advances. A bean-sized mass of inspissated sebum (smegma) that may be present in the urethral fossa needs to be removed and the urethral process, glans penis and diverticula carefully cleansed and examined.

---

### Lesions found on the penis and prepuce

- nodules or cutaneous pustules associated with coital exanthema
- granulomas from *Habronema* sp.
- papillomas
- sarcoids
- squamous cell carcinomas.

Scarring, abrasions, or the presence of a hematoma are indicative of trauma.

---

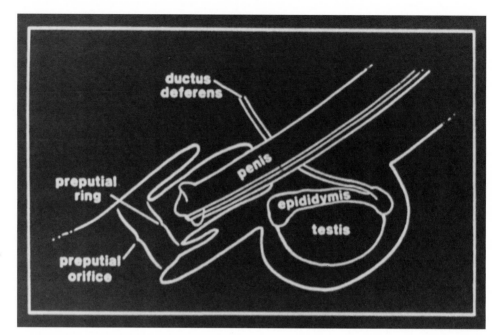

**Fig. 22.17**
Configuration of the stallion's prepuce and related structures. Taken from Varner et al, 1991.

The skin of the prepuce should be thin and pliable, with no evidence of inflammatory or proliferative lesions.

If a stallion is being examined for fertility potential the testes are measured with either calipers (scrotal width) or ultrasonography (testes volume; see Ultrasonography) because testicular size is related to daily sperm output. Scrotal width is measured by grasping the neck of the scrotum with one hand above the testes and pushing the testes down into the scrotum. The ends of the calipers (Lane Manufacturing, Denver, CO; Fig. 22.18) are then placed on the widest part of the testes and closed so that

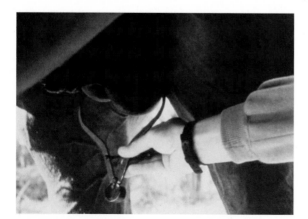

**Fig. 22.18**   Measurement of scrotal width in a stallion using calipers.

there is slight pressure on the scrotum. The width between the two ends of the calipers is measured with a tape. Total scrotal width of mature stallions with normal fertility ranges from 95 to 120 mm.

## EXAMINATION OF INTERNAL GENITALIA

The internal genitalia are not always examined because of the highly excitable and aggressive nature of stallions. If there is evidence of a problem, such as pus, bacteria, or inflammatory cells in the ejaculated semen, or there is no semen in the ejaculate, evaluation of the accessory glands is warranted. Stallions that are to be evaluated may need tranquilization. If an α-agonist drug is to be given it should be used in combination with another drug such as butorphenol to reduce hypersensitivity through the hindquarters and the horse's tendency to kick.

The stallion has four distinct accessory sex glands

- the paired ampullae which surround the terminal segment of each deferent duct
- the bilobed prostate
- the paired bulbourethral glands
- the paired vesicular glands (seminal vesicles) (Fig.22.19).

The glands are dynamic in nature in that they change shape and size with sexual excitation. All four glands contribute to the watery fluids that are secreted at ejaculation, whereas the gel is only from the vesicular glands. Although readily accessible, it is difficult to accurately identify all four glands by rectal palpation owing to their texture. Therefore, if pathology is suspected it is best to ultrasound the glands per rectum using a 7.5 MHz probe and culture the seminal fluids that pass through a catheter placed 15–20 cm into the urethra after the stallion has been exposed to an estrous mare.

## Ampullae

The ampullae are paired tubular glandular thickenings of the distal ductus deferens located dorsal to the bladder. They are easily located by rectal palpation by moving one's hand cranially along the pelvic urethra until the two ductus deferens are palpated near the neck of the bladder. There is a palpable widening of the ductus deferens, 20–25 cm in length, 2–4 cm cranial to the bifurcation. These are the ampullae. Anatomically the ampullae have a central fluid-filled lumen surrounded by an inner glandular layer and an outer muscular layer. Ultrasonographically

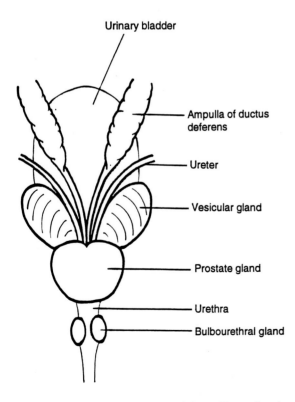

**Fig. 22.19**   Accessory sex glands of the stallion – dorsal view.

- the lumen appears dark (echolucent)
- the glandular parenchyma appears gray
- the muscular layer appears bright (echogenic).

The diameter of the ampulla averages 13 mm. The luminal diameter of the ampulla doubles in size following teasing and decreases to resting values following ejaculation. The prominent size of the ampullae and the large cross-sectional area of the glandular tissue creates the potential for excessive accumulation of sperm and glandular secretions. This may result in distension of the glandular portion and possible blockage of the duct and azoospermia.

## Prostate gland

The prostate gland is located dorsal to the intersection of the pelvic urethra and the bladder neck. It is entirely external to the urethra and is divided into a narrow central isthmic portion and two lobular portions that follow the lateral edges of the pelvic urethra. It is soft and difficult to palpate via the rectum and is best identified ultrasonographically. The interior of the prostate contains gray glandular parenchyma and narrow bands of dark fluid. The prostate gland increases in size and fluid content following teasing and decreases to sexually rested values following ejaculation.

## Bulbourethral glands

The bulbourethral glands are ovoid organs located dorsolateral to the pelvic urethra in the vicinity of the ischial arch. They are difficult to identify by rectal palpation because of their thick muscular covering. Ultrasonographically, the bulbourethral gland contains homogeneous gray parenchyma and small (1–2 mm) pockets of dark fluid. The border is highly echogenic due to the muscular covering. They average 28 mm long and 19 mm wide. They do not change significantly in size or shape with teasing and ejaculation.

## Vesicular glands

The vesicular glands are elongated, pyriform sacs with a central lumen located on either side of the bladder neck. Their long axes radiate cranially and laterally from the origin at the proximal pelvic urethra. To locate them via the rectum one locates the urethra on the floor of the pelvis and moves the hand cranially until the bifurcation of the ductus deferens is palpated. The examiner then rotates the wrist laterally, opens the hand and gently gropes along the lateral wall of the pelvic inlet. If the vesicular gland is filled with fluid, a long, soft, spongy structure is palpable. Inflamed vesicular glands may be enlarged and firm, and occasionally have a lobulated texture and irregular borders. They are rarely painful except in acute stages of disease.

## Clinical Pointer

The vesicular glands can be difficult to palpate per rectum unless they are filled with fluid or inflamed.

The semen of stallions with seminal vesiculitis has varying quantities of neutrophils with clumps of purulent material. Bacteria may be seen on microscopic examination. Ultrasonographically the vesicular glands are irregular in shape with thin, bright walls and a dark central lumen. The vesicular glands of sexually rested stallions are dorsoventrally flattened pouches with gray muscular walls and a dark central lumen. The lumen increases in diameter following teasing, and decreases or disappears following ejaculation.

### Inguinal regions

The inguinal rings are most commonly explored by rectal palpation to determine the location of a retained testis and to evaluate the contents of the inguinal canal in horses with inguinal or scrotal hernia. To identify the location of a retained testes, both the superficial inguinal ring and the deep inguinal ring on the side of the retained testis need to be palpated.

1. The superficial inguinal ring can be located by palpating the ventral abdominal wall between the penis and the medial aspect of the thigh. If the examiner is having difficulty in identifying the inguinal ring on the side of the undescended testis, the spermatic cord of the descended testicle can be palpated and followed up to the superficial inguinal ring to estimate the other ring's location in relationship to the thigh and penis. The opening of the superficial inguinal ring is 2–3 cm in diameter and the canal is 10–12 cm long. The ring is directed laterally, cranially, and slightly ventrally from the edge of the prepubic tendon.
2. The deep inguinal rings (also referred to as vaginal rings) are identified on rectal palpation as slit-like openings ventrolateral to the pelvic brim. To locate them the examiner clears all feces out of the rectum as far cranially as can be reached, and then passes a well lubricated hand just cranial to the pelvic brim, moving it ventrally and laterally until contact is made with the abdominal wall. The examiner then sweeps the hand medially and

laterally while slowly retracting it caudally. During the procedure the hand will come into contact with either vessels entering the inguinal ring, or with the ring itself. The stallion must be adequately restrained during this procedure to permit an accurate evaluation.

Cryptorchidism is categorized as either complete or incomplete abdominal retention, depending on the location of the undescended testis and its associated structures. In incomplete abdominal retention the testis is usually located in the abdomen and the vaginal tunic and its contents (epididymal tail, gubernaculum, and vas deferens) are palpable in the inguinal region. The testis is close to the deep inguinal ring and has less potential mobility than is found with complete abdominal retention. In complete abdominal retention the testis usually lies close to the deep inguinal ring, though it may become mixed up with coils of intestine and may lie dorsal to the rectum or lateral to the bladder. In exceptional cases it is adherent to the wall of the abdomen or to other organs, such as the spleen, and may then be exceedingly difficult to identify. A testis found within the abdomen is small and characteristically flabby.

## BREEDING SOUNDNESS EXAMINATION

The Society of Theriogenology has established guidelines for evaluating fertility potential. The Breeding Soundness Examination (BSE) is used to make recommendations on the number of mares that a stallion may mate successfully each season. Stallions are rated as unsatisfactory, questionable, or satisfactory breeders. Stallions that pass the examination are expected to render at least 75% of 40 or more mares pregnant when bred naturally, or 75% of 120 mares when bred artificially in one breeding season, when under good management and given fertile mares. In addition, stallions with genetic defects are identified and owners are alerted of potential problems.

The BSE includes

- identification
- physical examination
- evaluation of external genitalia
- libido
- mating ability
- semen quality, and
- testis size.

In the BSE two semen samples are collected 1 hour apart after the stallion has had a week of sexual rest. If the two samples are representative, the total number of live, progressively motile, morphologically normal, sperm in the second ejaculate is a fairly accurate assessment of daily sperm output. A sample is representative if the second ejaculate contains between 30% and 70% of the total sperm numbers seen in the first ejaculate. The number of live, progressively motile, morphologically normal, sperm needed for a stallion to pass the BSE differs between months and is presented in Table 22.3.

## Semen collection

Semen can be collected by having the stallion mount an estrous mare, a phantom or, in some cases, by manual stimulation while he is standing on the ground. Prior to collection the stallion should be teased with a mare in behavioral estrus to stimulate erection. Once erect, the penis and associated external genitalia need to be inspected for lesions and the penis cleansed to minimize contamination of the ejaculate with bacteria, dirt, and epithelial debris. The penis is routinely rinsed with water only because repeated cleansing with soap scrubs removes the normal bacterial flora and may allow overgrowth of potentially pathogenic organisms. After it is washed the penis should be dried with paper towels, as water may be spermicidal. The washing procedure can be performed in the center of the breeding shed or, if the stallion is fractious, with the animal backed into a corner.

Prior to semen collection it is important that individuals involved are well versed on the procedure. All personnel involved in collecting the semen should wear helmets. The person collecting the semen normally stands 2–3 feet behind the handler as the stallion attempts to mount the phantom or mare. Once he has mounted, the penis should be deflected to the left and introduced into the artificial vagina (AV). If the stallion is reluctant to thrust it may be necessary for the semen collector to

- change the pressure or temperature of the water in the water jacket
- place warm, wet compresses at the base of the penis, or

- use slight manual pressure ventrally and laterally at the base of the penis.

Ejaculation is recognized by the appearance of fluid in the collection receptacle, by urethral pulsations, or by the stallion flagging its tail. If the stallion is difficult to handle or has never been used for semen collection a fourth person may be needed to assist. This person will stand to the right of the collector, facing the stallion's hip and, if needed, will place manual pressure on the stallion's hip to keep the horse up on the mount. This person will also monitor the behavior of the stallion and mare, and if a problem occurs will pull the collector out of harm's way.

There are a number of AVs commercially available for semen collection, each with its own attributes and peculiarities. Basically, models have an outer rigid tube and an inner soft liner, with the space between the two filled with warm water. The collecting system is arranged so that semen contacts the latex liner for the shortest time possible. A model that is widely used in the USA is the Missouri Model AV (Nasco, Fr Atkinson, WI; Fig. 22.20). It has fairly good heat retention and, because the glans penis should extend beyond the water jacket at the time of ejaculation, the internal temperature of the AV may exceed the 45–48°C spermatozoal tolerance threshold without causing heat-related injury to ejaculated sperm.

The AV should be prepared immediately before attempting semen collection. It needs to be filled with warm (48–50°C) water to provide an internal temperature of 44–48°C. The inner surface needs to be well lubricated with a non-spermicidal lubricant (Priority Care, Gilberts, IL) before the penis is inserted. The luminal pressure should be adjusted so that the penis fits snugly within the AV, but not to the extent that it is

| Table 22.3. Minimum number of morphologically normal, progressively motile sperm by month | | | | | |
|---|---|---|---|---|---|
| *Number X 10⁹ per ejaculate* | | | | | |
| Jan. | Feb. | Mar. | Apr. | May | June |
| 1.2 | 1.7 | 1.8 | 1.8 | 2.0 | 2.2 |
| July | Aug. | Sep. | Oct. | Nov. | Dec. |
| 1.8 | 1.7 | 1.2 | 1.2 | 1.2 | 1.0 |

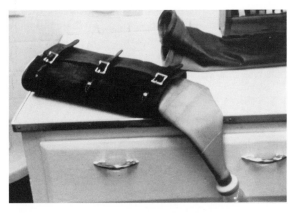

**Fig. 22.20** The Missouri Model artificial vagina for collecting semen from stallions.

difficult for the stallion to penetrate it. The penis needs to be inserted into the AV at the first thrust so that 50% or more of the shaft enters the AV. Otherwise, the glans penis may bell (dilate) near the AV opening and the penis will be too large for the shaft to be inserted, resulting in ejaculatory failure.

The receptacle used for semen collection should contain a filter for trapping the gel portion of the ejaculate. Separating the gel from the gel-free fractions maximizes the number of spermatozoa in the collection. The filter with its contained gel should be removed immediately upon collection of the semen to prevent seepage of gel into the gel-free portion of the ejaculate. During semen collection and transport to a laboratory, the receptacle should be protected from light and air and kept at body temperature to prevent cold shock of the sperm. Transport time should be minimal – less than 5 minutes. Some of the semen, 3–5 ml, should be reserved for evaluating concentration and motility. The remaining semen is extended in a prewarmed (37°C) milk-based extender (Kenney Milk Base Extender) at a ratio of 1:10 to 1:20 semen to extender and placed in an incubator set at 37°C. It appears that the greater the dilution factor, the better the spermatozoal survival rate.

## Semen evaluation

The quantity and quality of sperm produced is influenced by many factors, including

- season of year
- frequency of ejaculation
- thermal shock
- drug administration
- stress of performance
- age.

In general stallions produce more sperm in the summer than in the winter, with intermediate numbers found in the spring and autumn.

Semen parameters that are routinely evaluated in an ejaculate are the color, volume, motility (total and progressive), morphology, and concentration. Additional procedures include measuring pH, staining semen

> ### Clinical Pointer
>
> Unlike cattle and small ruminants there is no clear-cut link between semen quality and fertility in stallions, most probably because stallions placed at stud are chosen on past performance not on reproductive capability.

samples to identify bacteria or inflammatory cells, and longevity studies. All findings need to be recorded. A typical BSE form is presented in Figure 22.21.

Normal semen is pale white or skimmed milk-like in color. Mean volume is 60–70 ml (range 30–300 ml) per ejaculate. The volume will depend to some extent on the volume of the gel. Concentration of sperm will range from $100–800 \times 10^6$/ml, with a total output of $1–20\ 10^9$ sperm in each ejaculate. At least 50% of the sperm should be progressively motile (able to swim in a forward direction) and at least 50% should be morphologically normal.

The equipment for semen evaluation should be assembled before collection. It does not need to be elaborate but should include a microscope (a phase-contrast microscope with a heated stage is preferable), a hemacytometer or densitometer, slides, coverslips, pipettes, formal buffered saline, a receptacle for measuring volume, stain for assessing morphology, (e.g. nigrosin/eosin), semen extender, and a water bath or incubator to keep the sample at 37°C. All slides, coverslips, and extenders that come in contact with the semen also need to be maintained at 37°C. This can be accomplished by placing them in an incubator or on a slide warmer.

## *Motility of sperm*

> ### Clinical Pointer
>
> Sperm motility must be evaluated within 5 minutes of collection.

Both initial motility and the longevity of undiluted and extended semen should be assessed and recorded. Assessment of motility is subjective, but the same observer can become very consistent. A technique for evaluating motility is to place a drop of raw semen onto a warmed (37°C) slide, coverslip it and evaluate the motility of at least 50 sperm under 40 × power. Five sperm per field are chosen and the number of those five sperm that are moving, i.e. the total motility, are counted. The examiner then counts how many of the five sperm are swimming across the slide, this number represents progressive motility. Ten or more fields are evaluated to determine the percentage of total motile and progressively motile sperm in the raw sample. The procedure is then repeated using the samples diluted in semen extender. The longevity of spermatozoal motility is determined on raw semen samples and on samples diluted in various extenders during stored refrigeration (4–5°C) at 8, 12, 24, 36 and 48 hours after collection.

Association Offices
P.O. Box 2118
Hastings, NE 68902-2118

Telephone(402)463-0392
Facsimile(402)463-5683
Date: _____

**Society for Theriogenology**
**Stallion Breeding Soundness Evaluation Form**
Form Number: **A 02556**

**Stallion Information:** _____
Name: _____
Age: _____ Breed: _____ Color: _____
Lip Tatoo #: _____ Registration #: _____
Markings/Brands: _____
_____

Present Breeding Status:
☐ Sexually rested    ☐ Actively breeding
☐ At daily sperm output
Intended Use: _____
_____
_____

**Owner/Agent:** _____
Address: _____
_____
_____
Telephone: _____
Facsimile: _____
**Referring Veterinarian:** _____
Telephone: _____
**Veterinary Examiner:** _____
Address: _____
_____
_____
Telephone: _____

**History:** _____
_____
_____
_____
_____

**Physical Breeding Condition:** _____
_____
_____
_____
_____

**External Genital Examination:**    Method(s) Used    ☐ Palpation    ☐ Ultrasound    ☐ Other _____

| | Left | Right |
|---|---|---|
| **Testis:** | | |
| L x W x H (cm): | _____ | _____ |
| Volume (cm$^3$): | _____ | _____ |
| Consistency: | _____ | _____ |
| **Epididymis:** | _____ | |
| **Spermatic Cord:** | _____ | |

- **Prepuce:** _____
- **Penis:** _____
- **Scrotum:** _____
- Total Width (cm): _____
- **Other Findings:** _____
_____

**Internal Genital Examination:**    ☐ Performed    ☐ Not performed
Method(s) Used:    ☐ Palpation    ☐ Ultrasound    ☐ Other _____

| | Left | Right | | Left | Right |
|---|---|---|---|---|---|
| **Inguinal Ring (size)** | _____ | _____ | **Ampulla:** | _____ | _____ |
| **Vesicular Gland:** | _____ | _____ | **Prostatic Lobe:** | _____ | _____ |

**Behavior and Breeding Ability:**

| Temperament | Libido | Erection | Mounting | Intromission | Ejaculation |
|---|---|---|---|---|---|
| | | | | | |

**Other Examination Findings:** _____
_____
_____

**Additional Diagnostic Tests:**

| Test | Date Performed | Results |
|---|---|---|
| _____ | _____ | _____ |
| _____ | _____ | _____ |
| _____ | _____ | _____ |

Page 1 of 2 (please turn page)
© Copyright 1992 Society for Theriogenology
FOR USE BY LICENSED VETERINARIANS ONLY

**Fig. 22.21**  Breeding Soundness Evaluation form developed by the Society for Theriogenology.

Society for Theriogenology
Stallion Breeding Soundness Evaluation Form
(Page 2 of 2)

Stallion Name: _____     Date: _____

| Semen Evaluation: | Ejaculate | | |
|---|---|---|---|
| | 1 | 2 | 3 |
| Collection Time: | | | |
| Collection Method: | | | |
| Number of Mounts/Time to First Mount (min): | | | |
| Volume (ml) - gel free/gel: | | | |
| Gross Appearance: | | | |
| Seminal pH/Seminal Osmolarity: | | | |
| Motility % (total progressive): ☐ raw ☐ extended | | | |
| Velocity (0-4 or microns/second): ☐ raw ☐ extended | | | |
| Concentration (x $10^6$/ml) - Method use: _____ | | | |
| Total Number of Sperm (x $10^9$): | | | |
| Total # Sperm x % Progressively Motile (x $10^9$): | | | |

**Sperm Morphology:** ☐ Buffered Formal Saline  ☐ Phase Contrast Microscopy  ☐ Bright Field Microscopy
☐ Stain _____     ☐ Other _____

| | | | |
|---|---|---|---|
| % Normal Sperm: | | | |
| % Abnormal Acrosomal Regions/Heads: | | | |
| % Tailless Heads: | | | |
| % Proximal Droplets: | | | |
| % Distal Droplets: | | | |
| % Abnormally-shaped/Bent Midpieces: | | | |
| % Bent/Coiled Tails: | | | |
| Premature (Round) Germ Cells: | | | |
| Other Cells (WBC, RBC, etc.): | | | |
| Total # Sperm x % Morphologically Normal (x $10^9$): | | | |

**Longevity (Viability) Test:** Reported as Storage Time (hours) / % Prog. Motile Sperm:

| | | | |
|---|---|---|---|
| _____ Raw at ___ °C: | | | |
| _____ Extender (10:1) at ___ °C: | | | |
| _____ Extender (10:1) at ___ °C: | | | |
| _____ Extender (25 x $10^6$ sperm/ml) at ___ °C: | | | |
| _____ Extender (25 x $10^6$ sperm/ml) at ___ °C: | | | |

**Culture and Sensitivity:**

| | | | |
|---|---|---|---|
| Pre-Wash Urethra | | | |
| Pre-Wash Penile Shaft | | | |
| Pre-Wash Fossa Glandis | | | |
| Post-Ejaculate Urethra | | | |
| Other: _____ | | | |
| _____ | | | |
| _____ | | | |

**Classification:** Based on the intended use of this stallion and interpretation of data resulting from this examination, the above stallion is classified as a (an):

Satisfactory Breeding          Questionable Breeding          Unsatisfactory Breeding
Prospect ☐                     Prospect ☐                     Prospect ☐

☐ See attached letter     Date: _____          Signature: _____
                                                     ☐ Member of Society for Theriogenology

                                                     Clinic Name: _____

## Spermatozoal morphology

Sperm can be evaluated as stained smears using standard bright-field microscope optics or as wet mounts using either phase-contrast microscopy or differential interference-contrast microscopy. Stains currently used include

- India ink
- eosin–nigrosin
- eosin–aniline blue
- Giemsa
- Wright.

To make a stained smear, one drop of semen is mixed with one to two drops of stain at one end of a glass slide. A second glass slide is placed at 45° in the middle of the first slide and pushed slowly towards the mixture of semen and stain. Once the stain–semen mixture has flowed under the edge of the top slide, the top slide is pulled slowly over the bottom slide. Poor technique results in artifactual changes, primarily an increase in the number of detached heads, kinked tails, head shape abnormalities, and clumping.

Wet mounts are made by fixing a few drops of semen in 3–5 ml of buffered formal saline or buffered 4% glutaraldehyde solution. A few drops of the fixed sample is placed on a slide, coverslipped and examined at 1000 × magnification. Artifactual changes are negligible using wet mounts. It may be difficult, however, to evaluate sperm heads owing to the three-dimensional field and the tendency of the cells to roll or float in the wet mount preparation.

A minimum of 200 sperm should be evaluated to accurately assess morphology. Normal sperm, as well as those with acrosomal, head, midpiece, and tail defects, and the presence of droplets need to be recorded (Fig. 22.22). Traditionally, abnormal sperm were categorized as having primary, secondary, or tertiary abnormalities

- primary abnormalities are associated with a defect in spermatogenesis and are therefore testicular in origin, they include defects in the head, acrosome, and midpiece, and severely coiled tails
- secondary abnormalities occur in the excurrent duct system and include kinked tails and proximal and distal cytoplasmic droplets

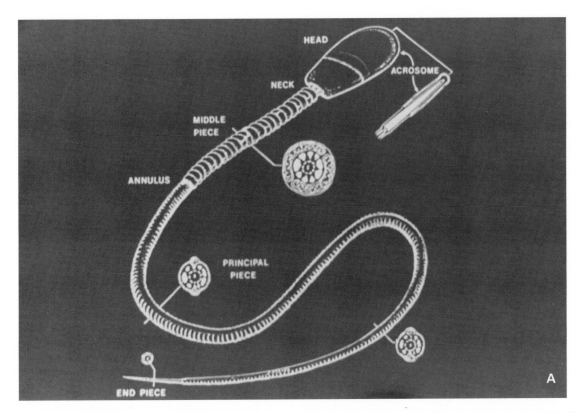

**Fig. 22.22** **(A)** Anatomy of equine spermatozoa. **(B)** Normal sperm (right) and one with a distal cytoplasmic droplet (left); **(C)** kinked tail; **(D)** folded acrosome. Adapted from Varner et al, 1991.

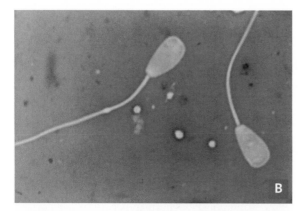

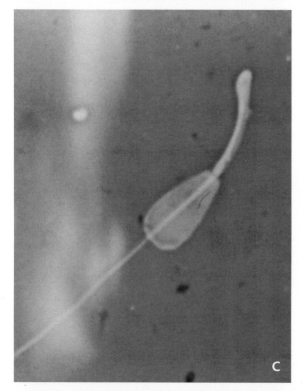

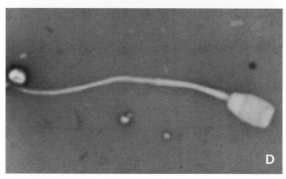

**Fig. 22.22 B,C and D**

- tertiary abnormalities develop in vitro as a result of improper semen collection or handling procedures, and include detached heads and kinked tails.

The classification of specific defects is considered superior to the traditional system because it reveals more specific information regarding a population of sperm.

### Spermatozoal concentration

The sperm concentration of gel-free semen can be measured with a properly calibrated hemacytometer or densimeter. A technique for counting sperm numbers with a hemacytometer is to add 50 μl of raw semen to 5 ml formal buffered saline and mix well. One drop of the solution is placed on the grid of the chamber and coverslipped. The fluid is allowed to settle for 3–5 minutes. The heads of sperm in either five small squares in the large central square of the hemacytometer (Neubauer chamber) or in all 25 small squares are counted. To determine the number of sperm per ml of ejaculate, the number of sperm counted is multiplied by $5 \times 10^6$ if only 5 squares are counted, and by $1 \times 10^6$ if all 25 squares are counted.

### pH and osmolarity determination

The pH of gel-free semen should be determined using a properly calibrated pH meter. The pH of normal semen is slightly basic, with a reported range of 7.2–7.7. The pH of normal stallion semen can be altered by

- season of the year
- frequency of ejaculation
- spermatozoal concentration.

Abnormally high pH can be associated with contamination of the ejaculate by urine or soap, or with inflammatory lesions of the genital tract.

### Clinical Pointer

Accurate measurement of sperm concentration is critical because total sperm number in an ejaculate is derived by multiplying sperm concentration and semen volume.

## ULTRASONOGRAPHY

Ultrasonography is helpful in

- assessing the accessory sex glands (see earlier) and scrotal contents
- measuring testicular volume to determine daily sperm output
- identifying the location of an undescended testis.

**Clinical Pointer** ✳

It is important, if any ultrasonographic abnormalities are noted, to evaluate the contralateral testis.

### Scrotum and testes

A 5 MHz transducer is most commonly used to measure testicular volume and to locate an undescended testis, whereas a 7.5 MHz transducer is used for scanning the accessory sex glands.

Ultrasonographically, normal testes have a homogeneous, echogenic appearance. In the center is a small (2–3 mm) circular non-echogenic area that corresponds to the central vein (Fig. 22.23). The epididymis has a mottled appearance ultrasonographically as it contains many echogenic and non-echogenic areas owing to fluid within the convoluted seminiferous tubules. Pathological conditions affecting the scrotum that may be visualized ultrasonographically include

- testicular neoplasia
- abscesses
- hematocele
- orchitis
- scrotal hernia, and
- hydrocele.

Testicular neoplasia may be differentiated from normal testicular tissue by its decreased echogenicity, but cannot be differentiated from orchitis or testicular

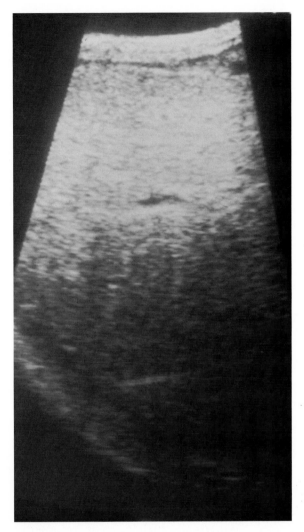

**Fig. 22.23** Ultrasonic image of normal testes. The black center corresponds to the central vein.

abscess as they may have a similar parenchymal pattern.

The scrotum should be free of fluid and any tissue other than the testes, epididymis, and spermatic cord. A transudate within the scrotal sac is non-echogenic, whereas a hematoma may have fibrin strands that create a spider-web appearance on ultrasound (Fig. 22.24). Pus within the scrotal sac cannot be differentiated ultrasonographically from free blood, as both may have echogenic flecks floating within a non-echogenic fluid.

Recent work indicates that measurement of testicular volume is a more accurate indicator of daily sperm output than testicular size. Testicular volume can be estimated by measuring the testicular length, width, and height either with calipers or by ultrasonography. It is calculated with the formula

$$V = \pi \times (D/2) \times L \times 0.9$$

where V = volume, D = diameter and L = length. The constant, 0.9, corrects for the fact that the testis is not cylindrical but oval. Linear regression equations then can be used to predict daily sperm output from testicular volume. The height and width of the testes is determined by placing a 5.0 MHz ultrasound probe horizontally on the ventral surface of the scrotum, perpendicular to the longitudinal axis of the testis. The probe should be positioned until the screen image appears circular and yields the largest cross-sectional area (Fig. 22.25). An oblong image indicates incorrect probe alignment. The length is determined by placing the probe vertically on the caudal aspect of the scrotum directly at the caudal aspect of the testis and directing the beam cranially. The probe is rotated until the distance between the tunica albuginea on the cranial and caudal poles is greatest.

### Undescended testes

The location of a retained testis can be determined ultrasonographically using both a transabdominal and

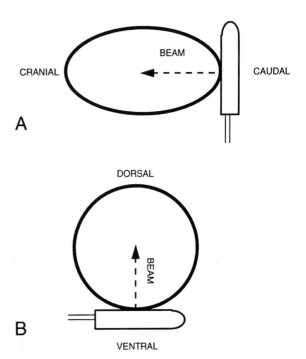

**Fig. 22.25** Placement of the ultrasound probe for measurement of (A) length and (B) cross-sectional area to measure the width and height of the testes.

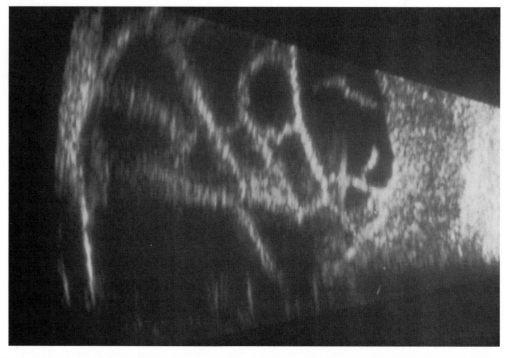

**Fig. 22.24** Ultrasonic image of a coalescing hematoma in the scrotum. Note the spider-web appearance.

a rectal approach. Ultrasonographic scanning of normal descended testes is recommended to acquaint the operator with the ultrasonographic appearance of testicular tissue prior to attempting the diagnosis of cryptorchid testis. To determine whether the testis is retained within the inguinal canal, the ultrasound probe is placed longitudinally on the skin over the external inguinal ring. If it is in the canal the testis will be visualized as a small, rectangular to oblong homogeneous mass. To determine the location of a testis retained in the abdomen, the caudal abdomen is examined rectally, by palpation and by ultrasonography. The examiner first cleans the rectum of feces and performs a thorough examination by rectal palpation of the deep inguinal rings and the caudal abdomen to try and locate the testis. The transducer is then introduced into the rectum. The pelvic brim and caudal abdomen are scanned by moving the transducer cranially in a to-and-fro pattern between midline and the lateral abdominal wall. The retained testis will be small, ranging in size from 2–4 × 3–6 cm. It is soft and less dense than a normal descended testis. If it is retained in the abdomen it is most frequently located directly over or within 6 cm of the deep inguinal ring.

## CULTURE FROM THE MALE REPRODUCTIVE TRACT

Equine semen contains a variety of bacteria. The majority are non-pathogenic, but others are capable of causing infection in mares. Bacteria considered to be pathogenic are *Taylorella equigenitalis*, *Klebsiella pneumoniae* (capsule types 1, 2, and 5) and some strains of *Pseudomonas aeruginosa*. Cultures of the urethra prior to and after semen collection, and of the semen itself, are taken routinely when conducting a BSE. Prior to the collection of samples for bacterial isolation, the penis and prepuce are washed thoroughly with a surgical scrub. Particular attention is given to removing debris from the glans penis and fossa glandis. The penis should be scrubbed at least twice, rinsed with warm water and dried with towels. Briskly rubbing the glans during the washing process usually stimulates the secretion of clear fluid (presperm fraction of the ejaculate) into the urethral lumen. A cotton swab is then inserted 3–5 cm into the urethral orifice. The procedure is repeated post ejaculation. The results from cultures of semen and pre- and postejaculation urethral swabs are compared to identify the quantity and the predominance of an individual organism. If there is heavy growth of a pathogenic bacterium such as *Pseudomonas* or *Klebsiella*, the stallion may be harboring the bacteria in the accessory sex glands and

a thorough examination of the internal genitalia should be performed (see earlier).

There are two venereally transmitted viruses in horses: coital exanthema (equine herpesvirus 3), a self-limiting disease, and equine viral arteritis (a RNA pertivirus of the Togaviridae family). Diagnosis is based on clinical signs, virus isolation and, in the case of EVA, serologic tests.

### Equine viral arteritis (EVA)

To determine whether a stallion is an EVA carrier, semen for virus isolation and serum for titer determination are needed. Once collected, samples should be refrigerated and shipped to the appropriate laboratory (The Gluck Center, Lexington, KY, the Diagnostic Laboratory at Cornell University, Ithaca, NY or the Animal Health Trust, Newmarket, UK) by overnight mail. The sale of stallions shedding the virus is prohibited in certain countries.

# Ruminants

## INTRODUCTION

Abnormalities of the reproductive systems of the cow, doe, and ewe may be suggested by abnormal behavior such as prolonged or otherwise irregular estrus, or elevation of the tail and straining, likened to tenesmus or dysuria. Other signs may be physical in nature, such as abdominal enlargement, abnormal discharge or malodor from the reproductive tract, retained fetal membranes, eversion or prolapse of the vagina or uterus, or abortion. More subtle signs of reproductive abnormalities may be discerned only by the watchful husbandryman or discovered during a review of health records. Examples of these include the absence of estrous activity or unobserved estrus, and failure to conceive or repeat breeder syndrome.

Male ruminants also manifest abnormalities of the reproductive system in behavioral or physical abnormalities or poor reproductive performance. Different types of impotence are indicated by lack of libido or failure to produce an erection or achieve intromission. Persistent straining as if to urinate is another behavioral sign potentially related to diseases of the reproductive tract. Physical signs of abnormalities include

- paraphimosis or inability to retract the penis
- eversion or prolapse of the prepuce
- diffuse or localized swelling of the sheath
- scrotal asymmetry.

Failure to produce a sufficient pregnancy rate in otherwise fertile females is a sign of subfertility, which is possibly the most common manifestation of abnormalities of the reproductive tract in males.

## GENERAL ASPECTS

The signalment of mature females should include parity and current reproductive status, including lactation. In males, the manner and management of history should be noted. Points of interest in the anamnesis related specifically to the reproductive system include any behavioral or physical signs and reproductive performance, as mentioned above. Information regarding any pharmacological or other human interventions, including manipulations of the estrous cycle or breeding season, may prove to be valuable. Any drugs or other treatments, including vaccinations, administered by the producer or other persons should be noted in the medical record. Some hormones may affect the reproductive tract (e.g. oxytocin), and hence the results of its examination. A history of proper immunization, or lack thereof, may influence the differential diagnosis of conditions that potentially affect the reproductive tract (e.g. leptospirosis). In short, any intervention preceding the examination may influence its course or findings. The producer might also be queried about related (potentially genetic) conditions in other members of the herd, especially the ancestors, offspring, and siblings of the subject.

### Female

A record of recent estrous activity is often useful in assessing the reproductive system of the female. The estrous cycle of the cow is normally about 21 days in length, and that of the heifer approximately 20 days. Estrus, the period of receptivity, normally lasts 12–18 hours. Standing to be mounted is the only primary sign of estrus in cattle. Discharge of clear, viscous, stringy mucus and anxiousness or restlessness are signs suggestive of estrus. Pink-tinged to blood-red mucous discharge from a cyclic cow's reproductive tract is termed metrorrhagia and occurs early in metestrus, usually 2 days after estrus. No outward signs of diestrus, the progestogenic or luteal phase, are displayed. Cows in any phase of the reproductive or estrous cycles may mount other cows, but those in proestrus are appar-

ently more compelled to be so active. Although any of the above observations may be useful, they may also be confusing or misleading: many cows experience physiological estrus and ovulation with no outward display or no human observation, and pregnant cows will occasionally stand to be mounted.

Most sheep and goats are seasonally polyestrous, with activity beginning about the time of the autumnal or vernal equinoxes in the temperate latitudes of the northern or southern hemispheres, respectively. Nearer the equator they may maintain estrous cycles throughout the year. After the estrous cycle is established and regular, its length is about 21 days in the doe, with standing estrus of 12–24 hours; that of the ewe is about 18 days, with standing behavior exhibited for 24–36 hours. Producers should be questioned about any manipulations of the reproductive or estrous cycles. Artificial lighting, hormones, and buck or ram management may be used for control or manipulation of reproduction.

Reproductive status should be ascertained, as certain conditions occur more frequently in particular phases of the reproductive cycle. The reproductive cycle is the series of events marked at the beginning and end by parturition. It consists of

- parturition
- postpartum anestrus and involution of the uterus
- estrous cycle activity
- gestation.

---

### Parity

Parity refers to the number of complete gestations, and includes the delivery of term or near-term fetuses. Embryonic and early fetal losses are not counted.

- in dairy cows parity and lactation number are virtually the same
- abortion, which initiates a new lactation, should be considered an increase in parity
- multiple births (e.g. twins) do not constitute additional parities, although their occurrence should be noted because of the generally detrimental effects on involution of the bovine uterus.

Parity may be given a number (parity 3) or a prefix on the root '-parous'. Females which have had no offspring are nulliparous, but during their first gestation and parturition are called primiparous. Those having completed one, two or three gestations are uniparous, biparous, or triparous, respectively. Alternatively, females having completed two or more gestations may simply be termed multiparous.

It also consists of lactation and a 'dry' (non-lactating) period. Thus, dates of calving, estrus, breeding, and pregnancy diagnosis may be useful, as well as status of lactation and, in the dairy cow and doe, the amount of milk produced.

## Male

The breeding history of the male should include the time of year and duration of the breeding period, and the number of females to which the animal was exposed. The presence of other males in the breeding pasture (a multiple-sire system) should be noted. If semen has been collected and frozen for artificial insemination, the frequency and method of collection may be useful information. In either case some measure of fertility, usually a direct or indirect estimate of pregnancy rate, will be reasonably representative of the health of the sire's reproductive system at the time of breeding or semen collection. This may not be representative of the state of the tract during the examination at hand. If the animal has been recently observed with females in estrus, the owner or herdsman could be questioned about the libido and success in mounting and serving those females.

---

### The effects of photoperiod on ruminant breeding

- changes in photoperiod have little effect on the breeding behaviour of bulls
- bucks and rams usually experience decreased libido during periods of increasing and prolonged daylight
- semen quality in small ruminants is affected by photoperiod, with notable variations in this effect between breeds and between individuals, semen quality in male ruminants is usually adversely affected in hot weather.

---

## EXAMINATION TECHNIQUES

### Inspection

Changes in the shape and size of the abdomen may be caused by

- distension with fluid (e.g. urine)
- distension or displacement of the abdominal viscera (which includes the gravid uterus), or
- changes in the abdominal wall or integument.

Hydrops and multifetal gestations predispose to rupture of the prepubic tendon (Fig. 22.26). Prodromal signs of rupture of the prepubic tendon must be differ-

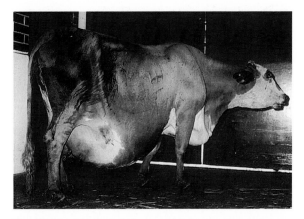

**Fig. 22.26**    Rupture of the prepubic tendon in a cow.

entiated from mammary hematoma or severe peripartum edema of the udder in females, and rupture of the penile urethra with subcutaneous accumulation of urine in males.

Grossly apparent abdominal enlargement caused by distension of the uterus is usually the result of hydrops of the allantoic or amniotic cavities (hydrallantois or hydramnios, respectively)

- hydrallantois is most common, with rapid onset late in gestation, it is usually associated with defects of placentation
- hydramnios is usually associated with defects of the fetus and develops more slowly.

There are sometimes advantages in observing the external genitalia before restraining an animal for close physical examination of the reproductive tract. If possible, the genitalia should be observed with the animal at rest and in motion. Mild forms of prolapse of the vagina and prepuce may be observed in relaxed, recumbent subjects. Carriage of the genitalia of males in motion may indicate pain or dysfunction. The scrotum of the male ruminant should be pendulous during warm weather, with an obvious narrowing of the 'neck' of the scrotum between the testes and the body

---

### Clinical Pointer

The distension caused by hydramnios may only become apparent late in gestation, care must be taken to differentiate it from hydrallantois

- hydrallantois → the abdomen becomes rounded and tense
- hydramnios → the abdomen is pear-shaped and less tense.

wall. Symmetry of the testes and scrotum allows the examiner to presumptively rule out unilateral conditions (e.g. inguinal hernia). In heifers and cows the term 'springing' refers to the visible inward traction on the perineum, and its recoil, while walking. This motion is due to the bouncing weight of the near-term gravid uterus and, perhaps, the attendant relaxation of the pelvic ligaments.

## Palpation

Palpation of the reproductive tracts of ruminants yields a great deal of information to the experienced examiner. Additional descriptions of rectal palpation of the reproductive tracts of cows and heifers are available (Settergren 1980, BonDurant 1986, Roberts 1986b), as are descriptions of palpation of the accessory genitalia of bulls (Larson 1986, Ott 1986). The neophyte is encouraged to practice under the tutelage of a qualified veterinarian. Digital rectal palpation of small ruminants is less rewarding and seldom practiced.

### Females

For rectal palpation of cows and heifers, a plastic sleeve is used and obstetric lubricant applied to the hand and arm. After removing feces from the caudal rectum, the bovine uterus is located by first identifying its cervix, usually on the cranial floor of the pelvis or just over the brim. The 'open' (non-gravid) uterus or that in early pregnancy (less than about 75 days' gestation) may be drawn into the pelvic canal, if not already located there. The process of bringing the uterus into the pelvic canal and raising the ventrally coiled uterine horns into an accessible position is called 'retraction'. Direct retraction is possible when, after traction on the cervix, the ventral intercornual ligament is directly accessible. Traction on this ligament allows the remainder of the uterus to be elevated into the pelvis and the coiled horns to be identified and palpated. More commonly, the ventral intercornual ligament is not easily reached and indirect retraction is necessary. In this technique the cranial edge of the broad ligament is identified beside the uterus (on the same side as the arm the palpator is using). After gentle traction on the cranial edge of the broad ligament, which draws the horn of that side of the uterus laterally, the fingers are turned medially and the horn is identified and followed to the ventral intercornual ligament. Completion of retraction follows as in direct retraction, above. The ovaries are identified near the cranial edge of the broad ligament, just lateral to its attachment to the uterus. Later pregnancies and early postpartum tracts may be too large to allow these maneuvers. In any case, all of the uterus that is accessible

should be examined for its consistency and content, and in non-gravid females the ovaries should be examined for the presence of cyclic ovarian structures.

Vaginal palpation is not often performed in cattle except during obstetric examination. When indicated, the perineum should be thoroughly washed and the sleeved, well-lubricated arm introduced as aseptically as possible. The arm is introduced in a dorsocranial direction, as with the vaginal speculum, unless the express purpose is to examine the external urethral orifice or suburethral diverticulum. The vaginal portion of the cervix may be palpated as it protrudes from the cranial vaginal wall. During late gestation fetal parts may be palpable through the cranial vaginal wall. In such cases care should be exercised in vaginal palpation, especially of the cervix, as partial dilation of the cervix may make the fetal membranes accessible. Obstetric examination, however, is a specialized procedure which has been described elsewhere (Schuijt & Ball 1980, 1986, Roberts 1986c,d,e).

## Vaginoscopy

Vaginoscopy is used to visualize the vaginal vault and vaginal portion of the cervix. The animal's tail should be restrained and the perineum thoroughly washed. A speculum of appropriate size is lubricated and inserted, dorsocranially at first to avoid the urethral orifice, then in a more horizontal and cranial direction. A light is directed into or through the speculum and the vaginal vault is explored visually. Observations that may be useful include

- the color of the vaginal walls
- the character of the mucus
- the position and character of the cervix
- any acquired or congenital abnormalities.

### Males

Rectal palpation of the accessory genitalia and internal inguinal rings of the bull is easily performed, given adequate restraint, usually in a cattle chute. A heavy bar or post should be placed behind the bull for the safety of the examiner, especially during rectal palpation, and for restraint, because head gates will not hold many bulls whose necks are wider than their heads. The lubricated, sleeved hand is introduced through the anal sphincter and feces are removed. With the palpator's wrist drawn caudally into the anus, the ischiocavernosus and bulbospongiosus muscles are just beneath the palm of the hand and the urethralis muscle is beneath the extended fingers; these muscles often contract rhythmically in response to palpation. The body of the prostate is a firm, ring-shaped ridge at the cranial end of the urethralis; the disseminate part of the prostate is not palpable. The vesicular glands are thumb-sized or larger, lobulated, spongy, and positioned cranial to the prostate, against the bony pelvis or obturator foramen. The ampullae are paramedian on the cranial floor of the pelvis between the vesicular glands, and are pencil-sized in diameter. The internal inguinal rings may be identified just over the brim of the pelvis and about a hand's breadth from the midline. They may be identified as folds of peritoneum or semilunar depressions in the caudoventral abdominal wall. The paired bulbourethral glands, which are virtually embedded in the ischiocavernosus and bulbospongiosus muscles, are not palpable unless enlarged.

Palpation of the external genitalia of the bull may be performed in a cattle chute with removable panels that expose the underside of the bull. Rams and bucks may be adequately restrained manually, in a sitting position or with a halter. The haired sheath may be palpated for swelling, fibrosis, or pain involving the prepuce and penis. Beginning at the preputial orifice and working caudally, the penis will be encountered, usually before reaching the neck of the scrotum. A slight thickening may be recognized about 12 cm behind the glans penis in bulls: this is the reflection of the internal preputial epithelium on the free portion of the penis. If the shaft of the penis is palpated as it passes the neck of the scrotum it may be followed to the sigmoid flexure, of which the distal portion is palpable, and may be used to assist in extrusion of the penis. The scrotum, testes, epididymides, and spermatic cords should be examined for their shape, size, symmetry, and consistency. The testes should move dorsoventrally in the scrotum without adhesions or pain.

## LABORATORY EVALUATION

Of the many tests that are supported by laboratory assistance, only a few which are relatively specific to the reproductive tract are mentioned here. However, other procedures more often applied to other body systems should not be forgotten. The range of examples might include the relatively conservative (e.g. fine-needle aspiration and cytology of masses of undetermined etiology) or the more aggressive (e.g. laparoscopy or laparotomy for observation of otherwise inaccessible potential lesions).

### Abortion

Examination of the female is seldom the key to diagnosis of the cause of abortion. Submission to a diagnostic laboratory of the whole placenta and fetus

in a chilled (not frozen) state, or submission of placental and fetal specimens according to the laboratory's instructions, are the best methods for obtaining a diagnosis for the cause of abortion. The importance of such specimens cannot be overemphasized to the producer, who must usually be the one to retrieve and properly store the abortus. Paired sera from the dam is a poor alternative sample compared to the fresh placenta and fetus. Single serum samples and microbial culture seldom provide useful information in the diagnosis of abortion.

> ### Clinical Pointer
>
> Abortion is a manifestation of a variety of diseases which together constitute one of the greatest losses to the livestock industry.

### Females

Bacteriological culture and identification of organisms from the uterine lumen, and in vitro tests of antibiotic sensitivity of the isolated organisms, are not often beneficial when balanced against their cost. The subject has been addressed elsewhere (deBois & Manspeaker 1986). Because the cow has a normal flora in her uterine lumen during certain phases of the reproductive cycle, the isolation of organisms should be viewed accordingly. Specific organisms might be sought (e.g. *Campylobacter fetus*), or the potential pathogenicity of isolates might be considered in light of the results of uterine cytology (e.g. the presence or absence of neutrophils).

Using a rapid 'cowside' test such as the milk progesterone enzyme-linked immunosorbent assay may be useful in determining the presence of a functional, progesterone-producing ovarian structure (corpus luteum or luteal cyst). When the presence or absence of such a structure is critical to the diagnostic process (e.g. pyometra, luteal versus follicular cysts), such a test may be beneficial. Radioimmunoassay is also available and provides a more quantitative result, but requires considerably more time for submission, analysis, and return of the results.

Biopsy and histopathological examination of the endometrium of female ruminants has not enjoyed the widespread popularity of the procedure as practiced in the mare. It may be useful in the assessment of relatively valuable animals, repeat breeders, those apparently unable to carry a fetus to term, and the like. This subject is discussed at greater length elsewhere (deBois & Manspeaker 1986). As with many tests involving the submission of samples for laboratory analysis, consultation with the supporting laboratory's personnel may be advisable.

## Males

Microscopic examination of semen is an integral part of breeding soundness examinations. Fresh, incubated, undiluted semen is examined under low-power magnification for its mass motion. Diluted (usually with warmed saline) semen is examined under a coverslip at about 400 × magnification for the progressive linear motility of individual cells, which is usually expressed as an estimated percentage of the total. Spermatozoal morphology is examined using eosin/nigrosin-stained air-dried preparations under oil-power magnification. Usually 100 cells are counted and the number with normal morphology is expressed as a percentage.

Testing for certain specific infectious diseases in the bull has been discussed elsewhere (Larson 1986). Microbial culture may be useful in the identification of causative organisms in cases of

- orchitis
- epididymitis
- vesiculitis
- balanoposthitis, or
- infectious infertility.

Quantitative culture of the various fractions of the ejaculate (vesicular, sperm-rich, and postejaculatory fluids) may be useful in this regard.

## FEMALE REPRODUCTIVE ORGANS

The reproductive tracts of the female ruminants have in common

- most anatomical features
- cotyledonary placentation (although the cotyledons of the bovids are concave and those of the small ruminants convex), and
- some pathological problems such as prolapse of the vagina.

The great difference is the accessibility of the entire bovine tract to rectal palpation, which is not possible in the doe and ewe.

## Cow

### External genitalia

In the peripartum state the vulva, composed of the right and left labia, becomes enlarged and edematous.

---

### Lacerations

Lacerations through the dorsal commissure of the vulva sometimes occur during parturition. Episiotomy is performed by a veterinary obstetrician to release the tension of the vestibular constriction and prevent such lacerations. The scarring that results from these lacerations or other injuries may cause poor apposition of the labia and incompetence of the vulvar seal against contamination. Lacerations are classified as

- first-degree if they involve only the vestibulovaginal epithelium
- second-degree if the rent extends into the perineal body
- third-degree if the tear extends into the anus and/or rectum.

---

The slope of the vulvar cleft from its dorsal to ventral commissures may be affected by the body condition of the animal: because it is primarily fat that fills the ischiorectal fossa, the anal sphincter and perineal body may be drawn cranially into the pelvic canal in females of lesser body condition. A more horizontal slope from the anal sphincter along the length of the vulvar cleft predisposes to fecal contamination.

Asymmetry, lacerations, or other trauma may affect the apposition of the labia at the vulvar cleft.

The proportion of the vulvar cleft that lies dorsal to the ischial arch may be estimated by palpating the floor of the pelvis through the skin lateral to the labia. If the examiner's thumbs or fingers are placed against the skin lateral to the labia, or the lateral borders of the labia are gently grasped, the vulvar cleft can be opened.

The vestibular mucous membranes can also be observed: this location for assessment of the character of the mucous membranes may be less subject to outside influences (except parturition) than the gingiva or conjunctiva. The glans clitoridis is located inside the ventral commissure of the vulva, and the body of the clitoris may be palpable through the skin. In postpartum cattle the vestibule should be observed for contusions or lacerations, especially of the perineal body dorsally.

---

### Clinical Pointer

An inrush of air when the vulvar cleft is opened indicates questionable competence of the constrictor vestibuli muscles and the potential for pneumovagina.

### Vulvovaginitis

- infectious vulvovaginitis is the genital form of the infectious bovine rhinotracheitis (herpes) virus, the pustules are painful, may cause dyspareunia, and have a mucopurulent discharge
- granular vulvovaginitis is typified by small granular lesions.

### Clinical Pointer ✳

- prolapse of the uterus is a postpartum accident – the organ hangs down to the hocks and caruncles are visible (Fig. 22.27)
- vaginal prolapse is usually a prepartum event – variable amounts of tissue protrude but seldom hang below the level of the stifle (Fig. 22.28).

If the vestibule can be sufficiently dilated, the common opening of the suburethral diverticulum and external urethral orifice may be observed at the cranial limit of the floor of the vestibule. In the females of some species (especially mares) the vestibulovaginal junction is marked by a distinct hymen, or its remnants the transverse folds. In heifers and cows, however, these are relatively rare. Patches of lymphoid tissue exist in the epithelium of the vestibule and may be grossly visible. Major vestibular glands (Bartholin's glands) are located in the walls of the vestibule and may become cystic. They may also become so enlarged that they protrude from the vulva, and must be differentiated from minor (first- or second-degree) vaginal prolapse. Minor vestibular glands may be visible alongside the external urethral orifice. Cows may have either or both types of vestibular glands, but the major vestibular glands are more common. Pustules, ulcers, or neoplasia may be noted on the labia or vestibular mucous membrane.

Any discharge from the reproductive tract should be differentiated from that of metritis or endometritis. As noted previously, clear viscous stringy mucus is indicative of estrus. Metrorrhagia is indicative of early metestrus, but must be differentiated from lochia. Ulcers may be a manifestation of mucosal disease in the cow, or may be neoplastic in origin. Neoplasia of the vulva may be ulcerative or proliferative.

When the uterus or vagina protrudes from the vulva it is actually everted (turned inside out), although the term 'prolapse' has been adopted through common usage; the urinary bladder may be everted or prolapsed. At its largest extreme, vaginal prolapse may be vaginocervical eversion with exposure of caudal cervical annular rings and the bladder positioned within the everted vagina. In less serious cases less tissue protrudes from the vulva, or protrudes only when the cow is recumbent or straining. Lesser degrees of vaginal prolapse must be differentiated from rarer conditions, such as

- cysts of the major vestibular (Bartholin's) glands
- prolapse of the bladder through rents in the vaginal floor, or
- eversion of the bladder through the urethra.

### Internal genitalia

The vagina may be explored visually or manually. During vaginoscopy the color and other characteristics of the vaginal walls should be noted. They are pale, with small amounts of thick, off-white mucus during diestrus and pregnancy. The vagina is more hyperemic in non-luteal phases. Fluid accumulation (urine, pus)

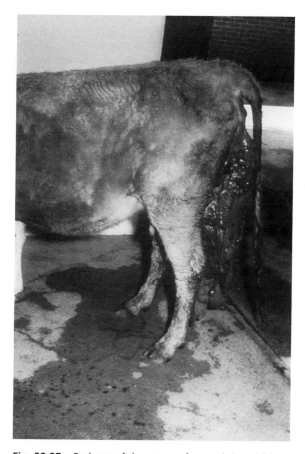

**Fig. 22.27** Prolapse of the uterus of a cow is invariably a postpartum event. Although the placenta obscures the view of the caruncles to which it is attached, they are apparent on closer examination of the organ.

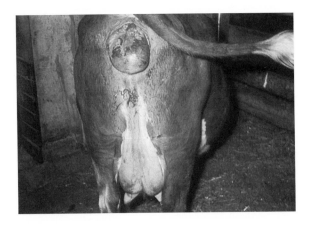

**Fig. 22.28** Prolapse of the vagina, which in cattle is considered hereditary, usually occurs shortly before parturition. A dried, leathery surface indicates a prolapse of some duration.

may be noted on the floor of the cranial vagina or discharged from the cervical os. Contusions commonly result from coitus and parturition. A variety of other anomalies (e.g. uterus didelphys), acquired lesions (e.g. transvaginal adhesions), foreign bodies (e.g. semen straws), and traumatic lesions (e.g. cervical lacerations) may also be observed during vaginoscopy.

Vaginal palpation allows manual assessment of the vaginal portion of the cervix and other structures or abnormalities which are palpable. In heifers the vaginal cervix is small and firm, but that of cows may be larger owing to the eversion of some of the caudal annular rings. Some of the abnormalities mentioned under vaginoscopy may also be identified by vaginal palpation. A variety of foreign bodies have been removed from the vagina of cattle, including incompletely expelled abortuses and foreign objects left after acts of perversion or sadism. Vaginal rents may result from these acts, or from exposure to bulls with excessive penile length.

The cervix is most thoroughly assessed through rectal palpation, with the exception of the vaginal portion, which is better examined per vaginam. In parous cows with everted cervical rings the caudal end of the cervix often feels enlarged, such that the cervix seems mushroom-shaped or conical, but almost invariably maintains its competence. Otherwise, irregularities of the shape may be caused by paracervical abscesses, fibrous lesions resulting from cervical laceration, and the like.

The remainder of the uterus is palpated as described above. The goal of palpation of the reproductive tract of the cow or heifer is to answer the following questions

- is she pregnant?
- if so, in which (or both) uterine horn(s)?
- what is the gestational age?

Asymmetry of the uterine horns, fluid content, the presence of a functional corpus luteum, and fremitus in the middle uterine artery are the secondary signs or indications of pregnancy. The presence of an amnionic vesicle, chorioallantoic membranes, placentomes, or a fetus are the positive or cardinal signs of pregnancy.

1. If the animal is not pregnant, has she begun or returned to the estrous cycle? If so, in which phase is she? The ovaries are located near the cranial edge of each broad ligament, lateral to each uterine horn. They may contain cyclic ovarian structures (follicles, corpora hemorrhagica, and corpora lutea) which usually allow the experienced examiner to determine the phase of the estrous cycle.
2. Do congenital or acquired lesions or pathological processes exist? Some examples include segmental aplasia, which is a common congenital abnormality among freemartins. Metritis usually becomes clinically apparent between the third and twelfth postpartum days, and retained fetal membranes predispose to the condition. Uterine torsion is an accident of late gestation in the cow, and a spiralling of the tract cranial to the cervix may be appreciated on rectal examination. The horns of the uterus are usually palpable on rectal examination of cows with hydrallantois, but the placentomes and fetus are not; the converse is true in cases of hydramnios. Cystic ovarian degeneration is the most common diagnosis for enlarged ovaries, especially in dairy cows, in which the condition is associated with high milk production. The small, serpentine uterine tubes, which are normally not palpable in the broad ligaments between the ovaries and uterine horns, may become enlarged and palpable if inflamed (salpingitis) or filled with fluid due to aplasia or blockage (tubal obstruction).

## Doe

### External genitalia

The labia of some individual does becomes edematous and hyperemic during estrus. Also, the mucus of late estrus is purulent in appearance. These signs are shared by some cases of genital caprine herpesvirus infection and granular or ulcerative vulvovaginitis in the doe. The season of the year and the behavior of the doe in the presence of a buck may suggest the possibility of estrus. The vesicles or erosions of genital herpesvirus infection, or the lesions for which the other vulvovaginal conditions are named, may suggest one of these diagnoses. Ectopic mammary tissue located in the vulva has been described and should be differentiated from inflammation (Smith & Sherman, 1994b).

Intersex states are especially common in polled goats (Fig. 22.29). In animals that appear phenotypically female

- an enlarged clitoris
- increased anogenital distance
- hypospadias
- infertility, or
- male behavior and odor

are suggestive of the intersex condition.

Tissues that may be found protruding from the vulva of the doe include retained fetal membranes, prolapsed (everted) vagina, and prolapsed uterus. Fetal membranes should be readily apparent and, if not expelled within 12 hours of delivery of the fetus, are considered pathologically retained. The cervix of the doe closes rather rapidly, such that membranes may be trapped in the uterus within days of parturition.

Prolapses of the vagina or uterus in the doe are similar to those in the cow. Vaginal prolapse occurs most commonly in the prepartum period and tends to recur in subsequent gestations. It varies from the mild form, in which little tissue protrudes from the commissure of the vulva and only when the doe is recumbent, to more severe forms such as vaginocervical prolapse. The urinary bladder may be contained in the everted tissue, with such a reflection of the urethra that urination is not

possible. Uterine prolapse occurs in the immediate postpartum period. Both horns of the prolapsed uterus are usually apparent and the organ is longer than the prolapsed vagina, such that it will hang down to, or below, the hocks. The caruncles visible on the endometrial surface of the prolapsed uterus are concave, rather than convex as in the cow.

### Internal genitalia

Vaginoscopy reveals a more hyperemic and moist vaginal vault at the time of estrus than during other periods. The appearance of the vaginal mucus changes from clear to cloudy to purulent through the course of estrus. The paired longitudinal ducts of the epoophoron (Gartner's ducts) may be observed on the floor of the vagina and may be distended with mucus. Evidence of trauma (e.g. postpartum), foreign bodies (e.g. progesterone-releasing intravaginal devices, which are usually sponges), and polyps or neoplasia are other potential findings. Inability to insert the vaginal speculum could be the result of an intersex state or freemartinism, persistent hymen, or vaginal adhesion or stricture. Palpation of the reproductive tract of the doe is limited to digital vaginal palpation, except in some obstetric examinations.

Further examination of the reproductive tract of the doe may include techniques that are prohibitively invasive or expensive. Thorough visual or manual examination of the uterus and ovaries requires laparoscopy or laparotomy, respectively. Pregnancy and pseudopregnancy (below) may be identified and differentiated with real-time ultrasonography, but such equipment is expensive.

Real-time ultrasonography using a linear array probe or sector scanner is the most accurate means of diagnosing pregnancy in the doe. Transrectal imaging for early pregnancy diagnosis (20–30 days' gestation) is possible using a linear array probe attached to a rigid extension. Either type of scanner may be used transabdominally to identify the fluid, fetus, and placentomes of later pregnancy. Less sophisticated ultrasound machines, abdominal palpation, ballottement of the fetus using a rigid rod inserted in the rectum, failure to return to estrus, and hormonal assays have also been used, but are generally less accurate.

Postpartum infections of the uterus are usually indicated by malodorous or purulent discharge from the reproductive tract. Pyometra occurs later in the reproductive cycle and, in the absence of apparent discharge, must be differentiated from pregnancy and hydrometra (pseudopregnancy). Acute metritis usually occurs early in the postpartum period, and consists of a less purulent but more voluminous and malodorous

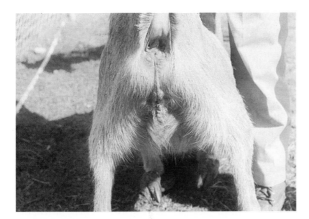

**Fig. 22.29** Intersex state in a goat. Note the enlarged clitoris, increased anogenital distance, and apparent development of a scrotum.

> ### Pseudopregnancy with hydrometra in the doe
>
> This is probably caused by prolonged luteal function and may be accompanied by signs of pregnancy and parturition, including failure to return to estrus. It may be differentiated from pregnancy using laparotomy or ultrasonography to identify voluminous fluid in the uterus, in the absence of fetal parts and placentomes. The expulsion of the fluid (if observed) is called 'cloudburst' by the layperson.

> ### Clinical Pointer
>
> The incidence of retained placenta in ewes is low and may indicate the presence of an undelivered fetus in the uterus.

discharge than chronic metritis/endometritis. The doe with acute severe metritis may also be febrile and anorexic, indicating the severity of the disease through systemic illness. The chronic form, which might also be termed endometritis, is marked by a purulent to mucopurulent discharge indicating a prolonged leukocytic response. This condition stands as a risk factor for infertility, but the doe is probably not systemically ill (at least not from the endometritis).

Ovarian cysts have been diagnosed in the doe, usually in seeking an explanation for nymphomaniac behavior. Definitive diagnosis is possible using ultrasonography, laparoscopy, or laparotomy to identify persistent follicular structures larger than the diameter of the normal ovulatory follicle (about 1 cm). A presumptive therapeutic diagnosis might also be obtained if treatment with human chorionic gonadotropin or gonadotropin-releasing hormone alleviates the condition within a few days.

### Ewe

#### External genitalia

The vulva of the ewe shows little change through the estrous cycle. In the peripartum period edema and relaxation of the labia occur. Vulvovaginitis may be suggested by edema of the vulva and the presence of additional lesions, such as vesicles, ulcers, papules, or the like. The parapoxvirus of contagious ecthyma (orf) has been implicated in cases of vulvovaginitis (with the attendant zoonotic potential), as have a variety of microbial etiologies. Attempts to identify the causative organism are often not successful. The condition may be initiated or aggravated by myiasis, which in turn may be predisposed by short docking of the tail.

Tissues emanating from the reproductive tract of the ewe are most commonly retained fetal membranes or prolapsed vagina, the differentiation of which should not be difficult. As in the cow and doe, prolapsed vagina occurs most commonly in late gestation.

#### Internal genitalia

Physical diagnosis of conditions of the internal genitalia of ewes is for the most part limited to pregnancy diagnosis. However, two metabolic diseases that occur in the ewe, pregnancy toxemia and hypocalcemia, occur commonly in the late pregnant and peripartum periods, respectively. Therefore, the diagnosis of pregnancy (and, in cases of pregnancy toxemia, the diagnosis of multifetal gestation) may be important in the assessment of the ewe.

A variety of methods of pregnancy diagnosis in the ewe have been practiced with varying degrees of accuracy and limited ability to identify multifetal pregnancies

- radiography after 80 days' gestation is probably the most accurate in both regards, but is limited by expense and inconvenience
- real-time ultrasonography in the hands of a skilled operator is quite practicable, but such equipment is expensive (Fig. 22.30)
- rectoabdominal palpation is quite accurate in the diagnosis of pregnancy, but less so in identifying multiple fetuses: using a lubricated rod inserted in the rectum of the ewe in dorsal recumbency, fetal parts are 'palpated' through the end of the instrument
- laparotomy and laparoscopy are intensive and invasive, and laparoscopy may not permit the diagnosis of multiple fetuses.

Diagnosis of multifetal gestations is unlikely with any of the remaining techniques. These include less sophisticated ultrasonographic techniques, progesterone assay, vaginal biopsy, abdominal ballottement/palpation, and non-return to estrus.

## MALE REPRODUCTIVE ORGANS

An excellent review of the reproductive anatomy of the bull is available and contains additional discussions of other aspects of the examination and testing of breeding bulls (Larson 1986, Ott 1986). Similar discussions regarding the examination of bucks (Smith 1986b) and rams (Bruere 1986) are available in the same text.

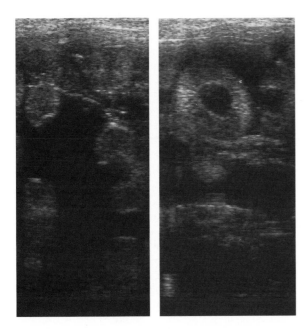

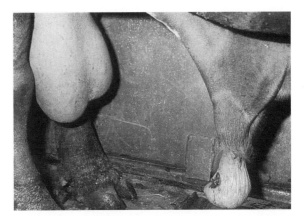

**Fig. 22.31** Prolapse of the prepuce of a bull. Note the enlargement which prevents retraction, and the resultant scab or crust due to drying and/or trauma. This bull also has a degree of periorchitis.

**Fig. 22.30** Ultrasonographic images of placentomes of the ewe, often described as 'Cs' and 'donuts'. **(a)** A reversed C-shaped image is apparent in the middle of the right side of the ultrasonograph. **(b)** A typical donut-shaped image and a less obvious reversed C are visible at the top of the image.

## Bull

### External genitalia

The sheath should be observed and palpated for signs of trauma or disease. In the bull, localized to widespread swelling of the prepuce may be caused by a retropreputial abscess or penile hematoma and may cause prolapse (eversion) of the internal, non-haired prepuce through the preputial orifice (Fig. 22.31). Bulls sometimes allow normal eversion of the prepuce for brief periods (e.g. during urination), but the development of edema (usually caused by trauma) prevents its retraction into the preputial orifice. The pendulous nature of the prepuce of *Bos indicus* bulls and their hybrids may make them more susceptible to the causes of preputial prolapse (Hudson 1986a). Polled bulls may also be predisposed because the genetic tendency for weak or vestigial retractor prepuce muscles is closely associated (usually inherited) with the gene for polledness.

Examination of the extended penis is most easily accomplished in bulls which relax the retractor penis muscles during rectal palpation and expose part of the free portion of the penis. The penis may thus be grasped with the aid of a gauze sponge (to prevent slippage) and extended. Alternatively, an electroejaculator may be used in an attempt to extrude the penis, as usually occurs with electroejaculation during the breeding soundness examination (discussed below). This should not be done if penile hematoma is suspected. In either approach assistance may be provided by grasping the distal portion of the sigmoid flexure and moving it cranially, thus counteracting the effects of the retractor penis muscles. The extended penis should be examined for signs of

- disease, e.g. fibropapillomas (Fig. 22.32)
- trauma, e.g. lacerations, and
- congenital defects, e.g. persistent frenulum (Fig. 22.33).

Phimosis may be the result of a variety of conditions including peripenile adhesions, stenosis of the preputial orifice, or incomplete epithelial separation of the penis from the internal prepuce.

The scrotal skin may reveal signs of trauma, frostbite, or other insult. The consistency and symmetry of the testicular parenchyma and epididymal heads and tails should be noted. Signs of inflammation may be indicative of orchitis and/or epididymitis. Fluid in the potential space between the visceral and parietal vaginal tunics (periorchitis, Fig. 22.31) should be differ-

---

### Clinical Pointer

Care must be taken to differentiate fat in the neck of the scrotum ('cod fat') from loops of bowel (inguinal hernia).

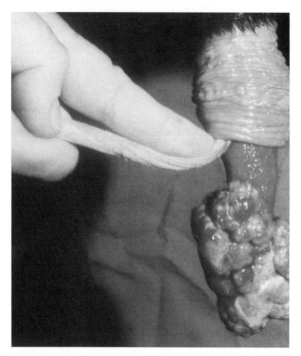

**Fig. 22.32** A fibropapilloma surrounding the glans penis of a bull.

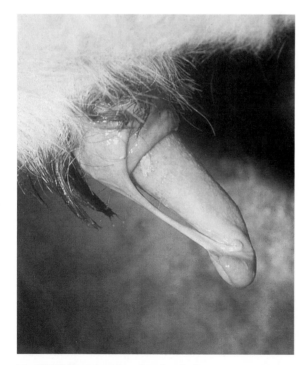

**Fig. 22.33** Persistent frenulum in a bull.

entiated from extreme softening of the testicular parenchyma (testicular degeneration), although these may occur concurrently. The spermatic cords consist of cremaster muscles, testicular vessels, and nerves, ductus deferentia and mesoductus. They may be palpated in the neck of the scrotum for the presence of hydrocele, hematocele, or spermatocele.

### Internal genitalia

Tenesmus, pain during urination or defecation, and even lameness in the hindquarters of bulls are potentially caused by inflammation of the vesicular glands, and the latter of these also by orchitis. Because orchitis and vesiculitis may occur concomitantly or in succession in bulls, the possibility of each should be investigated.

Of the several structures palpated during rectal examination of bulls, the vesicular glands and inguinal rings are the most telling. Signs of inflammation in the accessory genitalia are most commonly and palpably manifested in the vesicular glands. Heat, pain, and swelling, which leads to the loss of palpable lobulation, are signs of acute vesiculitis; if semen is collected, many neutrophils are present in the ejaculate. Chronic vesiculitis is marked primarily by fibrosis and the intermittent or inconsistent presence of white cells in the ejaculate. Individual lobules of the vesicular glands will occasionally become quite firm, perhaps owing to ductular obstruction, with no apparent ill effects.

> ### Clinical Pointer
>
> Enlargement of the inguinal rings indicates a predisposition to inguinal herniation of the bowel. If the internal inguinal ring of the bull is readily apparent it should admit no more than one to one and one-half phalanges of two or three digits of the palpator's hand.

## Buck

### External genitalia

The penis of mature bucks can usually be extended manually. Alternatively, an electroejaculator may be used in an attempt to extrude the penis, as usually occurs with electroejaculation during the breeding soundness examination. The penis and prepuce should be examined for

- congenital (hypospadias, persistent frenulum), or
- acquired (hair rings, hematomas)

abnormalities, with special attention given to the urethral process (villiform appendage), in which urethral calculi sometimes lodge. Balanoposthitis may be bacterial or viral in origin.

The penis may not be completely epithelialized and separated from the prepuce until after puberty. Therefore, the penis of the prepubertal buck may be impossible to extrude. The glans penis of juvenile bucks, if visible, has an irregular surface.

The scrotum and its contents should be examined with special attention to the testes and epididymides. Other than hypospadias, indications of the intersex state in an apparent male may be found therein. Testicular hypoplasia and cryptorchidism are two such indications. Obstruction of the epididymis by sperm granuloma and segmental aplasia of the epididymis have also been reported in bucks. Orchitis and epididymitis may be caused by a variety of microorganisms, including trypanosomes and *Brucella melitensis*. Neoplasias and hematomas, though rarer, are additional abnormalities that may be found in the scrotum.

### Internal genitalia

Examination of the accessory genitalia of the buck is seldom practical or indicated. Smith (1986b) has indicated that rectal examination may be possible if the buck is very large and the examiner's hand very small. Some indication of vesiculitis (e.g. leukocytes identified in the semen during breeding soundness examination) might justify such examination or transrectal ultrasonography to support the diagnosis.

## Ram

### External genitalia

As with the buck, the penis of the ram can usually be extended manually or examined during electroejaculation. Also as in the buck, uroliths commonly lodge in the villiform appendage. Phimosis, balanoposthitis ('pizzle rot') and injuries to the villiform appendage during shearing are other common abnormalities.

The scrotum may be affected by trauma, abscesses, and mange mites, and in severe cases these conditions can affect the organs within. The scrotum should be shorn in breeds with wool on the scrotum, as the insulating effect may otherwise adversely affect testicular thermoregulation.

As in the other ruminant species the testes of the ram should be

- large
- firm

### Epididymitis

This is a particularly important and detrimentally widespread condition in rams. Palpable enlargement and/or fibrosis of parts of the epididymis is grounds for culling most rams from the breeding flock without further consideration. The condition may be caused by a variety of bacteria, the two most common are *Actinobacillus seminis* in ram lambs and *Brucella ovis* in adults.

- symmetrical, and
- mobile in the scrotum.

Cryptorchidism, testicular hypoplasia and/or atrophy, and varicocele in the spermatic cord are common problems in rams.

### Internal genitalia

As in the buck the accessory glands of the ram are relatively inaccessible. Should an indication for examination of the internal genitalia present itself, digital rectal examination or transrectal ultrasonographic imaging using a linear array probe might be attempted.

## ANCILLARY DIAGNOSTIC TESTS

### Ultrasonography

Ultrasonography has emerged as one of the most practicable technological innovations of late. Transrectal imaging of the tubular tract of cows and heifers has been addressed (Hanzen & Delsaux 1987, Pierson & Ginther 1987). Ultrasonography has also been used to localize and measure fluid in the scrotum and lesions in the testes.

### Other imaging techniques

Several imaging techniques have been used in attempts to define or diagnose lesions in the reproductive tract of bulls. Radiological contrast studies ('cavernosograms' or 'penograms') have been used to demonstrate cavernosal shunts. Thermography has been used to demonstrate loss of thermoregulation in the scrotum.

### Test matings

Test matings involve the observation of sexual behavior and physical attempts at coitus in relatively natural surroundings with a female in heat (Fig. 22.34). Some aspects of libido testing in bulls (Chenoweth 1986a) and in rams (Holmes 1986) and sexual behavior in bulls (Chenoweth 1986b) bucks, (Smith 1986b) and rams (Holmes 1986) have been addressed. Test matings are not commonly performed as a part of the physical examination of bulls, nor as a part of the breeding soundness examination unless history or other indications warrant.

Another test sometimes also called a test mating, but not to be confused with that described above, involves the mating of a potential sire suspected to be the carrier of some genetic defect. The male in question is mated to several females known or suspected also to be carriers of the defect. The number of matings is adjusted to maximize the odds of phenotypic expression of the defect in the resultant offspring.

## SAMPLING REPRODUCTIVE TRACTS

### Female

Intrauterine culture and endometrial biopsy are possible, especially in the cow, using any of a variety of long, guarded swabs and biopsy instruments. These are passed through the cervix, as are artificial insemination and embryo transfer instruments. Such sampling of the tracts

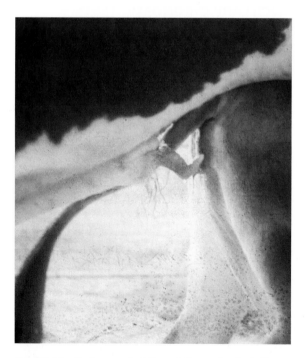

**Fig. 22.34** Corkscrew deviation of the penis of a bull discovered during test mating.

of the doe and ewe is less feasible, except during the puerperal period. The most problematic aspect of culture and biopsy of the ruminant uterus is the interpretation of results. With notable exceptions (e.g. *Tritrichomonas fetus* in cattle) bacteria may be incidental flora and biopsy results inconclusive or unrepresentative.

### Male

Collection of semen from male ruminants may be accomplished with an artificial vagina and another animal estrogenized or restrained to be mounted. Alternatively, a phantom may be used for mounting but this, like all aspects of collection using an artificial vagina, requires training. Semen samples may also be collected from the bull through rectal massage of the accessory genitalia.

---

### Electroejaculation

This simple and relatively safe technique requires little time and no training of the animal from which the semen is to be collected

- a cylindrical probe with a conical tip and raised, longitudinal electrodes is lubricated and inserted into the rectum of the restrained male
- a cord connects the probe to a power source with some means of control of the current amplitude
- electrical pulses of increasing amplitude are thus created around the genital musculature, bringing about emission and ejaculation, albeit artificial in character and volume.

---

Lavage of the proximal urethra using a sterile urinary catheter has been suggested for the identification of the causative organisms of vesiculitis in the bull. Methods for collection of samples from the penis and prepuce include swabbing, flushing or lavage of the preputial cavity, or scrubbing of the penis with collection of the rinse (usually normal saline).

## BREEDING SOUNDNESS EXAMINATION

### Female

Breeding soundness examination, as practiced in the male ruminants and the females of some other species (i.e. the mare), is not well defined for female ruminants. The criteria for breeding soundness are not so well established as in the male, because any such measures thus far conceived are not reliable or repeatable in so far as they relate to the ability to conceive, carry to term, and deliver healthy offspring.

## Male

The breeding soundness examination of males entails

- a general physical examination
- a thorough examination of the genitalia (as above)
- the collection and examination of semen.

The breeding soundness examination is intended to select bulls, bucks, or rams for success in pasture breeding programs, but tests for libido, mating ability, or infectious diseases are not included unless indicated. Breeding soundness examinations have been discussed in numerous books, articles and chapters, only a few of which are noted here (bull: Ott 1986; buck: Refsal 1986; ram: Bruere 1986; Martin 1986).

The male must be free of physical defects that would impede the searching and mounting activities of the herd sire. During the general physical examination particular attention is given to the eyes, feet, and legs. Conformation and body condition are also considered. Serious physical defects and heritable conditions are grounds for classification as an unsatisfactory potential breeder without further consideration.

If the candidate demonstrates no serious flaws in the general physical examination, the genitalia are examined closely. Again, they must be free of defects and heritable conditions.

Semen is collected by one of the methods described above and examined microscopically for progressive motility and normal morphology. Because estimates of individual progressive motility are fairly subjective, and as the value of motility in predicting fertility is unproven, considerable latitude is allowed in rating motility as acceptable. On the other hand, morphological defects can be very reliably and repeatably determined and linked to infertility. Usually 100 cells are counted and a minimum acceptable percentage of normal cells of 70% or 80% is established.

Males that satisfy all aspects of the breeding soundness examination are classified as satisfactory potential breeders. Those with problems or defects so serious and irreparable that the examiner believes that no aid or convalescence will suffice are classified as

unsatisfactory potential breeders. A third category for animals which may recover or improve (variously called 'questionable', 'deferred', 'recheck', or the like) is employed for those animals that require some convalescence before re-examination. If the defect appears to be one of spermatogenesis, 60 days are usually allowed for one spermatogenic cycle and epididymal transport of newly formed spermatozoa.

# Swine

## INTRODUCTION

Modern integrated hog production is an industry based on goal-oriented production and health management. To this end producers seek to optimize reproductive performance. In gilts and sows the most common manifestations of suboptimal reproductive performance are delayed or unobserved estrus or, when they are discovered in estrus and bred by fertile boars, failure to conceive or small litter sizes. The analogous problems in boars include the various forms of impotence, or in terms of suboptimal production, subfertility, including failure to produce conceptions or to produce litters of sufficient size.

Physical manifestations of disease in the female reproductive tract include abnormal discharge, which during the postpartum period must be differentiated from normal lochia. Common visible lesions caused by trauma to the external genitalia of the female include vulvar hematomas and lacerations. Vaginal or uterine prolapse and abortion occur in swine, as they do in other species.

Scrotal and penile lacerations occur in boars, usually as a result of attack by other animals. Other signs of injury or disease include hematuria or other hemorrhage from the preputial or urethral orifice. Eversion or prolapse of the prepuce also occurs in boars. Injury or disease of the testes or scrotum may be indicated by scrotal asymmetry. Orchitis in its acute and chronic forms may be indicated by testicular swelling or fibrosis, respectively.

## GENERAL ASPECTS

Signalment and anamnesis, including management practices, are particularly important in the assessment of the reproductive system of swine. For instance, age, weight, and breed composition affect the onset of

---

### Scrotal circumference

This is an indirect but highly correlated measure of sperm-producing capacity. The testes are gently drawn to the bottom of the scrotum and a measure is taken of the circumference of both testes together (the 'scrotal circumference'). Minimum acceptable scrotal circumference varies by species and age, and sometimes by breed.

puberty. Manipulations of the estrous cycle and certain mating practices have attendant risks and advantages in so far as reproductive health is concerned. Vaccinations, hormonal therapy, and other pharmacological interventions may also be integral to the understanding of reproductive health and disease. Effective record keeping in modern swine production systems may also allow investigation of the heritability of defects along genetic lines.

## Female

The onset of puberty in gilts is variable, but usually occurs between 5 and 9 months of age. The estrus cycle is approximately 21 days in length, with normal variation of 3 or 4 days on either side of this mean. Estrus, the period of receptivity, is 1–3 days in duration.

---

### Clinical Pointer ✳

Most females in estrus acquire a solid, immobile, standing posture when pressure is applied to their back. However, not all females respond to this test when performed by humans, and the odor or presence of a boar may be necessary to elicit this response.

---

Gestation is approximately 114 days in swine, and piglets may be weaned 3–4 weeks after birth. Under these circumstances sows return to estrus and may be rebred within 7–10 days of weaning. Thus, intensive reproductive management may allow a sow to produce an average of more than two litters per year during her productive life. Maximization of the number of pigs in each litter is also important in modern swine production.

## Male

The process of puberty in young boars is rather gradual, and culminates in the production of an ejaculate that is capable of producing conceptions in fertile females. This usually occurs no earlier than 5 months of age and no later than 10 months. After this age the breeding history of males may be sufficient to rule out problems of the reproductive tract: boars which are willing and aggressive breeders and produce acceptably large litter sizes are probably free of abnormalities. Likewise, an accurate and complete history of a boar's reproductive performance will usually aid in the identification of problems which are not otherwise obvious.

# EXAMINATION TECHNIQUES

## Inspection

Inspection of the reproductive tracts of swine is limited for the most part to the vulva of the female and the scrotum and sheath of the boar. Soundness of the feet and legs, and the symmetry and number of glands in the mammary chain are also important in the assessment of breeding soundness, but these are covered elsewhere. Useful observations may be made during breeding, but further visualization of the genitalia (i.e. the penis) is unlikely because the boar obtains intromission at the time of extension of the penis, with the preputial orifice in close apposition to the vulva of the female. Thus, examination of the penis usually requires its redirection away from the vulva during breeding attempts.

## Vaginoscopy

Vaginoscopy has been described as an aid in the differentiation of urogenital infections. The signs of vaginitis or observation of discharge from the urethral orifice or external cervical os may help determine the source of discharges from the urogenital tract. It has also been suggested that uterine cultures may be obtained through the speculum if the cervical canal is patent.

## Palpation

Palpation per rectum has been described as a means of pregnancy diagnosis in large sows (Buddle 1986). Indications of pregnancy include

- fremitus in the middle uterine artery
- enlargement of the uterus and thinning of its walls
- the presence of corpora lutea on the ovaries about 21 days after breeding.

Palpation per vaginam is usually limited to obstetric examination and manipulations. Palpation of the testes, epididymides, and scrotum is an important part of the physical examination of the reproductive tract of the boar, and manual examination of the sheath and/or preputial diverticulum is sometimes indicated. In any event, adequate restraint is necessary for a thorough examination and for the safety of the examiner and subject.

## Pregnancy diagnosis

In the several weeks after breeding, and especially 18–24 days after service, gilts and sows that do not display a return to estrus in response to either the back pressure test or a teaser boar may be presumed to be pregnant. This is one of the earliest methods of diagnosis of non-pregnancy and allows immediate rebreeding if desired. Rectal palpation, when feasible, may also detect pregnancy and non-pregnancy relatively early in gestation. Several types of ultrasonography (amplitude–depth, Doppler, real-time) are available. In the hands of experienced examiners they are accurate, but only after about 30 days and before about 90 days of gestation. Vaginal biopsy has been used to demonstrate returns to estrus, because the vaginal epithelium displays a distinct thickening during estrus compared to that under progestogenic influence. Likewise, progesterone assay may be used to presumptively diagnose non-returns to estrus 21 ± 3 days after breeding. Estrone sulfate, which is produced by the conceptus, may be measured in the plasma of the dam, peaking between 23 and 30 days after breeding. Pregnancy diagnoses by laparotomy or laparoscopy are generally restricted to research applications.

## Slaughter examination

The inaccessibility of the internal genitalia of gilts and sows necessitates examination of the excised tract, usually at slaughter. Identification of the animal from which the tract was collected is necessary in order to correlate findings of the examination with clinical signs. The severed caudal end of the tract may be tied closed with string to preserve its contents and flora, after which it may be placed in an individual container (e.g. plastic bag), labeled, and placed on ice. Tracts may thus be transported to a place where a thorough gross examination may be performed and appropriate samples collected for further evaluation.

## Test mating

Examination of a boar during his interactions with a sow or gilt in estrus allows evaluation of libido and mating ability. After the boar mounts the female, and during his attempts at extension and intromission, the penis may be redirected for examination and, if desired, the collection of semen.

## Collection of semen

A physiological ejaculate from boars is most easily obtained by redirecting and grasping the glans penis in a gloved hand as the boar mounts and attempts to breed a female in heat. The grip of the hand apparently simulates the engagement of the glans in the cervix of the female, which seems to be the stimulus for ejaculation in this species. The semen is collected in an insulated vessel, usually with a gauze filter to reduce the amount of the gelatinous portion of the ejaculate contained in the sample. An artificial vagina, or the combination of an artificial vagina and the gloved hand method, has also been successful in obtaining physiological ejaculates. Electroejaculation of the boar requires general anesthesia, but also allows the collection of a representative sample.

## LABORATORY EVALUATION

### Fetal wastage

Fetal wastage in swine occurs in many forms. These include

- abortion
- mummification
- stillbirth
- weakness of the neonate.

Cutler (1986) has suggested that normal herds experience

- abortions in 2% of sows
- mummification of 0.5% of fetuses
- stillbirths in 6–8% of piglets delivered.

If any of these figures show a twofold or greater increase, pursuit of a diagnosis may be justified. Along with a comprehensive history and astute clinical observations, submission to a diagnostic laboratory of placentae, if possible, and fetuses and/or weak neonates is most helpful.

| Clinical Pointer  |
| :--- |
| When a pattern of fetal wastage is emerging in a herd it is essential to submit entire litters, or groups of three or more fetuses/piglets from affected litters, for laboratory analysis. The submission of samples from isolated cases of individually affected fetuses seldom results in a definitive diagnosis and may even be misleading. |

### Females

Samples for microbial or histopathological evaluation are usually collected during slaughter examination of the female reproductive tract. Alternatively, the cranial vagina may be sampled for microbial culture with a guarded swab, but such samples may still be contaminated, less representative, or otherwise less useful. The details of preparation of samples for shipment are best discussed with the laboratory personnel who will receive and analyze the samples.

## Males

Thorough evaluation of boar semen involves evaluation of motility and morphology, as in the ruminants, but also includes estimation of volume and concentration of the ejaculate. The gross motility of raw, undiluted semen is observed under low magnification for its swirling action. The percentage of individual progressively motile sperm is estimated during observation of diluted semen under a coverslip at higher magnification (usually 400×). The percentage of morphologically normal sperm is obtained through a count of 100 stained cells observed under oil-power magnification (approximately 1000×). Measures of volume and concentration of the ejaculate are necessary because the size or volume of the testes is not easily measured in boars (as it is in ruminants), although testicle size has been correlated with sperm-producing capacity. Concentration is multiplied by volume to arrive at an estimate of total sperm per ejaculate.

Microbial culture of semen may be indicated if leukocytes are observed in the ejaculate or there are other signs of infection of the reproductive tract. *Brucella* spp. and some streptococcal species are venereally transmitted in swine.

## FEMALE REPRODUCTIVE ORGANS

### External genitalia

Examination of the external genitalia of the sow and gilt is for the most part limited to observation of the vulva and any tissue or discharge emanating from the reproductive tract. During estrus the vulva becomes edematous and hyperemic. These characteristics may also be indicative of estrogenic mycotoxicosis if they occur in the vulvae of groups of females that have not been otherwise synchronized. Mammary development may also accompany this condition. In the peripartum period the vulva becomes somewhat enlarged and relaxed.

Small, underdeveloped or 'infantile' vulvae are characteristic of prepubertal gilts or, less commonly, intersex states. Vulvae that are tilted dorsally, sometimes called 'skyhooked' because the ventral commissure curls dorsally, also occur in prepubertal

and intersex conditions. When this conformation remains in postpubertal females intromission may be difficult for boars because of the angle of the commissure.

Lacerations and hematomas of the vulva occur most

---

**Prolapse of the genitalia**

- uterine prolapse occurs early in the postpartum period and may contain the urinary bladder
- vaginal prolapse occurs most commonly during the last few days of gestation
- some degree of prolapse of the rectum may result from any condition that causes straining on the part of the sow
- 'lateroflexion' of the urinary bladder into the space between the vaginal and pelvic walls appears much like vaginal prolapse and usually occurs at the same time (in late gestation), but is unilateral; because the bladder may not be emptied in this position, this condition also causes straining, which may result in secondary prolapse of the vagina.

---

commonly as a result of fighting and farrowing, respectively. Certain management (e.g. housing and feeding) practices predispose to bite injuries of the vulva as sows vie for position in the pen or at the feed trough. Hematomas or hemorrhage resulting from farrowing injuries will obviously be observed during or soon after parturition.

Abnormal discharges from the vulva must be differentiated from normal discharge, which for the most part is limited to lochia expelled during the several days after farrowing. Abnormal discharge may emanate from the urinary or reproductive tracts and thus may be the result of

- cystitis
- pyelonephritis
- vaginitis
- metritis, or
- endometritis.

Urinalysis, vaginoscopy, and slaughter examination may allow the source of the discharge to be further defined.

### Internal genitalia

Antemortem examination of the reproductive tract of female swine is limited by its inaccessibility. Some specific techniques are available (see above) for the diagnosis of pregnancy (rectal palpation, ultrasonography) and visualization of the vaginal vault (vaginoscopy). However, in many cases slaughter examination is necessary to obtain a definitive diagnosis.

Infertility or subfertility may be the only clinical sign of several conditions most easily diagnosed at slaughter examination. Congenital lesions such as segmental aplasia and cervical anomalies may be discovered in this way. Adhesions may occur in a variety of anatomical locations with no disruption of the estrous cycle. Cystic ovaries cause anestrus or other irregularities of the estrous cycle, but they are confirmed at slaughter examination, as are infantilism and intersex conditions.

Slaughter examination allows differentiation of the inflammatory diseases of the female reproductive tract, with or without suggestive clinical signs (e.g. purulent discharge).

---

### Inflammatory conditions of the internal genitalia

Microbial culture or histopathological assessment in the laboratory can confirm the diagnosis

- metritis is inflammation of the several layers of the uterine wall (mucosa, muscularis and, perhaps, serosa)
- endometritis is more superficial and involves only the endometrium
- vaginitis is inflammation of the vaginal vault
- salpingitis is inflammation of the uterine tube.

---

## MALE REPRODUCTIVE ORGANS

### External genitalia

The scrotum and its contents may be palpated in the adequately restrained boar. The scrotum is a common site of injury, usually in the form of lacerations caused by fighting or sharp objects in the boar's environment (e.g. nails or other sharp metal). The testes are situated with the long axis nearly vertical, the head of the epididymis on the cranioventral pole, and the tail caudodorsad. The testes and epididymides should be examined for symmetry, consistency, and any signs of acute or chronic inflammation. Cryptorchidism, in which one or both testes fail to migrate to the scrotum, occurs in the boar. Testicular asymmetry may be the result of shrinkage or hypoplasia, in which the smaller testis is probably fibrotic with a prominent epididymis,

or swelling in the larger testis, usually accompanied by pain and hyperthermia associated with acute orchitis. An extremely soft consistency of the testicular parenchyma is indicative of testicular degeneration, the diagnosis of which may be supported by the identification of a high proportion of abnormal sperm in the ejaculate. Enlargement or fibrosis of parts of the epididymis are indicative of epididymitis. The sheath and preputial orifice of the boar may be examined for signs of trauma or hemorrhage, and the preputial diverticulum explored digitally. Hemorrhage may be the result of breeding injuries or attacks, damage to the urethra from uroliths, or other erosive lesions in the urogenital tract. Accumulation of smegma in the preputial diverticulum is often associated with signs of discomfort. The prepuce of the boar is most easily examined at the same time as the penis, but preputial prolapse is easily diagnosed beforehand.

---

### Clinical Pointer

If the moist epithelium of the prepuce is everted for a prolonged period, drying and trauma prevent its retraction.

---

The penis of the anesthetized boar may be extended manually or with forceps, but is more easily examined by deflecting it from the vestibule of the female during breeding attempts, usually during the process of semen collection. The source of any hemorrhage from the tract may thus be investigated. Possible sources are lacerations, including urethral fistulae, abrasions and the like. Hematuria may have been noted in the history, but hemospermia may be observed only during collection of semen. Persistent frenulum and hypospadias are congenital lesions that may be discovered during examination of the penis. Phimosis in the boar may be the result of immaturity or adhesions, whereas apparent phimosis may result from impotence or diversion of the penis into the preputial diverticulum. The latter is also a method of masturbation in the boar.

### Internal genitalia

The accessory glands of the boar are seldom examined directly, although rectal palpation of large boars is feasible. More commonly, a presumptive diagnosis of inflammatory conditions of the accessory genitalia is based on the observation of leukocytes in the ejaculate in the absence of signs of orchitis and epididymitis.

# BREEDING SOUNDNESS EXAMINATION

## Female

Criteria for the prospective evaluation of breeding soundness in sows and gilts do not exist as they do in the male. Rather, breeding soundness is judged retrospectively through detailed examination of past reproductive performance.

## Male

Breeding soundness examination of the boar consists of

- identification
- history
- general physical examination
- examination of the genitalia
- collection and evaluation of semen.

The history should include health maintenance procedures and past reproductive performance, as well as any abnormalities, injuries and diseases. The general physical examination should include an assessment of general condition, soundness and conformation of the feet and limbs, and the symmetry and adequacy of numbers of teats in the mammary chain. Examination of the genitalia and collection and evaluation of semen have been described above, see also (Gibson & Thacker 1986; Larsen 1986; and Larsson 1986).

The volume of the gel-free ejaculate is normally 100 ml or more, with total numbers of sperm per ejaculate of $10-100 \times 10^9$. Suggested minimum acceptable values for these measures are 50 ml of gel-free semen and $10 \times 10^9$ sperm per ejaculate. Progressively motile sperm should meet or exceed 70% of the total. Maximum acceptable numbers of specific morphological defects have also been suggested, but in general morphologically normal sperm should comprise 70% of the total. Abaxial attachment of the midpiece and distal cytoplasmic droplets are not considered abnormal in the boar.

# REFERENCES AND FURTHER READING

Adams GP, Kastelic JP, Bergfelt DR et al. Effect of uterine inflammation and ultrasonically-detected uterine pathology on fertility in the mare. Journal of Reproduction and Fertility 1987; Suppl. 35: 445–454.

Allen WE. Fertility and obstetrics in the horse. Oxford: Blackwell Scientific Publications, 1988; 125–144.

Amann RP. A review of anatomy and physiology of the stallion. Equine Veterinary Science 1983; May/June: 83–105.

Ames TR, Geor RJ (eds) The horse: diseases & clinical management. Philadelphia: WB Saunders, 1995; 914–918.

Asbury AC, LeBlanc MM. Diagnosis of reproductive diseases in the mare. In: Kobluk CN, Ames TR, Geor RJ. The horse: diseases and clinical management. Volumes 1 & 2, 1995. WB Saunders, Philadelphia.

Bjurstrom L, Linde-Forsberg C. Long-term study of aerobic bacteria of the genital tract in breeding bitches. American Journal of Veterinary Research 1992; 53(5): 665–669.

Bollwahn W. Surgical procedures on boars and sows. In: Morrow DA (ed) Current therapy in theriogenology 2. Philadelphia: WB Saunders, 1986; 1071–1082.

BonDurant RH. Examination of the reproductive tract of the cow and heifer. In: Morrow DA (ed) Current therapy in theriogenology 2. Philadelphia: WB Saunders, 1986; 95–101.

Brook D. Uterine cytology. In: McKinnon AO, Voss JL (eds) Equine reproduction. Philadelphia: Lea and Febiger, 1993; 246–255.

Bruere AN. Examination of the ram for breeding soundness. In: Morrow DA (ed) Current therapy in theriogenology 2. Philadelphia: WB Saunders, 1986; 874–880.

Buddle JR. Pregnancy diagnosis in swine. In: Morrow DA (ed) Current therapy in theriogenology 2. Philadelphia: WB Saunders, 1986; 918–923.

Chenoweth PJ. Libido testing. In: Morrow DA (ed) Current therapy in theriogenology 2. Philadelphia: WB Saunders, 1986a; 136–142.

Chenoweth PJ. Reproductive behavior of bulls. In: Morrow DA (ed) Current therapy in theriogenology 2. Philadelphia: WB Saunders, 1986b;148–152.

Cooper WC. The effect of rapid temperature changes on oxygen uptake by and motility of stallion spermatozoa. Proceedings of the Annual Meeting of the Society for Theriogenology 1979: 10–13.

Couto MA, Hughes JP. Sexually transmitted (venereal) diseases of horses. In: McKinnon AO, Voss JL (eds) Equine reproduction. Philadelphia: Lea and Febiger, 1993; 845–854.

Cox JE. Developmental abnormalities of the male reproductive tract. In: McKinnon AO, Voss JL (eds) Equine reproduction. Philadelphia: Lea and Febiger, 1993; 895–903.

Cutler R. Diagnosis of reproductive failure in sows manifested as abortion, mummified fetuses, stillbirths and weak neonates. In: Morrow DA (ed) Current therapy in theriogenology 2. Philadelphia: WB Saunders, 1986; 957–961.

deBois CHW, Manspeaker JE. Endometrial biopsy of the bovine. In: Morrow DA (ed) Current therapy in theriogenology 2. Philadelphia: WB Saunders, 1986; 424–426.

Dee SA. Porcine urogenital disease. Veterinary Clinics of North America (Food Animal Practice) 1992;8: 641.

Doig PA, Waelchli RO. Endometrial biopsy. In: McKinnon AO, Voss JL (eds) Equine reproduction. Philadelphia: Lea and Febiger, 1993; 225–233.

Easley J. External perineal conformation. In: McKinnon AO, Voss JL (eds) Equine reproduction. Philadelphia: Lea & Febiger, 1993; 20–24.

Ellington JE. Diagnosis, treatment, and management of poor fertility in the stud dog. Seminars in Veterinary Medicine and Surgery (Small Animal) 1994; 9(1): 46–53.

Feldman EC, Nelson RW. Canine and feline endocrinology and reproduction. Philadelphia: WB Saunders, 1987.

Freshman JL. Clinical evaluation of infertility in dogs. The Compendium of Continuing Education for the Practicing Veterinarian, 1988; 10(4): 443–460.

Freshman JL. Clinical approach to infertility in the cycling bitch. Veterinary Clinics of North America (Small Animal Practice) 1991; 21(3): 427–435.

Freshman JL, Amann RP, Soderby SF, Olson PN. Clinical evaluation of infertility in dogs. The Compendium of Continuing Education for the Practicing Veterinarian, 1988; 10(4): 443–456.

Gibson CD, Thacker BJ. Physical examination of new boars introduced to the herd. In: Morrow DA (ed) Current therapy in theriogenology 2. Philadelphia: WB Saunders, 1986; 967–969.

Ginther OJ. Mobility of the early equine conceptus. Theriogenology 1983; 19: 603–611.

Ginther OJ. Ultrasonographic imaging and reproductive events in the mare. Cross Plains, WI: Equiservices, 1986.

Hanzen C, Delsaux B. Use of transrectal B-mode ultrasound imaging in bovine pregnancy diagnosis. Veterinary Record 1987; 121: 200.

Hinrichs K. Ultrasonographic assessment of ovarian abnormalities. Proceedings of the Annual Convention of the American Association of Equine Practitioners 1990; 36: 31–40.

Holmes RJ. Sexual behavior of sheep. In: Morrow DA (ed) Current therapy in theriogenology 2. Philadelphia: WB Saunders, 1986; 870–873.

Hudson RS. Diseases of the penis and prepuce. In: Howard JL (ed) Current veterinary therapy, food animal practice 2. Philadelphia: WB Saunders, 1986a; 801–803.

Hudson RS. Diseases of the internal genitalia of males. In: Howard JL (ed) Current veterinary therapy, food animal practice 2. Philadelphia: WB Saunders, 1986b; 799–800.

Hudson RS. Diseases of the testicle and epididymis. In: Howard JL (ed) Current veterinary therapy, food animal practice 2. Philadelphia: WB Saunders, 1986c; 800–801.

Jann HW, Rains JR. Diagnostic ultrasonography for evaluation of cryptorchidism in horses. Journal of the American Veterinary Medical Association 1990; 196: 297–300.

Johnson C. Reproductive disorders in small animals. In: Willard MD, Tredden H, Turnwald GH (eds) Clinical diagnosis by laboratory methods. Philadelphia: WB Saunders, 1989; 283–296.

Johnston SD. Examination of the genital system. In: Bistner SI (ed) Veterinary Clinics of North America (Small Animal Practice) 1981; 11: 543–559.

Johnston SD, Olson NS, Root MV. Clinical approach to infertility in the bitch. Seminars in Veterinary Medicine and Surgery (Small Animal) 1994; 9(1): 2–6.

Johnston SD, Olson PNS, Root MV. Clinical approach to infertility in the bitch. Seminars in Veterinary Medicine and Surgery (Small Animal) 1994; 9(1): 41–45.

Kenney RM. Clinical fertility evaluation of the stallion. Proceedings of the Annual Convention of the American Association of Equine Practitioners 1975; 336–355.

Kenney RM, Hurtgen J, Pierson R et al. Manual for clinical fertility evaluation of the stallion. Journal of the Society for Theriogenology 1983; 9: 7–100.

Kobluk CN, Ames TR, Geor RJ (eds). The horse: diseases and management. Vols 1 & 2, 1995. WB Saunders, Philadelphia. 926–932.

Larsen RE. Semen collection from the boar. In: Morrow DA (ed) Current therapy in theriogenology 2. Philadelphia: WB Saunders, 1986; 969–972.

Larson L. Physical examination of the reproductive system of the bull. In: Morrow DA (ed) Current therapy in theriogenology 2. Philadelphia: WB Saunders, 1986; 101–116.

Larsson K. Evaluation of boar semen. In: Morrow DA (ed) Current therapy in theriogenology 2. Philadelphia: WB Saunders, 1986; 972–975.

LeBlanc MM. Vaginal examination. In: McKinnon AO, Voss JL (eds) Equine reproduction, Philadelphia: Lea & Febiger, 1993; 221–224.

Lindsay FEF. The normal endoscopic appearance of the caudal reproductive tract of the cyclic and non-cyclic bitch: post-uterine endoscopy. Journal of Small Animal Practice 1983; 24: 1–15.

Little TW, Woods GL. Ultrasonography of accessory sex glands in the stallion. Journal of Reproduction and Fertility 1987; Suppl. 35: 87–94.

Lofstedt RM. The estrous cycle of the domestic cat. The Compendium of Continuing Education for the Practicing Veterinarian, 1982; 4(1): 52–58.

Love CC, Garcia MC, Riera FR, Kenney RM. Evaluation of measures taken by ultrasonography and caliper to estimate testicular volume and predict daily sperm output in the stallion. Journal of Reproduction and Fertility 1991; Suppl 44: 99–105.

McKinnon AL, Squire EL, Voss JL. Ultrasonic evaluation of the mare's reproductive tract. Part 1. The Compendium on the Continuing Education of the Practicing Veterinarian 1987; 9: 336–345.

McKinnon AL, Squire EL, Voss JL. Ultrasonic evaluation of the mare's reproductive tract. Part 2. The Compendium on the Continuing Education of the Practicing Veterinarian 1987; 9: 472–482.

McKinnon AO, Squire EL, Harrison LA et al. Ultrasonographic studies on the reproductive tract of post-partum mares: effect of involution and uterine fluid on pregnancy rates in mares with normal and delayed first postpartum ovulatory cycles. Journal of the American Veterinary Medical Association 1988; 192: 350–353.

McKinnon AO, Voss JL, Squires EL et al. Diagnostic ultrasonography. In: McKinnon AO, Voss JL (eds) Equine reproduction. Philadelphia: Lea and Febiger, 1993; 266–302.

Martin ICA. Semen collection and evaluation. In: Morrow DA (ed) Current therapy in theriogenology 2. Philadelphia: WB Saunders, 1986; 880–883.

Neely DP, Liu IKM, Hillman RB. Evaluation and therapy of genital disease in the mare. In: Hughes JP (ed) Equine reproduction. Princeton Junction: Veterinary Learning Systems 1983; 53–55.

Olson PN. Clinical approach for evaluating dogs with azoospermia or aspermia. Veterinary Clinics of North America (Small Animal Practice) 1991; 21(3): 591–608.

Olson PN, Thrall MA, Wykes PM, Neft TM. Vaginal cytology Part I. A useful tool for staging the canine estrous cycle. The Compendium of Continuing Education for the Practicing Veterinarian, 1984; 6(4): 288–298.

Ott RS. Breeding soundness examination of bulls. In: Morrow DA (ed) Current therapy in theriogenology 2. Philadelphia: WB Saunders, 1986; 125–136.

Pascoe RR. Observations on the length and angle of declination of the vulva and its relationship to fertility in the mare. Journal of Reproduction and Fertility 1979; 27 Suppl: 299–305.

Peter AT, Steier JM, Adams LG. Diagnosis and medical management of prostate disease in the dog. Seminars in Veterinary Medicine and Surgery (Small Animal) 1995; 10(1): 35–42.

Pickett BW. Factors affecting sperm production and output. In: McKinnon AO, Voss JL (eds) Equine reproduction.

Philadelphia: Lea and Febiger, 1993; 689–704.

Pierson RA, Ginther OJ. Ultrasonographic appearance of the bovine uterus during the estrous cycle. Journal of the American Veterinary Medical Association 1987; 190: 995.

Post K. Canine vaginal cytology during the estrous cycle. Canadian Veterinary Journal 1985; 26: 101–104.

Refsal KR. Collection and evaluation of caprine semen. In: Morrow DA (ed) Current therapy in theriogenology 2. Philadelphia: WB Saunders, 1986; 619–621.

Ricketts SW, Young A, Medici EB. Uterine and clitoral cultures. In: McKinnon AO, Voss JL (eds) Equine reproduction. Philadelphia: Lea and Febiger, 1993; 234–244.

Roberts SJ. Veterinary obstetrics and genital diseases, 3rd edn. Woodstock, VT: Published by the author 1986.

Roberts SJ. Diseases and accidents of the gestation period. In: Roberts SJ. Veterinary obstetrics and genital diseases (theriogenology), 3rd edn. Woodstock, VT: published by the author, 1986a; 123–244.

Roberts SJ. Examinations for pregnancy. In: Roberts SJ. Veterinary obstetrics and genital diseases (theriogenology), 3rd edn. Woodstock, VT: published by the author, 1986b; 14–37.

Roberts SJ. Procedures preliminary to the handling of dystocia. In: Roberts SJ. Veterinary obstetrics and genital diseases (theriogenology), 3rd edn. Woodstock, VT: published by the author, 1986c; 287–297.

Roberts SJ. Obstetrical operations. In: Roberts SJ. Veterinary obstetrics and genital diseases (theriogenology), 3rd edn. Woodstock, VT: published by the author, 1986d; 298–325.

Roberts SJ. Diagnosis and treatment of various types of dystocia. In: Roberts SJ. Veterinary obstetrics and genital diseases (theriogenology), 3rd edn. Woodstock, VT: published by the author, 1986e; 326–52.

Root MV, Johnston SD. Basics for a complete reproductive examination of the male dog. Seminars in Veterinary Medicine and Surgery (Small Animal) 1994; 9: 1, 2–6.

Rynbeck A, deVries HW. Medical history and physical examination in companion animals. Dordrecht: Kluwer Academic, 1995.

Sack O, Habel RE. Rooney's guide to the dissection of the horse. Ithaca, NY: Veterinary Textbooks, 1982; 65–70.

Samper JC. Diseases of the male system. In: Kobluk CN, Ames TR, Geor RJ (eds) The horse. Philadelphia: WB Saunders, 1995; 947–955.

Schuijt G, Ball L. Delivery by forced extraction and other aspects of bovine obstetrics. In: Morrow DA (ed) Current therapy in theriogenology 2. Philadelphia: WB Saunders, 1980; 247–257.

Schuijt G, Ball L. Physical diagnosis during dystocia in the cow. In: Morrow DA (ed) Current therapy in theriogenology 2. Philadelphia: WB Saunders, 1986; 214–219.

Schumacher J, Varner DD. Neoplasia of the stallion's reproductive tract. In: McKinnon AO, Voss JL (eds) Equine reproduction. Philadelphia: Lea and Febiger, 1993; 871–877.

Sertich PL. Cervical problem in the mare. In:McKinnon AO, Voss JL (eds) Equine reproduction. Philadelphia: Lea & Febiger, 1993; 404–407.

Settergren I. Physical examination of the bovine female reproductive system. In: Morrow DA (ed) Current therapy in theriogenology 2. Philadelphia: WB Saunders, 1980; 159–164.

Singleton WL. Physical examination of the sow and gilt. In: Morrow DA (ed) Current therapy in theriogenology 2. Philadelphia: WB Saunders, 1986; 897–901.

Smith MC. The reproductive anatomy and physiology of the female goat. In: Morrow DA (ed) Current therapy in theriogenology 2. Philadelphia: WB Saunders, 1986a; 577–579.

Smith MC. The reproductive anatomy and physiology of the male goat. In: Morrow DA (ed) Current therapy in theriogenology 2. Philadelphia: WB Saunders, 1986b; 616–618.

Smith MC, Sherman DM. Urinary system. In: Smith MC, Sherman DM (eds) Goat medicine. Philadelphia: Lea & Febiger, 1994a; 387–409.

Smith MC, Sherman DM. Reproductive system. In: Smith MC, Sherman DM (eds) Goat medicine. Philadelphia: Lea & Febiger, 1994b; 411–463.

Thompson DL, Pickett BW, Squires EL, Amann RP. Testicular measurements and reproductive characteristics in stallions. Journal of Reproduction and Fertility 1979; Suppl. 27: 13–17.

Varner DD, Shumacher J, Blanchard TL, Johnson L. Diseases and management of breeding stallions. Goleta, CA: American Veterinary Publications, 1991.

Weber JA, Woods GL. Ultrasonographic studies of accessory sex glands in sexually rested stallions and bulls, sexually active stallions and a diseased bull. Proceedings of the Annual Meeting of the Society for Theriogenology 1989; 157–165.

West DM. Pregnancy diagnosis in the ewe. In: Morrow DA (ed) Current therapy in theriogenology 2. Philadelphia: WB Saunders, 1986; 850–852.

Wingfield-Digby NJ. The technique and clinical application of endometrial cytology in mares. Equine Veterinary Journal 1978; 10:167–170.

# 23
# Clinical Examination of the Mammary Glands

*J. Tyler*

## CLINICAL MANIFESTATIONS OF DISEASES OF THE MAMMARY GLANDS

**Abnormal lymph node** The supramammary lymph node may be enlarged, indicating the presence of inflammation of the mammary gland.

**Abnormalities of secretion** Abnormal secretions may be clinical and visible with the naked eye, or subclinical requiring the use of field tests. **Gross or clinical** changes in the secretions or milk include the presence of clear watery fluid, serous secretions, clots, flakes and pus, waxy plugs (ceruminous exudate), red-tinged secretion or blood in the milk, and a foul odor.

- **Subclinical changes** are usually due to increased somatic cell counts, which are detectable with the California Mastitis Test, a field test. **Colostrum** is present at parturition and is much thicker than milk and yellowish, and gradually becomes milk within a few days.

**Abnormalities of size** The mammary gland may be grossly enlarged symmetrically or asymmetrically because of udder edema, engorgement with milk, tumors or inflammation as in mastitis. Rupture of the suspensory ligament in cattle results in dropping of the udder, which is swollen and hard and swings laterally with each step when the cow walks. Atrophy of the mammary gland is the terminal stage of chronic mastitis: the gland is smaller than normal and on palpation little mammary tissue remains.

- **Palpable abnormalities** Palpable abnormalities of the mammary gland include increased temperature due to acute inflammation; a decreased temperature and coldness indicating the presence of gangrene and avascular necrosis, as in some cases of peracute mastitis in cattle and sheep. Increased firmness

indicates acute inflammation. Fibrosis is characterized by varying sizes of nodular tissue palpable in affected glands. Diffuse pitting edema occurs in udder edema. Firm masses either deep or superficial in the gland indicate abscesses or tumors. Slackness of the mammary gland occurs in sudden onset of agalactia, regardless of the cause. Subcutaneous emphysema commonly accompanies gangrene of the skin of the udder and teats in some cases of peracute mastitis. Single or multiple nodules in one or more glands in small animals suggests the presence of mammary tumors.

**Agalactia (lack of milk secretion)** Agalactia is the absence of milk secretion, which may be primary, secondary to systemic disease, or due to specific causes such as ergotism. Primary agalactia or hypogalactia may occur in animals fed an inadequate diet during pregnancy.

**Blind or non-functional glands** are characterized by lack of milk, usually as a result of severe mastitis; commonly the gland is increased in size, firm to hard, and almost no secretion can be milked out of it. A small amount of purulent material may be present.

**Failure of milk letdown** is any circumstance causing excitement or severe pain, and severe udder edema at the time of parturition. With failure of letdown the udder is distended; this can usually be corrected with oxytocin.

**Hungry neonate** Nursing newborn animals which are unable to obtain milk because of agalactia, failure of milk letdown, or blocked teats will make repeated unsuccessful attempts to suck their dams. Examination of the udder will reveal the problem.

**Leaky teats or leakers** These are cows that drip milk continously or after stimulation of milk letdown.

**Pain** may be detected on palpation of inflamed glands, palpation of enlarged inflamed supramammary lymph nodes, or alteration of gait because of painful glands.

**Teat and udder skin lesions** may be visible on the skin of the teats and udder. They include focal or diffuse *erythema, papules, linear* and transverse teat *chapping, pustules, vesicles, ulcers, scabs, nodules* and *fibropapillomas (warts), necrotic and sloughing skin, gangrenous areas* with a line demarcation, and diffuse inflammation of the lateral aspects of the skin of teats, as in photosensitization. (see Chapter 13)

**Teat-end lesions** are usually associated with the teat orifice. There may be teat canal eversion, teat canal prolapse, prolapse of the meatus, and teat orifice erosion. Teat-end lesions are classified as *proliferative ring lesions; smooth, chronic ring-smooth* ring of tissue around the teat orifice; *rough, chronic ring-proliferative* ring of tissue around teat orifice; acute-ulcerative or hemorrhagic appearance of teat orifice, with or without a scab; *unclassified*–teat ends disfigured by trauma or warts.

- **Black spot lesions** occur at the teat end and are characterized by deep crater-shaped ulcers with raised edges and a black spot in the center.

**Teat fistula** A fistula into the teat cistern allowing milk to drip through the teat wall.

**Teat necrosis** Abrasions of the teats of piglets raised on rough floor surfaces resulting in inverted teats, non-functional teats and glands when the pigs mature and farrow for the first time.

**Teat obstructions or blocked teats** are usually due to obstructions of the teat cistern or teat canal by waxy plugs, or fibrous tissue due to chronic inflammation. The teat cistern is distended with milk and attempts to empty the teat are impossible or difficult because of the obstruction in the canal.

**Teat stenosis** is characterized by a marked narrowing of the teat orifice or streak canal (or both), which makes milking difficult.

**Thelitis** (mammillitis) Inflammation of the lining of the wall or skin of the teat. The wall of the cistern is thickened, hardened and painful, and in chronic cases the internal lining can be felt as a dense vertical cord in the center of the teat..

**Traumatic** wounds may occur anywhere on the teat or udder. Superficial wounds involve the skin. Deep wounds may extend to the teat or gland cistern.

## CLINICAL ANATOMY OF THE MAMMARY GLANDS OF FARM ANIMALS

### Number and position of mammary glands in domestic mammals

- the dog, cat, and pig have multiple pairs of mammary glands and teats symmetrically placed on either side of the ventral midline in two rows along the length of the thorax and abdomen
- horses, sheep, and goats have a single pair of mammary glands located in the inguinal region between the pelvic limbs
- cattle have two co-joined pairs of mammary glands likewise located in the inguinal region.

The development of skin glands which produce milk for the nutrition of neonates is most specialized in the mammals.

In cattle, sheep, and goats the teat has a single opening, the teat sphincter, which communicates with the teat cistern. The teat cistern opens into the gland cistern. Lactiferous ducts which arborize into smaller and smaller ducts drain milk from alveolar glands, which are arranged in lobules within the mammary gland parenchyma and empty into the gland cistern. In the mare and sow each teat has two separate orifices. Each opening serves an anatomically distinct duct and gland system located within the single mammary gland. Each gland has 2–3 duct/gland systems.

Normal anatomical structures of the mammary gland which should be examined in the course of a clinical examination include the

- teats
- streak canal
- teat cistern
- gland cistern
- udder parenchyma
- supramammary lymph nodes, and
- vascular supply.

## CLINICAL EXAMINATION OF THE MAMMARY GLANDS OF FARM ANIMALS

The mammary gland should be inspected both visually and manually for symmetry and consistency.

**Clinical Pointer**

An asymmetrical udder may be caused by either unilateral increases or unilateral decreases in the size of a mammary gland.

Active inflammation, edema, and abscessation will often cause enlargement of the udder. However, edema will typically be symmetrical. End-stage fibrosis caused by chronic infection may cause atrophy of single or multiple mammary glands. Affected glands are usually firm and fibrotic. Of the common intramammary pathogens of cattle, diffuse glandular atrophy and fibrosis is most consistent with *Staphylococcus aureus* mastitis. In herds with endemic *Staph. aureus* mastitis 'blind-quartered' or 'three-teated' cows are often presumptively diagnosed and classified as *Staph. aureus* infected.

Changes of temperature in the mammary gland should be noted during physical examination, particularly if they are restricted to a single gland or half of the udder

- inflamed glands are often warm
- glands undergoing avascular necrosis or gangrene are cool or cold.

When gangrene is present a clear border of erythema and warmth often defines the border of necrotic and viable udder parenchyma. Gangrenous mastitis is most commonly caused by peracute *Staph. aureus* or, alternatively, clostridial infection.

Clostridial infections tend to produce a dry gangrene because the toxins released by bacteria compromise the arterial blood supply to the mammary gland. In direct contrast, gangrenous mastitis caused by *Staph. aureus* tends to cause a weeping of serum-like material from the tissues. This wet gangrene results from the destruction and occlusion of the venous drainage of the affected gland. Clostridial infections of the udder result in the production of a mammary secretion which has a strong fetid odor.

Areas of localized fibrosis and abscessation are readily identified on deep palpation of the mammary gland, ranging in size from microscopic to several centimeters in diameter. Abscesses are usually roughly spherical and surrounded by a firm capsule. Superficial abscesses may be visible beneath the skin of the gland. Lesions of this type are usually associated with chronic pyogenic infections, the most common being *Staph. aureus* mastitis, although *Mycoplasma* sp., *Actinomyces pyogenes* and other bacteria have been associated with intramammary abscesses. Fibrotic areas are readily recognized because adjacent normal parenchymal tissue provides a direct and distinct contrast. Diffuse increases in firmness are often seen in sheep and goats following

- caprine arthritis–encephalomyelitis virus, and
- ovine progressive pneumonia

infections that have been associated with 'hard bag' syndromes, in which interstitial mastitis causes agalactia or hypogalactia and a diffuse firmness of the udder.

The **skin of the udder** also should be examined closely. Several viral diseases have been associated with vesicular or erosive lesions of teats and udder. Recognition of such lesions warrants closer examination and diagnostic testing. The skin of the clefts formed between the right and left halves of the udder and between the lateral surface of the udder and the medial surface of the pelvic limb is moist, warm, and relatively anaerobic. Superficial pyoderma is common in these areas, particularly in recently fresh cows with large udders or marked udder edema.

**Udder edema** also is readily recognizable on physical examination as a diffuse firmness and swelling of the mammary gland. On deep palpation edematous udders will 'pit', leaving hand or fingerprints in the palpated tissue. Edema may be either a normal physiological response, in periparturient first lactation heifers, or a pathological manifestation of disease. It often accompanies inflammatory responses to intramammary infection. The expected symmetry of normal edema may not be apparent in cows which are recumbent. In these circumstances the cow's weight may actually force interstitial fluid from the udder, eliminating edema in dependent portions of the udder.

**Clinical Pointer**

In cattle with clostridial mastitis intraparenchymal emphysema is often palpable. The interface of gas bubbles within tissue planes creates a sensation similar to that of crumbling a plastic wrap.

**Clinical Pointer**

- physiological or normal edema is usually symmetrical
- pathological edema is localized in inflamed quarters.

The bulk of **lymphatic drainage** in the ruminant mammary gland is through the supramammary lymph nodes. These are paired structures located within the parenchyma of the proximal mammary glands lateral to the median suspensory ligament. They are readily palpated by placing the thumbs in the furrow formed by the median suspensory ligament and the remaining four fingers of either hand on the lateral aspect of the mammary gland. Deep palpation reveals a flat bean-shaped structure approximately 7 × 5 × 2 cm. The supramammary lymph nodes are often enlarged in cattle, sheep, and goats with either chronic mastitis or multicentric lymphosarcoma. The prefemoral, internal iliac, and deep inguinal lymph nodes may also be enlarged in these diseases, but are less readily accessible during physical examination and consequently these changes may not be detected.

Palpation of an inflamed mammary gland will often elicit pain. Cattle will often attempt to kick, and sheep and goats will stamp their hind feet. Inflammation of the mammary gland will also often cause ruminants to have dramatic changes in their gait. The hindlimb ipsilateral to the affected gland is often abducted in an exaggerated fashion, particularly during protraction of the pelvic limb.

The examination of mammary gland secretions is a component of the clinical examination of all lactating animals. After washing the teats with soap and water if excessively soiled, the teat ends are swabbed with an alcohol-soaked gauze and the teat sphincters examined visually and by palpation. The **external orifice** is visually appraised for

- eversion of the streak canal
- traumatic lesions
- verrucous growths.

These disruptions of normal anatomical structure impair mammary gland defense mechanisms and may permit bacterial proliferation in situ. The streak canal is readily palpated by rolling the distal 1 cm of the teat between the thumb and forefinger. Although the canal is normally palpable in this manner, scarring and fibrosis of the teat is readily diagnosed when the clinician detects an increased firmness of this structure.

Cows are expected to have four functional teats and associated mammary glands.

The **teat sphincter** should be assessed for competency. Manipulation of the udder will often trigger an endogenous release of oxytocin and cause some cows to drip milk. This is a normal response. The spontaneous dripping of milk without external stimulation that occurs in some cows is abnormal and may be caused by an incontinent teat sphincter. In these circumstances a chronically open sphincter may permit environmental

bacteria to invade the mammary gland and cause severe clinical mastitis. Cattle affected with acute clinical coliform mastitis are purported to undergo endogenous oxytocin release. Consequently, inappropriate dripping of milk should be considered an indication for closer clinical examination.

Farm animals should be closely observed for prepartum dripping of colostrum or waxing. Because colostral immunoglobulins are transferred to the mammary gland well before parturition and the concentration of immunoglobulin is decreased in later secretions, the offspring of dams that wax are at a greater risk for failure of passive transfer of immunoglobulins, and consequently of neonatal septicemia.

---

### Clinical Pointer

Premature waxing and prepartum loss of colostral immunoglobulin can result in neonatal septicemia of offspring. This is more common in mares than in cows.

---

The inspection of mammary gland **secretions** or **milk** is a standard component of many clinical examinations of the udder and is of vital importance in the lactating ruminant. **Milk samples** are typically obtained by occluding the base of the teat with the thumb and forefinger and forcing out the milk trapped in the teat cistern by sequentially closing the remaining three fingers into a fist. With short teats, the base of the teat is occluded as previously described and the thumb and

---

### Some features of supernumerary teats in cattle

Supernumerary teats are

- additional to the four normal teats
- observed in one-third of dairy cattle
- most commonly located caudal to the four normal teats
- occasionally located between normal teats, cranial to a cranial teat, or attached to a normal teat
- non-functional
- usually smaller than normal teats
- often removed surgically when the animals are heifers
- sometimes removed later if they cannot be clearly differentiated from normal teats.

forefinger are slid down the teat, expressing the entrapped milk. Milk should be stripped on to a flooring surface or into a container, which is thoroughly cleaned and disinfected between cows. A strip cup equipped with flat black smooth recessed cover and a drainage hole is ideal for the gross examination of milk from mastitic mammary glands. The milk is streamed on to the recessed cover and the consistency, the presence of clots, purulent material, and other inflammatory debris can be easily visualized as the milk flows across the flat surface. Abnormal findings in mammary secretions that should be observed and recorded are

- clots
- abnormal color
- decreased opacity.

Watery or thin milk and clots are presumptive evidence of acute intramammary inflammation, usually infectious in origin. Inflamed glands will often produce a secretion which is either red or yellow tinged. Red discoloration may also be caused by udder trauma or postpartum hemorrhage in the udder. Postpartum hemorrhage causing bloodstained milk occurs frequently in dairy cows and usually resolves without specific treatment.

The **California Mastitis Test (CMT)** is a cowside clinical examination procedure often performed in lactating ruminants. The mammary gland secretion is mixed with an equal volume of detergent solution, releasing the chromosomal DNA contained by milk leukocytes. This DNA increases the viscosity of the milk–detergent solution. Inflamed glands will typically have increased concentrations of leukocytes, particularly neutrophils and macrophages. Consequently, the thickness of the gel observed in the assay is roughly equivalent to the severity of intramammary inflammation. Observed reactions are graded on a negative, trace, 1+, 2+, 3+ scale.

The CMT is usually performed on foremilk, the milk contained in the teat cistern. The cell count of foremilk is higher than that of composite or strippings, enhancing the sensitivity of the test procedure. The

CMT paddle contains four labeled recessed cups to hold samples from each quarter. The handle is held toward the cow's head and milk from each quarter is collected into the corresponding cup. Strict adherence to this sampling strategy will avoid confusion regarding which quarter or quarters have increased CMT reactions. This is particularly important in dairy herds, in which cows are commonly milked from either the right or the left side. After the collection of milk samples the paddle is tipped to a 45° angle and excess milk is permitted to run out. An equal volume of detergent solution is added to each cup. After mixing, the paddle is tipped from side to side and swirled in a circular pattern. Gel reactions are recorded using the classification in Table 23.1. Normal non-inflamed mammary glands will usually produce a secretion that generates a negative CMT reaction.

The CMT is also useful in small ruminants. In goats the procedure is probably preferable to electronic cell counting methods. Normal goats shed cytoplasmic droplets, which are erroneously recognized as inflammatory cells by cell counts. However, these structures contain minimal DNA. Unlike cattle, CMT readings of trace or even 1+ are usually considered normal in goats.

The structure of the mammary gland in **ewes** is similar to that of cows. One distinct difference is that sheep typically have two rather than four functional glands, and the teat cistern is proportionally smaller in sheep than in cattle. Goats also have two rather than four glands and the teat and teat cistern are similar in size to those of cattle. Clinical examination of the udder of the doe and ewe is similar to that done in cattle.

Mammary gland disease is less common in **horses** than in ruminants. Examinations are usually based on extrapolation of the previously outlined diagnostic approach, recognizing the clear differences in mammary gland anatomy.

## CLINICAL ANATOMY OF THE MAMMARY GLANDS OF DOGS AND CATS

The dog has four to five mammary glands on each side of the midline, extending from the ventral thorax to the inguinal region. Each teat may have as many as 20 distinct openings, each of which serves a separate and distinct system of ducts and glands. Glands are named either by

- number (1–5, with number increasing in a craniocaudal direction), or by
- anatomic location (cranial and caudal thoracic, cranial and caudal abdominal, and inguinal).

---

**Clinical Pointer**

Collection of milk into the examiner's hand for examination is strongly discouraged – either may be contaminated with contagious mastitis pathogens such as *Streptococcus agalactia*, *Staphylococcus aureus*, and *Mycoplasma* sp., thus potentiating the cow-to-cow spread of intramammary infections.

| Table 23.1. California Mastitis Test reactions and equivalent milk somatic cell counts in cattle | | |
|---|---|---|
| Test result | Reaction observed | Equivalent milk somatic cell count |
| Negative | The mixture remains fluid without thickening or gel formation. | 0–200,000 cells/ml |
| Trace | A slight slime formation is observed. This reaction is most noticeable when the paddle is rocked from side to side. | 150,000– 500,000 cells/ml |
| 1+ | Distinct slime formation occurs immediately after mixing solutions. This slime may dissipate over time. When the paddle is swirled fluid neither forms a peripheral mass nor does the surface of solution become convex or 'dome-up'. | 400,000– 1,500,000 cells/ml |
| 2+ | Distinct slime formation occurs immediately after mixing solutions. When the paddle is swirled the fluid forms a peripheral mass and the bottom of the cup is exposed. | 800,000– 5,000,000 cells/ml |
| 3+ | Distinct slime formation occurs immediately after mixing solutions. This slime may dissipate over time. When the paddle is swirled the surface of solution becomes convex or 'domed-up'. | > 5,000,000 cells/ml |

Half of all dogs lack one of the cranial abdominal glands. Cats have four pairs of mammary glands, the nomenclature is similar to that used in dogs.

Knowledge of the normal vascular supply and lymphatic drainage of the mammary glands is important for the interpretation of physical examination findings and for treatment planning in disease states, particularly in cases of neoplastic disease. The primary vascular supply to the mammary glands is the cranial and caudal superficial epigastric arteries. Additional blood supply to the abdominal and inguinal glands comes from the segmental and circumflex iliac vessels, penetrating arteries from the deep caudal epigastric artery, and branches from the perineal and perivulvar arteries. The thoracic glands are also supplied by the ancillary, intercostal, and penetrating branches of the internal thoracic arteries. Venous blood flow parallels the arterial blood flow, with the exception of superficial veins that cross the midline. Lymphatic drainage of the mammary glands in dogs and cats is primarily to the inguinal and axillary lymph nodes. Glands 1 and 2 drain to the axillary lymph node and glands 3, 4, and 5 drain to the superficial inguinal lymph nodes.

## Clinical Pointer ✳

Lymphatic drainage may cross the midline, but rarely crosses between cranial (1 and 2) and caudal (3, 4, and 5) glands.

## CLINICAL EXAMINATION OF THE MAMMARY GLANDS OF BITCHES AND QUEENS

Prior to examination of the mammary gland the signalment of the animal and a complete history, including details of

- whelping
- prior surgery or biopsy results
- the onset and duration of clinical signs
- breeding history

should be obtained from the owner. A complete general physical examination to assess overall health status should be undertaken first. Examination of the mammary glands of dogs and cats begins with visualization to determine gland number, size, color, and the presence of any overlying skin lesions or discharges. Any milk secretion should be evaluated visually for color and consistency, and examined cytologically when indicated. Visual examination is followed by manual examination of each gland, the associated lymph nodes, overlying skin and surrounding tissues. Swellings or nodules must be characterized in terms of

- size
- firmness
- attachment to surrounding tissues and overlying skin
- whether pain is elicited on palpation.

It may be difficult to differentiate between swelling of normal glandular tissue and the development of neoplasia. Neoplastic growths are less often painful than inflammatory disorders with the exception of inflammatory mammary carcinoma in the bitch.

If a mastectomy has been performed, biopsy results should be reviewed.

Abnormal findings of the mammary gland can generally be classified into four categories

- milk accumulation
- inflammation
- neoplasia
- hypertrophy/hyperplasia.

Some distinguishing features of each are presented here.

The abnormal collection of milk in the mammary glands is referred to as **galactostasis**. This may occur when the blood supply to the glands is greater than that which can be accommodated by the venous system, or in heavily lactating bitches on a high level of nutrition. Entrapped milk within the ducts results in inflammation with secondary edema and engorgement of the mammary glands. Palpation of the involved glands may produce a pain response. The glands may be palpably firm and warm, with teat inversion, and normal-appearing milk secretion. Pertinent history will include recent or current pregnancy or pseudocyesis (false pregnancy).

Inflammation of the mammary glands is characterized by erythema, swelling, pain, and warmth. Additional features noted on physical examination may include

- edema of the surrounding tissues
- green to yellow discoloration of the skin due to gangrene or abscessation
- viscous and discolored milk (yellow, pink, or brown)
- evidence of systemic illness, such as fever, listlessness, and loss of interest in pups.

The primary differential diagnoses for inflammatory mammary gland disease are mastitis and inflammatory mammary carcinoma.

1. **Acute mastitis** occurs most often in hot, humid weather and when bitches and queens are housed in unsanitary surroundings. In queens, mastitis may occur as early as 24 hours postpartum or may occur from 1 to 6 weeks after parturition, often owing to injury from the kittens' nails. Bitches or queens suffering from subclinical mastitis are presented because their offspring are failing to thrive or have signs of septicemia. Physical examination findings and the appearance of the milk may be normal and milk cytology is required to confirm the tentative diagnosis.

2. **Inflammatory mammary carcinoma** is a distinct neoplastic disease syndrome which is often misdiagnosed. In a report of 10 cases of canine inflammatory mammary carcinoma four were initially misdiagnosed as other inflammatory diseases, including mastitis, mammary gland abscesses, and dermatitis. Inflammatory mammary carcinoma is characterized by firm mammary masses, diffuse tumor infiltration of multiple glands, warmth, pitting mammary or limb edema, erythema, and pain. The overlying skin may be indurated, ulcerated, dimpled, and necrotic.

Mammary tumors are often detected by thorough physical examination during routine office visits. Therefore, palpation of the mammary glands and associated lymph nodes is indicated in all general physical examinations of dogs and cats.

Dogs have the highest incidence of mammary neoplasia of all mammalian species, with 50% of all canine neoplasia involving the mammary glands.

Palpation of the affected glands may reveal small, firm, painless nodules with or without attachment to underlying tissues. More chronic cases present with large, firm masses which may ulcerate. Occasionally, physical examination reveals hyperemia, edema, and pruritus, which may indicate the presence of an inflammatory carcinoma. The differential diagnoses in these cases should include

- glandular fibrosis or chronic inflammation
- skin tumors
- inguinal hernias
- galactoceles – foci of incomplete glandular involution.

---

### Abnormal number of teats in dogs and cats

- supernumerary teats are generally of no clinical significance
- fewer teats than normal indicates previous surgery.

---

### Clinical Pointer

The onset of clinical signs of both mastitis and inflammatory carcinoma is acute. Consider the breeding history and age of the animal to reach the most likely diagnosis.

If a mammary mass is palpated the axillary lymph nodes should also be palpated to assess for size and pain response. Normally the axillary lymph nodes are not palpable. Lymph node enlargement, especially with evidence of pain on palpation, is suggestive of mammary tumor metastasis.

The incidence of mammary tumors is less in cats than in dogs, but feline mammary masses are usually (70%) malignant.

Palpation reveals firm, non-painful masses that may adhere to the overlying skin, but rarely to the underlying abdominal wall. If the lymphatics are involved palpation will reveal subcutaneous linear, beaded chains.

A unique syndrome in cats is the **feline mammary hyperplasia/fibroadenoma complex**, in which rapid abnormal growth of mammary tissue occurs as a result of hyperplasia of epithelial and mesenchymal tissues. The disorder occurs in

- young cats in early pregnancy
- cycling queens, and
- neutered males or females receiving progestins, such as megestrol acetate.

The physical examination findings mimic mammary neoplasia. Masses are painless and involve one or more mammae. As with mammary neoplasia, the overlying skin may ulcerate.

Lactation which is not associated with pregnancy and parturition is referred to as galactorrhea. In the bitch this is the most common clinical manifestation of false pregnancy. Milk secretion is due to increased prolactin concentration, which may be stimulated by falling progesterone concentrations in late diestrus or following spaying during diestrus.

---

### Some features of feline mammary neoplasia

- mammary tumors have been reported in cats from 9 months to 23 years of age
- the average age at the time of diagnosis is 10–12 years
- 70% of feline tumors are malignant
- site predilection for feline mammary tumors is controversial, in two reports, glands 1 and 2 were most commonly affected, a third study reported that the distal glands were more frequently involved, with almost half arising in the caudal glands
- however, most cats have multiple gland involvement
- at least one-quarter of cases present with ulcerated masses.

---

### Clinical Pointer

Galactorrhea with pseudopregnancy is more common in dogs with hypothyroidism, due to stimulation of prolactin release by TRH, which is elevated in hypothyroidism.

---

### Some features of canine mammary neoplasia

- mammary tumors are most common in intact females or those spayed after 2 years of age
- the average age at the time of diagnosis is 10 years
- male dogs may be affected
- one-half of all canine mammary tumors are benign
- a combination of benign and malignant masses may occur in the same dog, therefore, if a nodule is palpated in the mammary tissue thorough palpation of all mammary and surrounding tissue is indicated
- the majority of canine mammary tumors occur in glands 4 and 5
- 40% of tumors affect the inguinal glands.

---

### Clinical Pointer

Since mammary tumours occur in the male dog, examination of the male mammary tissue must not be overlooked.

---

## FURTHER READING

Baker GJ. Treatment of malignant neoplasia: surgical management. Journal of Small Animal Practice 1972; 13(7): 373–379.

Barsanti JA. Abnormalities of the external genitalia. In: Lorenz MD, Cornelius LM (eds) Small animal medical diagnosis, 2nd edn. Philadelphia: JB Lippincott, 1993; 365–373.

Bostock DE. Canine and feline mammary neoplasms. British Veterinary Journal 1986; 142: 506–515.

Brodey RS, Goldschmidt MH, Roszel JR. Canine mammary gland neoplasms. Journal of American Animal Hospital Association 1983; 19: 61–90.

Concannon PW, Butler WR, Hansel W et al. Parturition and lactation in the bitch: serum progesterone, cortisol, and prolactin. Biology of Reproduction 1978; 19: 1113.

Hayden DW, Neilsen SW. Feline mammary tumors. Journal of Small Animal Practice 1971; 12: 687–697.

Hayes HM Jr, Milne KL, Mandell CP. Epidemiological features of feline mammary carcinoma. Veterinary Record 1981; 108: 476–479.

Mann FA. Canine mammary gland neoplasia. Canine Practice 1984; 11: 22–26.

Ogilvie GK. Feline mammary neoplasia. Compendium Continuing Education for the Practicing Veterinarian 1983; 5: 384–393.

Olson JD, Olson PN. Disorders of the canine mammary gland. In: Morrow DA (ed) Current therapy in theriogenology 2. Philadelphia: WB Saunders, 1986; 506–509.

Olson PN, Olson AL. Cytologic evaluation of canine milk. Veterinary Medicine 1984: 641–646.

Schalm OW, Carroll EJ, Jain NC. Bovine mastitis. Philadelphia: Lea & Febiger, 1971; 23–47.

Schneider R, Dorn CR, Taylor DON. Factors influencing canine mammary cancer. Journal of the National Cancer Institute 1976; 56: 779–786.

Silver IA. Symposium on mammary neoplasia in the dog and cat I. The anatomy of the mammary gland of the dog and cat. Journal of Small Animal Practice 1966; 7: 689.

Weijer K, Hart AAM. Prognostic features in feline mammary carcinoma. Journal of the National Cancer Institute 1983; 70: 709–716.

# Index

Entries in **bold** denote major discussions in the text